C000115660

Handbook of Dialysis Therapy

Handbook of Dialysis Therapy

5th Edition

Allen R. Nissenson, MD
Chief Medical Officer
DaVita Kidney Care
Emeritus Professor of Medicine
David Geffen School of Medicine at UCLA
Los Angeles, California

Richard N. Fine, MD
Professor of Pediatrics
Stony Brook Medicine
Stony Brook, New York

ELSEVIER

ELSEVIER

1600 John F. Kennedy Blvd.
Ste 1800
Philadelphia, PA 19103-2899

Notices

Knowledge and best practice in this field are constantly changing. As new research and experience broaden our understanding, changes in research methods, professional practices, or medical treatment may become necessary.

Practitioners and researchers must always rely on their own experience and knowledge in evaluating and using any information, methods, compounds, or experiments described herein. In using such information or methods they should be mindful of their own safety and the safety of others, including parties for whom they have a professional responsibility.

With respect to any drug or pharmaceutical products identified, readers are advised to check the most current information provided (i) on procedures featured or (ii) by the manufacturer of each product to be administered, to verify the recommended dose or formula, the method and duration of administration, and contraindications. It is the responsibility of practitioners, relying on their own experience and knowledge of their patients, to make diagnoses, to determine dosages and the best treatment for each individual patient, and to take all appropriate safety precautions.

To the fullest extent of the law, neither the Publisher nor the authors, contributors, or editors, assume any liability for any injury and/or damage to persons or property as a matter of products liability, negligence or otherwise, or from any use or operation of any methods, products, instructions, or ideas contained in the material herein.

Library of Congress Cataloging-in-Publication Data

Names: Nissenson, Allen R., editor. | Fine, Richard N., editor.
Title: Handbook of dialysis therapy / [edited by] Allen R. Nissenson, Richard N. Fine.
Description: 5. | Philadelphia, PA : Elsevier, [2017] | Includes bibliographical references and index.
Identifiers: LCCN 2016023558 | ISBN 9780323391542 (pbk. : alk. paper)
Subjects: | MESH: Renal Dialysis
Classification: LCC RC901.7.H45 | NLM WJ 378 | DDC 617.4/61059—dc23 LC record available at https://lccn.loc.gov/2016023558

Content Strategist: Maureen Iannuzzi
Content Development Specialist: Angie Breckon
Publishing Services Manager: Patricia Tannian
Project Manager: Ted Rodgers
Design Direction: Ryan Cook

Printed in the United States of America

Last digit is the print number: 　9　8　7　6　5　4　3　2

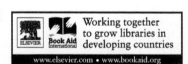

Working together
to grow libraries in
developing countries

www.elsevier.com • www.bookaid.org

This book is dedicated to the memory of my mother, Sylvia Nissenson, who died after a long and debilitating illness in 2013. Her love, charm, wit, and deep sense of caring for others still inspire me and motivate me to try even harder to help patients and contribute to the good of society. Though no longer here, she will always be a part of me.

Allen R. Nissenson, MD

I would like to dedicate this edition of Handbook of Dialysis to my wife of 44 years, Shawney, whose encouragement, support, and advice have made the journey to facilitate access to ESRD care for children of all ages possible, as well as our 4 children and 11 grandchildren, 2 of whom aspire to become physicians. They have tolerated my conflicting priorities over the years. I appreciate their continued understanding.

Richard N. Fine, MD

CONTRIBUTORS

Rajiv Agarwal, MBBS, MD, DNB, FAHA, FASN
Professor of Medicine, Division of Nephrology, Indiana University; Staff
Physician, Department of Medicine, Richard L. Roudebush VA Medical Center,
Indianapolis, Indiana

Alessio Aghemo, MD
Division of Gastroenterology and Hepatology, Maggiore Hospital and IRCCS
Foundation, University School of Medicine, Milano, Italy

Ali Al-Lawati, MD
Sultan Qaboos University Hospital, Muscat, Oman

Michael Allon, MD
Professor of Medicine, Division of Nephrology, University of Alabama at
Birmingham, Birmingham, Alabama

Walter S. Andrews, MD
Professor of Surgery, University of Missouri-Kansas City School of Medicine;
Director, Pediatric Transplant Surgery, Department of Surgery, The Children's
Mercy Hospital, Kansas City, Missouri

Rachel A. Annunziato, PhD
Associate Professor of Psychology, Fordham University, Bronx, New York;
Associate Professor of Pediatrics, Icahn School of Medicine at Mount Sinai,
New York, New York

Carlos E. Araya, MD
Assistant Professor, University of Central Florida; Division of Pediatric
Nephrology, Nemours Children's Hospital, Orlando, Florida

Arif Asif, MD
Chair and Professor of Clinical Medicine, Department of Medicine,
Jersey Shore Medical Center, Meridian Health, Neptune, New Jersey

Rose M. Ayoob, MD
Assistant Professor of Pediatrics, Director of the Pediatric Renal Dialysis Unit,
Nationwide Children's Hospital, The Ohio State University College of Medicine,
Columbus, Ohio

Rossana Baracco, MD
Assistant Professor of Pediatrics, Wayne State University School of Medicine,
Children's Hospital of Michigan, Detroit, Michigan

Joanne Bargman, MD, FRCPC
The Home Peritoneal Dialysis Unit, University Health Network, University of
Toronto, Toronto, Ontario, Canada

Gerald A. Beathard, MD, PhD, FASN
Clinical Professor of Medicine, University of Texas Medical Branch;
Co-Medical Director, Lifeline Vascular Access, Galveston, Texas

Antonio Bellasi, MD
Division of Nephrology, ASST-Lariana, Ospedale Sant'Anna, Como, Italy

William M. Bennett, MD
Medical Director, Legacy Transplant Services, Portland, OR

Jeffrey S. Berns, MD
Professor of Medicine and Pediatrics, Renal, Electrolyte and Hypertension
Division, Perelman School of Medicine at the University of Pennsylvania,
Philadelphia, Pennsylvania

Scott Bieber, DO
Clinical Assistant Professor of Medicine, University of Washington; Medical
Director, Scribner Kidney Center, Northwest Kidney Centers, Seattle, Washington

Geoffrey A. Block, MD
Director of Research, Denver Nephrologists, PC, Denver, Colorado

Paola Boccardo, BiolSciD
IRCCS - Istituto di Ricerche Farmacologiche Mario Negri, Clinical Research
Center for Rare Diseases "Aldo e Cele Daccò", Ranica (Bergamo), Italy

Andrew Brookens, MD
Nephrology Fellow, University of Washington, Seattle, Washington

Patrick D. Brophy, MD, MHCDS
Director, Pediatric Nephrology, Dialysis and Transplantation, Stead Family
Department of Pediatrics, Division of Nephrology, University of Iowa, Iowa City,
Iowa

Steven Brunelli, MD, MSCE
Vice President of Health Economics and Outcomes Research, DaVita Clinical
Research, Denver, Colorado

John M. Burkart, MD
Professor of Internal Medicine/Nephrology, Department of Internal Medicine,
Section on Nephrology, Wake Forest School of Medicine, Winston-Salem, North
Carolina

David Bushinsky, MD
Department of Medicine, University of Rochester School of Medicine and
Dentistry, Rochester, New York

Vito M. Campese, MD
Division of Nephrology, Keck School of Medicine, University of Southern California, Los Angeles, California

Celina Denise Cepeda, MD
Pediatric Nephrology, Rady Children's Hospital; Division of Nephrology, University of California, San Diego Medical Center, San Diego, California

Vimal Chadha, MD
Associate Professor of Pediatrics, University of Missouri-Kansas City School of Medicine; Director, Acute Kidney Injury Program, and Associate Director, Dialysis and Transplantation, Children's Mercy Hospital, Kansas City, Missouri

Christopher T. Chan, MD, FRCPC
Department of Medicine, Division of Nephrology, University Health Network, Toronto, Ontario, Canada

Deepa H. Chand, MD, MHSA, FASN
Associate Medical Director, Abbvie Research and Development; Visiting Associate Professor, Pediatrics, University of Illinois College of Medicine, Children's Hospital of Illinois, Peoria, Illinois

Anthony Chang, MD
Professor of Pathology, University of Chicago, Chicago, Illinois

Tara I. Chang, MD, MS
Instructor of Medicine, Division of Nephrology, Stanford University, Palo Alto, California

Chaim Charytan, MD
Clinical Professor of Medicine, Cornell University College of Medicine, New York, New York; Chief, Renal Division, New York Hospital Medical Center of Queens, Flushing, New York

Joline L.T. Chen, MD, MS
Health Sciences Associate Clinical Professor, Division of Nephrology and Hypertension, University of California Irvine, Irvine, California; Attending Physician, Nephrology Section, Department of Medicine, Long Beach Veteran Affairs Medical Center, Long Beach, California

Wei Chen, MD
Department of Medicine, University of Rochester School of Medicine and Dentistry, Rochester, New York

Ronco Claudio, MD
Department of Nephrology, Dialysis and Transplant, San Bortolo Hospital, International Renal Research Institute, Vicenza, Italy

Allan J. Collins, MD, FACP
Director, Chronic Disease Research Group, Minneapolis Medical Research Foundation, Minneapolis, Minnesota; Professor, Department of Medicine, University of Minnesota, Minneapolis, Minnesota

John H. Crabtree
Visiting Clinical Faculty, Division of Nephrology and Hypertension, Harbor-University of California Los Angeles Medical Center, Torrance, California

Lisa E. Crowley, MBChB, MRCP (UK), PhD
Post Doctoral Fellow, Kidney Clinical Research Unit, London Health Sciences Centre, London, Ontario, Canada

Daniel Cukor, PhD
Associate Professor of Psychiatry, SUNY Downstate Medical Center, Brooklyn, New York

Simon J. Davies, MD
Professor of Nephrology and Dialysis Medicine, Institute for Applied Clinical Sciences, Keele University; Professor, Department of Nephrology, University Hospital of North Midlands, Royal Infirmary, Stoke-on-Trent, Staffordshire, United Kingdom

Serpil Muge Deger, MD
Department of Medicine, Division of Nephrology, Vanderbilt University School of Medicine, Nashville, Tennessee

Thomas A. Depner, MD
Internal Medicine, Nephrology, University of California Davis, Sacramento, California

Jose A. Diaz-Buxo, MD, MS, FACP
Advisor, Fresenius Medical Care Renal Therapies Group, Waltham, Massachusetts; Chairman of the RRI Research Board, New York, New York

Lesley C. Dinwiddie, MSN, RN, FNP, CNNe
Senior Vice President, Institute for Clinical Excellence, Education, and Research, Wheaton, Illinois

Ramanath Dukkipati, MD
Division of Nephrology, Harbor-UCLA Medical Center and UCLA School of Medicine, Division of Nephrology, University of California at Irvine, Irvine, California

Sarah E. Duncan, MA
Clinical Psychology Doctoral Program, Fordham University, Bronx, New York

Fabrizio Fabrizi, MD
Staff Nephrologist, Division of Nephrology, Maggiore Hospital and IRCCS Foundation, University School of Medicine, Milano, Italy

Michel Fischbach, MD
Head of Pediatric Department and Professor of Pediatrics, Children Dialysis Unit, University Hospital Strasbourg, Strasbourg, France

Steven Fishbane, MD
Professor of Medicine, Hofstra Northwell School of Medicine; Chief, Division of Kidney Diseases and Hypertension, Department of Medicine, North Shore University Hospital and Long Island Jewish Medical Center, Great Neck, New York

William Henry Fissell IV, MD
Associate Professor, Nephrology and Hypertension, Vanderbilt University, Nashville, Tennessee

Bethany Foster, MD, MSCE
Associate Professor of Pediatrics, McGill University, Montreal, Quebec, Canada; Pediatric Nephrologist, Montreal Children's Hospital, Montreal, Quebec, Canada

Miriam Galbusera, BiolSciD
IRCCS—Istituto di Ricerche Farmacologiche Mario Negri, Centro Anna Maria Astori, Science and Technology Park Kilometro Rosso, Bergamo, Italy

F. John Gennari, MD
Emeritus Professor of Medicine, University of Vermont College of Medicine, Burlington, Vermont

Marc Ghannoum, MD
Associate Professor of Specialized Medicine, University of Montreal, Verdun Hospital, Montreal, Quebec, Canada

Sassan Ghazan-Shahi, MD, FRCPC
The Home Peritoneal Dialysis Unit, University Health Network, University of Toronto, Toronto, Ontario, Canada

Stuart L. Goldstein, MD
Director, Center for Acute Care Nephrology, Cincinnati Children's Hospital, Cincinnati, Ohio

Frank A. Gotch, MD
Associate Clinical Professor of Medicine, Division of Nephrology, University of San Francisco, San Francisco, California

Sharlene Greenwood, PhD
Consultant Physiotherapist in Renal and Exercise Rehabilitation, King's College Hospital; Honorary Senior Clinical Lecturer, Department of Renal Medicine, King's College, London, United Kingdom

Dieter Haffner, MD
Department of Pediatric Kidney, Liver and Metabolic Diseases, Hannover Medical School, Hannover, Germany

Rainer Himmele, MD, MSHM
Vice President Medical Information, Fresenius Medical Care Renal Therapies Group, Waltham, Massachusetts

Janet E. Holland, RN, CNN
Senior Clinical Research Manager, DaVita Clinical Research, Minneapolis, Minnesota

Jean L. Holley, MD
Clinical Professor of Medicine, University of Illinois, Urbana-Champaign; Carle Physician Group, Urbana, Illinois

Clifford Holmes, PhD
Renal Therapeutic Area, Baxter Healthcare, Deerfield, Illinois

Stephen R. Hooper, PhD
Pediatric Neuropsychologist, Associate Dean and Chair, Department of Allied Health Sciences, University of North Carolina School of Medicine, Chapel Hill, North Carolina

Daljit K. Hothi, MBBS, MRCPCH, MD
Consultant Pediatric Nephrologist, Nephrology Department, Great Ormond Street Hospital for Children, London, United Kingdom

Susan Hou, MD
Professor of Medicine, Loyola University Stritch School of Medicine, Loyola University Medical Center, Maywood, Illinois

Alastair J. Hutchison, MBChB, FRCP, MD
Clinical Professor of Renal Medicine, Manchester Academic Health Science Centre; Clinical Head of Division of Specialist Medicine, Manchester Royal Infirmary; Consultant Nephrologist, Renal Unit, Manchester Institute of Nephrology and Transplantation, Manchester, United Kingdom

T. Alp Ikizler, MD
Catherine McLaughlin-Hakim Professor of Medicine, Department of Medicine, Division of Nephrology, Vanderbilt University School of Medicine, Nashville, Tennessee

Bertrand L. Jaber, MD, MS
Division of Nephrology, Department of Medicine, St. Elizabeth's Medical Center, Boston, Massachusetts; Department of Medicine, Tufts University School of Medicine, Boston, Massachusetts

Sarbjit Vanita Jassal, MD
Staff Nephrologist and Director, Geriatric Dialysis Program, Division of Nephrology, University Health Network; Professor of Medicine, University of Toronto, Toronto, Ontario, Canada

Kamyar Kalantar-Zadeh, MD, MPH, PhD
Professor of Medicine, Pediatrics and Epidemiology, Division of Nephrology, Harbor-UCLA Medical Center and UCLA School of Medicine, Torrance and Los Angeles, California

Timothy Koh Jee Kam, MBBS, MRCP (UK), MMed(S'pore)
Department of Renal Medicine, Division of Medicine, Tan Tock Seng Hospital, Singapore

Mark Kaplan, MD
Vice President Medical Affairs and Clinical IT, DaVita Healthcare Partners

Pranay Kathuria, MD
Professor of Medicine; Director, Division of Nephrology and Hypertension; Program Director, Nephrology Fellowship, University of Oklahoma School of Community Medicine, Tulsa, Oklahoma

Jeffrey L. Kaufman, MD, FACS
Vascular Surgeon, Baystate Vascular Services, Department of Surgery, Baystate Medical Center, Springfield, Massachusetts

Ramesh Khanna, MD
Professor of Medicine, Division of Nephrology, University of Missouri-Columbia, Columbia, Missouri

Neenoo Khosla, MD
Assistant Professor of Medicine, Division of Nephrology and Hypertension, NorthShore University HealthSystem and University of Chicago Medical Center, Chicago, Illinois

Paul L. Kimmel, MD, MACP
Clinical Professor of Medicine, Division of Renal Diseases and Hypertension, George Washington University, Washington, D.C.

Laura Kooienga, MD
Denver Nephrologists PC, Denver, Colorado

Pelagia Koufaki, PhD
Research Fellow, School of Health Sciences, Queen Margaret University, Edinburgh, Scotland

Eugene C. Kovalik, MD, CM, FRCP, FACP, FASN
Associate Professor of Medicine, Department of Medicine, Division of Nephrology, Duke University Medical Center, Durham, North Carolina

Martin Kreuzer, MD
Pediatric Kidney, Liver, and Metabolic Diseases, Hannover Medical School, Hannover, Lower Saxony, Germany

Vinay Narasimha Krishna, MD
Clinical Scholar, University of Alabama at Birmingham, Birmingham, Alabama

Mahesh Krishnan, MD, MPH, MBA, FASN
International Chief Medical Officer and Group Vice President, Research and
Development, DaVita Healthcare Partners

Martin K. Kuhlmann, MD
Director, Department of Internal Medicine, Nephrology, Vivantes Klinikum im
Friedrichshain, Berlin, Germany

Ravi S. Lakdawala, MD
Division of Nephrology, Keck School of Medicine, University of Southern
California, Los Angeles, California

Danica Lam, MD
Nephrologist, Humble River Regional Hospital, Toronto, Ontario, Canada

Mark Lambie, MD, PhD
Senior Lecturer in Renal Medicine, Institute for Applied Clinical Sciences, Keele
University; Consultant Nephrologist, Department of Nephrology, University
Hospital of North Midlands, Royal Infirmary, Stroke-on-Trent, Staffordshire,
United Kingdom

Charmaine E. Lok, MD, MSc, FRCPC
Professor of Medicine, University of Toronto Medical Director, Renal
Management Clinics and Hemodialysis, UHN Senior Scientist, TGRI

John D. Mahan, MD
Professor, Department of Pediatrics, Nationwide Children's Hospital, The Ohio
State University College of Medicine, Columbus, Ohio

Harold J. Manley, PharmD, FASN, FCCP
Director, Medication Management and Pharmacovigilance, Dialysis Clinic Inc.,
Albany, New York

Kevin J. Martin, MB, BCh, FACP
Professor of Internal Medicine and Director, Division of Nephrology, Saint Louis
University, St. Louis, Missouri

Paul Martin, MD
Division of Hepatology, University School of Medicine, Miami, Florida

Piyush Mathur, DNB (Nephrology)
Santokba Durlabhji Memorial Hospital, Jaipur, Rajasthan, India

Christopher W. McIntyre, MBBS, DM
Professor of Medicine and Robert Lindsay Chair of Dialysis, Research and
Innovation, Department of Medicine, University of Western Ontario, London,
Ontario, Canada

Rajnish Mehrotra, MD, MS
Harborview Medical Center and Kidney Research Institute, Division
of Nephrology, Department of Medicine, University of Washington,
Seattle, Washington

Ravindra L. Mehta, MD, FACP
Professor of Clinical Medicine, Division of Nephrology, University of California
San Diego, San Diego Medical Center, San Diego, California

Federica Mescia, MD
Unit of Nephrology and Dialysis, Azienda Socio Sanitaria Territoriale Papa
Giovanni XXIII, Bergamo, Italy

Mark M. Mitsnefes, MD, MS
Pediatric Nephrology, Division of Nephrology and Hypertension, Cincinnati
Children's Hospital Medical Center, Cincinnati, Ohio

Gopesh K. Modi, MD, DM
Samarpan Kidney Hospital, Bhopal, India

Louise Moist, MD
Schulich School of Medicine and Dentistry, Western University, Kidney Clinical
Research Unit London Health Sciences Center, London, Ontario, Canada

Divya G. Moodalbail, MD
Pediatric Nephrologist, Nemours/Alfred I. duPont Hospital for Children,
Wilmington, Delaware

Michael L. Moritz, MD
Professor of Pediatrics, University of Pittsburgh School of Medicine; Clinical
Director of Pediatric Nephrology and Medical Director of Pediatric Dialysis,
Children's Hospital of Pittsburgh of UPMC, Pittsburgh, Pennsylvania

Alvin H. Moss, MD, FACP, FAAHPM
Professor of Medicine, Sections of Nephrology and Supportive Care, West
Virginia University School of Medicine; Director, West Virginia University
Center for Health Ethics and Law; Medical Director, Supportive Care Service,
West Virginia Hospitals, Morgantown, West Virginia

Federico Nalesso, MD, PhD
Department of Nephrology, Dialysis and Transplant, San Bortolo Hospital,
International Renal Research Institute, Vicenza, Italy

Sharon J. Nessim, MD
Nephrologist, Department of Medicine, Division of Nephrology,
Jewish General Hospital; Assistant Professor of Medicine, McGill University,
Montreal, Quebec, Canada

Shari K. Neul, PhD
Psychologist, Department of Neurosciences, University of California San Diego, La Jolla, California

Allen R. Nissenson, MD
Chief Medical Officer, DaVita Kidney Care; Emeritus Professor of Medicine, David Geffen School of Medicine at UCLA, Los Angeles, California

Ali J. Olyaei, PharmD, BCPS
Professor, Medicine and Pharmacy, Oregon Health and Science University, Portland, Oregon

David I. Ortiz-Melo, MD
Duke University Medical Center, Department of Medicine, Division of Nephrology, Durham, North Carolina

Biff F. Palmer, MD
Professor of Internal Medicine, Department of Internal Medicine, Division of Nephrology, University of Texas Southwestern Medical Center, Dallas, Texas

Suetonia C. Palmer, MB, ChB, PhD
Department of Medicine, University of Otago Christchurch, Christchurch, New Zealand

Patrick S. Parfrey, MD, FRCPC, OC, FRSC
Professor of Medicine, Memorial University of St. John's, Newfoundland and Labrador, Canada

Melissa Pencille, PhD
Brooklyn Health Disparities Center, SUNY Downstate Medical Center, Brooklyn, New York

Phuong-Chi T. Pham, MD, FASN
Clinical Professor of Medicine, Nephrology and Hypertension, Division of Nephrology, David Geffen School of Medicine at UCLA, Olive View-UCLA Medical Center, Sylmar, California

Phuong-Thu T. Pham, MD, FASN
Clinical Professor of Medicine, David Geffen School of Medicine at UCLA, Kidney Transplant Program, Division of Nephrology, Department of Medicine, University of California at Los Angeles School of Medicine, Los Angeles, California

Joanne D. Pittard, RN, MS
Nursing Education Consultant, Hemodialysis, Inc.; Co-Director, American Dialysis College Hemodialysis Nursing Program; Professor Emerita of Allied Health, Glendale Community College, Glendale, California

Giuseppe Remuzzi, MD, FRCP
IRCCS—Istituto di Ricerche Farmacologiche Mario Negri, Centro Anna Maria Astori, Science and Technology Park Kilometro Rosso, Bergamo, Italy; Unit of Nephrology and Dialysis, Azienda Socio Sanitaria Territoriale Papa Giovanni XXIII, Bergamo, Italy; Department of Biomedical and Clinical Sciences, University of Milan, Italy

Connie M. Rhee, MD, MSc
Department of Medicine, Division of Nephrology and Hypertension, University of California, Irvine School of Medicine, Irvine, California

Claudio Rigatto, MD
Associate Professor of Medicine, Chronic Disease Innovation Centre, University of Manitoba, Winnipeg, Canada

Darren M. Roberts, MD, PhD
School of Medicine, University of Queensland, Brisbane, Queensland, Australia

Rudolph A. Rodriguez, MD
Professor of Medicine, Division of Nephrology, University of Washington, Seattle, Washington

Claudio Ronco, MD
Director, Department of Nephrology, Dialysis, and Transplantation, International Renal Research Institute, St. Bortolo Hospital, Vicenza, Italy

Deborah Rosenthal, PhD
Brooklyn Health Disparities Center, SUNY Downstate Medical Center, Brooklyn, New York

John H. Sadler, MD
Retired Associate Professor of Medicine, Division of Nephrology, University of Maryland, Baltimore, Maryland; President and CEO, Independent Dialysis Foundation, Baltimore, Maryland

Scott G. Satko, MD
Nephrology Associates, PLLC, Winston-Salem, North Carolina

Franz Schaefer, MD, PhD
Professor, Division of Pediatric Nephrology, University Children's Hospital, Heidelberg, Germany

David T. Selewski, MD, MS
Division of Nephrology, Department of Pediatrics and Communicable Disease, C.S. Mott Children's Hospital, Ann Arbor, Michigan

Christine B. Sethna, MD, EdM
Division Director, Pediatric Nephrology, Cohen Children's Medical Center of New York, New Hyde Park, New York; Assistant Professor, Hofstra Northwell School of Medicine, Uniondale, New York

Hitesh H. Shah, MD
Associate Professor of Medicine, Hofstra Northwell School of Medicine; Director, Nephrology Fellowship Program, Division of Kidney Diseases and Hypertension, Department of Medicine, North Shore University Hospital and Long Island Jewish Medical Center, Great Neck, New York

Ron Shapiro, MD
Professor of Surgery; Surgical Director, Kidney/Pancreas Transplant Program, Mount Sinai Hospital-Recanati Miller Transplantation Institute, Icahn School of Medicine at Mount Sinai, New York, New York

Richard A. Sherman, MD
Professor of Medicine, Division of Nephrology, Rutgers—Robert Wood Johnson School of Medicine, New Brunswick, New Jersey

Rukshana Shroff, MD, FRCPCH, PhD
Renal Unit, Great Ormond Street Hospital for Children, NHS Foundation Trust, London, United Kingdom

Pamela Singer, MD, MS
Assistant Professor, Pediatric Nephrology, Cohen Children's Medical Center Hofstra Northwell School of Medicine, New Hyde Park, New York

Jodi M. Smith, MD, MPH
Associate Professor of Pediatrics, University of Washington, Seattle, Washington

Michael J.G. Somers, MD
Associate Professor of Pediatrics, Harvard Medical School; Clinical Director, Division of Nephrology, Boston Children's Hospital, Boston, Massachusetts

Euan Soo, MBBS, MRCPCH, FHKAM (Paed), FHKCPaed, PDipMDPath
Resident Specialist, Paediatric Nephrology Center, Princess Margaret Hospital, Hong Kong

Bruce S. Spinowitz, MD, FACP
Associate Director, Nephrology, Vice Chairman, Medicine, New York-Presbyterian Hospital Queens, Flushing, New York; Clinical Professor of Medicine, Weill Cornell Medical College, New York, New York

Deborah Stein, MD
Instructor in Pediatrics, Harvard Medical School; Assistant in Medicine (Nephrology), Department of Medicine, Boston Children's Hospital, Boston, Massachusetts

John C. Stivelman, MD
Emeritus Chief Medical Officer, Northwest Kidney Centers; Professor Meritus of Medicine, Division of Nephrology, Department of Medicine, University of Washington School of Medicine, Seattle, Washington

Giovanni F.M. Strippoli, MD, MPH, MM, PhD
Professor of Nephrology, Department of Emergency and Organ Transplantation, University of Bari, Bari, Italy; Adjunct Professor of Epidemiology, University of Sydney School of Public Health, Sydney, Australia

Lynsey Stronach, BSc, MSc
Nephrology Department, Great Ormond Street Hospital for Children, London, United Kingdom

Paweena Susantitaphong, MD, PhD
Division of Nephrology, Department of Medicine, Faculty of Medicine, King Chulalongkorn Memorial Hospital, Chulalongkorn University, Bangkok, Thailand

Cheuk-Chun Szeto, MD, FRCP
Professor, Department of Medicine and Therapeutics, Prince of Wales Hospital, The Chinese University of Hong Kong, Shatin, Hong Kong

Rebecca Thomas, MD
Senior Nephrology Fellow, Montreal Children's Hospital, McGill University Health Centre, Montreal, Quebec, Canada

Ashita Tolwani, MD, MSc
Professor of Medicine, University of Alabama at Birmingham, Birmingham, Alabama

Avram Z. Traum, MD
Harvard Medical School; Division of Nephrology, Boston Children's Hospital, Boston, Massachusetts

Tushar Vachharajani, MD, FASN, FACP
Chief of Nephrology, W.G. (Bill) Hefner VA Medical Center; Professor, Section of Nephrology, Edwards Via College of Osteopathic Medicine, Salisbury, North Carolina

Rudolph P. Valentini, MD
Chief Medical Officer and Clinical Professor of Pediatrics, Children's Hospital of Michigan, Wayne State University School of Medicine, Detroit, Michigan

René G. VanDeVoorde III, MD
Assistant Professor of Pediatrics, Monroe Carell Jr. Children's Hospital at Vanderbilt, Nashville, Tennessee

Anand Vardhan, MBBS, MD, DNB, FRCP, MD
Consultant Nephrologist and Clinical Lead for Peritoneal Dialysis, Manchester Institute of Nephrology and Transplantation, The Royal Infirmary, Manchester, United Kingdom

Thanh-Mai Vo, MD
Division of Nephrology, Saint Louis University, St. Louis, Missouri

Thor A. Wagner, MD
Assistant Professor of Pediatrics, University of Washington; Center for Global
Infectious Disease Research, Seattle Children's Research Institute, Seattle,
Washington

Bradley A. Warady, MD
Professor of Pediatrics, University of Missouri-Kansas City School of Medicine;
Senior Associate Chairman, Department of Pediatrics, Director, Division of
Pediatric Nephrology; Director, Dialysis and Transplantation, Children's Mercy
Kansas City, Kansas City, Missouri

Katherine Wesseling-Perry, MD
Division of Nephrology, Department of Pediatrics, David Geffen School of
Medicine at UCLA, Los Angeles, California

Spencer Westcott
Regional Operations Director, DaVita Healthcare Partners, Nashville, Tennessee

James B. Wetmore, MD, MS
Associate Professor of Medicine; Staff Nephrologist, Division of Nephrology,
Hennepin County Medical Center, Minneapolis, Minnesota

Keith Wille, MD, MSPH
Associate Professor of Medicine, University of Alabama at Birmingham,
Birmingham, Alabama

Mark E. Williams, MD, FACP, FASN
Associate Professor of Medicine, Harvard Medical School; Director of Dialysis,
Beth Israel Deaconess Medical Center; Director of Dialysis, Joslin Diabetes
Center, Boston, Massachusetts

Jay B. Wish, MD
Professor of Clinical Medicine, Indiana University; Medical Director, Out-Patient
Dialysis Unit, Indiana University Hospital, Indianapolis, Indiana

Farhanah Yousaf, MBBS
Department of Nephrology, New York-Presbyterian Queens, Flushing, New York

Ariane Zaloszyc, MD
Children Dialysis Unit, University Hospital Strasbourg, Strasbourg, France

Joshua Zaritsky, MD, PhD
Assistant Professor, Thomas Jefferson Medical School; Chief, Pediatric
Nephrology, Nemours/A.I. DuPont Hospital for Children, Wilmington, Delaware

PREFACE

The delivery and financing of dialysis care have continued to evolve rapidly throughout the world. The United States has seen the continued consolidation of the dialysis providers, with two large organizations now overseeing the care of two-thirds of all patients. In addition, younger as well as older and sicker patients are now surviving multiple chronic illnesses such as diabetes, hypertension, and congestive heart failure and congenital diseases and progressing through chronic kidney disease (CKD) to end-stage renal disease (ESRD), entering dialysis or seeking conservative care. This has led to advances in care delivery focusing on patient-centric, holistic care and emphasized the need for care coordination and true integration of care across providers and sites of care. In such an integrated, patient-centric world, an increasing number of providers are taking financial risk in ensuring quality outcomes. Elsewhere in the world, the rising middle class in countries such as India, China, and throughout the Middle East has seen the concomitant rise of "life-style" illnesses including obesity, hypertension, and diabetes, and ultimately CKD and ESRD, putting pressure on care providers and governments to deliver and pay for the care of millions of patients. The increasing affluence has also facilitated the extension of CKD and ESRD care to infancy and early childhood.

The objective of the initial edition of *Dialysis Therapy* was to enlist the involvement of preeminent individuals in areas of clinical dialysis to address, in a succinct fashion, the pertinent clinical problems encountered in adults and children undergoing dialysis. The intent was to provide a "how-to" approach to help the potential reader solve specific patient problems. *Dialysis Therapy* was developed to help nephrologists (pediatric and adult), nurses, technicians, and other members of the health care team resolve the myriad problems confronting the patients undergoing dialysis.

It has been almost a decade since the publication of the 4th Edition of *Handbook of Dialysis Therapy*, and the practice of dialysis continues to be modified to meet the increasing complexity of the patient population and the technical and pharmaceutical advances. Many of the contributors to this edition of *Handbook of Dialysis Therapy* have contributed to previous editions; however, there are over 60 new contributors and they have brought a new perspective to the clinical problems of dialysis.

Similarly, the format for this 5th edition has been updated. In addition to adding new chapters, we have paid particular attention to the readability of the text, tables, and figures. Resizing of the book to make it more portable and the abundant use of color are additional enhancements. And for the first time, the book is accompanied by access to a complete and searchable online text.

This book remains a problem-solving tool and is complementary to our larger, more comprehensive textbook *Clinical Dialysis*, the 4th Edition, which was published in 2006.

We wish to thank all of our contributors for their outstanding work and hope that this book will be a useful reference for physicians, nurses, technicians, dieticians, social workers, and administrators, all of whom assiduously attempt to optimize the clinical care of the dialysis population. The editors wish to thank Helene Caprari, Kellie Heap, Julia Roberts, and Angie Breckon, from Elsevier, whose invaluable assistance made the publication of this text possible.

Allen R. Nissenson, MD
Richard N. Fine, MD
Editors

CONTENTS

Section XI: Peritoneal Dialysis: Clinical Practice

Section XII: Peritoneal Dialysis: Infectious Complications

Section XIII: Peritoneal Dialysis: Noninfectious Complications

Section XIV: Peritoneal Dialysis: Intra-Abdominal Pressure-Related Complications

Section XXVII: Pediatric Dialysis

Section XXIX: Miscellaneous Areas of Clinical Importance

SECTION I

Demographics

CHAPTER 1

Demographics of the End-Stage Renal Disease Patient

James B. Wetmore, MD, MS • Allan J. Collins, MD, FACP

Introduction

Over the past decade, significant changes have occurred worldwide in the end-stage renal disease (ESRD) population receiving maintenance dialysis. The previous edition of this book reported data through 2004, whereas the current edition reports data through 2012 in most cases. While the dialysis population as a whole has continued to grow dramatically, complex trends are in evidence that defy simple characterization. Incidence rates have increased in most, but not all, developing countries, a phenomenon that will almost certainly continue as such countries undergo further economic development. In addition, incidence rates have continued to increase in some developed countries but have stabilized in others, most notably in the United States, home to nearly half of all maintenance dialysis patients. In developed countries, the growth in the dialysis population has been fueled primarily by an increase in prevalent patients, who are now living substantially longer than they did only a decade ago. Thus, the growth of the incident population in developing countries, which will face immense barriers to creating the infrastructure to meet patient needs, and of the prevalent population in developed countries, which will struggle to provide health care for ever-aging populations with multiple comorbid conditions, constitute major challenges to policy makers and public health officials worldwide. Government policies related to dialysis programs may need to increase efforts directed at prevention strategies, and confront difficult choices about whether conservative-care strategies may be most appropriate for some patients.

In this chapter, demographic data are reviewed from the United States and from other countries to provide background for subsequent chapters. Most US data are derived from the United States Renal Data System (USRDS) Annual Data Report (www.usrds.org) and the PEER Report (www.peer.org). International data are drawn from various sources.

Growth of the ESRD Population

International data on ESRD incidence and prevalence are provided annually in the USRDS Annual Data Report. Incidence rates and accompanying percentages of change are shown from 2006 to 2012 by country (Fig. 1.1). As noted, most but not all developing countries appear to be experiencing growth in the incident population; this seems particularly striking in certain Asian and Middle Eastern countries. In contrast, substantial differences exist among developed countries, where incident growth remains high in some (eg, Hong Kong, Singapore, the Republic of Korea,

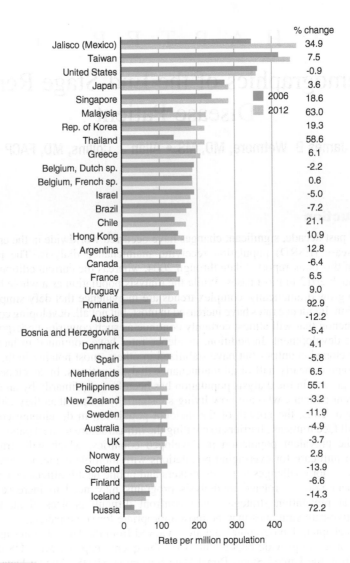

% change

Country	% change
Jalisco (Mexico)	34.9
Taiwan	7.5
United States	-0.9
Japan	3.6
Singapore	18.6
Malaysia	63.0
Rep. of Korea	19.3
Thailand	58.6
Greece	6.1
Belgium, Dutch sp.	-2.2
Belgium, French sp.	0.6
Israel	-5.0
Brazil	-7.2
Chile	21.1
Hong Kong	10.9
Argentina	12.8
Canada	-6.4
France	6.5
Uruguay	9.0
Romania	92.9
Austria	-12.2
Bosnia and Herzegovina	-5.4
Denmark	4.1
Spain	-5.8
Netherlands	6.5
Philippines	55.1
New Zealand	-3.2
Sweden	-11.9
Australia	-4.9
UK	-3.7
Norway	2.8
Scotland	-13.9
Finland	-6.6
Iceland	-14.3
Russia	72.2

■ 2006
■ 2012

0   100   200   300   400
Rate per million population

Figure 1.1

Incident Rates of ESRD, by Country. United States Renal Data System.
*2014 USRDS annual data report: Epidemiology of kidney disease in the
United States.* Bethesda, MD, National Institutes of Health, National Institute
of Diabetes and Digestive and Kidney Diseases, 2014. Data from Volume 2,
Chapter 10, Table 10.1. (Data available at http://www.usrds.org/2014/view/
Default.aspx.)

France, and Greece) but has stabilized or is declining in others (eg, the United States, United Kingdom, Canada, Australia, Belgium, Spain, Austria, and the Scandinavian countries).

Numbers of prevalent ESRD patient have continued to grow throughout the world. To better portray the worldwide burden, prevalent counts, rather than rates, are shown (Fig. 1.2). In the United States, the number of prevalent ESRD patients has increased to more than 600,000, almost all of whom are receiving maintenance hemodialysis. Of note, data are incomplete, and data quality is likely to vary substantially by country; as such, the data presented are unlikely to be definitive. Even acknowledging this caution, however, inferences about overarching trends can safely be made.

Trends in incidence and prevalence in the US dialysis population are shown in more detail in Fig. 1.3. The number of incident patients (Fig. 1.3A) appears to have stabilized beginning in approximately 2009, while the number of prevalent patients (Fig. 1.3B) rose unabated from less than 250,000 in 1997 to approximately 450,000 in 2012. Overall ESRD incident rates have been decreasing since 2007, with the sole exception of 2009 (Fig. 1.4A; to provide context, year-to-year percentages of change are superimposed in the incident count bars). Year-to-year changes in ESRD prevalent rates (Fig. 1.4B) have been relatively stable at approximately 2% since about 2003, but even this modest-appearing annual change has produced an approximately 33% increase from 1997 (fewer than 1400 cases per million) to 2012 (more than 1900 cases per million). The percentages of yearly increases in the prevalent rates have not changed substantially even in recent years (eg, since 2007), suggesting that the dialysis population will continue to grow at a brisk pace for the foreseeable future.

Incident rates and prevalent rates and their associated temporal changes are not evenly distributed geographically or demographically in the United States. For example, adjusted ESRD incident rates are highest in the Ohio River Valley, southern Texas, and southern California (Fig. 1.5). Although certain demographic changes can be hypothesized to underlie this finding in Texas and California, the same explanation seems unlikely to adequately account for the finding in the Ohio River Valley. Regarding age and race, ESRD prevalent rates are growing fastest in older populations (ages 65–74 and 75 years or older) and among African Americans (Figs. 1.6A and 1.6B). The latter finding is not surprising, as African Americans tend to survive longer on dialysis than members of other races, for reasons that remain uncertain. The former finding heralds a change in the dialysis landscape, however, as the growth of the elderly population receiving dialysis suggests that older, and likely sicker, patients are also surviving longer on dialysis.

Comorbidity, Expected Survival, and Causes of Death

Patients start dialysis with a substantial comorbidity burden (Fig. 1.7). In the United States, the Centers for Medicare & Medicaid Services Medical Evidence Report (Form CMS-2728) must be completed upon initiation of dialysis. It inquires about several comorbid conditions, lifestyle choices (eg, smoking, alcohol consumption, and use of drugs of abuse), and functional status measures (eg, inability to ambulate and transfer), and is the source of data shown here. Hypertension, as might be expected, is the most common comorbid condition, present in more than 85% of

(text continued on p. 11)

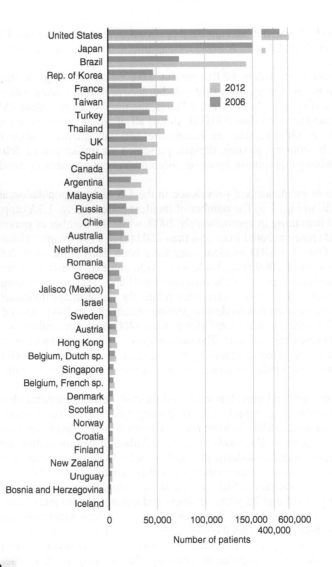

Figure 1.2

Prevalent Counts of ESRD Patients, by Country. United States Renal
Data System. *2014 USRDS annual data report: Epidemiology of kidney
disease in the United States.* Bethesda, MD, National Institutes of Health,
National Institute of Diabetes and Digestive and Kidney Diseases, 2014.
Data from Volume 2, Chapter 10, Table 10.2. (Data available at
http://www.usrds.org/2014/view/Default.aspx.)

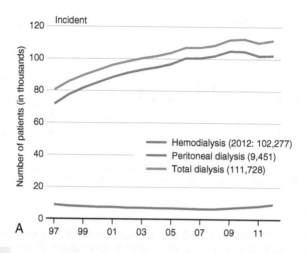

Figure 1.3A

Incident Dialysis Patient Counts. United States Renal Data System. *2014 USRDS annual data report: Epidemiology of kidney disease in the United States.* Bethesda, MD, National Institutes of Health, National Institute of Diabetes and Digestive and Kidney Diseases, 2014. Data from Volume 2, Chapter 1, Figure 1.1. (Data available at http://www.usrds.org/2014/view/Default.aspx.)

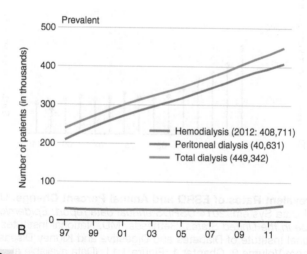

Figure 1.3B

Prevalent Dialysis Patient Counts. United States Renal Data System. *2014 USRDS annual data report: Epidemiology of kidney disease in the United States.* Bethesda, MD, National Institutes of Health, National Institute of Diabetes and Digestive and Kidney Diseases, 2014. Data from Volume 2, Chapter 1, Figure 1.10. (Data available at http://www.usrds.org/2014/view/Default.aspx.)

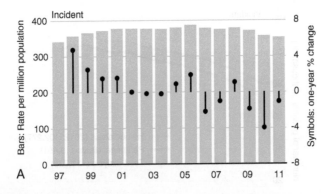

Figure 1.4A

Adjusted Incident Rates of ESRD and Annual Percent Change. United States Renal Data System. *2014 USRDS annual data report: Epidemiology of kidney disease in the United States*. Bethesda, MD, National Institutes of Health, National Institute of Diabetes and Digestive and Kidney Diseases, 2014. Data from Volume 2, Chapter 1, Figure 1.2. (Data available at http://www.usrds.org/2014/view/Default.aspx.)

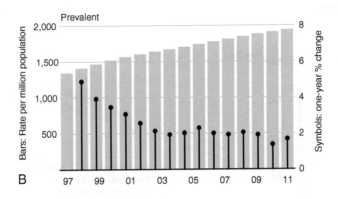

Figure 1.4B

Adjusted Prevalent Rates of ESRD and Annual Percent Change. United States Renal Data System. *2014 USRDS annual data report: Epidemiology of kidney disease in the United States*. Bethesda, MD, National Institutes of Health, National Institute of Diabetes and Digestive and Kidney Diseases, 2014. Data from Volume 2, Chapter 1, Figure 1.11. (Data available at http://www.usrds.org/2014/view/Default.aspx.)

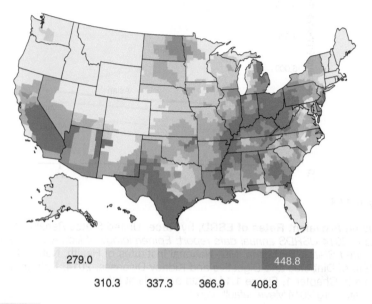

279.0				448.8
310.3	337.3	366.9	408.8	

Figure 1.5

Adjusted Incident Rates of ESRD, by Health Service Area, 2011 (Per Million Population). US Renal Data System. *USRDS 2013 Annual Data Report: Atlas of Chronic Kidney Disease and End-Stage Renal Disease in the United States.* Bethesda, MD, National Institutes of Health, National Institute of Diabetes and Digestive and Kidney Diseases, 2013. Data from Volume 2, Chapter 1, Figure 1.3. (Data available at http://www.usrds.org/atlas13.aspx.)

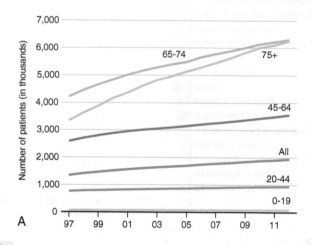

Figure 1.6A

Adjusted Prevalent Rates of ESRD, by Age. United States Renal Data System. *2014 USRDS annual data report: Epidemiology of kidney disease in the United States.* Bethesda, MD, National Institutes of Health, National Institute of Diabetes and Digestive and Kidney Diseases, 2014. Data from Volume 2, Chapter 1, Figure 1.13. (Data available at http://www.usrds.org/2014/view/Default.aspx.)

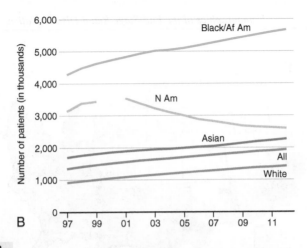

B

Figure 1.6B

Adjusted Prevalent Rates of ESRD, by Race. United States Renal Data
System. *2014 USRDS annual data report: Epidemiology of kidney disease in
the United States.* Bethesda, MD, National Institutes of Health, National
Institute of Diabetes and Digestive and Kidney Diseases, 2014. Data from
Volume 2, Chapter 1, Figure 1.14. (Data available at http://
www.usrds.org/2014/view/Default.aspx.)

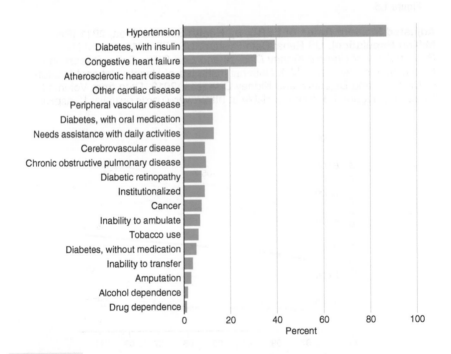

Figure 1.7

**Prevalence of Comorbid Conditions, According to the Medical Evidence
Report, 2011.** Weinhandl E, Constantini E, Everson S, et al. Peer Kidney
Care Initiative 2014 report: Dialysis care and outcomes in the United States.
Am J Kidney Dis. 2015;65(6):S30. (Data regraphed; data available at
http://www.peerkidney.org/report/download-peer-report.)

patients, and diabetes (requiring and not requiring insulin) is the next-most common at about 50%. Congestive heart failure is also relatively common, at about 33%. Despite this, mortality rates for incident dialysis patients have fallen substantially since about 2003 (Fig. 1.8A) and for prevalent patients since about 2001 (Fig. 1.8B). A conceptual representation of this is shown in Fig. 1.9, which standardizes patient counts and patient deaths to 1996 data (producing a dimensionless unit for the y-axis). The patient line and the death line diverged in about 2005, conceptually demonstrating how improved survival has contributed to the growth in the number of dialysis patients in the United States (and, potentially, in other developed countries). The expected remaining lifetimes (Fig. 1.10) increase substantially for prevalent dialysis patients across the age spectrum. While some of these increases may appear small, they nevertheless prolong life to a meaningful extent. For example, for a person aged 45–49 years with approximately 6 years of life remaining in 2003, an increase of 1.7 years over less than a decade represents a nontrivial improvement.

Sudden cardiac death is the largest single cause of death in each age group (Fig. 1.11) and, combined with other cardiovascular causes of death, accounts for more than 40% of all deaths in every age group except 80 years or older. As might be expected, dialysis withdrawal accounts for an increasingly larger proportion of deaths as age increases and is the cause of death for more than 20% of patients aged 80 years or older. Even for patients aged 18–44 years, however, withdrawal accounts for approximately 6% of deaths. Sudden cardiac death is particularly likely in the first 3 months of dialysis (Fig. 1.12). This could be because, as described above, newly initiated patients carry a high burden of cardiovascular disease; such patients

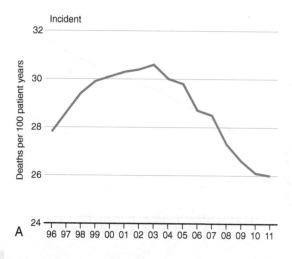

Figure 1.8A

Mortality Rates in Incident Dialysis Patients. Weinhandl E, Constantini E, Everson S, et al. Peer Kidney Care Initiative 2014 report: Dialysis care and outcomes in the United States. *Am J Kidney Dis.* 2015;65(6):S98. (Data regraphed; data available at http://www.peerkidney.org/report/download-peer-report.)

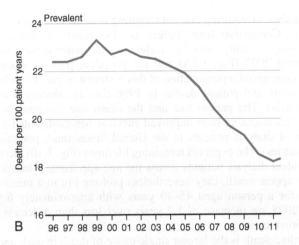

Figure 1.8B

Mortality Rates in Prevalent Dialysis Patients. Weinhandl E, Constantini E, Everson S, et al. Peer Kidney Care Initiative 2014 report: Dialysis care and outcomes in the United States. *Am J Kidney Dis.* 2015;65(6):S108. (Data regraphed; data available at http://www.peerkidney.org/report/download-peer-report.)

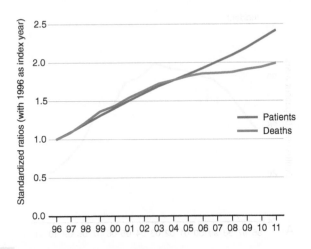

Figure 1.9

Prevalent Dialysis Patient Counts and Deaths. Weinhandl E, Constantini E, Everson S, et al. Peer Kidney Care Initiative 2014 report: Dialysis care and outcomes in the United States. *Am J Kidney Dis.* 2015;65(6):S112. (Data regraphed; data available at http://www.peerkidney.org/report/download-peer-report.)

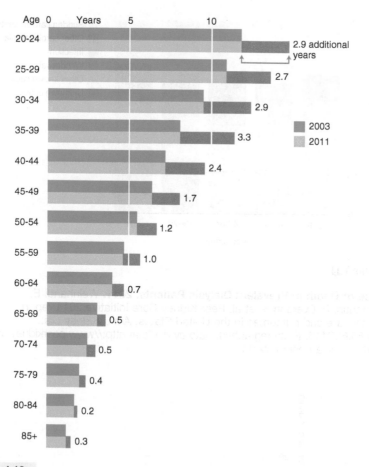

Figure 1.10

Expected Remaining Lifetimes in Prevalent Dialysis Patients. Peer Kidney Care Initiative, March flier on World Kidney Day. http://www.peerkidney.org/educational-materials/march-2015-world-kidney-day.

may experience great difficulty in adapting to the cardiovascular stresses that characterize dialysis in general and hemodialysis in particular. Dialysis patients experience wide swings in blood pressure, cardiovascular hemodynamics, and circulating concentrations of electrolytes (especially potassium), which likely contribute to high rates of early cardiovascular death. Possibly, after an initial period of adaptation during which the most vulnerable patients succumb, the increase in sudden cardiac death as the year progresses may be due to longer-term dialysis-induced changes such as development of left ventricular hypertrophy or the cardiotoxic effects of abnormalities in mineral metabolism related to secondary hyperparathyroidism.

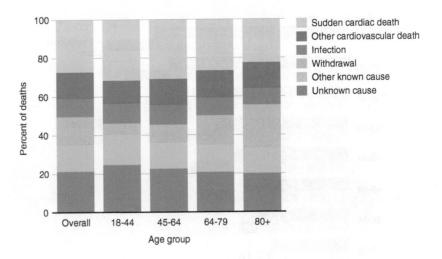

Figure 1.11

Cause of Death in Prevalent Dialysis Patients, 2011. Weinhandl E,
Constantini E, Everson S, et al. Peer Kidney Care Initiative 2014 report:
Dialysis care and outcomes in the United States. *Am J Kidney Dis.*
2015;65(6):S115. (Data regraphed; data available at http://www.peerkidney.org/
report/download-peer-report.)

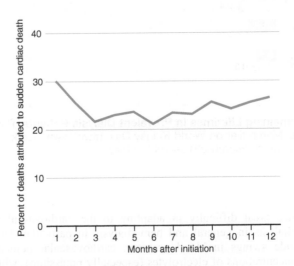

Figure 1.12

Sudden Cardiac Death in the First Year of Dialysis, 2011. Weinhandl E,
Constantini E, Everson S, et al. Peer Kidney Care Initiative 2014 report:
Dialysis care and outcomes in the United States. *Am J Kidney Dis.*
2015;65(6):S105. (Data regraphed; data available at http://www.peerkidney.org/
report/download-peer-report.)

Dialysis Initiation: Predialysis Care and Modality Selection

The transition from predialysis chronic kidney disease (CKD) to ESRD, and specifically to dialysis, is a time of increasing interest. In the United States, the percentages of CKD patients who see a nephrologist vary widely by geographic region. Overall, only 68% were receiving nephrology care as of 2011 (Fig. 1.13); this represents only a modest increase from about 65% in 2008 despite increasing efforts to implement automated laboratory reporting of estimated glomerular filtration rates (eGFRs). The percentage climbed to nearly 80% in New England as of 2011, and was lowest, at about 62%, in the West South Central region (Arkansas, Louisiana, Oklahoma, and Texas). If significant improvements in the care of CKD patients are to occur, overcoming barriers to nephrology care is imperative.

Dialysis initiation at higher eGFR levels has been a growing trend in the United States (Fig. 1.14). From 1997 to 2012, the percentage of patients initiating at eGFR 10–<15 mL/min/1.73 m^2 increased, as did the percentage initiating at ≥15 mL/min/1.73 m^2. This trend may be abating over the most recent years for which data are available, 2011–2012. However, efforts designed to promote initiation at lower levels, which confers many benefits such as increased time for fistula maturation, will likely also require efforts to improve access to nephrology care. Optimizing vascular access remains a vexing problem for most, if not all, countries; data from DOPPS show that even in the highest-performing countries, arteriovenous fistulas account for only about 75% to 80% of all accesses on a cross-sectional basis; the sole exception is Japan, where fistulas are used in more than 90% of hemodialysis patients, and use of tunneled dialysis catheters is virtually nonexistent (Fig. 1.15).

Hemodialysis remains the overwhelmingly most common modality by which ESRD care is delivered worldwide (Fig. 1.16). The largest proportions of peritoneal

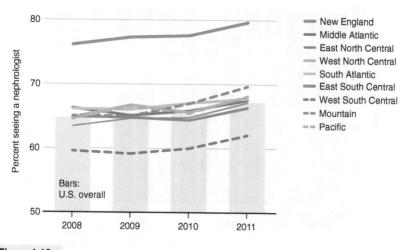

Figure 1.13

Nephrology Care Before Starting Dialysis. Weinhandl E, Constantini E, Everson S, et al. Peer Kidney Care Initiative 2014 report: Dialysis care and outcomes in the United States. *Am J Kidney Dis.* 2015;65(6):S28. (Data available at http://www.peerkidney.org/report/download-peer-report.)

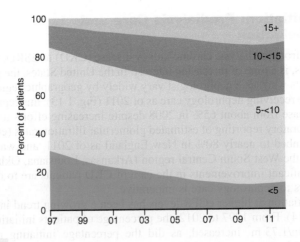

Figure 1.14

eGFR at Initiation. United States Renal Data System. *2014 USRDS annual data report: Epidemiology of kidney disease in the United States.* Bethesda, MD, National Institutes of Health, National Institute of Diabetes and Digestive and Kidney Diseases, 2014. Data from Volume 2, Chapter 1, Figure 1.1.22. (Data available at http://www.usrds.org/2014/view/Default.aspx.)

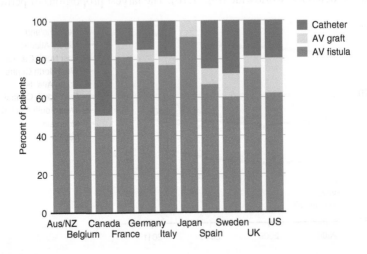

Figure 1.15

Vascular Access in Use, by Country. *2012 annual report of the Dialysis Outcomes and Practice Patterns Study: Hemodialysis data 1997-2011.* Ann Arbor, MI, Arbor Research Collaborative for Health. Downloaded from http://www.dopps.org/annualreport/html/vType_c_mostrec2011.htm.

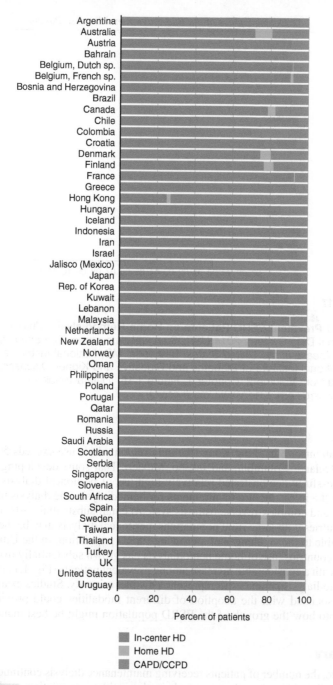

Argentina
Australia
Austria
Bahrain
Belgium, Dutch sp.
Belgium, French sp.
Bosnia and Herzegovina
Brazil
Canada
Chile
Colombia
Croatia
Denmark
Finland
France
Greece
Hong Kong
Hungary
Iceland
Indonesia
Iran
Israel
Jalisco (Mexico)
Japan
Rep. of Korea
Kuwait
Lebanon
Malaysia
Netherlands
New Zealand
Norway
Oman
Philippines
Poland
Portugal
Qatar
Romania
Russia
Saudi Arabia
Scotland
Serbia
Singapore
Slovenia
South Africa
Spain
Sweden
Taiwan
Thailand
Turkey
UK
United States
Uruguay

Percent of patients

■ In-center HD
■ Home HD
■ CAPD/CCPD

Figure 1.16

Prevalent Dialysis Patients, by Type of Therapy, 2012. United States Renal
Data System. *2014 USRDS annual data report: Epidemiology of kidney
disease in the United States.* Bethesda, MD, National Institutes of Health,
National Institute of Diabetes and Digestive and Kidney Diseases, 2014. Data
from Volume 2, Chapter 10, Figure 10.9. (Data available at
http://www.usrds.org/2014/view/Default.aspx.)

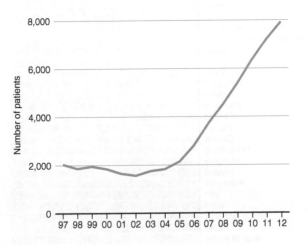

Figure 1.17

Number of Prevalent ESRD Patients on Home Hemodialysis. United States Renal Data System. *2014 USRDS annual data report: Epidemiology of kidney disease in the United States.* Bethesda, MD, National Institutes of Health, National Institute of Diabetes and Digestive and Kidney Diseases, 2014. Data from Volume 2, Chapter 1, Figure 1.18. (Data available at http://www.usrds.org/2014/view/Default.aspx.)

dialysis patients are in Hong Kong (the only region where use exceeds 50%); New Zealand; Iceland; Columbia; and Jalisco, Mexico. That some developing countries have successfully demonstrated relatively high use of peritoneal dialysis is important, since the infrastructure requirements for hemodialysis (the dialysis unit and its expensive and complex reverse osmosis system) entail substantial costs. For developing countries with large rural populations, peritoneal dialysis may be the modality most suitable to the challenges of a growing ESRD population. In the United States and other countries, use of home hemodialysis has grown substantially over the past 10 years, with a considerable increase among prevalent patients (Fig. 1.17); however, home hemodialysis patients still represent a distinct minority. Studies examining the factors associated with the adoption of different modalities could provide crucial insights into how the growth of the ESRD population might be best managed.

Summary

Worldwide, the number of patients receiving maintenance dialysis continues to grow. This is attributable primarily to growth in the incident population in developing countries and in the prevalent population in developed countries. For reasons that are uncertain, dialysis patients appear to be living substantially longer than they did just a few years ago, at least in the United States. As a result, governments in all countries will have to manage the immense economic and social costs of growing dialysis populations. Encouraging and facilitating patients to elect "self-care" modalities such as peritoneal dialysis and home hemodialysis might be a way to meet these prodigious anticipated needs. Likewise, governments will be challenged to improve access to predialysis care, which even in a developed country such as the United States is far from optimal. The trend toward initiating dialysis at ever-higher eGFR levels appears to be abating. Reducing deaths during the first 3 months of dialysis must remain a major focus for the nephrology community in the face of the major comorbidity burden that affects the dialysis population as a whole. These and many other topics are addressed in subsequent chapters.

SECTION II

Vascular Access for Hemodialysis

C H A P T E R   2

Vascular Access for Hemodialysis in Adults

Charmaine E. Lok, MD, MSc, FRCPC • Michael Allon, MD

Introduction

It is well established that dialysis cannot be provided without access; while this should not be taken for granted, such access can be achieved in a majority of cases. In contrast, the attainment and maintenance of a single *reliable, long-lasting* dialysis access with *minimal complications* continue to be challenging. Achievement of such an access is associated with optimal patient clinical outcomes, superior quality of life, and minimal costs. As such, a paradigm shift in thinking is needed that requires a focus on understanding the individual patient's short- and long-term needs as a *person* with end-stage kidney disease (ESKD). Such a focus requires a multidisciplinary team approach where all renal replacement therapy (RRT) options are understood and considered, in order for the patient to attain the potentially *multiple,* optimal access(es) at appropriate junctures in their ESKD lifetime. Such an approach thoughtfully considers patient transitions from one RRT modality to another, including conservative and palliative care, depending on individual needs. Clearly, the goals and abilities of a young man with glomerulonephritis as his cause of ESKD may differ from that of an elderly woman with multiple comorbidities and diabetes mellitus as her cause of ESKD; as such, these differences may be reflected in their dialysis access needs. This approach contrasts to a prior, more static approach where the goal was to attain an "ideal vascular access" for all patients for all time. Theoretically, such an ideal access would improve outcomes and limit costs, yet a one-size-fits-all approach may inadvertently have unintended negative consequences to both patients and health care systems. Thus, this chapter will discuss vascular access selection and review the pros, cons, and unique clinical applications of each key hemodialysis vascular access: the arteriovenous (AV) fistula (AVF), the arteriovenous synthetic graft (AVG), and the central venous catheter (CVC). In doing so, the reader will be better equipped to consider these accesses in the context of what is appropriate for each patient at different phases of his or her own unique ESKD lifetime. Newer vascular accesses on the horizon should be considered similarly. Further, while peritoneal dialysis (PD) is a clearly important RRT modality with its own access considerations, this chapter will not discuss PD access but will emphasize hemodialysis vascular access issues as they relate to a patient who may need to transfer to or from PD. Similarly, the importance of hemodialysis vascular access planning, creation, and maintenance in a patient transitioning from transplantation will be briefly discussed.

History of Vascular Access

The history of vascular access types reflects the changes in the ESKD population demographics and needs over time (Table 2.1).

Multidisciplinary Approach to Vascular Access

Strategy and Roles

Key members of the multidisciplinary vascular access team include the nephrologist, surgeon, endovascular interventionalists, vascular access coordinator, cannulator (typically nurse or technician), the patient, and his or her support system. The planning, creation, and maintenance phases of the vascular access have different emphases, and, as such, a different team member may "lead" where needed and appropriate. This requires a mutual respect and trust among team members where clear, timely, and effective communication between health team members, and between health team members and the patient and their support team, is critical for successful access care. Examples of team members and roles are in Table 2.2.

The vascular access coordinator facilitates communication and activities across all phases. The patient and his or her support system should be engaged to participate in informed decision making during all phases.

Education

Each member of the multidisciplinary team must coordinate educational efforts so that the patient receives nonconflicting and clear information about their chronic kidney disease (CKD), modality options, and the associated access. When patients and their family members are active participants in the decision-making process, adherence greatly improves. Optimal outcomes, such as initiating hemodialysis with a functioning access, are more likely when patients and their families receive high-quality, individualized CKD education. For example, in a nationwide study of >3000 patients, patients who received education about vascular access had an odds ratio of 2.06 for having an AVF or AVG placed compared with a CVC. Patients who receive education about vascular access also had reduced anxiety about receiving their AVF or AVG.

A key element to emphasize in the education of patients about hemodialysis vascular access is to preserve veins by protecting them against venopunctures, intravenous lines, central venous catheterizations, and pacemaker insertions on the side of the planned future hemodialysis vascular access. For example, when venous access is required, only the dorsal aspect of the hand should be used. Peripherally inserted central catheters, "PICC lines," should be avoided in patients with a potential future dialysis need and should be considered absolutely contraindicated in patients with stage 4 or 5 CKD. Patients already undergoing hemodialysis can have blood drawn during their hemodialysis session to preserve veins. This emphasis on vein preservation, as well as other important vascular access education, must be supported by health care workers and administration alike within the hospital or dialysis facility, in order for it to be effective. Optimal patient outcomes and lowered costs will reinforce the effectiveness of comprehensive modality and access education.

Table 2.1

Key Highlights in the History of Vascular Access

Year	Patient Demographics & Needs	Important Influences	Key Vascular Access Development	Impact
1945	Kidney failure fatal without hemodialysis	HD was the only RRT available	Single arterial and venous cut-down for single HD	HD truly limited by access sites
1960	Young patient with limited comorbidity	Ethics committee reviewed hemodialysis eligibility—provided at home	Scribner shunt	Maintenance HD became possible; infection and clotting were predominant issues
1961	Similar to 1960	Rapid access for dialysis required	First subclavian vein access for dialysis	Subclavian catheter approach became the preferred method for temporary access for the following 2 decades
1966	Young patient (<55 years old) with limited comorbidity	Diabetic individuals were not eligible for dialysis	Cimino-Brescia fistula	Longer patency and reduced complications; Primary failure rate <15% in original fistulas
1970	Patients with lack of or exhaustion of peripheral vessels; pediatric hemodialysis population with small vessels	A new method of access besides a shunt was required	Prosthetic graft	Thrombosis, infection remained a problem (as in shunts); aneurysms were linked with repeated cannulation
1973	Diabetic patient with greater comorbidity	Patients of all ages and etiologies of ESKD became eligible for dialysis	Prosthetic graft	Search for synthetic and biologic materials that would improve patency and reduce complications began and is ongoing
1993	As above	Need for repeated catheter insertions in the same patient	Chronic central venous catheter	Chronic HD with permanent CVC possible

Table 2.1

Key Highlights in the History of Vascular Access—cont'd

Year	Patient Demographics & Needs	Important Influences	Key Vascular Access Development	Impact
1994	As above + more home nocturnal dialysis patients		Uldall-Cook central venous catheter	Patients were able to provide dialysis of long duration overnight at home
2013	As above	Increasingly older patients with greater comorbidity and living longer; exhaustion of vascular access options and central venous occlusion	HeRO graft; a hybrid between synthetic graft (arterial component) and CVC (venous outflow)	Bypasses the central occlusion with the CVC portion and allows peripheral access via graft portion. Combined risks of graft and CVC exist, diligent care required

Planning and Choice of Vascular Access

Dialysis access planning should start in CKD stage IV (glomerular filtration rate [GFR] 15–30 mL/min), when education about CKD and modalities of RRT should be discussed. The rate of decline of GFR over time is perhaps the best predictive guide to timely referral and access placement. Recently, a CKD progression prediction model was developed and validated. This model and the patient's degree of proteinuria may help estimate the progression of CKD to ESRD. The components required for patient-focused access planning are as follows:
1. Timely and appropriate referral;
2. Education (above);
3. Patient history and physical examination;
4. Supportive investigations.

Timely and Appropriate Referral

Timely referral to a nephrologist and access surgeon for CKD management and surgical evaluation, respectively, increases the likelihood of placing a native vein AVF and reduces the likelihood of temporary CVC placement. Therefore, when GFR approaches 30 mL/min (CKD stage 4), patient education about CKD, and its potential progression to require RRT and dialysis access, must begin. In terms of the GFR "sweet spot" for AV access creation, this will depend on the patient's age, rate of CKD progression, and prognosis. For example, elderly patients have a slower rate of GFR decline, lower incidence of ESRD, and higher mortality rate and may suffer from an excessively high ratio of unnecessary to necessary permanent

Table 2.2

Hemodialysis Vascular Access Team Members and Primary Roles

Lead Team Member	Phase	Role
Nephrologist	Before VA created	Medical eligibility for RRT modality and vascular access: evaluates comorbidities, functional status, life circumstances and goals
Surgeon		Surgical eligibility of vascular access: vessel assessment ±mapping
Surgeon or interventionalist Nephrologist Surgeon	VA creation/insertion	Creates AV access or inserts catheter
	After VA creation	Assesses access for development, complications, and readiness for use
Surgeon Interventionalist		Facilitates or rectifies access issues in order to attain and/or maintain patency (e.g., AVF revision, AVG angioplasty, CVC exchange)
Cannulator Nephrologist		Assesses for readiness of cannulation Monitors for dialysis-related complications
Patient and support system		

access surgeries and interventions. Clinicians should aim to reduce the number of unnecessary procedures to attain functioning necessary AV accesses. An approach to access creation is illustrated in Fig. 2.1.

Patient and Vascular Access History

A "hemodialysis access–focused" history is unique and required in planning dialysis access. Such a history will shed light on potential complications that may occur, such as failure of an AVF to mature, potential for high cardiac output failure, or AVG-associated steal syndrome and will navigate the surgeon to either preemptive intervention or consideration of an alternate access. This "vessel-focused" history includes determining the type and nature of past access-affecting procedures (especially CVCs, PICC lines, and pacemakers), past accesses (interventions required to facilitate or maintain its patency and reason(s) for loss), breast and axillary dissection surgery, chest radiation, and emergency vascular cut-downs. Furthermore, a parallel "PD-focused" history should be pursued to help inform the choice of dialysis access. Factors that may affect the peritoneum, such as the presence of significant inflammatory bowel or active diverticular disease and prior abdominal surgeries, may lead one to exclude PD and focus on hemodialysis vascular access.

Physical Examination

The focused physical examination includes a detailed inspection of the neck, chest, abdomen, and extremities. The examination must take into consideration the significance of previous chest and abdominal surgeries (for PD), pacemakers, presence of edema, and collateral vein formation that may suggest central vein pathology. The vascular examination must assess both the arterial and venous systems.

The hemodialysis vascular access examination requires a relaxed patient in a comfortable environment. A cold room will cause vessel vasoconstriction and potentially underestimate the size of available vessels. The use of an upper arm tourniquet or warming the extremity (e.g., with hot water) followed by asking the patient to close and open his or her fists will help augment vessels for assessment. The arterial assessment includes evaluation of pulse quality, segmental blood pressure, and the Allen test. The venous system comprises a detailed inspection and palpation for vessel integrity, caliber, and size. Duplex ultrasound (DU) may be used to clarify or confirm concerns of vessel integrity and/or may be used to better define surgical and interventional anatomy.

Supportive Investigations

DU is particularly useful in the obese patient, but may not always add much to a careful and experienced physical examination (see "Physical Examination" section). Indeed, the quality of the DU examination is operator dependent; ideally, the surgeon should perform the DU or be present to direct the sequence of examination steps and mark the skin, documenting vessel size, intended surgery sites, and anatomic variations. The specific features assessed during DU are listed in Table 2.3.

Since DU findings need to be considered within the context of the other variables determined by the history and physical examination, caution should be given to using size criteria alone to determine vessel eligibility for the desired access. Doing so

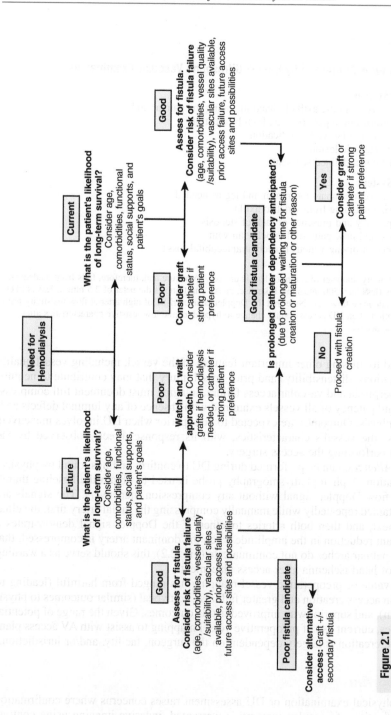

Figure 2.1

Algorithm for Considering Vascular Access Choice.

Table 2.3

Main Features Addressed by Duplex Ultrasound Vascular Examination

Arterial System
- Artery size from the axilla to hand including the palmar arch[a]
- Dual arteries in upper arm, i.e., high bifurcation
- Degree of arterial wall calcification
- Arterial stenotic lesions
- Blood flow at defined segments

Venous System
- Detailed venous anatomy in arm and leg as needed
- Vein size mapping from wrist to axilla
- Vein patency and presence or lack of stenosis
- Patency and flow pattern of subclavian vein
- Presence of diving venous branch at antecubital fossa

[a]A (radial) artery diameter of 2 mm or less is unlikely to mature and, therefore, fails from inadequate fistula flow (less than 500 mL/min). Likewise, an AV anastomosis diameter of 2.5 mm or less is likely to yield inadequate flow rate. Note that the Doppler characteristic of high arterial flow resistivity prior to the creation of an HD access should change to hyperdynamic low resistive characteristics after creating the access.

may lead to missing other important features of the vessel, including vessel quality (calcifications, distensibility) and prior vessel injury that may contribute to neointimal hyperplasia and vascular access failure. Imaging must document full compressibility and patency of all vessels examined with absence of any luminal defects and/or thrombosis. Outcomes are expected to be superior when DU involves maneuvers to assess the vessel's characteristics, with its response directly observed by the surgeon performing the access surgery.

The *Allen test* can be performed during DU to confirm findings found by physical examination. A photoplethysmography probe is used to obtain the baseline thumb arterial flow Doppler signal without any compression maneuvers. The signals are then obtained repeatedly while manually compressing the radial artery first, the ulnar artery next, and then both arteries together. If the Doppler signal demonstrates a significant reduction in the amplitude when the dominant artery is compressed, that is, both palmar arches do not communicate (Fig. 2.2), this should serve as a warning of risk of hand ischemia after access placement.

The value of preoperative vessel mapping has ranged from harmful (leading to delays in access creation and greater failures), equivocal (similar outcomes to physical exam), and superior with improved fistula outcomes. Given the range of potential outcomes, current use of preoperative vessel mapping to assist with AV access planning and creation is largely dependent on the surgeon, facility, and/or jurisdiction.

Angiogram

If the physical examination or DU assessment raises concerns where confirmation or clarification of vascular anatomy is warranted, invasive imaging using contrast dye or CO_2 angiography (as appropriate) is warranted. Ten to fifteen milliliters of dilute contrast dye has not been associated with accelerating the decline in GFR.

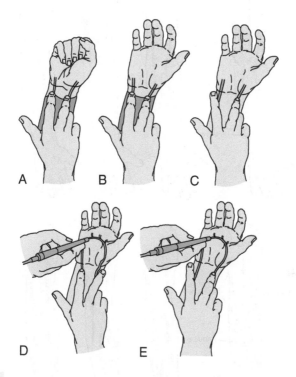

Figure 2.2

Allen's test is used to determine whether the arterial supply of the hands is adequate and whether the hand arch connects the ulnar and radial arteries. Arteries should not be ligated or occluded during an access procedure if the Allen's test shows poor collaterals.

Access Site Locations

In considering access location, there should be a carefully thought-out, systematic progression from one vascular access site to another, in an attempt to preserve and use every site available to extend the patient's ESKD "lifeline." An "upper extremity first," followed by a "distal to proximal" approach, maximizes potential access sites and takes advantage of the dilation effect of access procedures on the vasculature; this may lead to the development of veins and arteries at sites that were initially deemed suboptimal.

Upper Extremity

Fistulas

Fistulas are relatively simple to create, and different types of autogenous artery-vein anastomoses are possible, including end-to-side (end of the vein to side of the artery), terminalized side-to-side, laterolateral, and end-to-end (Fig. 2.3A).

Wrist. Snuffbox radiocephalic fistula: an anastomosis between the distal radial artery and cephalic vein (between the tendons of the extensor pollicis brevis and extensor pollicis longus in the anatomic snuffbox).

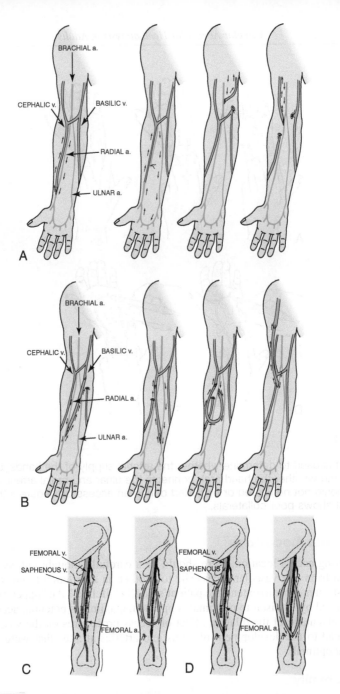

Figure 2.3

Optimal Progression of Access Procedures. The optimal progression of
access is from the nondominant upper extremity distally to proximally, using
autogenous veins (A). Next, the dominant arm should be used. Once all
autogenous veins have been exhausted, prosthetic graft should be used in
the same progression. When upper extremity access sites have been
depleted, the lower extremities can be used (C = autogenous fistula; D =
prosthetic graft). The progression suggested is based on the durability of the
conduit and likelihood of complications such as access thrombosis, steal
syndrome, and infection.

Forearm. Radiocephalic fistula: the Brescia-Cimino fistula connects the radial artery to the cephalic vein.

Radiobasilic transposition: the basilic vein in the forearm is also an excellent conduit for hemodialysis, although it needs to be transposed to the radial region for good function. Mobilization of the basilic vein, with retunneling, is a good alternative when the cephalic vein is not available in the forearm.

Upper arm. Brachiocephalic (a variant is the Gracz fistula): a brachial artery to cephalic vein anastomosis; or brachiobasilic: brachial artery and transposed basilic vein anastomosis.

Special circumstances

- Veins with adequate diameter but inadequate length: the addition of harvested veins, such as saphenous veins, can be used to provide extra length that may be required (as in transposed fistulas) and is an option. Tunneling and transposition of veins may allow the approximation required to create an arteriovenous anastomosis.
- Deep veins with inadequate diameter: a two-stage approach can be used in this situation. The first stage is to connect the artery and the vein. A period of time is given to allow the vein to "arterialize" or mature. If successful, the second stage is to transpose the matured vein to a subdermal location to allow for cannulation.

Grafts

An AV graft is a prosthetic interposition between an artery and a vein. Grafts are typically categorized as synthetic or biologic. There are a variety of graft materials, types, and configurations (Fig. 2.3B).

Wrist. Straight forearm: a straight graft from the radial artery to the median cubital vein.

Forearm. Loop forearm: a loop graft connecting the distal brachial artery or proximal radial artery to the median cubital vein.

Upper arm. Straight or curved upper arm: grafts of various configurations can connect the brachial artery with the basilic, brachial, or axillary vein.

CVC

Catheters are typically used in urgent or emergent situations that require hemodialysis. In such situations, the CVCs are typically noncuffed and untunneled. However, they may also be cuffed and tunneled within the subcutaneous tissue to reach the target vein. The right internal jugular vein is preferred to the left internal jugular vein because of a more direct route to the right atrium. Subclavian vein catheters should be avoided because of their high risk of central vein stenosis. The CVC tip should be placed in the mid right atrium. After insertion, the position should be checked by a chest radiograph in the upright position. The order of preference of CVC location is indicated in Table 2.4. Regardless of location, all insertions should be guided by ultrasound, using the Seldinger technique. It is important to use a dilator over the guidewire before inserting the catheter to minimize vessel trauma. Trauma to vessels increases the likelihood of central vein stenosis.

Lower Extremity

Femoral Region

When all upper extremity sites have been exhausted, lower extremity access (primarily femoral) may be the only option. As with upper extremity access, lower extremity

Table 2.4

Suggested order of location for CVC placement

Preference	Vein	Comments
1	Internal jugular[a]	Right preferred Postinsertion imaging required to check placement
2	Femoral vein	Ensure adequate catheter length
3	Subclavian	Lowest infection risk of all locations Trendelenburg position during insertion may decrease the risk of air embolism Postinsertion imaging required to check placement
4	Lumbar	A location of last resort when no other access site is available

[a]In a patient who is anticipated to require long-term dialysis, it may be preferable to use the femoral vein as the first choice of temporary access in order to preserve central veins in the neck for future AVF or AVG creation. Stenosis of internal jugular veins is more common than previously indicated (up to 30% or more) and may rival the rate of central stenosis found with subclavian veins. However, the risk factors, timing, and onset of central stenosis is currently not well understood. This approach to preserve neck veins is particularly important to consider in patients with good prognosis and/or an expected long-term survival (particularly if they are not transplant candidates). These patients would benefit from an AV access, but this may not be possible if a CVC in the internal jugular vein caused central vein stenosis, preventing successful AV access creation on the side of the CVC.

access is dependent on adequate arterial inflow and unobstructed outflow in a good quality vein. In such cases, AVFs and AVGs can be constructed in a similar manner to that of the upper extremity (Fig. 2.3C and D). Because of the higher flow rates through femoral vessels, there may be a greater risk of steal syndrome. There is also the potential risk of greater bacterial colonization and infection; careful access care using aseptic technique is required regardless of the location but special care is required in situations that put patients at high risk of access infection in the femoral region, such as diarrheal illness.

CVC can also be placed in the femoral region. Temporary requirements (e.g., when dialysis is needed while an AV access is being declotted) typically involve an uncuffed, untunneled femoral catheter that can be removed immediately after the dialysis session. More prolonged use requires the insertion of a cuffed, tunneled catheter. A randomized controlled trial and several meta-analyses have demonstrated equivalent thrombosis and infection rates using tunneled femoral catheters compared with internal jugular catheters. However, except when there are no other available access options, femoral catheters should only be used for limited time frames and only when necessary.

Unusual Locations
Axillary-axillary/femoral-popliteal: When all conventional access sites have been exhausted, the access surgeon must be creative to obtain a permanent access. Connecting an available and adequate large artery to any acceptable outflow vein can, in necessary situations, result in a functional chronic dialysis access. It is critical, *before* a dialysis access is created, to consider the "exit strategy," that is, what corrective options are available for the patient in case of complications and/or what *type* and *where* the next access will be created.

Overall Clinical Considerations

Fig. 2.1 provides an algorithm to assist in the clinical approach to a patient who needs vascular access.

Once the HD access is created, it should be routinely monitored by physical examination. The presence of a palpable thrill, pulse quality, and appearance of the overlying skin (i.e., redness, edema, skin quality) are essential components of the examination (see "On Dialysis Rounds" section).

This approach encompasses patients who have established CKD or ESKD. However, the patient who requires emergent or urgent hemodialysis deserves separate discussion.

Emergent patient: The emergent patient requires immediate hemodialysis to limit or prevent life-threatening complications such as hyperkalemia, pulmonary edema refractory to medical management, uremic seizures, uremic pericarditis, and uremic bleeding, especially prior to required surgeries. If such a situation arises and the patient is without a usable AV access, the only alternative is to provide a temporary access for hemodialysis. In most cases, a temporary uncuffed femoral catheter is the most appropriate access. After dialysis has been completed, more permanent access can be discussed, if required. Again the focus is on saving central veins if the patient is anticipated to require permanent dialysis in the future.

Urgent patient: The urgent dialysis start patient is typically a CKD patient who is in one or more of the following common situation(s): (1) the patient has established CKD with stable GFR who suffers an unexpected medical event that destabilizes the previously stable GFR; (2) hospital-admitted inpatient who develops or has newly diagnosed ESKD; (3) the patient arrives in the emergency room for an unrelated reason or with non–life-threatening symptoms, previously undiagnosed but has ESKD. Other situations exist; however, the common factor is that the patient does not fit the criteria of "emergent" dialysis and has limited time (1–3 weeks) before dialysis becomes critically necessary. These urgent start patients account for 30%–50% of new starts to dialysis. These patients deserve time to consider their ESKD life plan before rushing in to put in a temporary CVC access. Again, the principle is to preserve future access sites. All RRT modalities should be considered; if PD is appropriate, an "acute" PD catheter can be inserted by the surgeon, interventionalist, or at the bedside by the nephrologist (depending on the facility's available personnel and skillset). If hemodialysis is appropriate, an early cannulation graft can be placed and used within 72 hours. If this is placed in the forearm, it will avoid unnecessary central vein damage by a CVC, to facilitate future AV access success. Once the graft becomes problematic, a fistula can be created by the cephalic vein developed by the graft. On the other hand, if the surgeon assesses that an AVF can be created and matured within the time frame before dialysis is required, an urgent AVF creation is appropriate. This requires the coordinated teamwork and education discussed above.

Pros and Cons of Each Vascular Access Type

AVF

Pro

The undisputed benefit of a matured, carefully cannulated functioning fistula is that it can provide reliable, long-standing access for dialysis with minimal complications.

By extension, such a fistula should then offer the patient high satisfaction and good quality of life and be cost effective.

The minimal vascular requirements for a successful AVF are listed below:

1. Absence of central vein obstruction.
2. Segmental blood pressure differential of less than 20 mm Hg.
3. Lack of segmental stenosis of artery or vein.
4. Anastomosis luminal diameter of at least 2.5 mm.
5. Straight vein cannulation segment to allow at least 2.0 cm between 2 cannulation sites.
6. Vein cannulation segment less than 5 mm below the skin surface.
7. Matured vein diameter of at least 4 mm.
8. Flow rate of 500 mL/min or more (for typical North American dialysis patient and prescription)

At 6 weeks after creation, if the AVF has not dilated to 6 mm or has a blood flow >600 mL/min, the AVF should be investigated (e.g., duplex ultrasonogram or fistulogram) to identify correctable abnormalities, such as stenotic or collateral vessels that may be limiting flow through the vein.

Con

The most frequent AVF complications include maturation failure (20%–60%), thrombosis, aneurysm formation, and steal syndrome. Fistula infections are uncommon, but vary with cannulation technique. Buttonhole cannulation is associated with increased risk of infection and associated serious complications (septic emboli and metastatic seeding, e.g., endocarditis, osteomyelitis, infected mycotic aneurysms, fistula loss). Buttonhole cannulation should only be used in special circumstances such as those with short or limited cannulation length and convoluted and/or large aneurysmal fistulas.

Graft

Pro

Grafts have a lower early failure rate in comparison to AVFs and can be used soon after creation. The newer "early cannulation grafts" can be used within 24 hours of creation while the standard grafts can be used 2–4 weeks after creation (depending on extremity swelling). Recent data have indicated equivalent cumulative patencies, infection, and intervention rates compared with AVFs. Thus, in subsets of patients where AVFs are not possible, an AVG is a reasonable alternative.

A variety of synthetic and biologic materials can be used and/or are in development. Examples of synthetic compositions include expanded polytetrafluoroethylene (ePTFE) and variants (trilaminate compositions, polyurethaneurea and siloxane additives, elastomeric membranes, heparin bonding, etc.) and Dacron. Examples of biologic material–based grafts include bovine heterografts, bovine mesenteric vein, cryopreserved saphenous vein, human umbilical vein, and engineered human extracellular matrix compositions. There are a number of graft types (straight, tapered, spiral) and configurations that can be placed within the body (straight, loop, curve). Grafts can connect two vessels that may not otherwise be possible because of their distance. Thus, a graft can be used for almost any patient if he or she has acceptable receiving vessels.

Con

The most common complication of AVG is the development of neointimal hyperplasia that leads to recurrent stenosis and thrombosis. Multiple agents have been used to reduce stenosis and thrombosis such as warfarin, dipyridamole, sulfinpyrazone, ticlodipine, aspirin, dipyridamole and aspirin (Aggrenox), and fish oil. Only Aggrenox and fish oil have been found to be effective in reducing thrombosis and improving graft patency in randomized controlled trials. Other agents have either been ineffective or had a signal for harm (e.g., serious bleeding with warfarin). When hemodynamically significant stenosis (typically evidenced by clinical signs or symptom; see "On Dialysis Rounds" section) or thrombosis occurs, corrective endovascular or surgical intervention is needed to maintain or salvage graft patency.

Another important complication is infection. Previously, grafts have been shown to have a significantly greater infection risk than fistulas (up to 10-fold higher), but in recent data, they have shown equivalent infection risk. This may be due to more consistent perioperative antibiotic coverage, better attention to hygiene by patients, and use of aseptic cannulation technique by cannulators. Indeed, graft infection is a modifiable complication (see chapter on vascular access infections).

Lastly, pseudoaneurysms and aneurysms result from poor cannulation, such as "one-site-itis." Typically, pseudoaneurysms are resected when they reach a diameter 2 times greater than the graft width or increasing in size. Vascular steal syndrome and monomelic neuropathy are less common but serious complications, often necessitating ligation of the graft.

Catheter

Pro

Central venous catheters are widely available, can be quickly and easily inserted into various sites in the body, and can be used immediately for dialysis. There are a variety of CVC materials and configurations. The two most commonly used materials are silicone and polyurethane; both are biocompatible and durable. In an attempt to reduce bacterial colonization or improve flow, catheters have been coated with antimicrobial agents and anticoagulants; however, this protective effect typically dissipates by 2–3 weeks. There are a variety of port and tip designs to assist in reducing recirculation. Many catheters can provide excellent blood flow rates of >350 mL/min to achieve dialysis adequacy (KT/V >1.2 or PRU >66%). Many patients like the convenience of catheters, without the need for 2-needle cannulation or the need to wait for hemostasis after dialysis has been completed. Some patients prefer a catheter because it does not have the cosmetic disfigurement that can occur with fistulas or grafts, and one can hide the catheter under the clothing.

Con

Catheters are the vascular access type associated with the greatest risk of complications leading to significant morbidity, hospitalizations, and mortality. Complications can be short term (around the time of insertion: 5%–15%) or long term. Short-term insertion-related complications include arterial puncture, cardiac/pericardial puncture, hematoma, hemothorax, air embolism, pneumothorax, infection, malposition, mechanical problems, and malfunction (catheter kinking or fracture; intraluminal thrombosis). Long-term complications include infection (see chapter on vascular access infections), thrombosis, and stenosis of veins. Because of the serious consequences of catheter use, cuffed tunneled CVC use should be limited to the following situations:

- True exhaustion of all options to create an AV access (AVF or AVG), as determined by a qualified surgeon/interventionalist
- Use as a bridge access until an already created AVF or AVG matures
- Use as a bridge access until the time of a scheduled donor kidney transplant (within a reasonable time frame determined by the facility, e.g., 6 months)
- Use as a bridge when a patient requires hemodialysis due to a complication from peritoneal dialysis (e.g., "resting" of the peritoneal membrane after an episode of peritonitis, or in delayed graft function in a patient with a newly transplanted kidney)
- Limited life expectancy

As a result of some of the perceived benefits of catheters, some patients have a personal preference for CVC as their access of choice. However, it should be documented that the patient understands the risks of prolonged CVC use, especially when an alternate AV access is available. The benefits of other AV access (AVF or AVG) and their availability as an option should be made clear to ensure informed consent to using the CVC.

On Dialysis Rounds

Following are the key physical examination findings indicative of access problems:

- Swelling within the face, chest wall, shoulder, breast, or neck may be indicative of high venous pressure suggestive of central stenosis (e.g., superior vena cava or innominate vein). Collateral veins may also be evident on physical examination.
- Localized edema is indicative of potential infection or venous outflow impairment, for example, isolated forearm edema suggests a stenosis in the main draining vein.
- Palpably increased access pulsation: May be predictive of venous anastomotic stenosis and/or stenosis in the access body.
- Palpation may detect fibrotic stenotic lesions, for example, a "step" can be felt at the anastomosis.
- An overly strong (water hammer) pulse may be detected upstream to a stenotic lesion. The access downstream to the stenosis may collapse on arm elevation.
- High bruit pitch and/or short diastolic component may indicate stenosis; recall bruit should be heard throughout systole and diastole.
- Reduction in bruit intensity following arm elevation is indicative of arterial inflow abnormalities limiting flow.
- Prolonged bleeding time after needle withdrawal of >10 minutes or a change from current baseline with no change in anticoagulation: This should be measured and documented as a potential indicator for AVF or AVG stenosis and requires evaluation.
- Evidence of aneurysms or pseudoaneurysms, thinning of the skin over the access, superficial ulcers.

Dialysis staff should be aware of key findings indicative of access dysfunctions; such findings should be promptly brought to the rounding nephrologist's attention.

Similarly, nephrologists should themselves be vigilant in order to follow up with appropriate investigations or corrective procedures in a timely manner. Depending on how regularly a nephrologist rounds, part of or an entire dialysis round should be dedicated to identifying and evaluating vascular access–related issues. However, one should be mindful that the assessment of access stenosis might be problematic when the patient is connected to the dialysis machine. Thus, arrangements should be made for proper access evaluation when the patient is off dialysis.

The above hemodialysis vascular access strategies and decision-making processes require a coordinated teamwork approach, which encompasses a "continuum of care" model for CKD. The dialysis access strategy should be considered a "life plan" whereby the appropriate access is the one that aligns the modality for renal replacement therapy (dialysis or transplant) to help each patient achieve his or her life goals safely. As such, a dialysis access short- and long-term plan should be updated on a regular basis. With a proactive approach, future anticipated access problems can be addressed with the overall goal to avoid access complications, dialysis interruptions, temporary central venous catheter use, and associated morbidity.

CHAPTER 3

Central Venous Access for Hemodialysis

Louise Moist, MD • Tushar Vachharajani, MD, FASN, FACP

Vascular access plays a critical and crucial role while providing hemodialysis therapy. The three main types of dialysis vascular access commonly used in practice are arteriovenous fistula (AVF), arteriovenous graft (AVG), and central venous catheter (CVC). More recently, a hybrid catheter-graft device (HeRO device, Hemodialysis Reliable Outflow) has been introduced into clinical practice for a highly select group of patients, and clinical experience remains limited. Dialysis vascular access continues to remain a lifeline and an Achilles heel for patients with end-stage renal disease.

Despite the advantages of relatively easy placement and immediate use, CVC is not the preferred vascular access for maintenance hemodialysis in the majority of patients, because of the association with a higher incidence of morbidity and mortality compared to AVFs and AVGs. Unfortunately, 80% of incident chronic hemodialysis patients in the United States and Canada start dialysis with a CVC. On the other hand, CVC remains the only means of providing hemodialysis in an acute setting.

Types of Catheters

CVCs for dialysis can be classified as nontunneled or tunneled. Use of the terms "temporary" and "permanent" catheter should be avoided, as long-term use of CVC is associated with a higher incidence of infection, central venous stenosis, and inadequate dialysis therapy. Tunneled catheters are considered as "bridge access" until a functioning permanent access is available (Table 3.1).

Catheters differ by material, length, lumen size, lumen configuration, inlet/outlet holes, method of connection to bloodlines, and surface coating (Fig. 3.1), and a wide assortment is available.

Catheters are designed to accommodate easy insertion and appropriate positioning and to provide maximal blood flows to support adequate hemodialysis therapy. Nontunneled, noncuffed catheters are made of polyurethane, which is stiff at room temperature, to facilitate insertion but softens at body temperature to minimize vessel trauma. Tunneled cuffed catheters are primarily composed of silicone and silicone elastomers that are flexible and require a stylet and/or sheath for insertion. The Dacron cuff on a tunneled catheter fixes the catheter in the tunnel and also prevents migration of bacteria along the catheter wall from the exit site. The walls of the lumens of a silicone catheter must be thicker than a polyurethane catheter because silicone provides less structural support. Silicone and polyurethane are less thrombogenic than materials such as Teflon and polyvinyl used in the past.

Catheter lumen sizes range from 9 to 16 French (0.75–2.2 mm inner diameter). Catheter length varies greatly to accommodate proper positioning of the tip. In

Table 3.1

Table 3.1

Characteristics of Central Venous Catheters

Nontunneled	Tunneled
Acute indication to initiate dialysis	Bridge access until functioning arteriovenous access is available
Noncuffed catheter	Cuffed catheter
Placed at bedside	Placed in interventional radiology suite or operating room
Best performed with USG guidance	Performed with USG and fluoroscopic guidance

USG, ultrasonography.

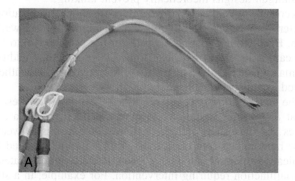

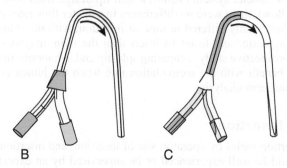

Figure 3.1

(A) Smooth curve seen on a catheter removed from right internal jugular vein. (B) Schematic representation of the smooth curve. (C) Cross-sectional schematic representation of the smooth curve. (From Atlas of Dialysis Vascular Access, by Tushar Vachharajani.)

general, nontunneled catheters inserted in the right internal jugular vein are 16 cm, in the left internal jugular vein are 20 cm, and in the femoral vein are 24 cm long to minimize recirculation and to reach the great veins. Tunneled cuffed catheters are much longer to accommodate the creation of tunnels and allow the tip to be placed in the right atrium or inferior vena cava as required. The length of the tunneled catheter is conventionally measured from the cuff to the tip. In an average-sized individual, the length of a tunneled catheter in the right internal jugular vein, left internal jugular vein, and femoral vein is 23, 28, and 32 cm, respectively.

The arterial and venous lumens can be completely separated (e.g., Tesio catheter), partially separated (Ash split catheter), or conjoined throughout their length with a symmetric tip with slots (e.g., Palindrome) or a step-tip (e.g., Dura-flow). The lumens of conjoined catheters can be configured as a shotgun design (e.g., Perm-cath), single round catheter with midline septum ("double D") Circle C, coaxial, and triple lumen design (e.g., Mahurkar). Inlet and outlet holes can be a single large hole or multiple small holes in various patterns or slots. The split tip and symmetric catheters are widely used in the United States, and twin catheters are mainly used in Europe. Traditionally, connector ports have been of Luer lock design. Midline septums or shotgun designs theoretically prevent kinking.

Catheters coated with either heparin or silver are another innovation seen in recent years. Catheters may be coated either on the outside wall, inner wall, or both walls of the lumen. Even though coating the catheter has been shown to reduce infection in intensive care units, it has not been shown to provide any additional benefit in the chronic maintenance dialysis population. Moreover, coated catheters are expensive compared to noncoated catheters.

Despite the myriad of designs and purported advantages, at present there is little evidence that one design is superior to others. Most catheters are tested in ideal circumstances and over short periods of time. Comparisons between devices have included few randomized controlled trials (RCTs) and have failed to show differences in clinically important outcomes such as solute clearance, rates of bacteremia, or catheter malfunction requiring intervention. For example, in a study comparing a twin-dialysis catheter system (Tesio), a split-tip design (Ash-Split), and a step-tip design (Opti-flow), there were no differences in catheter flow rates or rates of infection. The catheters only differed in time of insertion, with the split-tip and step-tip catheters being easier and faster to insert than the twin-dialysis system. Another randomized prospective study comparing split-tip and symmetric-tip catheters failed to show any benefit with the recirculation rate when the lumen connections were reversed during hemodialysis.

Catheter Insertion

Catheter insertion varies by operator, site of insertion, and insertion technique. The operator should be well experienced or be supervised by an experienced operator. In general, tunneled cuffed catheters are inserted in operating rooms or clean interventional suites under fluoroscopy—with the operator gowned, gloved, and masked. Full surgical drapes are used, and the patient is masked and given a combination of sedative and an analgesic. Nontunneled catheters are generally inserted at the bedside or in the dialysis unit, with full-barrier precautions consisting of a mask, sterile gloves, gown, and a large drape. The skin can be disinfected with chlorhexidine, povidone-iodine, or alcohol. Alcohol disinfects instantly, whereas povidone-iodine should be allowed to dry for 2–3 minutes to maximize the antibacterial effect. The preferred skin disinfectant recommended by the Centers for Disease Control and Prevention (CDC) is chlorhexidine.

Ultrasonographic (US) guidance for venous puncture is considered the standard of care, and all persons inserting CVCs should be trained in the US approach. US allows the trained operator to examine the vein for anatomic abnormalities and to directly visualize the venous puncture. US guidance has been shown to minimize insertion complications in both the internal jugular and femoral sites and results in a decrease in immediate catheter dysfunction. Using ultrasound guidance, inexperienced operators can increase their success rate to 95%. The NKF-K/DOQI (Kidney Disease Outcomes Quality Initiative) guidelines support this practice.

The preferred site of placement for both tunneled and nontunneled catheters is the right internal jugular vein. Catheters placed in the left internal jugular vein provide significantly less blood flow than right-sided catheters and are nearly four times as likely to require removal for malfunction. Catheters placed in the left internal jugular vein traverse through multiple curves in both lateral and anteroposterior planes compared to the right internal jugular vein catheters, resulting in loss of smooth lamellar flow (Figs. 3.1 and 3.2). If at all possible, catheter placement in the subclavian vein should be avoided. Although studies have shown a decrease in infection rate with the use of subclavian catheters, these catheters have been associated with an increase in central vein stenosis (which may compromise future permanent access creation in the ipsilateral arm). In a prospective study in which patients underwent routine venography after removal of their first subclavian catheter, 52% of patients had subclavian vein thrombosis/stenosis and only half of these recanalized at 3 months. Furthermore, the incidence of subclinical subclavian vein stenosis in patients with cardiac rhythm devices is well recognized.

In practice, thrombosis/stenosis of the subclavian vein is often subclinical until an arteriovenous access is placed in the ipsilateral arm, which results in increased venous blood flow and manifests with overt clinical signs like severe arm swelling. Treatment of the stenosis with angioplasty or stent is difficult and requires repeated procedures to maintain patency. Often the stenosis requires ligation of the permanent access and renders the arm unusable for future permanent access creation. Thrombosis/stenosis of the internal jugular vein is less frequent than the subclavian vein (approximately 6%–10% as reported in literature) and does not generally compromise future permanent arteriovenous access creation unless it extends to the superior vena cava.

Nontunneled catheters have a stiff conical tip, making it easy to advance the catheter over a guidewire into the vein. In contrast, a tunneled catheter requires a peel-away sheath of stiff stylets to advance the catheter over the wire.

Nontunneled catheters placed in the subclavian or internal jugular vein should have their position checked by chest radiograph or fluoroscopy before commencing dialysis. The tip of a nontunneled catheter should rest in the superior vena cava. Nontunneled catheters are commonly placed in the femoral vein in bed-bound patients, but the infection rate is higher than either of the neck locations. The tip of the femoral vein catheter should be placed in the common iliac vein and preferably in the inferior vena cava. Evaluation of a dysfunctional catheter placed in a femoral vein should include an abdominal radiograph to confirm the location of the tip to be at least above the pelvic brim for the common iliac vein or at L2–L3 lumbar vertebrae level for inferior vena cava placement.

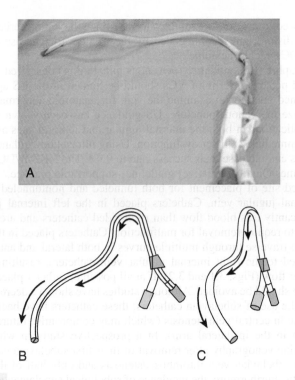

Figure 3.2

(A) Multiple curves on a left-sided tunneled catheter removed from left internal jugular vein. (B) Schematic representation of the additional angulation, as the catheter traverses mediastinum and is not visualized on frontal projection radiograph. (C) Schematic representation of the angulations caused by the left internal jugular vein, left brachiophalic vein, and superior vena cava. (From Atlas of Dialysis Vascular Access, by Tushar Vachharajani.)

Tunneled cuffed catheters may be placed in the femoral vein, and as a last resort the catheter may be inserted via the translumbar and transhepatic routes directly into the inferior vena cava.

Catheters can be dressed with either standard or adhesive dry gauze or breathable transparent dressings. Patients and caregivers may feel that an adhesive dressing better secures the catheter or better protects the exit site from contamination. The CDC has no definite recommendations for catheter dressing or use of exit-site antiseptic or antibiotic ointments. The key relevant precaution is to keep the dressing dry and clean, change it at least once a week, and the use of a mask both by the patient and the caregiver while handling the catheter.

Many complications have been associated with hemodialysis catheter insertion. Complications are seen often when the operator is inexperienced and venous puncture is performed blindly rather than under US guidance. Average rates and ranges of complications in the literature are outlined in Table 3.2.

Table 3.2

Complications From Hemodialysis Catheter Insertion

Complication	Mean (%)	Range (%)
Arterial puncture	4.4	0–11.9
Local bleeding	4.0	0–18.1
Aspiration	2.2	NA[a]
Recurrent laryngeal palsy	1.6	NA
Hemo/pneumothorax	1.35	0–3.0
Air embolism	1.2	0–2.2
Cardiac arrhythmia	1.1	NA
Hemomediastinum	0.74	0–1.2
Vessel perforation	0.7	0–1.3
Pericardial tamponade	0.56	0.5–0.6
Retroperitoneal bleeding[b]	0.06	N/A

[a]N/A = not available.
[b]Femoral catheterization only.

Catheter Malfunction

Catheter malfunction is defined as the inability to provide adequate dialysis. This generally occurs with a blood flow of <300 mL/min; however, patients with weights below 70 kg may have adequate dialysis with flows between 250 and 300 mL/min. The two primary mechanisms of malfunction are thrombosis and malposition of the catheter relative to the central veins. Catheter malposition is the most likely cause if adequate blood flows were never achieved (early malfunction). Malposition of the tip or kinking of the catheter has been reported in up to 68% of early malfunctions, and catheters should be imaged to diagnose malposition.

Late malfunction is more likely caused by thrombosis. Thrombosis can occur within the catheter lumen, at the catheter tip, or around the catheter (fibrin sheath), can involve the entire vein (mural thrombus), or can form in the right atrium. One-year patency rates for tunneled cuffed catheters are estimated at 30%–74%. Efforts to prevent thrombosis have been disappointing. Fixed mini-dose warfarin has not proved effective, and systemic anticoagulation is generally undesirable.

Regardless of the etiology of malfunction, simple measures—such as patient repositioning, flushing the catheter with saline, rotating the catheter (uncuffed catheters), and lumen reversal—are usually tried to improve blood flow. It is not clear how effective these interventions are, but they are commonly performed.

In an attempt to prevent CVC malfunction, interdialytic instillation with anticoagulant solutions or "catheter locks" have been employed. Heparin has been used for decades, in concentrations between 1000 and 10,000 U/mL, with a rate of CVC thrombosis between 4.0 and 5.5 episodes/1000 catheter days, and the rate of CVC loss due to malfunction is 1.8–3.6/1000 days. Recent alternatives, including citrate and recombinant tissue plasminogen activator (rt-PA), have been used to improve CVC patency. Several systematic reviews have compared outcomes between citrate and heparin with citrate with similar malfunction rates but improved safety from bleeding episodes. In an RCT, use of rt-PA once weekly, instead of heparin, reduced the risk of catheter malfunction by a factor of 2, with demonstrated cost effectiveness. Warfarin prophylaxis is not recommended, and the efficacy and safety of using antiplatelet agents alone for the prevention of CVC malfunction has not been adequately studied in well-designed, appropriately powered clinical trials.

Catheters that are refractory to simple measures are usually treated with a thrombolytic dwell as first line of treatment because it can be given in the dialysis unit. Currently available thrombolytics include streptokinase and rt-PA. Streptokinase is highly antigenic and has been largely replaced by rt-PA. During dwells, rt-PA is instilled into the catheter to fill the dead space in the lumen at doses of 1–2 mg/mL. The drug is usually left to dwell for 20 to 60 minutes, but dwells of 1 to 4 days also have been described. During the dwell, active drug can be periodically advanced toward the tip with saline. Larger doses of rt-PA (50 mg) have been infused to treat refractory catheter malfunction or specific thrombotic complications (e.g., right atrial thrombus). Despite the increased dose, only minimal effects on bleeding parameters have been shown.

Catheter malfunction may also be treated with guidewire insertion, fibrin sheath stripping, or exchange over a guidewire. The immediate success of most techniques is good. However, the effect is short lived and usually requires repeated intervention. Guidewire insertion has only been described in one report and is not recommended. Catheter exchange avoids femoral puncture, and any fibrin sheath may be disrupted at the time of the procedure with either a snare or balloon. One small study resulted in greater long-term patency rates for catheter exchange compared to fibrin sheath stripping. Catheter exchange does not increase the risk of subsequent infection. Therefore, catheter exchange is probably the best solution to catheter malfunction. However, this requires further investigation by rigorous well-designed and appropriately powered clinical trials.

Catheter-Related Infections

Use of tunneled and nontunneled CVCs is a well-recognized risk factor for infectious complications and contributes to increased morbidity, mortality, and costs. When compared to AV access use, there is an associated 15- to 33-fold increase in risk of a catheter related infection (CRI) in patients with end-stage kidney disease (ESKD), although the rate of CRI may be lower in the elderly. Catheters can be complicated by exit-site infections, tunnel infections, bacteremia, and distant infections, such as osteomyelitis and endocarditis. The exact definition of these infectious outcomes varies by source (see "Recommended Reading" for CDC definitions). A practical and simple definition of *exit-site infection* is "purulent drainage at the exit site." Redness, swelling, crusting, and pain may accompany this discharge, but these findings are more subjective than purulent drainage. Tunnel infections occur if inflammation extends 5 cm beyond the exit site or beyond the cuff. Bacteremia is defined by positive peripheral blood cultures in a patient with signs and symptoms of infection such as fever, chills, nausea, headache, hypotension, and elevated white blood cell count. Bacteremia is confirmed to be catheter related if no other source is found. Distant infections occur when organisms seed during bacteremia. The most common distant infections are endocarditis (3.9%–4.1%), osteomyelitis (0.5%–5.9%), and septic arthritis (1.0%–3.8%). Other reported complications are septic phlebitis, septic pulmonary emboli, spinal abscess, myocardial abscess, and septic death. Gram-positive organisms cause approximately 75% of catheter-related bacteremias, with an increasing incidence of methicillin-resistant *Staphylococcus aureus* (MRSA). The remainder are caused by gram-negative organisms, fungi, and mixed organisms. A similar spectrum of organisms is cultured from exit-site infections. Coagulase-negative staphylococci and diphtheria frequently cause CRI but can also be contaminants. Therefore, it is more likely that they are the true source if both blood culture bottles grow one of the organisms. The utility of cultures from catheters, cultures from dialysis lines connected to catheters, and surveillance cultures has not been established.

The rate of CRIs for nontunneled catheters is higher than for other types of catheters (4.8 vs 2.7 per 1000 catheter days). However, when comparing cuffed-tunneled catheters, femoral and internal jugular catheters had similar CRI rates. Duration of placement is the most consistent risk factor (i.e., the longer the use, the higher the incidence of infection). The high CRI rate prompted the National Action Plan for Reduction of Hospital-Acquired Infections and the CDC to develop a number of surveillance and core intervention programs to prevent CRI. The CDC Dialysis BSI Prevention Collaborative core interventions are listed in Box 3.1 (see Recommended

---

Box 3.1   CDC Dialysis BSI Prevention Collaborative Interventions

Core Interventions

Surveillance and feedback using NHSN: Conduct monthly surveillance for BSIs and other dialysis events and enter events into CDC's NHSN. Calculate facility rates and compare with rates in other facilities using NHSN. Actively share results with frontline clinical staff.

Chlorhexidine for skin antisepsis: Use chlorhexidine (>0.5%) with alcohol solution as the first-line agent for skin antisepsis, particularly for central catheter insertion and during dressing changes. Povidone-iodine, preferably with alcohol, or 70% alcohol are alternatives.

Hand hygiene surveillance: Perform monthly hand hygiene audits with feedback of results to clinical staff.

Catheter/vascular access care observations: Perform quarterly audits of vascular access care and catheter accessing to ensure adherence to recommended procedures. This includes aseptic technique while connecting and disconnecting catheters and during dressing changes. Share results with frontline clinical staff.

Patient education/engagement: Provide standardized education to all patients on infection prevention topics, including vascular access care, hand hygiene, risks related to catheter use, recognizing signs of infection, and instructions for access management when away from dialysis unit.

Staff education and competency: Provide regular training of staff on infection control topics, including access care and aseptic technique. Perform competency evaluation for skills such as catheter care and accessing at least every 6–12 months and upon hire.

Catheter reduction: Incorporate efforts (e.g., through patient education, vascular access coordinator) to reduce catheters by identifying barriers to permanent vascular access placement and catheter removal.

Supplemental Intervention

Antimicrobial ointment or chlorhexidine-impregnated sponge dressing: Apply bacitracin/gramicidin/polymyxin B ointment or povidone-iodine ointment to catheter exit sites during dressing change *or* use a chlorhexidine-impregnated sponge dressing.

Abbreviations: BSI, bloodstream infection; CDC, Centers for Disease Control and Prevention; NHSN, National Healthcare Safety Network.
Downloaded from CDC approach to bloodstream infection prevention in dialysis facilities, http://www.cdc.gov/dialysis/PDFs/Dialysis-Core-Interventions-5_10_13.pdf, accessed May 1, 2015.

Reading for further details). Use of this "bundled" set of interventions applied together, in conjunction with staff education, and a program monitoring for infection with real-time feedback has been shown to reduce access-related bloodstream infections by 54%.

Antimicrobial Locks and Catheter Surface Treatment

Antimicrobial locks instilled within the catheter lumen have been effective at reducing CRIs, with a recent meta-analysis of RCTs demonstrating a 69% reduction in CRI rate and a 32% reduction in exit-site infections. Importantly, however, the rate of CRI was not improved if the baseline rate of CRI was <1.15 per 1000 catheter days. Citrate is gaining favor over heparin for its extra antimicrobial and anti-biofilm effects, and decreased risk of bleeding, even with concentrations of 4%; however, the literature remains controversial as to whether this reduces the CRI or catheter malfunction rate. An RCT by Maki compared heparin locks with locks containing a mixture of sodium citrate, methylene blue, methylparaben and propylparaben (C–MB–P) with significantly fewer CRI and fewer discontinuations due to poor flow in the mixture group. The use of ethanol 60% alone or ethanol 30% with citrate 4% has been studied although early data suggest possible interaction with the catheter material. In fact, all locking solutions should be considered for compatibility with the catheter materials. Addition of antibiotics to either heparin or citrate have been associated with reduced CRI rates; however, there are additional concerns such as higher costs, practical issues related to the compounding of solutions, and, most importantly, the possibility of promoting antibiotic resistance. Prospective RCTs are needed to determine the most suitable locking solution to prevent CRI and minimize resistance. Use of recombinant tissue plasminogen activator (rt-PA) once weekly instead of heparin reduced the risk of a CRI by a factor of 3, with demonstrated cost effectiveness. Heparin coating of the tunneled catheter is associated with a lower CRI rate with no improvement in catheter malfunction, although larger, more robust studies are needed before adopting this practice.

Topical Antibiotic Ointments

The application of topical antibiotic ointments at the CVC exit site is associated with a 75%–93% reduction in the risk of CRI. However, some agents are incompatible with some catheters, and there has been concern regarding an increased rate of resistance. Mupirocin, povidone-iodine, polysporin triple antibiotic ointment (gramicidin + bacitracin + polymyxin B), and medical honey have been the most commonly studied ointments applied at the exit site. A Cochrane systematic review demonstrated that mupirocin ointment reduced the risk of CRI primarily by reducing CRI caused by *S. aureus*. However, only polysporin ointment had a significant reduction in CRI and all-cause mortality but had no effect on mortality related to infection.

Treatment of CRIs

Temporary catheters with exit-site infections should be removed immediately in light of the fact that the bacteremia rate is greater than 10% after 24 hours from the onset of exit-site infection. Exit-site infection from tunneled cuffed catheters may be treated with oral or topical antibiotics.

All other CRIs should be treated with antibiotic therapy, with empiric therapy providing broad-spectrum coverage for both gram-positive and gram-negative organisms. In units with a high prevalence of MRSA, empiric therapy should include coverage for MRSA. Patients found to have methicillin-sensitive *S. aureus* should be treated with cefazolin if there is no allergic contraindication. Empiric gram-negative coverage should be based on local antibiotic sensitivities, with subsequent antibiotics prescribed according to the identification and sensitivities of the isolate. Guidelines for treatment of CRI recommend 4–6 weeks of antimicrobial therapy for uncomplicated *S. aureus*, 7–14 days for gram-negative bacilli or enterococcus, and a minimum of 14 days for *Candida* species. Complicated CRB characterized by the presence of septic thrombophlebitis and/or endocarditis should be treated for 4–6 weeks, whereas osteomyelitis should be treated for a minimum of 6–8 weeks. Vancomycin and gentamicin can cause ototoxicity, and drug-level monitoring should be used for dosing adjustment if use is >1 week.

Catheter Management

Guidelines for CRI management are variable in their recommendations. Catheter removal with delayed CVC replacement is generally required in clinically unstable patients, when fever persists beyond 48 hours, with a tunnel infection, or if a metastatic infectious complication is present. In clinically stable patients, the strategies for CVC management in addition to systemic antibiotics include catheter salvage without antibiotic lock, catheter removal with delayed replacement, catheter exchange over wire, or catheter salvage with antibiotic lock. A recent systematic review of primarily observational studies suggests similar outcomes to catheter exchange or catheter salvage with antibiotic locks. Until there are more data from prospective RCTs, the recommendations are for catheter exchange if possible. Exit-site infections that do not respond to antibiotics should prompt review of the need for catheter removal or catheter rewire with a new tunnel/exit site.

Conclusions

Catheters are an essential form of vascular access in the patient with acute kidney injury or with vessels not suitable for an AV access. However, permanent catheter use remains high in both incident and prevalent patients on hemodialysis in many areas. Several factors have been identified that lead to lower catheter use, including early referral to a nephrologist, AV access creation at eGFR between 10–15 mL/min in patients expected to start dialysis, timely access to a surgeon and radiology services for creation and maintenance of the vascular access, education of the patient, use of a multidisciplinary team, and experienced nurse cannulators. However, there will be a continued need for catheters, and we must strive to better understand how to optimize catheter performance and minimize complications.

CHAPTER 4

Noninfectious Complications From Vascular Access

Jeffrey L. Kaufman, MD, FACS

Many complications from hemodialysis access sites are a local nuisance, mandating a brief daystay procedure for revision. They can also prove immediately life-threatening, expensive, or the cause of a prolonged hospitalization. They can provoke an end-of-life discussion when they are severe. Complications require careful attention because they often interrupt the normal dialysis schedule or decrease hemodialysis efficiency, leading to a decreased sense of well-being. They are labor-intensive for the entire dialysis support team. They are a frustrating imposition on the patient and his or her family. The patient may need to endure altered body image or sustain increased disability from some complications.

Autogenous arteriovenous fistulas are favored over prosthetic grafts because of their greater longevity, lower ongoing cost, and reduced risk of mechanical complications. Despite these advantages, all access constructions suffer "wear and tear" from use and degeneration and are associated with potentially serious problems stemming from infection, circulatory embarrassment, hemorrhage, thrombosis, edema, and seroma formation (Table 4.1).

Assessment of Extremity Perfusion and Fistula Flow at the Bedside and in the Vascular Laboratory

Complications relating to placement of dialysis access are often worse in the patient who starts with abnormal circulation in the extremity. This is not to imply that a patient with abnormal circulation in an extremity should be denied an attempt at access there, but prediction of the patient at risk for complications will facilitate planning if access failure occurs. The baseline vascular examination starts with palpating pulses, recognizing that distal occlusive disease may be masked by edema or effects of prior surgery in people with end-stage renal disease (ESRD). Capillary refill and skin color are inaccurate measures of perfusion. The arm with severe inflow disease in the subclavian-axilllary segment may have a lower brachial blood pressure compared with the opposite arm. A Doppler stethoscope can be used to determine blood flow patterns, but grading blood flow with this instrument is subjective unless one has special bidirectional equipment. A bedside Allen test using a Doppler stethoscope is not helpful in predicting steal, with the exception of identifying the occasional patient who has virtually all flow to the hand coming from the radial artery. This is a patient for whom a Cimino fistula can readily result in hand ischemia. The examination proceeds with an assessment of vein anatomy. Vein size is assessed with and without a tourniquet, and the arm is positioned as if it were being used for dialysis, so that the exposure of vein segments for puncture can be noted. The vein

Table 4.1

Complications From Permanent Hemodialysis Access

Failure of maturation
    small vein or vein with scar or
        stenosis
    arterial anatomic variation causing
        flow restriction
    venous insufficiency or segmental
        stenosis
    obesity causing excessive depth of
        puncture
Infection (see Chapter 5)
    catheter infection
    catheter-related septic central venous
        thrombosis
    localized graft infection, including
        primary blowout with skin
        erosion
    total graft infection
    mycotic aneurysm involving
        anastomoses
    endocarditis
    port infection or erosion with
        contamination
    metastatic infection
Emboli
    arterial
    venous (pulmonary embolism)
    septic pulmonary embolism
    air embolism
Thrombosis
    central venous thrombosis
    graft thrombosis
    arterial thrombosis adjacent to
        surgical anastomosis
    sleeve thrombosis around catheters
    superficial phlebitis
Hemorrhage
    perigraft hematoma
    perianastomotic hematoma
    false aneurysm
    conduit degeneration
    needle puncture bleeding
    ecchymosis, operative bleeding as
        effect of antiplatelet medication
    subfascial or intramuscular
        hematoma from extravasation

Ischemia/obstruction
    steal
    intimal flap
    neointimal fibrous hyperplasia,
        involving graft, native artery, outflow
        vein
    venous outflow obstruction/recirculation
    graft lumen stenosis/laminated
        thrombus
Aneurysm
    conduit degeneration
    enlargement related to outflow
        obstruction
    false aneurysm at anastomosis
Stenosis
    in conduit
    native vessel inflow
    outflow obstruction after central catheter
        or PICC
    outflow obstruction at cephalic arch,
        naturally occurring or after pacemaker
    progressive atherosclerosis
Stent complications
    erosion
    strut fracture
    in-stent stenosis: compression, bending,
        intimal hyperplasia
Seroma, lymphocele
Edema
Carpal tunnel syndrome
Neuralgia, hypesthesia, hyperesthesia,
    ischemic monomelic neuropathy
Wound- and site-related problems from
    surgery
    edge necrosis
    scar at site of necessary puncture for
        treatment
    misalignment of conduit, kinking, depth,
        too short, too long
    site inconvenient or uncomfortable for
        patient during treatment
Compartment syndrome
Cardiac failure, high output
Visible scarring or mass affecting body
    image, visible large collateral veins

is palpated to determine areas of scarring from previous intravenous catheter sites or phlebotomy.

In the vascular laboratory, duplex ultrasonography is the core method for assessment of anatomy and flow prior to and after access placement in an extremity. Pulse volume recordings are useful to document digital flow, in particular when Doppler occlusion pressures cannot be obtained because of vascular calcification. Ultrasonography will define vascular occlusions, stenoses, anatomic variation such as high brachial bifurcations, aneurysms, and flow abnormalities. Patients with highly abnormal baseline distal circulation should be considered at high risk for steal syndrome. They can have conventional access constructions performed, but their hand perfusion should be monitored closely thereafter in order to prevent irreversible ischemic changes in the digits. Although the most serious sign of steal is gangrene, patients may develop small nonhealing ulcers at the sites of fingersticks for glucose testing, digital stiffness, paronychias, or severe pain (globally in hand or as ischemic monomelic neuropathy). If these changes occur, the patient should have urgent conversion of the access site to a different configuration or access ligation. In addition, patients with arterial calcification may be at risk for acute arterial occlusion from fracturing of plaques at the time of access placement. Ready access to vascular laboratory equipment will facilitate the diagnosis of this problem should it occur. The assessment of venous anatomy in the vascular laboratory includes notation of size, compressibility, and interconnection of suitable veins. Many experienced access surgeons personally check the ultrasound-based configuration of veins, in particular prior to complex access procedures such as translocated basilic vein fistulae.

Based on the resting examination of an arm prior to placement of an access, it is difficult to determine overall arterial sufficiency that will allow high blood flow volumes in an access site. A minor stenosis of the inflow artery at rest may have no effect on distal blood pressure or flow in the arm, yet it may become very significant after placement of the conduit, where flow volumes can increase by 10 to 20 times.

Failure of Maturation

Technical success of an access site has two components, that it should be flowing at the time the patient leaves the operating room and in the first week or two after construction, and practical configuration and flow volume that will allow dialysis treatment to occur. KDOQI guidelines and the Fistula First program have targets for access site creation that reflect the reality that with the best vessel mapping and the most careful surgery, not all access constructions will work, and maturation is not guaranteed. The fistula that has poor flow at the first postoperative visit needs a careful assessment by duplex scanning to determine what is wrong and how the site can be salvaged. Catheter techniques for assisted maturation have been well described. If the site is realistically beyond salvage, a new procedure should be performed quickly in order to limit the amount of time the patient will live with a catheter.

Revision of a site that is not quite right for dialysis can be required for a variety of reasons. It is now very common for obese patients with upper arm fistulae to require liposuction or superficialization procedures to allow easier placement of needles. The patient with a fistula ipsilateral to a pacemaker or Automatic Implantable Cardiac Defibrillator (AICD) may develop venous hypertension with edema, and the outflow may need revision. After a period of maturation for forearm access sites, stenoses may become apparent at places where the patient had previous venipuncture.

Surveillance of Access Sites

Many complications relating to dialysis access are best evaluated using noninvasive testing in the vascular laboratory. KDOQI guidelines mandate regular surveillance of all access sites, at a minimum by careful examination. A site with abnormal function is then evaluated with duplex ultrasonography, which can provide flow characteristics, flow volume, and determination of the diameter of the flow lumen. Stenoses, false aneurysms, and other conduit abnormalities can be readily determined with duplex scanning. It is common to find that multiple segments of an established access site are abnormal. In some instances, CT angiography may be needed to assess for central (intrathoracic or intraabdominal/pelvic) vascular abnormalities. Many vascular interventions are now performed in the setting of a hybrid operating room, where diagnostic fistulography is part of a larger angiographic assessment. Catheter-directed repair or open revision can be performed in the same setting based on imaging or pullback pressure measurement.

Thrombosis

Thrombosis is the most common late complication. The diagnosis is often first made by the patient, who notes loss of a palpable pulse or thrill in the access. Examination of the site may reveal loss of a machinery bruit, and there may be aspiration of clot when the site is punctured. A Doppler stethoscope will demonstrate absence of a flow signal. If an outflow thrombus has acutely formed, the graft may have an accentuated pulsation without forward Doppler flow. It is important to recognize this situation, which is not common, because the patient can be quickly anticoagulated with heparin to avoid total graft thrombosis, and urgent mechanical lysis, balloon angioplasty, or surgery will be easier to perform on the site. For autogenous fistulae with multiple venous channels, thrombosis may be accompanied by increased flow volume in collateral veins or increased distal edema.

The mainstay technique to treat a clotted access site is mechanical lysis augmented by balloon angioplasty of luminal defects. In some institutions, thrombolysis with TPA has been preferred, but the results are in general no better than with saline alone. Lysis techniques also include the Angiojet. It is common for an outflow obstruction to require stenting in this circumstance. Angiographic procedures are generally very well tolerated, and most complications relate to volume overload from contrast administration or problems with excessive sedation for the procedure. Some clot from the graft will embolize to the lung during the washout procedure in most cases, but this is usually asymptomatic. Paradoxical embolization of this type of clot through a patent foramen ovale has occurred, and the clot has embolized distally to cause hand ischemia. The advantage of catheter techniques is that the anatomic defect causing thrombosis is both diagnosed and treated at the same setting. If the site is deemed to be hopeless, a dialysis catheter is placed, and the patient can be quickly prepared for construction of a new site. Ideally, a problem access site will have function restored in a manner that will allow elective revision of the problem as a daystay procedure. Because the goals of treatment for the clotted access site are safe restoration of flow, preservation of access sites for the future, and preservation of dialysis treatment continuity, it is important for interventional staff and surgeons to work together closely and communicate carefully with the dialysis unit staff. In addition, angiographic procedures can have associated complications that require surgery: Puncture sites may fail to seal, leading to significant hemorrhage. Balloon catheters can rupture, leading to fragment retention or embolization. Intimal flaps may be raised in arteries. Vessels may rupture. If there is a close working relationship between the surgeons and catheter intervention staff, complications will receive better treatment.

A large percentage of catheter-directed treatments for dialysis access sites are performed with minimal intravenous sedation, often in the setting of a freestanding access center. Dire cardiac events can readily occur during access procedures. For the patient thought to be at higher than average risk for an event or for the patient who needs deeper sedation or management of pulmonary issues (notably a history of sleep apnea syndrome), the access procedure should be performed under the care of an anesthesiologist, and this is often in a hospital setting where full monitoring and consultative medical services are available.

Open Thrombectomy and Revision

Despite the advances of catheter technology in treating thrombosed access sites, surgery is still commonly necessary for acute thrombosis. Often, such a site is known to have an anatomic problem, and a decision is made that it is of a nature that it will be repaired only when the site fails. Realizing this, surgeons treating these sites should perform the thrombectomy with revision of the flow defect, and if they cannot revise it, the site should be moved to a new anatomic region. Revision is most commonly necessary for a stenosis at the venous outflow, and this is invariably due to neointimal fibrous hyperplasia (NFH or "intimal hyperplasia"). Options include placement of a patch angioplasty to widen the venous anastomosis or interposition of a new conduit to a new venous outflow. Areas treated with previous stenting will require more major re-routing with a new section of conduit. If a prosthetic graft has degenerated with dilation to form an aneurysm, or if there are large false aneurysms, the extension to a new outflow can be combined with a longer segmental interposition comprising half the extent of the access site. If one leaves a segment of incorporated graft, one-third to one-half the access site length, it can be used acutely to maintain continuity of dialysis without need for a central venous catheter.

Laminated thrombus is commonly found to cause a stenosis within a synthetic conduit. This pale, leathery material can cause web-like stenoses or diffuse flow lumen narrowing. To remove this material, a surgeon can use a uterine curette or a special wire thrombectomy catheter. Red to tan, firm thrombus may be adherent across the arterial and venous anastomoses. On the arterial side, the meniscus of this material must be removed, or the construction will clot again. On the venous side, this material will adhere firmly to areas of NFH, and there will be a failure of back-bleeding when the thrombectomy is performed. In this circumstance, the surgeon must be careful to avoid repeated passage of balloon thrombectomy catheters into the outflow veins, which will suffer a diffuse intimal injury from instrumentation. This will lead to more NFH and recurrent failure. Ideally, a site freshly revised or thrombectomized will have intraoperative imaging to verify that no problem remains.

The complications of thrombectomy and revision of access sites are the same as those for primary access placement overall, but there is in addition the rare problem of embolization of clot into the inflow artery and its distal bed, causing a significant degree of ischemia. If there is any question about the quality of access site flow after an intervention, a central venous catheter should be placed, such that continuity of treatments is preserved.

Coagulopathy

Suspicion will arise that a patient is hypercoagulable based on repeated thrombosis of technically sufficient access sites. Before coming to this conclusion, one must be certain that repeated technical error by the surgeon is not the cause, nor is there arterial insufficiency causing low flow volumes in the constructions. Patients at risk for hypercoagulability include those:

- refractory to heparin
- who have known clotting abnormalities, such as a baseline subnormal prothrombin time
- who clot an access site despite a therapeutically elevated prothrombin time from warfarin
- with paradoxically excessive bleeding during surgery (possible platelet aggregation abnormality)
- who undergo "heparin-free" dialysis without clotting the dialyzer
- with repeated thrombosis of central vein catheters, even more so of the central veins themselves
- patients with a family history of thrombosis
- patients with a history of venous thrombosis, especially more than once (thrombophilia)

Theoretically, the population receiving dialysis should mirror the population at large in the incidences of factor V-Leiden and prothrombin G-20210a. There is no evidence supporting routine testing for these alleles before vascular access is constructed. For patients who repeatedly clot access constructions, these tests can be readily performed, as well as measurement of proteins C, S, and antithrombin III and anticardiolipin antibody levels (antiphospholipid antibody).

A pragmatic approach to the problem of repeated thrombosis requires the surgeon to verify adequacy of a construction's hemodynamics, such that flow is ideally more than 600 mL/min and there is no tendency to kink or occlude the construction by the patient's body habitus or position. If these are acceptable, the patient may require warfarin to keep the access flowing. Another alternative is for the surgeon to convert the site to a different and larger autogenous configuration, such as a translocated basilic vein. When erythropoietin was first used, many surgeons were concerned that the elevation of hematocrit would lead to an increase in viscosity of blood that would in turn cause access sites to clot. There is no evidence to support this contention. There are rare patients with a history of repeated thrombosis who will be forced to use central catheters long-term.

Excessive bleeding from puncture sites, until proven otherwise, must be attributed to venous outflow obstruction. Bleeding is also related to conduit degeneration with false aneurysm formation, skin erosion, and localized infection. Many dialysis patients take major antiplatelet agents, such as clopidogrel, which may lead to prolonged puncture site bleeding. Faulty puncture technique through and through the conduit or vein will lead to massive hemorrhage, which can also occur when the return needle is dislodged into subcutaneous tissues during a treatment. These hematomas usually require surgical evacuation. Poor puncture technique can also lead to longitudinal tears in a prosthetic graft, which are manifested as false aneurysms. The actual technique of access puncture remains a matter of much discussion and controversy. Some adherents favor "buttonhole" technique that puts the puncture always in the same place, whereas others advocate for a "stepladder" approach to move the punctures along the access site in an organized linear manner. There remain technical pros and cons related to each approach, and the method chosen will also depend on the access site configuration and comfort of the patient.

Circulatory Abnormalities

NFH is the commonest acquired access site lesion, more often on the venous side than arterial. There is no certain means to prevent these lesions, other than for the surgeon to use precise and gentle technique, preferably not injuring the vessel intima through excessive handling at the time of surgery. Some surgeons have found that use of anastomotic stapling will lower NFH rates in comparison with conventional suturing. In addition, excessively rough passage of balloon thrombectomy catheters will cause denudation of venous intima, leading to outflow destruction over time. On the arterial side, rough technique will lead to clamp injury, which will in turn cause a stenosis, problematic for access flow if it is on the afferent side of the anastomosis, and potentially a cause of severe ischemia to the hand or arm if it is on the efferent side.

Anatomic variation can also lead to blood flow abnormalities in an access site, often with sluggish flow and thrombosis. Between 7% and 15% of people will have a variant position of the brachial artery bifurcation. A surgeon finding a small "brachial" artery in the antecubital fossa or upper arm should consider that a high bifurcation may be present. The small artery diameter may predispose to low flow volumes and early thrombosis. Revision to a larger proximal artery inflow may be needed. Inflow abnormality can also occur when the ipsilateral brachial or radial artery has been used for cardiac catheterization, which can cause diffuse arterial scarring from NFH.

Central or venous outflow stenoses occur for many reasons, most often from prior ipsilateral central vein catheter placement. Fistulae based on the upper arm cephalic vein may become compromised from narrowing of the vein as it passes through the pectoralis major muscle to join the axillary vein system (cephalic arch syndrome). Any patient who has had intravenous therapy through a peripherally inserted central catheter (PICC) should be studied carefully by ultrasound prior to placement of an ipsilateral access site because of the possibility of an induced outflow stenosis or occlusion from prolonged trauma to the vein wall.

Vascular Steal

Although insufficient flow is problematic because it leads to thrombosis of an access construction, a more dangerous and increasingly common problem is steal, which can lead to significant dysfunction or damage in the affected extremity. In order for steal to occur, three factors must be present: disease in the inflow arteries, such that they cannot dilate to meet access flow demands; disease in the distal vessels, such that they have higher than normal resistance to flow; and a low-resistance access construction conduit. Symptoms can range from a hand that is cold or numb only during treatments, to mononeuropathy with intrinsic muscle weakness in the hand, to rest pain in the extremity with gangrene.

Predicting the patient who will develop steal is not always easy. Patients with diabetes and nonpalpable radial arteries are at primary risk, as are patients with obviously hardened palpable brachial arteries. An Allen test can be used to try to predict steal, but it is of poor predictive power. The effects of radial artery occlusion can be performed with a hand-held Doppler stethoscope, but there is no noninvasive test that can predict what will happen to hand flow when the ulnar artery feeds across the wrist into a high-flow fistula. Patients who have had the radial artery harvested for a cardiac bypass may be at higher risk for steal when access is based on the ipsilateral brachial artery.

The diagnosis of the steal phenomenon is possible at the bedside with only a Doppler stethoscope. One checks for baseline digital blood flow at the level of the proximal phalanges and compares subjective flow patterns before and after temporary access site occlusion. If occlusion causes flow to increase, especially if it goes from none to vigorous with visible hyperemia of digits, the diagnosis is certain. Further documentation of suspected steal is possible using pulse volume recordings of digits before and after fistula occlusion, or by using color-flow duplex ultrasonography to evaluate flow into the extremity. For minor steal, the access site can be followed, reserving repair or revision for the patient who does not demonstrate adaptation to the symptoms. For major steal that threatens the limb, an urgent procedure is indicated. This can range from local revision to a new arterial inflow site, bypass around the access site (the DRIL procedure), revision using distal inflow (RUDI), banding or flow limitation to the site, proximalization of inflow, or purposeful thrombosis or ligation of the site.

Arterial Occlusion

Acute arterial occlusion from access construction or revision is fortunately uncommon. Occlusion of a single branch artery in the forearm distal to a brachial access site is usually asymptomatic, unless there has been previous instrumentation with arterial thrombosis at the wrist, as might occur with a radial artery cannulation. Total brachial artery occlusion may result in severe symptoms of hand ischemia, especially if combined with an element of vascular steal. The etiology may be a clamp injury, an intimal flap from fracture of a calcified artery, or a technical error in suturing the conduit to the artery. Retrograde thrombosis may also very rarely occur as a complication of sudden outflow occlusion of a conduit while a patient is being dialyzed, where the clot is pumped by the dialyzer. Urgent repair is required in these cases. Thrombectomy of access sites can result in embolization of clot into the distal arterial runoff of an extremity, but this is fortunately rare. More often a problem is acute intimal injury from passage of the thrombectomy catheter or instruments, such as a curette, from the conduit into the native vessel. Again, immediate symptoms of ischemia should be recognized by the surgeon and immediately repaired if there is any question about the viability of the extremity.

Chronic arterial occlusion after access site construction is most often related to induced NFH. Any instrumentation of an artery (even more so, of veins) will lead to destruction of intima, with deposition and degranulation of platelets. The resultant release of platelet-derived growth factor and other less well defined stimulating kinins will lead to proliferation of subintimal fibroblasts and creation of a stenosis. This can progress to complete occlusion. The key time period for appearance of this disease in arteries is usually from 6 to 24 months after instrumentation, but NFH can occur in as few as 6 weeks in dialysis access sites. The treatment is primarily preventive, by keeping intimal injury to the minimum through careful technique and minimal manipulation of balloon catheters in the native vessels. Antiplatelet drugs also play a role in decreasing the risk of occurrence of this disease for coronary and peripheral vascular bypasses, but there are only a few reports that support improved patency in access sites if antiplatelet drugs are administered. If the distal extremity is symptomatic due to arterial lesions related to an access site, the treatment is conventional bypass or patch angioplasty of the affected vessel, and balloon angioplasty or stenting may prove alternatives in selected cases.

Early Perioperative Complications Related to Access Placement

Problems Relating to Wound Care During Surgery

Gentle tissue handling is extremely important in placing dialysis access conduits, and wound problems are even more an issue when reoperations are performed for access sites with complications. Skin preparation for surgery optimally includes a long-acting iodinated agent, such as Duraprep, or one containing chlorhexidine. All patients receive prophylactic antibiotics before procedures, except for those for whom minor autogenous constructions are planned. There is no evidence supporting antibiotics for a wrist Cimino fistula or antecubital vein-brachial fistula. The agent of choice according to U.S. surgical quality standards is a single dose of cefazolin, corrected for body weight. Antibiotics are often included in wound irrigation solutions. Infection risk also stems from poor tissue handling technique and problems in wound closure. Care must be taken to avoid hematomas and trauma to subcutaneous fat. Prolonged or forceful retraction can lead to fat necrosis, which is manifested later by drainage of cloudy fluid from a wound, as can excessively tight closure of subcutaneous fat. Electrocautery, especially for hemostasis, should be used with care in order to avoid fat necrosis. A dire complication of sloppy tissue handling is edge necrosis of a wound, which can lead to exposure of a conduit. These considerations are particularly important for translocated basilic vein constructions, especially in obese patients, where there may be substantial wound healing problems. Skin closure must be meticulous.

Neuralgia from access constructions occurs from several causes. First is direct injury to adjacent nerves at the time of access placement. Second is pain related to ligation or clipping of a small cutaneous nerve, where there is late development of a neuroma. This has been observed in the forearm and wrist, as there is a small cutaneous branch of the radial nerve that is prone to injury during creation of autogenous fistulas. Third, there is the problem of puncture into or near a cutaneous nerve overlying an access conduit. The patient with this problem will have severe pain from a dialysis needle, or there may be development of chronic pain and dysesthesias in the scar tissue that inevitably overlies an access conduit. Fourth is the problem of access conduits placed under or near surgical scars. Some patients experience significant pain when dialysis needle punctures are necessary through scars. For this reason, conduits are best routed away from prior areas of surgery if possible. Finally, neuralgia may be the major sign of early steal, and if this is not addressed, protracted ischemic neuropathy in the hand may result.

Hemorrhage

Intraoperative hemorrhage immediately after initiation of flow into a hemodialysis conduit is fortunately uncommon. Persistent bleeding from suture holes in polytetrafluoroethylene (PTFE) conduits is a nuisance in some patients. It is avoided by careful suturing technique, and some surgeons prefer PTFE suture rather than polypropylene with a belief that the holes in the graft are smaller yet better filled by the suture, leading to less bleeding. Bleeding is also prevented by avoiding too much heparin during the procedure, especially in patients on chronic warfarin therapy where anticoagulation reversal has been incomplete. When bleeding from suture holes occurs, the heparin effect can be reversed with protamine, but care must be taken to avoid hypotension from excessively rapid administration of this drug. Desmopressin is also useful in achieving hemostasis in these cases, as is topical recombinant thrombin. Hemorrhage at the venous anastomosis during a thrombectomy and revision procedure is not unusual, especially as a paradoxical problem in patients with a coagulopathy such as an anticardiolipin antibody, and bleeding can be a hint that there is an outflow venous obstruction. Faced with bleeding, a surgeon must achieve patient control of the problem, because a postoperative hematoma can lead to infection, skin necrosis, pain, or deformity at the access site.

Early hemorrhage along a PTFE conduit into the subcutaneous tissues is avoided by creating a tight tunnel with a small-diameter tunneling device. It is a problem more likely to occur when a plastic graft is tunneled for a new proximal site in an arm that has a patent autogenous fistula distally at the wrist. Compression of the arm with a gently applied elastic bandage can also control this diffuse oozing into the tunnel. In the past, peri-graft hemorrhage from puncture into a new PTFE access site was avoided by allowing a period of 4–6 weeks for the graft to incorporate into tissue. In more recent practice at many centers, this period of waiting has been shortened to 1–2 weeks, if the surgeon uses tight tunnels for routing the graft. Nevertheless, a peri-graft hematoma can be a major, disabling complication. It can cause skin breakdown that exposes the graft, and it can form a nidus for infection to occur. Peri-graft hemorrhage is best managed in consultation with the surgeon who initially placed the graft. Peri-graft hematoma causes reddening of skin overlying the conduit, so the differential diagnosis is an acute graft infection, or a small hematoma can become secondarily infected even several weeks after graft placement. The surgeon who placed the conduit must be involved in the decision making regarding these conduits, whether to give antibiotics and local care to the extremity or to remove the graft. New multilayer grafts have been designed for early puncture in order to avoid many of these complications.

Edema

Edema may occur soon after placement of a high-flow vascular access. Edema will occur when there is a stenosis or occlusion of veins central to the venous outflow, and swelling will be accentuated in patients with anasarca. Fistulograms, including imaging of the veins in the thoracic outlet through to the superior vena cava, are helpful in determining the best treatment for the swollen arm after access placement. Where there is a stenosis, balloon angioplasty may relieve venous hypertension. Although stents are commonly used for these lesions, they carry the drawback that intimal hyperplasia may be accelerated in the treated segment, causing early reocclusion. In some cases, veno-veno bypass will relieve edema from venous hypertension. Also in rare cases, intractable edema from fistula flow will require access ligation.

Edema may also occur merely from the fact of multiple access operations in an arm. Troublesome edema has occurred in the central tissues in the middle of a looped forearm or groin graft. Such edema may be a phenomenon of no clinical significance, but it may also herald subclinical graft infection. In such cases, the site should be rested without puncture, the extremity elevated, and consideration made to the use of gentle compression with elastic bandages.

Technical Problems and Miscellaneous Difficulties

Conduit malposition can hamper access function. Surgeons should become familiar with the patient's usual position in a dialysis chair, such that the access conduit is placed in a position that does not hinder puncture. In addition, the conduit must be positioned close to the skin but not too shallow. If a conduit is too deep to the skin, conventional needles may pop out of the conduit with patient movement, leading to a massive arm hematoma. If too shallow, skin erosion may occur with graft exposure. Translocated basilic vein constructions must be long enough to provide room for the dialysis needles, and this usually requires adequate mobilization of the vein. Some patients have limited shoulder mobility due to arthritis, stroke, or previous injury. Placing a conduit far to the medial volar aspect of such an extremity will prevent the conduit from being cannulated.

Peri-graft seroma is a troublesome complication generally limited to PTFE conduits. Plasma may be seen to "weep" through grafts that have come in contact with wetting agents (surfactants) such as povidone-iodine or alcohol. Seroma may be prevented by using barrier plastic draping or surgical technique that carefully avoids contact of the graft with prepped skin. Patients with low serum protein levels may also be prone to seromas. Some seromas may respond to careful aspiration drainage. Rather than risk infection of a graft from repeated manipulation, a persistent seroma may require wound exploration in order to ligate the leaking lymphatic channel and a careful reclosure, or it may require graft removal and replacement of the conduit in a new site. Seromas are an important complication after placement of groin grafts and are best avoided by careful technique with ligation of exposed lymphatics.

Aneurysms occur at anastomoses, within conduits as they degenerate, as a manifestation of graft sepsis, and as a result of chronic hemodynamic stress in the inflow artery or outflow vein. Aneurysms may cause pain or visible deformity in the extremity. When this occurs in a prosthetic site, a revision can eliminate the aneurysmal segment. This is most easily done by splicing a new conduit in parallel to the diseased segment, thereby allowing continuity of access site function. Fusiform aneurysms in an autogenous fistula can be mobilized, tailored to a smaller diameter, and then replaced in a position that will allow salvage of the access site. The most dangerous acute problem from aneurysmal change is skin erosion, especially when it is associated with localized sepsis in the conduit. The patient may have thinned skin over the access graft with damage due to repeated puncture in the same site. A small puncture eschar may fail to heal, leading to erosion and exposure of the conduit. Massive hemorrhage is usually preceded by a "herald bleed" controlled with local pressure. Dialysis nurses must be taught that eschars overlying grafts or bleeding erosions must be brought to the attention of a surgeon. Nurses must also learn to differentiate the appearance of skin where a "buttonhole" access puncture technique is used from skin that is threatening erosion. A shallow subcutaneous position of a conduit may predispose to erosion, as may be the case for patients taking therapeutic doses of steroids.

Surgical repair of exposed sites or erosions is aimed at maintaining access site function overall while rerouting blood away from the diseased segment and skin ulcer. Through the site of erosion, the diseased conduit can be removed, usually without making a massive skin incision. The area of contamination is locally drained or placed on wet dressings for secondary closure. In the case of a catastrophic hemorrhage, primary ligation and removal of the contaminated graft is often necessary, with temporary access by a central venous catheter. Local skin suture over a site of erosion is generally unsuccessful, leading to more extensive sepsis in the area. There have been a few case reports of rotational cutaneous flaps used to treat this type of graft exposure, with mixed results. A course of intravenous antibiotics is often necessary in the immediate perioperative period after such a graft catastrophe.

In the past, there has been no adverse effect on renal transplantation by the creation or maintenance of hemodialysis access. Recently, cryopreserved veins have become available for use as prosthetic conduits in vascular surgery, and some have been used for dialysis access. Some transplantation surgeons have been concerned about the possibility of these allogenic conduits causing immunosensitization. There is no evidence that xeno-conduits (bovine carotid) have an adverse effect on transplantation.

Anesthesia for Access Surgery

It is generally assumed that patients with ESRD are at higher than average risk for cardiopulmonary complications should general anesthesia be required for surgery. Therefore, multiple small procedures under local or regional anesthesia seem safer and better tolerated than extensive ones under general anesthesia. The ready availability of temporary central vein catheters to bridge periods of access failure facilitates this flexible approach.

Most procedures are performed on a daystay basis under local or regional anesthesia. Ideally, procedures are arranged for morning surgery time in order to allow for recovery from sedation, the performance of any necessary afternoon dialysis, and transportation to home. For short procedures, lidocaine suffices, but for longer operations, bupivacaine will allow 2–3 hours of anesthesia. Although many procedures are easily performed with true local anesthesia for the surgical field, some surgeons prefer regional blocks, also based on some studies that may have shown a higher patency for sites created that way. All of these procedures are facilitated by sedation with propofol, fentanyl, or midazolam. General or conduction anesthesia is necessary for central axillary/subclavian procedures or for groin grafts.

It is not unusual to find severe hyperkalemia or hyperglycemia in a patient with a clotted access site presenting for surgical thrombectomy. These abnormalities can occur even when the patient has never suffered a break in his or her usual hemodialysis schedule or a known decrease in the quality of hemodialysis prior to the thrombosis. The availability of point-of-care laboratory measurement of metabolic parameters theoretically improves the safety of urgent angioaccess procedures, because patients with significant abnormalities can be treated with an aggressive dialysis session using a temporary dialysis catheter prior to their revisional surgery.

The complications from dialysis access procedures include sudden cardiac death and acute ("flash") pulmonary edema. Perioperative myocardial infarctions are fortunately rare, but under the stress of a prolonged procedure with insufficient local anesthesia or sedation, induction of dysrhythmias and transient coronary insufficiency do occur. Medication reactions during surgery are also rare. Physicians in the OR nevertheless need to be cautious about rapid administration of protamine (best to avoid excessive heparin in the first place), inadvertent intravenous administration of bupivacaine, excessive doses of lidocaine, and excessive amounts of iodinated contrast for intraoperative fistulography.

Virtually all procedures are best performed under monitored anesthesia care (MAC). Strictly local anesthesia without monitoring can be used for removal of central venous catheters, placement of temporary nontunneled dialysis catheters, and ligation of access sites. In a young, cooperative patient, a Cimino fistula can be performed without sedation, as can a tunneled dialysis catheter.

Surgeons must be sensitive to the fact that some patients will experience severe discomfort after even a relatively minor access site revision, such that their pain is not well controlled using oral narcotic analgesics after surgery. To avoid complications from excessive sedation, and to prevent the patient or his family from having severe anxiety or anger about the process of access surgery, patients with severe pain should be observed overnight and treated with parenteral narcotics as necessary. In general, the need for major analgesia after access procedures is transient.

Uncommon Late Complications

There are three rare complications that stem from high-flow access constructions. First is excessive arterial dilation proximal to the access inflow. This induced arteriomegaly can be associated over time with thrombosis of native arterial segments, with resultant severe distal ischemia. Fortunately, there are no reports of gangrene or amputation from this phenomenon. Second and also rare is exacerbation of congestive heart failure from high cardiac output. Unless the underlying cardiac lesion can be repaired, the patient truly having this problem will require chronic central venous catheterization for dialysis rather than a high-flow access site. Finally, there is induced carpal tunnel syndrome from high-volume access flow across the wrist. This is a phenomenon that can occur when there is access inflow based on the radial artery and when the proximal radial artery side of the construction becomes narrowed. Flow is then dependent on collaterals from the ulnar artery coming across the carpal row and retrograde into the distal radial artery. If this collateralization is very large, it can compress the median nerve, causing symptoms. The diagnosis of this phenomenon can be made by compression of the ulnar artery, which almost immediately brings some relief to the hand, and flow across the base of the palm can be demonstrated by duplex ultrasonography. Definitive treatment is by revision of the access inflow anastomosis to eliminate the proximal stenosis.

Body image problems from dialysis access sites may occur. An aneurysmal autogenous fistula may provoke a discussion about repair, not because it is malfunctioning but because it is ugly. A renal allograft recipient with an unused fistula may ask for ligation and debulking of aneurysmal forearm veins. Old prosthetic conduits are benign, but they can be prominent. Patients will ask about removing them, and the reality to be explained is that removal will lead to even worse appearance. Some patients become concerned about visible collateral veins that can develop in the outflow of an access site. Unless these veins are associated with an outflow occlusion or stenosis causing access malfunction, they should be left alone.

The influence of the patient's age on selection of dialysis access has been a concern of some surgeons. In general, the preponderance of evidence is that any patient suitable for hemodialysis is suitable for the best autogenous access site possible. Tissue laxity and thinned skin may make cannulation of arm veins difficult for some dialysis technicians, and very elderly patients may be more prone to development of ecchymoses and periconduit hematomas. These problems are addressed by education and training of the dialysis center staff and not by placing dialysis catheters in this population.

CHAPTER 5

Infectious Complications From Vascular Access

Michael Allon, MD • Charmaine E. Lok, MD, MSc, FRCPC

Overview of Vascular Access-Related Infection

Infections are the second most common cause of hospitalization and mortality in hemodialysis patients. In the 1846 hemodialysis patients enrolled in the HEMO Study, 23% of all deaths and 25% of all hospitalizations were infection-related. Among all infection-related hospitalizations, 23% were considered access-related. Moreover, 44% of hospitalizations related to access infection resulted in death, an intensive care unit stay, or prolonged ($\geq$7 days) hospitalization. The rate of infection associated with central vein catheters (CVC) is much higher than that associated with arteriovenous grafts (AVG) or arteriovenous fistulas (AVF) (100–200, 8–10, and 1–4 infections per 100 patient-years, respectively). In a large single-center study of catheter-dependent hemodialysis patients, 88% of the infections were access-related, whereas only 12% were non-access-related. Thus, it is not surprising that patients with CVCs account for a disproportionate number of access infection hospitalizations. In the HEMO Study, 32% of access-related infections occurred in CVC-dependent patients, even though these patients accounted for only 7.6% of all vascular accesses used in the study. Likewise, in EPIBACDIAL, another multi-center prospective study of 988 hemodialysis patients, 36% occurred in CVC-dependent patients, even though this subset accounted for only 6% of the study population.

Arteriovenous Fistula-Related Infections

AVF infections should be exceedingly rare, given that there is no artificial material involved. For example, a single-center study of 389 AVF observed an infection in only one AVF (0.25%). Unfortunately, the use of "buttonhole" cannulation has markedly increased this risk. Standard "rope ladder" cannulation entails using sharp dialysis needles with rotation of the AVF cannulation sites. In contrast, buttonhole cannulation entails the creation of subcutaneous tracks between the skin and the AVF. Cannulation is performed with blunt needles inserted repeatedly into the AVF through these tracks, using the identical skin puncture sites at the identical angle. This technique has been associated with reduced needle infiltration and formation of pseudoaneurysms. The rope ladder technique requires a single antiseptic application to the skin prior to AVF cannulation. In contrast, buttonhole cannulation requires two separate antiseptic applications. A scab forms at the cannulation site and is a nidus for bacterial colonization. After swabbing the skin with chlorhexidine, the scab is removed, and then the skin is swabbed a second time with chlorhexidine. Failure to remove the scab and resterilize the skin prior to AVF cannulation may result in the introduction of bacteria from the scab into the bloodstream. Bacteria may also be colonized within the multiple subcutaneous tracks that may be created if buttonhole cannulation is performed incorrectly. While the buttonhole cannulation technique has been touted as an approach to decrease pain and improve the ease of cannulation, not all prospective studies have supported these claims and have instead uncovered a greater risk of infection.

A single-center study reported a cluster of 22 episodes of AVF-related bacteremia in 56 patients using the buttonhole cannulation technique. Ten of the bacteremic episodes were caused by *Staphylococcus aureus,* and four resulted in metastatic infections. A European dialysis center that used universal buttonhole AVF cannulation observed a spike of AVF-related bacteremia that resolved after intensive education of the dialysis staff about proper antiseptic technique for buttonhole cannulation. A Canadian randomized controlled trial (RCT) of 140 hemodialysis patients allocated patients to buttonhole or rope ladder AVF cannulation. The frequency of local AVF infection was more than twofold higher in patients using the buttonhole technique (5.0 vs 2.2 events per 100 dialysis sessions, $p = .003$). Moreover, use of the buttonhole technique did not improve AVF survival. Finally, a recent meta-analysis comparing buttonhole to rope ladder AVF cannulation reported a 3.3-fold higher risk of AVF infection with the buttonhole technique in four RCTs and a 3.2-fold increase in AVF infection after switching from rope ladder to buttonhole cannulation in seven observational studies. Taken together, these publications strongly suggest that the buttonhole AVF cannulation technique should be abandoned.

Arteriovenous Graft-Related Infections

Arteriovenous graft infections are caused by introduction of skin contaminants into the AVG at the time of cannulation. The typical clinical presentation includes fever, erythema, and tenderness over the AVG. There may also be a purulent discharge from the AVG access site. AVG infections are associated with major systemic complications in ~20% of cases. AVG infections occur most commonly within 6 months of AVG creation, but may occasionally be observed at later time periods. A cure usually requires AVG excision, in conjunction with systemic antibiotics. In a minority of cases with very localized infection, partial excision and placement of a jump graft may be sufficient. AVG infection is usually followed by a period of prolonged catheter dependence. Infection is more common with AVGs in the thigh, compared with those in the upper extremity, with frequencies of 14% versus 9%, respectively, in one large series. In a series of 209 thigh AVGs, the cumulative incidence of AVG infection was 21%, 27%, and 39% at 1, 2, and 5 years, respectively. Whereas upper extremity AVG infections are almost exclusively caused by gram-positive bacteria, about one-third of thigh AVG infections are due to gram-negative bacteria, presumably enteric organisms from the groin. This means that empiric antibiotics for treatment of suspected thigh AVG infection must include coverage for both gram-positive and gram-negative bacteria. Finally, metastatic infections are more common with thigh AVGs versus upper extremity AVGs (15% vs 3%), perhaps because of the delayed diagnosis of the former. The optimal antiseptic regimen prior to AVG cannulation has not been evaluated in RCTs. However, a large RCT that compared chlorhexidine to povidone-iodine for preoperative skin antisepsis in patients undergoing surgery observed a 60% lower rate of skin infection in those treated with chlorhexidine. Extrapolation from this study suggests that chlorhexidine is the preferred skin antisepsis prior to AVG cannulation.

Dialysis Catheter–Related Infections

As mentioned previously, CVC infections represent the overwhelming majority of vascular access–related infection. CVC-related infections fall into three categories: exit-site infection, tunnel infection, and catheter-related bacteremia (CRB). In non-tunneled CVC, used exclusively in the inpatient setting, there are two potential pathways for bacteremia: the bacteria can enter the bloodstream from the exit site along the outside of the catheter or they can be introduced from the catheter lumen. Tunneled CVCs, used routinely in outpatients, have a Dacron cuff around the sub-cutaneous portion. The cuff induces inflammation and fibrosis, thereby creating a mechanical barrier to entry of bacteria along the outside of the CVC. By largely eliminating one possible route of bacteremia, tunneled CVCs are associated with ~50% reduction of CRB, compared with nontunneled CVCs. The remainder of the discussion is focused exclusively on tunneled CVCs.

Exit-site infections present with erythema, tenderness, or exudate at the catheter exit site and are almost exclusively caused by *Staphylococcus aureus* or *Staphylococcus epidermidis* infection. Mild cases can be treated with exit-site antibiotic ointment or oral antibiotics. If the exit-site infection persists, or if it is associated with CRB, the tunneled CVC should be removed. Tunnel infections present with exquisite tenderness and erythema over the subcutaneous tunnel, and a large amount of purulence can be expressed by applying pressure to the overlying skin. They always require CVC removal and systemic antibiotics, usually in conjunction with incision and drainage of the tunnel.

The three major issues regarding management of CRB in CVC-dependent hemo-dialysis patients are (1) how to diagnose CRB; (2) optimal antibiotic therapy (type, dose, and duration); and (3) what to do about the CVC. CRB should be suspected and blood cultures obtained whenever a CVC-dependent hemodialysis patient pre-sents with signs of systemic infection (fever, unexplained hypotension, or rigors) without an obvious non-CVC source. Less commonly, patients may present with delirium, nausea, or vomiting. Approximately one-third of patients with documented CRB present with rigors in the absence of fever. In nondialysis hospitalized patients with suspected CRB, two sets of blood cultures are typically obtained: one from the catheter lumen and another from a peripheral vein. However, because of the logistic difficulties in obtaining cultures from peripheral veins in dialysis outpatients and the need to save veins for future vascular access creation, the second set of blood cul-tures is usually obtained from the dialysis bloodline, once the dialysis session has been initiated. The bloodline culture serves as a surrogate for the peripheral vein culture. If the symptoms occur during the dialysis session, the dialysis nurse obtains two separate bloodline cultures separated by about 10 minutes. The frequency of CRB varies substantially among centers, but most have reported a frequency of 2.5–5.5 episodes per 1000 catheter-days, and approximately 10% of cases are com-plicated by metastatic infection.

The likelihood of bacteremia in a symptomatic CVC-dependent hemodialysis patient is very high (59%–81%). Therefore, empiric systemic antibiotics should be initiated pending blood culture results. The choice of antibiotics is dictated by (1) knowledge of the typical organisms in dialysis patients with CRB, particularly in one's own dialysis facility, as well as (2) the desire to preferentially use antibiotics whose pharmacokinetics permit one to avoid the need to administer antibiotics between dialysis sessions. Examples of antibiotics that could be easily used to treat CRB include vancomycin, cefazolin, ceftazidime, and aminoglycosides. Although gram-positive bacteria are the most common cause of CRB, gram-negative infections may account for up to 40% of cases. Moreover, methicillin-resistant *Staphylococcus* is common in this population. Given these considerations, empiric antibiotics should be initiated with a combination of vancomycin or cefazolin and an antibiotic with broad-spectrum gram-negative coverage (third-generation cephalosporin or an aminoglycoside). Once the specific organism and its sensitivities are available, it is important to switch to a more narrow spectrum antibiotic, in order to minimize the risk of the development of antibiotic resistance. If the blood cultures grow a methicillin-sensitive *Staphylococcus*, the patient should be switched from vancomycin to cefazolin or another organism-sensitive antibiotic. Similarly, if the gram-negative organism is susceptible, the patient should be switched from a third-generation cephalosporin to a more narrow spectrum one, to avoid antibiotic resistance. Given their favorable pharmacokinetics in dialysis patients, all four discussed antibiotics (vancomycin, cefazolin, ceftazidime, and aminoglycosides) can be administered thrice weekly after dialysis. Table 5.1 provides the recommended doses of these antibiotics in hemodialysis patients. However, it is important to gain familiarity with other effective antibiotics that are locally and commonly used. To avoid prolonged vancomycin administration after the dialysis session ends, this drug can be infused during the last 1–2 hours of each dialysis session, as long as the infusion rate does not exceed 1 g/h. Most patients with CRB are treated with a 2- or 3-week course of antibiotics. However, in cases of complicated CRB (endocarditis, osteomyelitis, septic arthritis, or epidural abscess), the patient should receive a longer course of antibiotic therapy, and treatment may be guided by consultation with infectious diseases experts (depending on the degree of complications). Hospitalization for initial treatment of CRB is not indicated unless the patient has severe sepsis or evidence of metastatic infection. At one large dialysis center the overall frequency of hospitalization in 184 cases of CRB was 37%. This occurred primarily in patients with *S. aureus* CRB (53% hospitalization), and was much less likely in those with CRB due to *S. epidermidis* or gram-negative bacteria (23% and 17%, respectively).

Table 5.1

Recommended Intravenous Doses of Commonly Prescribed Antibiotics in Hemodialysis Patients

Vancomycin	20 mg/kg loading dose, then 1 gm IV during the last 1 hour of subsequent HD sessions
Ceftazidime	1 gm IV after each dialysis
Cefazolin	1 gm IV after each dialysis
Gentamicin	1 mg/kg after each dialysis (not to exceed 80 mg per dose)

HD, hemodialysis; IV, intravenous.

Systemic antibiotics alone are not sufficient in the management of CRB. Although they may temporarily treat the bacteremia, positive blood cultures recur in up to 75% of cases once the course of antibiotics has been completed. Given that the tunneled CVC is the source of CRB, some would advocate routine CVC removal in conjunction with systemic antibiotics. Unfortunately, such an approach creates significant logistic obstacles, namely, the continued need for an access to provide hemodialysis thrice weekly. If the tunneled CVC is removed, one places a temporary nontunneled CVC. Once the nephrologist is satisfied that the bacteremia has resolved, a new tunneled CVC can be placed. This strategy entails the need for at least three separate procedures in each case of CRB (removal of the infected CVC, placement of a temporary nontunneled CVC, placement of a new tunneled CVC). An alternative approach is to initiate systemic antibiotics, and if the fever and bacteremia resolved within 2–3 days, exchange the infected catheter for a new one over a guidewire in cases where the exit site and tunnel are non-purulent. This strategy has been effective in 70%–80% of CRBs in several series, and has the virtue of reducing the number of procedures from three to one.

A final approach to management of the infected CVC in hemodialysis patients with CRB was proposed on the basis of the observation that a bacterial biofilm rapidly forms on the inner lumen of all infected CVCs. If the bacteria in the biofilm could be eradicated, it might be possible to treat the source of bacteremia without removing the CVC. This can be achieved in many cases by instilling a concentrated antibiotic solution (together with an anticoagulant) into the catheter lumen ("an antibiotic lock"), in conjunction with systemic antibiotics (Fig. 5.1). The efficacy of this approach has been validated in 10 separate observational studies, which cumulatively demonstrated that CRB could be eradicated while salvaging the CVC in 410 of 546 (75%) episodes of CRB. Importantly, the success rate of an antibiotic lock in achieving a CRB cure is highly dependent on the infecting organism. It is most successful in patients with gram-negative or *S. epidermidis* infections, and least successful in those with *S. aureus* infections (Fig. 5.2). Regardless of the particular strategy used to manage CRB, a collaborative team approach is critical to ensure appropriate antibiotic prescription, patient and catheter management, and has been shown to improve patient outcomes, as compared to the usual physician-managed care.

Prevention of CRB

As mentioned previously, CVCs are routinely colonized by bacteria, which form a biofilm on the inner lumen of the catheter. These bacteria are in turn derived from organisms colonizing the skin around the exit site, and are introduced into the catheter lumen during almost any form of catheter manipulation, including connection and disconnection of the catheter to the dialysis tubing. Aseptic technique is paramount in reducing the transfer of skin flora to the catheter lumen by the dialysis staff, and has been shown to markedly reduce the frequency of CRB. Nevertheless, as a consequence of the high workload of dialysis nurses/technicians and lapses in aseptic technique, CRB continues to be a major problem leading to hospitalization and death among CVC-dependent HD patients.

One potential method to prevent CRB is the application of an antibiotic ointment at the CVC exit site after each dialysis session. Mupirocin (effective against gram-positive bacteria) and polysporin (effective against both gram-positive and

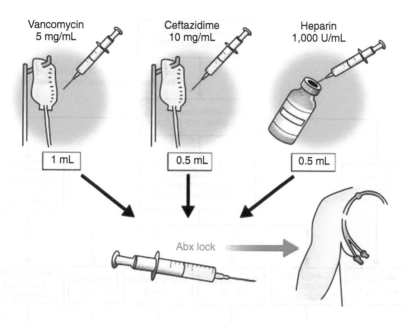

Vancomycin
5 mg/mL

Ceftazidime
10 mg/mL

Heparin
1,000 U/mL

1 mL

0.5 mL

0.5 mL

Abx lock

Figure 5.1

How to Administer an Antibiotic Lock in Patients With Catheter-Related Bacteremia. The dialysis nurse prepares the antibiotic lock by mixing an aliquot of antibiotic from the solution used for systemic administration with an aliquot of heparin into a single syringe. Note that the final antibiotic concentration in the lock is approximately 100-fold higher than therapeutic plasma antibiotic concentrations. The antibiotic-heparin lock solution is instilled into each catheter port at the end of the dialysis session and aspirated immediately before initiation of the next dialysis session. If the systemic antibiotic regimen is changed, then the antibiotic lock components are changed accordingly. Once the course of systemic antibiotics is completed, standard heparin locks are resumed. (Reproduced from: Allon M. Current management of vascular access. *Clin J Am Soc Nephrol.* 2007;2:786-800.)

gram-negative bacteria) ointments have been demonstrated in RCTs to markedly reduce CRB. Of some concern, prolonged prophylactic antibiotics may select for resistant organisms. Thus, instances of mupirocin-resistant *Staphylococcus* have been reported. Likewise, prolonged use of exit-site polysporin has been associated with exit site yeast colonization, which may potentially lead to fungemia. However, long-term follow-up has not found this to generally be the case. Nevertheless, prolonged prophylactic use of any form of antibiotic must be monitored carefully for adverse effects. A second alternative is to instill an antibiotic or antimicrobial solution into the catheter lumen after each dialysis session, in an attempt to prevent biofilm formation. Numerous RCTs have been conducted comparing the frequency of CRB in patients receiving an antimicrobial catheter lock, as compared to standard anticoagulant locks (heparin or citrate). These studies have employed several types of antibiotics (gentamicin, cefotaxime, cefazolin, and minocycline), as well as a

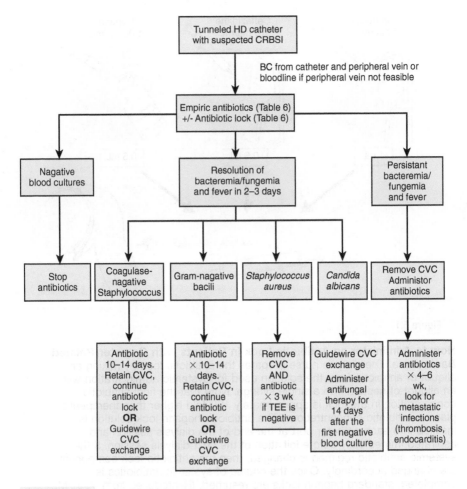

Figure 5.2

Recommended Management of Dialysis Catheter–Related Bloodstream Infection. (Reproduced from: Mermel LA, Allon M, Bouza E, et al. Clinical practice guidelines for the diagnosis and management of intravascular catheter-related infection: 2009 Update by the Infectious Diseases Society of America. *Clin Infect Dis.* Jul 1 2009;49(1):1-45.)

variety of nonantibiotic antimicrobial solutions (taurolidine, ethanol, 30% citrate, and methylene blue). The vast majority of these RCTS have demonstrated substantial reductions of CRB in the patients allocated to an antimicrobial catheter lock. A meta-analysis of seven RCTS found that each of these solutions reduced CRB by 50%–100%, as compared to the frequency observed in patients with standard heparin locks (Fig. 5.3). Overall, CRB was 7.7-fold less likely with antimicrobial locks than with heparin locks. Impressively, a recent multicenter observational study reported that, not only did prophylactic gentamicin locks reduce CRB by 73%, they were also associated with a 64% reduction in patient mortality.

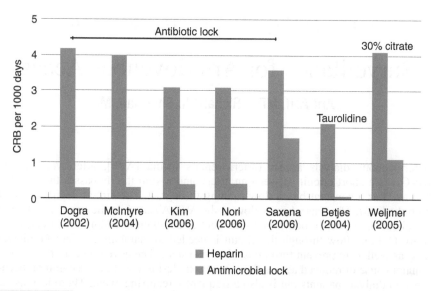

Figure 5.3

Summary of Frequency of Catheter-Related Bacteremia With Antimicrobial Locks Versus Heparin Locks in Published Randomized Clinical Trials. Five trials used an antibiotic lock, one used taurolidine, and one used 30% citrate. In each study, the catheter-related bacteremia frequency was 50%–100% lower in the group with antimicrobial lock compared with the heparin controls. (Reproduced from: Allon M. Prophylaxis against dialysis catheter-related bacteremia: A glimmer of hope. *Am J Kidney Dis.* 2008;51:165-168.)

The salutary effects of exit-site antibiotic ointments and antibiotic catheter locks are additive: in one RCT, the frequency of CRB was lower in patients receiving a gentamicin lock in conjunction with a polysporin exit-site ointment, compared with those treated with the polysporin ointment alone.

Notwithstanding the impressive reduction of CRB with antimicrobial locks, there are some concerns about the safety of their long-term use. A portion of the lock solution invariably leaks into the bloodstream and may cause toxicity. Thus, for example, gentamicin locks caused ototoxicity in one study, and 30% citrate solutions caused frequent paresthesias (presumably due to hypocalcemia) in another study. There is also a concern that prolonged antibiotic lock use may select for resistant infections, an effect that may have been missed in many RCTs with relatively short patient follow-up (~6 months). In this regard, a large observational study using gentamicin locks over 4 years documented the emergence of gentamicin-resistant CRBs, many of which were associated with substantial morbidity and mortality. In contrast, two other large studies with prolonged patient follow-up did not observe a similar problem.

Regardless of the prophylactic strategy used, it is important for the dialysis facility to know their baseline CVC infection rate, track their outcomes, and benchmark their progress against their own historical data and that of recommended standards.

C H A P T E R 6

Surveillance for Arteriovenous Access

Arif Asif, MD • Richard A. Sherman, MD

Arteriovenous dialysis access (arteriovenous fistula [AVF], arteriovenous graft [AVG]) is a short circuit between an artery and a vein that bypasses the capillary bed and has a constant blood flow running through it. The circuit begins and ends with the heart. The artery brings flow to the AVF/AVG while the venous outflow of the circuit transports blood flow to the central circulation, ending the circuit at the heart. Optimal flow through the circuit is needed to maintain an adequate dialysis dose as well as to prevent thrombosis in the system. The development of stenosis is a major cause of reduced access flow. A stenotic lesion is not only a common occurrence in dialysis patients but is also a frequently recurring event. These lesions can develop in any part of the access circuit; however, in AVG patients they are more prevalent at the vein-graft anastomosis whereas in AVF patients they are usually localized to the juxta-anastomotic area. Regardless of their location, stenotic lesions can limit flow through the access circuit and, when hemodynamically significant (flow limiting), can lead to vascular access dysfunction and eventual thrombosis.

Nearly one-third of hospitalizations in chronic hemodialysis (HD) patients are related to vascular access complications resulting in high expenditures (more than $1 billion annually). Although access infection is an important consideration, the development of stenosis (leading to access dysfunction and thrombosis) is the major factor leading to the complications of vascular access.

Based on the premise that vascular access stenosis limits flow, which can result in vascular access dysfunction and thrombosis, it seems reasonable to implement surveillance strategies that can preemptively diagnose stenosis before dysfunction develops or access thrombosis ensues. Features such as noninvasiveness, cost-effectiveness, and reliability are desirable elements for a surveillance tool. At the same time, such a tool should have a high sensitivity and specificity for preemptive detection of access dysfunction, lead to fewer emergent procedures, a decreased thrombosis rate, and less use of catheters; fewer hospitalizations and lower overall costs related to vascular access might also be anticipated. It is reasonable to expect that access survival should be prolonged following angioplasty of a stenotic but patent (flowing) access compared to that of an access that has already clotted and requires thrombolysis as well as angioplasty.

Commonly used surveillance techniques include static venous pressure, duplex Doppler ultrasonography, and blood flow measurements using the ultrasound dilution technique. Early studies found that implementing a surveillance program significantly reduced graft thrombosis. However, these studies were all observational in nature. Subsequent randomized studies have raised serious doubts about the validity of the results of the observational studies.

Ram and colleagues conducted a 28-month randomized trial in which 101 patients with AVG were assigned to one of three groups: control (n = 34), access flow (n = 32), or stenosis (n = 35). Although surveillance in the control group was limited to clinical examination, the access flow group underwent an ultrasound dilution test on a monthly basis and the stenosis group had duplex ultrasonography performed quarterly to assess the degree of stenosis. The following criteria were used to determine referral for angioplasty: (1) control group (clinical criteria); (2) flow group (Qa <600 mL/min or clinical criteria); and (3) stenosis group (stenosis >50% or clinical criteria). The study found that graft thrombosis was lowest in the stenosis group; however, the 2-year graft survival was similar for the control (62%), access flow (60%), and stenosis groups (64%) (p = .89). In essence, performing percutaneous transluminal angioplasty (PTA) for asymptomatic access stenosis detected by low access flow or by duplex ultrasonography was not superior to clinical examination in extending access survival.

In another study, 126 patients were subjected to either clinical monitoring alone (control group) or ultrasonographic surveillance every 4 months for graft stenosis in addition to clinical monitoring (ultrasonography group). The study reported no difference in the frequency of thrombosis between the two groups (control = 0.78, ultrasonography group = 0.67 events per patient-year, respectively; p = .37). In addition, the median time-to-permanent graft failure did not differ between the two groups (38 vs 37 months, p = .93). Significantly more procedures were performed in the ultrasonography group than the control group (ultrasonography = 1.05 vs control = 0.64 events per patient-year, p < .001). Thus, more graft stenosis was detected in the ultrasonography group, resulting in more frequent interventions but not prolongation of graft longevity or improvement in thrombosis-free graft survival.

Two additional randomized studies conducted by Dember et al as well as Moist and colleagues separately evaluated the role of static pressure ratios (intraaccess pressure/mean arterial pressure) and blood flow, respectively; both failed to demonstrate any benefit of surveillance. Indeed, the study by Moist et al reported more interventions in the blood flow group without an impact on the time to graft thrombosis, rate of graft thrombosis, or time to graft loss compared to the control group.

The value of monitoring patients for low (<750 mL/min) or falling (>20% drop from the baseline) access flow was assessed in a 5-year controlled cohort study evaluating 159 hemodialysis patients with mature AVF using ultrasound dilution every 1–4 months. The control group was followed by clinical criteria alone. The number of elective repairs of stenosis in the flow group increased (HR = 2.3, 95% CI = 1.2–4.4, p = .017), thromboses declined (HR = 0.27, 95% CI = 0.09–0.79, p = .017), and access survival tended to increase (HR = 0.35, 95% CI = 0.11–1.09, p = .071), significantly so in the short term (3 years). Importantly, access-related costs were $1213/AVF-year in the control and $743 in the flow group ($p$ < .001).

Although prolonging access patency is important, hospitalizations and cost of care are also key considerations in this fiscally responsible era. In their randomized study discussed above, Ram et al also assessed access-related hospitalizations and costs of care in the three groups. Because a catheter is often required in the event of thrombosis, the study also evaluated the use of catheters among the three groups. Significantly more hospitalizations were found in the control and flow group than the stenosis group (0.50, 0.57, and 0.18 per patient-year, respectively; p < .01). The stenosis group tended to require fewer catheters (0.44, 0.32, and 0.20 per patient-year, respectively; p = .20). The costs of care were higher in the control and flow groups than in the stenosis group ($3727, $4839, and $3306 per patient-year, respectively; $p = .015$).

Any interpretation of the conflicting data between observational and randomized studies must come down on the side of the more rigorous study methodology. Two meta-analyses shed further light on the issue and provide some additional guidance. First, Tonelli et al conducted an analysis of randomized clinical trials comparing access surveillance (using blood flow or ultrasonography) with standard care and failed to find a decrease in the risk of graft thrombosis or access loss in the surveillance group. Additionally, surveillance did not reduce the risk of fistula loss or decrease expenditures. One might expect surveillance to be of more benefit in AVG than in AVF in view of the more frequent development of stenosis and greater thrombotic tendency of the former. However, even when surveillance was limited to patients with AVG, the report found no evidence that blood flow or Doppler ultrasonography was of benefit. Nevertheless, limited sample size and inadequate power might be the reasons for not detecting the difference.

Very recently, Muchayi et al conducted a meta-analysis of randomized controlled trials of access surveillance using blood flow monitoring. Their hypothesis was based on the premise that blood flow surveillance lowers the risk of access thrombosis and that the outcome differs between arteriovenous fistulae and grafts. The results revealed a clinically and statistically insignificant benefit for blood flow surveillance: the estimated pooled risk ratio (RR) of access thrombosis was 0.92 (95% confidence limit [CL] = 0.71–1.18). The pooled RR for thrombosis were 0.65 (95% CL = 0.41–1.01) and 1.08 (95% CL = 0.80–1.47) in the fistula and graft subgroups, respectively. Although neither group clearly benefited from surveillance, the tendency for a possible benefit to accrue to the fistula group was surprising.

Although randomized trials have failed to demonstrate the benefit of surveillance, a number of limiting factors continue to surround these studies. The overall quality of these trials was, at best, poor to moderate. All suffered from a small sample size and inadequate power. In addition, the timing of intervention after the detection of access dysfunction was also not appropriately controlled or investigated. In the presence of these factors, one cannot conclusively reject or endorse the use of surveillance. A large, well-designed, multicenter, randomized study with adequate power is needed to conclusively settle the role of surveillance in patients with arteriovenous access. Until then, it is difficult to endorse the routine use of surveillance.

CHAPTER 7

Interventional Nephrology

Gerald A. Beathard, MD, PhD, FASN

Introduction

The dialysis vascular access is simultaneously both the "lifeline" and the "Achilles heel" of the chronic hemodialysis patient. The lifeline because it is the sine qua non for hemodialysis treatments, and the Achilles heel because it is imperfect and frequently associated with recurrent problems. Since the beginnings of hemodialysis, the involvement of nephrologists in dialysis vascular access has been critical, but varied. It has been both active and reactive. After a prolonged period of inactivity during the synthetic graft era, interventional nephrology (IN) began in the mid-1980s as a reaction to the fact that dialysis vascular access problems had come to be major contributors to patient morbidity and mortality and the leading cause of hospitalization in the end-stage renal disease (ESRD) patient population. Unfortunately, nephrologists often found that they were spending more time on the telephone trying to arrange for a surgical appointment than they were solving their patients' problems.

Interventional nephrology first appeared and was stimulated in its development as a reaction to a system that delivered poor medical care—excessive reliance on synthetic grafts, excessive use of catheters, poor vascular access management, fragmented medical care, and delays in medical procedures that compromised patient welfare. This new approach to vascular access began within the private practice sector, and even though academic training programs have appeared, it continues to exist and develop primarily within the private practice sector.

History of Interventional Nephrology

Nephrologists have been intimately involved with the development of the interventional aspects of the specialty from its very beginning (actually prior to its formal recognition as a separate medical specialty). The first hemodialysis shunt, first guidewire-directed percutaneous catheter, first double-lumen catheter, first arteriovenous fistula for hemodialysis, first arteriovenous fistula angiogram, first tunneled catheter for peritoneal dialysis, and first laparoscopically inserted peritoneal dialysis catheter can all be attributed to nephrologists.

The Practice of Interventional Nephrology

In practice, although some would want to broaden the definition, the term *interventional nephrology* has come to be defined as that branch of nephrology which deals with the establishment and maintenance of dialysis access, particularly arteriovenous access. A tabulation of the variety of procedures performed in a typical group of facilities is shown in Fig. 7.1. Most interventional nephrologists work in freestanding

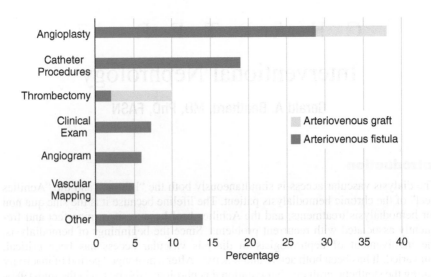

Figure 7.1

Case Distribution for Interventional Nephrology Facility. (Based on 100,000 procedures performed in 75 facilities for the year 2014.)

dialysis access centers (DACs), which carry a CMS place of service code 11 for doctor's office. These centers are generally built to Ambulatory Surgery Center specifications and are specifically designed, equipped, and staffed for the management of dialysis access problems. Many are accredited by the Joint Commission or other accrediting body, and several states require state licensure. Their primary goal is to provide an efficient and economical alternative for managing access dysfunction away from the hospital setting. Their efficiency allows for a patient with a thrombosed vascular access to receive therapy and return to the dialysis clinic within a matter of hours, thus avoiding missed treatments.

As the numbers of nephrologists performing dialysis access procedures and the numbers of procedures performed have increased, the numbers of DACs in operation have also multiplied (Fig. 7.2). The size of these centers varies according to the numbers of dialysis patients in the population served by the DAC (Fig. 7.3). It is of interest that paralleling the development of these types of dialysis access facilities, the dialysis patient hospitalization rate for vascular access problems has markedly decreased (Fig. 7.4).

Training in Interventional Nephrology

As with its development, training in IN has taken place primarily within the private sector. This consisted of training in the management of problems occurring with arteriovenous dialysis access, dialysis access catheters, and peritoneal dialysis catheters. In 2000, the American Society of Diagnostic and Interventional Nephrology (ASDIN) was established, published training guidelines and competency standards, and provided certification for those who met these requirements. ASDIN also developed and administered standards for the accreditation of IN training programs. The

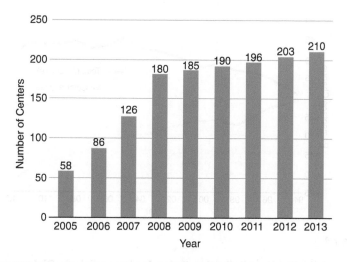

Figure 7.2

Numbers of Interventional Nephrology-Operated Freestanding Dialysis Access Centers in United States for Years 2005–2013.

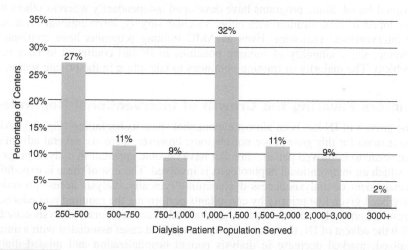

Figure 7.3

Percentage of Dialysis Access Centers According to Sizes of Dialysis Patient Populations Served.

primary obstacles to the development of these programs in academic medical centers (AMCs) have been a lack of qualified faculty and a lack of a dialysis patient population of the size necessary to support an active training program. However, these obstacles have been gradually disappearing.

As AMC training programs have developed, some have used the freestanding DAC model for their training facility whereas others have been completely

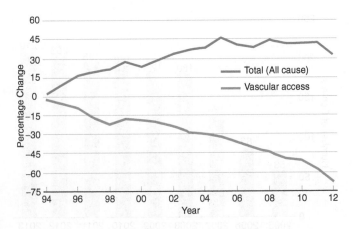

Figure 7.4

Trends in Adjusted Hospitalization Rates for Hemodialysis Dialysis Patient Population for Years 1994–2012. (From USRDS data.)

hospital-based. Some programs have developed independently whereas others have developed in collaboration with either vascular surgery, interventional cardiology, or interventional radiology. Even as AMC training programs have continued to develop, the availability of training positions in IN has continued to be a major problem. The majority of training continues to take place in the private sector.

Factors Favoring the Growth of Interventional Nephrology

The growth of IN has been almost exponential since its beginning (Fig. 7.5). All of the reasons for this growth are not obvious; however, there are several advantages that relate to improved patient care that have become apparent in dialysis programs in which an interventional nephrologist is involved. The first of these is expeditious management of dialysis access dysfunction. Typically, dialysis access procedures have been given low priority by consultants performing the required procedures. As a result, frequently patients require hospitalization and temporary dialysis catheters. With the advent of IN, these have become outpatient cases associated with a quickly realized, marked decrease in dialysis patient hospitalization and missed dialysis treatments.

A second advantage is individualized patient care. The dialysis patient is unique and has unique problems. A variety of issues can materially impact upon and influence decisions related to the patient's dialysis access. It has been suggested that an individual dealing with dialysis access management should possess three characteristics. They should have an understanding of dialysis patients and their problems, they should have in-depth knowledge of evidence-based principles relating to dialysis vascular access, and they should have the necessary procedural skills for the procedures required. The nephrologist trained as an interventionalist can provide the required individualized care and a prospective approach to the planning for future dialysis vascular access.

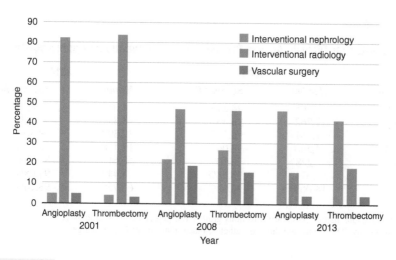

Figure 7.5

Change in Percentage of Dialysis Access Procedures Performed by Interventional Nephrology in Relation to Interventional Radiology and Vascular Surgery Over a 13-Year Period From 2001 to 2013.

An additional advantage relates to the opportunity for research and innovation that is offered by involvement in the management of the dialysis patient's vascular access. The NKF KDOQI Vascular Access Guidelines published in 2006 made it obvious that many of the recommended tenets of vascular access management are opinion based. They proposed questions to serve as a "stimulus to the nephrology community to begin to ask better questions regarding vascular access with a goal of better outcomes for our patients." Problems with dialysis vascular access contribute significantly to patient morbidity and mortality. This problem is of obvious paramount importance to the nephrologist providing care to these patients. The nephrologist who is well versed in the basic principles of dialysis vascular access and has the ability to manage these problems independently is in an advantageous position to conduct meaningful research and innovation in this area.

Quality of Care Provided by Interventional Nephrologists

Quality of medical care is of paramount importance regardless of the clinical problem. Early in the development of IN, concern was voiced by members of other specialties involved in the management of dialysis vascular access problems that treatment by a nephrologist would result in adverse outcomes. However, this concern has been dispelled by the publication of data to support both efficacy and safety of interventional procedures in the hands of trained nephrologists.

In a retrospective cohort study of 14,067 cases performed by 29 interventional nephrologists working in 11 freestanding DACs, a 96.18% clinical success rate was recorded. This study was based on prospectively collected data maintained in an electronic medical record and included six different procedures related to dialysis

Table 7.1

Success Rates for Dialysis Access Procedures for Interventional Nephrologists

	2004		2014	
Procedure	*Number*	*Success Rate*	*Number*	*Success Rate*
TDC-Place	1,765	98.24%	4,038	97.89%
TDC-Ex	2,262	98.36%	8,851	99.29%
AVF-PTA	1,561	96.58%	32,392	99.40%
AVG-PTA	3,560	98.06%	12,418	99.56%
AVF-T	228	78.10%	2,613	87.94%
AVF-T	4,671	93.08%	8,447	94.08%
Combined	14,067	96.18%	68,759	98.24%

AVF, arteriovenous fistula; AVG, arteriovenous graft; PTA, percutaneous angioplasty;
T, thrombectomy; TDC, tunneled dialysis catheter; Place, placement; Ex, exchange.

vascular access management. The clinical success rate and size for each of these individual procedures were tabulated separately and are shown in Table 7.1.

The data shown in Table 7.1 are reflective of the vascular access profile of dialysis patients in the period preceding 2004. With the advent of Fistula First, this profile has made a major shift toward arteriovenous fistulas with fewer catheters as reflected in Fig. 7.1. Although the number of published studies available for comparison with this report was somewhat limited, the success rate for these cases was equal or superior to the results that were available at that time.

Table 7.1 also shows data for 2014 from this same DAC group, expanded in number from 11 to 75 facilities. Over this 10-year span of time, the success rate for all procedures continued to be high. It is obvious that a shift from AVG to AVF use occurred during this period. Additionally, the success of dealing with AVF thrombosis improved by 10%.

Safety of Care Provided by Interventional Nephrologists

In addition to quality, the safety of the medical care provided is also of extreme importance. Dialysis patients represent a high-risk group for any type of interventional procedure. Published reviews of serious complications encountered in association with procedures performed by interventional radiologists have shown that hemodialysis access management procedures carried a greater risk than other interventional vascular procedures that are primarily arterial. There are three areas of concern related to the safety of interventional procedures: the incidence of procedure-related complications, complications related to sedation/analgesia used in association with the procedure being performed, and the risk of radiation injury related to the use of fluoroscopy in performing the procedures.

Procedure-Related Complications

As with any type of medical procedure, interventional treatment of dialysis vascular access dysfunction can result in procedure-related complications (PRCs). In general, a PRC for any given procedure is an adverse event that can be expected to occur.

The important issue is the rate at which it is observed. A background occurrence rate is to be expected; however, the rate should not exceed an acceptable norm. An excessive complication rate suggests the need for critical evaluation. The expertise and skill of the operator are major determinants of excessive PRCs.

In the cohort study of 14,067 cases discussed above, complications were classified according to the Society of Interventional Radiology (SIR) complication classification system. According to this system, complications are classified as none, minor, or major. In a general sense, minor complications are those that have no permanent sequelae and require no specific therapy. Major complications are those that require a change in medical management or have permanent sequelae. Complication rate thresholds have also been established. In this series of patients, the PRC rates (Table 7.2) were below the SIR thresholds and were less than those previously published from seller, but smaller studies. Table 7.2 also shows data for 2014 from this same DAC group, expanded in number from 11 to 75 facilities. In addition to reflecting the changes brought about by evolving from primarily synthetic grafts to primarily arteriovenous fistulas, the PRC rates are even lower, especially for arteriovenous thrombectomies.

In a more recent report, a review of serious complications occurring in a cohort of 84,669 hemodialysis access procedures performed by interventional nephrologists in freestanding DACs was presented. Serious complications were characterized as either a medical emergency (ME) or a cardiopulmonary arrest (CPA). For the purposes of this report an ME was defined as any change in cardiovascular status or mentation that required that the patient receive a higher-than-planned level of care, including, but not limited to, transfer to the hospital. A CPA was defined as a state of cardiac or pulmonary activity that required initiation of an advanced cardiac life support protocol or attempted intubation. Prospectively collected data revealed that the procedure success rate for this cohort was 98.5%. The patients treated in this series (IN group) were representative of the dialysis population at large. Although they were treated in freestanding outpatient facilities, patients were not selected on the basis of complexity or comorbidities. Patients who were transferred to the hospital at the time of evaluation before the procedure, not related to an ME or CPA, represented <0.1% of all encounters.

Table 7.2

Complication Rates for Dialysis Access Procedures for Interventional Nephrologists

Procedure	2004			2014		
	Number	Minor	Major	Number	Minor	Major
TDC-Place	1,765	1.36%	0.06%	4,038	0.42%	0.15%
TDC-Ex	2,262	1.37%	0.04%	8,851	0.19%	0.15%
AVF-PTA	1,561	4.29%	0.19%	32,392	1.24%	0.08%
AVG-PTA	3,560	1.04%	0.11%	12,418	0.64%	0.07%
AVF-T	228	6.07%	0.44%	2,613	4.13%	0.92%
AVF-T	4,671	5.99%	0.26	8,447	2.13%	0.41%
Combined	14,067	3.26%	0.28%	68,759	1.17%	0.16%

AVF, arteriovenous fistula; AVG, arteriovenous graft; PTA, percutaneous angioplasty; T, thrombectomy; TDC, tunneled dialysis catheter; Place, placement; Ex, exchange.

Table 7.3

Comparison of Dialysis Access–Related Procedure Complications

	AV Access Procedures							
	Thrombectomy		Angio/PTA		Total		Catheter	
	IR	IN	IR	IN	IR	IN	IR	IN
N	393	11,789	1,258	50,300	1,651	62,089	2,088	22,580
CPA	0.51%	0.102%	0.08%	0.016%	0.18%	0.031%	0.29%	0.013%
ME	0.76%	0.407%	0.32%	0.095%	0.42%	0.155%	0.24%	0.075%
All	1.27%	0.509%	0.40%	0.111%	0.61%	0.187%	0.53%	0.088%

AV, arteriovenous; IR, interventional radiology; IN, interventional nephrology; Angio/PTA, combined angiogram and angioplasty groups.

The incidence of serious complications as defined was compared with that from an Interventional Radiology report that was concurrently published. This was from a hospital-based program and included data on 38,927 procedures, 4132 of which were dialysis access related (IR group). A combined frequency of 0.61% for ME and CPA for arteriovenous access interventions (angioplasty and thrombectomy) was reported in this IR group (Table 7.3), whereas IN group data showed a frequency of 0.187%. The IR group had a rate of 0.53% for ME and CPA for dialysis catheter procedures whereas the IN group showed a rate of 0.088%.

Sedation/Analgesia-Related Complications

Pain management through effective sedation/analgesia (S/A) is important in the performance of dialysis access maintenance procedures. However, this aspect of management carries with it a degree of risk, especially considering the ages and comorbidities of the dialysis patient population. The question arises as to whether a nephrologist who is not specialty trained in anesthesia can administer S/A safely in this setting. To answer this question, data derived from a cohort of 12,896 hemodialysis patients undergoing dialysis access maintenance procedures performed by interventional nephrologists were analyzed to determine the safety of S/A drug administration in a freestanding DAC.

In this study, all medications were administered by the nephrologist performing the procedure who had specific training in S/A. Intravenous midazolam, fentanyl, or a combination of both were used. The S/A goal was moderate sedation as defined in all patients. All drug dosages were individualized and administered in small, incremental doses that were titrated to the patient's response. Doses were adjusted to account for patient size, age, and comorbidities at the physician's discretion.

A preprocedure evaluation was performed in all patients, and all patients were monitored during the procedure by a critical care nurse using continuous assessment of oxygen saturation, blood pressure, cardiac rhythm, pulse rate, and ventilation. All adverse events that were observed were recorded as complications. However, special attention was paid to complications that were felt to be directly related to the medications used for S/A. These were hypotension (persistent, requiring nominal or higher level therapy), a drop in oxygen saturation below 90% (persistent, lasting for more than 20 seconds), and apnea (absence of respiratory activity lasting for more

Table 7.4				

Complications Related to Sedation/Analgesia

Group	Number	Minor	Major	S/A Related
High Risk	5,415 (42%)	181 (1.40%)	57 (0.44%)	11 (0.085%)
Lower Risk	7,481 (48%)	123 (0.96%)	10 (0.08%)	6 (0.046%)
Total	12,896	304 (2.36%)	67 (0.52%)	17 (0.131%)

S/A, sedation/analgesia.

than 20 seconds). Oxygen via a nasal cannula was routinely used on all patients during the procedure.

All dialysis patients are considered to be at higher risk than normal for these types of procedures; however, within the cohort, an especially High Risk group was identified. This consisted of individuals who met one or more of the following criteria: age ≥80 years, symptomatic shortness of breath, airway problems, requiring oxygen to maintain an oxygen saturation ≥90%, or American Society of Anesthesiology Physical Status classification of 4 or greater. The remainder of the cases were grouped together as the Lower Risk group (all dialysis patients are at increased risk).

The total (all types) complication rate in this cohort of patients was 2.9%, 2.4% of which were minor complications. Complications felt to be directly related to S/A were 0.13% (17 cases). Two-thirds of these occurred in the High Risk group (Table 7.4). Two deaths occurred, but at a time remote from the procedure and not felt to be a related procedure (the duration of the complication-monitoring period is 30 days). The conclusion of this study was that S/A administered for these types of procedures by interventional nephrologists is a safe procedure even in very high-risk patients.

Radiation-Related Complications

Interventional procedures performed for dialysis vascular access management requires the use of fluoroscopy. Any time radiologic equipment is used by a nonradiologist, there are legitimate concerns about radiation exposure to the patient and health care team. The effects of radiation are cumulative. Most dialysis patients require repetitive procedures that are generally fluoroscopy guided. Most interventional nephrologists and the staff of the DAC spend a major portion of their work time in the procedure room and anticipate doing so for a number of years. Therefore, radiation safety must be of concern.

To analyze this issue as it relates to the interventional nephrologist, a study was conducted to assess the levels of radiation dosage involved with these procedures. Dosimetry information including dose–area product (DAP), reference point air kerma (RPAK), and fluoroscopy time (FT) was collected prospectively. Radiation dosage data were collected from 24 centers in various parts of the United States and reflected cases managed by 69 different interventional nephrologists. The data were tabulated separately for eight procedures: fistula angioplasty and thrombectomy, graft angioplasty and thrombectomy, tunneled catheter placement and exchange, vein mapping, and cases in which only angiographic evaluation was performed. The numbers of cases involved for each of these varied. The results are shown in Table

Table 7.5

Radiation Dosages for Procedures Performed by Interventional Nephrologists

Metric		AVF-PTA	AVF-T	AVG-PTA	AVG-T	Angio	Cath-Place	Cath Ex	Map
FT	Geo. Mean	54.3	90	47.7	88.3	30	24.8	22	50
(seconds)	N	6,126	513	2,876	2,098	1,808	810	2,043	978
RPAK	Geo. Mean	2.12	4.60	2.14	5.35	1.08	0.69	1.08	2.02
(mGy)	N	168	24	126	40	36	44	78	46
DAP	Geo. Mean	0.741	0.873	0.798	0.903	0.590	0.832	0.892	1.142
(Gy*cm^2)	N	6,128	513	2,876	2,098	1,808	810	2,043	978

FT, fluoroscopy time; RPAK, reference point air kerma; DAP, dose–area product; Geo. Mean, geometric mean; n, number of cases in group; AVF, arteriovenous fistula; AVG, arteriovenous graft; PTA, percutaneous angioplasty; T, thrombectomy; Angio, angiogram; Cath, tunneled dialysis catheter; Place, placement; Ex, exchange; Map, vein mapping.

7.5 as the number of cases reviewed for each procedure and each metric and the geometric mean (the distribution was non-Gaussian) for the group.

Biologic effects resulting from radiation exposure are traditionally divided into stochastic effects (primarily cancer induction) and deterministic effects (primarily skin injury). The radiation dose metric used to assess stochastic risk is DAP. Assuming a normal life expectancy, it has been estimated that this risk of experiencing a fatal malignancy is increased 0.5% for each 100 mGy of effective dose of x-ray radiation. The DAP values listed in Table 7.5 are in mGy*cm^2 (radiation dose in milligray multiplied by area exposed in centimeters squared). It is not possible to convert this information directly into effective dose of radiation; however, the values listed represent a minuscule stochastic risk.

Deterministic effects are characterized by a threshold dose below which they do not occur. In much the same way as sunburn resulting from sun exposure, deterministic effects do not occur until the dose threshold is reached and then their severity increases from that point on. The threshold for the earliest skin changes, erythema, has been established at 2 Gy. The radiation dose metric used to assess deterministic risk is RPAK. The RPAK values listed in Table 7.5 are in milligray, with the highest value for any of the eight procedures being 6.4 mGy for AVG thrombectomy. At this level, it would require more than 300 procedures to produce skin erythema, provided that the fluoroscopy machine was not moved at any time during the procedures.

Very little has been published in the literature concerning radiation dosage associated with dialysis vascular access maintenance procedures. Comparisons with the studies that are available are published by radiologists working in a hospital setting. These show a 3- to 8-fold greater radiation dose than in this study. It should be recognized that some of the decrease in dosage is related to the fact that interventional nephrologists working in DAC use a mobile C-arm whereas those in a hospital setting generally use a fixed C-arm fluoroscopy unit. The dose levels are considerably lower with a mobile C-arm because of the way it operates.

Clinical Value of Interventional Nephrology

The vascular access of a dialysis patient is prone to recurrent problems. It is important that these problems be managed effectively, efficiently, and timely. Not infrequently, there is an emergent situation that requires an emergent solution, defined as the absence of a functioning access for hemodialysis in a patient requiring emergent hemodialysis. The goal of dialysis access management should be to avoid missed dialysis treatments and avoid hospitalization. The effectiveness and safety issues discussed above speak to the clinical value of interventional nephrology; however, there are also published reports that address the overall value of an interventional nephrology program working in a freestanding DAC.

Using retrospective data, a study was conducted to compare hospitalization and missed dialysis treatment rates between two patient populations—a test group consisting of a cohort of approximately 6000 patients receiving dialysis access management at an interventional nephrology operated facility and a control group consisting of a national cohort of approximately 290,000 patients. This study looked at a period of 7 years. Interventional nephrology involvement was initiated during the fourth year, allowing for a comparison of data within the test group representing a period before and after the initiation of interventional nephrology involvement. During the first 3 years of the study period, there was no significant difference between the test and control groups. However, with the initiation of interventional nephrology in the test group, both metrics, hospitalization and missed dialysis treatment rates, declined markedly. By the end of the study period, hospitalization days per patient-year decreased 57% in the test group and missed dialysis treatments per patient-year decreased 29% in comparison with the control group ($p = .01$).

The clinical value of interventional nephrology nephrologist working in a DAC was further demonstrated by a prospective study designed to evaluate the efficiency and outcomes of emergent hemodialysis access procedures over a 3-month period in a high-volume facility. A total of 157 emergent procedures were performed during the period of the study. The procedure was successful in 95% of the cases, with 90% being completed within 24 hours of referral. Dialysis treatment was performed within 24 hours in 61% of the cases and within 48 hours in an additional 29%.

To evaluate the overall clinical effect of a DAC, Medicare claims data were collected representing incident and prevalent ESRD patients who received at least 80% of their dialysis vascular access managenment at either a DAC or a hospital outpatient department (HOPD) over a 4-year period. Using propensity score–matching techniques, cases with a similar clinical and demographic profile from these two sites of service were matched according to 47 different variables. Medicare utilization, payments, and patient outcomes were compared across the matched cohorts. This created a DAC group (n = 27,613) and a HOPD group (n = 27,613) for comparisons. Patients treated in the DAC (Fig. 7.6) had significantly better clinical outcomes ($p < .001$). This included fewer vascular access–related infections (0.18 vs 0.29) and fewer septicemia-related hospitalizations (0.15 vs 0.18). Mortality rate was lower (47.9% vs 53.5%).

Although this study was not able to make direct evaluations based on medical specialty, the data did indicate that interventional nephrologists were more likely and interventional radiologists were less likely to be providing the majority of the patients dialysis vascular access–related care in the DAC than in an HOPD.

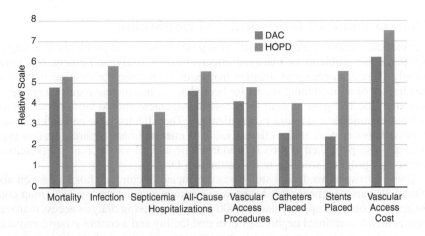

Figure 7.6

Clinical Value and Economy of DACs. Scale is relative, see text for actual values; for all values $p \leq .01$.

Economic Value of Interventional Nephrology

The Medicare claims data-based study listed above also examined the economic value of a freestanding DAC (Fig. 7.6). This study showed that matched patients treated in the DAC had fewer dialysis vascular access procedures than those treated in the HOPD (20.5 vs 23.9, $p = < .01$), less all-cause hospital admissions (2.3 vs 2.8, $p < .001$), fewer catheters placed (1.3 vs 2.0, $p < .001$), and fewer stents placed (0.6 vs 1.4, $p < .001$) despite having longer episodes and lower mortality rates.

Matched patients who received their care in a freestanding DAC had an average Medicare per member per month (PMPM) payment for dialysis vascular access services that was \$626 lower than those who received care in the HOPD (\$3162 vs \$3788, $CI = -\$736, -\$516; p < .001$). This represented a savings of \$7012 per patient per year or almost \$200 million per year for the total cohort of 27,613 patients studied.

Summary

Over the course of the past 20 years, Interventional Nephrology has developed as a subspecialty of nephrology specializing in the management of dialysis vascular access problems. Working primarily in freestanding, dedicated dialysis access facilities, interventional nephrologists have demonstrated an ability to provide effective, safe, and economical interventional vascular access management care to the dialysis patient population whom they serve. Interventional Nephrology has grown to the point that today it is providing the majority of these essential medical services.

CHAPTER 8

Cannulation of Hemodialysis Vascular Access: Science and Art

Lesley C. Dinwiddie, MSN, RN, FNP, CNNe • Janet E. Holland, RN, CNN

The objective and subjective quality of a hemodialysis treatment using a subcutaneous vascular access can be highly variable based on the cannulation experience. This is increasingly evident as practitioners, with the urging of the Centers for Medicare and Medicare Services, strive to attain an arteriovenous fistula (AVF) access rate of greater than 60%—the undisputed gold standard for vascular access worldwide. There are many explanations for the disparate data regarding achieving and maintaining functional AVFs in the United States, but one that causes a great deal of frustration for practitioners and patients alike is failure to effectively cannulate the outflow vein on a consistent basis. This chapter provides practical and actionable information on cannulation to increase the functionality of AVFs while reducing the number of cannulation errors in both AVFs and arteriovenous grafts (AVGs).

The entire vascular access team is responsible, through the continuous quality improvement (CQI) process, for all vascular access outcomes (including those related to cannulation). The seminal act of piercing the skin and threading the needle, usually performed by nurses and patient care technicians under their supervision, is but one step in the cannulation process. All members of the collaborative team must understand this entire procedure.

Steps of the Cannulation Process

Assessment

The predialysis subcutaneous vascular access assessment is both holistic and focused. Flow through the access vessel is the product of cardiac output and mean arterial pressure that will be affected by local anatomic variables such as vessel size, collaterals, stenoses, and aneurysms. If vital signs are normal for the patient, the cannulator asks about changes in the access and inspects the access limb for absence of swelling and the skin over the vessel for integrity, checks for the absence of inflammation, and assesses changes in aneurysms, if present. After inspecting and comparing the access extremity with the nonaccess extremity proximal to distal for color, swelling, and normal movement, the cannulator should then feel both extremities for temperature and palpate distal pulses.

Next, the cannulator feels for the access flow's thrill and notes the vibratory versus pulsation character. The cannulator then listens with a clean stethoscope over the entire length of the cannulated portion of the AVF or AVG for confirmation of flow (ie, the bruit) and for evidence of stenosis characterized by a change in amplitude and pitch. Absence of a thrill and bruit should be reported immediately.

Cannulating to assess for flow is unacceptable and can complicate interventions to lyse thrombus and restore flow.

Once the assessment of flow is complete, the cannulator identifies recent cannulation sites and asks the patient about those cannulation experiences (both positive and negative). If the patient does not have established buttonholes, the cannulator chooses the sites for both the arterial (afferent to the extracorporeal circuit) and venous (efferent) needles. Any area of skin break, with or without exudate, or inflammation must be reported to the nephrologist or advanced practice nurse (APN) prior to cannulation. Site choice involves decision making with regard to rotation of sites, avoidance of stenoses, aneurysms, and pseudoaneurysms, and proximity to anastomoses. Site of entry *and* site of needle tip postcannulation must be considered to ensure successful placement. Accesses bend; steel needles don't.

Needles, both cutting bevel for new sites and noncutting for buttonhole use, currently come in 0.6-, 1-, and 1.25-inch lengths and in sizes from 14- to 17-gauge. The arterial needle can be placed either retrograde or antegrade. Retrograde placement of the arterial needle should not position the needle tip in or near the anastomosis. Similarly, the tip for the venous needle (always antegrade) in an AVG placement should not be close to the anastomosis. Recent research at the University of Alabama shows that outflow from the venous needle significantly increases turbulence downstream, which might promote graft pathology such as neointimal hyperplasia.

Another consideration is needle placement to avoid recirculation. Cannulation lore holds that needle tips should be approximately 2 inches apart to prevent recirculation. This rule is somewhat arbitrary because recirculation is related to access flow rates in which the extracorporeal flow exceeds intra-access flow. However, in accesses where flow is less than 600 mL/min the greater the distance between needle tips the less risk there is of recirculation.

For the recently created fistula, the assessment is geared toward maturation following the Rule of 6s as stated in the NKF-K/DOQI guidelines (see Table 8.1). This is a hypothetical construct to assist in maturation assessment. Experienced nurses have been shown to correctly predict maturation suitable for cannulation through physical assessment 80% of the time. Whereas DOPPS (Dialysis Outcomes and Practical Pattern Study) data have shown that cannulation can be performed successfully at 4 weeks, the revised NKF-K/DOQI guidelines continue to advise longer maturation times of 6–8 weeks and early professional assessment. This conservative stance is supported by recent evidence that the two significant variables that lead to

Table 8.1

Rule of 6s for AVF Maturation

- The AVF should be expertly assessed within 6 weeks of creation for maturation.
- Flow through the vessel should exceed 600 mL/min.
- The vessel should be greater than 6 mm in diameter.
- The vessel should be less than 6 mm from the skin surface.

AVF, arteriovenous fistula.

a major fistula infiltration are advanced patient age and AVF age of less than 6 months.

Additional assessment is required to determine direction of flow. Normal fistula outflow is anatomically proximal to the central circulation, but exceptions do exist (surgically and by default) regarding retrograde flow through collateral vessel(s) when the intended outflow vein is occluded. If any doubt exists regarding the vascular anatomy, ultrasound mapping should be obtained before the first cannulation. Ultrasound can also measure the thickness of the vessel wall to determine if there is sufficient strength for cannulation (ie, maturation).

Cannulation readiness of an AVG is determined not only by the type of graft material but by the condition of the extremity. Generally, the synthetic polytetrafluoroethylene (PTFE) can be cannulated in 14 days or less according to manufacturers' directions. However, healing, swelling, and pain in the extremity take precedence in the decision to cannulate if a functional catheter is available for access. If these symptoms do not subside within 4–6 weeks postoperatively, an outflow obstruction may exist that requires intervention prior to cannulation. Biologic grafts, hybrids of the anatomic features of outflow veins, and PTFE must be assessed accordingly. The assessment method is the same as for any AVG, but the cannulation technique for a biologic graft is more like that for a native vein.

Skin and Patient Preparation

Washing of the patient's hands and access site upon entry to the dialysis unit should be mandatory. Following the assessment, the skin over the chosen sites is cleansed with agents per facility protocol—using strict aseptic technique. With the buttonhole technique, the skin is cleaned after stretching the skin away from the buttonhole and/ or soaking with a bactericidal solution to loosen the scab. The scab over the entry site is removed with a sterile piece of gauze or a sterile instrument (never the tip of the cannulating needle); hand hygiene and glove changes are performed prior to a second skin cleaning. For all AVF cannulation, regardless of vessel size, a tourniquet is placed proximal to the chosen cannulation sites—sufficient to engorge the vein without occluding flow. The tourniquet not only helps stabilize the vessel but increases the surface tension of the skin—promoting smoother needle entry. Hand hygiene and glove changes are performed between skin preparation and cannulation.

Cannulation frequently causes the patient anxiety—anticipating both the pain of needle entry and the uncertainty of successful placement. Preparing the patient requires professional reassurance of the cannulator's ability as well as ascertaining the need for local anesthetic. A relaxed and confident patient is easier to cannulate with less pain. Patients who routinely need local anesthetic should be prescribed, and self-administer, a cream containing lidocaine that numbs the skin. Alternatively, vapocoolant spray or intradermal lidocaine injection can be offered on a limited basis. Local anesthetic should be offered until the patient develops enough trust and scar tissue to safely discontinue it.

An important variable for successful cannulation is patience. The cannulator must take the necessary time to properly set up, assess the patient, prepare skin over the access, and establish confidence. As a patient once asked, "How is it that they have enough time to stick me two or three times when they miss but never enough time to do it right the first time?"

Cannulation

Specific techniques for both rope ladder—a pattern of site rotation that alternates needle sites from recent punctures (steps) while maintaining an effective distance between tips—and buttonhole cannulation are described in the revised NKF-K/DOQI guidelines.

"Rope ladder" cannulation technique was developed to ensure consistent cannulation needle site rotation to prevent aneurysm formation secondary to weakening of the vessel wall by repeated cannulation in a small area of the AVF or AVG. When performing rope ladder cannulation, anatomic assessment indicates the appropriate angle of needle entry. The texture of the vessel dictates the degree of force required to penetrate the entry wall while avoiding perforation of the back wall. It is generally thought that AVF cannulation requires a shallower angle of entry than that required for a PTFE graft. When vessel entry is confirmed by the flashback of blood, the cannulator pauses to prevent back wall damage and reorients the needle to follow the angle of the vessel in order to successfully thread the needle in the center of access flow. Needles do not need to be rotated 180 degrees (flipped) because an arterial needle with a hole in the back of its bevel (a back-eye) is a feature that allows optimal flow of blood into the needle. The venous needle does not require this feature.

The introduction of the buttonhole technique by Twardowski was greeted with much skepticism because it appeared to be directly contradictory to the preferred method of rotation of cannulation sites. Twardowski stated that in addition to maintaining the integrity of the vein wall cannulation with the buttonhole or constant-site technique was less painful—in addition to being quick and easy. He added that this method also virtually eliminates infiltrations and reneedling and the infection rate was not significantly higher than multisite cannulation. Marticorena et al. demonstrated the salvaging of function in aneurysmal AVFs using the buttonhole technique. However, recent literature indicates increased risks of bloodstream and local access site infections, lack of AVF survival benefits, no decrease in interventions, nor improved patient quality of life. MacRae et al. (2014) concluded: "AVFs with buttonhole needling did not have improved survival. The lack of survival benefit and higher risk of infection should be noted when promoting buttonhole needling." Wong et al. (2014) reviewed "1,044 identified citations, 23 studies were selected for inclusion … no difference in cannulation pain was found among randomized controlled trials … Buttonhole, as compared to rope-ladder, technique appeared to be associated with increased risk of local and systemic infections. Conclusions: Evidence does not support the preferential use of buttonhole over rope-ladder cannulation."

Buttonhole, also known as "Constant Site" cannulation, may be prescribed for the patient who has an AVF, but the outflow vein has limited cannulation sites. This method involves repeated cannulation into the exact same puncture site allowing a scar tissue tunnel tract to develop. The scar tissue tunnel tract allows the needle to pass through to the (outflow) vessel of the fistula following the same path each time.

Each patient may have two established sets of buttonholes, if possible, created by two different expert cannulators. After at least six sharp entries to establish each buttonhole, the cannulator can then switch to "dull" needles for all future cannulations. (Ball has reported that 6 is not enough and the number required can range anywhere from 8 to 12, with fewer for nondiabetic and more for diabetic.)

The technique needed to find the vein through the tunnel with a dull needle requires needle insertion into the buttonhole, using a twisting motion if necessary to approach the vein. It feels like the tip is bouncing on the vein wall. The cannulator should go 20 degrees forward or back until the needle "drops" into the vein. "When the cannulator goes by feel (not sight) you know they've 'got it.'"

Toma et al. (2003) confirmed this experience by noting that the angle of the scar tract changed over time, with the entry into the vein becoming more proximal. This Japanese group also developed a sterile peg device for holding the tunnel open interdialytically for the first 2 weeks to speed up the buttonhole development process. Other methods of forming the tunnel/track by leaving an object (e.g., an angiocath in situ) have been demonstrated to be successful. However no device has been approved for this use in the United States and the adverse event experienced in Canada with the angiocath method should inspire caution around using any unapproved innovation.

Needle Taping and Initiating Dialysis

Securing the needles to prevent dislodgement while maintaining easy flow is a necessary art. Usually a 1-inch-wide tape across the wings of the needle to anchor and a $\frac{1}{2}$-inch tape chevroned behind and across the wings is sufficient. It is important to be able to see the needle entry site for both needles throughout the dialysis procedure to be able to detect dislodgement or bleeding. Once both needles are secured, the loading dose of heparin can be given and the needles attached to the extracorporeal circuit. The cannulator should set the pump speed to no more than 200 mL/min and observe both of the needles, the prepump arterial pressure, and the venous pressure while filling the extracorporeal circuit with blood. Ascertaining the patient's comfort and confirming appropriate vital signs precede increasing blood flow to the prescribed level.

Needle Removal

All supplies necessary should be assembled before needle removal. Gentle removal of the tape precedes placing a hemostasis dressing over the needle entry site and the vessel entry site.

The caregiver then gets control of the needle and safety device. The needle should be withdrawn at the same angle it was inserted. Pressure is applied to both the skin and vessel entry site *only* when the needle is *all* of the way out. To do otherwise causes pain and can damage the vessel or buttonhole tunnel. The needle safety device is deployed and both needles are disposed of into a sharps container.

Removing one needle and having the patient hold pressure over the cannulation site is optimal. After hemostasis is achieved, the other needle is similarly removed. However, many elderly or disabled patients are unable to hold their sites. Spring-loaded clamps can be placed over the cannulation sites in those patients, but staff must be vigilant in checking the patient and the clamps frequently and removing them as soon as bleeding from the sites stops. The dressing used for post–needle removal bleeding is removed, the site is checked for hemostasis and a dry, sterile dressing of an adhesive bandage and gauze is applied for discharge. Tape is not applied circumferentially or pulled tightly across the access.

Patients and their families should be instructed to remove the gauze upon arriving home, and to remove the adhesive bandage the next morning. Additional instruction on achieving hemostasis, should bleeding recur, is also necessary.

Postdialysis Assessment

Postdialysis assessment should mirror the predialysis assessment for patency and access condition, noting any significant changes from the predialysis assessment. Specifically, the access should be observed for the presence of hematoma or pain, for length of time to hemostasis, and for character of the thrill and bruit.

Special Considerations in Cannulation
Initial Cannulations

Initial cannulations must be performed by the most skilled cannulators. Some cannulators' practice is to cannulate a new fistula, when the patient has a functioning catheter in place, using one 17-gauge needle for the arterial (or "pull") side, with return of dialyzed blood to the venous circulation through the catheter. This is sometimes referred to as the "one-and-one" method.

Attention needs to be directed to the use of heparin in the one-and-one circumstance. A lesser quantity for the loading bolus should be considered, as well as making sure that no heparin is given during the last hour of dialysis.

The lumen of the catheter not used for dialysis must be flushed and locked early in each treatment minimizing the amount of freshly circulating concentrated heparin at the end of dialysis. Progressing to using two needles and increasing needle gauge is prescribed by the physician based on the success of cannulations and the confidence of the patient.

If an infiltration occurs, subcutaneous bleeding should be quickly controlled and a "cold-pack" applied to the site. The access should not be recannulated until all pain and swelling is resolved. The next attempt to cannulate must be by a very experienced practitioner.

With regard to initial cannulation of a new AVG, general assessment is as previously described. To confirm direction of flow, especially with a forearm loop configuration, the surgical note should be consulted for the surgically altered anatomy. Assessment to confirm direction of flow of any access can be achieved by gently compressing at the mid-access and both listening and feeling for flow dynamics on either side with a pressure increase proximally (arterial) and decrease distally (venous).

Once healed, a new AVG may be cannulated with both arterial and venous needles of the standard size as prescribed. A PTFE graft has optimal flow and size when new and does not require the stepwise process commonly employed for patients with catheters and new AVFs.

Who Is the Cannulator?

Venotomy is a basic nursing skill, perfected by experience. However, many staff placing needles in the dialysis unit have limited experience in venotomy when hired to perform patient care in the dialysis unit. Training is "on the job" and the quality of that training is commensurate with the commitment and skill of the trainer. Ideally, all trainees should be subjected to a curriculum that involves detailed anatomy and physiology of the cardiovascular system in order to properly appreciate assessment of the access. Cannulation training tools such as a "training arm" should be used to familiarize the trainee with the feel of the needles as well as the movements necessary to successfully enter the vessel and thread the needle into position. Observing cannulation performed by more experienced staff can inform about technique as well as details of the procedure.

Matching the experience of the cannulator to the degree of difficulty ascribed to the access is also very important. Only those staff members considered expert cannulators should be assigned to cannulate new AVFs and AVGs, as well as accesses that continue to present cannulation challenges. Newly hired staff must complete competency testing prior to cannulating, even when they claim appropriate experience.

Self-Cannulation

Many patients are capable of cannulating themselves if the vessel is easily accessible. The benefits of self-cannulation are several, but primary is the increased control it gives the patient over the quality of his therapy. This method also reduces staff time requirements and cannulation errors. New patients should be assessed for the ability to self-cannulate, and strongly encouraged to do so if that assessment is positive. Buttonhole cannulation by its very nature lends itself as the technique of choice for the self-cannulator.

Summary

Cannulation of the hemodialysis vascular access is more an art than a science. Many current practices of cannulation need to be scientifically tested, and innovative techniques that will make cannulation easier must be researched for patient safety and satisfaction. Until proven otherwise, rope ladder cannulation, also known as "site rotation," is the preferred cannulation method as the buttonhole technique has not shown the benefits of pain-free, simplified cannulation in the AVF access. The risks for infection with the established tunnel to the bloodstream must not be minimized— and the learning curve for the staff to establish the buttonholes correctly remains quite steep.

The vascular access team must keep in mind that although the push is to create AVFs, its challenge is to maintain them. The patient-centered CQI process is essential in ensuring appropriate assessment and expert cannulation.

SECTION III

Peritoneal Access Devices

CHAPTER 9

Peritoneal Access Devices, Placement Techniques, and Maintenance

John H. Crabtree, MD, FACS

A functional and durable access to the peritoneal cavity is prerequisite to the success of peritoneal dialysis (PD) as renal replacement therapy. In the present era, access is obtained with a catheter device that bridges the abdominal wall to provide a cutaneoperitoneal fistula through which dialysis solutions can be exchanged. The two most common reasons for PD failure are infectious and mechanical complications of the access device. Knowledge of best practices in catheter placement and maintenance can minimize the risk of these complications and optimize the likelihood for successful therapy. To serve as a practical resource for the management of the adult renal failure patient, this chapter will focus on current practices, describing the most commonly used catheter types, procedures for matching the most appropriate device to the patient, placement methods, break-in procedures, and catheter care and maintenance. Investigational PD devices and techniques are not discussed. Pediatric dialysis is covered in Section 30.

Selection of catheter devices and insertion techniques often vary depending on whether the access is needed for acute or chronic PD therapy, geographic availability of material resources, and local provider expertise in placing catheters.

Acute Catheters

Acute PD access can be obtained with either rigid noncuffed catheters or soft cuffed catheters.

Rigid Noncuffed Catheters

Although the use of rigid noncuffed catheters has ceased in North America, their use continues in many parts of the world. These devices are composed of semirigid plastic in straight or slightly curved configurations with numerous side holes in the intraperitoneal segment. The rigid acute catheter is inserted by percutaneous puncture using an internal stylet. Typically, a 1-cm midline or paramedian skin incision is made approximately 2.5 cm below the level of the umbilicus. A hemostat clamp is used to spread down to the fascia. The stylet is inserted into the catheter until the pointed tip is exposed. With the patient tensing the abdominal musculature, the catheter-stylet assembly is advanced through the musculofascial layer with a twisting motion under constant controlled pressure until a sudden drop in resistance is sensed, indicating entry into the peritoneal cavity. The patient is allowed to relax the abdominal muscles. Holding the catheter in place, the stylet is withdrawn several centimeters to hide the pointed end. The catheter is gently advanced toward the pelvis without moving the stylet until satisfactory depth has been achieved. The stylet is removed and the administration set is attached to the catheter. The catheter is secured to the skin with a suture or catheter holder. Alternatively, the abdomen may be pre-filled with 1–2 L of dialysis solution before inserting the catheter-stylet. A 16–18-gauge intravenous cannula or a Veress needle (spring-loaded needle used to create a pneumoperitoneum for laparoscopic surgery) is inserted into the peritoneal cavity through the incision described above to perform the prefill.

During insertion of rigid noncuffed catheters, if the stylet of the catheter fails to enter the peritoneal cavity, the catheter may be unintentionally advanced into the preperitoneal space. Dialysis solution inflow will be slow and often painful. Outflow will be minimal and the effluent may become blood-tinged. If this occurs, as much fluid as possible is drained and the catheter is removed and inserted at another site.

There is no specific strategy to break-in acute rigid catheters. An incremental approach to increasing the peritoneal volume is advisable to minimize the risk of leakage. Because the risk of infection is high with rigid noncuffed catheters, the generally accepted period of maximum use is 3 days. Removal of the acute rigid catheter is performed by gently withdrawing it after draining the abdomen and cutting the retaining suture. It is recommended that the peritoneum be allowed to rest for a couple of days before placing a new catheter. Insertion sites for replacement catheters should alternate between medial and lateral locations, allowing a distance of at least 2–3 cm from the previous site. If a short course of peritoneal dialysis is anticipated or therapy must be initiated before a chronic catheter can be placed, the temporary rigid catheter remains an option.

Soft Cuffed Catheters

Most of the soft cuffed catheters for chronic PD (described more fully in the following section) can serve as acute peritoneal access devices. With the availability of self-contained sets permitting bedside placement using a percutaneous needle-guidewire approach to insert a peel-away catheter introducer sheath, soft cuffed chronic catheters have increasingly replaced the use of temporary rigid catheters. If it is anticipated that the need for peritoneal dialysis will be longer than a few days, a chronic catheter should be placed initially. While the trend for chronic catheters is to use two-cuff devices, one of the continuing demands for a one-cuff catheter is to provide acute access. Compared to the rigid catheter, the one-cuff soft tube can be left in place indefinitely, and it is easier to insert and remove than two-cuff chronic devices. If long-term dialysis is expected and the patient's clinical condition permits, consideration should be given to placing a two-cuff catheter. Catheter insertion, maintenance, and removal techniques for chronic soft-cuffed catheters are covered in later sections of this chapter.

Chronic Catheters

Currently, all chronic catheters are constructed of silicone rubber. A small percentage of catheters were previously fabricated from polyurethane rubber, but production ceased in 2010. Although the number of surviving polyurethane catheters is quickly diminishing, it is important to identify these devices because of the tendency for polyurethane rubber to develop stress fractures or to soften and rupture from chronic exposure to polyethylene glycol or ethanol present in certain topical antibiotic ointments and creams commonly used for long-term catheter exit-site prophylaxis. Polyurethane catheters can be recognized by a permanently bonded catheter adapter and characteristically show dark discoloration of the tubing after several years.

The most commonly employed PD catheter types are illustrated in Fig. 9.1. The standard double Dacron (polyester) cuff, coiled- and straight-tip Tenckhoff catheters and their "swan neck" variants with a preformed arc bend in the intercuff segment constitute the mainstay of PD access around the world (Fig. 9.1 A and B). The primary difference among these catheters is that the coiled-tip configuration and the preformed arc bend increase the cost of the device. No significant difference in functionality has been convincingly demonstrated between coiled- and straight-tip catheters with or without a preformed arc bend. The incidence of inflow discomfort is greater with straight-tip catheters because of the jet effect of the dialysate from the end hole of the catheter. Coiled-tip catheters provide for better dispersion of the dialysate during inflow. Standard abdominal catheters can be inserted by any of the implantation methodologies.

Fig. 9.2 depicts a chronic peritoneal catheter showing its relationship to abdominal wall structures. Catheters equipped with two cuffs provide for better immobilization of the tubing within the abdominal wall. The deep cuff is preferably implanted in the muscle to provide for firm tissue ingrowth and fixation of the catheter. The superficial cuff is positioned in the subcutaneous tissues 2–4 cm from the exit site. When properly positioned, the superficial cuff serves as an effective barrier to entry of cutaneous debris and bacteria into the subcutaneous track and minimizes the pistonlike motion of the catheter in and out through the exit site that can drive these contaminants into the track.

Extended two-piece catheters were originally designed to provide a presternal exit site (Fig. 9.1C). The extended catheter consists of a one-cuff abdominal catheter segment that attaches to a one- or two-cuff subcutaneous extension segment using a double-barbed titanium connector to permit remote location of the exit site to the upper chest. Extended catheters are also used to provide remote exit-site locations to the upper abdominal and back regions. The abdominal catheter can be placed by any insertion method. The subcutaneous extension catheter is implanted using a vascular tunneling rod or similar device supplied by the catheter manufacturer.

Most currently manufactured chronic catheters possess a white radiopaque stripe along the longitudinal axis of the tubing, which enables radiographic visualization. The stripe can also serve as a guide during implantation of the catheter to prevent accidental twisting or kinking of the catheter tubing. The majority of adult catheters have a 2.6 mm internal diameter. One catheter brand possesses a 3.5 mm internal diameter and can be identified by its blue radiopaque stripe. While the in vitro flow rate of the larger-bore catheter is faster, therapeutic advantage of this device has yet to be demonstrated in the in vivo state. The importance of recognizing the catheter bore size is to prevent accidental interchange of replacement catheter adapters that can result in a loose fit and separation.

Various modifications of the basic Tenckhoff catheter designs have been made in an attempt to address the common mechanical problems of tissue attachment, tip migration, and pericatheter leaks. However, none of these alternative configurations have been shown to outperform the standard Tenckhoff catheter design, but do increase the cost and difficulty of device insertion. Concerns for these common mechanical problems are more reliably addressed by proper implantation technique than by a catheter design.

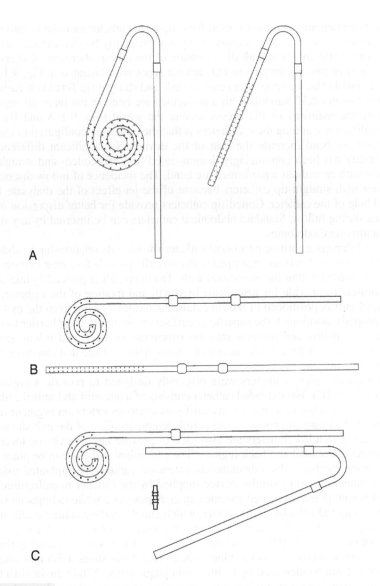

A

B

C

Figure 9.1

Commonly Used Peritoneal Catheters. (A) Tenckhoff catheters with preformed intercuff arc bend, two cuffs, and coiled or straight tips. (B) Tenckhoff catheters with straight intercuff segment, two cuffs, and coiled or straight tips. (C) Extended catheter with one cuff, coiled tip abdominal catheter, two-cuff extension catheter with preformed intercuff arc bend, and titanium double-barbed connector.

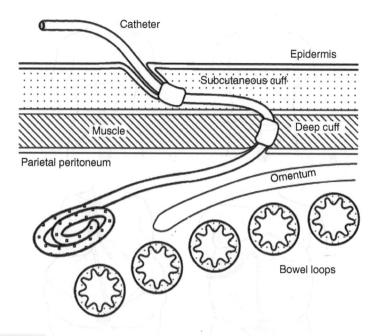

Figure 9.2

Schematic of a Coiled-Tip Tenckhoff Peritoneal Catheter Showing Its Proper Relationship to Adjacent Anatomic Structures.

Choosing a Chronic Peritoneal Catheter

Because patients come in all sizes and shapes with a variety of medical conditions, it is quite simplistic to expect that one catheter type should fit all. Choice of catheter type should take into consideration the patient's belt line, obesity, skin creases and folds, presence of scars, chronic skin conditions, incontinence, physical limitations, bathing habits, and occupation. The provider's familiarity with a basic inventory of catheter types is essential to enable customization of the peritoneal access to the specific needs of the patient and to afford maximum flexibility in exit-site location. An exit site that is located in an environmentally unfriendly zone or in a position that the patient cannot easily see or take care of predisposes to exit site and tunnel infection.

Fig. 9.3 illustrates how a basic catheter inventory might be applied. Patients who wear their belt lines below the umbilicus are usually best fitted with a catheter having a straight intercuff segment that is bent to produce a laterally directed exit site emerging above the belt line. Patients who wear their belt lines above the umbilicus are often best served with a catheter with a preformed arc bend that allows the exit site to emerge below the belt line. Individuals who have large rotund abdomens, severe obesity, drooping skin folds, intestinal stomas, feeding tubes, suprapubic catheters, urinary or fecal incontinence, yeast intertrigo, or desire to take deep tub baths are candidates for extended two-piece catheters to produce upper abdominal or presternal exit sites.

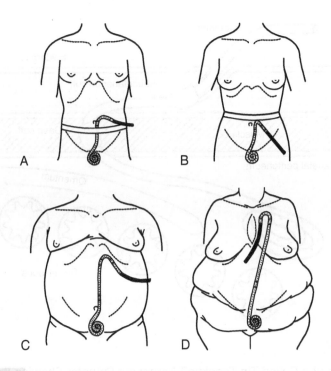

Figure 9.3

Practical Applications of a Basic Catheter Inventory. (A) Straight intercuff segment catheter with laterally directed exit site emerging above a low-lying belt line. (B) Preformed intercuff arc bend catheter with downwardly directed exit site emerging below a high-lying belt line. (C) Extended catheter with upper abdominal exit site for an obese rotund abdomen, lower abdominal skin folds, or incontinence. (D) Extended catheter with presternal exit site for severe obesity, multiple abdominal skin folds, intestinal stomas, or incontinence.

The most appropriate choice of catheter is the one that produces the best balance of pelvic location of the catheter tip, exit site easily visible to the patient, and can be inserted through the abdominal wall with the least amount of tubing stress. The catheter insertion site is the fulcrum of this best balance and will determine the pelvic position of the catheter tip and the range of reachable exit sites. Therefore, catheter selection begins with determination of the insertion site. With the patient in the supine position, the insertion site for each style and size of catheter is determined by marking the upper border of the deep cuff in the paramedian plane when the upper border of the catheter coil is aligned with the upper border of the pubic symphysis (Fig. 9.4). For straight-tip catheters, a point 5 cm from the end is aligned with the upper border of the pubic symphysis. During the catheter placement procedure, the deep cuff is implanted within the rectus muscle (or just below) at the level of the insertion incision. Using this convention to determine the insertion site will prevent the catheter tip from being implanted too low in the pelvis, producing

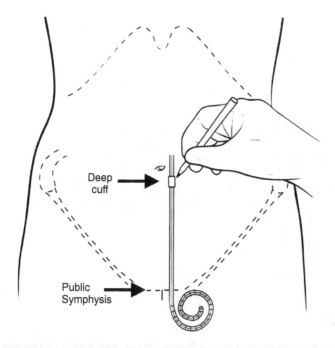

Deep cuff

Public Symphysis

Figure 9.4

Schematic of a Supine Patient Showing the Manner in Which the Catheter Insertion Site and Deep Cuff Location Are Selected to Achieve Proper Pelvic Position of the Coiled Catheter Tip. (Crabtree JH. Selected best demonstrated practices in peritoneal dialysis access. Kidney Int 2006; 70:S27-37, Figure 9)

pressure or poking discomfort, early termination of dialysate outflow, and severe end of drain pain.

After determining the catheter insertion site, the subcutaneous tunnel path and exit site location for catheters with a swan neck bend simply follows the configuration of the tubing, marking the skin exit site 2–3 cm beyond the superficial cuff. Catheters with a straight intercuff segment should assume a gentle arc in the subcutaneous tissues to produce more of a laterally directed exit site. Illustrated in Fig. 9.5 is a convenient three-step algorithm for catheters with a straight intercuff segment to design a laterally directed tunnel and exit site that minimizes creation of excessive tubing stress and shape-memory resiliency forces that can lead to catheter tip migration and superficial cuff extrusion. If the catheter needs to be bent more than a laterally directed exit site, a swan neck catheter should be used instead to eliminate these excessive forces. Upwardly directed exit sites should be avoided to prevent pooling of cutaneous bacteria and debris, perspiration, and shower water in the exit sinus, predisposing the patient to exit-site and tunnel infection.

After mapping exit-site locations, the patient assumes a sitting or standing position and the marked exit sites are checked to see which is best visualized by the patient and does not conflict with the belt line, skin creases, or apices of bulging

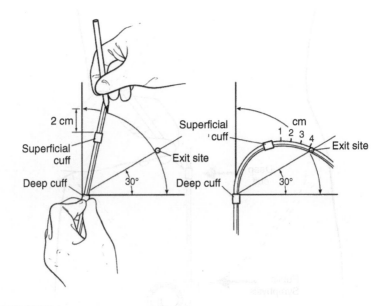

Figure 9.5

Three-Step Algorithm for Lateral Tunnel Track and Exit-Site Design. Step 1: Scribe arc from vertical to horizontal plane using catheter as compass from point 2 cm external of superficial cuff. Step 2: Mark exit site at junction of medial two-thirds and lateral one-third of arc. Step 3: Indicate tunnel track shape by bending catheter over from point 4 cm external of superficial cuff to exit site. (Crabtree JH. Selected best demonstrated practices in peritoneal dialysis access. Kidney Int 2006; 70:S27-37, Figure 10)

skin folds. If none of the marked exit sites for the standard abdominal catheters are satisfactory, the patient is then considered for an extended catheter to produce an upper abdominal or presternal exit-site location.

Some dialysis catheter manufacturers produce marking stencils for the most commonly used catheter designs. Properly constructed stencils contain critical catheter design information including the distance between the deep cuff and the coil, suggested subcutaneous tunnel configurations, and recommended exit-site locations relative to the position of the superficial cuff. Additional features of a well-designed stencil plate permit its precise orientation on the trunk region according to fixed anatomic landmarks, such as the pubic symphysis, representing the anterior upper border of the true pelvis, and the anatomic midline of the torso. Stencils permit accurate and reproducible association of the catheter design elements to these anatomic landmarks to help determine the best catheter style and insertion site that will produce optimal pelvic position of the catheter coil and ideal exit-site location. In addition to the preoperative evaluation, the marking stencil is used again at the time of the catheter placement procedure to retrace the previously determined insertion incision, tunnel configuration, and exit-site location. Be aware that some manufacturers produce impractical stencils that show only the cutout patterns of a swan neck bend but do not allow for proper alignment of the stencil plate on the abdominal or chest wall.

Chronic PD Catheter Placement Procedures

Independent of the catheter implantation approach, adherence to a number of universal details is required to ensure the best opportunity for creating a successful long-term peritoneal access. Best practices for preoperative preparation and peritoneal catheter placement are listed in Table 9.1. Omission of any one of these practices can lead to loss of the PD catheter. Some implantation techniques do not incorporate all of the best practices, such as percutaneous needle-guidewire approaches performed through the midline or positioning the deep cuff above the level of the fascia. It is essential that the practitioner be aware of deviations from recommended

Table 9.1

Best Practices in Peritoneal Catheter Placement

Patient Preparation
- Preoperative assessment to select the most appropriate catheter type, insertion site, and exit-site location
- Bowel prep the day before procedure: 2 L of polyethylene glycol solution, enema, or stimulant suppository
- Shower on the day of procedure with chlorhexidine soap wash of the planned surgical site
- Removal of body hair in the preoperative holding area, preferably with electric clippers
- Empty the bladder before procedure; otherwise, Foley catheter should be inserted
- Single preoperative dose of prophylactic antibiotic to provide antistaphylococcal coverage

Procedure Performance
- Operative personnel are attired in cap, mask, sterile gown and gloves
- Surgical site is prepped with chlorhexidine-gluconate scrub, povidone-iodine (gel or scrub), or other suitable antiseptic agent and sterile drapes applied around the surgical field
- Peritoneal catheter is rinsed and flushed with saline and air squeezed out of the Dacron cuffs by rolling the submerged cuffs between fingers
- Paramedian insertion of the catheter through the body of the rectus muscle
- Deep catheter cuff positioned within or below the rectus muscle
- Pelvic location of the catheter tip
- Catheter flow test performed to confirm acceptable function
- Skin exit site directed lateral or downward (not upward)
- Subcutaneous tunneling instrument should not exceed the diameter of the catheter
- Exit site should be smallest skin hole possible that allows passage of the catheter
- Position subcutaneous cuff 2–4 cm from the exit site
- No catheter anchoring sutures at the exit site
- Attach transfer (extension) set at time of procedure
- Exit site protected and catheter immobilized by nonocclusive dressing.

(Crabtree JH. Peritoneal dialysis catheter implantation: avoiding problems and optimizing outcomes. Semin Dial 2015; 28:12-5, Tables 1 & 2)

practices and be observant for the potential complications that may arise from such departures.

Percutaneous Needle-Guidewire Technique

Placement of catheters by blind percutaneous puncture is performed using a modification of the Seldinger technique. The convenience of this approach is that it can be performed at the bedside under local anesthesia using prepackaged self-contained kits that include the dialysis catheter. The abdomen is prefilled with 1.5–2 L dialysis solution instilled with an 18-gauge introducer needle inserted through a 1.5- to 2-cm infraumbilical or paramedian incision. Alternatively, a Veress needle may be used to perform the prefill. A guidewire is passed through the needle into the peritoneal cavity and directed toward the pelvis. The needle is withdrawn. A dilator with overlying peel-away sheath is advanced through the fascia over the guidewire. The guidewire and dilator are removed. Optionally, to facilitate insertion, the catheter can be straightened and stiffened by insertion of an internal stylet. The dialysis catheter is directed through the sheath toward the pelvis. As the deep catheter cuff advances, the sheath is peeled away. The deep cuff is advanced to the level of the fascia.

The addition of fluoroscopy to the procedure permits confirmation of needle entry into the peritoneal cavity by observing the flow of injected contrast solution around loops of bowel. The retrovesical space is identified by contrast pooling in the appropriate location. The guidewire and catheter are advanced to this site. Ultrasonography can be used in a similar fashion. The remainder of the procedure proceeds as described for blind placement. Although the radiopaque tubing stripe permits fluoroscopic imaging of the final catheter configuration, the proximity of adhesions or omentum cannot be assessed. Percutaneous guidewire placement techniques often leave the deep catheter cuff external to the fascia. After testing flow function, the catheter is then tunneled subcutaneously to the selected exit site.

Open Surgical Dissection

A transverse or vertical paramedian incision is made through the skin, subcutaneous tissues, and anterior rectus sheath. The underlying muscle fibers are split to expose the posterior rectus sheath. A small hole is made through the posterior sheath and peritoneum to enter the peritoneal cavity. A purse-string suture is placed around the opening. The catheter, usually straightened over an internal stylet, is advanced through the peritoneal incision toward the pelvis. Despite being an open procedure, the catheter is advanced mostly by feel, therefore, blindly, into the peritoneal cavity. The stylet is partially withdrawn as the catheter is advanced until the deep cuff abuts the posterior fascia. After satisfactory placement has been achieved, the stylet is completely withdrawn and the purse-string suture is tied. Encouraging the catheter tip to remain oriented toward the pelvis is achieved by oblique passage of the catheter through the rectus sheath in a craniocaudal direction. The catheter tubing is exited through the anterior rectus sheath at least 2.5 cm cranial to the level of the purse-string suture and deep cuff location. Attention to detail in placement of the purse-string suture and repair of the anterior fascia is imperative to prevent pericatheter leak and hernia. The catheter is tunneled subcutaneously to the selected exit site following a satisfactory test of flow function.

Y-TEC Procedure

The Y-TEC procedure is a proprietary laparoscopic-assisted technique of peritoneal catheter placement. A 2.5-mm trocar with an overlying plastic sleeve is inserted percutaneously into the peritoneal cavity through a paramedian incision. The obturator of the trocar is removed, permitting insertion of a 2.2-mm laparoscope to confirm peritoneal entry. The scope is withdrawn and 0.6–1.5 L of room air is pumped into the abdomen with a syringe or hand bulb. The scope is reinserted and the overlying cannula and plastic sleeve are visually directed into an identified clear area within the peritoneal cavity. The scope and cannula are withdrawn, leaving the expandable plastic sleeve to serve as a conduit for blind insertion of the catheter over a stylet toward the previously identified clear area. The plastic sleeve is withdrawn and the deep cuff is pushed into the rectus sheath. After testing flow function, the catheter is tunneled subcutaneously to the selected exit site.

Surgical Laparoscopy

Laparoscopy provides a minimally invasive approach with complete visualization of the peritoneal cavity during the catheter implantation procedure. The advantage of laparoscopic catheter placement over other approaches is the ability to proactively employ adjunctive procedures that significantly improve catheter outcomes. Laparoscopically guided rectus sheath tunneling places the catheter in a long musculofascial tunnel directed toward the pelvis and effectively prevents catheter tip migration, eliminates pericatheter hernias, and reduces the risk of pericatheter leaks. Observed redundant omentum that lies in juxtaposition of the catheter tip can be displaced from the pelvis into the upper abdomen and fixed to the abdominal wall (omentopexy). Compartmentalizing adhesions that may affect completeness of dialysate drainage can be divided. Intraperitoneal structures that siphon up to the catheter tip during the intraoperative irrigation test can be laparoscopically resected, including epiploic appendices of the sigmoid colon and uterine tubes. Previously unsuspected abdominal wall hernias can be identified and repaired at the time of the catheter implantation procedure.

Through a lateral abdominal wall puncture site remote from the point of intended catheter insertion, the abdomen is insufflated with gas through a Veress needle to create an intraperitoneal working space. A laparoscopic port and laparoscope are inserted. Under laparoscopic guidance, the catheter is introduced at a second puncture site and placed in a musculofascial tunnel oriented toward the pelvis, usually through the use of a port device that creates the rectus sheath tunnel. Some variations of the technique use a third laparoscopic port site to introduce laparoscopic forceps to assist in the catheter tunneling process. The catheter tip is directed into the true pelvis under visual control. The deep cuff of the catheter is positioned in the rectus muscle just below the anterior fascial sheath. A purse-string fascial suture is placed around the catheter at the level of the anterior sheath to minimize the risk of pericatheter leak. The pneumoperitoneum is released but laparoscopic ports are left in place until a test irrigation of the catheter demonstrates successful flow function. After any indicated adjunctive procedures are completed, the catheter is tunneled subcutaneously to the selected exit site.

Special Peritoneal Access Methods

Extended Two-Piece Catheters

The abdominal segment of two-piece extended catheters can be implanted by any of the above-mentioned insertion techniques. A secondary incision is made in the vicinity of the planned upper abdominal, presternal, or back exit site. A marking stencil is invaluable in devising the location of the secondary incision and exit site. The measured distance between the abdominal insertion incision and the secondary incision is used to calculate how much tubing length will be trimmed from one or both of the catheter segments in order to correctly span the distance. The trimmed catheters are joined with a double-barbed titanium connector and the linked catheter segments are tunneled on the surface of the fascia from the abdominal insertion site to the remote secondary incision with a tunneling rod. The extension catheter is then passed from the secondary incision through the exit site using a stylet to complete the procedure.

Catheter Embedding

Commonly referred to as the Moncrief-Popovich technique, catheter embedding consists of implanting a peritoneal dialysis catheter far in advance of anticipated need. Instead of bringing the external limb of the catheter out to the surface, it is embedded under the skin in the subcutaneous space. When renal function declines to the point of needing to initiate dialysis, the external limb is brought to the outside through a small skin incision (Fig. 9.6).

Because the catheter has been afforded extended healing time within the abdominal wall, the patient is able to proceed directly to full volume peritoneal dialysis without the necessity of a break-in period that ordinarily accompanies a newly placed catheter. Firm tissue ingrowth of the cuffs and absence of biofilm formation have been speculated to reduce catheter infection–related peritonitis. Another important attribute of catheter embedding is greater patient acceptance for earlier commitment to peritoneal dialysis by catheter placement ahead of time. The patient is not burdened with catheter maintenance until dialysis is needed. The need for insertion of vascular catheters and temporary hemodialysis can be avoided in patients previously implanted with an embedded catheter. The embedding technique permits more efficient surgical scheduling of catheter implantation as an elective nonurgent procedure and helps to reduce stress on operating room access. Disadvantages of the catheter embedding strategy include the need for two procedures (implantation and externalization) as opposed to one and the possibility of futile placement in the event of a change in the patient's condition during the time period that the catheter is embedded that precludes the use of PD.

Catheter embedding can be incorporated into any of the implantation approaches using any catheter device. The catheter is temporarily externalized through the future skin exit site prior to embedment. The exit-site scar serves as a landmark to know where to come back to for externalization. After acceptable flow function of the catheter is confirmed, the tubing is flushed with heparin, plugged, and buried in the subcutaneous tissue. To minimize the risk of hematoma or seroma and to facilitate subsequent externalization, the catheter should be embedded in a linear or curvilinear subcutaneous track using a tunneling stylet as opposed to curling the tubing into a subcutaneous pocket. Embedding should not be performed if the anticipated need for dialysis is less than 4 weeks. Externalization of embedded catheters is an office

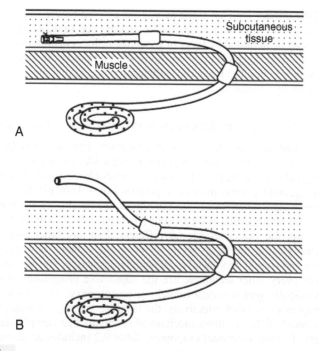

Figure 9.6

The Embedded Catheter Strategy. (A) External limb of the catheter tubing is embedded under the skin at the time of catheter placement. (B) External limb of the catheter is externalized when renal function declines to the point that dialysis is required.

procedure. Catheters have been embedded for months to years with an 85%–93% immediate function rate upon externalization. Catheter dysfunction is usually due to adhesions or intraluminal fibrin clots. Overall, 94%–99% are successfully used for dialysis after radiologic or laparoscopic revision of nonfunctioning catheters.

Acute Complications of Chronic Catheter Placement

Inadvertent preperitoneal position of the introducer needle, peel-away sheath, and catheter can occur during chronic peritoneal catheter placement using percutaneous needle-guidewire approaches. Inflow of dialysate will be slow and painful and the outflow minimal with the effluent often becoming blood-tinged. If preperitoneal placement is suspected, as much fluid as possible should be drained, the catheter should be removed, and the insertion process repeated.

In addition to preperitoneal catheter placement, blood-tinged outflow can represent injury to a blood vessel in the abdominal wall or mesentery. The return will usually clear with continued dialysis. Grossly bloody effluent, fall in hematocrit, or signs of hemodynamic instability signify large blood vessel injury. Urgent laparotomy is generally required. Unexplained polyuria and glycosuria suggests accidental puncture of the urinary bladder. If the needle has entered bowel, instillation of dialysate will be accompanied by pain and/or an urgent need to defecate. Unrecognized bowel entry may be heralded by feces or gas in the effluent or watery diarrhea having high glucose content. Surgical intervention is often necessary. If surgical exploration is planned, it is beneficial to leave the catheter in place so that the site of perforation can be more easily identified.

Catheter Placement Approaches and Best Outcomes

It is often argued that no single catheter placement approach has been shown to produce superior outcomes. Operator performance aside, when catheter implantation by open surgical dissection, percutaneous needle-guidewire with or without fluoroscopic imaging, and laparoscopy are compared side to side on identical study populations with equivalent adherence to best practices, the results are essentially equal. It should be of no surprise that if laparoscopy is used only to witness the position of the catheter tip, the outcomes are no different than any other catheter insertion method. Simply using the laparoscope to locate the catheter is underutilization of this modality and should be viewed as substandard practice. The advantages of laparoscopy over every other technique are the adjunctive procedures enabled by this method, principally rectus sheath tunneling, omentopexy, and adhesiolysis. When these techniques are applied effectively, the laparoscopic approach can both prevent and resolve most of the common mechanical problems that complicate insertion of PD catheters. To ensure optimal outcomes, Table 9.2 includes additional best practices that are specific for laparoscopy.

Care of the Chronic Peritoneal Catheter

Postoperative Catheter Immobilization and Dressings

Because no catheter-anchoring stitches should ever be used, it is important to immobilize the catheter on the abdominal wall with medical adhesive tincture and sterile

---

Table 9.2

Best Practices Specific for Laparoscopic Peritoneal Catheter Placement

- No midline abdominal entry points for laparoscopic ports
- Immobilize catheter toward pelvis by rectus sheath tunneling (no pelvic anchoring stitches)
- Omentopexy performed for redundant omentum
- Adhesiolysis performed to enable catheter placement and/or to eliminate recognized intraperitoneal compartmentalization that can impede dialysate drainage
- Laparoscopic port wound is not used as a catheter skin exit site
- Irrigation test completed before removal of laparoscopic ports in case additional interventions required
- Suture closure of all laparoscopic port sites regardless of port size if acute or urgent dialysis is anticipated

(Crabtree JH. Peritoneal dialysis catheter implantation: avoiding problems and optimizing outcomes. Semin Dial 2015; 28:12-5, Table 3)

adhesive strips. A nonocclusive barrier dressing of sufficient size to protect the exit site and surgical wounds and to further immobilize the catheter should be applied at the time of the placement procedure. In addition, the transfer set should be secured to the abdominal wall to prevent tugging on the catheter at the exit site. It is helpful to secure the transfer set to the abdominal wall separately from the main dressing so that the PD nurses have access to the tubing for catheter irrigations without having to disturb the dressing over the exit site. As long as the dressings are clean and intact and the exit site appears stable, dressings are changed on a weekly basis until such time that the patient is instructed on the protocol for chronic exit-site care. If at any time the exit site appears unstable, the frequency of exit-site care is modified according to the findings.

Catheter Irrigation

Catheters that are not used immediately should undergo irrigation with 1 L of solution (saline or dialysate) within 72 hours following insertion to wash out blood and fibrinous debris. If the effluent is particularly bloody, irrigation is repeated until signs of clearing are evident. To ensure patency, it is a good idea to repeat the irrigation weekly until such time that dialysis is instituted. Heparin added to the irrigant (1000 units/L) is helpful in preventing fibrin plugging of the catheter during the early postoperative period.

Catheter Break-in Procedures

Nonurgent Start

When feasible, delaying start of dialysis for 2 weeks following catheter insertion helps to reduce the risk of pericatheter leakage. Either continuous ambulatory peritoneal dialysis or automated peritoneal dialysis can be initiated after this period. Although most patients can begin dialysis with 2 L volumes, starting with lower volumes and increasing incrementally to target levels can be performed during the training period.

Urgent Start

PD catheters can be used immediately postimplantation if care is taken to create a tight seal at the insertion site. Although no standard dialysis prescription exists for patients starting urgent PD, a low volume, supine, intermittent PD protocol is advisable to minimize the risk of leak. Such an approach might consist of initiating automated exchanges using 1–1.2 L volumes and increasing the amount by 250–500 mL per week. The abdomen should be left dry during ambulatory periods for the first 2 weeks.

Long-Term Catheter and Exit-Site Care

Patients should limit themselves to nonstrenuous activities for 4–6 weeks following catheter placement to permit good wound healing. If exit site healing is uneventful, most patients are able to resume showering in 3–4 weeks. This usually coincides with implementation of the chronic exit site care routine. Most exit site care protocols involve daily cleansing with nonirritating, nontoxic, antiseptic agents and application of a prophylactic antibiotic ointment or cream such as mupirocin or gentamicin.

Sterile dressings over the exit site are encouraged. Tub bathing and swimming with immersion of the exit site are discouraged. Centers that permit swimming usually restrict the activity to properly chlorinated private pools or ocean water. It is recommended that an ostomy appliance or similar device cover the exit site and catheter during swimming and to perform routine exit site care after the activity. Patients should be reminded that the catheter is a "lifeline" and advised to consider the consequences of risking exposure of their peritoneal access to potential contamination during swimming.

Embedded Catheter Care

Patients who undergo catheter embedment may resume showering after 48 hours. Nonstrenuous activities are required for 4–6 weeks following catheter placement to permit good wound healing. Externalization of embedded catheters is a clinic procedure performed using sterile technique in a suitable treatment room under local anesthesia. If appropriate embedding technique was performed, the catheter tubing should be easily palpable at the incision scar created during the procedure while the catheter was temporarily externalized at the future exit site. In equivocal cases, ultrasound examination has been employed to identify the catheter tubing at the correct distance from the superficial cuff. Care is exercised in anesthetizing the skin and making the incision to avoid damage to the catheter. Hemostat dissection is used to identify and deliver the catheter from the embedment track. The plugged end of the tubing is amputated, catheter adapter inserted, transfer set attached, and flow function tested. The catheter may require brisk irrigation with a 60-mL syringe and saline to dislodge fibrin clots. Unsatisfactory flow function should be managed as described under the section on mechanical complications and management. Exit-site care following externalization of embedded catheters is the same as described for primarily externalized catheters.

Complications of Chronic Peritoneal Catheters

Mechanical and infectious complications are the two most common reasons for PD failure. With early and appropriate intervention, many catheters can be saved, often without interruption of therapy, or, in the event of catheter loss, the interval before return to PD can be minimized.

Mechanical Complications and Management

Mechanical complications of the catheter include pericatheter leaks and hernias, infusion and drain pain, flow failure, catheter tip migration, and superficial cuff extrusion.

Pericatheter Leaks and Hernias

Leakage around the catheter is usually related to catheter implantation technique, timing of initiation of dialysis, initial dialysate volumes, and strength of abdominal wall tissues. When dialysis is initiated, subcutaneous leakage may occur at the catheter insertion site and usually manifests itself as fluid appearing through the incision or at the exit site. Questionable leaks can be verified by a positive glucose dipstick indicating high glucose concentration in the leaking fluid. Delaying initiation of dialysis for 2 weeks following catheter placement minimizes the risk for developing a leak. Temporarily discontinuing dialysis for 1–3 weeks usually results in spontaneous cessation of an early leak. Dramatic early leaks may indicate purse-string suture failure or technical error in wound repair and compels immediate exploration. Leakage through the exit site or insertion incision leaves the patient susceptible to tunnel infection and peritonitis. Prophylactic antibiotic therapy should be employed. Persistent leaks necessitate catheter replacement.

Late pericatheter leaks are caused by pericannular hernia or occult tunnel infections with separation of the cuffs from the surrounding tissues. The occurrence of pericannular hernia is largely influenced by the location and degree of fixation of the deep cuff. At the parietal peritoneal surface, the mesothelium reflects along the surface of the catheter to reach the deep cuff. If the deep cuff was placed outside of the muscle wall or the cuff shifts outward because of weak midline fascial attachments, then the peritoneal lining actually extends above the fascial layer creating the potential for a subcutaneous sac filled with dialysate. This fluid-filled subcutaneous mass is referred to as a pseudohernia and can eventually lead to a pericatheter leak. If the abdominal wall is weak, a pericannular track may dilate and develop a true hernia. Most late leaks and pericatheter hernias are best managed by catheter replacement.

Infusion and Drain Pain

Pain during dialysate infusion is ordinarily observed in new patients initiating dialysis and is often transient in nature, gradually disappearing over several weeks. Persistent infusion pain is commonly associated with the acidity (pH 5.2–5.5) of conventional lactate-buffered dialysis solutions. Use of bicarbonate/lactate-buffered dialysis solutions (pH 7.0–7.4) can eliminate this pain. If buffered solutions are not available, manual addition of bicarbonate to each dialysis bag (4–5 mEq/L) can be performed to treat acid-related infusion pain. Alternatively, a 1% or 2% lidocaine solution added to the dialysate (5 mL/L) may be tried to lessen infusion discomfort.

Other causes of dialysate-related pain include hypertonic glucose solutions, aged dialysis solution, overdistention of the abdomen, or extremes in dialysate temperature. Compared to coiled dialysis catheters, straight-tip catheters appear to be associated with a higher incidence of mechanical inflow pain caused by the jet effect of the dialysate from the end hole of the tubing. Catheter malposition with the tip against the abdominal wall or tube restriction by attached tissues can produce both inflow and outflow pain. Slower infusion rates and incomplete drainage may diminish these symptoms; however, transluminal catheter manipulation or laparoscopic exploration should be considered for flow pain that is persistent or accompanied with flow dysfunction with or without associated catheter malposition.

Pain during outflow is common, especially toward the end of the drain phase, particularly in the early days after initiation of dialysis. As the intraperitoneal structures siphon up to the catheter tip during the drain, it causes the catheter to bump up against the exquisitely sensitive parietal peritoneum. The pain is frequently experienced in the genital or anorectal region. Drain pain is more often a problem with automated peritoneal dialysis because of hydraulic suction on the peritoneal lining. Catheters implanted too low on the abdominal wall can wedge tubing into the deep pelvis resulting in drain pain from early closure of pelvic viscera around the catheter tip. Similarly, constipation with crowding of the bowel around the catheter in the pelvis can cause or contribute to the severity of the symptoms. The drain pain sometimes resolves with time or with treatment of associated constipation. If persistent, it can be managed by avoiding complete drainage of the peritoneal effluent. In cycler patients, this can be achieved by performing tidal peritoneal dialysis. In resistant cases of drain pain, repositioning of the catheter may be attempted but even this does not always resolve the problem.

Flow Failure

Catheter flow dysfunction ordinarily manifests as outflow failure where the volume of drained dialysate is substantially less than the inflow volume and there is no evidence of pericatheter leakage. Outflow failure usually occurs soon after catheter placement, but it may also begin during or after an episode of peritonitis, or at any time during the life of the catheter.

The most common cause of outflow dysfunction is constipation. Distended rectosigmoid colon may block the catheter side holes or displace the catheter tip into a position of poor drainage function. Extrinsic bladder compression on the catheter due to urinary retention occurs less frequently. An abdominal radiograph is helpful to look for a fecal-filled colon and catheter displacement. Constipation is treated with oral administration of an emollient, such as 70% sorbitol solution, 30 mL every 2 hours until the desired effect is achieved. Polyethylene glycol solution, 2 L, ingested over a period of 4–6 hours is usually effective in persistent cases. Stimulant laxatives such as bisacodyl and saline enemas are reserved for refractory cases because chemical and mechanical irritation of the colonic mucosa has been associated with transmural migration of bacteria and development of peritonitis.

Mechanical kinking of the catheter tubing is usually accompanied by two-way obstruction. A flat-plate radiograph of the abdomen is often helpful in identifying a kink in the catheter tubing. Catheter revision or replacement will be required.

Another cause of two-way obstruction is fibrin plugging of the catheter. Heparin should be added to the dialysate whenever fibrin strands are visible in the effluent. Heparin is more useful prophylactically than therapeutically, preventing the formation of fibrin clots and extension of existing clots. Once outflow obstruction has occurred, dwelling the catheter with heparin is usually unsuccessful in recovering function. If flow function is not restored with heparin, thrombolytic therapy with tissue plasminogen activator (tPA) may be attempted. Failure to dislodge intraluminal debris by brisk irrigation of the catheter with saline is followed by instillation of tPA. If catheter obstruction is due to a fibrin clot, recovery of flow function with tPA has been reported at nearly 100%. Because of cost considerations, the dose of tPA (used in a dilution of 1 mg/mL) is based on the estimated volume of the catheter assembly; however, no adverse consequences have been documented for catheter overfill or repeat administration.

If treatment of constipation and fibrinolytic therapy are not successful in restoring drainage function and urinary retention and tubing kinks have been excluded, the catheter is presumed to be obstructed by omentum or other adherent intraperitoneal structures. Interventions to resolve catheter obstruction most commonly use radiologic and laparoscopic techniques.

Radiologic intervention by fluoroscopic guidewire manipulation has been used to redirect displaced and obstructed catheters. Stiff guidewire manipulation of catheters with a swan neck bend can be difficult to perform and painful to the patient. Forceful straightening of the subcutaneous tunnel can produce tissue trauma and infection. Transluminal manipulation is not possible for extended catheters because of the long tubing length. A preprocedure dose of prophylactic antibiotics to provide antistaphylococcal coverage is advisable. Particular attention must be given to antiseptic preparation of the catheter tubing in addition to creating a sterile surgical field for the procedure. The transfer set is disconnected and discarded. After catheter manipulation is performed, restoration of flow function is checked by syringe irrigation. Frequently, multiple, separate manipulation procedures are required, with long-term flow function restored in only 45%–73% of cases. Failure rates for fluoroscopic manipulation as high as 90% were observed when patients had an antecedent history of abdominopelvic surgery or peritonitis, suggesting that adhesions play a major factor in technical failures.

Laparoscopy has become an invaluable method of evaluating and resolving catheter flow obstruction. Because laparoscopy can reliably identify the source of flow dysfunction and provide a means for definitive treatment, it is often considered as the next step in the management sequence after other causes for obstruction have been excluded. The dialysis catheter frequently can be used to perform the initial gas insufflation of the abdomen because most catheter obstructions represent outflow problems. Alternatively, a Veress needle is used for insufflation or the initial laparoscopic port is placed by direct cut-down on the peritoneum. Laparoscopic exploration is performed to identify the source of obstruction. Additional laparoscopic ports for introduction of operating instruments may be required depending on the findings.

Omental attachment to the catheter coil with displacement of the tubing out of the pelvis is a common cause of outflow dysfunction. Omental entrapment is relieved by using laparoscopic grasping forceps to strip the omentum from the catheter. The catheter tip is temporarily exteriorized through one of the port sites to facilitate removal of residual intraluminal tissue debris. The omentum is laparoscopically sutured to the upper abdominal region (omentopexy) to keep it away from the catheter. Redundant epiploic appendices of the sigmoid colon and uterine fimbria may siphon up to the catheter coil and produce obstruction. Laparoscopic resection of the involved epiploic appendices and uterine tube prevents recurrent obstruction. Obstruction of the catheter by adhesive scar tissues can be treated by laparoscopically dividing the adhesions or simply pulling the catheter free of the adhesions if they are not too extensive. Adhesiolysis for poor drainage function, especially after peritonitis, is associated with a 30% failure rate secondary to reforming of adhesions.

Catheter Tip Migration

Migration of the catheter tip to a position of poor drainage function is frequently caused by shape-memory resiliency forces of a straight catheter bent into a configuration that imposes excessive stress on the tubing. Simply repositioning the catheter will be followed by recurrence of the migration in a high percentage of cases. Laparoscopic suturing of the catheter tip to a pelvic structure has an unacceptable rate of failure due to erosion of the suture. A more reliable approach is to laparoscopically place a suture sling in the suprapubic region through the abdominal wall and around the catheter. A sling will maintain the catheter toward the pelvis and not hinder catheter removal if required at a later date.

Superficial Cuff Extrusion

Erosion of the superficial cuff through the exit site can result from positioning the cuff too close (<2 cm) to the exit wound during catheter placement. In addition, excessive bending of the catheter with a straight intercuff segment to produce a downward exit direction can induce mechanical stresses upon the tubing. In combination with proximity of the cuff to the exit site, the shape-memory forces of a catheter bent into this configuration can lead to tube straightening over time with migration of the superficial cuff toward and through the exit site. Another cause for superficial cuff erosion that can eventually result in extrusion of the entire catheter is outer displacement of the tubing due to poor location and fixation of the deep cuff. Also, exit-site infection extending to the superficial cuff may cause it to separate from the surrounding tissues and extrude through the exit site.

An extruded cuff becomes a reservoir of bacteria within the vicinity of the exit wound. Aggravated by daily wetting of the cuff material during routine exit-site care, the presence of the infected cuff interferes with maintaining exit-site hygiene. Using a scalpel blade applied parallel to the cuff surface, the cuff is shaved in repetitive slices until all of the cuff material is removed. The blade should be changed frequently to ensure ease in performing the shave without applying undue pressure on the tubing. Care should be exercised when shaving the cuff of 3.5-mm-internal-bore catheters (identified by the blue radiopaque stripe). The thin-walled tubing can be easily damaged. If the cuff material cannot be safely removed, simultaneous catheter replacement, described below in the section on PD-related peritonitis, may be an alternative management strategy if the exit site remains unstable.

Catheter Infection and Management

Details of antibiotic treatment for catheter infections are discussed in Chapter 35. The eventual outcome of a chronic exit-site infection with superficial cuff involvement is a tunnel abscess or progression of the tunnel infection to the peritoneal cavity producing concurrent peritonitis. Early recognition of chronic exit site and tunnel infection is essential to providing the best opportunity for catheter salvage.

Exit-Site and Tunnel Infection

Exit-site infection presents as redness, swelling, and tenderness at the exit site. With tunnel involvement, the signs of infection extend along the subcutaneous course of the catheter. In most cases, exit-site and tunnel infections are accompanied by purulent discharge from the exit site. In chronic smoldering cases, the exit-site skin is loose around the catheter, granulation tissue is present at the skin exit sinus, and purulent material can be expressed through the exit orifice with pressure over the subcutaneous cuff or stroking the skin over the tunnel toward the exit site while gently tugging on the catheter. As long as the infection has not extended to the deep cuff, it is possible to resolve the problem without losing the catheter or interrupting therapy. Ultrasonography of the catheter tunnel is a useful preoperative tool to evaluate for deep cuff involvement, particularly in obese patients where physical signs are often unreliable. Patients found to have sonographic evidence of deep cuff infection should undergo catheter removal. Moreover, patients with concurrent peritonitis are not candidates for catheter salvage procedures, this condition suggesting that transmural spread of the infection has already occurred.

If the deep cuff is not involved, surgically opening up the subcutaneous tunnel and shaving the superficial cuff is an option. Unroofing the skin and subcutaneous tissue overlying the infected tunnel permits drainage of pus, debridement of granulation tissue, and removal of the cuff material. The catheter, including the shaved tubing segment, is directed out of the medial corner of the incision and stabilized in this position by securing it to the adjacent skin with medical adhesive tincture and sterile adhesive strips. The wound is left open with performance of once- or twice-daily wet to dry dressing changes with saline-soaked gauze and allowed to heal by secondary intention. Depending on the magnitude of the infection, the procedure can be performed in the treatment room or operating room under local or general anesthesia. Catheters with a 3.5-mm internal bore, identified by the blue radiopaque stripe, should undergo cuff shaving with great care because the thin-walled tubing can be easily damaged. The primary advantage of the unroofing-cuff shaving procedure is that dialysis is not interrupted.

An alternative surgical treatment approach for chronic exit-site infection that has not extended beyond the superficial cuff into the intercuff section is replacement of the infected external tubing segment by catheter splicing (Fig. 9.7). This may be the preferred salvage procedure for a badly chosen exit-site location that was placed in

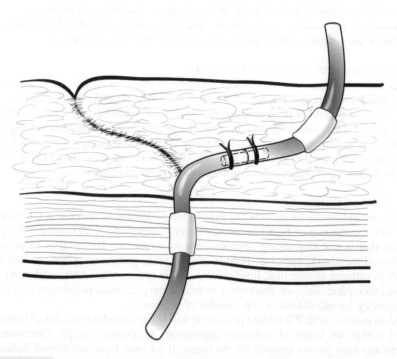

Figure 9.7

Catheter Splicing Procedure for Chronic Exit-Site Infection Permits Remote Routing of Tubing to New Location. Procedure also applicable for catheter tubing damage that is too short for external repair.

an infection-prone area, such as within a skin crease, on the apex of a flabby skin fold, or under the belt line. In this circumstance, performing only an unroofing-cuff shaving procedure may still result in an exit-site location that is predisposed to infection. The spliced catheter segment can be routed to a more stable exit-site location including the upper abdomen or chest region. Because the procedure requires more extensive dissection and tunneling, it is best performed in the operating room under local or general anesthesia.

After skin preparation, the infected exit site is isolated from the primary surgical field during draping and managed in the final step to prevent contamination of the new catheter and wound. An incision is made through the previous insertion site scar to expose the uninvolved intercuff segment of the catheter at the level of the fascia. The catheter is divided in the intercuff segment to preserve a 2.5-cm stump on the deep cuff side. A single- or double-cuff catheter with or without a preformed swan neck bend may be selected for the splicing segment. After trimming the new catheter to appropriate length, the segment is joined to the stump of the deep cuff end of the former catheter with a double-barbed titanium connector. The external segment of the spliced catheter is tunneled to a suitable exit location remote from the infected exit site. The wound is closed and dressings applied. In the final step, the external part of the old catheter is removed and the wound is debrided and packed open with saline wet-to-dry dressings. Antibiotics are continued for 2–4 weeks until the infected wound is healed. Peritoneal dialysis is continued uninterrupted.

Simultaneous catheter replacement, discussed under PD-related peritonitis, is another management strategy for chronic exit-site and tunnel infection.

Catheter Infection-Related Peritonitis

Progression of an exit-site and tunnel infection to the deep cuff can lead to concurrent peritonitis. Rarely, peritonitis can lead to chronic deep cuff infection and proceed in a retrograde fashion to manifest initially as a tunnel infection. Ultrasonography can be helpful in evaluating deep cuff involvement. Catheter infection–related peritonitis is best managed by catheter removal. Antibiotic treatment for peritonitis is covered in Chapter 36. Reinsertion of the dialysis catheter can be performed 4–6 weeks following completion of antibiotic therapy for peritonitis.

PD-Related Peritonitis

Diagnosis and antibiotic therapy for PD-related peritonitis is covered in Chapter 36. Importantly, there must be a low threshold for removal of the PD catheter for peritonitis that is not responding appropriately to treatment. The goal is to preserve peritoneal membrane function. Peritonitis can cause peritoneal adhesions that may result in catheter obstruction, limit the dialyzable space, or produce loculations that cause incomplete dialysate drainage. Fibrosis of the peritoneal membrane may affect its capacity for ultrafiltration and transfer of solutes.

Most patients with PD-related peritonitis will show considerable clinical improvement within 48 hours of initiating appropriate antibiotic therapy. Occasionally, symptoms may persist beyond 48–96 hours. If patients have not shown definitive clinical improvement by 96 hours, catheter removal should be performed. In patients with pseudomonas peritonitis, catheter removal should be performed by 48–72 hours if there has been no clinical improvement. Reinsertion of the dialysis catheter can be performed 4–6 weeks following completion of antibiotic therapy.

Table 9.3

General Guidelines for Simultaneous Catheter Replacement Without Interruption of Peritoneal Dialysis

- Procedure acceptable for peritonitis not due to mycobacteria, fungi, enteric organisms, or *Pseudomonas* species.
- Procedure acceptable for bacterial exit-site and tunnel infections.
- Clinical signs of peritonitis must be resolved and peritoneal leukocyte count is <100/μL.
- Continue appropriate antibiotic coverage perioperatively.
- Insert new catheter (clean step) before removal of old catheter (dirty step).
- Close watertight all penetrating points through musculofascial layers of abdominal wall.
- Utilize intermittent regimen of supine, low-volume peritoneal dialysis during interval of postoperative recovery; leave peritoneum dry during ambulatory periods.

(Crabtree JH, Siddiqi, RA. Simultaneous catheter replacement for infectious and mechanical complications without interruption of peritoneal dialysis. Perit Dial Int 2016; 36:182-7)

Often, an opportunity presents for simultaneous catheter replacement without interruption of PD for selected cases of PD-related peritonitis and exit-site and tunnel infection. When appropriately applied, the procedure spares the patient from a central venous catheter, a shift to hemodialysis, the ordeal of a change in dialysis modality, and a second surgery to insert a new PD catheter. General guidelines for simultaneous catheter replacement are outlined in Table 9.3.

Removal of Chronic Catheters

Because firm tissue ingrowth of the Dacron cuffs has occurred by 2–3 weeks, chronic catheters in place for a longer period will usually require removal by surgical dissection in the operating room or suitable procedure room, especially if the deep cuff was positioned in the rectus muscle. Fascial defects will require suture repair to prevent an abdominal wall hernia.

Secondary Embedding of Chronic Catheters

On occasion, catheter removal is performed because patients regain sufficient renal function to discontinue dialysis, but recovery is not expected to be permanent. An alternative to removing the catheter is secondary embedding. The inconvenience and cost of catheter maintenance can be eliminated for the interim by secondary embedding while still preserving a readily available peritoneal access that can be immediately employed to its fullest extent without the complications of new catheter placement, for example, flow dysfunction and pericatheter leak.

The procedure is performed similar to catheter splicing except that the spliced external segment is embedded. After skin preparation, the existing exit-site and catheter are isolated from the primary surgical field during draping and managed in the final step to prevent contamination of the spliced catheter and wounds. An incision is made through the previous insertion site scar to expose the intercuff segment of the catheter. The catheter is divided in the intercuff segment to preserve at least a 2.5-cm stump on the deep cuff side. A single- or double-cuff catheter with or without a preformed swan neck bend may be selected for the splicing segment. After trimming the new catheter to appropriate length, the segment is joined to the stump of the deep cuff end of the former catheter with a double barbed titanium connector. The external segment of the spliced catheter is temporarily externalized at the new exit site and then tunneled into a subcutaneous bed as described in the section on embedded catheters. After the wounds are closed and protected, the remaining external segment of the former catheter is removed and the old exit-site wound is excised and closed.

Mechanical Aspects
of Dialysis

CHAPTER 10

Water Treatment Equipment for In-Center Hemodialysis

Scott Bieber, DO

Introduction

During the provision of contemporary hemodialysis, the dialysate flows through the dialysate chamber of a dialyzer, which separates the toxic substances from the bloodstream into the dialysate via diffusion. The dialysate is composed of solute electrolytes in solvent water. In order to produce the final dialysate solution, a concentrated electrolyte solution is mixed with water. The ratio of concentrated electrolyte solution to water can vary based on many factors, including the type of concentration solution used and the proportioning system of the dialysis machine. In general, dialysate-proportioning systems mix around 1 part concentrate with 35–45 parts water. This final mixed dialysate is delivered to the dialyzer at a flow rate of 500–800 mL/min. Therefore, over a standard dialysis session, patients are exposed to vast quantities of water in the dialysate, that is, for a 4-hour session, anywhere from 120 to 192 L. To give you an idea of the magnitude of this volume, compare it with the estimated volume of total body water in a 70-kg man, which is around 42 L, with only 3.5 L of the total body water present in the plasma space. Therefore, dialysate water must be completely clear of potential contaminants to prevent injury to the patient during dialysis. Even contaminants found in dialysate water in small concentrations should be a cause for concern because their levels can reach toxic concentrations in the blood just by virtue of the vast quantity of water to which the blood is exposed. In addition, because of the absence of water contaminants in the blood, the diffusive pressure that can drive toxic solutes into the plasma space from the dialysate is high, and dialysis membranes do not offer selective protection to impede their entry from the dialysate into the bloodstream. Even contaminants in the dialysate that do not cross the dialysis membranes because of their size (e.g., bacteria) are found to be associated with systemic inflammation in dialysis patients. Systems that lack a separation of the blood from the treated water are available in some locations and demand an even higher level of water purity. For example, hemofiltration demands ultra-pure or sterile water produced "on-line" for infusion into the bloodstream as replacement fluid. These mentioned considerations, among others, highlight the obligatory need for water purification methods that are effective and reliable in order to provide a safe dialysis therapy.

This chapter serves to highlight common contaminants found in municipal water sources that can be harmful to dialysis patients; it reviews the equipment used to prepare product water for use in the production of dialysate, covers some of the maintenance, monitoring, and design considerations for water treatment systems as well as regulatory aspects that clinicians should be aware of when caring for dialysis patients. In addition, the reader is advised to consult guidelines published by the

Association for Advancement of Medical Instrumentation (AAMI)/International Organization for Standardization (ISO) as well as their local governmental guidelines and regulations when considering water treatment systems for their dialysis patients. For the purposes of this chapter, we will focus on the most recently available ISO/AAMI guidelines, which are a product of the latest available knowledge and expertise. The content within may differ from local or governmental regulations, which tend to lag behind ISO/AAMI recommendations.

Water Contaminants

Water used for production of dialysate fluid must meet a higher purity standard than what most municipal water supplies can provide. Because the production of dialysis water takes place in the dialysis facility, the responsibility for purification of water for dialysis rests on the dialysis provider. Common chemical contaminants in the water and their acceptable ranges are listed in Table 10.1. Contaminants can be present naturally in the water source, can be added to the water for specific purposes,

Table 10.1

Water Contaminant Acceptable Levels

Contaminant	Maximum Allowable Concentration
Contaminants With Documented Toxicity in Dialysis Patients (mg/L)	
Aluminum	0.01
Total chlorine	0.1
Copper	0.1
Fluoride	0.2
Lead	0.005
Nitrate (as N)	2
Sulfate	100
Zinc	0.1
Electrolytes Normally Found in Dialysate (mmol/L)	
Calcium	0.05
Magnesium	0.15
Potassium	0.2
Sodium	3
Trace Elements (mg/L)	
Antimony	0.006
Arsenic	0.005
Barium	0.1
Beryllium	0.0004
Cadmium	0.001
Chromium	0.014
Mercury	0.0002
Selenium	0.09
Silver	0.005
Thallium	0.002

ISO 13959, AAMI 2011

or can enter the water at the level of the dialysis facility. Each of these sources of potential contamination should be appreciated and monitored. Because the contaminants present in water can vary over time, dialysis providers are encouraged to establish a relationship with local water authorities so that they are apprised of any changes to the water supply contents. Examples of substances added to water by water authorities that can be toxic to dialysis patients include chlorine and chloramines for the control of microbiologic growth, fluoride for dental prophylaxis, and alum, which can be used as a flocculent to decrease water turbidity. Chloramines can also be naturally present in water. Occasionally, lime is added to acidic or ion-poor water to raise the pH and prevent damage to metal piping systems or lead leaching from older piping systems. Other trace elements, organic matter, agricultural products such as pesticides and fertilizers, and industrial products can also work their way into the water supply. Metals such as lead and copper can leach from plumbing systems. Microorganisms such as bacteria, fungi, protozoa, and endotoxins and other microbiologic fragments can also be present in water. Knowing the source of the water in your dialysis unit can help you anticipate which contaminants are more likely to be present. For example, water from surface sources such as rivers, lakes, and reservoirs is more likely to be ion poor (low conductivity) but is more prone to having organic surface contaminants present in it, such as particulates, pesticides, and others. Water that is derived from an aquifer or well tends to have more inorganic or ionic contaminants present (high conductivity), which the water accumulates as it percolates down through various sedimentary layers. Occasionally city water authorities issue boil water advisories when water is contaminated with microorganisms. Care should be taken to vigilantly monitor the water treatment system at this time. If the water treatment system is equipped with a reverse osmosis membrane, then dialysis can continue because this membrane will serve as a bacterial and endotoxin barrier. However, if a deionizing system is used, then ultrafilters or bacterial and endotoxin retentive filters downstream of the deionization (DI) system should be in place to prevent exposure to patients. Municipalities can often treat the water with higher concentrations of chlorine and chloramines during periods of infection, and care should be taken to make sure that the absorptive effect of the carbon tanks is not overwhelmed, thus causing spillover of chlorine and chloramines into the product water.

Exposure to these various contaminants in the water when in high concentrations can present in a catastrophic nature with multiple patients on dialysis being affected simultaneously. Sudden onset of illness in multiple patients, in particular, symptoms of hemolysis and intoxication, should prompt consideration of water or dialysate contamination. Episodes of hemolytic anemia involving multiple patients have been witnessed in dialysis units where carbon tanks were exhausted or overwhelmed, sometimes during times of system upgrades or increased water demands. Exhausted deionization systems have been linked to copper and fluoride exposures. Exposures to disinfectants such as hydrogen peroxide and formaldehyde can result from incomplete or improper rinsing of water treatment systems after the disinfection procedure. Deleterious exposure to metals such as copper, lead, or brass in piping, fittings, or valves or aluminum in pumps used to transfer concentrates has occurred in case reports. Although case reports highlight drastic incidents of water contamination, it should also be recognized that exposure to contaminants in lower concentrations can manifest in atypical and subtle ways, which can be missed by health care providers. For example, chronic exposure to bacterial fragments like endotoxin may present

Table 10.2

Signs and Symptoms of Water Contamination

Contaminant	Signs and Symptoms of Exposure
Aluminum	Intoxication, seizures, neurologic symptoms, bone disease, anemia
Calcium	Confusion, lethargy, nausea, vomiting
Copper	Hemolysis, acidosis, nausea, seizure, shock
Chlorine/chloramines	Hemolysis, methemoglobinemia
Fluoride	Intoxication, pruritus, headache, nausea, chest pain, ventricular fibrillation
Lead	Neuropathy, anemia, abdominal pain, confusion, seizure
Nitrate	Methemoglobinemia, cyanosis
Sodium	Hypertension, thirst, pulmonary edema, confusion, seizure
Sulfate	Nausea, vomiting, chills, fever
Zinc	Nausea, vomiting, fever, anemia

Table 10.3

Steps in Developing Specifications for a Water Treatment System

Step	Procedure
1	Determine applications for which water will be used. Estimate water consumption and required delivery pressures.
2	Define product water quality for each application.
3	Evaluate quality of feed water.
4	Compare feed water quality with required product water quality and determine the reduction needed for each contaminant.
5	List water purification options and determine the preferred system configuration.
6	Prepare request for bids.

with signs of systemic inflammation that are difficult to distinguish from other disease processes. Table 10.2 lists some of the common water contaminants and the symptoms that they can cause.

Water purification systems in dialysis units should take care to address each potential contaminant in the source water. Equipment used for water purification should be designed with knowledge of the contaminants that are present in the source water. Tables 10.3 and 10.4 contain some suggested steps to take when planning a new water system and considerations for water system design. Table 10.5 provides a list of considerations to take into account regarding the maintenance and monitoring of water treatment systems.

Equipment Used for Water Purification

Multimedia Filter (Fig. 10.1)

The purpose of the multimedia filter, also known as the sediment filter or depth bed filter, is to remove particulate matter from the source water. Plant debris, rocks, rust,

Table 10.4	

Questions to Be Considered in Configuring a Water Treatment System

Step	Procedure
1	What purification processes are needed to produce water of the required purity?
2	How should the processes be sequenced to maximize efficiency and minimize maintenance?
3	How should the feed water be pretreated to prolong the life of the major purification equipment?
4	Is a supplementary water heater needed to maintain feed-water temperatures in the winter?
5	Should the distribution system include a storage tank?
6	What is the planned method of sterilization of the water treatment system?

silt, clay, and other debris are removed from water as it passes through the multimedia filter. Multimedia filters are usually composed of layers of gravel, sand, and anthracite. The water passes from larger gravel to finer sand and anthracite as it moves through the filter tank. Bigger particulate matter is trapped in the initial gravel layers and smaller particulates are trapped in the finer layers of sand and anthracite. Most multimedia filters are capable of removing particulate matter down to 10 microns in diameter. In some ways, this mechanism of water filtration is similar to what happens in nature as ground water filters down through the water table into an underground aquifer. The multimedia filter is usually the first filter that source water passes through. It is a necessary component of the water treatment system for the protection of the downstream water treatment components. For example, if particulate debris is not removed from the source water, it can end up fouling or damaging the reverse osmosis membrane.

Monitoring the Multimedia Filter

- With use, the multimedia filter can become obstructed with debris. To prevent this, the filter is backwashed daily at a time when patients are not on dialysis.
- Pressure gauges should be present pre and post filter to measure the difference between the two. If the filter is occluded with debris, the pressure drop will increase. The pressure difference (delta) across the filter should be monitored regularly. Trends in pressure changes should be established and investigated if abnormal.
- Pressure delta of >10 mm Hg above baseline across the multimedia filter indicates a problem.
- If automated systems are used for backwashing of the filter, backwash timers should be monitored regularly to ensure that rinsing of the filter occurs during off hours, when patients are not on dialysis.

Water Softener/Brine Tank (Fig. 10.2)

Groundwater can accumulate calcium and magnesium as it percolates through deposits of limestone or chalk. Water that has large amounts of calcium and magnesium can leave behind hard residue or scale. One example of this left-behind

Table 10.5

Water System Monitoring

Test	Acceptable Level	Recommended Frequency of Measurement
Total chlorine	≤0.1 PPM	Measured at the start of the day and every 4 hours
Free chlorine	<0.5 PPM	Measured at the start of the day and every 4 hours
Chloramine	<0.1 PPM	Measured at the start of the day and every 4 hours
Hardness	<1 GPG (17 PPM)	Measured at the end of every day
Component inflow vs outflow pressure delta	>10 mm Hg above baseline	Daily, delta trends compared with previous measurements and with baseline/initial values
EBCT	>10 min	Monthly and with any change in flow or carbon volume
Loop flow velocity	>3 ft/s (indirect) >1.5 ft/s (direct)	Daily, measured at the end of the loop when operating under peak demand
Water analysis (source/tap water and treated water)	See Table 10.1	Quarterly (annually at a bare minimum) Whenever water authorities change the composition of water or when the source of the water changes When the RO is installed When RO membranes are changed When % rejection drops below 90% (When performing water analysis, always recalculate RO alarm set points)
Colony count/total viable microbial count (TVC)	See Table 10.6	From loop: first station and last station in loop monthly. All stations at least once annually. RO and storage tanks at least quarterly, monthly is preferred. Dialysate: At least 2 machines monthly, every machine at least once annually
Endotoxin	See Table 10.6	Same as for colony count
Percent rejection	Based on water analysis, usually >90%	Continuously measured by RO
Percent recovery	Depends on facility, based on trends	Continuously measured by RO
DI resistivity	>1 MΩ·cm	Continuously measured by DI resistivity meter
UV energy output	>30 mW·s/cm^2 (>16 mW·s/cm^2 if UV calibrated meter)	Monthly, more frequently if nearing end of life span of UV bulb

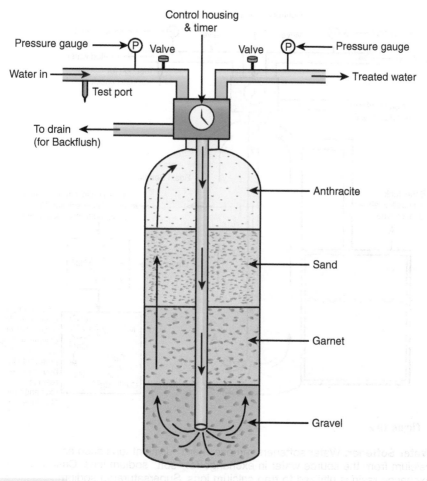

Figure 10.1

Multimedia Filter. The typical layout of a multimedia filter allows for the movement of water through a bed of particles of declining size. Multimedia filters are designed to trap particulate debris found in source water.

residue are water spots on a glass shower door. The hardness of water refers to its overall content of polyvalent ions that cause this scale, the major contributors being divalent calcium and magnesium. The process of "softening" the water is accomplished by the exchange of calcium and magnesium ions for sodium ions. Calcium and magnesium ions will be effectively removed through reverse osmosis (RO); however, the softening process is essential prior to water reaching the reverse osmosis unit to protect membranes from damage due to scaling. Additionally, in the case of systems that use deionization to form product water, presence of large amounts of divalent ions can overwhelm the deionizer resin beds leading to release of other toxic ions into the treated water. Water softener units are typically composed

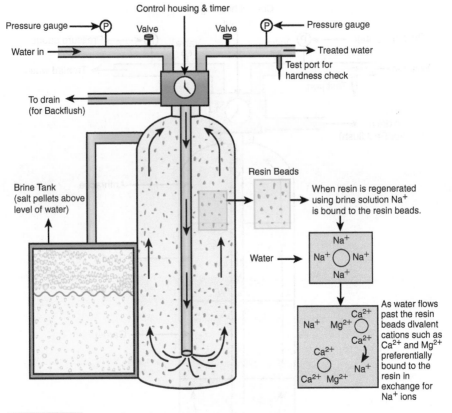

Figure 10.2

Water Softener. Water softeners remove "hard" divalent ions such as calcium from the source water in exchange for "soft" sodium ions. Cation exchange resin is ultilized to trap calcium ions. Supersaturated sodium solution from the brine tank is utilized to recharge the cation exchange resin.

of a tank that holds ion-exchange resin connected to a brine tank. As water moves through the softener tank, the resin releases sodium ions in exchange for higher-affinity divalent calcium and magnesium. The brine tank is used to hold a concentrated sodium chloride solution. Regeneration of the resin in the softener is accomplished by overcoming the affinity of the resin beads for polyvalent cations with a supersaturated sodium chloride solution from the brine tank. Recharging can be initiated on a timed basis or after a monitor, which measures a certain amount of water processed, indicates the need. Recharging should take place at a time when patients are not dialyzing to prevent accidental spillage of hypertonic sodium chloride solution into the water treatment system.

Monitoring the Water Softener

- Measurement of water hardness in grains per gallon (GPG) or parts per million (PPM) is used to monitor the efficiency of the water softener.

- Water hardness can be measured on site using colorimetric test strips. Personnel performing the testing should be able to distinguish between the colors on the test strips. There should be a well-labeled water sample port post water softener for the measurement of hardness.
- Source water hardness should be compared with treated water hardness periodically.
- After treatment by the water softener, the water should measure 1 GPG (17 PPM) or less.
- The hardness should be checked at the end of the day so that the capacity of the water softening system is fully appreciated.
- The brine tank should be checked daily to ensure that the solution is adequately supplied with sodium chloride (e.g., salt pellets are above the level of the water and are not forming a salt bridge).
- Pressure drop across the softener should be monitored regularly. Pressure change of >10 mm Hg above baseline suggests a problem with the resin bed.
- Regeneration of the softener resin should take place during a time when patients are not on dialysis.
- Timers set for automatic softener regeneration should be monitored to ensure that regeneration does not occur during facility operating hours. There is potential for high concentration of sodium to enter the water if regeneration occurs during dialysis treatments. Conductivity monitors on the RO system should sound an alarm if high sodium concentration is detected; however, they should not be relied upon exclusively.

Carbon Tanks (Fig. 10.3)

Activated carbon is used in water treatment systems to remove chlorine and chloramine from water. These agents are commonly added to the water supply by municipal authorities in small quantities in order to prevent microbiologic growth. Failure to remove chlorine and chloramines from treated water can lead to severe hemolytic anemia in patients on dialysis. Free chlorine has been known to degrade certain reverse osmosis membranes, leading to holes in the membranes and failure of appropriate filtration. Not all forms of carbon are equivalent. Powdered activated carbon has a large surface area in a smaller volume but is more prone to channeling and pressure problems, which reduce effectiveness. Granular activated carbon or catalytic carbon systems are more commonly used. Typically, water treatment systems are designed with a redundancy by placing two carbon tanks in series. The first tank is commonly referred to as the "worker" carbon. The second tank in series is known as the "polisher" carbon. The amount of carbon in the tanks must be considered in relation to the expected water flow through the tanks in order to ensure that there is a minimum of 5 minutes of contact time with the carbon for each tank or a total minimum of 10 minutes of contact time at the maximal expected water flows. Empty bed contact time (EBCT) can be used as an indirect way to estimate the contact time between the water and the carbon bed and is calculated using the following formula:

$$EBCT = V/Q$$

where V is the volume of carbon in the tank and Q is the flow rate. This equation can be used to calculate the EBCT in existing water treatment systems. Typically,

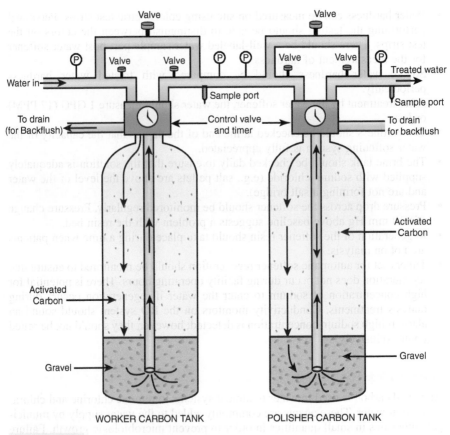

Figure 10.3

Carbon Tanks. The typical carbon tank layout has two tanks in series (worker followed by the polisher). The function of the carbon tanks is to remove chlorine and chloramines from the source water.

calculations would be done for a "worst case scenario" where every machine in the dialysis unit is in use, and demanding the maximum amount of water for production of dialysate and the Q in the equation would reflect the maximal flow needed to deliver water at the highest possible level of demand. In that way, even when water demands are stretched to capacity, EBCT of at least 10 minutes is ensured. Using units of cubic feet for volume and cubic feet per minute for flow, converting to gallons and solving for V yields the following equation:

$$V = (Q * \text{EBCT})/7.48$$

where 7.48 is the number of gallons in one cubic foot of water and Q is the flow rate in gallons per minute (GPM). This equation can be used when planning a water treatment system to estimate the volume of carbon you will need in the carbon tanks in order to achieve your EBCT goal of at least 10 minutes. Solving the above equation for EBCT, one can calculate the empty bed contact time under conditions of varying flow rates. This becomes important to do periodically because flow rates through RO membranes can change over time as the membranes age or with changing water conditions. For example, flows through RO membranes usually speed up in summer months as the water warms and becomes less viscous. This increase in flow through the RO can pull water through the carbon tanks more quickly and lead to decreased EBCT. EBCT must be calculated at least monthly to ensure changes over time are appreciated.

Monitoring the Carbon Tanks

- Testing for chlorine and chloramine is performed to monitor the function of the carbon tanks.
- The allowable limit for chlorine is 0.5 PPM and for chloramine 0.1 PPM.
- There is no way to directly test for chloramines. Indirectly, it can be measured by comparing the difference between the total chlorine and free chlorine.

chloramine level = total chlorine level – free chlorine level

- Most units do not check both free and total chlorine. It is acceptable and simpler to test only total chlorine with an allowable limit of <0.1 PPM.
- Chlorine tests are usually done with colorimetric strips. Personnel performing the tests should be able to distinguish differences in color change.
- Alternatively, on-line monitors can be used in accordance with manufacturer's specifications.
- The testing should be done after the first carbon tank (worker) from a well-labeled sample port. If the worker sample is not acceptable, then the water should be tested from a sample port following the second carbon tank (polisher). If the polisher sample is acceptable, then dialysis can continue but plans should be made to replace the failing worker carbon tank and consideration should be given to increasing the frequency of testing while running on a single tank. If the sample post polisher does not meet the allowable limit, then dialysis cannot continue until the problem is fixed.
- Testing should be performed at the start of the day and every 4 hours while patients are on dialysis.
- Testing at the start of the day should occur after allowing the system to run for 15 minutes.
- The carbon tanks must supply an EBCT of at least 10 minutes. The EBCT should be calculated periodically to ensure that the goal is met. In addition, changes in water flow (such as when adding stations to a unit) or carbon tank volume should prompt a recalculation of the EBCT.
- Pressure drop across each of the carbon tanks should be monitored with >10 mmHg difference above baseline, suggesting a problem such as fouling of the tank with particulate matter.
- Back-flushing of the carbon tanks should occur during hours when the facility is not in operation. Timers set for automatic back-flushing should be monitored regularly to ensure that they are set to the correct time.
- The risk for patient injury when the carbon tanks fail is high. Therefore, rigorous monitoring and routine recording and review of the function of the carbon tanks are mandatory.

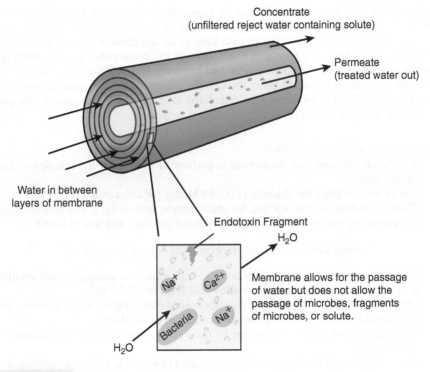

Figure 10.4

Reverse Osmosis. The reverse osmosis membrane typically has a tight
spiral configuration that allows water to pass but traps solute particles.
The permeate is the purified water, and the concentrate is the waste
or brine solution.

Reverse Osmosis (Fig. 10.4)

Reverse osmosis (RO) is a process by which pressure is used to force water through
a tight membrane that blocks passage of solute, particulate matter, bacteria, and endotoxins, among other things, to produce pure water. The water that is filtered by the
RO membrane is called product water, permeate, or filtrate; the leftover water and
solute that does not pass through the membrane is referred to as reject water, waste
water, or concentrate. The term *osmosis* describes the movement of water that occurs
when two compartments are separated by a semipermeable membrane whereby water
moves from an area of low solute concentration to an area of high solute concentration. During the reverse osmosis process, water is forced in the opposite direction or
against an osmotic gradient by using pressure, thus the term *reverse osmosis*. The
amount of energy or pressure needed to overcome osmotic pressure depends on the
ionic content (conductivity) of the source water. The RO system will require roughly
10 psi per 1000 ppm of solute. Thus, reverse osmosis is very reliant on energy to
produce a pressure gradient across the membrane, and the amount of energy required
will increase with increasing conductivity of the source water. RO systems typically
consist of pre-filters, pumps, flow and pressure controls, membranes (typically spiral-
wound membranes), and various monitors. As water flows parallel along the

membrane, a portion of the water is forced through the membrane and into the product water stream whereas the remainder that does not pass the membrane is directed to the drain or recycled. Orienting the flow of permeate and concentrate in this way allows for a natural process of continuous flushing of the membrane and avoidance of membrane fouling. Some RO systems will recycle the reject water stream and reroute it past the membrane to increase velocity through the membrane system and further prevent membrane fouling or failure. Reverse osmosis systems are very effective at producing water appropriate for dialysate production; however, they are complicated systems that require close monitoring and regular maintenance. Efficiency of the RO system is affected by a number of factors including pressure in the system, composition of the feed water, temperature of the feed water, and level of dissolved gases in the feed water. Often water treatment systems are designed with redundancy by placing two RO units in the water treatment system. This is known as a "double-stage" RO system. Whether or not a double- or single-stage RO system is necessary depends in large part on the quality of the source water. In most cases where source water is of reasonable quality, double-stage RO systems are not necessary to produce pure water but they are still desired for the purpose of supplying redundancy. In the event that one RO is not functional, the other RO can be utilized and patient care can continue. Alternatively, some water treatment systems will use reverse osmosis as the primary method of water treatment and deionization systems for polishing or as a backup in case of failure of the RO.

Monitoring the RO System

- Pressure and flow are measured at various points in the RO system to ensure proper function.
- Conductivity is used to monitor the removal of solute by the RO system. Conductivity describes the ability of the water to conduct electrical charge. If more dissolved solute is present, water will conduct electricity more readily.
- The conductivity of product water from the RO is monitored continuously during RO operation and often displayed as total dissolved solids or TDS.
- The percent rejection of an RO system describes the ability of the system to remove solute, thus reducing conductivity in the product water, and can be thought of as the percentage of solute that was removed from the water during reverse osmosis. The percent rejection is calculated using the following formula:

$$\% \text{ rejection} = [(\text{feed water conductivity} - \text{product water conductivity})/ \text{feed water conductivity}] * 100$$

- Modern RO systems will monitor and display the percent rejection in real time during operation.
- There is no absolute value that is desirable for the percent rejection. Rather, the dialysis facility should use the percent rejection to monitor the efficiency of the RO over time.
- The dialysis facility should take into account the source water composition, the percent nominal passage through the RO of each of the water contaminants with the given RO specifications from the manufacturer, the composition of the treated permeate water and, based on these values, calculate the lowest percent rejection at which the treated water still meets AAMI requirements as listed in Table 10.1. Alarms set points can then be established on the RO system when the desired % rejection is not achieved.

- Percent recovery (also known as the water conversion factor) can be used to monitor the performance of the RO system. The percent recovery can be calculated using the following formula, where Q is the flow rate:

$$\% \text{ recovery} = [\text{permeate } Q/(\text{permeate } Q + \text{reject } Q)] * 100$$

- The percent recovery does not inform water quality. Rather, it is useful for trending the performance of the RO membrane. Membranes that become fouled over time will drop their percent recovery. Permeate flow rate can vary due to changes in pressure and temperature as well. For example, a seasonal decrease in water temperature would be expected to decrease the percent recovery.
- The various measures of RO function—pressure, flow, conductivity, % rejection, % recovery, etc.—should be recorded in a daily treatment log for regular review and trending analysis.

Deionization (Fig. 10.5)

Deionization is a method by which water can be purified of cationic and anionic components using exchange resins. The resins in DI systems are essentially beads with either hydrogen (H^+) cations attached or hydroxyl (OH^-) anions attached. When higher-affinity cations from the feed water come in contact with the cation resin, H^+ ions are released and the higher-affinity cation is bound to the resin. Likewise, when anions in the feed water come in contact with the anion resin, OH^- anions are released and the anion is bound to the resin. Subsequently, H+ and OH^- are available to combine and form pure water (H_2O). Deionization systems can be set up in a two-stage process as dual-bed systems, where the cation and anion resins reside in separate tanks, or as mixed-bed systems, where the resins are combined in a single tank. Most commonly, deionizer systems consist of two mixed-bed systems in series with resistivity or conductivity monitors following each unit. The deionization system for dialysis water when operated and maintained correctly can provide product water of high quality. However, there are several limitations to deionizers. Deionizer systems have a limited life span. Once ionic resin sites are saturated, product water can become contaminated. This is because ions of lesser affinity which are not H^+ or OH^- can be released from the resin in exchange for higher-affinity ions. Multiple cases have been reported where anionic resin was depleted and fluoride (F^-) ions were released into product water as chloride (Cl^-) and other anions bound with the resin in higher affinity and displaced the F^- ions, leading to fluoride intoxication in the dialysis unit. Even partially exhausted DI resins can be a source of water contamination. Therefore, close monitoring of these systems is essential to protect patient safety. Exchange resins need to be regenerated periodically to prevent contamination from happening. During the regeneration process, strong acid and strong base is added to the ion beds to regenerate the resin with H^+ and OH^- ions and flush out previously bound ions. Unlike RO systems, deionization systems do not effectively remove particulate matter, bacteria, endotoxin, and other organic materials from the source water. Therefore, DI systems must be combined with other water treatment components. In particular, DI systems can serve as a breeding ground for bacteria. Deionizers that are used as backup systems can have absent or reduced water flow and are particularly prone to bacterial contamination. Downstream ultrafilters or cartridge filters capable of retaining endotoxin and fine resin

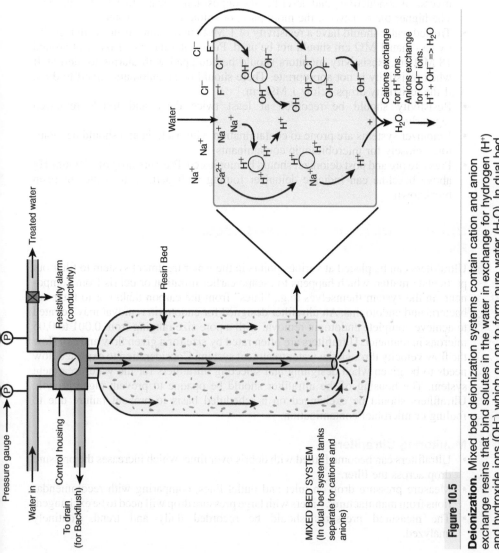

Figure 10.5

Deionization. Mixed bed deionization systems contain cation and anion exchange resins that bind solutes in the water in exchange for hydrogen (H^+) and hydroxide ions (OH^-) which go on to form pure water (H_2O). In dual bed systems (not shown) cation and anion exchange resins are in separate tanks.

debris should be in place to protect the loop from bacterial contamination originating in the DI tanks.

Monitoring the DI System

- Deionizers are monitored continuously using a resistivity meter. Resistivity is the inverse of conductivity and describes the opposition of water to electrical current. The higher the resistivity, the more pure, or solute-poor, the water.
- Treated water should have a resistivity of 1 MΩ cm or more. Water with resistivity less than 1 MΩ cm should not be used. Pure water has a resistivity of around 18 MΩ cm. Resistivity monitors should be equipped with alarms to alert staff when resistivity is not appropriate. There should be an automatic divert to drain if the resistivity drops below 1 MΩ cm.
- Resistivity should be recorded at least twice daily and trends reviewed regularly.
- Deionizer systems are prone to contamination with bacteria and should be monitored closely for microbiologic contaminants.
- Pressure pre and post deionizer should be monitored. Pressure drop of >10 mm Hg above baseline can indicate deionizer fouling with particulate matter or resin breakdown.

Ultrafilters/Cartridge Filters/Endotoxin Retentive Filters

Ultrafilters can be placed at various points in the water treatment system to filter out particulate matter, which happens to escape earlier filtration or debris from components in the system themselves (e.g., "fines" from the carbon tanks) or to filter out bacteria and endotoxins. An ultrafilter designed for endotoxin removal may be rated to achieve complete endotoxin removal with a pore size ranging from 0.001 to 0.05 microns in diameter. Ultrafilters are often rated by size for a given flow and can slow the flow velocity through the water treatment system. Consideration to expected flow needs to be given when designing and selecting ultrafilters for the water treatment system. The housing of the ultrafilter should be opaque to prevent algae growth. Ultrafilters should be exchanged on a scheduled basis to prevent failure due to fouling or microbial contamination.

Monitoring Ultrafilters

- Ultrafilters can become fouled with debris over time, which increases the pressure drop across the filter.
- Measure pressure drop on inlet and outlet lines, comparing with recommendations from manufacturer. Filters with large pressure drop will need to be exchanged.
- The measured pressures should be recorded daily and trends routinely analyzed.

Ultraviolet Lights

Ultraviolet (UV) light can be used in a water treatment system to control microbiologic growth. UV lights typically are composed of a quartz glass sleeve through which the water flows with a UV bulb overlying the sleeve. It is recommended that the UV light is applied at a wavelength of 254 nm and provides 30 mW·s/cm^2 of energy. UV light housings should be opaque. The UV lights are rated for flow. Thus, flow that is too fast may not allow for effective exposure of the water to UV light. When properly functioning, UV lights are capable of killing all potential free pathogens in the water stream, but it is important to recognize that UV light may not be effective in treating organisms imbedded in biofilm. UV lights should be followed by an ultrafilter that is capable of retaining bacteria and endotoxin.

Monitoring of UV Lights
- UV lights are monitored with a radiant energy meter that measures on-line energy intensity and is capable of alarming if the intensity is not sufficient.
- If the irradiator is not fitted with a calibrated ultraviolet intensity meter that is filtered to restrict its sensitivity to the disinfection spectrum, the dose of radiant energy provided by the lamp should be at least 30 mW·s/cm^2. If it does have a calibrated meter, the minimum dose of radiant energy should be at least 16 mW·s/cm^2. This requirement is meant to prevent development of microbial resistance.
- UV light intensity checks should be recorded daily and routinely reviewed.

Water Distribution Loop (Fig. 10.6)

The ideal water distribution loop would be composed of a biocompatible material that does not leach into the water, is smooth without ridges or gaps, and does not have any dead space where water is left stagnant. Accomplishing these criteria will promote flow velocity and prevent microbiologic adhesion and biofilm formation. Systems should be designed with the least amount of joints and fittings possible. Gradual bends are preferred over 90-degree turns. Flow through the loop ideally should be at least 3 ft/s to prevent bacterial biofilm formation. Piping systems and fittings can be made of polyvinyl chloride (PVC) or cross-linked polyethylene (PEX), among other materials. Care should be taken to understand the means of disinfection and how that affects the piping materials. For example, PVC is not compatible with heat sterilized disinfection systems. Water should run through the loop continually, and points of connection for the dialysis machine to the water source ideally would be designed as a loop with continuous flow and minimal dead space. Two types of water distribution loops include direct feed systems and indirect feed systems. Fig. 10.5 illustrates a direct feed system. With direct feed, there is no storage tank; water runs through the system directly to the loop. Water that is not consumed in the loop then returns back to the RO. In an indirect feed system, there is a storage tank that holds water, which is then pumped to the loop. Water not used in the loop then returns to the storage tank. The direct feed system can be simpler in that it does not require the storage tank and extra components that the storage tank demands; however, it has to be designed carefully with water needs in mind, and all components of the water treatment system need to be able to keep up with demand at peak times. Depending on the size of the unit, this sometimes makes direct feed systems impossible. In indirect feed systems, water can be produced and stored to meet demand at peak times, thereby overcoming this limitation. However, the presence of a large storage tank provides another source for microbiologic contamination of the loop.

Monitoring the Water Distribution Loop
- Flow velocity through the loop should be at least 3 ft/s for indirect systems and at least 1.5 ft/s in direct systems. Flow velocity is calculated using the following formula $V = Q/A$, where V is the flow velocity, Q is the flow, and A is the cross-sectional area of the pipe.

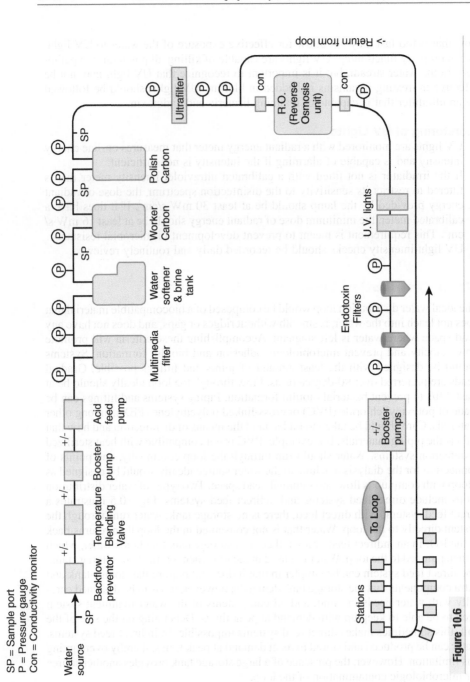

Figure 10.6

Water Distribution Loop (Direct Feed System). Potential layout of a direct feed system for water purification in a dialysis center. Indirect feed systems

- Flow rate should be measured at the end of the loop during peak usage.
- Regular flow rate measurements can be used to calculate flow velocity to ensure that the velocity is meeting requirements. Measurements should be documented for routine review.

Other Water Treatment Components

Backflow preventer: The initial component of the water treatment system, it consists of check valves that prevent water from moving backward from the water treatment system and into the plumbing of the building. This device is necessary to protect the plumbing of the building from contamination in the event of sudden loss of water pressure.

Temperature-blending valve: Decreasing temperature will increase the viscosity of water, which can have an effect on the efficiency of the RO membrane in the water treatment system. Temperature-blending valves can be used to maintain feed water temperature that is ideal for membrane performance. As an example, some RO membranes are rated for a temperature of 77°F, and the temperature-blending valve may be set between 60°F and 85°F to achieve best performance. The temperature-blending valve is more crucial in northern climates in the winter when dropping temperature may lead to the inability of RO to keep up with water demand. When temperature-blending valves fail, water temperature can rise quickly. Water temperature should be monitored and recorded at least daily when using temperature-blending valves. Trends in temperature fluctuation can indicate a failing valve.

Acid feed system: Water treatment components such as the RO and chlorine tanks function best at a pH of 7–8. Source water pH greater than 8.5 can be corrected with an acid feed system by adding inorganic acid to lower the pH. Conversely, systems to alkalinize the water can be added in cases where the pH is too low. Typically acidic water is not a problem because water municipalities will alkalinize the water to protect metal plumbing systems. When using acid feed systems, pH should be monitored with an on-line continuous monitor fitted with an alarm or tested at least daily if using test strips. The measured pH should be between 7 and 8.

Booster pumps: Booster pumps are often needed to maintain pressure and flow velocity throughout the system. Booster pumps are controlled by pressure or flow switches and activate when water pressure or flow drops below a set level. If city water pressure is not high enough, a booster pump may be required to feed the RO. Booster pumps should be monitored periodically to ensure that they are turning on and off at the appropriate pressures or flow rates.

Drain system: The drainage system must be capable of supporting maximal flow from all water treatment system components and should have an air break or some other means to prevent backflow of sewer water into the treatment system should there be an obstruction to flow in the sewer main. Drain systems can sometimes become malodorous. Acetate in spent dialysate can attract fruit flies. Treating the drain line with bleach can be an effective remedy.

Monitoring for Microbiologic Contamination

Water treatment systems for hemodialysis are under the constant threat of microbial contamination. Testing for bacteria and endotoxin in the water treatment system should take place at least monthly. Crucial components of the water treatment system such as the first station in the loop, last station in the loop, the RO, and storage tanks should be tested monthly. During times of contamination, when testing standards are not met, testing frequency should increase to at least weekly. Each dialysis station in the loop should be sampled at least annually. Samples should be collected just before scheduled disinfection and no sooner than 24 hours after disinfection. Samples from the loop should be collected in a "clean catch" manner after allowing the sample port to be rinsed for 1 minute. Loop sample ports should not be disinfected prior to sampling. Around 50 mL placed in a sterile endotoxin-free container is usually necessary. Dialysate from each dialysis machine should be collected at least annually with at least two machines sampled every month. Dialysate samples are drawn from a sample port in the dialysate line, which can be sterilized with alcohol and which is allowed to dry prior to placing a sterile syringe on the sample port and extracting 30 mL of dialysate for testing.

Special culture media should be used by the lab that is conducive to the growth of fastidious water-borne organisms (tryptone glucose extract agar or Reasoner's agar). Endotoxin levels are measured using the LAL assay. Methods used by the laboratory for culture count and endotoxin levels should be appropriately validated. All testing results should be recorded on a log sheet and trends analyzed regularly, in the context of the loop design, to identify and locate any problems that may exist with contamination of the water treatment components.

Bacteria and endotoxin levels should not exceed values listed in Table 10.6. If the action level is reached, the dialysis unit should have a plan in place to address the contamination, and subsequent testing should follow to ensure that the plan was effective. Corrective action for positive culture counts or high endotoxin levels can include:

- Increasing the frequency of water testing
- Increasing the number of sites tested
- Disinfection and cleaning of the RO
- Loop disinfection
- Increasing the frequency of disinfection
- Installing an endotoxin retentive filter
- Confirming that endotoxin retentive filters are not failing or contaminated
- Confirming that no dead spots exist in the loop plumbing
- Confirming that the water supply line connecting the machine to the loop is properly disinfected during loop disinfection.
- Ensuring that proper disinfection procedures are followed

Table 10.6

Recommended Maximum Allowable Levels for Total Viable Microbial Count (TVC, Also Known as Colony Count) and Endotoxins in Dialysis Water

	Maximum Allowable Level	Action Level	Ultrapure Dialysate
TVC	<100 CFU/mL	50 CFU/mL	<0.1 CFU/mL
Endotoxin	<0.25 EU/mL	0.125 EU/mL	<0.03 EU/mL

(ISO 13959, AAMI 2011)

Routine disinfection of the water treatment system must be performed at a minimum every month. Monthly disinfection of the loop should include a disinfection of the machine supply lines that are not routinely disinfected during the machine disinfection cycle. Water treatment systems can be heat sterilized or chemicals such as peroxide or formaldehyde can be used. If chemical disinfection is utilized, after the water treatment system is disinfected and rinsed, the water must be tested for residual chemicals. The disinfection process and testing should be clearly and completely documented and reviewed monthly.

C H A P T E R 1 1

Methods and Complications of Dialyzer Reuse

Paweena Susantitaphong, MD, PhD • Bertrand L. Jaber, MD, MS

Background and Rationale

Dialyzer reprocessing or reuse is a technique that has historically been employed in the United States for perceived potential benefits to the dialysis facilities and patients. The three main justifications for dialysis facilities include an economic benefit, the ability to use high-flux dialyzers, which historically have been more expensive, and a favorable environmental impact through decreased generation of biomedical waste. From the patients' standpoint, the conventional argument for reprocessing dialyzers has been to improve blood-membrane biocompatibility, particularly that of cellulose dialyzers, which have a high complement activation potential, and the prevention of first-use syndromes usually associated with the use of ethylene oxide–sterilized dialyzers. Such medical justifications are no longer applicable because the landscape of dialyzers and dialysis membranes has changed significantly over the past several decades. Unmodified cellulosic membranes are no longer used in the United States and have been replaced by dialyzers manufactured with more biocompatible (with lower complement activation potential) membranes, including substituted cellulose and synthetic polymers (eg, polysulfone and polyethersulfone), which can be sterilized using a number of new methods, rather than using ethylene oxide, including gamma irradiation, and steam and electron beam sterilization. Furthermore, substituted cellulose and synthetic dialyzer membranes are promoted by clinical practice guidelines, and the current widespread availability of cheaper high-flux dialyzers for single use, means that the traditional benefit of the ability to reuse such dialyzers no longer holds true. Although the medical arguments for dialyzer reprocessing no longer have validity, the economic considerations remain the driving force for the continued practice of dialyzer reuse in the United States, partly driven by a steady decline in reimbursement for provision of hemodialysis treatments.

Although dialyzer reuse remains a topic of ongoing controversy, it can be performed safely in accordance with the standards set by the Association for the Advancement of Medical Instrumentation (AAMI). Full compliance in a practical setting, however, is difficult to attain, and rigorous quality control standards are vulnerable to poor implementation.

This chapter reviews the current status of dialyzer reuse, dialyzer reuse methods, the effects of reprocessing on dialyzer performance, and a comparison of dialyzer reuse versus single use in terms of patient outcomes and environmental consequences.

Current Status of Dialyzer Reuse in the United States

The methods and frequency of dialyzer reuse have continuously evolved over the past three decades. In 1976, 18% of dialysis centers in the United States reprocessed dialyzers, using exclusively formaldehyde as the disinfectant or germicide and bleach as the cleaning agent. At that time, dialyzer reprocessing was largely performed manually (ie, without the use of an automated reprocessing machine). Between the early 1980s and the end of the 20th century, dialyzer reuse increased in popularity, peaking at greater than 80% of all dialysis facilities in the late 1990s. During that period, Renalin (a mixture of peracetic acid, acetic acid, and hydrogen peroxide) became the dominantly used germicide, and automated reprocessing machines became more common.

In the 2002 annual survey by the Centers for Disease Control and Prevention, 63% of dialysis facilities in the United Sates reused dialyzers, with 76% using peracetic acid, 20% using formaldehyde, and 4% using other methods of disinfection. In 2005, a study estimated that 61% of dialysis patients in the United States were treated with single-use dialyzers. Although there are no recent prevalence data on dialyzer reuse, since the early 2000, as integrated dialysis service providers started shifting toward single-use dialyzers, the proportion of for-profit dialysis facilities practicing reuse is estimated to have significantly declined.

Dialyzer Reuse Methods

The exact procedures used in the reprocessing of dialyzers depend on several factors. However, the basic essential steps are similar.

A schematic diagram describing these steps is shown in Fig. 11.1. A detailed step-by-step description of the reprocessing of dialyzers, including transportation

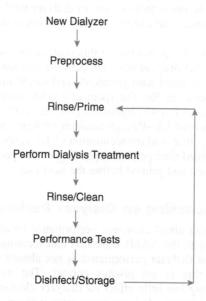

Figure 11.1

and handling, rinsing and cleaning, performance measurements, blood path integrity test, disinfection/germicidal process of the blood and dialysate compartments, dialyzer inspection, testing for residual germicide, and strict quality assurance, monitoring and recording is outside the scope of this chapter and can be reviewed in the AAMI standards.

The National Kidney Foundation clinical practice guidelines on hemodialysis recommend that each new dialyzer be preprocessed to obtain an accurate estimate of the total cell (or fiber bundle) volume of a given dialyzer before first use. Although this is not a routine practice at dialysis facilities, it is felt to be more reliable than trusting manufacturers' reported average volume or an average volume from a given batch of dialyzers—as there may be lot-to-lot variability in the total cell volume of dialyzers.

After preprocessing, the dialyzer is rinsed and primed. An important step in both preprocessing and reprocessing is to ensure that the residual germicide has been completely removed from the dialyzer before patient use. The dialyzer can then be connected safely to the patient and the dialysis treatment performed. Several technical factors that may cause thrombosis during or immediately after completion of the hemodialysis treatment can affect the number of times a dialyzer is reused. These include the dose of heparin, presence of air within the dialysis circuit, the blood level within the drip chambers, and appropriate placement of dialysis needles. After the end of the hemodialysis treatment, the dialyzer is rinsed and transported to the reuse room—where it is extensively rinsed. This rinsing and cleaning process may involve the use of a chemical agent, such as bleach or hydrogen peroxide.

The next step is to test the dialyzer to ensure that its performance is similar to that of a new dialyzer. The main performance test is to measure the total cell volume. If the total cell volume is between 80% and 120% of its initial value, small solute (eg, urea) clearances for this dialyzer are likely between 90% and 110% of their initial values. It should be noted that this test of dialyzer total cell volume does not evaluate other performance characteristics, such as middle-molecule solute clearances (see below).

A pressure/leak test is also performed at this stage to ensure that the integrity of the dialyzer is intact. If the dialyzer does not pass the required test, it is discarded. Otherwise, the dialyzer is filled with germicide and stored until the next use. The most common germicides are Renalin (peracetic acid concentration of 4%–6%, acetic acid concentration 8%–10%, hydrogen peroxide 20%–24%), formaldehyde or formalin (concentration of 1%–4%), glutaraldehyde (concentration of 0.8%), and heated water containing citric acid (concentration of 1.5%, reserved for polysulfone dialyzers). After a specified time period, depending on the germicide used, the dialyzer is ready to be rinsed and primed before the next use.

Effects of Reprocessing on Dialyzer Performance

Dialyzer reprocessing can affect clearance performance by altering the membrane permeability. According to the AAMI standards and recommended practices, it is commonly assumed that dialyzer performance is not altered when reprocessing is performed. However, this is not always correct. The available data suggest that dialyzer reprocessing has little effect on dialyzer clearance for small solutes. Heparin modeling can improve dialyzer reuse rates without compromising on the delivered dose of dialysis. The National Kidney Foundation Task Force on Reuse of Dialyzers recommends that for patients who reuse dialyzers, measurement of Kt/V_{urea} or determination of the urea reduction ratio be conducted at least monthly to estimate dialyzer performance. However, middle-molecule and large-solute removal by high-flux dialyzers may be substantially altered, with dialyzer performance changes varying as a function of both the dialyzer membrane and the reprocessing germicide.

Reprocessing Using Bleach

Reprocessing of high-flux dialyzers containing polysulfone membranes using bleach and formaldehyde has been shown to increase the removal of middle molecules and other large-molecular-weight substances as the number of reuses increases. One possible mechanism for altered dialysis membrane permeability is that bleach may lead to the loss of polyvinylpyrrolidone (PVP) from the dialyzer membrane. PVP, a wetting agent used as a copolymer in the production of some synthetic dialyzer membranes, imparts hydrophilicity to the membrane and constrains pore dimensions.

Loss of PVP (eg, when using bleach) potentially results in a more hydrophobic membrane with larger pores. The clearance of β_2-microglobulin (MW = 11.8 kilodaltons) increases approximately twofold after 10 bleach reuses of a high-flux polysulfone dialyzer compared to first use. Early studies also demonstrate that as the number of bleach reuses of a dialyzer containing high-flux polysulfone membranes exceeds a certain number (approximate 10 reuses), membrane pore size becomes so large that substances as large as albumin (MW = 66 kilodaltons) appear in the dialysate (with up to 20 g of intra-dialytic loss of albumin). It is no longer recommended that dialyzers containing high-flux polysulfone membranes tested in these early studies be reprocessed using bleach.

Subsequently, Fresensius Medical Care North America (FMC-NA) manufactured two different high-flux dialyzers for repeated use in the United States: the F80B dialyzer for reprocessing with bleach and the F80A dialyzer for reprocessing with other germicides. Similar different versions of more recent dialyzers (Optiflux 200B and 200A) are also available. Depending on the conditions during reprocessing, it is theoretically possible for dialytic albumin loss to occur. However, recent findings indicate that this is no longer a significant clinical concern. The specific disinfectant used in conjunction with bleach significantly influences the permeability changes of a high-flux dialyzer membrane. Data from a large trial (the HEMO Study) indicate that the increase in dialyzer membrane permeability occurring during successive bleach and formaldehyde reprocessing is similar when using bleach and Renalin (peracetic acid/acetic acid/hydrogen peroxide mixture) as the germicide, but not when using bleach and glutaraldehyde.

Reprocessing Using Peracetic Acid

Reprocessing using peracetic acid (without bleach) causes a decrease in the removal of middle molecules by high-flux dialyzers as the number of reuses increases. However, this effect is dependent on the type of dialyzer membrane. For example, the decrease in clearances of β_2-microglobulin observed in the HEMO Study was approximately 50% after four reuses for dialyzers containing high-flux cellulose triacetate membranes but insignificant for those containing polysulfone membranes.

This might be related to the failure of peracetic acid to remove proteins that have adsorbed to dialyzer membranes during contact with blood during dialysis. Proteins that adsorb to the membrane after each blood contact are fixed and can continuously accumulate within the membrane pore structure to increase the resistance to transmembrane transport of middle molecules.

The protein accumulation also decreases the water or hydraulic permeability of the dialyzer membrane but has little impact on small-solute clearances, suggesting that the adsorbed proteins foul or clog the pore structure but do not make the dialyzer membrane appreciably thicker. The resultant effect of protein adsorption, therefore, is a decrease in the removal of middle molecules. The effect of peracetic acid reprocessing on β_2-microglobulin clearances has been carefully studied in the HEMO Study because middle-molecule removal was one of the primary interventions during that trial.

Reprocessing Using Heat

The potential pitfalls encountered with chemical reprocessing of dialyzers have prompted the use of alternative reuse methods. Albeit used in only a small portion of dialysis facilities, reprocessing with heated water merits mention. To date, only dialyzers containing polysulfone membranes have been used in published studies using heat reprocessing. The first studies using heat alone (ie, 105°C for 20 hours) yielded concern for dialyzer integrity (eg, casing and resin leaks) at these high temperatures. The specific mechanisms for these findings are not known, although it is thought to involve the direct effects of heat on the casing and potting compounds of the dialyzer.

To better maintain membrane integrity, more recent studies have used modified heat reprocessing techniques—specifically, 1.5% citric acid in water heated to 95°C for 20 hours. Early studies concluded that heated citric acid reprocessing of dialyzers containing high-flux polysulfone membranes results in a modest increase in membrane permeability, thereby enhancing the removal of β_2-microglobulin without a corresponding increase in albumin loss. These findings were corroborated in the HEMO Study. A limitation of heat reprocessing is that the maximum number of reuses is limited to approximately 15 reuses, well below the typical values for other chemical-based reuse techniques. Consequently, the overall impact of heat reprocessing on dialyzer performance may also be less.

In summary, dialyzer reprocessing can alter dialyzer performance. Alterations in the clearance of small solutes as a result of dialyzer reprocessing are minor. Alterations in the clearance of middle molecules as a result of dialyzer reprocessing can be substantial. However, the clinical significance of these changes remains unclear.

Dialyzer Reuse Versus Single-Use Comparisons

Comparisons of clinical outcomes among patients using single-use dialyzers with those using reused dialyzers have been performed by numerous investigators over the past 30 years. Early comparisons in the late 1980s suggested that mortality was higher among patients who reused dialyzers with some germicides but not with others. Additional studies in the early 1990s, however, could not consistently reproduce these findings. Studies in the late 1990s suggested that mortality was lower in patients who reused dialyzers using bleach during reprocessing. These studies are not directly comparable because of differences in dialyzer reprocessing procedures and germicides, as well as differences in dialyzer membranes that have occurred over this time period.

In 2011, two observational studies comparing reused and single-use dialyzers reached distinctly different conclusions. In one study, abandoning peracetic acid–based dialyzer reuse was associated with improved patient survival, whereas the second study showed no impact of dialyzer reuse with peracetic acid on mortality. A recent systematic review of 14 observational studies was inconclusive regarding the safety of dialyzer reuse practices.

The differences in patient survival between reused and single-use dialyzers reported in observational studies are very small (less than 10%), and statistical significance was not achieved in all analyses. Potential biases inherent to these observational studies include lack of adjustment for possible confounders such as patient factors (eg, comorbid conditions, nutritional status, dialysis duration), and dialysis facility–related factors (eg, clustering of patients in various dialysis centers, dialyzer membrane type, and number of reuses).

Other differences between reused and single-use dialyzers are listed in Table 11.1. First, there is a concern over potential acute systemic toxicity of the infusion of chemicals into the patient. Reuse of dialyzers potentially exposes patients to residual amounts of germicides during each dialysis treatment, if not fully rinsed off, whereas single-use dialyzers potentially expose patients to very small quantities of leachable organic compounds that may not be completely removed during dialyzer manufacturing. These risks are small and are difficult to quantify because they will only likely become apparent after repeated exposure and there is no published data on these potential long-term consequences.

Second is the concern over the reliability of dialyzer sterility. The integrity of the reused dialyzer is the responsibility of the dialysis provider, whereas the integrity of the single-use dialyzer is ensured by the manufacturer. Several factors that are operative during dialysis place patients at risk for exposure to bacteria and/or bacterial products, including improperly reprocessed dialyzers. Clusters of bacterial infection in dialysis patients ascribed to bacterial contamination during dialyzer reuse are displayed in Table 11.2. The passage of endotoxin from the dialysate into the blood can occur by diffusion or convection. The use of high-flux dialyzers that have been reprocessed with bleach (which increases the permeability of the membrane) increases the risk of passage of bacterial endotoxin from the dialysate into the blood, which can produce transient febrile reactions. Reports of pyrogenic reactions with or without bacteremia (typically due to water-borne bacteria) due to dialyzer reuse have been attributed to improper disinfection procedures, inadequate potency of the

Table 11.1		
Differences Between Dialyzer Reuse and Single Use		
Concern	**Reuse**	**Single Use**
Acute systemic toxicity	Residual germicide	Leachable toxic substances
Dialyzer sterility/disinfection	Dialysis provider	Dialyzer manufacturer
Environmental disposal	Germicide waste	Plastic medical waste

Table 11.2

Pyrogenic Reactions and Reported Bacterial Infections Related to Dialyzer Reuse

Causative Agents	Identifiable Sources of Contamination	Manifestations
Bacterial Products		
Lipopolysaccharide	Dialysate backfiltration of soluble bacterial products in the setting of highly reprocessed high-flux dialyzers	Pyrogen reaction without bacteremia
Bacteria		
Klebsiella pneumoniae	Dialyzer O-ring (seal	Bacteremia
Acinetobacter species	between the end cap and	
Enterobacter species	the potting material)	
Bacillus species and	Low levels of disinfectant	
Achromobacter	Inadequate mixing of	
Stenotrophomonas maltophilia	disinfectant with tap water	
and *Burkholderia cepacia*	Inadequate potency of disinfectant despite standard measures	
	Highly reprocessed (15 reuses) dialyzers	
Mycobacteria		
Mycobacterium chelonae	Inadequate potency of	Mycobacteremia
abscessus	disinfectant despite	Soft tissue infection
	standard measures	Arteriovenous graft infection

solution used to disinfect the dialyzer, inadequate measures to disinfect the O-rings of dialyzers with removable headers, and the frequency of dialyzer reuse. In a survey by the Centers for Disease Control and Prevention in the United States, the incidence of pyrogenic reactions in the absence of bacteremia was reported by 19% of dialysis centers, and the use of high-flux reprocessed dialyzers was associated with a higher risk of these reactions. An outbreak of bacteremia among several patients involving a similar organism should prompt a thorough search for bacterial contamination of the dialysis equipment, as well as assessment of the integrity of the dialyzer reuse process. Recent data and commentary by the CDC suggests that dialysis providers should consider instituting less frequent reuse or non-reuse of dialyzers in the interest of patient safety. Facilities that continue to reuse dialyzers should maintain strict adherence to the AAMI standards on dialyzer reuse, carefully track and assess patient infection data, improve the documentation of reprocessing procedures, and establish more rigorous and standardized thresholds for disposal of reused dialyzers.

Third, environmental waste concerns differ for reused and single-use dialyzers. Using dialyzers only a single time creates considerable amounts of plastic medical waste, but dialyzer reprocessing frequently employs chemicals that cannot be readily environmentally degraded. These costs to the environment, therefore, are difficult to compare.

Summary and Conclusions

Reuse of dialyzers remains an essential method in many dialysis facilities throughout the United States to decrease hemodialysis-related treatment costs. Changes in dialyzer performance as a result of dialyzer reprocessing have been clearly identified. Routine measurement and maintenance of dialyzer total cell volume ensures adequate small-solute clearances with dialyzer reuse. In contrast, such measurements do not ensure constant dialyzer membrane permeability to middle molecules. Consequently, changes in middle-molecule and large-solute removal may go undetected clinically.

Future developments in dialyzer reprocessing would permit more complete cleaning of the dialyzer membrane (to maintain its permeability with only minimal exposure to bleach) and the development of simple tests for detecting changes in dialyzer membrane permeability during reprocessing to ensure the reliability and safety of dialyzer reprocessing. Dialysis providers, physicians, and patients should continuously update their knowledge of the economics and reliability of dialyzer reuse.

C H A P T E R   1 2

Dialysate Composition

Biff F. Palmer, MD

Introduction

Patients with end-stage renal disease (ESRD) depend on dialysis to maintain fluid and electrolyte balance. In hemodialysis, solutes diffuse between blood and dialysate such that, over the course of the procedure, plasma composition is restored toward normal values. The makeup of the dialysate is of paramount importance in accomplishing this goal. Individualizing the dialysate composition is of critical importance in improving tolerance to the procedure particularly given the number of comorbid conditions typically found in the ESRD patients.

Dialysate Sodium

As dialysis has evolved, there has been continued interest in adjusting the dialysate sodium (Na$^+$) concentration in an attempt to improve the tolerability of the procedure. In the early days of dialysis, fluid removal was accomplished by a process of osmotic ultrafiltration. High concentrations of glucose were placed in the dialysate in order to create an osmotic driving force for fluid removal since the coil dialyzers used at the time were unable to withstand high transmembrane hydrostatic pressures. In order to prevent the development of hypernatremia as water moved from plasma to dialysate the Na$^+$ concentration in dialysate was purposely set low, usually in the range of 125–130 mEq/L. With the development of more resilient membranes capable of withstanding high transmembrane pressures, osmotic ultrafiltration was replaced by hydrostatic ultrafiltration. Initially, a low dialysate Na$^+$ concentration continued to be used in order to avoid the problems of chronic volume overload such as hypertension and heart failure. With the institution of shorter treatment times volume removal became more rapid and symptomatic hypotension emerged as a common and often disabling problem during dialysis. It soon became apparent that changes in the serum Na$^+$ concentration, and more specifically changes in serum osmolality, were playing a role in the development of this hemodynamic instability.

The importance of a stable plasma osmolality in maintaining hemodynamic stability was first suggested when the hemodynamic profiles of ultrafiltration were compared to diffusional solute clearance. Ultrafiltration alone (the removal of isoosmolar fluid by exerting a transmembrane pressure across the dialyzer) decreases cardiac output primarily due to a reduction in the stroke volume but is accompanied by an increase in peripheral vascular resistance such that arterial pressure is maintained. By contrast, diffusional dialysis results in a fall in arterial pressure while peripheral vascular resistance remains the same. With conventional dialysis (ultrafiltration and dialysis), less volume removal can be achieved before hypotension occurs as compared to ultrafiltration alone.

In animal studies, both conventional dialysis and sequential ultrafiltration dialysis result in an ultrafiltrate volume that is less than the decrease in extracellular fluid volume consistent with a shift of fluid into the intracellular compartment. In addition, during sequential ultrafiltration hemodialysis, this shift only occurs during the diffusive phase. In the initial period of dialysis, the extracellular urea concentration rapidly falls, creating an osmotic driving force for water movement into the cell due to the higher intracellular urea concentration. With the advent of high-clearance dialyzers and more efficient dialysis techniques, this decline in plasma osmolality becomes more apparent as solute is more rapidly removed. Use of a low dialysate Na^+ concentration tends to further augment the intracellular shift of fluid as plasma tends to become even more hypoosmolar consequent to the movement of Na^+ from plasma to dialysate.

Raising dialysate Na^+ to between 139 and 144 mEq/L improves hemodynamic stability and general tolerance to the procedure. A high dialysate Na^+ concentration has been shown effective in maintaining a relatively constant plasma osmolality, thereby minimizing intracellular water movement during dialysis. By preventing a decrease in plasma osmolality, the higher Na^+ dialysate leads to mobilization of fluid from the intracellular space resulting in better preservation of plasma volume. As the dialysate to plasma Na^+ gradient increases, there is a greater contraction of the intracellular fluid compartment. The shift of fluid into the extracellular fluid space increases the hydrostatic pressure of the interstitium, thus increasing the capacity for vascular refilling during volume removal, resulting in a reduced frequency of hypotension and cramps.

The primary concern with use of a higher dialysate Na^+ concentration is the potential to stimulate thirst and cause increased weight gain and poor blood pressure control in the interdialytic period. Studies addressing this issue confirmed that a higher dialysate Na^+ modestly increased interdialytic weight gain. However, this excess weight was found to be readily removed with improved tolerance to ultrafiltration.

Sodium modeling refers to a strategy of varying the concentration of Na^+ in the dialysate during the procedure so as to minimize the potential complications of a high Na^+ solution while retaining the beneficial hemodynamic effects. A high dialysate Na^+ concentration is used initially with a progressive reduction toward isotonic or hypotonic levels by the end of the procedure. This method allows for a diffusive Na^+ influx early in the session to prevent the rapid decline in plasma osmolality resulting from the efflux of urea and other small molecular weight solutes. During the remainder of the procedure, when the reduction in osmolality accompanying urea removal is less abrupt, the lower dialysate Na^+ level minimizes the development of hypertonicity and any resultant excessive thirst, fluid gain, and hypertension in the interdialytic period. Unfortunately, despite the theoretical predictions of Na^+ modeling, the incidence of symptomatic hypotension during dialysis or the degree of interdialytic weight gain between fixed or variable Na^+ protocols have been difficult to demonstrate. In fact, the available data suggest that in most chronic dialysis patients, changing the dialysate Na^+ during the course of the treatment offers little advantage over a constant dialysate Na^+ of between 140 to 145 mEq/L.

The inability to clearly demonstrate a superiority of Na^+ modeling may be due to the fact that the time-averaged concentration of Na^+ was similar in many of the comparative studies. For example, a linear decline in dialysate Na^+ from 150 to 140 mEq/L will produce approximately the same postdialysis serum Na^+ as occurs when a dialysate Na^+ of 145 mEq/L is used throughout the procedure. In addition, the optimal time-averaged Na^+ concentration whether administered in a modeling protocol or with a fixed dialysate concentration is likely to vary from patient to patient as well as in the same patient during different treatment times. This variability is supported by studies demonstrating wide differences in the month to month predialysis Na^+ concentration in otherwise stable dialysis patients.

In a few, highly selected patients, Na^+ modeling may be of benefit (Table 12.1). Patients initiating dialysis with marked azotemia are often deliberately dialyzed so as to decrease the urea concentration slowly over the course of several days to avoid the development of the dialysis disequilibrium syndrome. The use of a high/low-Na^+ dialysate in these patients may minimize fluid shifts into the intracellular compartment and decrease the tendency for neurologic complications. Na^+ modeling may also be beneficial in patients suffering frequent intradialytic hypotension, cramping, nausea, vomiting, fatigue, or headache. In such patients, the modeling protocol can be individually tailored to minimize increased thirst, weight gain, and hypertension. Combining dialysate Na^+ profiling with a varying rate of ultrafiltration may provide additional benefit in particularly symptomatic patients. Use of this combined approach may be of particular benefit in ensuring hemodynamic stability in patients with acute kidney injury in the intensive care unit. It should be emphasized that when prescribing a Na^+ gradient protocol, it is important to monitor the patient for evidence of a progressive increase in total body Na^+ manifesting itself as large interdialytic weight gains and/or uncontrolled hypertension (Table 12.1).

Current research is focusing on ways in which the dialysate Na^+ concentration can be adjusted to more accurately match intradialytic Na^+ removal with interdialytic Na^+ intake. The ability to achieve zero Na^+ balance would enhance the ability to control hypertension in the interdialytic intervals and minimize the risk of hypotension during the dialysis procedure.

A recent special report emphasizes the need to prevent intradialytic Na^+ overload by recommending the dialysate Na^+ should be in the range of 134–138 mEq/L. To minimize the chance of hypotension and ensure adequate volume removal, the expected minimum duration of dialysis should be 4 hours in patients receiving thrice-weekly maintenance dialysis. Lastly, hypertonic saline and Na^+ modeling protocols should be avoided.

Table 12.1

Indications and Contraindications for Use of Na^+ Modeling (High/Low Programs)

A. Indications (Only Short-Term and in Highly Selected Patients, Should Generally Be Avoided)
- Intradialytic hypotension
- Cramping
- Initiation of hemodialysis in setting of severe azotemia
- Hemodynamically unstable patient (as in intensive care unit setting)

B. Contraindications
- Intradialytic development of hypertension
- Large interdialytic weight gain induced by high Na^+ dialysate
- Hypernatremia

With increased ability to individualize the dialysate Na^+ concentration, one can envision a scenario in which a patient initiated on hemodialysis is initially treated with a dialysate Na^+ concentration designed to achieve negative Na^+ balance. Once the patient becomes normotensive or requires minimal amounts of antihypertensive medications, the dialysate Na^+ can be adjusted on a continual basis to ensure that Na^+ balance is maintained. Achieving the optimal total body Na^+ content will likely become just as important as determining an accurate dry weight.

Dialysate Potassium

In most chronic outpatient dialysis centers, there is little individualization of the dialysate potassium (K^+) concentration. Rather, most patients are dialyzed with a K^+ bath that is prepared centrally and delivered with a concentration fixed at 1 or 2 mEq/L. When using a fixed dialysate K^+, it is difficult to predict the exact amount of K^+ that will be removed in a given dialysis session. Typically, one should not expect more than 80–100 mEq of K^+ removal even with the use of a K^+-free dialysate. In addition, there will be marked variability in the amount of K^+ removed from patient to patient despite similar predialysis K^+ levels and dialysis regimens. This variability can be explained by the fact that K^+ movement from the intracellular to the extracellular space and ultimately into the dialysate is influenced by several patient-specific factors.

The removal of excess K^+ by dialysis is achieved by the use of a dialysate with a K^+ concentration lower than that of plasma creating a gradient favoring K^+ removal; its rate is largely a function of this gradient. Plasma K^+ concentration falls rapidly in the early stages of dialysis, but as the plasma concentration falls, K^+ removal becomes less efficient. Because K^+ is freely permeable across the dialysis membrane, movement of K^+ from the intracellular space to the extracellular space appears to be the limiting factor in K^+ removal. Factors that importantly dictate the distribution of K^+ between these two spaces include changes in acid–base status, tonicity, glucose and insulin concentration, and catecholamine activity (Table 12.2).

The movement of K^+ between the intracellular and extracellular space is influenced by changes in acid–base balance that occur during the dialysis procedure. Extracellular alkalosis causes a shift of K^+ into cells, whereas acidosis results in K^+

Table 12.2

Factors Affecting K^+ Removal During Hemodialysis

A. Shifts K^+ Into Cell, Thereby ↓ Dialytic K^+ Removal
- Exogenous insulin
- Glucose containing dialysate vs glucose-free dialysate
- β-adrenergic agonists
- Correction of metabolic acidosis during dialysis

B. Shifts K^+ to Extracellular Space or Impairs K^+ Uptake, Increasing Dialytic K^+ Removal
- β-blockers
- α-adrenergic receptor stimulation
- Hypertonicity

efflux from cells. During a typical dialysis, there is net addition of base to the extracellular space, which promotes cellular uptake of K^+ and therefore attenuates the removal of K^+ during dialysis. The degree to which K^+ shifts into the cell is directly correlated with the bicarbonate concentration of the dialysate. However, with routine dialysis the change in blood pH is of small magnitude and the effect on K^+ removal is not profound. By contrast, dialysis in patients who are acidotic will result in less K^+ removal because K^+ is shifted into cells as the serum bicarbonate rises.

Insulin is known to stimulate the cellular uptake of K^+ and can therefore influence the amount of K^+ removal during dialysis. The use of a glucose-free dialysate results in greater amounts of K^+ removal when compared with use of a glucose-containing bath. The use of a glucose-free dialysate would be expected to result in lower levels of insulin. As a result, there is increased movement of K^+ to the extracellular space, where it becomes available for dialytic removal.

Changes in plasma tonicity can affect the distribution of K^+ between the intracellular and extracellular space. Administration of hypertonic saline or mannitol is sometimes used in the treatment of hypotension during dialysis. These agents would be expected to favor K^+ removal during dialysis because the resultant increased tonicity would favor K^+ movement into the extracellular space. There are no studies addressing whether there is any significant clinical benefit with this approach.

β-adrenergic stimulation is known to shift K^+ into cells and lower the extracellular concentration. Inhaled β-adrenergic stimulants have been reported to be effective in the acute treatment of hyperkalemia, so such therapy before dialysis may lower the total amount of K^+ removed during the dialytic procedure.

Alterations in serum K^+ concentration during dialysis can affect systemic hemodynamics. A decrease in serum K^+ concentration during hemodialysis would be predicted to increase systemic vascular resistance. Hypokalemia has been shown to increase resistance in skeletal muscle, skin, and coronary vascular beds, possibly through effects on the electrogenic Na^+/K^+-ATPase pump in the sarcolemmal membranes of vascular smooth muscle cells. In addition, decreased serum K^+ concentration may enhance the sensitivity of the vasculature to endogenous pressor hormones.

Changes in serum K^+ concentration during dialysis may also influence systemic hemodynamics through effects on myocardial performance. Dialysis is associated with an increase in contractility, which can be attributed to an increase in ionized serum calcium. Increased ionized calcium is most closely related to improved ventricular contractility, but modifying effects of concomitant decreases in K^+ may also be important.

An increase in peripheral vascular resistance secondary to the development of hypokalemia could have potential detrimental effects on dialysis efficiency. This decrease in efficiency would result from decreased blood flow to urea-rich tissues such as skeletal muscle and in effect increase the amount of bodywide recirculation. Although more studies are needed in this area, it is likely that any effect of a low dialysate K^+ concentration to decrease dialysis adequacy is small in magnitude. In addition, increasing the dialysate K^+ concentration to improve dialysis adequacy will increase the risk of hyperkalemia during the interdialytic period.

Most patients dialyzed with a fixed K^+ dialysate tolerate the procedure well and do not suffer from complications of hypokalemia or hyperkalemia. Nevertheless, there are clinical conditions in which an individualized dialysate K^+ concentration may be useful. Patients with underlying heart disease, particularly in the setting of digoxin therapy, are prone to arrhythmias as hypokalemia develops toward the end of a typical treatment. The risk of arrhythmias is also increased in the early stages of a dialysis session when the plasma K^+ concentration may still be normal but rapidly declining. The sudden reduction in the plasma K^+ concentration during the initial portions of the dialysis procedure has been shown to unfavorably alter the QTc (a marker of risk of ventricular arrhythmias) even in dialysis patients without obvious heart disease.

Setting the dialysate K^+ concentration to a higher value in any patient at risk for arrhythmias is not without risk. In an analysis of more than 80,000 maintenance hemodialysis predialysis serum K^+ values between 4.6 and 5.3 mEq/L were associated with the greatest survival whereas values <4.0 or ≥5.6 mEq/L were associated with increased mortality. Use of a higher dialysate K^+ concentration was associated with increased mortality in patients with predialysis K^+ values ≥5.0 mEq/L. A separate case-control study found the use of a low K^+ dialysate (<2.0 mEq/L) as an independent risk factor for the specific occurrence of in-center sudden cardiac arrest. Patients with cardiac arrest that were on low K^+ dialysate were noted to have lower predialysis serum K^+ than the control patients on low K^+ dialysate. Taken together, when considering the risk for cardiac death or mortality, predialysis serum K^+ should help guide the decision of the dialysate K^+ with caution to avoid excessively high or low serum K^+ levels.

Modeling the dialysate K^+ concentration in such a way as to minimize the initial rapid decline in the plasma K^+ concentration may be one way to minimize potential cardiac toxicity. This is accomplished by exponentially lowering the dialysate K^+ during the course of the procedure to maintain a constant blood-to-dialysate K^+ gradient. In addition to decreasing arrhythmias, maintenance of a constant blood-to-dialysate K^+ concentration may prove useful in patients who tend to develop worsening hypertension during the course of the dialysis procedure because of the effects of hypokalemia to cause increased vascular resistance as mentioned previously.

In summary, because of the kinetics of K^+ movement from the intracellular to the extracellular space, one can expect only up to 70–90 mEq of K^+ to be removed during a typical dialysis session. As a result, one should not overestimate the effectiveness of the dialytic procedure in the treatment of severe hyperkalemia. The total amount removed will exhibit considerable variability and will be influenced by changes in acid–base status, changes in tonicity, changes in glucose and insulin concentrations, and catecholamine activity. Studies examining the hemodynamic effect of K^+ fluxes during hemodialysis are limited. More importantly, deliberate alterations in dialysate K^+ concentration to effect hemodynamic stability would not be without risk. Use of low dialysate K^+ concentration may contribute to arrhythmias, especially in those patients with underlying coronary artery disease or those taking digoxin, and dialysate K^+ <2.0 mEq/L should generally be avoided. On the other hand, use of dialysate with high K^+ concentration may predispose patients to predialysis hyperkalemia. In patients who are at high risk for arrhythmias on dialysis, modeling the dialysate K^+ concentration so as to maintain a constant blood-to-dialysate K^+ gradient throughout the procedure may be of clinical benefit.

Dialysate Buffer

Bicarbonate is now the principal buffer used in dialysate. Producing bicarbonate dialysate requires a specifically designed system that mixes a bicarbonate concentrate and an acid concentrate with purified water. The acid concentrate contains a small amount of either lactic or acetic acid and all the calcium and magnesium. The exclusion of these cations from the bicarbonate concentrate prevents the precipitation of magnesium and calcium carbonate that would otherwise occur in the setting of a high bicarbonate concentration. During the mixing procedure, the acid in the acid concentrate will react with an equimolar amount of bicarbonate to generate carbonic acid and carbon dioxide. The generation of carbon dioxide causes the pH of the final solution to fall to approximately 7.0–7.4. This more acidic pH as well as the lower concentrations of calcium and magnesium in the final mixture allows for these ions to remain in solution. The final concentration of bicarbonate in the dialysate is generally fixed in the range of 33–38 mmol/L.

The use of a bicarbonate dialysate is associated with a number of potential complications. The liquid bicarbonate concentrate can be responsible for microbial contamination of the final dialysate largely because the bicarbonate concentrate is an excellent bacterial growth medium. This complication can be minimized by short storage time as well as filtration of the concentrate during the production procedure. Use of a bicarbonate cartridge can further minimize this complication. This device allows for the bicarbonate concentrate to be produced on-line by passing water through a column containing powdered bicarbonate. The concentrate is produced and proportioned immediately before mixing with the acid concentrate. Hypoxemia may occur during bicarbonate dialysis when high concentrations of bicarbonate are used. This complication appears to be the result of suppressed ventilation secondary to the increase in pH and serum bicarbonate concentration. In addition, excessively high levels of bicarbonate in the dialysate may result in acute metabolic alkalosis causing mental confusion, lethargy, weakness, and cramps.

The factors that determine bicarbonate requirements in hemodialysis patients include acid production during the interdialytic period, the removal of organic anions during the hemodialysis procedure, and the buffer deficit of the body. Because these factors are likely to vary from patient to patient, there is increasing interest in individualizing the dialysate bicarbonate concentration (Table 12.3). The optimal level of dialysate bicarbonate would be a concentration low enough to prevent significant alkalosis in the postdialytic period and yet be high enough to prevent predialysis acidosis.

A low predialysis serum bicarbonate level may contribute to protein-energy wasting and greater intradialytic electrolyte shifts, thus leading to higher mortality. Higher bicarbonate dialysate concentration has been associated with improvement in nutritional markers, bone metabolism, as well as hemodynamic stability. A recent publication from the Dialysis Outcomes and Practice Patterns Study (DOPPS) found that high dialysate bicarbonate concentration may be associated with increased morbidity and mortality likely through adverse effects related to postdialysis metabolic alkalosis; however, a causal relationship could not be proven given the observational design of the study.

The prescription of the dialysate bicarbonate is best tailored to the individual patient's acid–base status. Maintaining a predialysis total CO_2 concentration of at least 23 mEq/L is a reasonable goal. This can be achieved in most patients by individually adjusting the dialysate bicarbonate concentration. Substituting citric acid for acetic acid in the acid concentrate is also effective in improving the acidosis of chronic dialysis patients. Citric acid dialysate is associated with an increased delivered dose of dialysis, an effect postulated to be due to improved membrane permeability resulting from citrate's local anticoagulant effect. Improved membrane

Table 12.3

Considerations When Individualizing Components of the Dialysate

Dialysate Component	Advantage	Disadvantage
Na^+: Increased	More hemodynamic stability Less cramping	Dipsogenic effect Increased interdialytic weight gain ? Chronic hypertension
Decreased	Less interdialytic weight gain	Intradialytic hypotension and cramping more common
Ca^{2+}: Increased	Suppression of PTH, promotes hemodynamic stability	Hypercalcemia with vitamin D and Ca^{2+}-containing phosphate binders
Decreased	Permits greater use of vitamin D and calcium-containing phosphate binders	Potential for negative calcium balance, stimulation of PTH, slight decrease in hemodynamic stability
K^+: Increased	Less arrhythmias in the setting of digoxin or coronary heart disease, less rebound hypertension	Limited by hyperkalemia
Decreased (ramped dialysate K^+ ideal, prevents rapid initial decline in plasma K^+)	Greater dietary intake of K^+ with less hyperkalemia ? Improvement in myocardial contractility	Increased arrhythmias, may exacerbate autonomic insufficiency
HCO_3: Increased	Corrects chronic acidosis, thereby benefiting nutrition and bone metabolism	Postdialysis metabolic alkalosis
Decreased	Less metabolic alkalosis	Potential for chronic acidosis
Mg^{2+}: Increased	? Less arrhythmias ? Hemodynamic benefit	Hypermagnesemia
Decreased	Permits use of Mg^{2+}-containing phosphate binders	Hypomagnesemia
PO_4 (rarely added to dialysate)	Treats or prevents hypophosphatemia in malnourished or chronic disease state, overdose setting, daily dialysis	Hyperphosphatemia

PTH, parathyroid hormone.

permeability with greater diffusive flux of bicarbonate from dialysate to blood or metabolism of citrate to bicarbonate in liver and muscle are the most likely explanations for the improvement in bicarbonate concentration.

The bicarbonate concentration used in most dialysis centers is set at 35 mmol/L and rarely adjusted. Given the evidence that correction of chronic acidosis is of clinical benefit, consideration should be given to adjusting the bicarbonate concentration with the goal of maintaining the predialysis tCO_2 concentration of 23 mEq/L. In some patients, supplemental oral bicarbonate therapy will be required to achieve this goal. Substitution of citric acid for acetic acid in the acid concentrate is also a consideration. Further studies are needed to identify the optimal bicarbonate concentration at which hemodialysis patients experience the lowest rates of adverse clinical outcomes.

Dialysate Calcium

The calcium concentration in the dialysate can be varied extensively according to the individual needs of the patient. The most common concentrations used are 1.25, 1.5, and 1.75 mmol/L corresponding to 2.5, 3.0, and 3.5 mEq/L and 5.0, 6.0, and 7.0 mg/dL. In earlier times a higher end dialysate calcium concentration (typically 3.5 mEq/L) was widely used so as to provide a net flux of calcium into the patient. The substitution of calcium for aluminum-containing phosphate binders and the wider use of high doses of intravenous $1,25\text{-}(OH)_2$-vitamin D made the likelihood of hypercalcemia more common, leading to a progressive lowering of the dialysate calcium concentration.

Despite the enthusiasm for use of low-calcium dialysate, studies have emphasized that such an approach requires careful monitoring to ensure the patient does not develop negative calcium balance or worsening secondary hyperparathyroidism. In addition, a low-calcium dialysate can contribute to hemodynamic instability during the dialysis procedure. Raising the dialysate calcium concentration leads to an increase in ionized calcium concentration and an improvement in left ventricular contractility and less intradialytic hypotension. In patients prone to intradialytic hypotension who are at risk for hypercalcemia, dialysate calcium profiling can be used as a strategy to improve hemodynamic stability and yet minimize the potential for hypercalcemia.

Despite the favorable effects on hemodynamics, there is a concern that long-term use of a high dialysate calcium concentration may contribute to adverse effects on the cardiovascular system by promoting vascular calcification. A higher dialysate calcium concentration has been linked to progression of aortic calcification and increases in arterial stiffness. A final consideration in the selection of dialysate calcium is the rare occurrence of arrhythmias including sudden cardiac death. One case-control study evaluating more than 43,000 prevalent hemodialysis patients over the course of 4 years identified low dialysate calcium (<2.5 mEq/L) as an independent risk factor for the occurrence of in-clinic cardiac arrest. Further analysis established that a larger dialysate-to-serum calcium gradient was linearly related with the risk for cardiac arrest. These retrospective studies should heighten the awareness that independent of bone and mineral disease, there are some risks involved with excessively low dialysate calcium.

In summary, the dialysate calcium concentration has implications with regards to metabolic bone disease, hemodynamic stability, and long-term effects on vascular calcification. The most recent NKF-K/DOQI guidelines recommend a dialysate calcium concentration of 1.25 mmol/L as being a useful compromise between optimization of bone health and reductions in cardiovascular risk. However, as with the other dialysate constituents, the calcium concentration should be individually tailored to the patient. In patients who are prone to intradialytic hypotension a higher dialysate calcium concentration may be of benefit. On the other hand, the use of a lower calcium concentration in the dialysate will allow increased doses of $1,25\text{-}(OH)_2$-vitamin D to be used so as to reduce circulating levels of parathyroid hormone with less fear of inducing hypercalcemia. Further research is needed to define the optimal mix of dialysate calcium concentration, dose of vitamin D, amount of calcium- and non–calcium-containing phosphate binder, and use of the calcimimetic agent cinacalcet.

Dialysate Magnesium

The usual concentration of magnesium in the dialysate is 0.5–1.0 mEq/L and is only rarely manipulated. In an attempt to minimize the development of hypercalcemia associated with the use of calcium-containing phosphate binders and vitamin D, there has been some interest in using magnesium-containing compounds as a phosphate binder. Such a strategy requires a low dialysate magnesium concentration so as to avoid the development of hypermagnesemia.

Dialysate Phosphate

In patients with mild to moderate hyperphosphatemia, hemodialysis has been estimated to remove 250–325 mg/d of phosphorus when extrapolated to an average week. Because a diet that provides adequate protein may provide approximately 900 mg of phosphorus daily, it follows that dialysis cannot provide adequate control of phosphate by itself. Rather, management of hyperphosphatemia requires a combination of dietary restriction, oral phosphate binders, and dialysis.

The limited ability of dialysis to remove phosphorus is primarily related to the kinetics of phosphorus distribution within the body and not inadequate clearance across the dialyzer. In a typical dialysis session the rate of phosphorus removal is greatest during the initial stages of the procedure and then progressively declines to a low constant level toward the end of the treatment. This decline is due to the decrease in plasma concentration and the slow efflux of phosphorus from the intracellular space and/or mobilization from bone stores. Although dialysis membranes differ with respect to plasma clearance of phosphate, it is the slow transfer of phosphorus from the intracellular to the extracellular space where it becomes accessible for dialytic removal that is the most important factor limiting phosphorus removal.

There are only a few situations in which one might consider adding phosphorus to the dialysate. Hypophosphatemia can be an occasional finding in the chronic dialysis patient who is malnourished and suffering from some chronic disease state. In such patients, adding phosphorus to the dialysate may be an effective means to treat hypophosphatemia without having to use a parenteral route of administration. The phosphate must be added to the bicarbonate component of a dual proportioning system to avoid the precipitation of calcium phosphate that would result from addition to the calcium-containing acid concentrate.

Another situation in which addition of phosphate to the dialysate may be useful is in the setting of an overdose. In a patient with normal renal function and a normal serum phosphate concentration, use of a phosphate-free dialysate will commonly result in hypophosphatemia. In most circumstances, the hypophosphatemia is of short duration and is of little clinical consequence. However, some intoxications may increase the risk for complications of hypophosphatemia such that addition of phosphate to the dialysate may be warranted.

Finally, hypophosphatemia has been noted in patients treated with prolonged daily nocturnal hemodialysis. In this setting, adding phosphate to the dialysate may prove useful as a means to normalize the serum phosphate concentration.

CHAPTER 13

Safety Monitors in Hemodialysis

Joanne D. Pittard, RN, MS

Hemodialysis monitors include machines, devices, protocols, and personnel. The major goal is to ensure patient safety during the hemodialysis procedure. All tasks that check, observe, keep track of, and control the hemodialysis treatment are monitoring procedures. These important tasks are too often lightly dismissed.

This chapter focuses on the fluid delivery system and extracorporeal circuit, their respective monitoring devices, their functions, locations, performance standards, and management. Monitoring of the patient and hemodialysis prescription pre-, during, and post-dialysis are covered in other sections of this book. Incorporated are parts of the Conditions of Coverage (CfCs) dictated by the Department of Health and Human Services Center for Medicaid and Medicare Services (CMS), effective October 3, 2008, for end-stage renal disease (ESRD) facilities. The revised regulations update standards for delivering safe, high-quality care to dialysis patients. Specific regulations regarding dialysate (§494.40 Condition: Water and Dialysate Quality) are included. First-time regulations specific for dialysate include mixing, distribution, labeling, and use.

Definitions and Overview

The fluid delivery system is commonly called "the machine." The fluid delivery system prepares dialysate, a body temperature electrolyte solution. The dialysate flows through the dialysate compartment of the dialyzer where dialysis occurs. A blood pump circulates the patient's blood through the extracorporeal circulation to the blood compartment of the dialyzer and back to the patient. The two major categories to monitor are the dialysate circuit and blood circuit.

The blood circuit consists of a blood tubing set (arterial and venous), blood side of the dialyzer, intravenous (IV) normal saline and administration line, and heparin syringe and infusion line.

The blood and dialysate are separate circuits that interface at the dialyzer membrane. The machine design must involve extensive monitoring of both circuits. Specific warning alarms must be initiated when the machine's preset limits are exceeded and/or an unsafe condition exists.

Dialysate Solution

Dialysate solution or dialyzing fluid is a nonsterile aqueous electrolyte solution that is similar to the normal levels of electrolytes (Table 13.1) found in extracellular fluid

---

Table 13.1

Comparison of Normal Blood Values and Dialysate Composition

Electrolyte	Dialysate Level Range		Normal Blood Value Range	
Sodium	135–145	mEq/L	135–145	mEq/L
Potassium	0–4	mEq/L	3.5–5.5	mEq/L
Calcium	2.25–3.0	mEq/L	4.5–5.5	mEq/L
Magnesium	0.5–1.0	mEq/L	1.5–2.5	mEq/L
Chloride	100–115	mEq/L	95–105	mEq/L
Bicarbonate	30–40	mEq/L	22–28	mEq/L
Non-electrolyte				
Dextrose	0–200	mg/dL	80–120	mg/dL

From Pittard J, De Palma J. *Dialysate Monograph.* 1st ed. Glendale, CA: Hemodialysis; 2013.

with the exception of the buffer bicarbonate and potassium. Dialysate solution is almost an isotonic solution, with the usual osmolality of approximately 300 ± 20 milliosmoles per liter (mOsm/L). To ensure patient safety and prevent red blood cell destruction by hemolysis or crenation, the osmolality of dialysate must be close to the osmolality of plasma. The osmolality of plasma is 280 ± 20 mOsm/L. Dialysate solution commonly contains six (6) electrolytes: sodium (Na^+), potassium (K^+), calcium (Ca^{2+}), magnesium (Mg^{2+}), chloride (Cl^-), and bicarbonate (HCO_3^-). A seventh component, the nonelectrolyte glucose or dextrose, is invariably present in the dialysate. The dialysate concentration of glucose is commonly between 100 and 200 mg/dL. Freshly prepared dialysate solution circulates continuously to the dialyzer in the extracorporeal circuit. After making a single pass through the dialyzer, the effluent dialysate goes to the drain.

Fluid Delivery System

The vast majority of dialysis facilities in the United States use single-patient fluid delivery systems. This type of equipment is self-contained, preparing the dialysate only for the individual machine. Some dialysis facilities use central delivery systems with central manufacture of dialysate. Although that system is more economical, it is less safe than the individual machines. The discussion will focus on single-patient machinery. A few safety issues unique to a central delivery system are explored as well.

Control Panel and Monitor Display

All modern fluid delivery systems have a frontal control panel (Fig. 13.1) by which pressure and other limits may be set and system parameters may be viewed. The control panel and monitor display on the face of the machine will have audible and visual warning alarms as a mandatory part of safe dialysis monitoring.

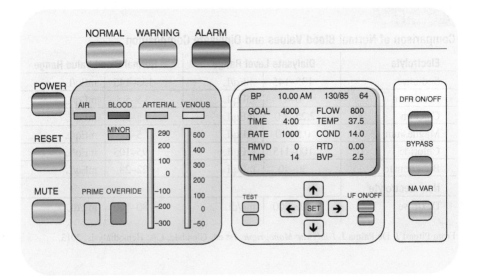

Figure 13.1

Control Panel and Monitor Display. (From Pittard J: Hemodialysis Nursing, Training Manual, 7th ed., version 7.0. Santa Monica, CA, 2003, with permission.)

Monitor Failure

Machine monitors are either mechanically or electrically operated, or a combination of both. All monitors can fail. Murphy's Law (if anything can go wrong, it will) should be remembered, and accepted as fact. Murphy's Law is attributed to an engineer working at the Los Alamos laboratories in the 1950s. The truth of this statement can be reworded to, "If you can think of a possible disaster with the present equipment, take the necessary precautionary steps immediately or it will happen." If one can access misadventure and incident reporting, virtually every possible projected failure of a monitor has occurred and has resulted in patient/staff injury or death.

Fail-Safe, a Misnomer

Machine monitors are frequently thought to be fail-safe devices, but they are not. A truly fail-safe device cannot be overridden to cause harm either by electronic or human intervention. By this narrow definition, there are no fail-safe dialysis machine monitors. Because all dialysis machine monitors can fail, they ought to be simple to operate and accurate—and should signal a warning when they are out of limits or not working properly. Any important factor requires dual monitoring: the machine monitor device and dialysis personnel. No machine, computer, or device can replace the continuous surveillance of the hemodialysis personnel.

Dialysate Circuit

Fig. 13.2 displays components of the dialysate fluid path. Dialysate monitoring includes prescription; composition (conductivity and pH); temperature; flow;

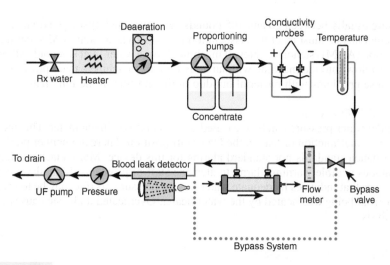

Figure 13.2

Fluid Pathway Simplified. (From Pittard J: Hemodialysis Nursing, Training Manual, 7th ed., version 7.0. Santa Monica, CA, 2003, with permission.)

pressure; effluent; absence of impurities (cleaning and disinfecting agents); potential pyrogenic agents; and microbiologic testing. Each monitor or control is discussed in order of the usual flow of fluid; from the water inlet solenoid valve to the effluent dialysate drain line.

Why Discuss the Details of Dialysis Machinery?

Each dialysis treatment exposes the ESRD patient's blood to hundreds of liters of dialysate. The dialysate should be of pharmaceutical grade, as dialysate is the equivalent of an intravenous (IV) solution. The machinery that manufactures dialysate can silently and quickly cause a patient serious injury or death because of contaminants or incorrect solute concentration. Even more distressing, if the machinery manufactures a substantially hypotonic fluid, but at a concentration that does not cause hemolysis, the patient may rapidly develop water intoxication, cerebral edema, seizures, and noncardiogenic pulmonary edema—signs and symptoms that the dialysis staff can easily misinterpret as requiring more ultrafiltration and more dialysis!

With current therapy using blood flow rates of 300 to 450 mL/min, the entire patient's circulating blood may be exposed to toxic chemicals or a hemolytic state in less than 15 minutes. Death can be both swift and the cause undiagnosed, even with postmortem examination. Each component of the dialysate circuit discussed, if it malfunctions, may induce hemolysis.

Water Inlet Solenoid

The water inlet solenoid permits the flow of treated water into the dialysis machine when the main power switch is activated and stops the flow when the main power is turned off. Treated water enters the machine via a water inlet valve with water pressure usually between 20 and 105 pounds per square inch (psi). The treated water for hemodialysis must meet the Association for the Advancement of Medical Instrumentation (AAMI) standards. Not all machines have a water inlet solenoid. Allowing water to flow into the machine without activating the machine's main power switch can cause problems with bacterial buildup in that portion of the fluid pathway.

Solenoid Monitoring

The inlet water pressure can be measured using a dial-type manometer. This mechanism may malfunction or leak in the On or Off position. There are neither published performance standards nor standard alarms for this device. Many machines have a continuous audible warning alarm, to alert the staff of problems. If an alarm condition exists that indicates inadequate water flow or pressure, its role may be to prevent water from being overheated by the water heater. Overheated dialysate causes gross hemolysis.

Dialysate Temperature

A heater raises the temperature of the incoming water to approximately body temperature. Heating partially degasses the cold water, which improves the mixing of water and dialysate concentrate. A thermistor feedback circuit usually controls the electrical heating elements. The heater may have a coarse adjustment control inside the machine and a fine adjustment control on the front panel. There may be a simple bimetallic dial thermometer within some machines that, though not alarmed, provides visual observation of its function.

The dialysate temperature is usually maintained between 37°C and 38°C (98.6°F and 100.4°F) throughout the dialysis treatment although recent research has suggested that somewhat lower dialysate temperature, as tolerated, may be beneficial and better maintain intradialytic cardiovascular stability. An internal temperature sensor (Fig. 13.3) monitors the dialysate temperature continuously. In some cases, the actual temperature reading is displayed on the front panel of the machine. Other machines have lights on the front panel that indicate an alarm condition. Most fluid-delivery machines have high and low temperature monitor alarms. Some older-model machines have only high temperature alarms. If the high or low internal temperatures exceed the preset internal limits, three actions result: an audible alarm, a visual alarm, and activation of the bypass mode.

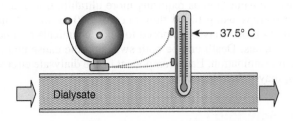

Figure 13.3

Dialysate Temperature. (From Pittard J: Hemodialysis Nursing, Training Manual, 7th ed., version 7.0. Santa Monica, CA, 2003, with permission.)

Heater and Temperature Monitoring

Internal, factory-set, controls should limit dialysate temperature to between 33°C (92°F) and 39°C (102°F). The fine adjustment control knob on the front panel of the machine should not be capable of overriding this setting.

Temperatures Greater Than 106°F

The usual causes of high dialysate temperature are either a malfunctioning water heater with a temperature controller or a water flow restriction. The internal high limit should be set at no higher than 41°C (105.8°F). Normal red blood cells (RBCs) begin to hemolyze at 42°C. Overheated dialysate has been known to precipitate cardiac arrhythmias.

Although it is true that the efficiency of diffusion during dialysis is increased with increased dialysate temperature, without excellent electronic temperature monitoring this is a dangerous way to increase dialysis efficiency. Under no circumstances should the high limit be adjusted above 41°C. Several articles in the literature suggest that the upper limits be set at 42°C (107.6°F), which is probably too high and may cause hemolysis. It should be remembered that uremic RBCs are more osmotically fragile and have a shorter half-life than normal RBCs. It is reasonable to assume that these uremic RBCs are more sensitive to all mechanical and thermal causes of trauma than normal RBCs.

Temperatures Less Than 98.6°F

Some nephrologists use lower-temperature dialysate in the belief that this promotes a more stable blood pressure response to high ultrafiltration. If low-temperature dialysate is used, the total dialysis time needs to be increased by about 8% for every 3°C below 98.6°F as that is the theoretical loss in diffusivity with temperature decrease. Low dialysate temperatures may induce venous vessel spasm and make it impossible to obtain maximum blood flows through the artificial kidney.

With dialysate temperatures below 98.6°F, patients may complain of being cold, ask for a blanket, and some will actually shiver in an attempt to increase their core body temperature. An increase in cardiac irritability in patients with coronary vessel disease may be observed if temperatures are too low.

Deaeration System

The deaeration system removes dissolved gases by exposing water to subatmospheric pressures generated by a vacuum pump. The gases coalesce, form bubbles, and are vented to the atmosphere by a bubble trap. Improper or inadequate removal of dissolved gases in dialysate can be a hidden cause of several serious dialysis problems, including false blood-leak alarms, false conductivity alarms, interference with volumetric control function, and decreased dialysis efficiency by air bubbles trapped on the dialyzer membrane that reduces functional dialyzer surface area. Microbubbles streaming from dialysate into blood have been reported to collect in the right atrium of the heart and cause air embolism without triggering an air-foam detector alarm. Exaggerated frothing and blood clotting in the drip bulb chamber with minute blood clots being carried to the right atrium may also be seen. A substantial number of all adults have a potentially patent foramen ovale. If the pulmonary artery pressure increases, the foramen ovale can shunt blood from the right to the left atrium. This can result in transfer of these small clots into the left heart and result in cerebral embolism. This set of conditions has occurred and is known as paradoxical embolism, which can be misdiagnosed as a transient ischemic attack (TIA) or other vascular insult and not embolic phenomenon.

Deaeration System Monitoring

Frequent false blood-leak alarms or rapid fluctuations in conductivity can indicate a malfunction of the vacuum pump. The machine should be removed from service and undergo maintenance. If the dialysate inflow and/or outflow lines are not correctly attached to the dialyzer, air can be pulled into the system. Proper technique by the dialysis staff who set up the dialysis machinery prior to dialysis and who secure the quick disconnects of the dialysate lines on the dialyzer dialysate ports will prevent this problem.

Mixing Device

The mixing device, also known as the proportioning system, proportions treated water and dialysate concentrate to create dialysate of the correct ionic concentration. The proportioning system ratio depends on the type of dialysate concentrate used and the type of fluid delivery system. Typical mixing ratios of water to dialysate concentrate are

- 34:1 or 44:1 for acid concentrate
- 20:1 or 25:1 for bicarbonate concentrate

The supply of treated water and dialysate concentrate generates dialysate flow rates between 500 and 1000 mL/min. The two basic types of proportioning systems are fixed-ratio mixing and servo-controlled mixing.

Fixed-ratio mixing uses diaphragms or piston pumps to deliver a set volume of water and concentrate to the mixing chamber. Servo-controlled mechanisms continuously monitor the dialysate composition with conductivity sensors that adjust the amount of concentrate mixed with water to maintain a variable or set composition.

In machines that add concentrate by a servo-controlled mechanism until the dialysate reaches a desired conductivity, a second independent conductivity and pH monitor must cause an alarm if the conductivity is incorrect. If acid and bicarbonate inputs are reversed, or if the wrong concentrates are used for a bicarbonate machine, the servo loops may make a solution of acceptable ionic strength (correct conductivity) but of lethal ionic composition. In this case, the pH monitor or concentrate pump speed monitor becomes critical. However, not all machines are equipped with pH monitors and this deadly event will not be diagnosed.

Mixing Device Monitoring

The conductivity and pH monitor will verify proper mixing with a fixed-ratio proportioning system. Equipment using servo-controlled mechanisms requires a diligent and trained staff to ensure that the proper dialysate concentrate is attached to the proper concentrate lines on the machine.

Composition and Conductivity of Dialysate

Analysis of the dialysate for the proper composition is necessary after it has been mixed and prior to exposing it to the dialyzer and patient. All modern fluid delivery systems have conductivity cells and meters. Total conductivity of dialysate is measured as a simple assessment and surrogate for dialysate ionic content. A conductivity cell is connected to a meter that displays the total ionic concentration of dialysate. Conductivity cells should be made of high-quality, corrosion-resistant materials. The conductivity of an electrolyte solution increases as the temperature increases. Conductivity cells used to monitor dialysate must be temperature compensated.

Measuring Conductivity

In dialysis, conductivity is usually measured using a two-electrode system. The electrodes are connected to a constant current and an ammeter (Fig. 13.4). An electric current is passed through the solution between the electrodes. The ammeter measures the flow of current (the inverse of electrical resistance) that passes through the solution between the electrodes. The conductivity measurement is an estimate of the total ionic content of the dialysate and does not measure or reflect specific ions or electrolytes.

The conductivity meters read the conductivity in millimhos per centimeter (mmhos/cm) or milliSiemens per centimeter (mS/cm). A range of 12.5–16.0 mS/cm is acceptable for a standard dialysate solution. Some facilities prefer a tighter range, that is, 13. 0–15.5 mS/cm. The range varies slightly from facility to facility depending on the dialysate formula in use.

Monitoring Conductivity

Conductivity meters on dialysis machines have external and internal limits set. Some machines may have three internal conductivity sensors set at different intervals of control. The conductivity, or dialysate ionic composition, is so important that this monitoring redundancy is a commonsense safeguard against single-monitor failure. The closest tolerance internal high-low limits are set at ±5%; the last set of conductivity monitoring may be set at 50% of normal conductivity. If the first two monitors

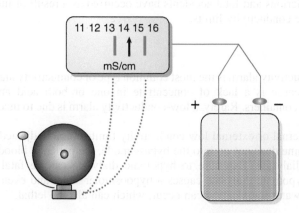

Figure 13.4

Conductivity Monitor. (From Pittard J: Hemodialysis Nursing, Training Manual, 7th ed., version 7.0. Santa Monica, CA, 2003, with permission.)

fail, the patient, without any alarms being triggered, will receive a massive infusion of hypotonic dialysate. Because different mixtures of ions have different conductivities, it is mandatory that the dialysate formulas determine the established conductivity setting.

It is now mandatory to perform and document an independent conductivity test prior to preparing the dialyzer for patient use and before the dialysis treatment is initiated. There are several methods available to perform an independent analysis of the machine's conductivity. The most common method is to use a portable conductivity meter that measures the total conductivity. Laboratory analysis that measures each electrolyte level can also be done.

When using independent analysis, be sure the reference conductivity meter is calibrated accurately prior to use. All standard solutions should be fresh and render acceptable readings.

If independent verification of the dialysate conductivity does not validate the conductivity meter, do not dialyze the patient with that machinery. A complete resolution of the problem is necessary before dialysis. Failure to resolve a problem prior to dialysis will only invite a potential disaster. It is best to bring in another dialysis machine and start over.

All facilities must have an established acceptable conductivity range, and this range must be publicly posted. Any deviation in the conductivity limits set should cause a conductivity alarm. A conductivity alarm causes three actions on the dialysis machine: an audible alarm, a visual alarm, and activation of the bypass system.

The bypass system diverts the dialysate to the drain before it can enter the dialysate inflow line leading to the dialyzer. Thus, exposure of the patient's blood in the dialyzer to an incorrect or unsafe dialysate composition is avoided.

No Intradialytic Conductivity Adjustments

Only a qualified and trained machine technician should adjust the external or internal conductivity limits. Under no circumstances should they be adjusted during the dialysis treatment. They must be properly adjusted and preset before the dialysis treatment. Serious and fatal accidents have occurred as a result of improper adjustments of the conductivity limits.

Low Conductivity

A low-conductivity alarm is the most common type of conductivity alarm (Fig. 13.5). The usual cause is a lack of concentrate in one or both acid and bicarbonate concentrate containers. Rarely, a low-conductivity alarm is due to incorrect dialysate concentrate.

If the internal or external low conductivity limits are not adjusted properly and/ or the machine does not go into the bypass mode, the patient's blood is exposed to hypotonic dialysate. Exposure to hypotonic dialysate can be fatal within a few minutes. Hypotonic dialysate causes a hypoosmolar state, and even without acute hemolysis, water intoxication can occur, which can also be lethal.

Low-Conductivity Monitoring

There must be an adequate amount of dialysate concentrate in the container(s) before starting dialysis. Dialysis staff should not rely on the conductivity meter to monitor dialysate concentrate supplies.

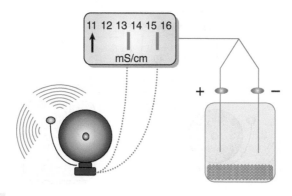

Figure 13.5

Low-Conductivity Alarm. (From Pittard J: Hemodialysis Nursing, Training Manual, 7th ed., version 7.0. Santa Monica, CA, 2003, with permission.)

True, if the dialysis machine goes into the bypass mode, there is no harm to the patient. But, when the dialysis machine is in the bypass mode, no dialysis is taking place and the time lost on dialysis is rarely, if ever, made up with a longer dialysis time the next dialysis session. If one accepts that the average dialysis in the United States comprises not the maximal amount of dialysis time, but probably the minimal amount of dialysis time, placing the dialysis machinery in bypass routinely will shorten the patient's life span.

Most new model fluid-delivery machines have timers that stop with a dialysate circuit alarm. This ensures that the patient receives their allocated time on dialysis.

High Conductivity

High-conductivity alarms (Fig. 13.6) can result from inadequate water flow to the proportioning system, untreated incoming water with an excess of calcium, or incorrect hook-up of dialysate concentrate to the dialysis machine (if using servo-controlled mechanisms) and sodium modeling. Newer-model fluid delivery systems will not go into conductivity with incorrect hook-ups.

With older machines, a common, serious cause of high conductivity occurs when two acid concentrate containers are connected to the dialysis machine instead of one acid container to the acid port and one bicarbonate container to the bicarbonate port. If the dialysis machine goes into bypass mode, there is no harm to the patient. However, if the internal or external high-conductivity limits have not been set correctly, the patient's blood is exposed to hypertonic dialysate and possibly hyperosmolar coma.

New model fluid-delivery systems have automatic built-in adjustment of conductivity limits for sodium variation, which causes an increase in conductivity. If sodium variation is done incorrectly, the patient will leave dialysis thirsty, in a hyperosmolar state, and attempt to relieve that thirst with free water. That will result in a marked expansion of their extracellular volume (ECV), and possibly malignant hypertension.

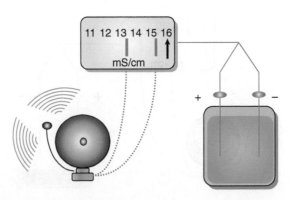

Figure 13.6

High-Conductivity Alarm. (From Pittard J: Hemodialysis Nursing, Training Manual, 7th ed., version 7.0. Santa Monica, CA, 2003, with permission.)

High-Conductivity Monitoring

If a conductivity alarm occurs during the dialysis treatment, the bypass mode is activated. While correcting the alarm condition, the dialysis staff must not adjust the external or internal conductivity limits. Adjusting the conductivity limits during an alarm condition overrides the bypass mode and endangers the patient's life. If the alarm situation cannot be corrected, the treatment must be stopped and the patient moved to another dialysis machine.

Acid–Base (pH) Control

Newer-model fluid-delivery systems will not go into conductivity if the pH is too high or too low. However, the majority of dialysis clinics perform independent pH tests before each dialysis. Fluid delivery machines using bicarbonate dialysate may or may not have pH monitors. There may be a pH meter on the front panel dialysis display with lights that activate when an alarm condition occurs.

Monitoring Acid–Base (pH)

The pH of dialysate is commonly checked by use of a pH paper test strip or bicarbonate pH test strips. With the pH paper test strips, the color change of the dialysate-soaked test strip is compared with a list of colors for various pH values. The bicarbonate pH test strips interpret the results by comparing the indicator pad to the color chart on bottle label. Acceptable range for test results is a pH of 7.5 ± 0.5 (7.0–8.0). If the pH is below or above the acceptable limits and the conductivity meter is within acceptable limits, the dialysis should not be carried out. Both the pH and conductivity must be in acceptable limits before initiating dialysis.

Bypass System

The bypass system diverts dialysate (Fig. 13.7) directly to the drain away from the dialyzer to avoid exposure of the patient's blood to unsafe dialysate. The dialysate

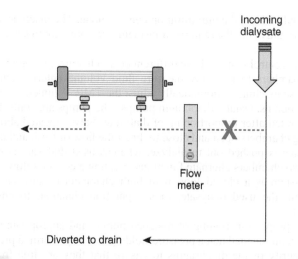

Figure 13.7

Bypass Valve Activated. (From Pittard J: Hemodialysis Nursing, Training Manual, 7th ed., version 7.0. Santa Monica, CA, 2003, with permission.)

bypass valve, located in the incoming dialysate circuit predialyzer, is activated by high/low conductivity, high/low pH, or high/low temperature. It is imperative to have the dialysis staff verify and check that the bypass valve diverts the dialysate to drain.

Bypass System Monitoring

There is no monitor for bypass system failure or function on most machines. A light on the front panel of the machine indicates when the machine is in the bypass mode. Also, an audible alarm usually occurs. If there is a float located in the dialysate inflow line, indicating flow, the float will drop to the bottom of the indicator. There usually is a manually operated control to initiate the bypass mode. Failure of the bypass valve during dialysis is a critical and dangerous situation.

Rinse Mode

The rinse mode on dialysis machines overrides the bypass system. It allows rinsing and disinfection of the entire fluid pathway. It should never be activated while a patient is on dialysis. In new-model machines, the blood pump cannot be activated when the machine is in the rinse mode.

Dialysate Pressure Monitor

The dialysate pressure monitor monitors ultrafiltration pressures. It is a critical function of dialysis therapy that ensures accurate and safe fluid removal from the patient. One method to regulate the patient's ultrafiltration is by application of transmembrane pressure (TMP). Newer machine models have ultrafiltration/volumetric control circuits. The dialysis personnel set the goal for the desired fluid removal, set the duration of dialysis, and activate the ultrafiltration control mode. The machine will automatically calculate and apply the required transmembrane pressure to achieve the desired ultrafiltration.

Volumetric control systems have different design features. A common design uses balancing chambers to precisely measure fluid volume entering and leaving the dialyzer. These machines automatically adjust the TMP. Volumetric control systems use matched pumps, usually diaphragm pumps. The pumps are controlled by valves and are integrated after proportioning of dialysate. Valves located above and below the balancing chambers open and close to direct the flow of fresh and used dialysate. Fresh dialysate is pushed out to dialyze, whereas used dialysate is pushed out to drain. The two chambers alternate functions, creating a constant flow of fresh dialysate. The system is a closed loop with both chambers exactly balanced. Air is removed from the used dialysate, in a separation chamber, to ensure accurate measurement.

To ensure proper functioning of matched pumps and appropriate sealing of the valves, it is recommended that a pressure-holding test be performed predialysis. This tests the integrity of the diaphragms to ensure that they are free from defects or flaws. Bad valve seals can cause inaccurate ultrafiltration that is potentially catastrophic with high-flux dialyzers. These tests can be performed manually or automatically, depending on the machine model.

Blood-Leak Detector

This monitor functions by transmitting filtered or unfiltered light through a column of effluent dialysate that has exited the dialyzer (Fig. 13.8). Tears or leaks in the dialyzer membrane cause RBCs to leak into the dialysate, interrupting the light transmission. The machine response to a blood leak alarm is an audible alarm, a visual alarm, the blood pump stops, and the venous line clamp engages.

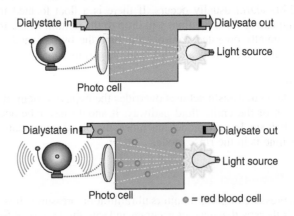

Figure 13.8

Blood-Leak Detector. (From Pittard J: Hemodialysis Nursing, Training Manual, 7th ed., version 7.0. Santa Monica, CA, 2003, with permission.)

It is recommended to have a blood-leak detection threshold set at 0.25–0.35 mL of whole blood per liter of dialysate. False blood-leak alarms can be caused by the presence of air bubbles in the path or by cloudy or dirty optical lenses.

Blood-Leak Detector Monitoring

If the machinery indicates this alarm, a stat Hemastix (benzidine test strip) must be taken at the dialysate drain line. A positive Hemastix test indicates a blood leak. If the Hemastix is weakly positive and the patient is on a hollow-fiber dialyzer, it is possible to closely monitor the patient, observe the dialysate outflow for increased turbidity (indicates air bubbles or RBCs), and wait a few minutes. The leaking fibers may seal or clot off. During this time, remove the ultrafiltration, decrease the blood flow rate, and attend the patient on a one-to-one ratio. If the patient cannot be continuously monitored, the dialyzer should be replaced.

If the repeat Hemastix is negative, dialysis can be continued. If the blood-leak alarm continues, or if blood is visible in the dialysate lines, the dialysis should be stopped and the dialyzer changed per unit protocol. The dialyzer should be discarded.

After a blood leak, it is important to clean the optical path of the blood leak detector. Always maintain a narrow range of sensitivity. Do not dialyze a patient with a faulty blood-leak detector. A major blood leak can be fatal.

Dialysate Flow

The dialysate flow rates may be preset or adjustable. The usual dialysate flow rate for conventional dialyzers is a minimum of 500 mL/min. For high-efficiency and high-flux dialyzers, it is usually 700–800 mL/min. It is counterproductive and provides an inefficient dialysis to use high blood flow rates with a high efficiency or high-flux dialyzer with a dialysate flow of less than one and one-half the blood flow rate. Adequate dialysate flow is essential for an efficient dialysis.

Dialysate Flow Monitoring

These alarm conditions include low incoming water pressure to the machine, dialysate pump failure, and obstruction in the flow path and power failure.

Most machines have a continuous audible alarm with these conditions. There usually are no alarms that alert the staff when the dialysate flow rate is set too low, for example, at 500 mL/min instead of at 800 mL/min. Dialysis personnel must be diligent in monitoring this aspect of care.

Effluent Dialysate Line

Dialysis personnel must monitor the dialysate effluent line to the drain to ensure that it is not obstructed and that it is properly placed in the drain. An obstruction can cause backpressure into the dialysate compartment and may decrease the dialysate flow rate.

Electrical Safety

Dialysis machines pose a risk of electrical shock to a patient or staff member. All electronic equipment must be inspected and tested on a periodic basis. The staff members, most frequently in the patient care areas, must accept responsibility for identifying and reporting any potential hazardous conditions. All electric components should be adequately isolated from liquid leaks and the outside of equipment shielded from liquid spills. Electric components must be plugged into the correct socket, and grounded plugs used. Electrical safety classes and safe use of equipment is mandatory for all dialysis personnel.

Other Areas to Monitor in the Dialysate Circuit

Additional areas requiring monitoring include correct prescription, absence of impurities (cleaning and disinfecting agents), microbiologic count, and absence of potential pyrogenic agents.

Dialysate Prescription

Dialysis personnel must confirm that the physician's orders prescribing the dialysate content match the delivered prescription of dialysate. The dialysate prescription is not static. Some physicians model and individually tailor sodium, potassium, calcium, magnesium, and dextrose. A major problem with using many individualized dialysate formulas in one facility is the increase in risk for error by personnel. The more variables that exist in a dialysis unit, the greater the inherent risk of staff errors increases as the variables increase in a dialysis unit.

Dialysate Prescription Monitoring

Staff must check and verify all dialysate concentrate containers for the appropriate content. Each container must be clearly labeled. No unlabeled dialysate concentrate container should be used. Labels must include each electrolyte; the amount, time, and date mixed; and the name of the person performing the task. All additives must be properly recorded on the labels. This is especially important for the bicarbonate concentrate, which must be used within a 24-hour period after mixing. The 24-hour precaution reduces the risk of bacterial growth and calcium and magnesium precipitation. The correct dialysate concentrate must be attached to the correct concentrate port on the dialysis machine.

Sterility and Impurities

The dialysate solution is very clean, but not sterile. Most dialysis facilities in the United States use reverse osmosis (RO) systems to filter the feed water. Theoretically, the product water should be sterile. But, as the water courses through the plastic piping of the dialysis unit to the dialysis machine and traverses through the fluid pathway, it comes in contact with bacteria, endotoxins, pyrogens, and other impurities.

All fluid pathways in the dialysis machines must be routinely rinsed, cleaned, and disinfected. The rinsing and cleaning process keeps the internal environment of the dialysis machine clean and free of cellular debris or deposits for proper operation. The disinfection eliminates bacterial growth and prevents the risk of pyrogen reactions. Each dialysis facility uses different techniques to achieve this end.

Inadequate cleaning and disinfection of the water treatment system, dialysate delivery system, and dialysate concentrate containers leads to high bacterial counts. Inadequate disinfection can be due to lack of frequent disinfection, too low concentrations of cold chemical disinfectants, and inadequate contact time of the disinfectant.

AAMI requires a minimum of once a month testing. The testing is to validate the proper disinfection of equipment. The sample for testing the fluid delivery system is taken "at the termination of dialysis at the point where dialysate exits the dialyzer." Industry standards recommend additional sampling. Samples from dialysate concentrate containers and mixing tanks should be taken after the longest period in between disinfection of these containers and after the longest storage time for the concentrate.

All test results must be documented.

Microbiologic Testing

Microbiologic monitoring is to check for the presence of live bacteria. The number of living bacteria in a set volume is reported as the colony count or colony-forming units per milliliter (CFU/mL). Bacterial testing requires that the total viable microbial count is not to exceed 200 colony-forming units per milliliter (Table 13.2). Microbial test results must be documented. Microbial counts exceeding the industry standards require analysis and a more frequent and vigorous disinfecting routine. It is recommended to take action if levels exceed 50 CFU/mL. "Action" is to disinfect the system and repeat cultures at several sites. The action may be to repeat the culture, particularly if only one in a set of cultures was above the action limit.

Bacteria in Bicarbonate Concentrate

The acid dialysate concentrate is bacteriostatic, inhibiting growth or multiplication of bacteria. However, bicarbonate powder used to make bicarbonate concentrate can be contaminated with bacteria, molds, and/or pyrogens. Failure to properly clean and disinfect all areas where water and dialysate travel leads to bacterial growth, often with *Pseudomonas,* in the fluid pathways.

Test for Endotoxins

Endotoxins are bacterial lipopolysaccharides. They are substances released from cell walls when a microorganism is broken down or dies. Their origin is usually from

Table 13.2

AAMI Microbiologic Standards

Fluid	Bacteria Maximum Action Level	Endotoxin Maximum Action Level
Water to prepare dialysate, to reprocess dialyzers, and prepare germicides	<200 CFU/mL ≥50 CFU/mL	<2.0 EU/mL ≥1 EU/mL
Dialysate	<200 CFU/mL ≥ CFU/mL	<2.0 EU/mL ≥1 EU/mL
Bicarbonate concentrate	<200 CFU/mL ≥50 CFU/mL	<2.0 EU/mL ≥1 EU/mL
Minimum frequency	Monthly	Monthly

(From Pittard J, De Palma J. *Dialysate Monograph.* 1st ed. Glendale, CA: Hemodialysis, Inc.; 2013.)

gram-negative bacteria. The presence of endotoxins is measured using the limulus amebocyte lysate (LAL) assay. The LAL concentration should be less than 2 endotoxin units (EU) per milliliter (<2 EU/mL). It is recommended to take action if levels exceed 1.0 EU/mL.

Pyrogens

High bacterial counts predispose to pyrogen reactions. The most common type of pyrogen is from fragments of dead bacteria. However, any type of cellular debris, even if it is sterile, can cause pyrogen reactions. An increase in pyrogen reactions is associated with the use of high-flux dialyzers and bicarbonate dialysate.

The lack of adequate removal of bacteria and bacterial end products from the dialysate solutions and/or fluid pathway of the dialysis machines is invariably the principal cause of these pyrogenic reactions. Dialysis facilities that practice scrupulous water disinfection and control, even with reuse of dialyzers, have virtually no pyrogenic reactions.

Some literature invokes the increased porosity of the high-flux membrane to whole bacteria as a substantial cause of pyrogen reactions. However, even in dialysis units using reprocessed high-flux dialyzers, correcting the high microbial counts of the feed water and delivered dialysate invariably eliminates all pyrogen reactions.

Ultrapure Dialysis Fluid

The term *ultrapure* has been in use since the early 1990s. The microbiologic quality of dialysis fluid dictates the definition of ultrapure dialysis fluid. Composed of ultrapure dialysate and water, this fluid should contain a bacteria count less than 0.1 CFU/mL and endotoxin levels less than 0.03 EU/mL. These levels, established in the European community, have much stricter standards for microbiologic testing as compared to the standards in use in the United States.

The European Best Practice Guidelines for Hemodialysis recommend the use of ultrapure dialysis fluid as a goal for all patients and all modalities along with recommendations on testing to validate the purity of the fluid. Evidence suggests that the use of "ultrapure" dialysate diminishes inflammatory processes seen in the dialysis patient population improving the overall morbidity and mortality rates.

Innovative approaches are currently in use in the United States. Bacterial and pyrogen filters for manufacturing ultrapure dialysis fluid are being integrated into the fluid delivery systems.

Cleaning and Disinfection

It would seem to be obvious that cleaning and disinfection of the dialysis machinery should only be done after all patients have been completely disconnected. Though obvious, there are several reported instances of patients being "bleached" or "cooked" when the respective cleaning procedure was begun before all patients were disconnected.

Central System Hazard

A central fluid-delivery system that services more than one room carries the enormous risk of this lethal misadventure. A careful and thorough bed and chair check by two individuals must be performed to verify that no patient is on dialysis in that setting.

Routine Cleaning

Routine cleaning of fluid delivery systems is accomplished by rinsing with purified water (AAMI standard) and acid cleaning of the fluid pathway on a daily basis. Acid cleaning minimizes the buildup of calcium precipitate that is associated with bicarbonate dialysate. Acid cleaning does not disinfect the machine. Acid cleaning is accomplished with the use of acetic acid (5%) or vinegar, citric acid, peracetic-based disinfectants, and acid concentrate. A minimum of a 5-minute water rinse is recommended before acid cleaning.

A thorough rinse of the dialysis machine must be done before patient use or chemical disinfection. Acetic acid can easily be tested for residuals by using pH test paper.

Fluid Delivery System Disinfection

Disinfection of the fluid delivery system is done by heat and/or chemical disinfection. Chemical disinfection is done usually once each week, or more often if necessary. Frequency of disinfection depends on routine bacterial counts and the orders of the medical director. Samples for bacterial counts should be taken before disinfection.

Heat Disinfection

Certain models of fluid delivery machines are equipped to use heat disinfection. In most cases, this is done on a daily basis. Heat disinfection occurs with water heated to about 85°C in the internal fluid pathway of the dialysis machine. The average length of heat exposure is about 30 minutes. It is important to follow the manufacturer's recommendations. If the machine is to be used following heat disinfection, it is critical to allow the proper cooling down cycle before patient use. Most machines using heat disinfection have a built-in safety feature that will not allow the machine to go into the "dialyze" mode until the temperature has dropped below 42°C.

Chemical Disinfection

Chemical disinfection may be done with a variety of chemicals. The most common chemical disinfectants in use are sodium hypochlorite, peracetic acid, and formaldehyde. A thorough water rinse is essential when using corrosive chemicals for disinfection. When using chemical disinfectants, it is important to remember that all disinfectants require a certain amount of contact time. High microbial counts in water require longer contact times.

Fluid pathways that have dead spaces, blind loops, or inactive dialysis stations that are improperly shunted to drain are especially hazardous. All dead spaces are difficult to disinfect.

All machines require labeling with a sign indicating the presence of the chemical disinfectant and the need for residual testing before the disinfection is deemed complete.

Sodium Hypochlorite

Sodium hypochlorite (bleach) is a cold disinfectant. It is available in different concentrations ranging from 5% to 10%. The advantages of sodium hypochlorite are its low cost, its effectiveness, and its safety. Free chlorine is a strong oxidant. It effectively cleans and eliminates any cellular debris in the fluid pathway that may interfere with the machine operation.

Residual testing for sodium hypochlorite is simple and done with chlorine reagent test strips that test down to 0.5 parts per million (ppm). The residual test is very sensitive. Sodium hypochlorite in minute amounts greater than 1 : 25,000 produces hemolysis. Some dialysis units clean their bicarbonate concentrate plastic containers with bleach but do not carefully rinse or test for residual chlorine before refilling with bicarbonate concentrate. This allows bleach to be dialyzed into the patient, causing a low-level persistent hemolysis that is ignored or attributed to functional iron deficiency. Failure to perform residual testing will result in acute hemolysis or slow hemolysis that may go undetected.

Formaldehyde

Formaldehyde is a cold sterilant that effectively kills all microorganisms, including spores and resistant viruses, when used in proper concentrations and given adequate contact time. There are several reports of serious to deadly septicemia, with inadequate formaldehyde concentrations being used to disinfect the fluid path of dialysis machinery. It is the most common periodic disinfectant used for fluid-delivery systems. It is an inexpensive and stable solution with a long shelf life.

Formaldehyde is a gas that is dissolved in water to form the compound formalin. Formalin is the saturated solution of formaldehyde in water. A 100% formalin solution is equivalent to 37%–40% formaldehyde. In dialysis, a 4% formaldehyde (11% formalin) concentration is used.

Concentrations lower than 4% formaldehyde do not adequately kill *Mycobacterium chelonae* in water. The formaldehyde gas is irritating to the eyes and has an offensive odor. Gloves must always be worn when handling formaldehyde to prevent dermatitis and allergic sensitivities. The room must be well ventilated. Any splashing must be minimized. A face shield gives total protection to the face. Minimally, eye protection (goggles) must be worn when handling formaldehyde.

Formaldehyde has no cleaning properties. Formaldehyde denatures protein and fixes most cellular debris. Therefore, before its use, the fluid pathway requires water rinsing and use of another chemical substance to remove any existing cellular debris and deposits. The fluid pathway of the fluid-delivery machines is filled with formaldehyde after cleaning to destroy any and all microorganisms. Generally, the formaldehyde is left in the machine overnight for effective contact time.

Sensitive residual testing is now available. Indicator test strips are now on the market to test for residual formaldehyde to a sensitivity of 1.0 ppm. The same principles apply to this cold sterilant as described for peracetic acid. In the past, safety tests for formaldehyde called for the use of Schiff reagent. Schiff reagent will test to 5 ppm. The newer indicator test strips are more sensitive.

There have been several outbreaks of feed water being contaminated with residual formaldehyde, which led to a number of dialysis patients on single patient machines becoming seriously ill with shock, coma, and semilethal consequences.

Peracetic Acid

The use of a stabilized mixture of peracetic acid, hydrogen peroxide, and acetic acid is probably the cold sterilant of choice for fluid delivery systems. Unlike formaldehyde, this mixture leaves no toxic residues. It decomposes into oxygen and acetic acid after reacting with organic material. The odor is pungent, similar to the smell of vinegar.

The mixture of peracetic acid, hydrogen peroxide, and acetic acid acts as a cleaning agent in addition to a cold sterilant. The mixture is a strong oxidant that readily cleans all cellular debris and precipitates or scale in the machines when used routinely. As a cold sterilant, it is effective with an 11-hour contact time. Because it is a strong oxidant, the manufacturer's recommendations must be followed carefully so that materials in the machines will not be adversely affected.

Test strips are available to check for the presence or absence of the peracetic acid mixture. Indicator test strips ensure the presence of this cold sterilant in the machines. After the peracetic acid mixture is rinsed from the machine, residual test strips test for the absence of the peracetic acid mixture. The residual testing is very sensitive, testing down to <1 ppm.

Because the peracetic acid mixture is a strong oxidant, its handling requires careful attention to avoid chemical burns. Gloves and face protection are mandatory. Accidental contact exposure to this chemical requires water flushes and medical attention similar to those described for formaldehyde.

Regardless of the type of cleaning or disinfecting agent used in the facility, a thorough water rinse must be done before adding chemicals and after cleaning and disinfection. Safety tests must be done after the final rinse to validate the absence of the chemical used. It is dangerous to rely on a timed rinse without the use of a valid safety test. Residual testing prevents patient injury due to chemical exposure.

General Principles for Chemical Disinfection

Time is an important factor in chemical disinfection. Total disinfection requires adequate time exposure of the chemical to the organisms to be killed. The concentration of the chemical, temperature, and the number of organisms to be killed determines the amount of exposure time. The greater the number of organisms to be killed, the longer is the exposure time needed. Organisms such as spores require longer exposure time than bacteria.

Chemical disinfectants need to remain moist for effectiveness. A chemical disinfectant that dries up is no longer effective. The concentration of the chemical must be in accordance with the manufacturer's recommendations. Lower concentrations may not be effective in killing all microorganisms, whereas concentrations that are higher may not be more effective. Blood and organic matter decrease the effectiveness of the chemical disinfectant. Chemical disinfectants should not be mixed, as mixing can alter their activity.

Dialysate systems must not have any dead spaces. A poorly designed dialysate system with dead spaces is impossible to disinfect adequately. To assess adequate chemical disinfection, monitor the equipment with cultures.

Additional principles include the following: (1) do not use chemical disinfectants beyond their expiration date, (2) always label equipment that contains a chemical disinfectant, and (3) perform an adequate water rinse prior to and after all chemical disinfection and perform the appropriate safety test after all chemical disinfection to ensure absence of the chemical (do not rely on a timed rinse).

Documentation of Dialysate Monitoring

Document the performance and results of all safety tests on the patient Daily Dialysis Record and/or the machine or log sheet. Documentation or charting of all activities

Table 13.3

Risks to Patients With Inadequate Monitoring

Problem	Potential Risk to Patient
Wrong prescription	Electrolyte imbalances, especially with potassium, leading to cardiac arrhythmias and cardiac arrest
Conductivity low	Hemolysis—death
Conductivity high	Hyperosmolar coma—death
High temperature	Hemodialysis—death
Dialysate flow rate absent	No dialysis with risk of serious electrolyte imbalances, especially hyperkalemia, cardiac arrhythmias, and cardiac arrest
Dialysate flow rate low	Inadequate and inefficient dialysis
Residual chemicals (bleach, formaldehyde, peracetic acid)	Hemodialysis—death
High bacterial count	Mild to severe pyrogen reaction

(From Pittard J, De Palma J. *Dialysate Monograph*. 1st ed. Glendale, CA: Hemodialysis, Inc.; 2013.)

in dialysate monitoring is critical for patient safety. Do not initiate dialysis until all of the appropriate checks are complete and recorded according to the established policies in the facility.

Education of all staff members is critical to a safe and well-run dialysis unit. In-service education must be given for any new dialysate concentrates, preparation of dialysate concentrates, safety tests, and fluid delivery systems. There are many risks (Table 13.3) to the patient's well-being with inadequate monitoring of the dialysate compartment prior to or during the dialysis treatment.

The Blood Circuit

The blood (extracorporeal) circuit (Fig. 13.9) monitors pressures in the arterial and venous blood lines, and the integrity of the circuit for the presence of air and blood leaks. The four main blood circuit monitors (Fig. 13.10) are the arterial pressure monitor, venous pressure monitor, air-foam detector, and blood-leak detector.

The blood-leak detector acts as a blood-circuit alarm but is entirely incorporated within the dialysate circuit and has already been described. The machinery responds to blood-circuit alarms by activating an audible alarm, a visual alarm, stopping the blood pump, and engaging the venous line clamp to stop the blood flow through the blood circuit.

Additional areas to monitor in the blood circuit are blood flow rate, heparin therapy, and normal saline supply.

Arterial Pressure Monitor—Pre-Blood Pump

The arterial pressure monitor measures the pressure in the arterial blood line between the patient's arterial access and the blood. With the blood pump set to blood flow

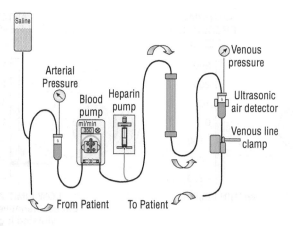

Figure 13.9

Blood (Extracorporeal) Circuit. (From Pittard J: Hemodialysis Nursing, Training Manual, 7th ed., version 7.0. Santa Monica, CA, 2003, with permission.)

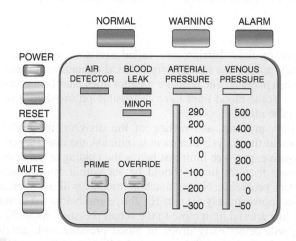

Figure 13.10

Blood Circuit Monitors. (From Pittard J: Hemodialysis Nursing, Training Manual, 7th ed., version 7.0. Santa Monica, CA, 2003, with permission.)

rates greater than 200 mL/min to as high as 450 mL/min, the pressure in this blood tubing segment is commonly subatmospheric to negative. This portion of the blood circuit can be a source of air entry into the blood circuit and is considered a high-risk area.

The arterial pressure monitor is leak-free with adjustable high/low limits (Fig. 13.11), which reads negative and positive pressures in millimeters of mercury (mm Hg; 10% accuracy). This monitor requires a filter to prevent viruses, bacteria, or blood from being refluxed back into the arterial pressure monitor. This filter is essential, as viral hepatitis has been transmitted by contamination of air devices.

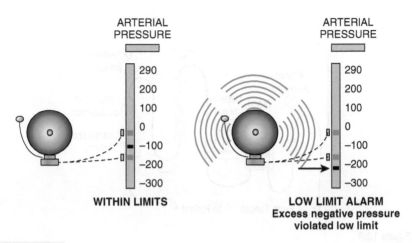

Figure 13.11

Arterial Pressure. (From Pittard J: Hemodialysis Nursing, Training Manual, 7th ed., version 7.0. Santa Monica, CA, 2003, with permission.)

These filters or fluid barriers are called isolators and/or transducer filters/ protectors. They protect the monitor from blood contamination and the spread of infection between patients. The pressure monitor lines must be unclamped and patent during dialysis. Some blood lines have collapsible pillow-shaped segments, which can initiate a false alarm.

During set-up, priming, and rinsing of the dialyzer, the high-low limits are opened. As soon as the dialysis treatment is initiated, the dialysis personnel must set the low, or negative, pressure limit just below the reading at the desired blood flow. Upper and lower monitor limits should be set within 50–100 mm Hg of actual reading to detect problems. Newer machine models will automatically adjust the high/low limits approximately 50 mm Hg above and below the actual pressure.

Setting the low arterial limit close to the actual pressure, about 50 mm Hg below that pressure, will detect early drops in blood pressure with arteriovenous (AV) fistulas. Some units limit the minimum arterial limit to –100 mm Hg.

The greater the vacuum, the greater the risk of air entering this tubing segment from any crack, improperly glued or fitted joint, sample port, saline infusion line, or the patient's access. It is advisable to set the high limit just below zero, which will pick up a disruption of the arterial blood line from the fistula needle.

Arterial Pressure Monitoring

The usual causes of a low-limit arterial pressure alarm are a drop in blood pressure (only with AV fistulas), a kink in the arterial blood line between the access and blood pump, malpositioned arterial needle or problem with arterial access, and a clotted arterial line. The circuit should always be checked for air bubbles.

The usual causes of a high-limit arterial pressure alarm are bloodline separation (only if the upper limit is set below 0 mm Hg), the saline infusion line is unclamped, an increase in patient's blood pressure, a leak in the circuit between the patient and monitor, and torn blood tubing in the pump segment. It is important to check for leaking blood.

The appropriate response to pressure alarms is to, first, mute the audible alarm; second, investigate the problem; third, correct the problem; and fourth, restart the blood pump by pressing the reset/restart button. Do not restart the blood pump until the problem is corrected for patient safety. Failure to correct the problem will cause the alarm to reoccur.

Venous Pressure Monitor

The venous pressure monitor, located postdialyzer, monitors pressure at the venous drip chamber, the segment between the drip chamber and the patient's venous access, and the added intra-access pressure. The resistance to the blood flow entering the venous access causes the pressure to be positive (Fig. 13.12), above 0 mm Hg.

The venous pressure monitor's structure and standards are similar to those described for the arterial pre-blood pump monitor. This pressure monitor requires protection by a filter or transducer fluid barrier.

Venous Pressure Monitoring

Causes of a high venous pressure alarm are a kink in the venous blood line between the drip chamber and patient's venous access, a clot in the venous drip chamber and/or downstream to the patient, and a malpositioned venous needle or problem with the venous access device.

Causes of a low venous pressure alarm are blood line separation or disruption of connections between the blood pump to and including the venous access; a kink in the blood line postdialyzer and pre–venous drip chamber; a clotted dialyzer; and a lowering of the blood-pump speed. Note that setting the low limit close to the

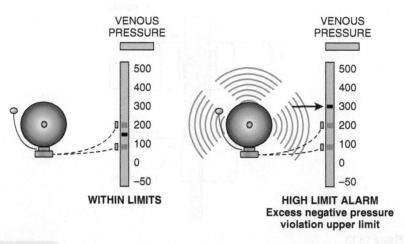

WITHIN LIMITS

HIGH LIMIT ALARM
Excess negative pressure
violation upper limit

Figure 13.12

Venous Pressure. (From Pittard J: Hemodialysis Nursing, Training Manual, 7th ed., version 7.0. Santa Monica, CA, 2003, with permission.)

operating pressure of the venous drip chamber can alert to a disruption of the blood circuit between the blood pump and venous access site. With a disruption of the circuit, the venous pressure will drop to 0 mm Hg.

It should be remembered that the venous pressure monitor reflects P_{BO} in the equation $TMP = P_{BO} - P_{DO}$. High venous pressures can result in too high ultrafiltration rates unless an ultrafiltration-controlled machine is being used.

Air-Foam Detector

The air-foam detector monitors blood in the venous tubing (Fig. 13.13) for the presence of air, foam, and microbubbles. It must be reemphasized that with almost all internal AV fistulas/grafts and all venovenous dialysis, a significant subatmospheric pressure exists between the arterial access and the roller pump. There are many junctions and heat-sealed joints in this portion of the circuit. If the heparin infusion line is in the negative-pressure segment rather than post blood pump, it may increase the risk for air entry. After the blood pump, the blood circuit is at considerable positive pressure and air can enter only by pumping or injecting it into the remainder of the circuit. Air embolism is a preventable and very serious dialysis misadventure.

Two types of air-foam detectors are in use: the ultrasonic and the reflected light detectors. It is believed that only the ultrasonic device is currently being sold. Nevertheless, many of the reflected light-type devices are still in use. Surprisingly, there are no standards for permissible detection of air because either type of detector readily identifies gross air displacement of blood in the venous drip chamber when properly armed and functioning. Microbubbles from 5 to 500 μm in diameter represent a different problem as they stream along with the blood flow. These microbubbles are entrained in the bloodstream.

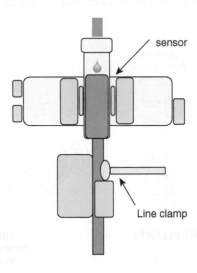

Figure 13.13

Air-Foam Detector. (From Pittard J: Hemodialysis Nursing, Training Manual, 7th ed., version 7.0. Santa Monica, CA, 2003, with permission.)

Although both types of monitors can detect microbubbles, their guaranteed detection requires a sensitivity setting that may result in many false alarms because of turbulence in fluid flow. The compromise is a sensitivity adjustment of the ultrasonic devices such that some false alarms occur that require the attention of dialysis personnel. In certain situations, microbubbles can go undetected and cause clinical air embolism. The current standards for these devices require response to air in blood, a blood and saline mixture, or saline. Only the ultrasonic device can meet this requirement. A dangerous aspect of the reflected light device is that it is effective only when sensing the whole blood of the patient. It cannot be accurately armed during priming, initiation, or rinsing.

Venous Line Clamp

An air detector alarm must activate the venous line clamp (Fig. 13.13). The venous line clamp must completely occlude the venous blood line and withstand an intraluminal pressure of 800 mm Hg. The venous line clamp should be constructed as to not damage the blood lines, and should not restrict the blood tubing when in an open position. The venous line clamp circuitry must interface with and stop the blood pump. Most integrated air-foam detectors meet all of these standards.

There are dialysis machines, which are unsafe as they include the ability to dialyze with both the air-leak detector and venous line clamp disarmed and only some marginal indication of this disarmed state.

Air-Foam Detector and Venous Line Clamp Monitoring

With an air-foam detector alarm state, identify that the venous line clamp is engaged and that the blood pump is stopped. Visually inspect the entire blood circuit from the venous access backward to the arterial end for the presence of air, foam, or microbubbles. Check the level in the venous drip chamber—it should be three quarters full. Check that the venous drip chamber is properly placed in its holder, the level detector door is closed and latched, and the mesh in the drip chamber is below the air detector. Also, check if the air sensors are clean. Always validate the absence of air before restarting the blood pump and disengaging the venous line clamp. If air is present, disconnect the patient from the extracorporeal circuit.

Before beginning dialysis, make sure that the air-foam detector is turned on and operational and that the venous blood line is properly placed in the line-clamp holder. Ultrasonic devices are usually activated during priming of the circuit. Reflected light devices cannot be activated until whole blood at full hematocrit is in the venous tubing.

Because each brand of detector varies in its operation, ensure that dialysis personnel are aware of the type of device used in the facility and are in-serviced on its unique features and operation. Unfortunately, when staff pushes the RESET/RESTART button in responding to this alarm condition, the blood pump restarts. This can be a potentially deadly response. Microbubbles that may not be visible to the naked eye can then flow into the patient. I advise staff to manually turn off the blood pump when responding to an air in blood alarm. After all inspections are complete, pushing the reset button will not automatically start the blood pump. However, if the problem is not corrected, the alarm will reoccur with no harm to the patient.

Four alarm conditions are outlined here for general information.

Alarm Condition 1. Careful inspection reveals that the blood-air level in the venous drip chamber is normal and that there are no microbubbles (foam) in any portion of the line or dialyzer. This is a false alarm—release the line clamp and reset the detector.

Alarm Condition 2. The blood level in the venous drip chamber has fallen. In response, check for upstream bubbles; if none is present, return the blood-air level to normal in the drip chamber with the usual technique, release the line clamp, and reset the alarm.

Alarm Condition 3. There are microbubbles (foam) in the venous line. In response, clamp the venous line and the venous access line, directing attention to the patient in the event that emergency management of air embolism is necessary. Another person should remove the line from the air detector clamp, disconnect the patient from the blood circuit, and aseptically join the arterial and venous ends of the blood circuit for recirculation. Remove ultrafiltration, and open the saline to remove air from the blood circuit and to collect it in the venous drip chamber. If this measure is successful, place the venous line into the air-detector line clamp and rearm the air-foam detector. If no further alarm is activated, reconnect the blood circuit lines to the patient and reinitiate dialysis.

Alarm Condition 4. Gross air and bubbles fill the entire blood circuit, including the dialyzer. In response, clamp the "venous" line and direct attention to the patient for emergency management of air embolism. Dispose of the entire blood circuit, including the dialyzer, and set up a new one to reinitiate dialysis.

Heparin Infusion Pump

The heparin infusion pump is usually located in the post–blood pump segment. A heparin infusion line attaches to a syringe filled with heparin. This allows for the infusion of heparin during dialysis. An electric motor drives a piston to move the heparin plunger forward to infuse the heparin. Dialysis personnel must turn the heparin pump on and set the correct hourly infusion rate. No alarms occur if the pump is not turned on or if an incorrect hourly infusion rate is set. Most machines have an audible alarm when the heparin level in the syringe is very low.

Heparin Infusion Pump Monitoring

Personnel must make sure they are using the correct-size syringe based on the way the heparin pump is calibrated. Make sure the syringe and plunger are placed properly in the holder. Check that the pump is on and the variable hourly rate is set correctly. Implement hourly checks to ensure the correct infusion of heparin therapy. Newer machine models allow the personnel to program the heparin bolus, infusion rate, and length of time for the infusion.

Blood Flow Rate

The blood flow rate is an important parameter that influences the efficiency of dialyzer clearance. All blood pumps have an on/off switch and an adjustable variable speed pump. There are no machine alarms if the desired blood flow rate is not set correctly.

Blood Flow Rate Monitoring

Double-check that the blood flow rate is properly set. A qualified person must calibrate blood pumps to ensure that the actual blood flow is comparable to the blood-flow setting. The facility must use appropriate blood-tubing size for proper occlusion of the roller pump. Inadequate occlusion causes back flow, foaming, and possibly hemolysis. Overocclusion causes tubing damage, blood leaks, and the potential for hemolysis.

Blood Pump and Blood Lines

Narrowed Blood-Pump Tubing Segment

In 1998, 30 patients in three different states in the United States developed hemolysis with or without chest pains, shortness of breath, nausea, or abdominal pain while undergoing hemodialysis. Two patients died. All of these catastrophes were due to a manufacturing defect in a small portion of the blood-pump segment of the blood tubing. The staff did not notice the defect when inserting the blood-pump segment. A marked narrowing of this segment induced massive hemolysis in these patients, which initially was unexplained and required a formal investigation by the Centers for Disease Control and Prevention (CDC).

Kinked Arterial Blood Lines

In a 1-year period, from December 1989 to December 1990, a total of 10 hemolytic reactions occurred in an outpatient hemodialysis unit. Eight patients were hospitalized and one died. All patients developed severe abdominal or back pain an average of 2.5 hours into a 4-hour hemodialysis session using bleach-formaldehyde reprocessed hollow-fiber Cuprophan dialyzers. All had visible hemolysis in a spun hematocrit; 7 had a significant decrease in hematocrit; and 6 developed pancreatitis. Hemolytic reactions continued despite changing to 15-gauge needles, removing bleach from the reuse procedure, and stopping reuse of the dialyzers.

Investigation of each episode failed to find an abnormality in dialysate temperature or tonicity; dialysate or water levels of copper, zinc, nitrates, chloramine, or formaldehyde; or blood pump or venous alarm. On the eighth hemolytic episode, a dialysis staff member noted a kink in the arterial blood line. Two subsequent hemolytic reactions occurred; in each, kinks were found in the arterial blood line, either in the excess tubing between the blood pump and drip chamber, or in the predialyzer segment. No further hemolytic reactions occurred after changing to a new arterial blood line without redundant tubing and securing all lines.

IV Saline Infusion

Access to normal saline (0.9% NaCl) into the extracorporeal circuit occurs via the saline administration line located at the beginning of the arterial blood circuit. Normal saline is used to prime the dialyzer and blood tubing for patient use, to replace volume in the patient during dialysis, and to rinse the red blood cells at the conclusion of dialysis.

IV Saline Infusion Monitoring

Personnel must make sure an adequate amount of normal saline is available for immediate use during the dialysis treatment. Normal saline drips should be discouraged. Although normal saline comes in collapsible plastic bags, if these accidentally empty during dialysis, a few hundred milliliters of air will enter the blood circuit, possibly causing an air embolism.

Conclusion

The world of dialysis has undergone many changes. The fluid delivery systems are much more sophisticated and dialyzers more efficient. No amount of electronic machinery, fail-safe devices, flashing lights, sirens, dials, or protocols can take the place of an alert and well-trained dialysis staff member. Non–registered nurses or patient care technicians (PCTs) perform 75% of direct patient care of ESRD patients in the United States, and it is essential that they understand potential alarm situations and are thoroughly trained to ensure safe dialysis treatment.

C H A P T E R   1 4

Methods of Hemodialysis Anticoagulation

David I. Ortiz-Melo, MD •
Eugene C. Kovalik, MD, CM, FRCP, FACP, FASN

Introduction

During hemodialysis and continuous renal replacement therapies (CRRT) blood is constantly flowing between the patient's vascular access and the dialyzer. This extracorporeal circuit exposes blood to surfaces with variable degrees of thrombogenicity. To prevent thrombosis and malfunctioning of the circuit, some form of anticoagulation is usually required. End-stage renal disease patients are also at increased risk of bleeding due to platelet dysfunction related to the uremic milieu. Therefore, the ideal anticoagulant for use in these patients should efficiently prevent thrombosis during hemodialysis therapy while at the same time not increase the risk of intra- and interdialytic bleeding. Moreover, the anticoagulation agent used during hemodialysis should also be simple to administer with minimal or no monitoring requirements, be cost-effective, and be well tolerated with no or negligible adverse effects.

Various anticoagulation protocols have been described and are currently available, including (1) full systemic anticoagulation, (2) anticoagulation of the extracorporeal circuit with minimal systemic effects (regional anticoagulation), and (3) anticoagulation-free dialysis. Strategies to minimize the risk of bleeding include the use of low-dose heparin or no-heparin hemodialysis protocols, such as use of heparin-grafted membranes, regular saline flushes, or predilution hemodiafiltration. Regional anticoagulation with citrate, prostacyclin, or heparin-protamine has been used with varying success. Other agents such as argatroban, recombinant hirudin, and heparinoids have also provided effective anticoagulation and represent a valid alternative in selected patients. In this chapter, we will discuss these agents, different protocols of hemodialysis and CRRT anticoagulation, as well as important considerations in various clinical scenarios.

Systemic Anticoagulation

Standard Heparin Anticoagulation

Unfractionated heparin (UFH) is the most commonly used anticoagulation agent during hemodialysis. UFH binds to antithrombin, inducing a conformational change that leads to an increased activity of this natural anticoagulant. This binding results in accelerated inactivation of coagulation factors, such as factor Xa and thrombin (Fig. 14.1). Unfractionated heparin is affordable, reliable, easily reversible, and

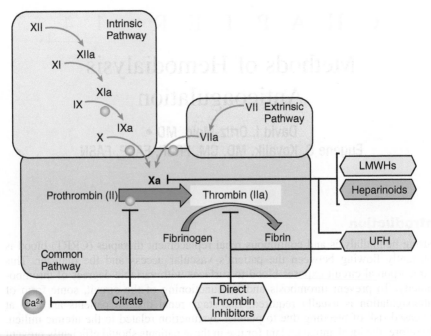

Figure 14.1

Schematic Representation of the Coagulation Cascade and Targets of Different Anticoagulants. Unfractionated heparin (UFH) binds to antithrombin and indirectly inhibits both factor Xa and thrombin. Low-molecular-weight heparins (LMWHs) and heparinoids only inhibit factor Xa. Direct thrombin inhibitors, such as argatroban and recombinant hirudin, directly bind and block thrombin, the key enzyme that converts soluble fibrinogen into insoluble fibrin. Citrate chelates calcium (Ca^{2+}, circles), a key cofactor of many reactions in the coagulation cascade.

requires minimal staff intervention after a patient's heparin dose is determined. UFH can also be safely used during pregnancy, since it does not cross the feto-placental barrier. Although heparin is relatively well tolerated, there are certain known risks and complications associated with its use, including increased risk of bleeding, heparin-induced thrombocytopenia (HIT) type I and type II, hypertriglyceridemia, hypersensitivity reactions, pruritus, and osteoporosis.

Unfractionated heparin has a rapid onset of action and relatively short half-life (approximately 1 hour in dialysis patients). It is important to keep in mind, however, that there is interpatient variability in heparin metabolism during hemodialysis. Heparin activity is highly determined by patient weight, and other variables such as dialyzer membrane adsorption, erythropoietin dose, thrombogenicity of the extra-corporeal circuit, blood flow, and length of the hemodialysis treatment, among others.

Anticoagulation with UFH during hemodialysis can be monitored by the deter-mination of activated partial thromboplastin time (aPTT), which is targeted to 1.5–2 times above the baseline value. However, this method requires frequent testing, leading to increased cost and repeated blood draws. Another option is the determination of activated clotting time (ACT), which can be obtained at the bedside with point-of-care devices. ACT is typically targeted to 80% higher than the baseline value. However, ACTs are used infrequently because of the need for rigorous standardization, resulting in quality assurance and regulatory issues. In general, most outpatient dialysis units do not routinely measure anticoagulation parameters unless there is clinical evidence suggesting excessive dialyzer clotting (i.e., visual clots, increased extracorporeal circuit pressures) or signs of over-anticoagulation, such as prolonged bleeding at needle puncture sites following dialysis. Except on rare occasions, we do not regularly monitor anticoagulation levels in the inpatient and outpatient facilities of our institution.

Currently there are no standardized heparin dosages for anticoagulation during hemodialysis in the United States. A number of empirically based protocols exist to address the competing issues of clotting and postdialysis bleeding from vascular access puncture sites. These methods require minimal staff intervention and are standard in most outpatient hemodialysis units; they are, however, unsuitable for patients with significant bleeding risks. Typically, the administration of heparin during hemodialysis requires an initial loading bolus, followed by a maintenance dose that can be given either as repeated separate boluses or as a continuous infusion. These strategies ensure systemic anticoagulation throughout the dialysis treatment. A routine repeated bolus regimen consists of an initial bolus of UFH (usually about 40–50 IU/kg body weight, or 2000–4000 IU) administered into the venous access needle, followed by a midtreatment dose of 1000–2000 IU. Alternatively, heparin modeling can be performed using an initial bolus followed by a constant fixed infusion of heparin (usually 10–15 IU/kg body weight/h, or 1000–2000 IU/h) to maintain an activated clotting time of 200–250 seconds (normal ≈ 90–140 seconds). Heparin infusion should be terminated 30–60 minutes prior to the end of treatment to reduce postdialysis vascular access puncture site bleeding. Some other protocols include the use of a single initial bolus dose with no maintenance doses, and the administration of a high bolus heparin dose (i.e., greater than 5000 IU) with decreasing infusion rates, as the treatment proceeds, to minimize postdialysis bleeding. Furthermore, in facilities that practice dialyzer reuse, incorporation of a pharmacodynamic approach to heparin modeling has also been shown to increase dialyzer reuse rate. The three most common standard anticoagulation regimens using UFH are summarized in Table 14.1. A simplified heparin anticoagulation protocol used in our institution is depicted in Table 14.2.

Low-Dose Heparin

The use of minimum-dose heparin is an alternative anticoagulation strategy for patients with a high bleeding risk who are unable to complete heparin-free hemodialysis as a result of frequent clotting. Currently there are no standardized dosages for this protocol. Initially, the extracorporeal circuit is rinsed with 2000–5000 IU of UFH followed by a saline rinse to remove the unbound anticoagulant. Generally, patients receive boluses of 500 IU of heparin every 30 minutes to keep the activated clotting time no higher than 40% above baseline (>150 but <200 seconds). Alternately, a continuous infusion of heparin with frequent ACT monitoring can be used to achieve the same degree of anticoagulation. Low-dose heparin protocols have been shown to reduce bleeding complications in high-risk patients when compared

Table 14.1

Commonly Used Standard Anticoagulation Regimens Using Unfractionated Heparin (UFH)

Regimen	Advantages	Disadvantages
Initial bolus 40 IU/kg, repeated bolus 1000–2000 IU midtreatment	Ease of administration, less postdialysis bleeding	Less effective for longer dialysis times
Initial bolus 40 IU/kg, continuous infusion 10–15 IU/kg/h	Steady-state anticoagulation	May require monitoring, prolonged postdialysis bleeding
Initial bolus >70 IU/kg, tapered continuous infusion	Steady-state anticoagulation, less postdialysis bleeding	May require monitoring, not suitable for patients with high risk of intradialytic bleeding

Table 14.2

Simplified Regimens Using Unfractionated Heparin (UFH) in Our Institution

Regimen	Doses
Standard	Initial bolus: 2000 IU Maintenance dose: 500 IU/h
Mini	Initial bolus: 1000 IU Maintenance dose: 500 IU/h
Tight	Initial bolus: 1000 IU (once)
No heparin	Saline flushes, no heparin

to regional anticoagulation with heparin and protamine neutralization. The major advantage of this technique is its simplicity. The main disadvantage is that some degree of systemic anticoagulation still occurs, necessitating careful monitoring. In addition, because it involves the use of heparin, this method of anticoagulation should be avoided in patients with heparin-induced thrombocytopenia.

Low-Molecular-Weight Heparins

Low-molecular-weight heparins (LMWHs) are derived from chemical or enzymatic depolymerization of commercial UFH. LMWHs are about one-third of the molecular weight of UFH (4000–5000 daltons vs mean 15,000 daltons for UFH). Like unfractionated heparin, LMWHs inactivate factor Xa (see Fig. 14.1). Because LMWH molecules do not contain enough saccharide units to form the ternary complex required to simultaneously bind thrombin and antithrombin, their ability to inhibit thrombin activity is significantly less. Another important difference from UFH is that the anticoagulation effect of LMWHs is not reliably reversed by protamine sulfate. Anticoagulation monitoring also differs from UFH, in that the aPTT is not accurate with LMWHs; heparinoid or anti–factor Xa activity must be measured to assess their anticoagulant activity. Currently, the recommendations are to aim for an anti-Xa activity of 0.4–0.6 IU/mL in the venous port of the extracorporeal circuit and <0.2 IU/mL at the end of hemodialysis therapy. However, routine monitoring is typically not required, and it is only recommended in those patients at increased risk of bleeding.

LMWHs have been proposed to cause less bleeding and less thrombocytopenia than UFH. The LMWH dalteparin is used widely in European countries; however, the use of LMWHs for hemodialysis anticoagulation in the United States is very limited. Although LMWHs have been demonstrated to be as safe and efficacious as UFH, they have generally not been found to be superior to heparin in terms of dialysis-related bleeding, and the increased cost may not justify the preferential use over UFH. It is also important to note that even though the incidence of HIT is lower than with UFH, LMWHs should not be used as a safe substitute in these patients, because of the extensive cross-reactivity (>90%) between LMWHs and standard UFH.

LMWHs can be used to decrease the thrombogenicity of the extracorporeal circuit itself by covalently coupling LMWH to all surfaces. Preliminary studies have shown that this strategy can be safely used without any additional agents, but the clinical and cost effectiveness of this approach to prevent thrombosis and bleeding compared with regional and no-heparin strategies has yet to be examined.

Recombinant Hirudin Anticoagulation

Hirudin directly binds and inhibits thrombin via the formation of a noncovalent complex (see Fig. 14.1). Recombinant hirudin (lepirudin) has been administered either as a single bolus at the start of hemodialysis or as a continuous infusion. Lepirudin is an effective anticoagulant and may result in less prolongation of the ACT than heparin. Lepirudin is primarily excreted by the kidneys, and for this reason it should be used carefully in hemodialysis patients, as its prolonged half-life (>35 hours) may lead to bleeding complications with repetitive use. There is no antidote available to reverse its anticoagulant effects. Lepirudin is recommended as an alternative hemodialysis anticoagulation agent in patients diagnosed with HIT.

Argatroban

Argatroban is a direct thrombin inhibitor derived from arginine approved for the anticoagulation of the hemodialysis circuit in patients diagnosed with HIT or with other contraindications to heparin. Argatroban reversibly binds to the catalytic thrombin active site, consequently preventing fibrin formation and inhibiting activation of factors V, VIII, and XIII (see Fig. 14.1). As opposed to recombinant hirudin products, argatroban is mainly metabolized by the liver; therefore, it should be used with caution in patients with liver disease. It can be given as an initial bolus of 100–250 µg/kg followed by a maintenance infusion of 0.5–2.0 µg/kg/min adjusted to an aPTT 1.5–3 times of the baseline value. As with most hemodialysis anticoagulation methods, argatroban infusion should be discontinued ~30 minutes before the end of therapy, to avoid excessive bleeding from cannulation sites.

Heparinoids: Danaparoid and Fondaparinux

Heparinoids are glycosaminoglycans derived from heparin. The experience with these agents as alternatives for hemodialysis anticoagulation is very limited.

Danaparoid contains heparin sulfate, dermatan sulfate, and chondroitin sulfate. Similar to heparin, its anticoagulation effects are mainly mediated by inhibition of factor Xa (see Fig. 14.1). Danaparoid is currently not available in the United States. For monitoring, aPTT is not helpful and anti–factor Xa activity has to be measured. There are no antidotes available. Danaparoid contains heparin-like compounds, and cross-reactivity with HIT antibodies has been reported in up to 10% of cases.

Fondaparinux is a pentasaccharide that also binds to antithrombin, causing indirect inhibition of activated factor X (see Fig. 14.1). This agent is not currently approved for hemodialysis anticoagulation, and it should be used with extreme caution in end-stage renal disease patients, because the half-life is significantly increased, which at times can lead to interdialytic systemic anticoagulation.

Regional Anticoagulation

Regional Anticoagulation With Protamine Reversal

The earliest method described to reduce hemodialysis-associated bleeding was regional anticoagulation with protamine reversal. This procedure involves the constant infusion of heparin into the dialyzer arterial line (predialyzer) and the simultaneous constant infusion of the neutralizing agent, protamine, into the venous (postdialyzer) limb of the circuit to prevent systemic anticoagulation (Fig. 14.2). The infusion pump rates are adjusted to keep the whole blood activated clotting time in the dialyzer circuit at 250 seconds and the blood returning to the patient at its predialysis baseline. Because of the technical difficulties and the release of free heparin from the protamine–heparin complex back into the general circulation 2–4 hours after the termination of dialysis (resulting in rebound bleeding), protamine reversal has been largely abandoned. In addition, simpler regimens consisting of minimum-dose and no-dose heparin as well as citrate regional anticoagulation have subsequently been developed that offer a lower incidence of bleeding complications.

Regional Citrate Anticoagulation

The regional citrate regimen that has been adopted in many institutions involves the continuous infusion of isosmotic trisodium citrate solution (102 mmol/L) into the arterial limb of the dialyzer. Citrate chelates calcium, a key cofactor required for various steps in the coagulation cascade (see Fig. 14.1). The fall in the free plasma calcium concentration induced by binding to citrate prevents the progression of the coagulation cascade in the extracorporeal circuit. A calcium-free dialysate is used, and some of the citrate–calcium complex is then removed across the dialyzer. The citrate infusion rate is adjusted to keep the ACT above 200 seconds in the arterial limb. Normocalcemia and regional anticoagulation are achieved by the infusion of 5% calcium chloride into the venous return line at a rate of 0.5 mL/min. This rate is constantly adjusted according to frequent measurements of plasma calcium concentration to prevent hypocalcemia or hypercalcemia. A modification of this technique uses hypertonic trisodium citrate (1.6 mmol/L) and dialysate containing 3 mEq/L of calcium in an attempt to minimize the amounts of replacement calcium needed via venous infusion (see Fig. 14.2). Citrate is converted to bicarbonate in the liver, which may lead to metabolic alkalosis, especially when used with CRRT.

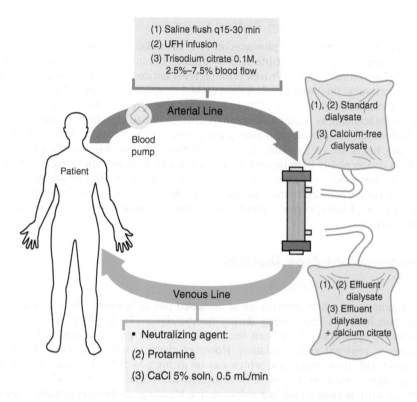

Figure 14.2

Schematic Representation of Hemodialysis Anticoagulation Modalities for Patients at Increased Risk of Bleeding. The modalities depicted are (1) no heparin/saline flush; (2) regional heparin anticoagulation with protamine reversal; and (3) regional citrate anticoagulation.

For this reason, it is recommended to use a dialysate with a lower concentration of bicarbonate. At times, the metabolic alkalosis is severe enough that it may require treatment with a hydrochloric acid infusion.

Comparative trials have shown a reduced incidence of bleeding with citrate-based regimens compared to standard heparin protocols, so it is recommended as an alternative method for patients with a high bleeding risk. Apart from technical complexity and the intensity of monitoring, the major problems with regional citrate anticoagulation are the possibility of hypocalcemia, hypercalcemia, hypernatremia (due to the hypertonic sodium citrate solution), and metabolic alkalosis (due to bicarbonate generated during hepatic metabolism of citrate). Patients with liver insufficiency are especially at risk for metabolic complications. Citrate infusion can also affect the function of cellular elements of the blood, including leukocyte activation and platelet function via its hypocalcemic effects. If closely monitored, however, the complication rate is relatively low.

Prostacyclin Regional Anticoagulation

The arachidonic metabolite prostacyclin is a vasodilator and inhibitor of platelet aggregation. Its in vitro half-life is 3–5 minutes because of rapid metabolism by endothelial smooth muscle. Prostacyclin regional anticoagulation involves the infusion of prostacyclin into the dialyzer circuit at 4–8 ng/kg per minute. This method is rarely recommended because of its unfavorable side effect profile, including headache, lightheadedness, facial flushing, hypotension due to vasodilation, and cost.

Nafamostat is a prostacyclin analog associated with less adverse effects on blood pressure, but is not yet available in the United States. It may, however, be associated with an unacceptably high incidence of clot formation. In one study using nafamostat, clot formation was observed in up to 36% of dialyzers despite adequate prolongation of the activated partial thromboplastin time (aPTT). In addition, nafamostat cannot be used with polyacrylonitrile membranes due to adsorption onto the membrane surface.

Anticoagulant-Free Dialysis

Heparin-Free Dialysis

In circumstances where patients are at increased risk of bleeding, the use of anticoagulation becomes challenging during hemodialysis (Table 14.3). A number of alternative approaches have been used in these at-risk patients, such as low-dose heparin or regional anticoagulation. However, there is still an associated risk of bleeding with these strategies, which can be as high as 50%. The use of regional citrate anticoagulation is generally restricted to specialized units. Therefore, in patients with increased bleeding risk or active bleeding, no-heparin hemodialysis is the preferred method of anticoagulation. This is also a reasonable alternative for patients with HIT or other contraindications to heparin. In this protocol, the dialyzer and tubing are pretreated with 2000–5000 IU of heparin contained in 1 L of normal saline. The heparinized saline is flushed from the extracorporeal lines before the start of the dialysis treatment so that heparin is not administered to the patient. Extracorporeal blood flows are rapidly increased to 250–500 mL/min and maintained throughout the treatment, and 25–30 mL saline flushes are administered every 15–30 minutes into the arterial (predialyzer) limb to minimize hemoconcentration and to wash fibrin strands from the dialyzer into the bubble trap. Of note, the volume of

Table 14.3	
Categorization of Bleeding Risk	
Medium Risk	**High Risk**
Pericarditis	Bleeding diathesis
Recent bleeding <48 hours	Clotting factor disorder
Recent placement of tunneled catheter <24 hours	Actively bleeding
Minor surgery <72 hours	Eye or major surgery <72 hours
Eye or major surgery within 3–7 days	Intracranial hemorrhage <7 days

(Modified from Saltissi D Management of anticoagulation for hemodialysis. In Nissenson AR Fine RN. *Dialysis Therapy*. Philadelphia: Hanley and Belfus, 2002)

saline administered must be removed during the dialysis to prevent volume overload. One-to-one nursing is required for administration of saline flushes and careful monitoring of the arterial and venous pressure alarms to detect early extracorporeal circuit clotting.

Using this technique, about 90% of ICU patients with increased risk of bleeding who require hemodialysis can be successfully dialyzed, with only a 2% clotting rate in the extracorporeal circuit. No significant loss of clearances has been reported compared to patients on standard anticoagulation. In approximately 5% of the cases, conversion to minimum-dose heparin or treatment discontinuation is required.

Disadvantages of this technique include the associated increased ultrafiltration rate required to maintain volume status, which can promote hypotension and increase dialyzer circuit clotting and thrombosis. An additional problem with the no-heparin technique is that blood transfusions cannot usually be given through the dialyzer circuit because of the increased risk of clotting, which may pose difficulty for patients with limited peripheral access. A potential solution, which has been successfully used, is to use a large-bore stopcock to transfuse blood into the venous limb (postdialyzer) of the circuit. An additional disadvantage is the increased technician labor required and the need for close observation, which can potentially elevate dialysis costs. For these reasons, no-heparin strategies are not recommended as a long-term anticoagulation therapy for outpatient hemodialysis.

Heparin-Grafted Dialyzers

Another alternative to no-heparin hemodialysis is the use of heparin-grafted dialyzers, which have been successfully used alone (without saline flushes) or in combination with a citrate-enriched dialysate. These dialyzers are coated with a substance that binds heparin. The clotting rate associated with these dialyzers seems to be between 15% and 30%. Preliminary studies suggest that heparin-grafted dialyzers are noninferior to current standard heparin-free dialysis, easy to use, and a reasonable choice for hemodialysis anticoagulation in patients with high bleeding risk.

Citrate Dialysate

Similar to regional citrate anticoagulation, this strategy utilizes the calcium-inhibiting effects of citrate to block different steps in the coagulation cascade (see Fig. 14.1). The citrate-enriched dialysate replaces the acetate normally used for acidification, instead utilizing citric acid at a relatively low concentration (2.4 mEq/L, 0.8 mmol/L). This results in reduced clotting formation locally in the extracorporeal circuit, which allows a dialysis treatment with either no or only a very low dose of heparin for anticoagulation. Importantly, citrate dialysate lowers serum calcium sufficient to interfere with the clotting cascade, but not enough to cause symptomatic hypocalcemia. Thus, calcium replacement is not necessary, as opposed to regional citrate anticoagulation.

Anticoagulation for Continuous Renal Replacement Therapy

Continuous renal replacement therapy (CRRT) has become a cornerstone for the management of renal failure in critically ill patients. This dialysis modality typically involves very slow blood flow rates, which are associated with an increased risk of thrombosis and lower filter life span. No-heparin hemodialysis, though used in very select patients, is usually discouraged when using this modality. Adequate anticoagulation allows for a more continuous therapy, minimizing the interruptions due to clotting, which results in less blood loss and more efficient total dialysis time.

Continuous hemodialysis therapy increases the likelihood of complications with prostacyclin or protamine. Therefore, minimal-dose heparin is generally the preferred approach in patients on continuous venovenous hemodialysis (CVVHD) or hemofiltration (CVVH). The alternative for patients with increased risk of bleeding is regional citrate anticoagulation.

Heparin

Unfractionated heparin is the most common anticoagulant used in CRRT. Similar to intermittent hemodialysis, there are no well-established guidelines regarding dosage. Typically, a bolus dose of 1000–2000 IU of UFH is given initially followed by a continuous infusion into the arterial limb of the circuit of 300–500 IU/h. The aim is to maintain the aPTT in the venous limb at 1.5–2 times control. The heparin dose may be drastically reduced in patients with disseminated intravascular coagulation or thrombocytopenia. Unfortunately, there is some systemic anticoagulation with this technique and it may be contraindicated in patients at high risk of bleeding. The heparin dose and aPTT goal can be adjusted downward in these patients, at the expense of a higher rate of extracorporeal clotting.

Regional Citrate Anticoagulation (RCA)

CRRT is usually performed in critically ill patients, and it is not uncommon that these patients are either actively bleeding or have an increased bleeding risk because of significant thrombocytopenia or coagulopathy from sepsis or other illness, recent surgery, or trauma. In these circumstances, systemic anticoagulation with heparin is contraindicated. Regional anticoagulation with citrate is recommended instead. Most recently, RCA has also been suggested to be the anticoagulation approach of choice for CRRT, even in the absence of such bleeding risk factors. Despite heparin being the preferred agent in terms of side effect profile and simplicity, evidence from several randomized controlled trials suggest that regional citrate may improve the survival rate of hemofilters and lower bleeding risk compared with heparin in continuous renal replacement therapies.

The principles and potential side effects of regional citrate anticoagulation in CRRT are the same as those in standard hemodialysis. Some protocols use a fixed dose of citrate in relation to blood flow according to an algorithm, whereas others measure postfilter ionized calcium and adjust the citrate dose and/or calcium infusion accordingly. Regional citrate can also cause calcium abnormalities, hypernatremia, and metabolic alkalosis. The possibility of alkalosis may be lessened in part by using an anticoagulant citrate dextrose formula as replacement fluid, which produces less bicarbonate compared with hypertonic trisodium citrate. RCA should be used with caution in patients with liver disease, as these patients have an inability to metabolize citrate, predisposing them to citrate toxicity. This is characterized by an elevated calcium gap >2.5, indicative of low ionized calcium with a disproportionate increase in total calcium, hypercitric academia with elevated anion gap, and hypotension.

Management includes discontinuation of citrate infusion, increase in dialysate flow rate, and correction of hypocalcemia with calcium supplementation.

Further studies in a larger number of patients are required to more accurately define the relative benefits and/or risks and cost-effectiveness of heparin versus citrate-based anticoagulation. Currently, the *Kidney Disease: Improving Global Outcomes (KDIGO) Clinical Practice Guideline for Acute Kidney Injury* recommends the use of regional citrate anticoagulation for CRRT, even in the absence of high bleeding risk. Although citrate is somewhat more complicated for nursing staff, appropriate protocols should simplify procedures, and citrate has slowly become the preferred anticoagulation approach in continuous renal replacement therapy. The protocol we use in our institution is shown in Fig. 14.3.

Regional Prostacyclin and LMWHs Anticoagulation

There are only limited data on the use of these anticoagulants with continuous dialytic techniques. One study found that prostacyclin decreased bleeding episodes and was superior to heparin in maintaining circuit integrity during CRRT, without inducing significant hypotension. Combinations of both prostacyclin and low molecular weight heparin have also been described. However, these favorable outcomes are at odds with studies performed during standard hemodialysis and must be interpreted with caution. Larger clinical trials with these agents are needed to establish their role in continuous renal replacement therapies. Current indications for the use of prostacyclin or LMWHs are similar to those in standard hemodialysis.

Heparin-Induced Thrombocytopenia

Unfractionated heparin can cause a modest reduction in platelet count (<100,000/mL), which is usually reversible (heparin-induced thrombocytopenia type I). In approximately 5%–10% of the patients treated with heparin, there is an immunologic reaction characterized by the formation of antibodies against the complex of heparin and platelet factor 4. This leads to platelet activation and consumption leading to severe thrombocytopenia (usually 30%–50% below baseline), known as heparin-induced thrombocytopenia type II. The main clinical concern in this disorder is a high incidence of arterial and venous thrombosis, rather than bleeding. Given overall safety and reasonable ease of use, no-heparin hemodialysis should be the first option among those with heparin-induced thrombocytopenia. If heparin-free dialysis cannot be performed, then the patient should be anticoagulated with regional citrate or in certain situations even converted to peritoneal dialysis. Another option would be the administration of one of the three drugs that appear to be effective in patients with HIT: danaparoid, recombinant hirudin (lepirudin), and argatroban. Melagatran is a novel long-acting direct thrombin inhibitor, which is currently available only in Europe. Feasibility studies using these agents have been conducted in hemodialysis patients, and they appear to be effective in preventing thrombosis without excess bleeding risk, but there is no published experience concerning melagatran use in patients with HIT. Overall, the experience with these drugs is limited.

Importantly, as long as the platelet count remains low in HIT and there is clinical evidence of active disease, systemic (and not regional) anticoagulation is mandatory. Table 14.4 summarizes the recommendations for use of these agents based on currently available data.

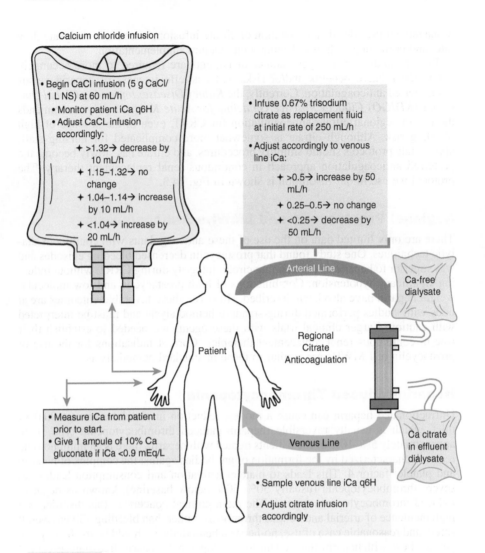

Calcium chloride infusion

- Begin CaCl infusion (5 g CaCl/ 1 L NS) at 60 mL/h
  - Monitor patient iCa q6H
  - Adjust CaCL infusion accordingly:
    + >1.32→ decrease by 10 mL/h
    + 1.15–1.32→ no change
    + 1.04–1.14→ increase by 10 mL/h
    + <1.04→ increase by 20 mL/h

- Infuse 0.67% trisodium citrate as replacement fluid at initial rate of 250 mL/h
- Adjust accordingly to venous line iCa:
    + >0.5→ increase by 50 mL/h
    + 0.25–0.5→ no change
    + <0.25→ decrease by 50 mL/h

Arterial Line

Patient

Regional Citrate Anticoagulation

Ca-free dialysate

Ca citrate in effluent dialysate

Venous Line

- Measure iCa from patient prior to start.
- Give 1 ampule of 10% Ca gluconate if iCa <0.9 mEq/L

- Sample venous line iCa q6H
- Adjust citrate infusion accordingly

Figure 14.3

Schematic Representation of Regional Citrate Anticoagulation Protocol With Continuous Renal Replacement Therapy (CRRT). After initial measurement of patient serum ionized calcium (iCa) levels, CRRT is begun with citrate replacement fluid and a calcium infusion via central line. Patient and machine iCa levels are monitored every 6 hours, and infusion rates are adjusted accordingly. Calcium infusion rates should be accounted for when targeting ultrafiltration rates.

Table 14.4

Anticoagulation for Dialysis-Dependent Patients With HIT

Parameter	Danaparoid	Lepirudin	Argatroban*	Melagatran
CRRT				
Infusion rate	2500 U anti-FXa bolus, then 600 U/h × 4 hours, then 400 U/h × 4 hours, then 200–600 U/h based on levels[‡]	Initiate at 0.005–0.01 mg/kg/h	Initiate at 0.5–1.0 µg/kg/min and dose adjust to aPTT	ND
Monitoring test	Anti–FXa level	aPTT	aPTT	aPTT
Target result[†]	0.5–1.0 U anti-FXa	1.5–2.0× mean of the normal pool	1.5–2.0× mean of the normal pool	ND
Hemodialysis				
Bolus therapy	3750 U anti-FXa bolus prior to first two HD treatments, then dose adjust using levels	0.15 mg/kg bolus prior to HD	0.1 mg/kg bolus prior to HD	Bolus IV dose of 2 mg, add to dialysis fluid for concentration of 0.2 mg/L
Infusion therapy	—	—	0.1–0.2 mg/ kg/h	ND
Monitoring test	Anti–factor Xa level	aPTT	aPTT	aPTT
Target result[†]	0.0–0.4 U anti FXa pre-HD	2.0–2.5× mean of the normal pool	1.5–3.0× mean of the normal pool	ND
Catheter lock				
Concentration/ volume	750 U in 50 mL saline, then 5–10 mL per port	5 mg/mL per port[††]	ND	ND

Anti–FXa, anti–factor Xa; CRRT, continual renal replacement therapy; HD, hemodialysis; HIT, heparin-induced thrombocytopenia; ND, no data available at this time.

*Argatroban should not be administered without first verifying normal liver function. Dose needs to be adjusted for hepatic insufficiency.

[†]Target results for the aPTTs are based on individual coagulation laboratory mean values. Do not exceed 100 seconds.

[‡]Use lower bolus dosing if weight is <50 kg.

[††]Must be aspirated prior to hemodialysis.

Modified from O'Shea, SI, Ortel, TL, Kovalik, EC. Alternate methods of anticoagulation for dialysis-dependent patients with heparin-induced thrombocytopenia. *Semin Dial* 2003;16:61.

Catheter Lock in Patients With HIT

Hemodialysis catheter lock options in patients with heparin-induced thrombocytopenia are to pressure bag the catheters (which is impractical for outpatients) or to instill either tissue plasminogen activator or urokinase. Highly concentrated (47%) citrate has also been used, but is not FDA approved because of concern over accidental systemic injection and arrhythmia. Studies with lower concentration citrate solutions (4%–7%) indicate that this strategy is safe and similarly effective for the maintenance of long-term interdialytic patency of hemodialysis catheters. A study using a 30% citrate locking solution found no increase in adverse events and also found a decreased risk of catheter-related bacteremia as compared to a standard heparin locking solution.

SECTION V

Home Dialysis

CHAPTER 15

Home Preparation and Installation for Home Hemodialysis

Timothy Koh Jee Kam, MBBS, MRCP (UK), MMed(S'pore) •
Christopher T. Chan, MD, FRCPC

Introduction

Home hemodialysis has been available as a modality of renal replacement therapy since the 1960s. The interest in home hemodialysis has been increasing over the past years because of its flexibility and benefits (which will be further discussed in the following section). Historically, home hemodialysis accounted for about 40% of the dialysis population in the United States in the 1970s and decreased in popularity in the 1980–90s. It is currently experiencing a resurgence in several countries, especially with the interest in more frequent or intensive hemodialysis. The USRDS 2014 Annual Data Report indicates that of the 49,000 prevalent dialysis patients undergoing dialysis at home, 7923 were treated with hemodialysis, with an increasing prevalence since the late 2000s. In fact, there was a 5-fold increase in patients undergoing home hemodialysis in 2012 (n =7923) versus in 2002 (n = 1563).

Basis for Home Hemodialysis

Home hemodialysis offers several benefits as compared to conventional facility based hemodialysis. These include improvements in patient outcomes (Blagg et al, 2006), increased freedom of time, cost reduction, as well as an improved quality of life. Improvements in patient outcome with more frequent or intensive home hemodialysis include improved survival (Weinhandl et al, 2012), blood pressure control (Chan et al, 2003), left ventricular geometry (Culleton et al, 2007), phosphate control and mineral metabolism (Walsh et al, 2010), quality of sleep (Hanly et al, 2001), and fertility (Barua et al, 2008). Home hemodialysis offers more control from a patient's perspective over dialysis treatment scheduling and may afford greater flexibility in terms of employment. As compared to facility-based hemodialysis, home hemodialysis is cost-effective or cost-saving (Walker et al, 2014) due to lower staff costs and likely medication cost and may have better health outcomes in kidney disease–related quality of life and survival (Van Eps et al, 2010).

Requirements

There are several prerequisites that need to be addressed before commencing on a home hemodialysis program. A home visit should be conducted prior to further discussion of home dialysis to determine its feasibility and assess the necessary modifications. The availability of a checklist for the home visit may facilitate the process (Table 15.1).

Table 15.1

Home Hemodialysis Initial Home Assessment Record

	Checklist (to Circle Appropriately)		
Plumbing			
Water source	Well	City	Others
Water conductivity			
Total chlorine			
Type of piping material used in plumbing			
Water pressure (psi) in home			
Source of water to RO	Wash room	Basement	Others
Type of drain pipe	ABS	Copper	Cast iron Others
Drainage to city or septic system	Flow open		Flow closed
Can system above handle RO and machine reject water	Yes		No
Electrical			
Space available on breaker panel	Yes		No
Type of panel (name)			
Storage space			
Appropriate area selected for storage	Yes		No
Area free of pest infestation	Yes		No
Dampness/water damage present	Yes		No
Room for stock rotation	Yes		No
Adequate space for dialysis room	Yes		No

There are multiple domains of requirements, including:

A. Legal

The local legal requirements regarding water supply, as well as land and housing, should be established to ascertain if home hemodialysis is feasible. There should be no legal restriction to the use of the building for the purpose of home hemodialysis. In addition, legal requirements concerning waste disposal, sewage, and electrical supply should also be established before the consideration of home hemodialysis. Consideration should be given toward specific policies regarding potentially biohazardous waste.

A unit policy should ideally be in place to decide who is financially responsible for the needed modifications to the home that may be necessary in terms of plumbing and/or electrical renovations.

B. Water Preparation, Standards, and Plumbing

Home hemodialysis, as compared to conventional in-center hemodialysis, is potentially a more water-intensive procedure, with larger volumes of water being necessary to reconstitute the dialysate (except for the mobile platform). The total dialysate volume can range between 110 and 150 L for a 6- to 8-hour session of dialysis, as compared to 120 L for a typical conventional session. This makes water preparation and quality measurement critically important.

Table 15.2

Water Quality Standards for Dialysis Water*

	Microbiologic Level	
	AAMI	**ISO**
Dialysis Water		
Colony-forming units (CFU)	<100 CFU/mL	<100 CFU/mL
Endotoxin units (EU)	<0.25 EU/mL	<0.25 EU/mL
Ultrapure Water		
Colony-forming units (CFU)	<0.1 CFU/mL	<0.1 CFU/mL
Endotoxin units (EU)	<0.03 EU/mL	<0.03 EU/mL

*Data from AAMI (Association for the Advancement of Medical Instrumentation) 13959:2014 and ISO (International Organization for Standardization) 13959:2014.

The water supply can come from various sources, for example, municipal water, feed water. Various water quality standards exist depending on where the dialysis is performed (International Organization for Standardization [ISO], Association for Advancement of Medical Instrumentation [AAMI]; Table 15.2), and the prevailing standards should be adhered to. It is important for a full chemical analysis of the water for dialysis to be conducted to determine the degree of water purification necessary.

The plumbing system modifications should also take into consideration the level in the home in which the dialysis is done. Should dialysis take place on higher floors, additional components, for example, pump systems and feeder tanks, may be needed to provide the necessary water pressure for the reverse osmosis unit and dialysis machine to function properly.

Depending on the local water conditions and regulations, other modifications like backflow preventers and blending devices may also be necessary.

C. Electrical Considerations Including Backup Power Supply

A stable power supply is necessary to conduct home hemodialysis. Typical electrical requirements for dialysis machines are 115 V AC at 20 amperes. There should also be an overcurrent device installed at the service panel board equipped with a 20-ampere fuse. The dialysis machine should also be connected to a separate branch circuit that does not supply any other outlets. For locations that may experience regular power failures, a backup power supply with its accompanying equipment is recommended. The power supply should be compatible with the dialysis equipment, and it may be necessary for an electrician to review for an outlet for the machine with a dedicated circuit to the circuit breaker. Most, if not all, dialysis machines should have their own circuit breaker. It is important to take into consideration measures to manage hemodialysis in the event of power failure, for example, manual wind-back functions of the machine. Lastly, it is essential to establish the local electricity safety regulations and adhere to them.

D. Dialysis Machine Choice and Other Equipment

There are different dialysis machines currently available for home hemodialysis. Some offer the advantage of mobility; however, any machine in general is able to provide effective and good home dialysis. The choice of machine should also be tailored to the patient's individual requirements and preference. In general, a home dialysis machine should be easy to operate and understand, as this facilitates the learning process for the patient and/or the caregiver.

The choice of dialysis machine would also determine the ease of dialysis fluid preparation. Some machines require water filtration systems, while others come with pre-packaged dialysate, or are able to generate on-line dialysis solutions.

The NxStage System One is available for home hemodialysis. To prescribe dialysis with this system, one would need to decide on the following parameters:

i. Frequency of dialysis per week, as well as the target spKt/V (per session as well as per week)
ii. Dialysate volume
iii. Dialysate composition
iv. Blood flow rate
v. Target flow fraction
vi. Ultrafiltration rate
vii. Heparin (initial bolus and additional bolus if necessary)

The dialysate volume and composition would depend on whether the PureFlow SL Dialysate Preparation System is used, or if prepackaged dialysate bags are used. The PureFlow system allows ultrapure product water to be produced from tap water, which is then mixed with the sterile concentrate to produce dialysate solution. It is available in 40–60 L preparations, while the prepackaged solutions come in 5-L bags.

A comparison of the different types of dialysis regimens is listed in Table 15.3.

A dedicated dialysis chair can be considered for home dialysis. This allows for an adjustable headrest that will allow the patient to be comfortable sitting up for the entire duration of the dialysis process and also allows the patient to recline. This should also allow the patient to assume a supine position quickly in the event that symptomatic hypotension occurs.

E. Space Considerations and Siting of Dialysis Machine

Patients will need storage space, for example, a cabinet/closet to store their dialysis equipment. This includes items like needles, filters, tubings, weighing scales, etc. Some patients may also choose to store their dialysis machines when not in use. The space considerations will also determine the choice of dialysis machine and vice versa. The conventional dialysis platforms will generally be larger and less mobile, whereas users of mobile batch dialysis equipment (e.g., NxStage) will have greater flexibility in terms of choosing the dialysis location.

The choice of the dialysis room is an important component of home hemodialysis. The dialysis room should allow for the dialysis session to be conducted safely and should also allow for maintenance to be conducted regularly. It should also be uncluttered and ideally have furnishing that is easy to maintain.

Table 15.3

Home Hemodialysis Regimens

			Dialysis Regimens		
	CHD	NxStage	Short Daily Hemodialysis	Long Hemodialysis[a]	Long Frequent[a]
Frequency (sessions/ week)	3	5+	5+	3–4	5+
Duration (hours/ session)	4		2.5–3.5	2.5–3	>5.5	>5.5
Dialysate flow (mL/min)	500–800	400	500–800	300–500	300–500
Blood flow (mL/min)	200–400	150–200	400	200–400	200–300
Standardized K_t/V_{urea}[b]	2.50 (12 hours/week)	–	3.75 (13.5 hours/ week)	3.75 (26.8 hours/ week)	5.83 (40.2 hours/ week)

[a]Can be performed as nocturnal hemodialysis.
[b]Adapted from the Frequent Hemodialysis Network analysis of solute clearance. Clearances reflect median weekly values and are model-based calculations for provided weekly treatment times. Tennankore et al, 2014.

The following items should be taken into consideration when choosing the dialysis room:
  i. Does the patient want to conduct dialysis privately or in the same room as family members?
 ii. What does the patient want to do during dialysis?
iii. The machine needs to be close to a water supply as well as drains.
 iv. Is the patient doing nocturnal dialysis? If so, the bedroom would be a suitable choice for locating the dialysis machine
  v. Proximity to a telephone is essential

Storage space is also necessary to house the supplies needed for the dialysis treatment. Once patients become familiar with the amount of supplies they need during a particular time period, they may be able to adjust their delivery schedule to better suit their space and storage requirements.

Water treatment units are an important component of the home hemodialysis system. The choice of the dialysis location should also take into consideration the space necessary for the water treatment unit. This area should ideally have water-resistant flooring in case of leaks and also have sufficient servicing and drainage access. The noise generated from the reverse osmosis unit will also need to be taken into consideration for locating the unit. The patient may also consider placing a protective vinyl sheet or a tray under the dialysis machine and water treatment unit as an additional safety measure in case of a water leak.

F. Hygiene and Noise

The surroundings in which the dialysis is conducted should be clean so as to prevent infections from occurring during home hemodialysis. Dirty clothing should be avoided during the dialysis process. Proper hand hygiene is also of importance, and proper handwashing techniques should always be adhered to, including the use of soap or alcohol rubs.

Pets may pose a hygiene problem during dialysis. In general, pets should not be allowed during the dialysis process, as they may pose both a hygiene and safety problem. Even if the pet is supervised, the pet should be kept out of the room during treatment initiation.

These hygiene requirements should extend to both the patient as well as any family member who may be assisting with the dialysis process. The participation of the family should also be assessed as part of the home visit prior to the consideration of home hemodialysis.

G. Safety

All dialysis machines should be equipped with monitors to detect exact arterial and venous pressures, with settings to narrow alarm ranges. The alarm type is usually sound based but may need to be light based in special circumstances (e.g., patients with hearing impairment). Leak detectors should be placed around the vascular access site, under the dialysis machine, as well as the water treatment system, to detect either blood, dialysate, or water leaks. Needles should be doubly secured with tape and plaster. For catheters, special connectors or catheter safety lock boxes can be used.

Alternative standby light sources are also necessary. Flashlights should be kept within easy reach so that the patient has an alternative light source in the event of a power failure to allow termination of treatment.

Twenty-four-hour access to the supporting dialysis care facility or technical support should be available in the event of emergencies. The relevant contact numbers for the dialysis unit and technical support should also be within easy access in the dialysis room.

H. Medical Staff and Technical Support

Machine breakdowns may occur, for example, due to electrical or water problems. Patients should be taught how to perform emergency dialysis termination. The dialysis unit supporting the patient should also be informed if a machine breakdown occurs so that the appropriate advice can be given and the technical staff directed to the home to service the machine.

I. Disposal of Waste

For most patients, disposal of the effluent via the sewage system provides the best option. Appropriate drainage systems should be taken into consideration during the planning process. All sharps should be collected in a dedicated sharps container for proper disposal. The other waste can be disposed of with the general waste, but should be double-bagged. Recycling of plastic waste can also be considered, given that the dialysis process has a high amount of plastic waste production. The patient should check with the dialysis unit providing the dialysis support regarding any extra waste disposal requirements.

J. Storage of Medication

As intravenous medications, for example, erythropoietin-stimulating agents (ESAs), iron, vitamin D analogs, are administered within the home, these drugs would need to be stored in the appropriate conditions.

Conclusion

Medical and technical support is essential for the development of a home hemodialysis program and training. With proper preparation, the establishment of home hemodialysis can be facilitated safely and efficiently and allow the patient to benefit from this treatment modality.

C H A P T E R 1 6

Peritoneal Dialysis Cyclers and Other Mechanical Devices

Jose A. Diaz-Buxo, MD, MS, FACP • Rainer Himmele, MD, MSHM

The development of peritoneal dialysis (PD) cyclers has come a long way from empirically designed basic mechanical machines to highly integrated devices that interact with the patient, provide pertinent treatment data to nurses and physicians, and can potentially communicate with a network of other medical devices.

Peritoneal dialysis cyclers were initially designed for intermittent PD to perform many frequent and short dialysate exchanges within a hospital setting. Following the introduction of continuous cycling PD (CCPD) and variations thereof, the cycler underwent modifications that allowed use of these regimens and laid the foundation for its success as a home therapy device. Further improvements in the performance, safety, and convenience of modern cyclers have increased the utilization of auto-mated PD (APD), which in various countries has become the predominant peritoneal dialysis modality. Although the emphasis during the early years was mainly on optimizing hydraulics and mechanical aspects, the current development goes far beyond filling the abdomen and draining the dialysate. Modern cyclers are highly integrated devices that are designed to communicate and exchange data with other devices. They have the potential to directly interact with the caregiver by transferring patient and prescription data and actively guiding the patient step-by-step through the treatment, enhancing the user's experience and ensuring adequate use of the device. Potential characteristics of cyclers are summarized in Table 16.1.

Mechanical Aspects and Hydraulics

Peritoneal dialysis cyclers are designed to automatically deliver multiple exchanges of dialysate solution. The dialysate flow is regulated by a central control unit that may include pumps, weigh scales, occluders, manifolds, electronics, and other mechanical components. An integrated heating system ensures adequate dialysate temperature. A display screen and control board is needed to enter patient treatment parameters and monitor treatment success. The filling of the abdomen and draining of the dialysate can be performed by gravity- or pump-based systems. Mechanically, cyclers can be categorized as devices that exclusively use gravity, combine gravity and pumps, or use pumps only.

Gravity-Based Cyclers

This type of cycler uses gravity to deliver the solution from the dialysate bags, through sterile tubing to a volume control unit and heater module, and into the peritoneal cavity (Fig. 16.1A). Alternatively, the dialysate bags may rest on a heating

Table 16.1

Potential Features of a Modern Cycler

Functionality
- Meets the needs of home and acute care setting
- Performs all prescriptions (e.g., CCPD, PD Plus, TPD, IPD, adapted PD) with programmable treatment time and broad options for fill, dwell, and drain
- Ability to vary each exchange regarding volume, dwell time, and solution used
- Allows extended treatment options to accommodate special patients:
  - High total volume of dialysate (>50 L) and large number of cycles with one setup
  - Maximal fill volumes (>4 L) for large adults
  - Minimal fill volumes (50 mL) and delivery of dialysis solutions in small increments (10–20 mL) for infants
- Automatic priming of the patient line and flush-before-fill as part of setup
- Fast and efficient warming of solutions
- Features optimized fill and drain logic allowing fast drainage (> 200 mL/min), intelligent end of drain detection, including established criteria to prevent overfill
- Last bag option
- Ability to pump effluent to either bags or drain
- Lock-out option to prevent unauthorized setting changes

User Interface
- Large color touchscreen control panel that is easy to read and use
- Variable voice and alarm volume
- User-friendly menu with easy-to-follow step-by-step instructions and video tutorials in multiple languages
- Integrated camera for real-time video assistance

Information Technology
- Comprehensive data capture and storage of all relevant patient treatment parameters
- Connectivity through Bluetooth, USB ports, WLAN, LAN with secured data communication, including help feature with online access to service
- Automatic wireless data import from scale and blood pressure monitor
- Interface and automatic data exchange with clinic management software
- Full therapy and patient data management, including prescription modeling, administrative module, and upgradable training courses

Mechanical
- Low weight, with custom-made travel case for ease of portability
- Small enough footprint to fit on average nightstand
- Stability to hold a broad range of bag sizes (up to 6 L) without tipping, and with locking wheels and nonslip feet to prevent rolling and sliding
- Able to withstand extreme temperatures with adequate performance at sea level and high altitudes
- Constructed of material that is easily disinfected with common agents and sealed outer case to prevent trapping of foreign matter and liquids from penetrating into the unit
- Noise level <40 dBA while running at maximum pumping speed
- 120 and 240 V AC power choices
- UL/CSA/CE approval

Disposables
- Single-use, sterile components
- One-step loading (cassette)
- Advanced connectology with elimination of clamps
- Adequate organizer for operator's use

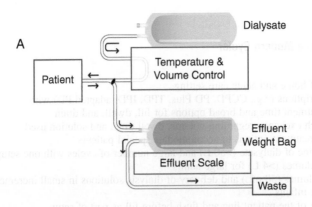

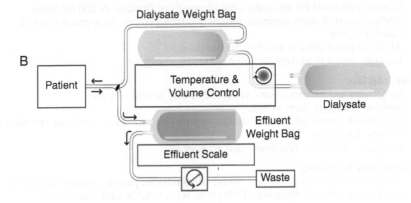

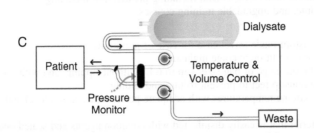

Figure 16.1

Flow Diagrams for Different Types of Cyclers. (A) Gravity-based cycler; (B) combined gravity- and pump-based cycler; (C) pump-based cycler. (Courtesy of Fresenius Medical Care North America.)

tray; from there the solution is then transferred to the volume control module and then to the patient. In either case, the cycler ensures that the fluid is heated to body temperature and the exact prescribed volume of dialysate is delivered to the patient. After the prescribed dwell period, the spent dialysate flows by gravity through the patient line into a weigh bag where the volume is measured to ensure complete drain and determine ultrafiltration. The dialysate is then either collected in an additionally attached drainage bag or disposed directly into the sewage. The transfer of dialysate into the sewage line can be accomplished by gravity or via a pump.

The control panel controls temperature and dwell time and monitors drain time and drainage volume. Most cyclers simply ensure that a predetermined percentage of inflow volume is drained before a new cycle takes place. Most cyclers are capable of precisely monitoring ultrafiltration. Inflow volume is determined and measured by a volume control unit or heating cabinet.

Combined Gravity- and Pump-Based Cyclers

There are various systems that combine one or multiple active pumps and gravity-based transport of the dialysate. In the simplest setup, one pump is added to a gravity-based system to help drain the dialysate effectively from the weigh bag to the drainage bag or sewer. The same or a second pump can be used to transport dialysate to the volume control bag and heater module prior to infusion into the patient's peritoneum. With any option of combined gravity- and pump-based cyclers, the fill and drain of the patient is performed by gravity only. One example of the dialysate flow is shown in Fig. 16.1B: The system pumps the exact dialysate volume for each fill into a measuring bag that typically rests on a plate above the heater and volume-controlling unit. The adequate volume of heated dialysate is determined by a weight transducer and will then be delivered into the patient's peritoneal cavity by gravity. After completion of the dwell, the inflow lines are occluded and the fluid is passively drained into a weigh bag mounted on a second weight transducer. Once drainage is accomplished, the pump voids the spent dialysate into a drain bag or sewer. All these functions are integrated by a control cabinet using microprocessors that allow precise control of inflow volume, ultrafiltration monitoring, dwell time, drain time, and number of cycles. Selection of dialysate osmolality and volume for the diurnal cycle of CCPD (last cycle) is also possible with some of these devices. The incorporation of active transfer of dialysate to a measuring unit located above the patient level allows for the design of simpler tubing sets and the practical use of larger volumes with a potential reduction in cost of therapy.

Pump-Based Cyclers

Various systems have been designed to actively infuse and drain dialysate. The simplest and most economical is the use of two peristaltic or roller pumps (Fig. 16.1C). The first actively infuses warmed dialysate into the patient, and the second generates negative pressure to drain the spent dialysate.

A more ingenious alternative is the use of an integrated cassette design for easy setup of the cycler. The exact measurement of fluid volume flowing through the cassette can be used for volumetric control and eliminates the need for weigh scales. Current systems contain fluid chambers that serve as pumps and a series of channels for solution flow (Fig. 16.2A).

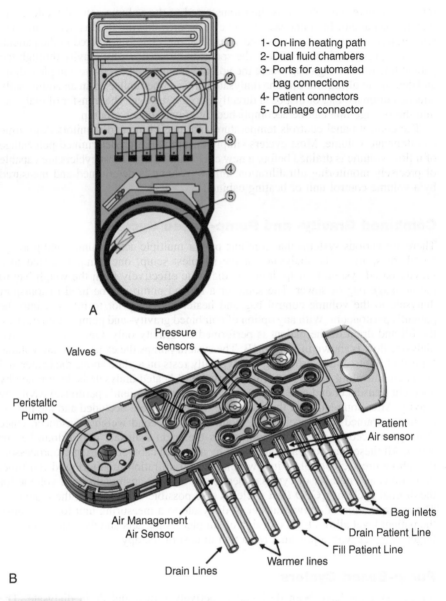

1- On-line heating path
2- Dual fluid chambers
3- Ports for automated
   bag connections
4- Patient connectors
5- Drainage connector

Figure 16.2

Integrated Cassette Systems. (A) Cassette with heating path, dual fluid chambers, ports for automated bag connectors, and drainage lines. (B) Integration of a peristaltic mechanism with valves and pressure sensors into a disposable fluid management cassette system. (Courtesy of Fresenius Medical Care North America.)

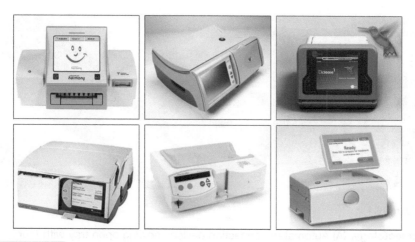

Figure 16.3

Contemporary Cycler Design. Examples of contemporary cyclers shown for educational purposes only and are not available or approved in all countries. (Bottom center and right images courtesy of Baxter International Inc. All other images courtesy of Fresenius Medical Care North America.)

Although gravity-based cycler systems are still available in a number of countries, recently developed cyclers mostly feature pump-based systems. Examples of modern cycler designs are provided in Fig. 16.3.

Connectology

Connectors may be required between the cycler tubing set, the patient's catheter, and the solution bags. Various connectors have been used, including spikes, Luer locks, and threaded male–female connectors with recessed pathways. Dialysate bags with integrated patient and drain lines add more convenience for the patient due to fewer connections. Connections can be manually performed or facilitated by automated spiking (Fig. 16.4A). Automated connections use a stationary manifold and a moving tray (connection rail) to attach the bag lines to the cassette. This technology simplifies the procedure and reduces the risk of touch contamination by the patient. In addition, the cycler's connecting device may incorporate a bar code scanner that identifies the specific solution connected to each port in the manifold by reading the printed bar code on the bag connector (Fig. 16.4B).

Upon termination of the cycling session, the patient line can be disconnected and capped using sterile technique, external occlusion, or with connectors that automatically occlude the lumen of the tubing with a pin to prevent leakage of dialysate or contamination (Fig. 16.5).

Information Technology and Connectivity

Modern cyclers have incorporated new functions as a result of continuously advancing electronics, computer systems, and connectology. Some cyclers feature memory

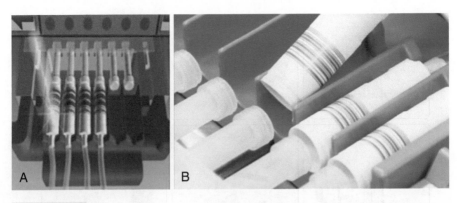

Figure 16.4

Connectology. (A) Automated connection device showing open tray with four bag lines connected to the cycler and bar-code reader. (B) Bag connector with printed bar code. (Courtesy of Fresenius Medical Care North America.)

cards or USB sticks to record treatment data or download new prescriptions whereas others are designed to transmit data without the need for an external drive. Color touchscreens, direct interface with central computers in medical centers or dialysis facilities, and accessory programs allow comprehensive record keeping and easy access to patient and prescription data. The main features of such software are provided in Table 16.2.

With this information readily available, the renal team can monitor adequacy of the dialysis treatment, provide feedback to the patient based on his or her clinical parameters and documented treatment compliance and incorporate changes in the prescription. In some cases, the dialysis prescription may be downloaded in the clinic to an external memory device that is reinserted into the cycler by the patient at home and the cycler is automatically reprogrammed with the new prescription. Data encryption with various levels of user rights ensures that only authorized individuals can access and/or modify part or all available information. Data provided by the cycler can also be used by technical support teams to troubleshoot and diagnose potential malfunctions of the device.

User Interface and Ease of Use

Much effort has been put into enhancing usability and user experience of modern cyclers. Technology advances include user interfaces with large graphical touch-screen displays, large soft buttons in selectable colors, and soft keypads for entering numerical values. The user-friendly screens allow for easy selection of regimen, times, and volumes. Patients may be guided at all times through on-screen video and audio instructions in the language of his or her choice. Dialysate fluid bag connections and patient line connections are illustrated in a stepwise manner and explained on the display for easy operation. The incorporation of bar codes has been used to automatically identify the type of solution employed. This information is transmitted to the cycler software, compared with the prescription and accepted or

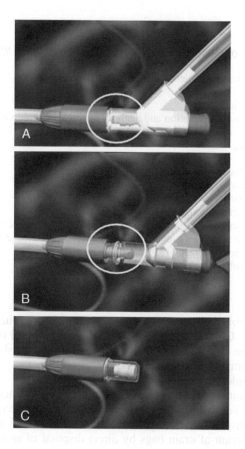

Figure 16.5

PIN Technology. PIN technology in APD for automatic occlusion of line lumen upon disconnection. (A) Normal position during treatment. (B) The pin is inserted into the catheter extension. (C) Final position with cap. (Courtesy of Fresenius Medical Care North America.)

rejected accordingly. This feature ensures selection of the correct dialysis solution based on the latest prescription. Other approaches to enhance ease of use are integrated voice commands, visual and audio feedback, and alarms.

Cost Considerations

The many models of cyclers on the global market reflect the requirements of different regimens, prescriptions, and availability of funds devoted to renal replacement therapy in different countries. The convenience and safety offered by the state-of-the-art cycler technology is impressive but not essential to the delivery of adequate care. Compared with manual peritoneal dialysis, the use of a cycler necessarily increases the cost of therapy. However, the overall cost of peritoneal dialysis is, in

| Table 16.2 |

Potential Features of Modern Information Systems to Be Used With PD Cyclers

- Management system for patient's personal and medical data
- Dialysis adequacy module
- Dialysis prescription module
- Advanced module for evaluation and analysis of single or multiple patient treatment data
  - Treatment data
  - Trends
  - Distribution histograms
  - Cross-correlations
- Data export module
- Graphics and special reports
- Administration module—customizable for the needs of the physician or administration
- Language module that allows immediate translation of downloaded data and cycler-generated data into other languages
- Online help module

general, considerably less than hemodialysis treatments despite the use of modern cycler technology. Costs can potentially be further minimized or contained by:

1. Using fewer but larger-volume dialysate bags manufactured with less expensive material and simplified packaging;
2. Designing simpler tubing sets;
3. Reducing the number of necessary connections and other steps that require additional, often expensive materials to maintain an aseptic environment; and
4. Reduction of disposables through reutilization of solution bags as drainage bags and the elimination of drain bags by direct disposal of spent dialysate into the sewage lines.

Current and Future Developments

Mechanical developments include integration of miniaturized peristaltic mechanisms with valves and pressure sensors into a disposable fluid management cassette system, leading to a smaller, more compact cycler design (see Fig. 16.2B). The disposable cassette may load automatically with silicone membrane valves that can be independently opened and closed using a pin and a small motor to fill or drain the dialysate. The miniaturized cassette plus the high degree of integration of the components can allow a cycler weight below 10 pounds with a very small footprint, which may significantly mitigate its intrusiveness in the patient's home and travel limitations.

Some cyclers already offer more flexible prescription options to individualize each single dialysate exchange. This is applied in adapted PD, where different exchanges within one treatment vary in volume, dwell time, and solution used. This allows an optimized, more patient-specific prescription of these parameters.

New possibilities emerge through increasing wireless connectivity of medical devices using Wi-Fi or Bluetooth. Although currently many patient parameters have to be entered manually for performing the daily treatment, the cycler has the possibility to expand the network and automatically integrate other important medical measurements, including daily weight, blood pressure, or blood glucose levels in diabetic patients, from various approved medical instruments.

Since home care means that assistance may be needed at any time, enhanced connectivity and integrated cameras may allow video-conferencing capability with direct and timely access to the dialysis nurse or the nephrologist at the touch of a button.

Conclusions

PD cyclers have evolved into systems that provide much more than automated exchanges for APD. Recent advances allow much improved usability and integration of information from multiple sources to facilitate comprehensive management of the peritoneal dialysis patient. Modern cyclers have come a long way to become interactive, user-centered medical devices that partner with the patient and physician in delivering a highly individualized dialysis treatment and user experience.

SECTION VI

Dialyzers

Selecting a Dialyzer: Technical and Clinical Considerations

Federico Nalesso, MD, PhD • Ronco Claudio, MD

Introduction

Membrane performance, as determined by the effectiveness of solute clearance and biocompatibility, is of greatest concern when choosing a dialyzer. Technological advances in membrane design, chemical composition, and sterilization methods have led to enhanced performance and versatility to the extent that dialyzer choice may reduce morbidity and prolong survival.

The membrane is the core of the dialyzer, and the dialyzer is the core of the extracorporeal treatment. According to this concept, it is clear the importance of the dialyzer to obtain the best blood purification for each individual clinical need. There is currently a wide selection of dialyzers in terms of type of membrane, surface, characteristics of surface, and method of sterilization.

The membrane is the "device" that allows one to obtain the processes of diffusion, convection, and adsorption required to purify the blood in the extracorporeal circulation.

The membrane allows one to broaden the spectrum of uremic toxins that can be removed depending on its chemical and physical characteristics. Thus, bioengineering advances over the last decade have resulted in the introduction of a wide spectrum of hemodialyzers and filters together with a multitude of different membranes that are currently available commercially.

The first major distinction, between the types of membranes, can be made by dividing the membranes into cellulosic and synthetic as shown in Table 17.1.

The polymer used in the dialysis membrane essentially determines the chemical and physical behavior of the membrane and its possible uses in the extracorporeal purification. The ideal polymer for use in dialysis should enable the production of a biocompatible membrane family whose members are of considerable physical strength, have excellent diffusive and convective properties, and have performance and biocompatibility profiles that are resistant to all chemicals and sterilizing agents. It is also vital that modern hemodialysis membranes should adsorb endotoxins at the outer surface, as this provides added protection against transfer of bacterial derivatives from the dialysis fluid to the patient in case of microbial contamination of the dialysis fluid. Nowadays, this event is rare but it can occur when the quality of water is not optimal or in case of system failure of the water production from the main's water.

Dialyzer Construction

The ideal dialyzer should be highly effective regarding solute removal, exhibit constant performance over the entire treatment time, have a small blood priming volume,

Table 17.1

Cellulosic and Synthetic Membranes

Cellulosic		Synthetic		
Regenerated Cellulose	**Modified Cellulose**	**Polysulfones**	**Polyarylethersulfones**	**Others**
Cuprophan	CDA, DICEA	Fresenius Polysulfone	PEPA	AN69 AN69ST
Cuprammonium rayon	CTA, Tricea	Helixone	Polyamix	PAN
SCE	Hemophan	Alfa polysulfone	DIAPES	PMMA
GOP DIAFIL	SMC	Toraysulfone	Arylane	EVAL
	PEG-Rc	APS		Polyamide
	Excebrane			

and contain a biocompatible membrane. To be absolutely safe, it has to be sterilized by steam in order to avoid the hazards of sterilization products such as residual ethylene oxide (ETO). The dialyzers are available either as parallel-plate or, more commonly, as hollow-fiber devices. In parallel-plate dialyzers, several layers of flat sheet membranes are stacked, supported by thin plates. This type of dialyzer does not contain polyurethane and can be more easily sterilized by ETO.

The parallel-plate dialyzers present a reduced thrombogenicity compared to their hollow-fiber counterparts as the shear stress experienced by the blood is lower in plate dialyzers. New hollow-fiber dialyzers have similar shear stress compared to plate dialyzers, so this advantage is no longer important. In summary, plate dialyzers have no real advantage over hollow-fiber devices; thus their usage has continued to decline year by year.

A modern hollow-fiber dialyzer consists of a housing containing a single-membrane fiber bundle that is embedded at both its ends in polyurethane (PUR) that also fixes it within the casing. To ensure a minimal activation of humoral and cellular systems in the blood, it is necessary to use a special cutting process to form a smooth end surface. Both of these end surfaces are covered by end caps that contain the blood inlet and outlet ports. In each type of dialyzer, the size and design of the fiber bundle determine the performance; the blood compartment has to be as low volume as possible, and each fiber should be surrounded by a uniform stream of dialysate during dialysis. The number of fibers and the fiber bundle density increase with surface area until performance has reached a maximum.

The composition of the potting compound has changed over the years in order to minimize risks associated with toxic substances that may be seen after sterilization of the PUR. Now it is known that irradiation with beta- or gamma-beams may lead to the fission product 4-4′-methylenedianiline that has a putative role in the carcinogenic processes. Polycarbonate and silicon rings were introduced to reduce the PUR of hollow-fiber dialyzers.

The quality of the bundle is a major determinant of the performance of the dialyzer. Nowadays, the fiber structure is uniform and several bundle configurations have been introduced to improve dialysate flow around the fibers. The blood volume of most dialyzers is smaller than that of the line sets, which is important in making the best dialyzer choice in patients with low blood volume (such as children). In the dialyzer, the priming procedure is influenced by the geometry and shape of the header, which determines the blood distribution within the housing.

Sterilization

Common sterilization methods are generally based on the use of ethylene oxide gas (ETO), irradiation (gamma or beta), or heat. The method by which a dialyzer is sterilized is of clinical interest and relevance when patient-specific sensitivities occur, which is why the same dialyzers are available sterilized in more than one way.

In Table 17.2, the type of sterilization for membrane polymers is explained. ETO sterilization is an inexpensive and relatively safe method of sterilization. In fact, dialysis membrane performance characteristics appear to be unaffected by exposure to this method because of low physical and thermal stress. Bacteria are killed by alkylation of sulfur-containing proteins in concentration, time, temperature, humidity, and pressure dependency. In the past, residues of ETO were identified as a common cause of allergic reactions in dialysis patients because of the adsorption and inadequate or slow release of ETO by some specific membrane polymers and by the potting material used (polypropylene, polyurethane, and PMMA). The introduction of organizational and technical measures at the manufacturing sites now ensures minimal residue levels of ETO in the devices. Additional precautionary measures are the intensive dialyzer pre-rising procedures and avoidance of infusion of any priming volume in order to allow a safe use of devices sterilized by ETO.

Radiation sterilization is obtained by exposing the dialyzers to either gamma or beta rays. This results in ionization of atoms by the high energy and the formation of free radicals resulting in dimerization of DNA bases and scission of the sugar-phosphate backbone that prevents bacterial replication. This procedure is safe and simple. Today the accelerators for beta radiation have a penetrating power similar to that of gamma radiation. The only advantage of beta radiation over gamma

Table 17.2
Sterilization Methods for Common Dialysis Membranes

Membrane Polymer		Gamma Irradiation	ETO	Heat
Cellulose-based polymers	Cellulose and modified cellulose (all except cellulose acetate)	+	+	+
	Cellulose acetate	+	+	−
Polysulfone-based polymers	Polysulfone	+	+	+
	Polyarylethersulfone	+	+	+
	PES	+	+	+
	Polyamide	+	+	+
	PEPA	+	+	+
Other synthetic polymers	PAN	+	+	−
	PMMA	+	+	−
	EVAL	+	+	−
	Polycarbonate	+	+	−
	Polyamide	+	+	−

radiation is the possibility to more precisely dose and target the sterilization. It is common to use gamma irradiation for heat-sensitive and higher-density materials while exposure time is shorter with beta irradiation with less material damage. The degree of sterilization is related to the amount of radiation adsorbed that is measured in gray (Gy). The devices to be sterilized are placed close to the radiation source for the right time (seconds for beta radiation and minutes or hours for gamma radiation). Membrane degradation is present with increasing dosage and time of radiation. The damage, caused by ionizing radiation, is based on crosslinking and chain scissions. In order to reduce this damage, stabilizers must be added to react with the first radicals blocking follow-up reactions. The stabilizers can also be a toxicological risk factor. In acrylic monomers (PAN) the gamma radiation can increase the permeability to higher-molecular-weight molecules, in cellulose it can determine chain scission. In polyamide one can see crosslinking and transient bluish discoloration after the irradiation. In PMMA it is common to find chain scission and reduction in permeability to higher-molecular-weight molecules. During the radiation in EVAL, crosslinking and aldehydes can be formed. Polycarbonate can darken with radiation. PVC and housings in polyvinylchloride are subjected to chain scission, darkening, leaching of decomposed additives, and release of hydrochloric acid and may release unpleasant odors and demonstrate accelerated ageing. The polyurethane can release mutagenic compounds as well.

With thermal sterilization, the bacteria are destroyed by heat denaturation of the cell walls and proteins. This method is free from chemical residuals, is effective, and avoids any changes to the dialyzer materials caused by gamma and beta rays. It is considered as the best sterilization method.

When using steam, the dialyzers are placed in an autoclave at 1–2 bar at a temperature around 121°C for 30–90 minutes. When using dry heat sterilization, a higher temperature (180 °C) and longer time are necessary to obtain sterilization. Following this type of sterilization, dialyzers must be rinsed with saline before use to ensure the removal of destroyed bacteria.

Not all dialyzer membranes can be sterilized by each of these procedures. Heat or steam sterilization appears to be superior to ETO or gamma irradiation sterilization. Unfortunately, not all dialyzers and casings are sufficiently thermostable and thus they can be sterilized by ETO or gamma irradiation. Today we can consider ETO sterilization safe, with negligible levels of residues of sterilization.

Dialysis Membrane Structure and Characteristics

As previously mentioned, the membrane can be divided into two families: membranes derived from cellulose and membranes derived from synthetic polymers. These two families can be further divided into subfamilies depending on the chemical and physical characteristics of the polymers and their process of production.

According to this classification membranes present common characteristics and can be classified as described below.

Cellulosic membranes are relatively thin (6.5–15 μm) in order to achieve high diffusive solute transport and have a uniform (symmetric) structure of the fiber wall. The uniform structure determines the symmetry of the membranes. The synthetic membranes present a membrane thickness of 20 μm and more and a structure that may by symmetric, such as in AN69, AN69ST, PMMA, or asymmetric such as in the Fresenius polysulfone or polyamide.

Thus in the synthetic family membrane, fibers are either symmetric or asymmetric and this characteristic can be seen in their cross-sectional views. Symmetric membranes are derived either from cellulose or entirely from synthetic polymers. These types of membranes have a homogeneous configuration throughout the membrane wall with both the inner and outer layers usually containing similar pore sizes. Conversely, asymmetric membranes are derived from synthetic polymers only and present a thin inner selective layer and an outer thick support layer. Typical membranes of this family are polysulfone or polyethersulfone. Whereas cellulose-derived fibers are naturally wavelike, synthetic fibers may be crimped to produce a rippled pattern that more evenly distributes the dialysate flow. This allows for better matching of blood and dialysate flows across all sections of the fiber bundle.

For each membrane, one can identify a molecular weight cut-off for the largest molecule that can pass through it. This parameter allows the removal of solutes of particular concern in an individual patient. Today the range of this cut-off is from 3000 Da to more than 15,000 Da. There is also a new generation of super high-flux membranes that have a cut-off closer to 65,000 Da.

Thanks to nanotechnology, we can obtain membranes with a superior uniformity of pore size, in contrast to earlier membranes that had a wide range of pore sizes with fewer large pores resulting in limited removal of middle-molecular-weight uremic toxins. Applying these concepts, membranes with homogeneous pore size and a narrow pore size distribution present a sharper cut-off in the sieving coefficient, leading to improved passage of low-molecular-weight proteins and a reduced loss of albumin.

Cellulose-Based Membranes

In this family, we can identify the regenerated cellulose membrane (Fig. 17.1) as the first progenitor membrane.

This membrane has specific characteristics: low hydraulic permeability and good diffusive performance for low molecular weight clearance because of its small membrane wall thickness. It can be sterilized by all common sterilization procedures (ETO, irradiation, steam).

Unfortunately, these membranes have poor biocompatibility and are generally unable to adsorb small bacterial products.

The substitution of some hydroxyl groups of the cellulose by N,N,-diethylaminoethyl (DEAE) produces a subtype of membrane named Hemophan in which the

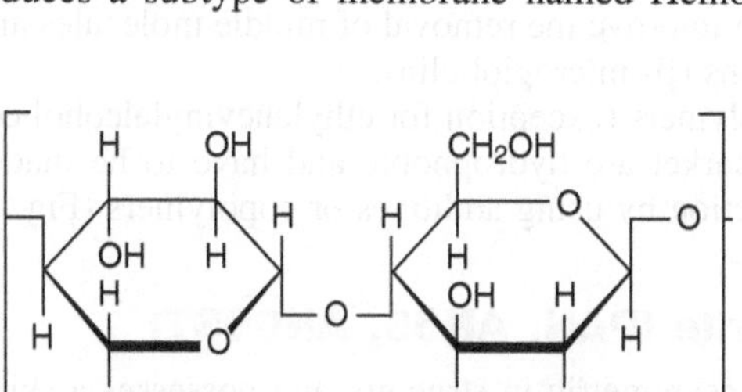

Figure 17.1

Regenerated Cellulose (RC).

positively charged groups constitute hydrophobic regions on a hydrophilic surface and sterically hinder the interaction of complement factors with the membrane resulting in improved biocompatibility compared with the first cellulose membrane.

It is also possible to create hydrophobic domains on a hydrophilic membrane surface by the substitution of less than 1% of the hydrophilic hydroxyl groups by hydrophobic benzyl groups through ether bonds. In this way, one can create a benzyl cellulose membrane (SMC).

All of these membranes are not completely biocompatible because of the hydrophilicity of their surface that can activate complement, platelets, and leukocytes. An improvement of cellulosic membrane biocompatibility was achieved by grafting the cellulosic backbone of cuprammonium rayon with a polyethyleneglycol (PEG) layer (AM-BIO membrane, Asahi).

The PEG chains form a hydrogel layer on the cellulosic surface (thickness 2.4 nm); this may act as a buffer zone between the cellulosic backbone and blood, hindering the direct contact of plasma proteins with the membrane surface leading to a reduction in platelet adhesion and complement activation.

Based on the concept that during the extracorporeal purification the interaction between membrane and blood can activate complement, platelets, and leukocytes, resulting in oxygen radical production and oxidative stress, bioengineering attempts to create a "bioreactive" dialysis membrane by the development of a vitamin E (D-α-tocopherol)–coated cellulosic membrane (Excebrane, Terumo, Japan) have been ongoing. In this regenerated cellulose graft membrane (Excebrane), the desirable performance properties of a highly porous cellulosic membrane are combined with the needed biocompatibility features of a synthetic copolymer resulting in reduction of oxidative stress due to the radical scavenger vitamin E.

Finally work has been carried out with a diacetate of cellulose membrane (CDA). In this membrane, at least two (substitution grade 2) of three hydroxyl groups of the cellulosic glucose monomer are replaced by acetyl groups. If the grade of substitution is 3, one has a cellulose triacetate membrane (CAT). CDA (grade of substitution from 2.4 to 2.0) are low-flow membranes, CTA (grade of substitution 3.0) are available in both low and high flux versions.

Synthetic Membranes

The main purpose of developing synthetic membranes was to create more porous membranes which could better simulate the filtration process of the natural kidney. In this way one can improve the removal of middle molecules and higher molecular weight uremic toxins (β_2-microglobulin).

All synthetic polymers (exception for ethylenevinylalcohol copolymer [EVAL]), currently on the market are hydrophobic and have to be made more hydrophilic during their production by using additives or copolymers (Fig. 17.2).

Polyacrylonitrile (PAN, AN69, AN69ST)

This membrane is asymmetric in structure and possesses a skin layer with a wide range of pore size (density of medium-sized pores). These characteristics determine the sieving properties of the membrane.

AN69 was believed to be one of the most biocompatible dialysis membranes available. It is not sterilizable by heat, however. The major problem with this membrane was anaphylactoid reactions when used in patients receiving

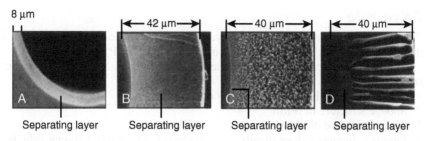

Figure 17.2

(A) Regenerated cellulose. No visible structure, homogeneous, symmetric. (B) AN69ST. Homogeneous, symmetric. (C) Fresenius polysulfone. Foamlike, asymmetric. (D) Polyamide. Microreticular, anisotropic, asymmetric.

angiotensin-converting enzyme (ACE) inhibitors that can stimulate the generation of vasoactive substances such as bradykinins.

In order to overcome problems with anaphylactic reactions, a new type of AN69 was developed by coating the polyacrylonitrile flat sheet membrane with poly(ethyleneimine) (PEI) that is a polycationic polymer. In fact, AN69 exhibits a high adsorption capacity for proteins due to its microstructure and its surface electronegativity; this is particularly evident for complement factor D and β_2-microglobulin.

Polymethylmethacrylate (PMMA)

This membrane is not a polar polymer and presents hydrophobic proprieties. Thus, the membrane is symmetric and almost homogeneous and isotropic. This membrane was the first membrane γ-ray sterilized. It is composed of 9 subtypes of different membranes. The PMMA presents a strong adsorbing property that may not always be of advantage. In fact, this characteristic may result in an undesirable adsorption of platelets, with an effect on fibrin formation that can decrease the efficiency of the dialytic process during the time of treatment.

Ethylenevinylalcohol Copolymer (EVAL)

This membrane is naturally hydrophilic as a result of the presence of hydroxyl groups. It exhibits a much better biocompatibility than membranes made from regenerated cellulose. EVAL is available in three different types according to the pore size: D-, C-, and M-type.

The hydrophilic property of the membrane can reduce the interaction between the blood and the membrane surface resulting in less cell activation and heparin need for anticoagulation.

EVAL EVOH is a synthetic polymer having both hydrophilic and hydrophobic segments. The hydrophilic segments attract water, creating a dynamic water structure at the membrane surface, which is considered to reduce blood–membrane interaction. It also has a unique surface that prevents adsorption of not only proteins and platelets but also medication, including anticoagulants.

Polyamide

Polyamide membranes consist of a hydrophobic, aromatic-aliphatic copolyamide that is blended with hydrophilic polyvinylpyrrolidone (PVP).

This structure results in an asymmetric membrane with three distinguishable regions:
1. A thin skin of 0.1–0.5 μm on the blood side
2. Sponge structure of 5 μm
3. Finger structure of about 45 μm
4. Pore size increases dramatically from the blood side to the dialysate side, being smallest at the skin layer at around 5 nm. The result of this structure is low complement activation and low cell activation with lower oxidative stress.

Polysulfones

According to the chemical definition, the term *polysulfone* comprises simply a group of polymers containing a sulfone group and alkyl- or aryl- groups. Only all such polymers, which additionally contain isopropylidene groups, are termed polysulfones (Fresenius polysulfone, Helixone, Asahi polysulfone, Toraysulfone, α-polysulfone). Conversely those dialysis membrane polysulfones that do not contain isopropylidene groups are termed polyarylethersulfones or polyethersulfones (DIAPES, Arylane, Polyamix).

Polysulfone and poly(aryl)ethersulfone membranes can be sterilized with all common methods, demonstrate excellent biocompatibility, and have high physical strength and chemical resistance. Both the low-flux and the high-flux versions exhibit good performance characteristics, and the high-flux type removes considerable amounts of β2-M by filtration. In addition, polysulfones, but not poly(aryl) ethersulfone, are suitable for use as endotoxin adsorbers because of their structure.

With the application of nanotechnology, an improved version of the original Fresenius polysulfone was developed and introduced as the Helixone membrane, in which hollow fiber wall thickness (35 nm) and inner diameter (185 μm) are reduced. By the nanotechnology process the nominal average pore size was increased from 3.1 in Fresenius polysulfone to 3.3 nm in Helixone. In this way, it was possible to create a uniform pore distribution at the dense innermost layer as well as a homogeneous pore size, which results in a sharper molecular weight cut-off.

Polyarylethersulfones (PEPA, Arylane, DIAPES, Polyamix)

To complete the description of polysulfones we have to introduce the PEPA that is a blend of polyethersulfone and polyarylate and is the only polyarylethersulfone membrane that does not contain PVP. The Arylane is a polyarylethersulfone/PVP. The Polyamix is a blend of polyarylethersulfone, PVP, and small amounts of polyamide. The DIAPES is a blend of polyarylethersulfone and PVP.

Clinical Implication of Membranes, Structure and Characteristics

Generally, the material used to make hollow fiber membranes includes polysulfones, polyethersulfone, cellulose triacetate, polymethylmethacrylate, ethylene vinyl alcohol, or polyacrylonitrile. Nowadays, the use of poorly biocompatible unmodified cellulose dialyzer membranes is discouraged. In fact, most dialyzers are made from synthetic polymers from the family of polysulfone/polyethersulfone.

Cellulose Triacetate: This type of membrane presents a high solute permeability that can remove β_2-microglobulin by diffusion. The efficiency in diffusion is very high as the fibers are thin and the structure results in a uniform dialysate flow distribution. Clinical benefits have been reported related to high antithrombogenicity, impact on lipid metabolism, and reduction of homocysteine and glycation end products. The phenomenon of albumin adsorption on the membrane surface suggests that this family of membrane may offer the potential for a lower activation of the coagulation cascade than polysulfone membranes.

Polyacrylonitile: This family of membrane is hydrophilic and attracts water to form a hydrogel structure that confers high diffusive and hydraulic permeability. The surface structure is able to adsorb basic, medium-sized proteins. The permeability to fluid is high and the membrane presents a broad spectrum of uremic toxins with a very high biocompatibility. An interesting characteristic of this family is the possibility to introduce membranes coated with polyethylene glycol or vitamin E in order to decrease the migration and activation of monocytes and granulocytes with improved biocompatibility. From the point of view of performing extracorporeal treatment in patients with a high risk of bleeding, this family of membranes was modified on the surface to bind heparin.

Polymethylmethacrylate: This family of membranes has high adsorptive properties because of its homogeneous structure, in which the entire membrane contributes to the adsorption. This type of membrane has been shown to adsorb intact PTH and to improve pruritus.

Ethylenevinylalcohol: This family consists of hydrophilic and uncharged membranes with a smooth surface that retains water resulting in less plasma protein adsorption and weak blood cells interaction. Based on these characteristics the long-term use of EVAL membranes may reduce oxidative stress and inflammation.

Polyamide: This family consists of an asymmetric membrane with 3 regions. The pore size increases dramatically from the blood side to the dialysate side, being smallest at the skin layer at around 5 nm. The result of this structure is low complement activation and low cell activation, resulting in lower oxidative stress.

Polysulfones: These membranes have the capacity to remove a broad range of uremic toxins and effectively retain endotoxins. Thanks to their structure, these membranes provide intrinsic biocompatibility and low cytotoxicity. They present a higher sieving coefficient with an increased hydraulic permeability that promotes efficient transport by convection. The original polymer can be blended with other polymers to give specific attributes to the membranes; for example, one can increase the hydrophilicity by adding polyvinylpyrrolidone (PVP). Finally, there are significant differences among polysulfone membranes because of variations in both the relative amounts of copolymers used in a particular blend and the fiber-spinning process employed.

Polyethersulfones: The new generation of this type of membrane has been developed through an advanced fiber-spinning process able to create large, uniform, and densely distributed pore size. Because of these characteristics, one sees improved selectivity. Polyethersulfones are therefore known for achieving outstanding middle molecule removal with minimal loss of albumin. In addition, their biocompatibility and endotoxin retaining are among the highest available.

Polyarylethersulfones: This family of membranes is a combination of polysulfones and polyarylate. There is only a single structure: three layers comprise the entire inner surface skin layer: A porous layer lies within the membrane, another skin layer covers the outer surface. The skin layer on the inner surface controls the water and solute permeability. The outer skin can block endotoxins from the dialysate side; thus, it can be used as an endotoxin filter. The amount of PVP added to the structure can control the albumin loss and β_2-microglobulin removal.

Biocompatibility

Biocompatibility is one of the most important elements to be considered in the choice of a dialyzer. In fact, the level of complement activation is a significant determinant of membrane compatibility. In general, all membranes activate complement and leukocytes to some extent; the most potent activators are unmodified cellulose membranes even if they are considered biocompatible. The activation of complement determines the production of anaphylotoxins, which may cause allergic reactions during dialysis and they can also lead to acute intradialytic pulmonary hypertension, chronic low-grade systemic inflammation, and immune dysregulation.

In every extracorporeal treatment, a significant amount of platelet activation can occur, resulting in clotting of the dialyzer. Platelets can also adhere to the membrane and become activated while blood flows within the dialyzer, and the extent to which air can be removed from it during priming can impact clotting according to the intrinsic membrane characteristics. Another important element that can determine platelet activation is the fibrinogen bond on the membrane surface. Biocompatibility is also influenced by the other dialyzer components such as the housing.

Bisphenol A (BPA) can be eluted from dialyzers made of polycarbonate and enter the bloodstream, where it can be present at elevated levels because of reduced excretion in chronic kidney disease and end-stage renal disease. For this reason, some manufacturers have developed dialyzers that contain no BPA. FDA has also reported that di(2-ethylhexyl)phthalate (DEHP) may have a putative role in health risk; thus, some manufacturers have removed it from their products.

Polyurethane is used to secure the hollow fiber at both ends of the dialyzer. This material has a high affinity for the sterilizing agent ethylene oxide (ETO). When ETO accumulates in the potting material, it can diffuse into the blood and cause anaphylactic reactions. Polycarbonate and other similar polymers used for the housing may be gas permeable and adsorb ETO during sterilization. For these reasons, the use of ETO is now less common, having been replaced with steam and gamma radiation.

Solute Removal

During the extracorporeal purification, solute removal occurs through a combination of diffusion, convection, and adsorption, depending on the type of treatment. The uremic solutes removed by the extracorporeal purification are divided into three main categories: small water-soluble compounds (such as urea) with an upper molecular weight less than 500 Da that can removed by any dialysis membrane through diffusion; larger middle-molecular-weight molecules ranging from 500 to 15,000 Da that can removed by dialyzer membranes with an enhanced transport capacity and large enough pores (this is typical in the high-flux dialyzers); finally protein-bound molecules mostly with a molecular weight of 500 Da but larger and more difficult to remove because of their binding to proteins.

The solute removal efficiency is dependent on the surface area of the dialyzer and the mass transfer coefficient. The convective separation of solutes and low-molecular-weight proteins from large serum proteins and blood elements is achieved with high-flux dialyzers by increased porosity and efficient mass transfer.

The process of adsorption is the process by which macromolecules and proteins can adhere to the membrane surface without penetration into the membrane structure. This process is primarily depending on the internal pore structure and the hydrophobicity of the membrane. A moderate level of protein adsorption combined with the ability to bind protein bound uremic toxins appears to be recommended and may increase biocompatibility.

The clearance (urea clearance) must be considered the most important parameter of a dialyzer as it is then a critical factor in the dialysis prescription.

Enlarging membrane pore size (beyond conventional low-flux dialyzers) leads to increased clearances for β_2-microglobulin. Because of its molecular weight of 11,000 Da, β_2-microglobulin clearance can be used as a marker of middle molecule removal and a surrogate marker for membrane flux.

Dialyzers are considered high flux if the ultrafiltration coefficient is greater than 15 mL/h/mmHg and the ability to clear β_2-microglobulin is more than 20 mL/min. If the β_2-microglobulin clearance is more than 50 mL/min, the membrane is considered super high flux and its cut-off can be close to 65,000 Da. This type of membrane allows an efficient removal of middle- and large-size uremic toxins, and inflammatory cytokines.

When considering all of these concepts, it is important to understand that back-filtration almost never occurs in low-flux dialysis, and its occurrence during high-flux treatments depends on the transmembrane pressure. This point is crucial for the safety of the treatment because any contamination of dialysate or wash-out from the membrane can reach the blood side.

Dialyzer Choice and Prescription

It is typical practice for nephrologists to follow an empiric model when devising the hemodialysis prescription. In general, patients are placed on the largest dialyzer that is affordable, and the longest amount of time tolerated by the patient, with the highest blood flow rate guaranteed by the vascular access. After this first prescription, nephrologists check the Kt/V and, if it is not as desired, they can attempt some corrective actions in order to improve clearance such as extending treatment time, increasing dialysate flow rate, increasing blood flow rate, or using a larger dialyzer. It is the clinician's challenge to find the optimal dialyzer based on the patient's size, years of dialysis, hemodynamic status, tolerance to treatment time, and tolerance to blood and dialysate flow rate. It is also important to analyze the residual renal function and comorbidities and the performance of the vascular access, the latter being a potential weakness of dialysis treatment even if all other parameters are optimized. From the point of view of other comorbidities, it is important to consider the need for removal of particular molecules, minimizing albumin losses if a higher cut-off membrane is used. Clinicians must also choose a membrane that will ensure the best impact on quality of life if long-term complications, such as dialysis-related amyloidosis, can be lessened through the use of specific high-performance membranes.

A low–priming volume requirement allows the use of the patient's blood to prime the circuit without serious hypovolemic effects. Thus, knowledge of the volume of priming for each dialyzer and the effective blood volume of the patient are important elements in the choice of the dialyzer. In a typical adult patient the priming volume may be of little consequence, but it could be important for children or small adults. There is an increasing demand in dialysis therapy for new measures of biocompatibility, such as reducing intradialytic blood pressure variability, decreasing oxidative stress, and delaying the onset or progression of complications.

Single-use dialyzers provide the advantage of reducing the cost of personnel, and technician training on dialyzer reuse, reuse record keeping, room maintenance for safety and sterilization, and quality assurance programs. The policy of single use also benefits patients by decreasing reuse syndromes caused by residual germicides. It is now known that synthetic membranes have reduced first use syndromes, especially since sterilization with ETO has been replaced with gamma radiation, electron beam radiation, and steam.

Dialyzers that are reused must be reprocessed following the Association for the Advancement of Medical Instrumentation (AAMI) Standards and Recommended Practices for reuse of hemodialyzers. Dialyzers intended for reuse should have a blood compartment volume not less than 80% of the original measured volume or a urea clearance not less than 90% of the original measured clearance.

Conclusions

Currently on the market there is a large series of dialyzers that differ in the characteristics of the membrane, and as a result the range of molecules that they can remove. The specific cut-off and hydraulic permeability allow the use of such filters in different configurations such us HD, HDF, HFD, AFB, and HFR (and their variants). The different dialyzer surfaces allow one to obtain the desired clearances in relation to the blood flow rate and patient's size. With these considerations, the nephrologist can choose and prescribe the best treatment for each patient in relation to his or her clinical needs. In case of intolerance or allergy to some dialysis components, nephrologists can choose among different membranes with equivalent features. Therefore the knowledge of the characteristics of each membrane allows the nephrologist to use the best device for the individual clinical needs, customizing the dialysis treatment and providing patient-centric care.

SECTION VII

Adequacy of Dialysis

CHAPTER 18

Uremic Toxicity

Thomas A. Depner, MD

"The clue, doctor, is that there are too many clues."
—Hector Poirot, in *Murder on the Orient Express* by Agatha Christie

Uremic Toxicity: The Modern Definition of Uremia

The renal excretory system is responsible for eliminating both nonvolatile waste solutes generated from endogenous metabolism and unwanted solutes that enter the body from absorption across the gastrointestinal epithelium. Most of these solutes are normally found in the urine. The term *uremia*, which literally means "urine in the blood," was first used by Piorry in 1847 to describe the clinical syndrome observed in patients with advanced kidney failure. Despite their limited knowledge of clinical chemistry, clinicians in that early era correctly assumed that toxic urinary solutes accumulated in patients with kidney damage, accounting for the syndrome. However, the uremic syndrome was assumed to encompass all aspects of the disease state, including fluid accumulation, hormonal derangements, and malnutrition. In the modern era, the advent of dialysis has tended to limit the definition of uremia to the symptoms and signs that respond to removal of solutes from the blood. Although anemia and malnutrition are important treatable aspects of the disease, they are viewed as separate from the toxic effects of retained solutes that are reversed by toxin removal. Meyer and Hostetter in their Medical Progress review of uremia state, "Today the term uremia is used loosely to describe the illness accompanying kidney failure that cannot be explained by derangements in extracellular volume, inorganic ion concentrations, or lack of known renal synthetic products. We now assume that uremic illness is due largely to the accumulation of organic waste products, not all identified as yet, that are normally cleared by the kidneys."

Clinical Syndrome of Uremia

Few organ systems escape the toxic effects of accumulated uremic retention products. The symptoms of uremia are initially vague and diverse, often expressed as fatigue, listlessness, and inability to mentally concentrate. The patient may lose the sense of taste or develop a metallic taste (dysgeusia), and the uremic breath has a fishlike odor. Loss of appetite progresses to nausea and vomiting, subjecting the patient to malnutrition. Itching sensations are accompanied by dry and flaky skin that has a sallow yellowish tan color, and in advanced cases crystals of urea known as *uremic frost* may appear where sweat has evaporated, especially in the intertriginous areas (Fig. 18.1). Biochemical abnormalities include hyperkalemia, acidosis, phosphorus accumulation, calcium malabsorption, and impaired cellular immune responses. As the kidneys continue to fail, fluid may accumulate, causing edema,

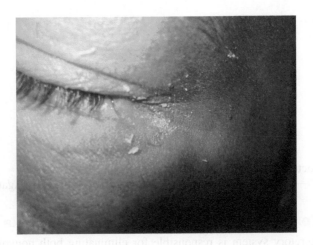

Figure 18.1

Uremic frost in dried lacrimal secretions from a 53-year-old man with chronic urinary obstruction. Blood urea nitrogen 256 mg/dL, serum creatinine 31.9 mg/dL.

hypertension, and respiratory compromise accompanied by a bat wing or butterfly infiltrate seen on chest radiograph. Prolonged toxicity may be expressed as uremic osteodystrophy (see Section 22, Uremic Osteodystrophy) including growth retardation in children, a stocking-glove peripheral neuropathy, and/or uremic encephalopathy that may eventually progress to uremic coma and death. Death occurs within 5–7 days after complete loss of renal function, and in the absence of fluid overload is usually painless and silent. However, even in advanced stages of uremic coma, recovery after institution of dialysis has been reported, indicating that many aspects of uremic toxicity are reversible simply by removing the offending (dialyzable) toxins.

Although a wide variety of diseases can impair kidney function, as the kidney disease progresses to near end stage the clinical manifestations are similar, indicating that they are largely due to the kidney failure itself, not the underlying disease. In fact, the clinical presentation is so monotonous that it led physicians for over a century to consider it a single disease that bore the name of the pioneer Richard Bright who described what became known in the late 19th and early 20th century as Bright's disease.

The full-blown syndrome of uremia is much less common today than in the predialysis era prior to 1943, despite the greater prevalence of end-stage renal disease (ESRD), including many anephric patients. The widespread availability of dialysis and transplantation together with frequent assessments of kidney function, especially in older patients, has allowed timely intervention to nearly eliminate the advanced stages of the syndrome. Choice of an optimal time to begin dialysis treatments has recently been clarified by a controlled clinical trial that showed no advantage to early presymptomatic intervention. Improvements in dialysis have also mitigated some of the more subtle aspects of uremia, including neuropathic and cutaneous disorders that were commonly experienced in earlier years. Such improvements include establishment of higher standards for small molecule clearance, substitution of bicarbonate base for acetate in the dialysate, use of more biocompatible membranes, increasing use of high-porosity (high-flux) membranes, and use of fewer neuropathic drugs. Some or all of these changes probably account for the better quality of life enjoyed by today's dialysis-dependent patients.

Dialysis reverses the life-threatening aspects of uremia, allowing survival in some cases for more than 30 years even with no urine output. It has been called the most significant advancement in medical treatment to be introduced during the last century. However, the probability of survival is much lower than in the general population; fewer than 50% are alive after 5 years of dialysis in the United States (see Chapter 1, Demographics of the End Stage Renal Disease Patient). In addition, the patient's quality of life is compromised in several ways, not the least of which is the burden of dialysis itself.

The Residual Syndrome

Having escaped the threat of encephalopathy, neuropathy, and death, ESRD patients suffer to varying degrees from a constellation of biologic and clinical abnormalities that have collectively been named the *residual syndrome*. Symptoms vary from patient to patient, but the most important feature of the syndrome is a higher than expected all-cause mortality rate, with cardiovascular events heading the list of causes as shown in Fig. 18.2. Note that the mortality rate in younger patients is as much as three orders of magnitude higher than in subjects of the same age without kidney disease. Some of the subjective and objective elements of the residual syndrome are depicted in Table 18.1, including growth retardation in children, features of malnutrition, inflammatory diseases, vascular disease due to accelerated atherosclerosis, hypertension, valvular heart disease, etc., and legacy disorders from the patient's original kidney disease such as diabetes, crystalline nephropathy, autoimmune disease, etc. The residual syndrome includes irritating disorders such as occasional nausea, dysgeusia, poor physical and mental stamina, and pruritus. These symptoms can be found in patients who appear otherwise well dialyzed. However, despite the improvements in dialysis, including increases in solute clearances, there are lingering concerns about incomplete removal of uremic toxins and the potential adverse effects of dialysis itself (see the section Adverse Effects of Dialysis in this chapter).

Uremic Toxins Defined

By definition, uremic toxins can be identified only in patients with kidney failure. Although some substances found in healthy people can also be found in kidney patients, they would not be recognized as uremic toxins were it not for their accumulation and toxic effects in patients with kidney failure. The higher concentrations achieved in uremic patients are therefore essential to their identity as toxins. Excluded from the list of toxins are vital substances such as sodium, potassium, calcium, magnesium, phosphate, and chloride, some of which can accumulate and cause illness, but their accumulation is more appropriately considered a failure of regulation, since the kidney is entrusted with the task of maintaining their physiologic concentrations rather than total elimination. Inorganic phosphate is an example of an anion that must be maintained within a set range to support bone and energy metabolism in muscle and other organs. As kidney function deteriorates, phosphate tends to accumulate but normal levels are maintained because native kidneys, under

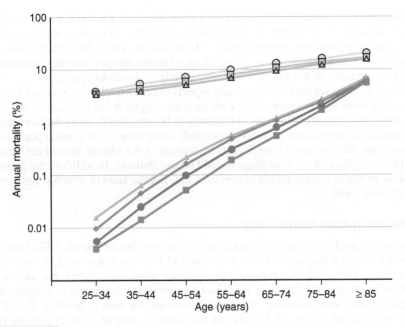

Figure 18.2

Mortality from cardiovascular disease (arrhythmias, cardiomyopathy, cardiac arrest, myocardial infarction, atherosclerotic heart disease, pulmonary edema) in the general population (GP) and in the dialysis population.◆, GP male; ■, GP female; ▲, GP black; ●, GP white; ◊, dialysis male; □, dialysis female; △, dialysis black; ○, dialysis white. (Adapted from: Foley RN, et al: Clinical epidemiology of cardiovascular disease in chronic renal disease, Fig. 1, Am J Kidney Dis 32(5) Suppl 3:S112-S119, 1998.)

the influence of parathyroid hormone (PTH), reduce the rate of tubular reabsorption (normally about 80%) to much lower levels, which maintains the elimination rate without the need for higher blood and tissue levels. This mechanism fails when the average adult's glomerular filtration rate falls below 30 mL/min, and phosphate begins to accumulate, ultimately contributing to metabolic bone disease.

Note also that elimination of foreign substances not commonly found in uremic patients, or in a list of uremic toxins, can be markedly impaired. Accumulation of these substances can cause serious illness, even death, in patients with compromised kidney function, but exposures may be well tolerated in individuals with normal kidney function. Examples of these include aluminum, once a major cause of death in some dialysis settings, certain drugs such as penicillin or aminoglycoside antibiotics, iron, potassium, and star fruit neurotoxin. Toxicities of this nature are not generally considered part of the uremic syndrome. Note also that some inorganic gases and organic compounds with high vapor pressures can accumulate, elimination of which is primarily by the lungs. For the most part, these are not considered here.

Table 18.1

The Residual Syndrome

Subjective
- Poor stamina
- Postdialysis lethargy, poor tolerance of hemodialysis
- Poor appetite
- Intermittent nausea, feeling sick
- Insomnia, sleep disturbance
- Impaired sexual function
- Reduced capacity for mental concentration, impaired cognitive function
- Depression, reduced ambition, sometimes leading to voluntary discontinuation of treatment

Objective
- Prolonged recovery from infection, illness
- Impaired inflammatory response
- Delayed wound healing
- Impaired cellular immune response
- Inhibition of leukocyte phagocytosis
- Altered membrane transport functions: Na^+, H^+, K^+
- Resistance to insulin, erythropoietin, parathyroid, and other hormones
- Infertility
- Decreased protein binding of small ligands
- Hypothermia
- Hypertension
- Hyperphosphatemia
- Intermittent vomiting
- Frequent congestive heart failure, cardiovascular disease

Source of Toxins: Nitrogen Compounds

The term *azotemia* refers to increased concentrations of nitrogen-containing substances in the blood, most of which are products of protein catabolism, more than 90% of which is urea (Fig. 18.3). Other nitrogen-containing compounds that accumulate in the blood and tissues include creatinine, guanidines, peptides, methylamines, and other aliphatic and aromatic amines, most of which depend on the kidney for elimination. The liver plays a role by detoxifying the ammonia produced endogenously from amino acid catabolism, converting it to urea; and by various conjugating mechanisms, for example, glucuronidation, sulfation, and N-acetylation, that serve to detoxify solutes and allow more efficient elimination by the kidneys. The liver also synthesizes serum albumin, the most abundant serum protein, which in addition to its oncotic function binds many waste solutes. Some of the latter compounds are hydrophobic and poorly soluble in aqueous bodily fluids, so binding to albumin increases the potential for renal elimination by tubular secretion (see the section Protein-Bound Solutes in this chapter). Albumin also serves as an antioxidant to limit damage by free radicals and other oxidative products of metabolism.

Prior to the advent of dialysis, physicians treated kidney failure with dietary protein restriction to reduce the burden of nitrogen elimination by the kidneys. Symptoms such as anorexia, nausea, vomiting, lethargy, and somnolence improved

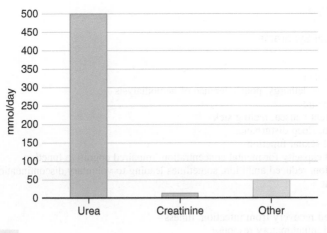

Figure 18.3

Urinary excretion of organic compounds. The "Other" category is the total excretion of about 90 compounds. (Graphic derived from data published in Geigy Scientific Tables, Vol 1, CIBA-GEIGY, 1981: Composition of the urine.)

significantly, prolonging survival in patients with low clearance levels. Ultimately, the combined effects of anorexia and dietary restriction led to malnutrition, which in some cases was severe and eventually contributed more to death than uremic toxicity. In the modern era, native kidney function is monitored closely and intervention is scheduled to avoid the need for protein restriction and attendant risks of malnutrition. Once maintenance dialysis is initiated, the emphasis has shifted to maintaining nutrition, including adequate protein intake (see Section 16, Nutritional Management of Dialysis Patients).

In view of recent data suggesting an enteric origin of some uremic toxins, it is possible that protein restriction also reduces the *generation* of toxic compounds by intestinal flora. Colon-derived toxic compounds such as indoxyl sulfate and para-cresol sulfate are also protein-bound (see the section Protein-Bound Solutes in this chapter) and therefore less easily removed by dialysis. Reducing the generation and/ or enteric absorption of such compounds using probiotics and oral sorbents offers promise as a method to delay or treat uremic toxicity.

Mechanisms of Toxicity

Many substances have been identified as retained in patients with chronic kidney disease (CKD) but few have been positively linked to toxicity. Perhaps most of the compounds identified in uremic serum by mass spectrometric analysis of gas and liquid chromatographic eluates cannot be designated as toxins because a definite link to one or more toxic phenomena has not yet been established. In the absence of such evidence, these substances are more properly called *retention solutes* rather than uremic toxins. In addition, linking serum levels of newly discovered retention solutes with the levels of established toxins cannot be used as evidence for toxicity, nor can linking levels with subjective or objective features of the uremic syndrome, including death, provide convincing evidence for toxicity. Patients with symptomatic uremic toxicity are likely to have higher levels of both toxic and nontoxic retention solutes. To establish a cause–effect relationship, the solute in question must be examined in isolation, either by in vitro studies or by administering it alone to animals or people. Unfortunately, such studies are difficult, expensive, and sometimes risky to perform. Furthermore, a toxic effect cannot be entirely ruled out with a negative study because of a possible synergistic effect of toxins each at a subtoxic level when studied in isolation. In vitro testing must also take into consideration protein binding of the solute and its free concentration, which is considered to be the active form of the molecule. Frustration with these obstacles probably stimulated Jonas Bergstrom, a renowned investigator of uremia, more than 30 years ago to remark, "despite more than 150 years of research, it has not been possible to explain all uraemic toxic manifestations by accumulation of known compounds. Accordingly the search for uraemic toxins continues" (Bergstrom 1983).

Proposed mechanisms of uremic toxicity parallel that of xenobiotic toxicity including competitive and noncompetitive blocking of vital receptors, disruption of cell signaling, inhibition of enzymes, interference with membrane transporters, and activation of inflammatory pathways. Analogous to glycosylation (posttranslational derivatization) of hemoglobin and other proteins from hyperglycemia, carbamylation of protein epsilon amino groups can occur in the uremic environment as a result of high urea concentrations. Solutions of urea exist in equilibrium with very low concentrations of cyanate, a reactive substance that can combine with free epsilon amino groups of proteins (Fig. 18.4). The resulting posttranslational carbamylation of long-lived proteins such as serum albumin has been associated with resistance to erythropoietin, cardiovascular events, atherosclerosis, and mortality in dialyzed patients. A cause-and-effect relationship, however, has not been definitely established, and the U-shaped correlation of urea levels with outcome (both high and low concentrations suggest poor outcomes) raises questions about the pathogenesis.

Another toxic mechanism in patients with advanced uremia is related to the production of ammonia from ureolytic bacteria in the mouth and lower gastrointestinal tract. Locally produced ammonia can cause mucosal ulcerations that can predispose to infection and contribute to bleeding.

Hormonal derangements are well described, including insensitivity to insulin, deficiencies of both erythropoietin and activated vitamin D, and excesses of hormones, for example, PTH, gastrin, and melanocyte stimulating hormone. Mechanisms responsible for hormone excess include impaired renal degradation of

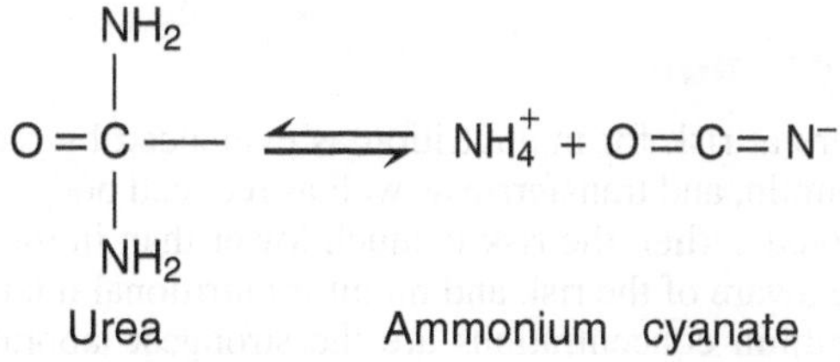

$$\underset{\text{Urea}}{\overset{\displaystyle NH_2 \atop |}{O = C \underset{|}{\overset{}{}} \atop NH_2}} \rightleftharpoons \underset{\text{Ammonium \ cyanate}}{NH_4^+ + O = C = N^-}$$

Figure 18.4

The reaction that forms cyanate from urea heavily favors movement to the left.

Table 18.2

Uremic Disorders Not Directly Linked to a Toxin

- Synergistic or additive effect of multiple toxins each at individual subtoxic levels could explain the failure to identify a single toxin for each single toxic effect
- Inhibition of normal detoxifying mechanisms, for example, binding to albumin by retention solutes that are otherwise relatively nontoxic, or saturation of hepatic detoxifying mechanisms
- Blockade of RES or hepatic excretory mechanisms by retention products that have no other intrinsic toxicity but contribute to the accumulation of toxins not normally excreted by the kidneys
- Hormonal excess or deficiency (e.g., anemia and erythropoietin deficiency, incomplete activation of vitamin D, parathyroid hormone excess)
- Malnutrition
- Inflammation, linked to low albumin concentrations in ESRD patients
- Psychological depression, unfortunately augmented by the burden of dialysis
- Legacy from the primary kidney disease (e.g., amyloidosis, diabetes, cystinosis)

polypeptide hormones, compensatory responses to another uremic disorder (e.g., PTH excess), and inhibition of endocrine and paracrine receptor activity (e.g., insulin). Loss of kidney synthetic tissue accounts for important deficiencies. Hormone deficiencies obviously cannot be corrected by dialysis, but supplementation of erythropoietin has added measurably to the average patient's quality of life, as has reversal of the long-term devastating effects of hyperparathyroid bone disease by calcitriol replacement. However, neither of these replacements prevents death from uremia, so they must take a second seat to the dialytic removal of small solutes as the primary mechanism for reversal of uremia.

The pathway to morbidity may be indirect (see Table 18.2); for example, susceptibility to infection, a frequent cause of death in patients with advanced kidney disease, may not be the direct consequence of a retained toxin but more a consequence of protein–calorie malnutrition. As noted above, malnutrition was a more frequent problem in the predialysis era, a consequence of both uremia-induced anorexia and attempts at therapeutic dietary restriction. Another indirect cause of morbidity not directly linked to a specific toxin is psychological depression, a reaction to dependency and/or ill health that can lead to suicide, an unfortunate common cause of death in the dialysis population.

Role of Malnutrition

Dialysis patients are at risk for malnutrition as evidenced by reduced serum levels of albumin, prealbumin, and transferrin as well as reduced body cell mass and physical function. As noted earlier, the risk is much lower than in the predialysis era but caregivers must be aware of the risk and monitor nutritional intake, especially in the elderly. Serum albumin concentrations are the strongest laboratory correlate with mortality, and although low albumin concentrations in many patients probably reflect inflammatory states, recently demonstrated increases in albumin concentrations in response to protein–calorie supplements given during dialysis strongly suggest a role for malnutrition as well. The recommendation to encourage or restrict protein intake achieving a high versus low urea generation rate should likely depend on the starting level. Similar to urea clearance, a ceiling is probably reached above, which further protein intake offers no advantage and may do harm by generating more nitrogenous end products and potentially stimulating the production of toxins by intestinal flora. Targeting an adequate but not excessive intake is the current recommendation.

Role of Inflammation and Oxidative Stress

In the average dialysis patient, serum indicators of inflammation such as C-reactive protein (CRP) and other acute phase proteins are continuously elevated and are periodically increased by episodes of inflammation that are accompanied by decreases in negative acute phase proteins such as albumin, prealbumin, and transferrin. In addition, chronically elevated levels of inflammatory markers such as C-reactive protein (CRP) and interleukin-6 (IL-6) in patients with CKD suggest that inflammatory events are common in CKD patients, or that inflammation is a component of the uremic syndrome, or that native kidneys are responsible for clearing inflammatory mediators. Once dialysis is started, however, the high concentrations of oxidative stress markers are not reduced.

The pathogenesis of vascular injury, a well-established consequence of kidney failure, is not completely understood, but is known to be mediated at least in part by oxidative stress due to inflammation. The balance of oxidation/reduction in patients with advanced kidney failure favors oxidation. Elevated serum concentrations of proinflammatory cytokines, particularly IL-6, and acute phase reactants such as C-reactive protein (CRP) and serum amyloid-A are highly associated with the high cardiovascular morbidity and mortality in dialysis patients shown in Fig. 18.2. The normal complex protective mechanisms that prevent tissue injury by reducing reactive oxygen species (ROS) are also impaired in uremic individuals, potentially contributing to endothelial damage. However, efforts to restore this protection by administering antioxidants to dialysis patients have been disappointing.

Role of Anemia

The contribution of anemia to the residual syndrome was highlighted in the past by patients who reported feeling much better after receiving transfusions in preparation for kidney transplants. When recombinant erythropoietin first became available to treat the anemia of kidney disease, patients echoed these salutary effects after their hemoglobin levels rose above 10 g/dL for the first time. Over the next 10 years, iron toxicity from multiple transfusions was nearly eliminated, further improving the lot of dialysis patients around the world. Patients with marginal cardiac status became eligible for dialysis, which probably accounted for the minimal improvement in mortality rates during the years that followed. However, more aggressive treatment with intent to restore hemoglobin to normal levels proved deleterious, in part due to facilitated thrombosis. Today clinicians recognize hemoglobin levels of 10–12 g/dL as the optimum range.

Magnitude of Toxicity

Lack of knowledge about the identity of critical uremic toxins has actually helped to simplify the measurement of dose and adequacy. We know that dialysis works, that it can reverse even advanced life threatening uremic toxicity within hours, restoring a relatively comfortable life often for many years. We also know that the only therapeutic effects of dialysis are removal of small (dialyzable) solutes and removal of water, the first by diffusion and the latter by convection. The convective effect is easily measured as a volume removed but the diffusive effect requires a measurement of clearance.

Note that measurement of solute levels in the patient are confounded by the solute generation rate; for example, if the generation rate falls, the level will fall regardless of the performance of the dialyzer. If treatment is based on the serum levels of a toxin generated from dietary intake, uremia-associated anorexia will cause the level to fall, giving the false impression of improvement, which could lead to a vicious cycle. So the effectiveness of dialysis is best measured as a clearance, which is essentially the ratio of the generation (equivalent to elimination in a steady state) to the concentration level, and as such is a measure of dialyzer performance independent of the generation rate or level.

Investigators of uremic toxicity have borrowed from the field of toxicology to quantify the purging of toxins by dialysis. The term Kt/V_{urea}, widely used to express the dose of dialysis, is derived from the basic pharmacokinetic expression of the time (t)-dependent exponential fall in concentration (C) of a drug or toxin caused by a first-order elimination mechanism:

$$C = C_0 e^{-kt}$$

where C_0 is the initial concentration (after loading) and k is the elimination constant, which is the constant fractional rate of fall in concentration for first-order processes like diffusion. The elimination constant (k) can also be expressed as K/V, where K is the clearance and V is the solute's volume of distribution. K/V is the fractional clearance, which can be easily calculated from the exponential fall in concentration during dialysis. The reason for targeting urea clearance, as explained in Chapter 19, is the success of dialysis itself, which removes small, easily dialyzed solutes like urea almost exclusively.

A perhaps disappointing conclusion from the above logic is that we can accurately measure the life-saving effect of dialysis but we have poor measurements of the uremic state itself, the target of dialysis. Current and future efforts to identify the causes of each aspect of uremia can extend knowledge about the syndrome with the promise to develop additional specific treatments.

Classification of Uremic Toxins

Several excellent reviews of suspected and confirmed uremic toxins have appeared in the literature and are periodically updated. The European Uremic Toxin Work Group (EUTox) created in 2000 by the European Society for Artificial Organs has continually updated a list of retained solutes that have potential toxicity, including detailed descriptions of each solute, levels identified in uremic compared to normal individuals, evidence for toxicity, and methods for analysis. The reader is referred to these comprehensive reviews listed at the end of this chapter for further information.

Today, well over 200 retained compounds have been identified; most but not all are easily removed by therapeutic dialysis. The beneficial effect of dialysis confirms our understanding of uremia as a reversible toxic state and also serves as the basis for the most popular classification of uremic retention solutes: those that dialyze easily and those that don't dialyze easily. Solutes in both categories are tagged as "uremic" when measured serum concentrations are significantly higher than concentrations found in people without kidney disease. Classification as a toxin, however, requires both a higher concentration than normal and a demonstration of toxicity using a variety of in vivo and in vitro methods. For solutes that accumulate but are poorly dialyzable, demonstration of toxicity is especially critical since failure of removal by dialysis despite recovery from uremia implies a lack of toxicity. Some of these solutes may contribute, however, to the subacute residual syndrome discussed above. The poorly dialyzed solutes have been further divided by EUTox into larger poorly diffusible solutes and protein-bound solutes. The latter diffuse easily across dialyzer membranes in free form, but overall removal is impeded by substantial binding to serum macromolecules, principally albumin.

Examples of well-established toxins in each category are listed in Table 18.3.

Small Water-Soluble (Dialyzable) Solutes

Except for urea, the guanidino compounds shown in Table 18.3 are quantitatively the most abundant solutes to accumulate when the kidneys fail. Among these, creatinine is usually the most abundant but others are potentially more toxic, including guanidine, guanidinosuccinic acid (GSA), methylguanidine (MG), and both symmetric and asymmetric dimethylarginine. In dialysis patients', creatinine usually accumulates to 1–20 times normal levels whereas GSA and MG accumulate to 100–200 times normal levels, although at lower concentrations. All are derived from the metabolism of the amino acid arginine, and all are found in the serum, cerebrospinal fluid, and brain, where they may have significant neurologic toxicity, contributing to encephalopathy and polyneuropathy by a variety of suspected mechanisms, including interference with amino acid receptors and neurotransmitters, demyelination, and oxidative injury. Symmetric and asymmetric dimethylarginine have also been shown to cause vasoconstriction by inhibiting nitric oxide. In vitro and in vivo animal studies have focused on the neuroexcitatory properties of the guanidine compounds, alluding to seizures that are occasionally seen in patients suffering from advanced uremia. However, most descriptions of terminal uremia describe a state of CNS depression, progressing to coma before death; seizures are more often blamed on medication overdoses, most notoriously penicillin and its derivatives. But as a whole and perhaps in concert, the guanidine compounds may be the most important contributors to the severe life-threatening aspects of uremia that are reversed by dialysis and appears to be without permanent sequelae in most patients.

Recently, trimethylamine oxide (TMAO), a product of the intestinal microbiome, has been linked to cardiovascular mortality in patients with normal and impaired kidney function and is linked to progression of kidney disease in animal models. TMAO is a small easily filtered and dialyzed molecule derived from dietary choline; elimination is dependent on both glomerular and tubular kidney function. Levels are markedly elevated in hemodialyzed patients but in contrast to normal and CKD patients in whom significant morbidity has been demonstrated, no correlation with cardiovascular disease or all-cause mortality has been found in the dialysis population.

Most of the myriad solutes identified by sensitive methods such as high-performance liquid chromatography (HPLC) and mass spectrometry are found in

Table 18.3

Examples of Proposed Uremic Toxins

	MW	Concentration[a]	Units
Small water soluble compounds (MW < 500 Da)			
Urea	60	100–3000	mg/L
Uric acid	168	30–150	mg/L
Myoinositol	180	10–100	mg/L
Pseudouridine	244	0.5–15	mg/L
Arabinitol	152	<0.6–15	mg/L
Oxalate	90	0.3–4.0	mg/L
Sorbitol	180	0.5–3.0	mg/L
Hypoxanthine	113	1.5–2.5	mg/L
Xanthine	152	0.5–1.5	mg/L
Methylmalonic acid	118	30–120	µg/L
Trimethylamine oxide	75	0.1–5.0	mg/L
Guanidines			
Creatinine	113	10–250	mg/L
Creatine	131	4.0–200	mg/L
Guanidinosuccinic acid	175	0.03–6.5	mg/L
Asymmetric dimethylarginine	202	0.2–7.0	mg/L
Methylguanidine	73	8.0–800	ug/L
Larger compounds—all peptides (MW > 500 Da)			
Beta-2 microglobulin	11,800	2.0–55	mg/L
Parathyroid hormone	9,225	<0.06–1.2	µg/L
Leptin	16,000	2.5–8.0	µg/L
Gastrin		25–160	ng/L
Hepcidin	2789	40–125	µg/L
Interleukin-6	24,500	5.0–90	ng/L
Peptide-linked AGEs[b]	50–400+	0.3–1.7	mg/L
Protein-bound compounds			
Indole derivatives			
Indoxyl sulfate	251	0.6–53	mg/L
Indole-3-acetic acid	175	0.02–1.5	mg/L
Melatonin	232	0.025–0.20	µg/L
Phenol derivatives			
p-Cresol sulfate	188	0.5–20	mg/L
p-Cresol glucuronide	283	0–0.4	mg/L
Phenol	94	0.6–2.7	mg/L
Hydroxyquinone	110	0–50	µg/L
Hippuric acid	179	<5–250	mg/L
Homocysteine	135	<1.5–8.0	mg/L
CMPF[b]	240	8.0–60	mg/L

[a]Approximate concentrations range from normal to high levels found in uremic patients.
[b]AGE, advanced glycation end products; CMPF, 3-carboxy-4-methyl-5-propyl-2-furanpropionic acid.
Adapted from Neirynck et al and other sources.

tiny concentrations of 1 ppm (1 μg/mL) or less. Of course many drugs and vital cofactors as well as hormones exert their effects at very low concentrations, so toxicity is not ruled out simply because the substance is present in tiny amounts.

Larger Solutes (Molecular Weight > 500 Da)

Larger less-well-dialyzed solutes likely contribute to the residual syndrome, but the magnitude of their contribution is debated. Advocates of high-flux hemodialysis and hemofiltration that are known to remove larger molecules point to the association of β2-microglobulin (B2M) levels with mortality and other adverse outcomes as shown in Fig. 18.5. However, rigorous controlled clinical trials designed to show a benefit of these methods, using B2M (molecular weight 11,800 Da) as a surrogate, have been disappointing at best. The observation that older cellulosic membranes that had an absolute molecular weight cutoff of ~10,000 Da did not remove larger molecules including B2M but successfully reversed advanced life-threatening uremia demonstrates the greater importance of small solutes as perpetrators of the uremic syndrome. However, larger solutes such as B2M, advanced glycosylation end products (AGEs), adipokines (leptin), and other larger peptides, examples of which are listed in Table 18.3, continue to be eyed suspiciously by investigators as possible agents responsible for suboptimal long-term patient outcomes (see the section The Residual Syndrome in this chapter). Accumulation and polymerization of B2M causes dialysis-related amyloidosis, a complication of both hemodialysis

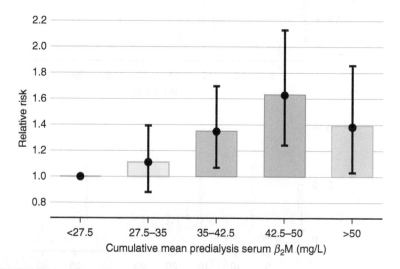

Figure 18.5

Time-dependent Cox regression showing the association of beta-2 microglobulin levels (β₂M) with risk of mortality in the HEMO Study (n = 1813 patients; p < .001). Data were adjusted for demographic factors and multiple other potential confounders at baseline. (Adapted from Cheung A, et al: Serum beta-2 microglobulin levels predict mortality in dialysis patients: results of the HEMO study. Fig. 5, J Am Soc Nephrol 17: 546-555, 2006.)

and peritoneal dialysis that has waned in frequency over the past several decades, possibly due to more frequent use of high-flux membranes. In several studies of high- versus low-flux membranes, secondary analyses of patient subgroups (diabetic kidney disease, low serum albumin concentrations, longer dialysis vintage) suggest a benefit, but overall mortality rates have not been improved by either high-flux dialysis or hemofiltration. Perhaps future more sophisticated separation techniques will be able to identify a toxic fraction in the larger-molecular-weight spectrum that will justify removal efforts.

Protein-Bound Solutes

Binding to macromolecules lowers the concentration of the free, presumably toxic fraction, which is also the driving force for diffusion across dialysis membranes. Although only a handful of protein-bound ligands in higher than normal concentrations in uremic fluids have been chemically defined, many undefined peaks can be seen in chromatography spectra from extracts of uremic serum proteins (Fig. 18.6). Several are indoles derived from gut-derived bacterial action on tryptophan, and

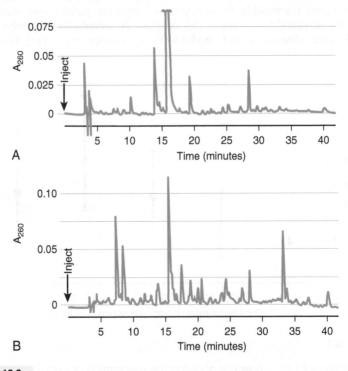

Figure 18.6

Column elution pattern of a protein-bound extract from (A) normal serum and (B) one-fifth the volume of uremic serum. (Adapted from Gulyassy PF, et al: Isolation of inhibitors of ligand–albumin binding from uremic body fluids and normal urine. Fig. 1, Kidney Int 24 (Suppl 16):S238-S242, 1983.)

others are phenyl derivatives derived from ingested foods. In contrast to urea levels, which average about 4 times the concentration in normal compared to patient serum, the concentration of some protein-bound solutes can reach as high as 100 times the concentration found in people without kidney disease.

Nearly all of the binding occurs relatively loosely to albumin, the most abundant and widely studied circulating protein. Serum albumin has several nonspecific binding sites to accommodate a variety of ligands, most notably fatty acids and bilirubin, but also the amino acid tryptophan, and a variety of drugs including salicylate and phenytoin. Bound solutes tend to have a nonpolar attribute as shown in Fig. 18.7. Accumulation in patients with kidney failure shows that native kidneys eliminate them, but since binding limits filtration, elimination is primarily by tubular secretion, which also favors solutes with nonpolar moieties. Passage through the renal peritubular capillaries releases the ligands most likely by pure diffusion across the huge capillary surface area followed by active transport across the tubular basement membrane. The robust anionic and cationic transporters positioned in the basolateral membranes of the proximal tubule puzzled investigators in the past who postulated a need to eliminate very toxic substances. More likely they serve to maintain a low but continuous concentration gradient across the capillary membranes. The rate of dissociation from albumin far exceeds the transport rate, so the removal rate can be substantial. For example, the free concentration of a bound ligand, 3-carboxy-4-methyl-5-propyl-2-furanpropionic acid (CMPF) (Fig. 18.8) is so low in the blood that dialysis and hemofiltration fail to remove it, yet it is

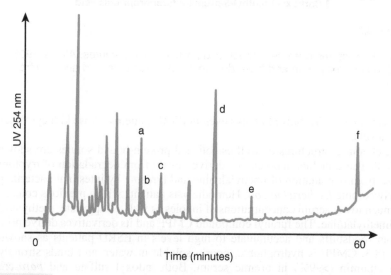

Figure 18.7

Compounds bound to serum albumin tend to have a nonpolar attribute. The chromatogram shows the sequential appearance of solutes from an ultrafiltrate of uremic serum loaded onto an HPLC column and eluted with increasingly nonpolar solvents. a = indoxyl sulfate, b = tryptophan, c = hippuric acid, d = indole-3-acetic acid, e = CMPF, f = internal standard. (Adapted from Dhondt A, et al: The removal of uremic toxins. Fig. 2, Kidney Int 58 (Suppl 76):S47-S59, 2000.)

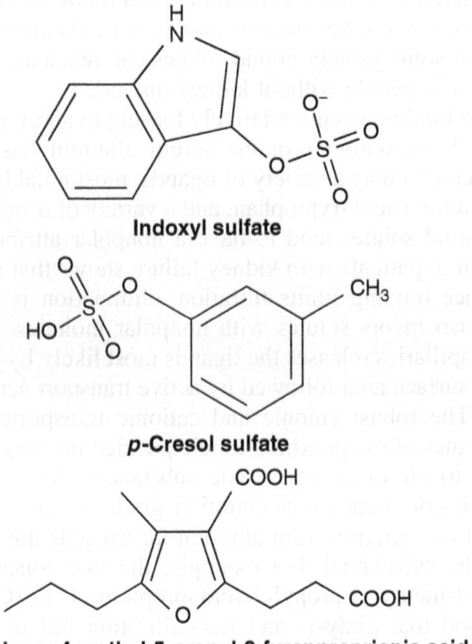

Indoxyl sulfate

p-Cresol sulfate

3-Carboxy-4-methyl-5-propyl-2-furanproprionic acid

Figure 18.8

Chemical structures of three well-studied protein-bound solutes. All are >90% bound to serum albumin and have demonstrated toxicity in vivo and in vitro.

effectively cleared by native kidneys even in ESRD patients whose kidneys function at low levels.

The chemical structures of well-established protein-bound solutes are shown in Fig. 18.8. These include indoles that derive mostly from degradation of tryptophan but also from degradation of phenylalanine and tyrosine by intestinal bacteria, particularly colonic *Escherichia coli*. Hemodialysis patients with a previous colectomy have much lower serum concentrations of indoles as well as hippurate, methylamine, and dimethylamine. The furanyl compound CMPF and its derivatives derive primarily from foodstuffs and accumulate to high levels in ESRD patients as shown in Table 18.3. CMPF is hydrophobic, poorly soluble in water, and binds strongly to serum albumin (>99%) in uremic serum. Both indoxyl sulfate and *para*-cresol sulfate are >90% bound to serum albumin, derive from colonic intestinal flora, accumulate in ESRD patients to high levels, and have demonstrated toxicity in vitro. Although elevated, concentrations are lower in serum from PD compared to HD patients possibly because of lower intestinal generation rates or losses of the albumin-bound fraction in the peritoneal dialysate.

As noted above, dialysis caregivers today encourage protein-energy intake to maintain nutrition, assuming that the toxic byproducts of protein intake are removed by dialysis, which also improves appetite. Outcome studies also show lower survival rates in patients with low protein intakes. However, in more recent times, restricting protein intake as well as use of prebiotics and probiotics has re-emerged as a method to reduce the availability of substrate for production of potential uremic toxins by intestinal microflora. High concentrations of *p*-cresyl sulfate and indoxyl sulfate, for example, as well as other retention solutes identified by HPLC in uremic serum have correlated positively with the patients' net protein catabolic rates and can be reduced by treatment with oral agents. By quantitatively reducing the generation of the most abundant bound solutes, the binding of other ligands, some of which may be very toxic, is shifted to the left, reducing their toxicity indirectly by enhancing their binding.

Sequestered Solutes

Sequestered solutes are usually small and easily dialyzed but their removal by dialysis is impeded by delayed diffusion within body compartments. All solutes exhibit this property, including urea, which has the least sequestration. During dialysis, concentrations of solutes other than urea fall more rapidly because the solute is extracted from a relatively small dialyzed compartment that equilibrates slowly with remote compartments. The dialyzed compartment in most cases is the extracellular or intravascular compartment, and the remote compartment is often the intracellular space. The behavior of sequestered solutes during hemodialysis has been used to explain the inefficiency of intermittent dialysis. Solute profiles coincide with those predicted by the peak concentration hypothesis (see Chapter 19, Urea Kinetic Modeling for Guiding Hemodialysis Therapy in Adults), which adds support for the concept of standard *Kt/V*, a measure of dialysis that attempts to express the dose as a continuous equivalent measurement. A familiar example of solute sequestration is seen in the kinetics of serum phosphorus during hemodialysis. Fig. 18.9 shows the rapid decline in phosphorus concentrations followed by a huge rebound lasting 4 hours immediately postdialysis. Other solutes show a similar larger rebound than urea but not as large as phosphorus. If the critical uremic toxins behaved like phosphorus, dialysis would not be successful, because adequate removal of phosphorus requires supplemental treatment with oral phosphate binders. Sequestration of otherwise easily dialyzed drugs like digoxin explains the inability of dialysis to reverse the toxicity of digoxin and similar sequestered compounds.

Markers of Uremic Toxicity: Role of Urea

Identifying a marker toxin has been the holy grail of investigators for more than a century. The required properties of a marker solute that can reliably denote the severity of uremic toxicity are listed in Table 18.4. To qualify, its accumulation must depend on native kidney function for elimination, and levels must correlate with other toxins and their toxicity. Because of the latter requirement, it is unlikely that concentrations of a single compound would apply at all times to all individuals. Because the concentration of retained solutes depends on both their generation and elimination, it would be necessary to monitor the levels of each toxin on a frequent basis to tailor the dialysis for control of each. The required frequency of measurement would depend on the toxin generation rate, which could vary from time to time and from patient to patient. Focus on just one toxin might leave some of the others at toxic levels if the generation rates differ. Today, lacking such a compound, clinicians rely on measurements of solute clearance.

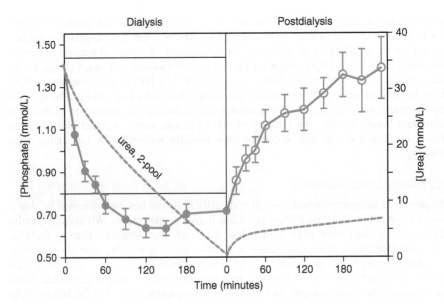

Figure 18.9

Serum phosphate levels during and following a 4-hour hemodialysis treatment. Urea concentrations predicted by a 2-pool model are shown for comparison. The horizontal lines represent the upper and lower boundaries for serum phosphate concentrations in normal people. (Adapted from DeSoi CA, Umans JG: Phosphate kinetics during high-flux hemodialysis. Fig. 1, J Am Soc Nephrol 4:1214-1218, 1993.)

Table 18.4

Properties of an Ideal Marker of Uremia

- Retained in renal failure
- Eliminated by dialysis
- Easily measured
- Proven dose-related toxicity
- Generation and elimination representative of other toxins

Urea satisfies the first three requirements but complies poorly with the last two. Because of the last requirement, probably no one single substance would qualify as ideal. Generation would likely differ in each patient and from time to time.
From Vanholder R, et al. Hippuric acid as a marker. In: Ringoir S, Vanholder R, Massry S, eds. *Uremic Toxins*, New York: Plenum Publishing Co.;1987.

Urea is a poor candidate for a marker of uremic toxicity, as it fails to meet all of the requirements listed in Table 18.4. In past experiments, when urea was added to the hemodialysate to prevent its removal, recovery from uremia still occurred. Normal kidneys apparently do not consider urea very toxic either, because they reclaim most of it by reabsorption along the tubule and use it as a medullary osmotic agent to assist with water conservation. Elasmobranchs, such as sharks, have also employed urea as an osmotic agent to combat the rising salinity of the oceans, often achieving concentrations in their blood over 1000 mg/dL, without apparently suffering any harmful toxicity.

Other easily dialyzed solutes such as creatinine or cystatin-c could be used to measure dialyzer clearance, but urea happens to be available in high concentrations and is easily measured by all clinical laboratories. Urea diffuses easily across dialyzer membranes and across the patients' cell membranes, so changes in serum concentrations during dialysis are sensitive indicators of the effect of dialysis on the patient (delivered clearance). Measurement of urea clearances using mathematical modeling programs also gives a measure of urea generation that can be directly translated to net protein catabolism, a measure of the patient's nutritional intake (see Chapter 19, Urea Kinetic Modeling for Guiding Hemodialysis Therapy in Adults).

Role of Salt and Water Accumulation

Fluid accumulation is not an essential feature of the uremic syndrome but frequently accompanies it. If urine output matches input, patients may progress to an advanced stage of uremia or even succumb to it without accumulating fluid. Conversely, restoration and maintenance of fluid balance are not enough to reverse uremia, so it must be considered as adjunctive therapy, albeit a vital one in most patients. Accumulation of fluid is increasingly recognized as a major component of the residual uremic syndrome, contributing to hypertension, peripheral and pulmonary edema, ventricular hypertrophy, and congestive heart failure.

Intermittent hemodialysis (e.g., thrice weekly), especially in anuric patients, usually obligates an abrupt reduction in extracellular volume that is unprecedented in nature and may itself cause harm to the patient as noted in Table 18.5. More frequent dialysis can reduce the fluctuations in ECV and dialysis-induced hypotension while preventing or reducing ventricular hypertrophy.

Adverse Effects of Dialysis

It is important to distinguish the residual syndrome from the potential adverse effects of dialysis listed in Table 18.5. For example, nephrologists have become increasingly aware of myocardial and cerebral ischemia caused by excessively rapid ultrafiltration during hemodialysis. The resulting myocardial and cerebral stunning can be exacerbated by warm dialysate and hemoconcentration because of overzealous treatment with erythropoiesis-stimulating agents. Dialysate warmed to 37°C can effectively warm the patient because the average core temperature of well dialyzed patients is approximately 0.5°C below the normal average, and ultrafiltration-induced vasoconstriction prevents heat loss. Medication side effects are especially important to anticipate and detect because, in the absence of native kidney function, higher levels are achieved that persist longer in the blood and tissues. Glucose added to peritoneal dialysate in high concentrations can lead to the formation of highly reactive degradation products (GDPs) that can modify proteins or DNA and potentially contribute to peritoneal sclerosis. Nonthermal methods of sterilization, use of icodextrin or amino acids in place of glucose, or proposed adsorption methods for removing GDPs offer hope for avoiding this cause of peritoneal sclerosis and other toxic effects of GDPs.

Table 18.5

Potential Adverse Effects of Dialysis

Inflammation/infection resulting from:
  Pyrogens and pathogens introduced by the dialysis equipment
  Membrane activation of WBCs, platelets, complement and inflammatory mediators
Allergic reactions to the dialyzer membrane
Myocardial and cerebral ischemia from:
  Volume depletion due to rapid fluid removal by ultrafiltration
  Vasodilation due to warming from heated dialysate
  Hemoconcentration due to:
    Ultrafiltration
    Overzealous treatment with erythropoiesis stimulating agents
Bleeding from anticoagulants given to prevent clotting in the dialyzer
Hemolysis from the action of blood roller pumps, kinking of blood tubing, interaction with
  dialysis membranes
Potential depletion of vital substances, e.g., hormones and amino acids
Toxicity and/or reactions to medications, e.g., aluminum phosphate binders, vitamin D,
  iron, antihypertensives
Formation of GDPs and AGEs from heat sterilization of glucose-containing peritoneal
  dialysate

Renal Toxicity From Uremic Toxins

There is increasing evidence for an adverse effect of retained indoxyl sulfate and
TMAO on the kidney itself. In theory, uremia-induced renal toxicity would generate
a vicious cycle of renal damage leading to more renal damage. In animal as well as
human studies, indoxyl sulfate accelerates the progression of CKD by stimulating
production of ROS in renal tubular and mesangial cells, and contributes to CVD by
a similar action in cardiomyocytes, vascular smooth muscle cells, and endothelial
cells. A proinflammatory effect of indoxyl sulfate as well as *p*-cresol sulfate and
TMAO has also been demonstrated as a possible mechanism for glomerular and
tubular damage. Although initial efforts met with success, a recent controlled clinical
trial designed to prevent this damage in humans with oral charcoal sorbents to reduce
the absorption of gut-derived toxins has failed to show a benefit.

Elimination of Uremic Toxins

How Much Removal?

The native kidney eliminates filtered foreign substances by simply ignoring them as
they flow through the renal tubules and are washed into the urine. The vital constituents of the plasma filtrate such as glucose and amino acids are recovered by active
reabsorption during transit through the renal tubule. Therapeutic dialysis attempts
to accomplish this feat by nonselective diffusion against a dialysate that contains the
vital blood components, a much less efficient but effective method that involves a
theoretical risk of depleting unidentified vital solutes. Amino acid losses are substantial but fortunately represent a small fraction of the usual daily intake generated
from dietary protein.

Several controlled clinical trials including the NIH HEMO Study and the more recent Frequent Hemodialysis Network trial suggest that increasing dialyzable solute clearance above currently established minimum levels confers little benefit to the patient. However, when kidney function is restored by transplantation, even well-dialyzed patients report significant improvements in well-being, despite the need for immunosuppression. Release from the burden of dialysis, the euphoric effect of glucocorticoids, and the restoration of a normal or near normal hemoglobin level may be more important to the sense of well-being than solute removal, especially in the past when higher doses of steroids were given and pretransplant anemia was more severe. It is difficult therefore to judge the significance of improved toxin removal. Other possible benefits provided by the transplanted organ include endocrine and paracrine secretions and continuous volume control, which avoids the dialysis-induced abrupt shifts in blood pressure and tissue perfusion noted above. Restoration of tubular secretion may also assist with removal of protein-bound toxins as discussed above.

Removal of Poorly Dialyzed Solutes

The success of dialysis in preventing death from uremia (usually within 5–7 days in anephric patients) gives testimony to the toxic effects of small easily dialyzed solutes. Other effects of dialysis such as fluid removal, endotoxin adsorption, and large molecule clearance cannot be given credit for this life-sustaining effect of dialysis, although they may add measurably to the long-term benefit. Table 18.6 shows a list of proposed methods for removing solutes that are less well-dialyzed than urea. Some small solutes such as phosphate dialyze easily but have limited access to the dialyzer because of sequestration in remote compartments (see Fig. 18.9). They can be removed effectively by prolonging the treatment or by increasing its frequency to allow for the slow transport into the blood compartment from remote locations in the body. Short infrequent treatments require supplemental methods, usually by intestinal adsorption, to remove phosphate and prevent long-term accumulation that may eventually be life threatening. The removal of protein-bound solutes can be augmented by increasing the dialyzer membrane surface area, analogous to the first (diffusional) step in their removal by native kidneys across the huge peritubular capillary surface. Other methods with demonstrated efficacy for removing protein-bound solutes include increasing the dialysate flow relative to blood flow

Table 18.6

Currently Proposed Methods to Improve the Clearance of Solutes Other Than Urea

Method	Target
Hemofiltration	Larger toxins
Larger, high flux membranes	Larger and bound toxins (membrane dependent)
Higher dialysate/blood flow rates	Bound toxins
More frequent dialysis	Sequestered toxins
More prolonged dialysis	Sequestered and bound toxins
Oral sorbents and probiotics	Indoles and other gut-produced toxins
Hemoperfusion using sorbents	Bound toxins

and adding a sorbent such as charcoal to the dialysate. Experimental methods include separation and extraction of or discarding plasma proteins as well as addition to the blood of nontoxic competitive inhibitors of binding. Removal of protein-bound solutes by dialysis is not affected by membrane pore size and is minimally affected by convective filtration.

Effect of Residual Kidney Function

The remnant kidney contributes measurably to removal of uremic toxins, perhaps more so than is apparent to the patient and clinician. The correlation of residual kidney urea clearance with patient survival as shown in Fig. 18.10 is difficult to ignore despite its observational nature. Even very low clearances, in the range of 0 to 3 mL/min appear to afford much longer survival, an observation that has prompted efforts to preserve renal function after initiating dialysis. For protein-bound toxins, the effect is magnified by the contribution of renal tubular secretion, a supplemental purging mechanism that could account for the survival advantage.

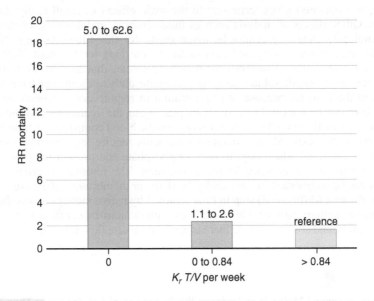

Figure 18.10

Effect of residual kidney function measured as urea clearance (K_rT/V) on the relative risk (RR) of mortality in hemodialysis patients during the Netherlands Cooperative Study on the Adequacy of Dialysis (NECOSAD) study. Data adjusted for age, primary kidney disease, comorbidity, subjective assessment of quality of life, and body mass index. (Adapted from Termorshuizen F, et al: Relative contribution of residual renal function and different measures of adequacy to survival in hemodialysis patients: an analysis of the Netherlands Cooperative Study on the Adequacy of Dialysis (NECOSAD)-2. J Am Soc Nephrol 15:1061-1070, 2004.)

Patient Variability

Patients may vary with regard to their accumulation of toxic compounds and need for dialysis. We know that variations in the diet can alter the need for phosphate binders, fluid removal, dialysate potassium concentrations, and influence acid–base balance, so there is reason to consider that accumulation of uremic toxins might vary in patients based on diet, body composition, genetics, physical activity, and perhaps other unknown factors. Population studies that report average results and recommendations based on average outcomes give the impression that everyone is the same with respect to the need for dialysis and other treatments for ESRD. Clinicians should be alert to the possibility of outliers and give more dialysis to patients exhibiting symptoms and signs of uremia. The well-recognized need for more dialysis during pregnancy supports this notion of patient variability.

Summary and Future Directions

Therapeutic dialysis as currently practiced can quickly reverse uremic encephalopathy and eventually eliminate many aspects of the uremic syndrome including the neuropathy, anorexia, malnutrition, etc., restoring life, sometimes with near normal functionality. The remarkable reversibility of the uremic state demonstrated by dialysis helps us to understand uremia in a way that differs from our predecessors who might have considered such near-death patients as suffering from an irreversible illness. It is likely that those witnessing the first reversals of uremic toxicity would have considered the treatment near miraculous.

Failure of higher doses and more frequent dialysis to improve morbidity and mortality should cause one to pause and consider that accumulation of dialyzable toxins is not the cause of the rampant cardiovascular disease and inflammatory states that contribute to the demise of patients with ESRD. This doubt is further extended by the failure of treatments that remove larger molecular species. Clinicians are left in an unsatisfactory and puzzling quandary in their attempts to explain and ultimately prevent the problems experienced by patients dependent on dialysis, and that thousands of caregivers wrestle with daily. One thing we can be certain of: The solution is not obvious.

For the future, the importance of seeking out and positively identifying each retention solute cannot be overemphasized. Efforts to individualize patient care may require repeated profiling of retention products in each patient using metabolomics or other methods to measure multiple solutes simultaneously. The scatter seen in the concentrations of retained solutes suggests that each patient is different with respect to generation and accumulation of different solutes, some of which are likely more toxic than others. Future therapeutic methods could allow targeting each toxic solute by modifying the dialysis prescription as well as the patient's diet and/or seeking to alter the patient's microbiome. Now that we have the means to keep such patients alive and functioning, it remains for future clinicians and investigators to further improve the patients' quality of life by identifying and treating those aspects of uremic toxicity that are not completely reversed by dialysis.

CHAPTER 19

Urea Kinetic Modeling for Guiding Hemodialysis Therapy in Adults

Frank A. Gotch, MD

This chapter addresses the use of urea kinetic modeling (UKM) in prescribing and monitoring the adequacy of dialysis. Optimal use of UKM requires the use of a computer urea kinetic modeling program because the mathematical routines are too complex for realistic manual or calculator solutions. The purposes of this chapter are to describe UKM, define the role it has had in determining adequacy of dialysis, and indicate some reliable approximation equations for UKM.

Blood Urea Concentration, Normalized Protein Catabolic Rate, and Fractional Clearance

There are only two randomized studies of dialysis dose, and both were guided with UKM (which remains the only generalized dialysis dosing model validated for correlating dose of dialysis with clinical outcome). Although urea is the modeled solute, it has been shown using UKM that uremic toxicity is not directly proportional to blood urea nitrogen (BUN) concentration. However, it has also been shown that the level of uremic toxicity is strongly related to the fractional clearance of urea (dialyzer urea clearance [K] times treatment time [t] divided by urea distribution volume [V], or Kt/V—which can be used to quantify the dose of dialysis and ensure that it is adequate. These relationships, which were discovered with the National Cooperative Dialysis Study (NCDS), are not intuitively obvious and were not well understood for several years after they were reported.

NCDS Domains of Adequate and Inadequate Dialysis Doses

The NCDS was a National Institutes of Health (NIH)–sponsored multicenter study of outcomes with randomized doses of dialysis. Its results were plotted on BUN and normalized protein catabolic rate (NPCR) axes, as shown in Fig. 19.1A. The urea model was used to prescribe and monitor therapy in the NCDS, which had four treatment arms: groups I and III had low BUN, with long treatment time (t) in I and short t in III; groups II and IV had high BUN, with long t in II and short t in IV. There was not a significant effect of t on outcome, but as seen in Fig. 19.1A the therapy failure rate (incidence of clinical uremic complications) was 52% in groups II and IV and 13% in groups I and III. However, there was an unanticipated fifth outcome (group V, shown in Fig. 19.1A).

The group V patients all had a low NPCR (g/kg/day) of 0.60–0.80 g/kg/day. In this group, there was a very high incidence of failure (75%)—irrespective of the

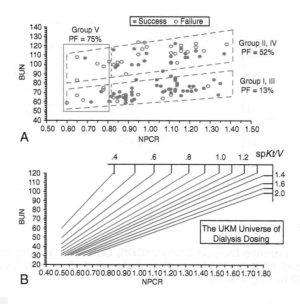

Figure 19.1

(A) Results of National Cooperative Dialysis Study (NCDS). (B) Solution of Urea Model.

BUN. These dichotomous results with respect to BUN were very puzzling. They seemed to imply that with normal protein intake, uremic symptoms resulted from underdialysis, whereas the same uremic symptoms were unresponsive to dialysis (expressed only as BUN) with low protein intake. Fig. 19.1B shows a generalized solution of the urea model for BUN as a function of NPCR at constant levels of dose expressed as single-pool Kt/V (spKt/V) ranging from 0.4 to 2.0. When Kt/V is constant, BUN increases linearly with the urea generation rate (its analog, NPCR)— as plotted in Fig. 19.1B. This plot might be considered the "UKM universe of dialysis dosing."

Fig. 19.2 depicts superimposition of the urea model solutions (Fig. 19.1B) on a map of clinical outcome groups (Fig. 19.1A). It is readily apparent in Fig. 19.2 that all groups with high failure rates (II, IV, and V) have spKt/V <.8, whereas group I and III patients with low failure rate are all distributed over the spKt/V range of 0.80–1.45. Thus, the mechanism common to all of the high-failure groups was a low dose of small solute clearance expressed as the fractional urea clearance (Kt/V). Note that the level of BUN is virtually irrelevant to the definition of an adequate dose because a BUN of 75 can represent low NPCR and very low spKt/V or can represent high NPCR and high spKt/V. The results shown in Fig. 19.2 indicate that uremic symptoms are not proportional to urea concentration, that the generation rate of uremic toxins is not proportional to Gu (group V patients had very low NPCR), and that urea serves only as a generic solute for modeling the fractional clearance of low-molecular-weight (LMW) toxins.

The NCDS outcome data in Fig. 19.2 are further explored in Fig. 19.3. In Fig. 19.3A, the domains of inadequate and adequate dialysis defined by that study are

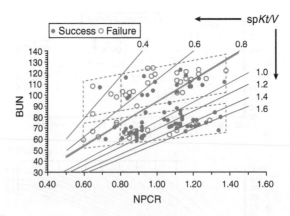

Figure 19.2

National Cooperative Dialysis Study (NCDS) Outcome Results With Superimposed *Kt/V* Grid Indicate That Outcome Failure Was Virtually Eliminated When *Kt/V* > .80.

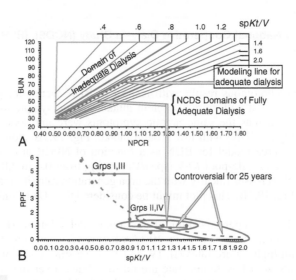

Figure 19.3

Two Views of Outcome in the National Cooperative Dialysis Study (NCDS).

depicted on the UKM Dialysis Dosing plot. In Fig. 19.3B, the NCDS data are shown as relative risk of failure in all patients stratified as a function of mean sp*Kt/V* achieved. Note that RPF was uniformly high in groups II and IV patients and uniformly low in group I and III patients. A step function was fitted to the data. This function defines the domains in Fig. 19.3A, reflecting the randomization of doses in the study (groups II and IV vs groups I and III).

The step function was used to construct the modeling line for adequate dialysis in Fig. 19.3, but both the step function and an exponential relationship were reported in the NCDS analysis. Over the subsequent 25 years, these two interpretations of the data were hotly contested. The step function indicated that no outcome benefit would occur with spKt/V >1.00, whereas the exponential relationship suggested that an outcome benefit would continuously occur with spKt/V doses as high as 2.00.

The HEMO Study

Because of ongoing controversy and uncertainty about the adequate dialysis dose, the NIH organized a second randomized trial of hemodialysis (HD; HEMO) beginning in 1994. The initial design in the pilot study called for a standard dose arm targeted for spKt/V 1.10–1.20 (which would overlap the middle of the high-dose arm in NCDS) and for a high-dose arm with spKt/V >1.45. However, a number of observational studies suggested that the minimal adequate dose of dialysis should be an spKt/V >1.40. Thus, when the HEMO study started, the design was changed to targeted doses to 1.40 and 1.75 in the two arms.

These relationships are shown in Fig. 19.4, where it can be seen that the final design of HEMO addressed only the very high-dose part of the NCDS controversy (spKt/V 1.4–1.8) but did not address the controversy about adequacy of spKt/V over the range 1.0–1.4. HEMO did clearly show that there was no improvement in outcome between spKt/V 1.4 and 1.85 but shed no light on the outcome with spKt/V 1.1–1.4.

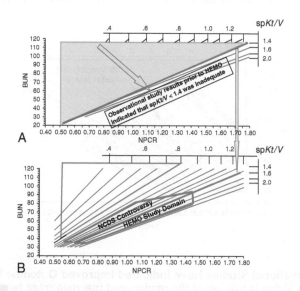

Figure 19.4

The Effect of Observational Study Results on Design of the HEMO Study.

Observational and Randomized Studies

Fig. 19.5 depicts the results of observational studies based on analyses of USRDS and CMS (Centers of Medicare and Medicaid Services) data, showing that relative risk of mortality (RRM) continues to fall as spKt/V increases to 2.00 (which must be interpreted to indicate that spKt/V less than 2.00 is inadequate therapy). It is quite remarkable, as illustrated in Fig. 19.5, that the observational studies indicate that all of the doses studied in both randomized trials (NCDS and HEMO) are inadequate. How can these profoundly different dose responses be reconciled?

The most likely explanation is shown in Fig. 19.6B, where the two arms of HEMO are shown individually stratified by quintiles of spKt/V and associated RRM normalized to the highest dose in each arm. This was originally done in the standard arm because of safety committee concern about patients who might not be reaching the target spKt/V of 1.4, judged to be the minimal adequate dose by observational data. The results for the standard arm in Fig. 19.6B were very alarming and jeopardized continuation of the study because the data strongly suggested that the lower doses in this arm were inadequate. However, the same analysis was done on the high-dose arm and (as also depicted in Fig. 19.6B) the identical relationship was observed over a range of doses that were clearly adequate.

The relationships in Fig. 19.6B provide striking examples of dose targeting bias resulting from unrecognized risk factors interfering with achievement of the targeted doses in nonrandomized observational studies. These factors cannot be interpreted as dose responses. Note that the higher the dose range studied the higher the apparently adequate dose becomes. The dose response becomes a self-fulfilling prophecy that seriously compromises the validity of dose-targeted observational studies. The outcomes in both arms of HEMO were equal, which is also shown in Fig. 19.6B (with RRM 1.0). So what can be concluded regarding the adequate dose of dialysis? There is clearly no benefit gained with spKt/V >1.4, and it remains unknown whether

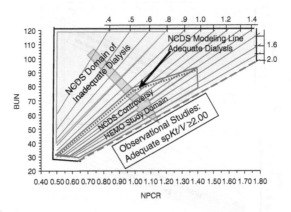

Figure 19.5

Recent Observational Studies Have Indicated Improved Outcome With spKt/V = 2.00. If this is true, all of the randomized trial data must be construed to be inadequate dialysis. Is there any way to reconcile these highly contradictory conclusions about an adequate dialysis dose?

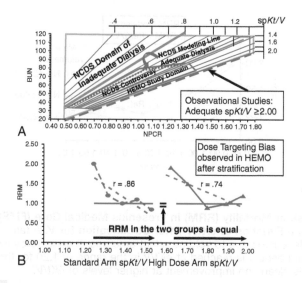

Figure 19.6

Reconciliation of Observational Studies With Randomized Trials.

an spKt/V of 1.4 is better than spKt/V = 1.0 because of compromise of the original HEMO study design (as discussed previously).

Volume as an Independent Predictor of Outcome

It has recently been reported that V per se is inversely correlated with RRM in dialysis patients, which adds complexity to analysis of the clinical outcome response to Kt/V. It is unknown why large patients with larger V have lower RRM, but in view of this relationship it is essential to stratify outcome data over a range of constant levels of V when examining RRM as a function of Kt/V (because both Kt/V and V may independently influence outcome).

Cross-sectional observational analyses have suggested that Kt is a better parameter of dosage, but analyses with V held constant have shown the interacting effects of V and Kt/V on RRM (Fig. 19.7). The curves in Fig. 19.7, where RRM is shown as a function of eKt/V over three tertiles of constant volume, show the strong inverse relationship of RRM to V but also indicate no improvement by increasing Kt/V in any of the groups. Similar relationships were found in the HEMO study. This puzzling relationship requires further research. At present there is no evidence that smaller patients require larger doses of dialysis expressed as Kt/V.

Role of UKM in Dialysis Therapy

A computer modeling program is required for full clinical use of UKM. There are simplified equations now available (Daugirdas 1993 and Tattersall 1996) that are quite reliable for calculation of Kt/V. The approximation equations of Tattersall provide highly reliable estimates of double-pool effects on the single-pool V

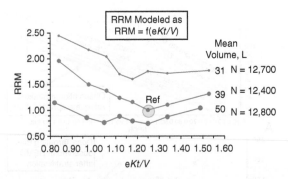

Figure 19.7

Relative Risk of Mortality (RRM) in Fresenius Medical Care (FMS) Data Modeled as a Function of e*Kt/V* After Stratification for *V*. A family of nearly parallel curves due to volume effect emerges. It appears by inspection that maximum benefit is reached at e*Kt/V* in the range of 1.20 for three strata of *V*. There is clearly no improvement at higher levels of e*Kt/V*.

calculation and are often combined with computer-based UKM analyses. In view of these considerations, it is important to ask what need there is for UKM in clinical dialysis.

There are four major advantages that accrue with the use of UKM. First, the delivered dose of dialysis is more reliably measured with UKM than with the approximation equations (i.e., a higher level of quality assurance is achieved). With UKM, the kinetic equations are solved to calculate V—and any errors in delivery of the dose (recirculation, flow, or time errors) are clearly manifest in errors observed in the calculated V (which should be relatively constant over time). Thus, a high spKt/V may be calculated with an approximation equation in the case of recirculation and faulty sampling technique (not uncommon). However, UKM would show a very small V and clearly indicate technical error.

A second advantage of UKM is that an accurate estimate of PCR (protein catabolic rate, g/day) is calculated, which is equal to dietary protein intake in relatively stable patients. The PCR is a very useful quantity for the renal dietitian, providing her or him with a reliable measure of actual protein intake and month-to-month variability in intake.

It is useful to plot the monthly BUN, NPCR, and Kt/V points on a graph (Fig. 19.1B) for each patient. Inspection of the graph over time with the patient can be a valuable educational tool. In patients on protein supplements, the PCR provides a method of evaluating the effect on nitrogen balance. If a plot such as that shown in Fig. 19.1B has been used, when protein supplements are seen to simply increase the NPCR and BUN proportional with the amount of supplement, probably little has been achieved.

UKM provides for calculation of individualized dialysis prescriptions, which is not possible using approximation equations. An individualized dialysis prescription requires a kinetically determined mean urea distribution volume for the patient (and solution of the dialyzer transport equations over a range of blood and dialysate flows and treatment times) in order to select the best combination of dialyzer, blood, and dialysate flows and treatment time for the patient. UKM computer programs permit archiving of treatment data and as such are also very useful for managing the therapy database for a patient population. Thus, the distributions of spKt/Vs, eKt/Vs, and NPCRs and comparison of delivered versus prescribed Kt/V are valuable analyses readily available with the archived data in UKM programs.

Role of UKM in More Frequent and/or Continuous Hemodialysis Therapy and With Residual Renal Function

There is a strong resurgence of interest in more frequent chronic hemodialysis, including short daytime and long overnight hemodialysis six times per week. In acute renal failure, the spectrum of therapy ranges from continuous to variable-frequency intermittent hemodialysis. There is also interest in starting dialysis at higher levels of residual renal function, and it has been recommended by NKF-K/DOQI that in such cases the combination of continuous ambulatory peritoneal dialysis (CAPD) or intermittent dialysis with continuous renal function be quantified with UKM. The most rational approach to these relationships is transformation of intermittent clearance to an equivalent level of continuous clearance. In the steady state with continuous clearance, the relationships among concentration of urea (C), clearance (K), and generation rate (Gu) are given by

$$G = K(C).$$
$$\text{(19.1)}$$

Solution of Eq. 19.1 for K gives

$$K = G/C.$$
$$\text{(19.2)}$$

Eq. 19.2 can be used to calculate a value for continuous clearance from G and a specified concentration point (C) on the concentration profile resulting with any therapy schedule. The mean predialysis BUN has been used to define an equivalent standard K (std$K$) and stdKt/V. The stdKt/V is the only model shown to predict identical adequate doses of both continuous CAPD and thrice-weekly HD (as shown in Fig. 19.8, where a generalized solution for weekly stdKt/V as a function of eKt/V delivered each dialysis and the number of dialyses per week are shown). Note the continuous clearance line, which is simply 7 times the values for eKt/V on the abscissa (i.e., each eKt/V is given continuously every day).

The two points on the plot show that a weekly Kt/V for CAPD of 2.0 corresponds well with the stdKt/V of 2.0, which is calculated for thrice-weekly dialysis with eKt/V 1.05 each treatment. The uniform flattening of each of the curves in Fig. 19.8 as eKt/V increases is due to the decreasing efficiency of solute removal in each individual dialysis as the fractional clearance of body water increases and solute concentration falls to very low levels.

It might be predicted from the shape of the curves in Fig. 19.6 that clinical benefits would increase minimally as eKt/V increases beyond 1.05—because of decreasing dialysis efficiency and minimal increase in stdKt/V in this range. The converse is also true. The curves in Fig. 19.6 suggest that increasing frequency of dialysis may result in substantial increase in clinical benefit because of the increase in stdKt/V, which can be raised to a new unexplored domain with 6-times-weekly dialysis.

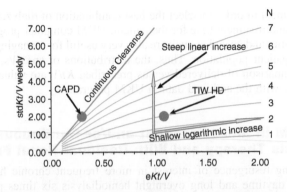

Figure 19.8

Results of Solution of std*Kt/V* Model Over Wide Ranges of e*Kt/V* and *N*.
Note that by inspection std*Kt/V* appears to increase linearly as *N* increases,
and logarithmically with e*Kt/V*. The dose of adequate continuous ambulatory
peritoneal dialysis (CAPD) and thrice-weekly hemodialysis (HD) are the same
with this model (weekly std*Kt/V* 2).

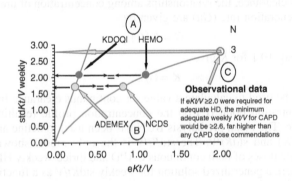

Figure 19.9

**Comparison of std*Kt/V* for Continuous Ambulatory Peritoneal Dialysis
(CAPD) and Three Sets of Hemodialysis (HD) Data.** The Ademex study
defined adequate std*Kt/V* = 1.7, which agrees well with the National
Cooperative Dialysis Study (NCDS) recommendation for adequate HD.
NKF-K/DOQI is based on the HEMO recommendation for sp*Kt/V* 1.4, which
results in std*Kt/V* values for both HD and CAPD of about 2.1. The
observational studies recommend e*Kt/V* 2.0, which would equate with std*Kt/V*
2.6 (far higher than recommended for CAPD).

Dosing Recommendations for Adequate HD per CAPD Dosing

Three sets of data are illustrated in Fig. 19.9. Set A depicts the recommendations
from HEMO for HD and from NKF K/DOQI for CAPD. These are highly consistent
and recommend an adequate std*Kt/V* = 2.1 for both therapy modalities. Set B shows

the recommendations of the ADEMEX study for CAPD and of the NCDS for HD. Note that these two studies are also highly consistent (recommending stdKt/V = 1.75 for both CAPD and HD). Data set C shows the recommended eKt/V = 2.0 for HD from observational studies. This would require a weekly stdKt/V of ≥2.6 for CAPD, which is far higher than any clinical recommendations.

So what can we conclude about dosing in CAPD and a thrice-weekly HD? It would seem clear that the observational studies give false levels of required stdKt/V. The reason for this appears to be dose targeting bias. The ADEMEX findings fit with the NCDS data very well, and both may provide fully adequate doses of dialysis. Because there are some uncertainties in all of these data sets, it would seem safest to use the average of NKF-K/DOQI and ADEMEX and the average of NCDS and HEMO to model the adequate dose for stdKt/V at about 1.9 and for eKt/V at about 1.05.

CHAPTER 20

The Dialysis Prescription

Steven Brunelli, MD, MSCE

Perhaps the most fundamental prescriptive question is how much dialysis is enough. On the surface, this question is seemingly simple. At essence, however, this question proves overly simplistic and its answer elusive and influenced by a myriad of considerations. The deceptive simplicity of the question stems from the bounded nature of the function. On the low end, zero dialysis is clearly insufficient and patients rapidly succumb to kidney failure. On the high end, there exist a finite number of hours per week during which patients can possibly be dialyzed. However, lurking just beneath this veneer is a series of much harder corollaries. (1) What are the direct objectives of dialysis? (2) How does one incorporate patient preferences? (3) Is there a threshold of "enough" or are relationships continuous? and (4) How are these answers impacted by temporal changes in sentiment and available technologies?

Question 1 is philosophical in nature. It is unclear that a consensus answer exists among stakeholders. It too is simplistic in that it does not account for the potential need to tradeoff among objectives (e.g., maximizing survival versus creating the least burden on quality of life). Question 2 extends uncertainty further in that generally accepted precepts at the population level likely do not pertain to an individual patient and certainly do not pertain to all individual patients. Often biologic systems behave on a threshold basis, and that function is un- or minimally impacted provided this threshold is met. However, question 3 reminds us that threshold effects are not universal in biology and may not pertain at all when one considers the intersection of biologic and technological systems; there may in fact not be an "enough" but rather an "enough is enough." Finally, question 4 reminds us that whatever the correct answer is—assuming there is a correct answer at a particular time in a particular context—may evolve and change over time.

Perhaps because these issues are so complex and interdependent research and practice in dialysis have found the need to invoke simplifying paradigms and to ask more directive, research-ready questions with empiric answers. In this chapter, we will explore how this line of reasoning has evolved, what it implies for contemporary practice, and how it may change in the future. However, be reminded that even this—the best available line of empiric data and data-driven practice—is by nature a shadow on the wall of Plato's cave and the reader is encouraged to harken back to earlier, more fundamental questions that may not have objective answers but nonetheless point to truth.

Philosophy of Dialysis Adequacy

Science is quantitative and clinical medicine at least semiquantitative. Therefore, in determining how much dialysis is enough, one must define the means by which dialysis can be quantified. The National Cooperative Dialysis Study was the first rigorous attempt to do so. The trial was begun in the mid-1970s at a time when dialysis had recently become "universally" available in the United States and where recent technological advances had made possible more efficient delivery of dialysis. At this time, there was no systematic tracking of patient survival (the abysmal survival rates among dialysis patients would not be fully recognized until the late 1980s) but providers recognized that many patients continued to feel uremic despite treatment adherence. In this setting, the obvious question was: How does one provide dialysis to patients in order that they not be uremic—the latter operationally defined based on terminal withdrawal from dialysis or hospitalization events. Investigators considered two metrics of dialysis dose: time-average blood urea concentration (50 vs 100 mg/dL) and time on dialysis (2.5–3.5 vs 4.5–5 hours) and randomized patients accordingly using a 2 × 2 factorial design. The former metric was meant as an index of small-molecular-weight toxemia and the latter as a proxy for a host of other factors. Upon trial termination, time-average blood urea was clearly associated with patient outcomes whereas time on dialysis did not bear statistical significance. With the benefit of hindsight, one may question whether a p value of .056 in the context of a trial that was stopped early and never met target enrollment was truly indicative of "no association." Nevertheless, it was clear that lower time-average blood urea nitrogen clearly led to preferable outcomes. In addition, a urea-based metric benefited from other obvious advantages: (1) it corresponded to a decade-long legacy of basic uremia research that had used urea as a marker, (2) it was readily measurable, and (3) a single unified measure of dialysis adequacy was more readily implementable than one that considered multiple domains (i.e., urea *and* treatment time). On this basis, small-molecular-weight solutes in general and urea in particular became the currency by which dialysis adequacy came to be measured, a legacy that persists through the present day.

Kt/V

Leveraging data from the National Cooperative Dialysis Study, Gotch and Sargent introduced the concept of *Kt/V* in 1985. *Kt/V* is the mathematical relationship between the rate of urea removal (K) times treatment duration (t) divided by the volume of distribution for urea (V). *Kt/V* was at essence part of the emerging urea-centric tradition but broke from the existing paradigm in two key respects. The first distinction was that *Kt/V* attempted to balance urea removal (the numerator, $K*t$) to physiologic need (the denominator, V). The second distinction is subtle but nonetheless important: It changed the paradigm by which urea was considered from how much is there in the body to how much is removed during dialysis. In typical mid-1980s circumstances, this distinction would have been academic: Technologies were reasonably homogeneous, and nearly all hemodialysis patients were dialyzed according to a thrice-weekly hemodialysis schedule. However, as we shall see later, interim changes in dialyzer efficiency and greater use of quotidian hemodialysis regimens have necessitated subsequent adaptations.

To be technically precise, Gotch and Sargent's original concept of *Kt/V* has subsequently been dubbed single-pool *Kt/V* (sp*Kt/V*). This name derives from the conceptual kinetic model through which the equations were derived, which are largely analogous to first-order elimination kinetics. Within the original paper, and more so subsequently in later papers, there are a number of mathematic equations by which spKt/V can be calculated. Perhaps the most popular of these is the Daugirdas formula, which states,

$$\text{sp}Kt/V = -\log(R - 0.03) + [(4 - (3.5 * R)) \times (\text{ultrafiltration volume/body weight})]$$

where R is the ratio of postdialysis to predialysis blood urea nitrogen.

The use of closed-form equations to calculate Kt/V has largely been supplanted by iterative computer algorithms—the most popular of which is termed *urea kinetic modeling*—the Daugirdas equation is nonetheless revealing as to the constituent components of spKt/V. The first term in the equation (quantitatively the most important) describes the amount of urea that is removed from the start to the end of a dialysis treatment; this is an alternative mathematical formulation of the urea reduction ratio, which will be discussed in the next section.

The second term in the equation corrects for urea generation during the dialysis treatment itself. To understand this term, consider that the typical thrice-weekly in-center hemodialysis patient spends approximately 7% of the time (12 of 168 hours) on dialysis; therefore one would anticipate that at least 7% of urea is generated during dialysis itself (perhaps more if one considers the catabolic nature of hemodialysis). The effect of this is that the change in body urea content will underestimate the amount of urea being removed, an effect for which this term attempts to compensate.

The third term in the equation accounts for urea that is removed convectively through ultrafiltration. Because urea is freely permeable across the dialysis membrane, it exists in essentially equal concentration in the blood as in ultrafiltrate. Therefore, although urea is removed in the process of ultrafiltration, this is not otherwise reflected in blood urea concentration.

The latter two terms are necessary because the prevailing paradigm is to measure urea removal on the patient-side (i.e., by changes in blood chemistry) rather than on the drain-side (i.e., by analysis of spent dialysate). (This is the only practicable solution: It is far easier to collect and analyze 14 mL of blood than 100+ L of spent dialysate.) However, as a thought experiment, consider a counterfactual circumstance where urea removal was assessed drain-side: In this circumstance, no correction would be needed for urea generation or for convective clearance. Both terms are similar in that they upwardly adjust spKt/V for factors not reflected directly in blood urea concentration change.

Urea Reduction Ratio

Urea reduction ratio (URR) is a measure of the proportionate reduction in blood urea nitrogen over the course of dialysis. It is calculated as:

$$\text{URR} = 100\% \times (\text{predialysis BUN} - \text{postdialysis BUN})/\text{predialysis BUN}$$

It is an alternative expression of the R term in the Daugirdas equation for spKt/V. For example, if a patient started dialysis with a BUN of 100 mg/dL and finished dialysis with a BUN of 30 mg/dL, R would equal 0.3 and URR would equal 70%. As thereby implied, there is an inherent mathematic correlation between URR and spKt/V. Discrepancies between URR and spKt/V derive from three primary sources: (1) URR is not directly indexed to body size, (2) URR does not directly account for urea generation during dialysis, (3) URR does not account directly for convective urea losses. Nonetheless, the two are largely considered interchangeable, and both are endorsed by guideline committees as valid markers of dialysis adequacy.

Thresholds for sp*Kt/V* and URR

In the initial description of sp*Kt/V* by Sargent and Gotch, they considered a cutoff sp*Kt/V* of 0.9 as that which best distinguished between treatment failure and success. Recall that success and failure were defined in that study as hospitalization or terminal withdrawal from dialysis.

Beginning in the early 1990s, there was a proliferation of observational studies that looked at the association between achieved urea removal and mortality. Survival was incrementally improved at higher URR up to 65% and at higher sp*Kt/V* up to 1.2. Ultimately, guidelines were issued that espouse sp*Kt/V* of 1.4 and/or URR of 70% (buffers added to guard against inadvertent "missed") as indicative of minimally adequate dialysis.

At the time these initial studies were conducted, comparatively few patients had sp*Kt/V* much greater than 1.4 or URR much greater than 70%. Therefore, these studies could not assess with precision whether upstream URR or sp*Kt/V* may have led to even greater survival advantage. In parallel, technological changes to dialyzers greatly improved the efficiency of urea removal. By the mid-1990s, it had become tenable to achieve greater urea removal in the context of thrice weekly in center hemodialysis than had previously been the case. The HEMO Study was launched to explore whether targeting higher *Kt/V* led to incrementally better survival. Patients were randomized to higher versus lower *Kt/V*; technically, *Kt/V* was defined based on equilibrated *Kt/V* (which will be discussed below) but was functionally equivalent to sp*Kt/V* of 1.25 versus 1.65. (Also, the HEMO Study randomized according to high-versus low-flux dialyzers in a factorial design, but that is beyond the scope of this chapter.) The HEMO Study found no survival benefit for higher versus lower *Kt/V* target, which served to reinforce existing *Kt/V* targets.

Equilibrated *Kt/V*

Use of urea as the currency for small-molecular-weight dialytic clearance is based on the notion that urea is freely permeable across membranes. Urea is small (molecular weight 60 Da) and uncharged, which are ideal characteristics for promoting passive diffusion across lipid bilayers. When one considers the local environment only, indeed urea is rapidly transferred across cellular membranes ($K_{flux} = 1 \times 10^{-7}$ mmol/cm^2/s [6,411,854]) and similarly across dialyzer membranes.

However, in in vivo systems, the picture is more complex. Individual vascular beds are differentially perfused. Urea present in less perfused tissues has less access to the central circulation and thereby is less available for dialytic removal. Moreover, there are vascular beds for which perfusion decreases during dialysis (in response to circulatory stimuli and the neuroendocrine milieu). Together, these regions form a reservoir for urea and other otherwise-freely transferrable solutes. In other words, small molecule clearance from these regions is kinetically limited.

sp*Kt/V*, and typically URR as well, is calculated based on urea concentrations measured at the end of the dialysis treatment. These levels reflect well the behavior of urea in the blood at other highly perfused tissues; however, they do not reflect the behavior of urea in more inaccessible tissues. Thereby, spKt/V and URR tend to overestimate total body urea clearance.

In fact, if one serially samples blood urea after the end of dialysis, one observes a "rebound" in blood urea levels that represents the reequilibration of urea across body fluids. Equilibrated Kt/V (eKt/V) is a metric used to account for the overestimation inherent to spKt/V and is derived by sampling postdialysis blood 30 minutes following dialysis as opposed to immediately at the end of treatment.

eKt/V may be a superior measure of total body clearance of low-molecular-weight solutes. However, there is no empiric evidence to suggest that outcomes are superior when eKt/V—as opposed to spKt/V—is used to gauge dialysis adequacy. Moreover, there are logistical barriers to sampling blood 30 minutes after dialysis, including considerations of shift turnover and patient travel. Perhaps for these reasons, eKt/V has not seen widespread clinical adoption in the United States. Current guidelines do not provide a benchmark level for eKt/V. However, for adherents, it may be possible to convert spKt/V thresholds to eKt/V: eKt/V is typically between 0.15 and 0.25 lower than spKt/V.

Middle Molecule Clearance

Up to this point, we have considered dialysis adequacy only in terms of low-molecular-weight solute clearance, or more accurately, solutes whose kinetic behavior mimics that of urea. In contrast, "middle molecules" are a group of compounds that are biologically relevant but that are removed less efficiently by dialysis. The name *middle molecules* harkens to the molecular weight of many such compounds that are middling in nature: falling between that of urea and other compounds readily cleared across dialytic membranes and that of proteins and glycoproteins that are typically too large to dialyze off. However, middle molecules also encompass low-molecular-weight compounds that are inefficiently removed during dialysis either due to polyvalence (which limits dialytic membrane flux), protein binding, or intracellular sequestration.

The effects of certain middle molecules such as phosphate and β_2-microglobulin have been extensively studied. For these, it is clear that accumulation is pathogenic. Emerging evidence suggests that metabolic byproducts such as *p*-cresol sulfate, indoxyl sulfate, methylamine, and dimethylamine may be relevant uremic solutes, but these have received comparatively less study. It is clear, however, that despite nearly four decades of research, there is no comprehensive litany of middle molecules. Nor is it certain—and, in reality, it is unlikely—that all middle molecules will behave similarly to one another with respect to dialytic removal. At present, there is no reliable means by which to consider middle molecules into the calculus of dialysis adequacy. Additional research in this area is sorely needed.

Fluid Removal

All too often, canonical dialysis "adequacy" (meaning low molecular weight clearance) and fluid removal are considered in parallel. Textbooks draw the distinction between solute clearance, which is predominantly diffusive in nature, and fluid removal which is convective. Trainees are typically taught that treatment time is determined by Kt/V considerations and fluid status by specification of target weight.

In a bygone era, this simplistic heuristic was seemingly reasonable. Solute clearance was very inefficient by today's standards, which afforded plenty of time for fluid removal. (In practice, fluid removal did not always go so smoothly, but this was more a consequence of inaccuracies in monitoring ultrafiltration volumes more so than due to implied time constraints.) Over decades, dialyzer technologies have evolved markedly. As a result, urea removal goals could be achieved increasingly more rapidly. This is evidenced by the trend in mean dialysis treatment times in the United States, which fell from 6 hours or more in the early 1970s to 3 hours by the late 1980s.

Greater dialyzer efficiency coupled with a urea-centric paradigm for determining treatment times implies the need for more rapid ultrafiltration during dialysis. Greater ultrafiltration rate portends both labile blood pressure during dialysis and frank intradialytic hypotension, which, in turn, are associated with transient interruptions in end organ perfusion. Until recently, it was believed that such phenomena were clinically relevant only inasmuch as they triggered overt clinical events or patient symptoms. However, converging lines of research indicate that the accumulation of subtle insults from subclinical events is of importance. For example, recent work demonstrates that low blood pressure during dialysis (e.g., <90 mm Hg; <100 mm Hg) is associated with increased risk of all-cause and cardiovascular mortality, and, in fact, this relationship is not potentiated when only symptomatic episodes are considered. Additional data demonstrate that transient interruptions in perfusion, often asymptomatic in nature, contribute substantively to transient myocardial stunning and white matter damage, which in turn are associated with cardiovascular events and neurocognitive deficits, respectively.

Viewed in this light, it is not surprising that more rapid ultrafiltration is associated with a greater risk of mortality, particular cardiovascular mortality. In theory, such observations could be confounded because greater interdialytic weight gain both implies more rapid ultrafiltration and independently associates with poor prognosis. However, matched-pair analysis indicates that even if patients are exactly matched on interdialytic weight gain (and body weight), those with the higher ultrafiltration rate (i.e., those with lower treatment time) have a higher adjusted risk of death.

Importantly, ultrafiltration rate is defined above in terms of volume removed per unit time per kilogram of body weight. Associations between absolute ultrafiltration rate, defined as volume removed per unit time—not indexed to body weight—is less clearly associated with clinical outcomes (unpublished observation). In essence then, the relevant parameter is related to how rapidly fluid is being removed relative to total body water (perhaps more accurately to extracellular volume although dedicated studies in this regard have not been conducted). This construct fits well into the framework of interruption of end-organ perfusion. As well, this may partially underlie the body weight paradox of dialysis whereby smaller patients consistently demonstrate poorer survival than larger patients. Differences in interdialytic weight between smaller and larger patients are comparatively less than differences in time needed to achieve spKt/V targets; thereby, smaller patients tend to have higher ultrafiltration rates on average than do larger patients.

Best available evidence suggests that risk begins to inflect when the ultrafiltration rate crosses 10 mL/h/kg body weight and becomes statistically significantly elevated when in excess of 13 mL/h/kg body weight. Further evidence is needed to confirm (or refute) precise thresholds vis-à-vis safe ultrafiltration rates. At present, several bodies are suggesting that guidelines for maximal Kt/V rate be incorporated into assessment of facility quality and remuneration.

Of note, ultrafiltration rate has been studied as an average rate for dialysis sessions: net fluid removal divided by total treatment time indexed to body weight. There has been no directed study of whether techniques in which ultrafiltration rate is varied over the course of treatment, such as ultrafiltration profiling, sequential ultrafiltration-hemodialysis, or biofeedback technologies, modulate associations.

The sobering reality is that patients do not want more dialysis whether in the form of longer or more frequent treatments. In a recent survey, fewer than one-quarter of respondents indicated a willingness to extend treatment time by 30 minutes and fewer than one-eighth indicated that they would increase the frequency of dialysis. Clearly, additional patient education is needed to underscore the benefits of mitigating implied fluid removal rates.

A number of potential adjuvant therapies lurk on the horizon. These include wearable ultrafiltration devices and drugs that block the uptake of sodium from the gut. Although such therapies are unlikely to fundamentally alter the association between ultrafiltration rate and outcome, they hold promise to reduce the net need for ultrafiltration during dialysis, which may enable reduction in treatment times in a safe and tolerable level. However, rigorous studies are needed to delineate the safety and efficacy of such treatments and to determine how they are incorporated into the fabric of clinical care.

Conclusion

In conclusion, urea kinetics—specifically the achievement of a spKt/V of 1.2 and/ or a URR of 65%—are a necessary component of adequate dialysis. Emerging evidence indicates that the prescription should also imply a tolerable ultrafiltration rate—optimally less than 10 mL/h/kg but certainly no more than 13 mL/h/kg. Available data do not inform with respect to how best to incorporate middle-molecule clearance into the dialysis prescription, but the reader is advised to monitor the literature for advances in this regard. Finally, as in all of clinical medicine, care should be tailored to individual patients based on circumstances and preferences rather than in a cookie-cutter approach.

Improving Outcomes in
Dialysis Patients

C H A P T E R 2 1

Improving Outcomes for End-Stage Renal Disease Patients: Shifting the Quality Paradigm*

Allen R. Nissenson, MD, FACP

Since the implementation of the End-Stage Renal Disease (ESRD) program entitlement in 1973, the program has been under the microscope, and rightfully so. Initially envisioned to provide needed coverage for a few thousand patients through Medicare, it was anticipated that the program would not only provide life-sustaining dialysis therapy but would also result in patients returning to full, active, productive lives, including a return to employment. Over the past 40 years, however, the evolution of the ESRD program has been quite different, a fact that has been documented by the United States Renal Data System (USRDS) as well as the recently developed Peer initiative, a database and analytical engine developed by the Chief Medical Officers of U.S. dialysis organizations in collaboration with the Chronic Disease Research Group in Minneapolis, Minnesota. In 2012, there were more than 430,000 patients on various forms of dialysis, and although the growth rate of this population may be slowing, the complexity of the patients receiving this high-cost, technically complex treatment is increasing. The majority of patients have three or four comorbid conditions in addition to ESRD, with diabetes and hypertension causing ESRD in nearly two thirds of patients, and cardiovascular disease highly prevalent. Patients are receiving 8 to 10 different medications daily, and the current most common form of dialysis, thrice-weekly in-center hemodialysis, replaces the equivalent of 10% to 14% of small-solute removal compared with natural kidneys. The ability of conventional dialysis to remove the full range of toxins necessary to optimize health, including salt and water, is inadequate.

As shown in the Peer report, mortality and hospitalization rates have improved significantly in ESRD patients over the past decade. Unfortunately, however, ESRD patients continue to have high mortality and morbidity. Mortality remains greater than 18% annually overall and nearly 40% for patients new to dialysis, with an average of nearly two hospitalizations still occurring per patient per year. Although late-stage chronic kidney disease (CKD) and ESRD patients comprise just over 1% of all Medicare patients, they consume nearly 10% of the overall costs of Medicare, nearing $45 billion.

Recent publications have pointed out the need to reexamine the approach that has been taken to improving clinical outcomes and constraining costs for this vulnerable

---

*Modified with permission from Improving outcomes for ESRD patients: shifting the quality paradigm. *Clin J Am Soc Nephrol.* 2014;9:430-434.

population. Largely because of the USRDS, Peer report, and provider consolidation with development of comprehensive administrative databases, U.S. ESRD patients are the most data-dense chronic disease population in the world. To date, quality improvement has been largely focused on biochemical or surrogate outcomes, as has been attempted with other disease states. However, there is an urgent need to move beyond such outcomes to focus on more patient-centric care, as emphasized by the Patient Centered Outcomes Research Institute (PCORI). Clearly, reorganization of the care delivery system, focusing on care coordination can be effective in this population as demonstrated by a recently completed Centers for Medicare & Medicaid Services (CMS) demonstration project. Ironically, despite the clear value shown in the demonstration project for certain interventions such as oral nutritional supplements in selected patients, such supplements remain an uncovered benefit in the current reimbursement system and must be provided by dialysis facilities at their own expense. The Center for Medicare and Medicaid Innovation (CMMI) has recognized the potential for improving outcomes in ESRD patients through system reengineering by announcing the Comprehensive ESRD Care Initiative. Through a request for proposal (RFP) process, applications to form an ESRD Seamless Care Organization (ESCO) will be reviewed, and up to 15 such programs will be awarded. Unfortunately, however, the small number of programs, small patient size of each program designated in the RFP, lack of specificity of quality metrics, and concerns over baseline rate setting make participation and success in this program challenging. In addition, results will not be available for 3 to 5 years, and, in the meantime, hundreds of thousands of ESRD patients will continue to have suboptimal outcomes.

The nephrology community should not wait for the results of the CMMI ESCO initiative to act; these vulnerable patients deserve action now, which will improve outcomes as well as provide the good stewardship of resources of this largely public program that the public expects. Recent publications show wide agreement within the nephrology community that care coordination incorporating nephrologist leadership is a promising approach to significantly improving outcomes. Care coordination as a delivery model is fundamental to improving outcomes by itself it will not ensure the goal—improving the lives of patients with kidney disease—without consensus on the key clinical targets and metrics to drive to this goal.

Although there is widespread recognition of the areas of clinical focus that are most likely to improve survival, morbidity, the patient experience, and overall quality of life, the ability of providers to deliver on these areas has been stymied by the lack of a unified conceptual framework for quality for ESRD patients and a well-meaning CMS Quality Improvement Program (QIP) which, unlike the approach advocated by VanLare and Conway at CMS, used primarily laboratory indicators, which in and of themselves are no longer the key drivers to significantly improve the primary clinical outcomes. Outcomes related to hospitalizations and mortality use standardized ratios, comparing actual with "expected" outcomes. The latter, however, are not based on transparent adjusters, and reliance on comorbidity data from the 2728 Medical Evidence forms adds to the inaccuracy.

We have, therefore, developed a patient-focused needs hierarchy meant to better describe and encourage the approach to patient outcomes that is the most likely to significantly improve the lives of patients with kidney disease (Fig. 21.1). As Stephen Covey, the business leader and author pointed out: "Begin with the end in mind." For patients with advanced kidney disease, the "end" is improving the quality

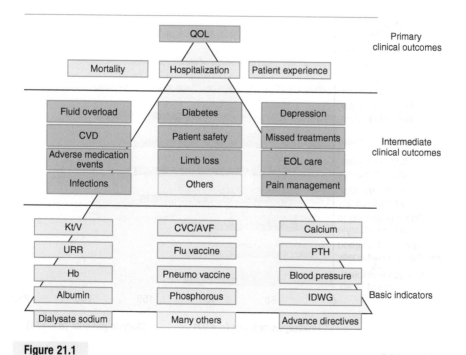

Figure 21.1

The patient-centered quality pyramid. Fundamental outcomes are necessary but not sufficient to climb the pyramid through complex programs to achieve lower mortality rates, fewer hospitalizations, and enhanced patient experience of care. Ultimately, if successful, patients will achieve an improved quality of life (QOL). *AVF,* arteriovenous fistula; *CVC,* central venous catheter; *CVD,* cardiovascular disease; *EOL,* end-of-life; *Hb,* hemoglobin; *IDWG,* interdialytic weight gain; *PTH,* parathyroid hormone; *URR,* urea reduction ratio.

of their lives. It should be noted that we use "quality of life" in this hierarchy because it is the term generally used as a key primary outcome in health care, although for the proposed paradigm, we define this somewhat more narrowly as aspects of improving the life of kidney patients that can be impacted through improving mortality, lowering hospitalizations, and enhancing patients' experiences with treatment. Although some patients may state that they cherish length of life more than anything, the vast majority focus on the quality rather than the quantity of life as most important. We recently had an independent group carry out a survey of 271 patients (DaVita Healthcare Partners data on file, 2011); some on dialysis, some with advanced CKD. Fig. 21.2 clearly shows that patients want to live long lives, but more important, they want to have a high quality of life and be treated with compassion and respect. The value of specific clinical outcomes is less important to patients because they assume that competent dialysis facilities will provide safe and effective treatment or they would not be allowed to function by Medicare. A study from Australia focused on patient priorities for research in CKD is consistent with these data.

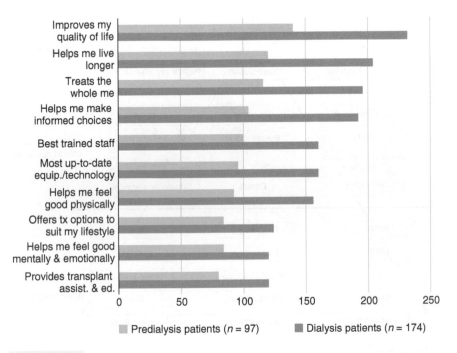

Figure 21.2

Survey of patients demonstrating that quality of life is the most important outcome to them. *Tx, treatment.*

So if one starts with the top of the hierarchy—the overarching goal to improve the lives of patients with kidney disease—it is necessary, if one is to accomplish this, to improve survival, decrease hospitalizations, and optimize the patient experience with care, which are on the highest tier of our pyramid as primary clinical outcomes. Moving further down the hierarchy, there are a constellation of potential intermediate clinical outcomes, complex clinical areas that if optimized are most likely to drive the desired improvements in primary clinical outcomes. In the case of hospitalizations, for example, recent analysis of claims data taken shows that cardiovascular disease, much caused or worsened by acute or chronic fluid overload, infection, and diabetes, accounts for the majority of hospitalizations (Fig. 21.3). Additionally, we believe that appropriate medication management is clearly critically important if hospitalizations are to be avoided, but quantifying the contribution of medication errors and complications is not possible to tease out from claims data. Other potential intermediate clinical outcomes, such as depression and missed treatments, have been shown to impact primary outcomes as well. These intermediate clinical outcomes are the areas of care that currently drive hospitalizations, rehospitalizations, and mortality and contribute to a suboptimal patient experience.

The basic indicators form the lower layer of the hierarchy and are the ones that have largely preoccupied the renal community and regulators over the past decades. What we propose is that poor performance on these basic indicators will ensure poor

	Percent of Total Admissions
Fluid excess (directly and indirectly related)	30.4
■ CVD (controllable)	9.9
■ Fluid overload	6.5
■ Hypertension	5.3
■ CHF	4.0
■ Fluid and electrolyte disorders	2.7
■ CVD (non-controllable)	2.1
Infection (directly related)	19.9
■ Vascular access	10.4
■ Septicemia	5.5
■ Vaccine preventable pneumonia	4.0
Diabetes (directly related)	5.1
■ Diabetes	4.3
■ Diabetes-related amputation	0.9
Other	0.3
■ Depression	0.3
Total listed above	55.7
All additional causes (e.g., brain aneurysm)	44.3
Grand total	100.0

Figure 21.3

The most common causes of hospitalizations in patients with end-stage renal disease based on claims data. *CHF*, congestive heart failure; *CVD*, cardiovascular disease. (2009 USRDS data; DVA patients. Courtesy of Dr. Steven Brunelli.)

intermediate clinical outcomes. However, excellent performance on these indicators, as is currently the case for a number of these for most providers of care, has not resulted in significant improvements in intermediate or primary outcomes. Thus, excellent performance on the basic indicators is necessary but not sufficient to lead to excellent primary outcomes. The intermediate outcomes are more complex than the basic indicators, requiring systematic, organized clinical programs; multiple indicators; and often-fundamental changes in the culture of the dialysis facility and dialysis team if they are to be successfully improved.

How could this conceptualization of the clinical hierarchy for ESRD patients be put to practical use to drive quality improvement in a dialysis clinic as well as inform policymakers responsible for oversight of the ESRD program as well as the overall public programs, Medicare and Medicaid, that focus disproportionate resources on the complex, chronically ill? In the dialysis clinic, the interdisciplinary team, including nurses, dietitians, social workers, technicians, and the medical director, needs to be the engine that drives clinical quality. To this team, the hierarchy can help organize thinking and action by drawing an analogy to a basketball team, the ultimate goal for which is to win the game. The team must start with skilled players and execute on the fundamentals namely the basic indicators—dribbling, passing, shooting, blocking. But mastering these fundamentals in no way ensures the game will be won. Instead, the players need to build on the fundamentals and evolve into more complex interactions—plays, offense, and defense. When these plays come together, the result is more offensive points, fewer defensive points, and ultimately the goal—the game is won. The analogy to this in the ESRD world is that when a facility has excellent scores on the basic indicators, it is time to move up to the big leagues by organizing the fundamentals into complex intermediate clinical initiatives on the way to achieving lower mortality rates, fewer hospitalizations, and better patient experiences and ultimately improving patients' lives.

Two major observations have significantly affected the way we perceive the basic, largely laboratory indicators in ESRD. First, we have a number of large prospective clinical trials that show us that what we may have observed about the achievement of certain basic biochemical markers and primary outcomes such as mortality and morbidity were not correct. Second, we have noted that many facilities have reached "clinical optimization" for many of the basic indicators. We use this term to indicate facility-level performance for a given indicator when the mean value is well into the target range and the performance variation is minimal among patients. Hemodialysis adequacy is a good example of clinical optimization based on recent QIP data with nearly 98% of facilities achieving optimization using CMS definitions. Although it will remain important going forward to maintain clinically optimized performance on the basic indicators, future focus and investment in clinical programs should move up the pyramid to intermediate outcomes if we are truly to drive to improving patients' lives. What does this mean practically within a large dialysis organization? We have developed and successfully implemented programs to drive the basic indicators. As these basic indicators have moved to a state of clinical optimization, the corporate support shifts from program development to active surveillance of performance across the organization to a focus on outliers to ongoing watchful monitoring to prevent deterioration in performance. Proactive program development and resource allocation now go to the areas of intermediate outcomes that are the most impactful, in particular fluid management, infection management, diabetes management, and medication management. The latter derive from claims data analyzed and published by Peer and the USRDS. This practical application of the conceptual pyramid drives other strategic decision making within the organization. For example, investment in new technology that specifically drives the key intermediary outcomes would have a higher priority than technology that addressed other aspects of care. In addition, areas of the organization that support the clinical care delivered such as clinical laboratories and information technology are using the clinical hierarchy prioritization scheme as they consider how best to provide the support needed to drive up the pyramid.

At the facility level, the hierarchy provides a powerful tool to ensure that the interdisciplinary team fully understands and embraces this new way of thinking about clinical outcomes. An example relates to a focus on the key secondary outcome of fluid management. This is a complex area on the surface, and because of its many components, it would be overwhelming to most dialysis facilities. By breaking it down using the hierarchy, however, it begins to be easier for facilities to tackle. In fact, for each such complex clinical program, we have built a program-specific pyramid, again emphasizing that each program can be thought of as composed of fundamental and more complex components. An example of a program-specific pyramid is provided in Fig. 21.4. We would use the generic pyramid and then the fluid-specific pyramid in the following way:

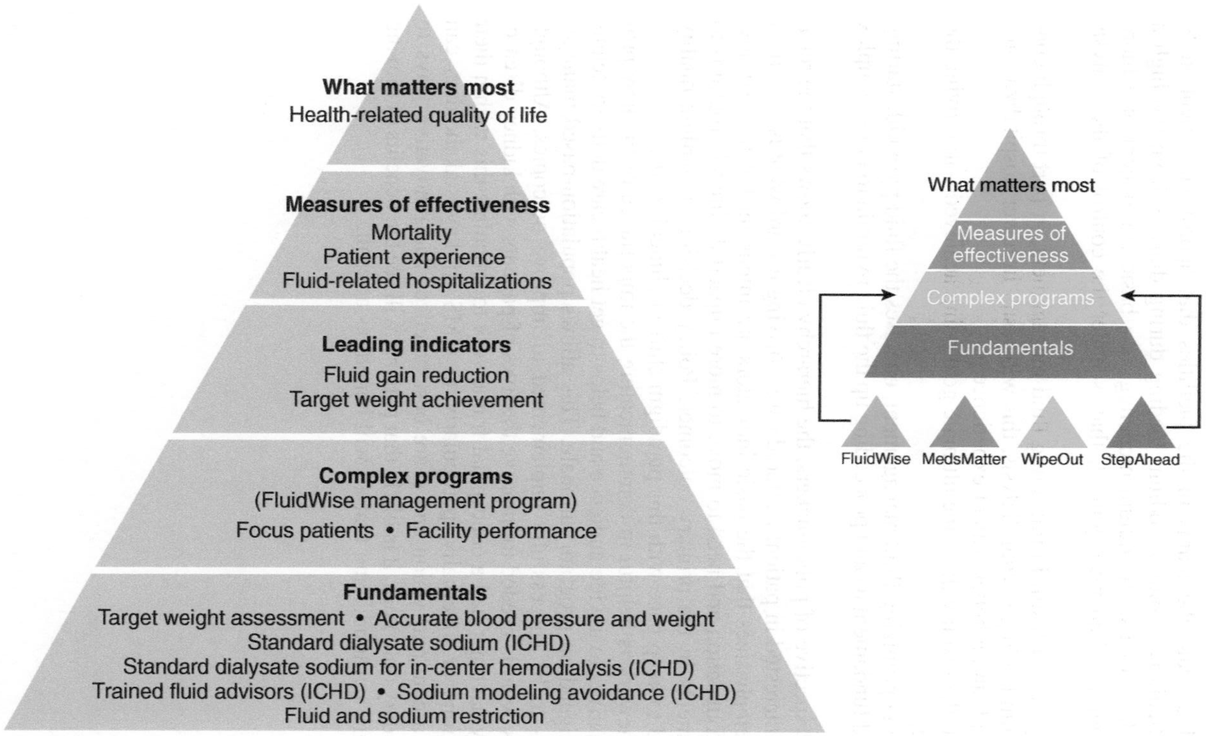

Figure 21.4

The quality pyramid for fluid management. *ICHD*, in-center hemodialysis. (DaVita HealthCare Partners, Inc., with permission.)

1. Explain and educate the teams in the facilities that appropriate attention to sodium, particularly avoiding sodium loading during dialysis from too high a dialysate sodium or use of sodium modeling, is a basic component of a more complex program, fluid management, that is under the control of the dialysis facility.
2. If the facility is successful in impacting fluid management, in part through controlling sodium loading during dialysis, this will result in fewer hospitalizations, better survival, and a better patient experience.
3. If successful, the result will be the ultimate goal being achieved—improving the patient's life.
4. To succeed in optimizing fluid management, one uses the fluid pyramid, starting with the fluid fundamentals and proceeding up the fluid pyramid to more complex actions.

From the perspective of policymakers, the hierarchy clearly shows that the renal community is interested in patient-centered care—driving toward what is important to patients. It emphasizes that the basic indicators are important but that we now have a strong foundation and need to move to more impactful clinical programs to drive improvements in the primary outcomes. Policy decisions regarding quality incentives need to keep pace with this paradigm shift in clinical focus.

Such a framework is helpful in communicating the importance of the new programs and initiatives to a wide audience and helps to get health care delivery teams and patients aligned on program rationale. This allows population-based management programs to be successfully implemented to improve outcomes. Although clinicians know what is needed to improve the lives of patients with kidney disease, up to now, they have not had a conceptual framework to articulate this within their own organizations or externally, particularly to CMS. If key stakeholders can embrace such a common vision and share best practices and innovative ways to drive the secondary outcomes, it is likely that patients will see the benefits of moving the focus "up the pyramid," and that all will benefit as a result.

CHAPTER 22

Quality, Safety, Accountability, and Medical Director Responsibilities

Jay B. Wish, MD

Introduction

The challenges found in end-stage renal disease (ESRD) facilities in the United States mirror fundamental shortcomings in the American health care system in general, as described in the Institute of Medicine (IOM) 2001 report *Crossing the Quality Chasm: A New Health Care System for the 21st Century*. The IOM concludes that "the American health care delivery system is in need of fundamental change." The IOM proposes six key goals for the 21st-century health care system: safe, effective, patient centered, timely, efficient, and equitable.

The IOM points out that much of the quality "chasm" that currently exists in health care delivery is due to misaligned incentives between health care systems, payers, medical professionals, patients, technology, education, and legal liability. Multiple interrelated dimensions of health care delivery must be addressed, improved, and aligned to improve the quality chasm. Several of these dimensions have immediate relevance to the care of dialysis patients and include quality, safety, and accountability.

Quality

Quality in health care has taken on increased importance over the past 2 decades as payers, regulators, and patients have all demanded an improved product from health care providers. In the 1980s and early 1990s, the emphasis was on *quality assurance*. However, traditional quality assurance activities were never embraced by physicians because quality assurance departments in hospitals were generally staffed by nurses involved in risk management and utilization review, which fostered the concept that quality assurance was a burdensome and intrusive function with little impact on patient outcomes. Although industry had successfully applied the principles of quality improvement for many years because of the opening of worldwide markets that forced manufacturers to focus on quality, American health care providers had been immune from competitive pressures until the increased penetration of capitated payment plans forced health care providers to lower costs and improve quality.

The principles of quality improvement are so intuitive that it is difficult to understand why physicians have been so resistant to embracing them. Table 22.1 summarizes the benefits of quality improvement. Quality improvement is similar to the differential diagnosis of a medical problem. First, one builds a list of possible etiologies ("rule-outs"). Then one initiates testing or therapy to rule out each possibility until the diagnosis is confirmed. Finally, one checks the patient for evidence of improvement to validate that the diagnosis and choice of therapy were correct.

Table 22.1

Benefits of Quality Improvement

Improved Patient Outcomes
- Decreased morbidity and mortality
- Improved quality of life
- Improved satisfaction

Improved Facility Outcomes
- Increased patient census
- Fewer absences for hospitalization
- Decreased mortality
- Increased market share
- Decreased costs
- Increased efficiency
- Improved employee retention and productivity
- Improved risk management
- Fewer regulatory hassles

Improved System-Wide Outcomes
- Decreased hospitalization expenses
- More cost-effective care
- Improved rehabilitation
- Contribution to evidence-based literature

In quality improvement, a multidisciplinary team at the provider level examines an issue in which there is an opportunity for improvement. This might be a structural issue (e.g., staffing ratios or the water treatment system), a process issue (e.g., the drawing of postdialysis blood urea nitrogen levels or the administration of influenza vaccine), or an outcome issue (e.g., a high percentage of patients with low Kt/V or with dialysis catheters). The team then brainstorms to list the "differential diagnosis" classified by category, such as procedures, equipment, policies, staff factors, and patient factors. The team develops consensus on which one or more of these causes might be responsible for the suboptimal performance and then develops and implements a change in process to test whether this improves performance. Data collected before and after the process change are compared. If significant improvements in performance occur after the change, the process change is incorporated more widely.

Thus, the fundamental principles underlying quality improvement are (1) all work can be described as a process, (2) variation exists in every process, (3) the performance of processes can be measured, (4) measurement requires comparison, and (5) the goal is to reduce variation within acceptable limits by testing and validating the processes that will produce the best results. Although the advancement of evidence-based medicine and the proliferation of clinical practice guidelines have begun to clarify which care processes are likely to produce the best clinical outcomes, all providers have unique barriers to process improvement that must be identified at the facility level by individuals who know the processes best.

Ultimately, "care" represents a linkage of many processes, and the success of quality improvement initiatives requires the empowerment of those individuals "in the trenches." An obstacle to the successful implementation of a quality improvement culture is management failing to relinquish power to its employees and to trust its employees to effectively use the resources that have been put at their disposal to improve processes of care and patient outcomes. Quality improvement has been described as both "bottom up" and "top down." The top-down aspect means that management must commit itself at the highest level (e.g., board of directors, chief executive officer) to a quality improvement culture and to allocate the resources necessary for a quality improvement program to succeed.

Successful quality improvement requires appropriate data management infrastructure to track processes and outcomes, education and training of staff in the principles and application of quality improvement techniques, providing employees with the protected time necessary to attend quality improvement meetings and to manage quality improvement data, and individuals in leadership positions emphasizing their commitment to quality improvement through their own actions and words. The bottom-up aspect of quality improvement means that it is ultimately the workers who execute the care processes on a daily basis and who are best qualified to examine which processes of care are most effective—identifying the barriers to improving outcomes and ultimately implementing changes in processes to overcome those barriers and to benefit patients.

Although the IOM has developed a somewhat arcane definition of health care quality ("the degree to which health services for individuals and populations increase the likelihood of desired health outcomes and are consistent with current professional knowledge"), many health care providers (including physicians) may find it easier to relate to health care quality as a product delivered by a provider to a customer. This customer could be identified as the patient or the payer. As in other markets, the customer can and should articulate whether or not the product meets expectations.

The expectations of a payer such as Medicare are very clear and are contained in the Conditions for Coverage (CfC) for dialysis facilities. However, satisfying the CfC is merely meeting a minimum standard of care required of all dialysis providers and is quality assurance, not quality improvement. Because the ultimate goal of quality improvement is to improve outcomes for patients, the patient's perspective must be considered—and the use of patient satisfaction and quality-of-life instruments has become increasingly important to identify opportunities for process improvement, especially in the context of the ongoing paradigm shift to a more patient-centered health care delivery environment.

The development of a data management infrastructure is essential to the ability to compare a provider's own performance with others and with itself over time. Data are a cornerstone of quality improvement. An adequate data management infrastructure is essential to repeated measurement of indicators over time and to inferences made about causality and the improved decision making that is ultimately based on evidence.

Another cornerstone of quality improvement culture is respect for the individual. Quality improvement projects succeed because they are owned and championed at the process level rather than at the executive level. The culture of quality improvement requires a paradigm shift from management to leadership, from control to coaching, from resistance to openness to change, from suspicion to trust, from an internal focus to a customer focus, and to seeing people as resources rather than as commodities.

Physicians have traditionally resisted quality activities as second guessing by nonexperts and have almost invariably delegated quality activities to a head nurse

Table 22.2

Barriers to Quality Improvement

- Management does not allocate sufficient resources for data infrastructure, employee training, and protected staff time
- Management behavior is not consistent and sends mixed message to employees
- Management fear of employee empowerment
- Lack of physician buy-in
- Failure to identify and train effective team leaders
- Failure to identify a "champion" for a specific project
- Discouragement or impatience regarding an unsuccessful project
- Assignment of blame

or quality assurance coordinator. Quality improvement cannot be delegated. All individuals, especially those in leadership positions, must embrace it for it to succeed. The commitment of the nephrologist is particularly vital for quality improvement to succeed in the dialysis facility because the physician is a respected leader who sets an example by his or her own actions and because the physician is a central figure for many of the care processes that ultimately impact patient outcomes. The failure of physician buy-in is a common barrier to the successful deployment of quality improvement at the provider level.

Table 22.2 summarizes some of the other barriers. It is easy to become discouraged about quality improvement because it does not always work on the first try. In a differential diagnosis of a medical problem, sometimes many tests with negative results are performed before a positive test result ultimately identifies the nature of the problem. The same is true for quality improvement. Physicians, in particular the medical director of the dialysis facility, must have the patience to champion the quality improvement approach through several unsuccessful cycles until its inevitable success converts the skeptics and is integrated into the facility's culture.

Improvement of physician buy-in to quality improvement can be achieved by giving physicians their own individual data (they are scientists and they love data), by giving physicians comparative data (they are competitive and love to "win"), and by inducing physicians to attend quality improvement meetings by providing refreshments (physicians are busy and most likely to attend meetings if they are concurrent with a meal). The medical director of a dialysis facility should provide leadership for staff physicians by identifying their individual interests and recruiting them as champions of specific quality improvement projects. The medical director is also in the best position to provide liaison among a dialysis facility's management, management staff, and medical staff, providing advocacy leadership for the quality agenda and access to the evidence-based literature that may provide a template for process improvement.

The design and implementation of a quality improvement project is relatively straightforward. The leadership of the facility must first make a commitment to adopting a quality improvement culture and providing the data, personnel, and educational resources necessary to its implementation. This could be a clinical outcome such as anemia management, a patient satisfaction issue such as waiting time to begin dialysis, an internal cost effectiveness issue such as dialyzer selection, or a regulatory issue such as hepatitis testing. Next, an interdisciplinary team (IDT) is

Table 22.3

Key Features of Health Care Quality

Methods
- Internal and external customer driven
- Management by fact
- Respect for people
- Teamwork
- Disciplined problem-solving process

Results
- *Appropriateness:* Balancing benefit and risk
- *Effectiveness:* Ability of intervention to achieve desired outcome in population
- *Efficiency:* Ability to provide effective care at lowest possible cost
- *Safety:* Minimizing adverse effects of interventions
- *Consistency:* Minimize variability of process and outcome
- *Patient satisfaction:* Ability to meet or exceed expectations

constituted with interest and expertise in the project. Any literature regarding the issue should be gathered and shared among team members. The team should ascertain whether standards for this issue already exist and whether they can be used as a template for process improvement.

The next step is to determine the scope of the data collection activity, including the sources of data, data collection tools, logistics of data collection, and methods of data analysis. The data are then managed to analyze the processes involved and to identify sources of variation. After the analysis of process has been completed, causes of process variation are identified, and an intervention opportunity is selected. An improvement trial is designed and implemented, and follow-up data are collected and analyzed to determine whether the process change resulted in decreased variation and improved outcomes. Ultimately, the results of the project are reported back to team members—and if the intervention was successful, process change is implemented on a wider scale with continued cycles of follow-up for validation.

It is essential that there be no assignment of blame throughout this quality improvement process. When a problem is identified, it should be determined how the system failed the individual rather than how the individual failed the system. Improvements to the system almost invariably lead to improvements in individual performance and the "ownership" of the process by those responsible for implementing the process improves consistency, employee morale, and employee retention. The key features of quality improvement in health care are summarized in Table 22.3.

Patient Safety

In 2000, the IOM published its landmark report *To Err Is Human: Building a Safer Health System*, which noted that between 44,000 and 98,000 patients in the United States die each year as a result of medical errors. This makes medical errors the eighth leading cause of death and results in additional national costs of 17 to 29 billion dollars, of which health care costs represent more than half. In addition to economic costs, morbidity, and mortality, medical errors result in a loss of trust by patients in the health care system, loss of morale among health care professionals, loss of worker productivity by employers, and reduced school attendance by children.

The authors note that the decentralized and fragmented nature of the health care delivery system contributes to unsafe conditions for patients, yet licensing and accreditation processes have focused limited attention on the issue. Health care organizations and providers have not focused on patient safety because of issues regarding liability risk exposure when efforts to uncover and learn from errors are successful. Medical errors can be of omission or of commission. The types of medical errors are summarized in Table 22.4.

The IOM report noted that health care services represent a complex and techno-logical industry prone to accidents, especially because many of its components are not well integrated. Nonetheless, much can be done to make systems more reliable and safe because the failure of large systems is due to multiple faults that occur together. One of the greatest contributions to accidents in any industry (including health care) is human error. Humans commit errors for a variety of known and complicated reasons, but most human errors are induced by system failures. Rede-signing the system to prevent human errors is more productive than assigning blame.

Latent errors are more insidious because they are difficult for people working in the system to identify. (They may be hidden in computers or layers of management, and people become accustomed to working around the problem.) Latent errors can and should be identified long before an active error. These errors pose the greatest threat to safety in a complex system because they lead to operator errors. Current

Table 22.4

Types of Medical Errors

Diagnostic
- Error or delay in diagnosis
- Failure to use indicated tests
- Use of outmoded tests
- Failure to act on results of tests

Therapeutic
- Error in performance of an operation, procedure, or test
- Error in administering a treatment
- Error in the dose or method of using a drug
- Use of outmoded therapy
- Avoidable delay in treatment or in responding to an abnormal test result
- Inappropriate (not indicated) treatment

Preventive
- Failure to provide prophylactic treatment
- Inadequate monitoring or follow-up of treatment

Other
- Failure of communication
- Equipment failure
- Other system failure

Adapted from Leape L, Brennan AG, Troyen A, et al. Preventing medical injury. *Qual Rev Bull* 1993;19:144.

error reporting and response systems tend to focus on active errors, but discovering and fixing latent errors and decreasing their duration is more likely to have a greater effect on building safer systems because it will prevent active errors before they occur. The IOM report made a number of recommendations to federal agencies and health care providers to improve patient safety.

After the release of the IOM report on patient safety, the Renal Physicians Association, Forum of ESRD Networks, and National Patient Safety Foundation cosponsored a consensus conference of stakeholders in ESRD to establish a patient safety agenda for the ESRD community. Representatives from the large dialysis chains were surveyed to determine which safety issues were of greatest concern at their facilities. These are summarized in Table 22.5. This collaborative effort led to the articulation of 47 action options to improve ESRD patient safety, many of which parallel those of the IOM in the *To Err Is Human* report.

At the individual provider level, efforts will be required to raise awareness about the magnitude of the patient safety issue and the need for change—along with a change in the culture of the provider to a blameless one in which staff regularly report "near misses" without fear of retribution. Systems must be implemented to track errors and adverse events such that patterns can be identified and systems can be improved. Because medical errors occur at the operator level, it is essential that a dialysis unit's staff be trained in the safety sciences and that errors and adverse events are viewed as opportunities for prevention rather than as evidence of individual failure.

Table 22.5

Top Dialysis Patient Safety Issues

Patient falls
Medication errors, including:
• Deviation from prescription
• Allergic or other adverse reaction
• Omissions
Access-related events, including:
• Clots
• Infiltrates
• Difficult cannulation
• Poor blood flow
Dialysis errors, including:
• Incorrect dialyzer
• Incorrect line
• Incorrect dialysate
• Dialyzer or dialysis equipment–related sepsis
Excessive blood loss, including:
• Separation of blood lines
• Improper hookup
• Prolonged bleeding from needle sites

Adapted from Forum of End Stage Renal Disease Networks, National Patient Safety Foundation, Renal Physicians Association. *National ESRD Safety Initiative: Phase II Report.* December 2001.

Patient safety officers should be designated to stay current with the patient safety literature, which is rapidly expanding, so that proven safety practices can be implemented in the facility without delay. As with quality improvement, the key to success in improving patient safety is the cultural change at the organizational level to promote a blameless environment. Health care providers must receive education in the safety sciences, particularly with regard to the importance of error detection and reporting. In addition, a data collection and reporting infrastructure must be developed to track and eliminate latent errors and near misses before they become active errors and adverse events.

The tensions between the tort system and patient safety demand that the adversarial dispute resolution paradigm in health care be reexamined. Although it is possible that appeals to physicians' ethical commitments to patient welfare and the demonstrated successes of industry-based models of systemic quality improvement may gradually yield buy-in to safety initiatives, the success of this approach is doubtful because the conflicts between the tort system and error reduction programs are fundamental and severe. In addition, physicians' concerns about being sued and losing their liability insurance have escalated considerably in recent years. A tort reform strategy may allay some of these concerns by health care providers, but even though it reduces economic exposure, tort reform does not create a more efficient system.

In a no-fault system, an injured patient would only have to demonstrate that a disability was caused by medical management as opposed to the disease process. There would be no need to prove negligence. Such an approach would be better aligned with the blameless philosophy of patient safety and quality improvement, which emphasizes evidence-based analysis of systems of care. A no-fault approach to patient injury would also align incentives for risk reduction, especially if hospitals and their medical staffs are insured by the same entity and all efforts to prevent medical errors are undertaken jointly. Blame and economic punishment for errors that are made by well-intentioned people working in the health care system drive the problem of patient safety underground and alienate people who are best placed to prevent such problems from recurring.

On the other hand, failure to assign blame when it is due is also undesirable because it erodes trust in the medical profession. Although it is important to meet society's needs to pursue legal justice when appropriate, this should not be a prerequisite for compensation as the current tort system requires. Ultimately, for patient safety efforts to succeed, patients, health care providers, and the legal system must understand the distinction between blame-worthy behavior and the inevitable human errors that result from the systemic factors that underlie most failures in complex systems.

Accountability

Even if an ideal blameless culture for patient safety and quality improvement were achieved, there must be accountability. There is a hierarchy of accountability within each dialysis unit organization, between chain facilities and their corporate parent, and among dialysis providers (including nephrologists), payers, regulators, and patients. Because primarily Medicare funds are used to pay for ESRD services in the United States and these funds are appropriated by Congress, Congress holds the

Centers for Medicare & Medicaid Services (CMS) accountable for ensuring that the dialysis services purchased with these funds are of high quality.

The mortality rate for ESRD patients in the United States has consistently been higher than that in Europe, Japan, and Australia, and although some argue that this is caused by differences in case mix, data from the United States Renal Data System (USRDS) and from the Dialysis Outcomes and Practical Patterns Study (DOPPS) suggest that this is not entirely the case. The progressive consolidation of dialysis interests in the United States, dominated by the for-profit dialysis chains, has raised concerns reported in the public press that quality of care has been compromised to maximize stockholder returns, although the data supporting these concerns have been criticized because of unaccounted confounding factors.

The most recent version of the CfC for ESRD facilities, released in 2008, is a 116-page document that specifies the minimum standards of operation including governance, patient safety, and patient care with an emphasis on the use of a formalized quality assessment and performance improvement (QAPI) program by the provider. Adherence to the CfC is monitored by surveyors from individual state Departments of Health, which contract with CMS to perform onsite surveys of dialysis facilities on an average of every 3 years but more often if triggered by patient grievances or other quality or safety concerns. The state surveyors use as their template the "Interpretive Guidance" of the CfC, a 304-page document also released in 2008, which includes hundreds of "V tags." These V-tags are specific "must" criteria, and if the facility fails to satisfy all of these criteria, it is required to develop a corrective action plan and undergo a resurvey to assure that the deficiencies have been corrected. Because the CfC and Interpretive Guidance went 32 years between revisions, within the Interpretive Guidance is a "Measures Assessment Tool" (MAT) that can be updated more frequently in response to changes in evidence or standards of care. The patient-level indicators in the current MAT are summarized in Table 22.6. It is expected by the state surveyors that dialysis providers will devote a substantial portion of their QAPI activities to the indicators in the MAT and the surveyors will seek written evidence to that effect.

Research has shown that variation in patient outcomes such as dialysis adequacy is largely attributable to factors at the facility (e.g., its policies governing patient care, associated practice patterns, and attention to individual patient outcomes as opposed to patient-specific causes). Facility-specific data regarding modality, hemoglobin, dialysis adequacy, transplantation, hospitalization for infection, patient influenza vaccination, vascular access, and hypercalcemia—along with facility-specific standardized ratios for mortality, hospitalization, and transfusions—are compiled each year by the Kidney Epidemiology and Cost Center (KECC) at the University of Michigan for every dialysis facility under contract with CMS. The facility-specific profiles are sent to the respective ESRD Networks for distribution to individual facilities and to state surveyor agencies, and some of the data are posted in a "consumer-friendly" form on Medicare's Dialysis Facility Compare (DFC) website (www.medicare.gov/Dialysis/Home.asp).

The KECC facility-specific profiles provide standardized mortality (SMR), hospitalization (SHR), and transfusion (STR) ratios that use a similar methodology, adding up patient deaths, hospitalizations, and transfusions, respectively, for each of the patients in the cohort (corrected for days at risk) and then dividing it by the expected number of events based on patient-specific factors, including

---

Table 22.6

Patient-Level Indicators in the Measures Assessment Tool

Dialysis adequacy
- HD duration (>3 hrs)
- HD Kt/V (>1.2)
- PD weekly Kt/V (>1.7)

Nutrition
- Albumin (>4.0 g/dL)
- Body weight

Anemia
- Hemoglobin level
- Iron indices

Mineral and bone metabolism
- Calcium
- Phosphorus
- Parathyroid hormone

Medical errors

Infection control
- Trends
- Immunizations

Vascular access
- Arteriovenous fistulas (prevalent >65%)
- Catheters (<10% >90 days)
- Thrombosis
- Infections
- Patency

Reuse (if applicable)

Patient satisfaction and grievances
- In-Center Hemodialysis Consumer Assessment of Healthcare Providers and Systems
- Grievances

Health Outcomes
- Kidney Disease Quality of Life survey
- Patient survival

Patient education and rehabilitation

HD, hemodialysis; PD, peritoneal dialysis.

---

demographics, cause of ESRD, and comorbidities. Starting in 2015, the SMR, SHR, and STR, as well as adequacy, vascular access, and hypercalcemia data are being used to calculate a 1- to 5-star rating for each dialysis facility on the DFC website. A 1-star rating is given to the bottom 10% of facilities, a 2-star rating to the next 20% of facilities, a 3-star rating to the middle 40% of facilities, a 4-star rating to the next 20% of facilities, and a 5-star rating to the top 10% of facilities. A summary of the measures used on the DFC website is provided in Table 22.7.

In 2012, as part of the bundled payment system for chronic dialysis that began in 2011, CMS initiated a quality incentive program (QIP), which was mandated by legislation in 2008. The legislation provides for withholding up to 2% of a dialysis facility's Medicare payments for a calendar year based on its performance with regards to anemia management; patient satisfaction; and, to the extent feasible, iron

Table 22.7

Measures Reported on the Dialysis Facility Compare Website

- Adequacy of hemodialysis
- Adequacy of peritoneal dialysis
- Arteriovenous fistula prevalence
- Central venous catheter prevalence >90 days
- Hypercalcemia ≥3 months
- Standardized mortality ratio
- Standardized hospitalization ratio
- Standardized transfusion ratio

management, bone and mineral metabolism, and vascular access. The legislation also requires that such measures be endorsed by the entity under contract for endorsement of clinical performance measures (currently the National Quality Forum [NQF]) or by a consensus organization identified by the Secretary of Health and Human Services. As the data infrastructure for the collection of such measures has evolved from Medicare claims (which included only hemoglobin, urea reduction ratio (URR), and vascular access type) to a web-based network that allows for batch data transmission in real time (CROWNWeb) and more performance measures have been endorsed by NQF, the number of measures included in the QIP has increased from 3 in payment year 2012 to 15 in payment year 2018. The QIP measures are classified as clinical measures, for which the dialysis facility is given a performance score and an improvement score for each measure based on national norms and awarded the better of the two, and reporting measures, for which the dialysis unit is awarded a score based on a percentage of reporting periods for which data are provided. The scores for the individual measures are weighted, and a total performance score (TPS) is scaled from 0 to 100 points. For payment year 2018, which is based on performance in 2016 compared with national norms in 2015, a TPS of below 60 will lead to a payment reduction, with lower scores leading to greater payment reduction up to 2%. The QIP measures for payment year 2018 are listed in Table 22.8.

The use of the same data for internal quality improvement activities and for external quality oversight and consumer choice raises several concerns. Traditionally, quality data shared between a health care provider and its respective peer-review organization (or specifically between a dialysis facility and its ESRD Network) have been confidential and nondiscoverable so that there is the highest probability that the data will be valid and free of "gaming." Such data can be used to drive internal quality improvement processes at the facility level and allow the respective ESRD Network to target the outlier facilities for confidential and collegial quality improvement intervention activities. As soon as quality data become public (through their release to Medicare state survey and certification agencies, to the DFC website, or to other patient-accessible media), there is inevitably a temptation for "gaming" that can undermine the effective use of these same data for internal quality improvement activities.

Another major concern regarding the public release of performance data is that of "cherry picking" of the most compliant and healthiest patients to make a facility's performance measure profile appear more favorable, masking process deficiencies and undermining the quality improvement process. Although most of the community

Table 22.8

Quality Incentive Program Measures for Payment Year 2018

Clinical Measures
- Adult HD Kt/V >1.2
- Adult PD weekly Kt/V >1.7
- Pediatric HD Kt/V >1.2
- Prevalent arteriovenous fistulas
- Prevalent central venous catheters >90 days
- Serum calcium >10.2 mg/dL $\geq$3 months
- Bloodstream infections
- Standardized readmission ratio
- Standardized transfusion ratio
- ICH-CAHPS scores

Reporting Measures
- Anemia management (Hb, ESA dose)
- Mineral metabolism (calcium, phosphorus, PTH)
- Pain assessment and follow-up
- Depression screening and follow-up
- Healthcare personnel influenza vaccination

ESA, erythropoiesis stimulating agent; HD, hemodialysis; Hb, hemoglobin; ICH-CAHPS, In-Center Hemodialysis Consumer Assessment of Healthcare Providers and Systems; PD, peritoneal dialysis; PTH, parathyroid hormone.

recognizes the need for public accountability by health care providers, there is considerable evidence that patients do not use these data consistently to make choices among health care providers and health care plans. Nonetheless, the public reporting quality data has sensitized health care providers to their opportunities for process and outcome improvements and in that sense has improved the overall quality of health care delivery.

It has been recommended by physician organizations that payment for performance systems start with process measures because these are the most actionable by providers. Outcome measures are used to capture the effect of an intervention on health status or patients' perceptions of care. Although outcome data are often much easier to capture (through a system such as CROWNWeb) than process data, analysis of outcome data and use of outcome data as performance measures requires much more statistical sophistication (e.g., case-mix adjustment) than process data.

The renal community supports the continued development and application of validated clinical performance measures derived from evidence-based clinical practice guidelines. Nonetheless, many providers fear the advent of "cookbook" medicine in which the training and experience of the practitioner are devalued. Evidence-based clinical practice guidelines, which are designed as clinical decision-making tools, have a misguided tendency to evolve into standards of care. Quality oversight activities then become inappropriately oppressive and cross the line to become the practice of medicine by the regulator.

This is a scenario that ESRD payers, providers, and the patient community must avoid at all costs because it stifles the innovation that leads to quality improvement, returns to the outlier focus of quality assurance, and may ultimately limit access to care as providers begin to cherry-pick patients to avoid the perception of underperformance. The development of a national data infrastructure to allow for provider-specific data collection and provider-specific profiling to drive internal quality improvement activities holds great promise for process and outcome improvement. However, the use of these same data for public accountability carries many concerns that must be addressed because it may undermine the success of the quality improvement partnership between ESRD Networks and dialysis providers. A system of public accountability implemented by CMS must include case-mix adjustment strategies to minimize patient selection bias and to encourage facilities to accept high-risk patients without fear that their adverse outcomes may negatively impact on their public facility profiles.

Medical Director Responsibilities

The responsibilities of the medical director of a dialysis facility are clearly specified in the CfC §494.150 and constitute V-tags 725 to 733 in the interpretive guidance. However, because medical director's responsibilities encompass all policies and procedures related to patient care, the failure of the medical director to be knowledgeable and actively involved in the clinical operation of the dialysis facility may lead to V-tag deficiencies in many domains, particularly safety, staffing, education, adverse events, care planning, QAPI, modality selection, infection control, water quality, and admission and discharge policies. The broad responsibilities of the medical director are summarized in Table 22.9.

The CfC require that every facility must develop, implement, maintain, and evaluate an effective data-driven QAPI program with participation by key members of the facility staff and led by the medical director. Such staff members should include the nurse manager or facility administrator, dietitian, social worker, and any other stakeholders in the processes being addressed. The QAPI is designed to achieve measurable improvements in health outcomes and reduction in medical errors by using measures that are tracked over time. QAPI activities are prioritized based on the prevalence and severity of problems and their impact on clinical outcomes and patient safety. The QAPI team is responsible for educating facility staff in QAPI objectives, communicating with the governing body, and evaluating the effectiveness of the QAPI program. State surveyors focus on the data and records of QAPI

Table 22.9

Medical Director Responsibilities

- Leading quality improvement team
- Facility staff training and education
- Infection control
- Water quality
- Dialyzer reuse
- Ensuring patients' rights
- Reviewing adverse events and outcomes
- Developing, reviewing, and implementing patient care policies and procedures
- Reviewing and approving involuntary patient discharges
- Reviewing clinical performance measure data

activities, review improvements, and interview staff. The QAPI program will be deemed inadequate by the state surveyor if the facility has failed to recognize and prioritize problems or has failed to develop and follow a written plan for correction.

The medical director is responsible for assuring that each patient's primary nephrologist participates in the IDT care planning for each patient. The IDT must consist of at least the patient or designee, RN, physician treating the patient, social worker, and dietitian. The IDT must provide each patient with individualized and comprehensive assessment of his or her needs and develop each patient's treatment plan and expectations of care. If the patient's nephrologist is not fulfilling his or her obligations regarding IDT care planning, there must be evidence that the medical director is aware of the situation and has developed a corrective action plan with the nephrologist.

The medical director is responsible for water quality in the dialysis facility and is expected to be familiar with components of the water treatment system. The medical director should have basic knowledge of maintenance procedures and triggers for intervention, should review and sign off on monthly testing of water system and dialysis machines, and should lead QAPI activities regarding water quality as appropriate.

The medical director is chief infection control officer of the facility and must be familiar with its infection control program. The medical director must review all infection control reports, must document action to address problems, and is ultimately responsible for reporting adverse event clusters to public health authorities. Infection control issues in the CfC with which the medical director should be knowledgeable are listed in Table 22.10.

Other medical director responsibilities include approving the training program for patient care dialysis technicians; developing, reviewing, or approving patient care policies and procedures; signing off on all involuntary discharges and transfers; and incorporating reports regarding quality metrics from external agencies into the QAPI. Such reports include the dialysis facility report from KECC, QIP data, DFC data, ESRD Network data, patient quality of life and experience of care data, and national comparatives from the USRDS and the Dialysis Outcomes and Practice Patterns Study.

Table 22.10

Infection Control Responsibilities of the Medical Director

- Isolation of hepatitis B–positive patients
- Contact precautions for skin wounds and fecal incontinence
- Strict hand hygiene
- Environmental cleaning and disinfection of dialysis stations
- One-way flow of supplies and medications
- Routine serologic testing of hepatitis B and C
- Immunization for hepatitis B, influenza, and pneumococcus
- Infection control training of staff and patients
- Infection surveillance (e.g., catheter-related bacteremias)

In summary, the CfC make the medical director the "captain of the ship" for quality in the dialysis facility with responsibilities that are far reaching and time consuming and that may require political and administrative skills that are not intuitive. Nonetheless, Medicare has acknowledged that the nephrologist is best suited for the job, which has become increasingly complex as the emphasis on quality and safety have evolved to affect not only facility survey and certification but also payment and public reporting. In recognition of the importance of this role, many professional societies have developed medical director curricula at their national meetings, and the *Clinical Journal of the American Society of Nephrology* has published a series of articles addressing the responsibilities and challenges facing medical directors.

C H A P T E R 2 3

Initiation of Dialysis Therapy

Scott G. Satko, MD • John M. Burkart, MD

Historical Criteria for Dialysis Initiation

For patients with acute kidney injury (AKI), the decision-making process involved in the proper timing of dialysis initiation is usually fairly straightforward. In these patients, the need for dialysis is typically heralded by clinical signs and symptoms such as evidence of intractable volume overload, uremic encephalopathy, pericarditis, gastrointestinal distress, pruritus, or bleeding diathesis. Laboratory data suggestive of an impending need for dialysis in these patients often includes metabolic derangements such as intractable hyperkalemia, worsening hyperphosphatemia, or severe metabolic acidosis.

This chapter focuses primarily on the indications and process of initiating dialysis in patients with progressive chronic kidney disease (CKD). In these patients, the decision-making process is usually not as straightforward as in patients with AKI. In patients with slowly progressive CKD, the typical uremic symptoms commonly seen in patients with acute renal failure are often absent. Although subtle signs of uremia such as anorexia, weight loss, early malnutrition, and decreased energy level may be present, their onset is often so insidious in nature that patients are able to compensate without much difficulty. As a result, these patients may not relate these problems to the physician, or otherwise the physician may not recognize their presence. Before 1997, when the National Kidney Foundation released its first set of evidence- and opinion-based guidelines on this subject, no real consensus existed within the nephrology community regarding the optimal time to initiate dialysis.

Evidence-Based Criteria for Dialysis Initiation

In 1997, the National Kidney Foundation Dialysis Outcomes Quality Initiative (NKF-DOQI) publication outlined the first set of comprehensive guidelines for initiation of dialysis and reviewed the evidence supporting these guidelines. Since that time, these guidelines have undergone several revisions, the latest of which (Kidney Disease Outcomes Quality Initiative [K/DOQI] Clinical Practice Guidelines and Recommendations for Peritoneal Dialysis Adequacy and Hemodialysis Adequacy) were released in 2006. This chapter provides an in-depth summary of the current recommendations from KDOQI and discusses some of the relevant literature that has been published since 2006.

Preparation for Dialysis

For a patient with CKD to begin dialysis in a timely manner, careful consideration needs to be given to access placement, well in advance of the time at which dialysis is initiated. Patients who have reached stage 4 CKD (defined as an estimated glomerular filtration rate [eGFR] of 15–29 mL/min) should receive education regarding the various options available for renal replacement therapy. These options should include kidney transplantation (for suitable candidates), hemodialysis (HD) (both in-center and home modalities), and peritoneal dialysis (PD). This education is usually best performed in a multidisciplinary fashion. At our center, the educational process begins with an in-depth discussion between the nephrologist and patient about the natural history of CKD and the need for timely initiation of renal replacement therapy. Involvement of family members in this discussion is often beneficial for the patient. The next step in the educational process involves referral to the outpatient dialysis center, where patients and their families are able to meet with other health care providers, including dialysis nurses, renal dietitians, and social workers. Having the opportunity to meet with multiple dialysis-care professionals, tour the dialysis unit, and meet with other CKD patients during these predialysis educational sessions usually helps to alleviate some of the fears and concerns that patients often have at this point in time. It has been our observation that patients who have received extensive predialysis education are more likely to be able to make an educated decision regarding dialysis modality.

To guide clinicians with the decision-making process, K/DOQI has developed a classification scheme for stratifying CKD patients based on their level of residual renal function (Table 23.1). Although patients with all stages of CKD should receive education regarding the natural history of their disease and the likelihood that they may eventually progress to end-stage renal disease (ESRD), efforts at education should be greatly intensified when the patient reaches stage 4. It is during this stage that the dialysis modality should be chosen because patients who elect to start HD will need an appropriate vascular access placed at this time.

Timing of Dialysis Initiation

Prior KDOQI guidelines have recommended that when the level of residual renal function, as measured in units of Kt/V urea, declines to less than 2.0/wk, initiation of dialysis should be considered when certain criteria are met (see Fig. 23.1 for calculation of residual renal Kt/V). This threshold was extrapolated from morbidity and mortality data in the PD patient population as reported in the CANUSA

Table 23.1	

Stages of Chronic Kidney Disease

CKD Stage	GFR (mL/min/1.73 m²)
Stage 1	≥90 (with urinary abnormalities, e.g., hematuria, proteinuria)
Stage 2	60–89
Stage 3	30–59
Stage 4	15–29
Stage 5	<15 (or dialysis)

CKD, chronic kidney disease; GFR, glomerular filtration rate.
Modified from National Kidney Foundation. http://www2.kidney.org/professionals/KDOQI/guidelines_ckd/p4_class_g1.htm. Accessed July 8, 2016.

Kt = urea clearance from 24-hour urine collection (mL/min) x 10.08 to convert to L/wk.

V = urea volume of distribution, or volume of total body water (L).

For women, estimate V as total body weight (kg) x 0.55.

For men, estimate V as total body weight (kg) x 0.60.

Figure 23.1

Calculation of residual renal Kt/V.

(Canada–U.S.A.) and ADEMEX studies. In CANUSA, a prospective, multicenter cohort study of 680 incident PD patients, an inverse relationship was found to exist between the level of total small solute clearance and mortality rate. Over a 2-year period, every 0.1-unit/wk increase in total Kt/V was found to correspond to a 6% decrease in the relative risk of death. The total Kt/V value that corresponded to a 78% 2-year survival rate was 2.1/wk. In ADEMEX, Mexican continuous ambulatory peritoneal dialysis (CAPD) patients were randomized to a standard dialysis prescription (4 daily exchanges of 2 liters) or a modified prescription (adjusted to maintain a target peritoneal clearance of 60 L/wk/1.73 m^2). Although mean total weekly Kt/V differed between the two groups (1.80 in the standard group vs 2.27 in the modified prescription group), the two groups had identical survival after 2 years of follow-up (69.3% vs 68.3%, respectively). In these patients, the level of peritoneal small-solute (urea and creatinine) clearance had very little impact on mortality, suggesting that the level of residual renal function may be a more important prognostic factor. Based on these data as well as data from other, smaller studies, the minimally acceptable total Kt/V target for CAPD patients was chosen by prior KDOQI Work Groups to be 2.0/wk.

However, the most recent KDOQI update from 2006 recommends evaluating residual renal function in terms of glomerular filtration rate (GFR) because this method is generally simpler for clinicians to follow compared with calculating residual Kt/V. Residual kidney GFR can be measured (with 24-hour urea and creatinine clearances, taking the average of the two to estimate GFR) or estimated (with either the Modification of Diet in Renal Disease [MDRD] equation or the Cockcroft-Gault equation). When the GFR declines to a level below 15 mL/min, the patient should be followed closely for evidence of uremic symptoms, volume overload, intractable acid–base or electrolyte derangements, malnutrition, and other signs that would indicate prompt initiation of dialysis. In most cases, a dialysis access should be placed at this time.

In addition to consideration of the laboratory parameters already discussed, the K/DOQI Work Group has also recommended using other clinical information to help guide the decision regarding timing of initiation of dialysis. If a patient has residual renal function below 15 mL/min but otherwise appears clinically well and is free of uremic signs and symptoms, it is acceptable under certain circumstances to monitor the patient closely and delay initiation of dialysis. In this situation, it is also necessary to ensure that the patient has evidence of an adequate nutritional state. It is important to ascertain that the patient has stable or increasing edema-free body weight, lean body mass greater than 63%, and stable or increasing serum albumin concentration within the normal range. Another helpful recommended tool is the

Subjective Global Assessment (SGA), which evaluates nutritional status based on four criteria: recent weight change, anorexia, subcutaneous tissue, and muscle mass, scored on a 7-point Likert scale. Evidence of malnutrition by any of the above criteria in a patient with eGFR less than 15 mL/min suggests the need to initiate dialysis.

Timing of Dialysis Access Placement

An important consideration when planning initiation of dialysis, one that is unfortunately too often forgotten, is the proper timing of placement of dialysis access. Ideally, this issue should be discussed with the patient by the nephrologist as early as possible, even as early as the initial clinic visit, with all patients with a history of progressive CKD. Much of the apprehension experienced by patients about dialysis can be alleviated if frank discussions about the need to prepare for the eventuality of dialysis are carried out well in advance of the time when it becomes necessary to initiate therapy. It should never be assumed that a patient will choose one modality of dialysis (i.e., HD or PD) over another. Patients in general seem to have an easier time adjusting to the idea of starting dialysis when they are given appropriate education about both major modalities of dialysis, including the risks and benefits of choosing one modality over another. In the absence of any compelling medical indications for choosing a particular modality over another, patients should be allowed to make their own decision regarding modality selection, with appropriate guidance from their nephrologist and multidisciplinary (e.g., nursing staff, social worker, dietitian) care team.

For patients who choose to perform HD, it is of paramount importance to make early arteriovenous fistula (AVF) placement a high priority. A native AVF should ideally be placed in all suitable patients with CKD when their GFR declines to less than 25 mL/min or at the time when it is estimated that ESRD will be reached within the next 6 to 9 months. The rapidity of decline in residual renal function should be taken into account. A patient who has demonstrated a pattern of maintaining a stable GFR slightly below 25 mL/min for a period of several years can often be followed closely and undergo access placement at a later point in time.

Early placement of a native AVF should give adequate time for this fistula to fully mature before the occurrence of ESRD. If this fistula does not mature within 6 to 8 weeks, early placement should also give ample time to consider angiography of the AVF to rule out stenoses that may be amenable to angioplasty or rule out issues that may require surgical revision of the fistula (e.g., large accessory vessels diverting flow away from the access or poor perfusion of the AVF from a diseased feeding artery), placement of a new upper arm AVF, or placement of a polytetrafluoroethylene (PTFE) arteriovenous graft (AVG) if no suitable veins are found to support a native AVF. For patients who are deemed not to have suitable vasculature to support a native AVF, the HD access of second choice is an AVG. Because these AVGs tend to thrombose or succumb to infection more often than native AVFs, they should not be considered the access of first choice in the majority of patients. However, a recently published study by Drew et al has suggested that the benefit-to-risk ratio of placing an AVF instead of an AVG or tunneled central venous catheter was not as great in patients with lower a priori likelihood of developing a mature AVF. This subset of the incident ESRD population included older patients (80 years of age or older) and women with diabetes.

Ideally, an AVG should be placed approximately 3 to 6 weeks before the time of initiation of dialysis. If placed too early, there is a high likelihood that the AVG may thrombose before the first use. A tunneled, cuffed internal jugular catheter should typically only be considered for the first dialysis access in patients who have no suitable vascular access for either a native AVF or AVG, patients who are uremic and in need of dialysis at the time of initial presentation, and possibly in patients who are deemed to have an extremely limited life span (<6–12 months). Tunneled, cuffed catheters are recommended over nontunneled, cuffed catheters for patients requiring catheter-based vascular access of over 3 weeks' duration. Because of the high risk for infectious complications, it is recommended that an intravascular catheter not be placed until the time when dialysis is initiated. For patients who need urgent dialysis at the time of presentation and initiate dialysis through a catheter, it is important to remember that this catheter should in the overwhelming majority of cases only serve as a "bridge" to a more permanent access. Placement of a more permanent access must be given a high priority and should be done as soon as the patient is medically stable to undergo this procedure.

For patients who choose to perform PD, a Tenckhoff catheter is usually placed between 2 and 4 weeks before the time of dialysis initiation. This approach is to allow optimal healing and sealing of the PD exit site before use. However, it is important to note that a PD catheter could be used starting on the day it is placed with minimal risk of leak if placed properly. Another approach some are advocating is to bury the external portion of the PD catheter subcutaneously at the time of insertion so that it "matures" in a sterile environment. The distal portion is then exteriorized in a simple outpatient procedure and immediately ready for use. Anecdotal data suggest it is safe to have these catheters in place 6 to 12 months before starting dialysis so the patient is ready with a natural access when time to start renal replacement therapy has arrived. No data exist to show that earlier placement of a curled-tip PD catheter is associated with an increased risk of complications or technique failure.

Although the majority of patients who initiate dialysis without an access previously placed do so with a tunneled internal jugular catheter, many of these patients could just as well have a peritoneal catheter placed as their first dialysis access. One barrier to this has traditionally been the availability of a skilled surgeon to place a peritoneal catheter on short notice. As more interventionalists (both nephrologists and radiologists) have become adept at performing this procedure, this barrier is becoming less of an issue in many centers across the United States and Canada. Also, many nephrologists have traditionally been reluctant to prescribe PD until a patient's catheter has been in place for at least 2 weeks to minimize the likelihood of peritoneal leak or hernia development. It has been our center's experience that initiating dialysis using low dwell volumes (usually no more than 1.0–1.5 L) using a cycler while the patient is supine greatly reduces the chance of such an adverse event occurring.

There may be financial advantages to urgent-start PD as well as clinical advantages. A recent paper from Liu et al found a 15% cost reduction ($16,398 for urgent-start PD vs $19,352 for urgent-start HD) during the first 90 days of ESRD therapy.

Conservative Management of End-Stage Renal Disease

Finally, it should be recognized that initiation of dialysis is not necessarily in the best interests of every patient with advanced CKD, especially for older patients who are relatively asymptomatic and have a limited expected life span because of other comorbid conditions. Many of these patients are at risk for experiencing a significant decline in their quality of life after initiating dialysis. Therefore, it is important to have frank discussions with patients and their families about the risks and benefits of dialysis therapy, as well as their expectations about what dialysis will and will not do. A recent paper from Brown et al described a cohort of 467 older patients with advanced CKD, 122 of whom chose to forego dialysis. Interestingly, the median survival time of patients who had decided to forego dialysis was 16 months, with a 53% 1-year survival rate. The median survival of this group was 13 months past the point when eGFR declined to a level less than 15 mL/min. These findings are even more impressive given the fact that the group that had decided to forego dialysis was older (mean age, 82 years vs 67 years) and had more comorbid medical conditions, including a 14-fold higher incidence of dementia. Although patient-reported symptoms were more frequent and quality of life lower on the initial clinic visit for the patients who declined dialysis, the rate of progression of symptoms or decline in quality of life in this group did not exceed that in the group that decided to initiate dialysis.

Writing an Initial Dialysis Prescription: "Full Dose" versus "Incremental"

When writing an initial dialysis prescription, it is important to take into account the amount of residual renal function present. For patients who meet the criteria for initiation of dialysis, as outlined earlier, dialysis could be initiated with a "full-dose" prescription, ignoring the residual renal component, or alternatively, with an "incremental" prescription, in which the dialysis dose is increased as residual renal function decreases, maintaining a total equivalent standardized weekly Kt/V urea greater than 2.0 at all times if on HD and greater than 1.7 if on PD. For patients with significant residual renal function (weekly Kt/V urea >1.0), the initial dialysis prescription can be either "full dose" or "incremental." In this group of patients, there are no data to show which of these two methods of prescription management is associated with a better outcome. For patients with minimal residual renal function (weekly Kt/V urea <1.0), it may be more practical to recommend that a "full-dose" prescription be used at the time of initiation of dialysis.

Writing an Initial Dialysis Prescription: Peritoneal Dialysis

Whether dialysis is initiated using a "full-dose" or an "incremental" prescription, frequent monitoring of the delivered dialysis dose is necessary to ensure adequacy of small solute clearance. For PD patients, the K/DOQI guidelines recommend measuring total solute clearance (as weekly Kt/V urea) two to three times within the first 6 months of initiating dialysis. If the PD prescription remains unchanged, it is recommended that both 24-hour dialysate and urine collections for clearance be obtained every 4 months, with urine collections every 2 months until the residual renal urine volume declines to less than 100 mL/day. After the residual renal volume has declined to a negligible level, only 24-hour dialysate collections are necessary, and they should ideally be performed every 4 months in stable patients. A 24-hour dialysate collection for measurement of peritoneal Kt/V urea should be performed within 1 month of any change in dialysis prescription or after any significant change in the patient's clinical status. The dialysis prescription for PD patients should then be adjusted with the goal of keeping total (dialysis + residual renal) solute clearance as measured by Kt/V urea at greater than 1.7/wk.

The patient's body size as well as residual renal function must be taken into account when deciding on the initial dialysate exchange volume and number of daily exchanges. For patients with body surface areas (BSAs) less than 1.8 m², an initial exchange volume of 2000 mL or less is usually appropriate. For those with BSAs of 1.8 to 2.0 m², depending on the amount of residual kidney function, larger instilled volumes may be needed, and when the patient is anuric, instilled volumes of 2500 mL will likely be needed. For larger patients with BSAs greater than 2.0 m², when the patient is anuric, exchange volumes of 3000 mL will likely be needed. For patients in whom an "incremental" approach to prescription management is taken, our protocol for deciding on the appropriate number of exchanges per day and their instilled volume per exchange is based on the amount of residual renal function at the time of initiation, as follows:

BSA (m²)	<1.8	1.8-2.0	>2.0
Initial number of exchanges per day	Residual renal GFR (mL/min)		
1	10	11	12
2	7	8	9
4	5	6	7

BSA, body surface area; GFR, glomerular filtration rate.
Modified from Burkart JM, Satko SG. Incremental dialysis: one center's experience over a two-year period. *Perit Dial Int* 2000;20:418-422.

For example, a patient with BSA of 1.9 m² and residual renal GFR of 8 mL/min could be placed on a prescription of two daily exchanges of 2500 mL to achieve an adequate total weekly Kt/V.

Writing an Initial Dialysis Prescription: Hemodialysis

As is true for PD patients, HD patients can also initiate therapy with either a "full-dose" or "incremental dose" prescription based on their level of residual renal function. For a patient with no residual renal function, the goal is to obtain a per treatment single-pool Kt/V urea of 1.2 or greater for each of three treatments a week. Patients with a significant amount of residual renal function (K_rt/V urea ≥ 1.0) may be able to perform dialysis with a less intense schedule (e.g., once or twice a week initially). As a matter of practicality, however, most HD patients initiate therapy with a "full-dose" prescription because residual renal function is usually lost fairly rapidly when HD is initiated. The 1997 NKF-DOQI document reviewed the suggested formula for prescription adjustment for HD patients performing "incremental" dialysis. HD is an intermittent therapy compared with the continuous nature of residual renal function. For this reason, Kt/V from dialysis (K_dt/V) cannot simply be added to K_rt/V urea to obtain the total weekly Kt/V, as can be done for PD patients. In this case,

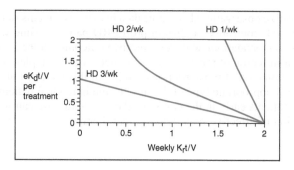

Figure 23.2

Estimated delivered eKdt/V per HD treatment needed if prescribing incremental HD in an incident patient based on frequency (per week) of the HD treatments and the patients residual Kidney function. eK_dt/V = equilibrated, double-pool Kt/V per hemodialysis (HD) treatment. K_rt/V = weekly residual renal Kt/V. (Modified from National Kidney Foundation. *NKF-DOQI clinical practice guidelines for peritoneal dialysis adequacy*. New York, Author, 1997, p. 104.)

one should target a weekly total "standardized" Kt/V of greater than 2.0. Fig. 23.2 demonstrates the per treatment K_dt/V urea necessary to maintain an "equivalent" total weekly Kt/V urea of 2.0 in patients with any given level of K_rt/V urea, performing HD once, twice, or three times weekly.

When HD is initiated, the first two or three treatments are often performed at a lower than usual blood flow rate and for a shorter than normal duration of time. This practice is performed to reduce the risk of "dialysis disequilibrium," which can occur in patients who are severely azotemic before being dialyzed. In these patients, the serum urea nitrogen level is a significant component of the total serum osmolality, and overly aggressive dialysis can abruptly decrease the serum osmolality before solute equilibration between the intravascular and extravascular fluid compartments can occur, particularly in the intracellular compartment. This can result in the sudden shift of fluid into cells, with the most serious side effect being that of cerebral edema. To replace some of the intravascular osmotic load that is removed with dialysis, it is standard practice at our center to give mannitol 12.5 g intravenously after the first hour of the first one or two dialysis sessions. A typical HD prescription for the first treatment session would be 2 hours at a 200 mL/min blood flow rate and then 2.5 to 3 hours at a 250 to 300 mL/min blood flow rate for the second session. Depending on the patient's tolerance of the first two sessions, subsequent sessions are usually performed with a full dialysis prescription, 3 to 4 hours at a blood flow rate of at least 300 mL/min, adjusted so that the total single pool Kt/V urea per treatment meets the current recommended guidelines of at least 1.2.

Conclusion

Considerable changes have occurred in the recommended approach to initiation of dialysis over the past decade. Although a great deal of evidence exists to support these changes, it is important to remember that much of this evidence is extrapolated from retrospective observational outcome data in dialysis patients rather than derived from randomized, controlled studies in pre-ESRD patients. Time will tell whether the current recommendations will truly improve outcomes in the ESRD population. The subject of initiation of renal replacement therapy is a complex one and involves not only determination of the appropriate timing of this therapy but also determination of the most appropriate type of therapy for the individual patient. Only through education of patients early in the course of their renal disease can we hope to attain timely initiation of effective renal replacement therapy.

Complications During Hemodialysis

C H A P T E R   2 4

Common Clinical Problems During Hemodialysis

Neenoo Khosla, MD

Background

The pattern of intradialytic complications has clearly changed over the past 25 years. The significant progress made in hemodialysis (HD) technology (especially the safety control systems integrated in HD machines), dialysate preparation (improved water standards, more frequent use of bicarbonate dialysate), and membrane bio-compatibility (synthetic membranes) have resulted in a reduction of intradialytic complications caused by technical problems. Today, cardiovascular complications such as intradialytic hypotension (IDH) and muscle cramps (MCs) prevail.

The reasons for this development are the changing demographics of dialysis populations (increasing age and number of comorbidities) and shortened dialysis times with higher ultrafiltration rates (UFRs). Today, close to half of incident patients have diabetes mellitus—and these patients are particularly prone to intradialytic cardiovascular complications.

Intradialytic Hypotension

Intradialytic hypotension is the most common intradialytic complication, with an incidence of 5% to 40% of treatments (depending on the definition of IDH, which varies from an asymptomatic percentage decrease in systolic blood pressure to symptomatic hypotension requiring active treatment). Hypotensive episodes may result in subclinical myocardial ischemia (myocardial "stunning") with detectable electrocardiographic (ECG) ischemia effects, suggesting that attention must be paid to reducing this incidence (which may be seen in 10% to 30% of dialysis sessions). Subclinical myocardial ischemia was implied by the finding of regional wall motion abnormalities detected by serial echocardiography. The wall motion abnormalities improved by 30 minutes postdialysis.

Women, older patients with isolated systolic hypertension, patients with diabetes, and those with documented autonomic neuropathy are at increased risk (Table 24.1). In healthy subjects, as much as 30% of the blood volume may be removed with maintenance of blood pressure. In the dialysis population, the combination of auto-nomic dysfunction, ventricular dysfunction and decreased venous return, and increased body temperature impairs the body's ability to cope with the hemodynamic stress caused by ultrafiltration (UF). Because of the reduced compensatory range, blood pressure falls earlier, and eventually IDH may occur.

Major factors determining the hemodynamic response are the UFR, the plasma refilling rate (PRR), and their instantaneous difference. The UFR is related to ultra-filtration volume (UFV) and the ultrafiltration time (t). Under most circumstances,

Table 24.1

Risk Factors for Intradialytic Hypotension

Diabetes mellitus
Cardiovascular disease: left ventricular hypertrophy, diastolic dysfunction with or without
    congestive heart failure, left ventricular systolic dysfunction and congestive heart failure,
    valvular heart disease, pericardial disease (constrictive pericarditis or pericardial
    effusion)
Poor nutritional status and hypoalbuminemia
Uremic neuropathy or autonomic dysfunction
Severe anemia
High-volume ultrafiltration caused by high IDWG
Predialysis systolic blood pressure <100 mm Hg
Age 65 years or older
Female gender
Unrecognized dehydration, especially in patients losing weight rapidly

IDWG, intradialytic weight gain.

the weight after the preceding dialysis equals dry weight (DW), and UFV equals intradialytic weight gain (IDWG).

$$UFR = IDWG/t$$

Obviously, prolongation of the procedure to permit slow filtration is possible. However, this is usually impractical. Advantages of longer UF times have been reported. Increase in frequency of dialysis increases total fluid removal with reported regression of left ventricular mass, but use of this technique has been infrequent. The PRR is the per time unit difference between filtration (Fil) and absorption (Abs) of plasma water in the capillary bed plus the lymphatic flow (Lym).

$$PRR = (Abs + Lym) - Fil$$

Fluid dynamics in the capillary bed can be described by the Starling forces, with the plasma oncotic pressure as a main absorptive factor. The threat of IDH can be reduced by two fundamentally distinct approaches. The first is a reduction of the UFR (by reducing the interdialytic weight gain and thus the UFV or prolongation of UF time, t). The second is by supporting the body's ability to deal with the hemodynamic challenges caused by UF (e.g., by improving vasoconstriction, therapy of congestive heart failure [CHF], or raising the serum albumin concentration).

Mean arterial pressure (MAP) is the product of cardiac output (CO) and total peripheral resistance (TPR):

$$MAP = CO \, \mu \, TPR.$$

CO is the product of stroke volume (SV) and heart rate (HR).

Cardiac output and TPR may be affected adversely in a variety of conditions (Table 24.2). During dialysis, UFR exceeds PRR frequently from the extracellular (and to a lesser extent, the intracellular) space. This results in a reduction in circulating blood volume. In healthy subjects, this reduction in intravascular volume is compensated for by constriction of peripheral arteries and venous capacitance vessels and in an increase in heart rate. Patients with diastolic dysfunction have particular difficulty in tolerating this hemodynamic stress. Diastolic dysfunction results from impaired myocardial relaxation and reduced distensibility of the left ventricle. This condition can be assumed when heart failure occurs in the presence of normal systolic function (left ventricular ejection fraction = 45%). In patients with diastolic dysfunction, even small reductions in blood volume can reduce end-diastolic filling pressures and thus provoke blood pressure falls.

Systolic dysfunction is in most cases due to myocardial ischemia on the basis of coronary artery disease (CAD). Consequent diagnosis of CAD and appropriate treatment both medically and with vascular interventions (percutaneous transluminal coronary angioplasty or bypass surgery) is recommended. Autonomic neuropathy is frequently present in patients with diabetes, and adequate metabolic control should be aimed at in the hope of preventing further deterioration. Therapy with drugs interfering with vasoconstriction and other hemodynamic responses to UF should be avoided immediately before or during HD.

Another approach to hypotensive problems has been the use of dialysate sodium increase (ramping, or "modeling") during dialysis, with the objective of maintaining blood volume during UF. Undoubtedly, the procedure of increasing the dialysate sodium concentration to 150 mmol/L at the beginning of the treatment is effective in reducing hypotensive episodes and maintaining blood pressure. However, the price paid is an increase in interdialytic weight gain and in blood pressure and in aggravation of the problems of overhydration. In general, this approach should be avoided.

What can be done to reduce interdialytic weight gain that would reduce UF needs and make it possible to remove all necessary fluid within a reasonable time? One possibility is a low-salt diet of no more than 3 g Na+/day (Fig. 24.1). This approach has been successfully used by the Tassin group for years. The value of salt restriction was shown in a cross-sectional study in which a strategy consisting of salt restricted diet (5 g/day) and intensive UF to maintain predialysis blood pressure below 140/90 mm Hg without antihypertensive medication significantly reduced interdialytic weight gain and IDH.

Iatrogenic salt loading results from a dialysate sodium concentration exceeding the plasma sodium concentration or from application of intravenous saline solutions during dialysis. It is helpful to align the dialysate sodium to the patient's own serum sodium concentration. This proposal relies on the supposition that the serum sodium is constant in an individual and that the use of dialysate sodium higher than the patient's own results in diffusion of sodium into the patient with an increase in sodium body content and in sodium plasma concentration. After the treatment is completed, the patient is thirsty because of the relative hypernatremia and drinks enough fluid to bring the sodium down to the initial set level. In general, the dialysate sodium in most patients should be 138 mEq/L or less.

Monitoring of relative blood volume (BV) changes by BV monitor (BVM) helps to estimate PRR in relationship to UFR. Changes in BVM can be tracked by changes in hemoglobin or protein concentration at the arterial port using optical photometry.

Table 24.2

Intradialytic Hypotension Causes and Preventive Strategies

Problem	Cause	Prevention Strategy
Reduction of Cardiac Output		
Reduced SV	Diastolic dysfunction: ischemic heart disease, ventricular hypertrophy; HCM (CMP), valve disease, restrictive CMP, pericardial effusion	Reduction of congestive state, prevention of tachycardia (calcium channel blockers, beta-blockers), conversion of AF antihypertensive drugs, promote regression of LVH (ACE inhibitors, ARBs)
	Systolic dysfunction: ischemia, dilated CMP, arrhythmia, hypocalcemia caused by low dialysate Ca, arrhythmias	Investigate for CAD, drug therapy of CAD, PTCA, bypass surgery, ACE inhibitors, ARBs, BB, platelet inhibition, avoid negative Ca balance during dialysis, avoid IDH
	Reduced venous return: UFR grossly exceeds PRR, blunted constriction of venous capacitance vessels, hypoalbuminemia	Reduction of UFR with prolonged treatment time, improve hypoalbuminemia; avoid mesenterial vasodilatation (no eating during HD), dialysate sodium $\geq$ plasma sodium, counseling on low sodium intake, avoid warm dialysate, apply isothermic dialysis by BTM
Reduced effective HR	Arrhythmia (AF most common), drugs (BB), autonomic neuropathy (especially in diabetes), tachycardia	Cardioversion (electrical or medical) with AF, reduction of BB, glucose control in diabetes, achieve adequacy targets
Reduction of TPR	Autonomic neuropathy, tissue ischemia, food intake (mesenteric vasodilatation), vasodilators, sympathicolytic agents, warm dialysate, anemia, hypoxia	Glucose control, achieve adequacy targets; achieve target Hct, avoid food during HD, predialysis midodrine, avoid warm dialysate, apply isothermic or cool dialysis, improve hemoglobin (ESAs) and oxygen saturation (treatment of concomitant lung disease), oxygen sympathicolytic agents after dialysis
High UFR		
High UFV	High IDWG (most important is salt input), wrongly low DW	Dietary counseling; avoid intradialytic salt loading; periodic reevaluation of DW
Short treatment time	Organizational time constraints, noncompliance, missed treatments	Prolonging dialysis time, more frequent dialysis, counseling on noncompliance, avoiding missed treatments, recognition of DW

ACE, angiotensin-converting enzyme; AF, atrial fibrillation; ARB, angiotensin receptor blocker; DW, dry weight; ESA, erythropoiesis-stimulating agent; HCM, hypertrophic cardiomyopathy; Hct, hematocrit; HR, heart rate; IDH, intradialytic hypokalemia; IDWG, interdialytic weight gain; LVH, left ventricular hypertrophy; PRR, plasma refilling rate; PTCA, percutaneous transluminal coronary angioplasty; UFR, ultrafiltration rate; UFV, ultrafiltration volume.

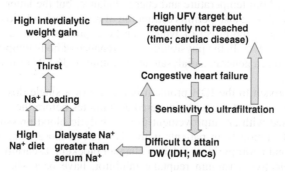

Figure 24.1

The relationship between salt, intradialytic weight gain (IDWG), and cardiac disease. A high dietary Na$^+$ intake or Na$^+$ loading during hemodialysis may result in postdialysis thirst and consequent drinking and weight gain. The high ultrafiltration volume (UFV) is frequently difficult to remove. With chronic fluid overload, congestive heart failure may ensue. Heart failure increases the patient's sensitivity to ultrafiltration and promotes intradialytic hypotension (IDH) and muscle cramps (MCs). These complications in turn are frequently treated by increasing the dialysate Na$^+$ concentration, which completes the circle. DW, dry weight.

A decrease of BV greater than 15% during an HD session sharply increases the risk of IDH. On the other hand, IDH is unusual with a BV decrease of less than 5%. BVM-guided feedback UF control is associated with reduced frequency of IDH. A randomized controlled trial to test whether BVM-guided UF adjustments results in reduction in IDH episodes is ongoing.

Maggiore first reported the biologic effects of cooling dialysate on systematic hypotensive episodes during dialysis. Increase in body core temperature occurs routinely during the dialytic procedures. Although initially considered the result of heat retention caused by vasoconstriction after fluid removal, this may not be the only major factor involved. Increased core temperature may cause centrally initialed vasodilatation, resulting in blood pressure decrease.

It was concluded from a systematic review of the clinical effects of reducing dialysate fluid temperature that IDH occurred 7.1 times less frequently with cool dialysis and that postdialysis MAP was higher with cool-temperature dialysis by 11.3 mm Hg. Is there an advantage to maintaining or reducing the core temperature by an automated feedback device (BTM, Fresenius Medical Care) as opposed to arbitrary reductions of dialysate temperature, the effect of which is variable depending on blood flow, UFR, plasma volume, the initial temperature of the patient, and possibly norepinephrine response? One major randomized trial provides evidence of effectiveness of increasing energy loss to maintain core temperature, with the percentage of hypotensive episodes reduced by 50%.

It was concluded that active control of body temperature by BTM can significantly improve intradialytic tolerance in hypotension-prone patients. Cooling dialysate temperature arbitrarily to one level could actually reduce core temperature too much, with consequent shivering and discomfort. The BTM at present provides the ability to change both temperature and energy balance, but the latter is not as clinically useful. The device also permits estimation of access recirculation by automated cooling of dialysate, the effect of which can be expressed as a rate of arterial to venous decreases. Overall, the physiologic maintenance of body temperature appears to be a useful tool. In general, a dialysate temperature of 36.5°C or less, as tolerated, should be used.

Another approach to the IDH problem is the use of a single dose (5–10 mg) of midodrine, an α_1-agonist drug administered 30 minutes before the dialysis session. This is associated with an improvement in intradialytic blood pressure. Midodrine should be used cautiously in patients with CHF and in those using beta-blockers, digoxin, and nondihydropyridine calcium channel blockers. L-carnitine therapy and sertraline, a selective serotonin reuptake inhibitor, have been shown to improve hemodynamic parameters in patients with IDH. However, these are not commonly used in clinical practice.

Symptomatic IDH should be treated promptly by reduction of UFR and bringing the patient to the Trendelenburg position. If despite this maneuver symptomatic IDH persists, 200 to 500 mL of 0.9% NaCl or 100 mL of 20% albumin (expensive but highly efficient) should be given. Most symptomatic episodes can be effectively treated with these interventions. If severe IDH persists, hypovolemia may not be the underlying cause, and an extended investigation (including physical examination, ECG, emergency echocardiography, and laboratory studies) is warranted. Arrhythmia, myocardial infarction, pericardial tamponade, hemorrhage, hemolysis, pulmonary embolism, and air embolism should be considered as differential diagnoses.

Muscle Cramps

Muscle cramps occur during 5% to 20% of HD sessions, leading to significant patient discomfort and occasionally HD termination. The etiology of HD-associated cramps is largely related to intravascular depletion and hyponatremia, but carnitine deficiency, hypomagnesemia, and elevated levels of leptin, a middle molecule, are implicated in the development of MCs. In the majority of cases, MCs represent potential precursors of IDH. MCs respond well to a single bolus of hypertonic saline (e.g., 10 mL 20% NaCl solution given over 2 to 4 minutes) or glucose (e.g., 20 mL 30% glucose solution given over 2 to 4 minutes). MCs are frequently observed in patients with DW targets below their "real" DW and thus have relatively high UFR. Preventive measures are similar to those discussed for IDH.

Dialyzer Reactions

There are two distinct types of dialyzer reactions, termed type A and type B. A type A reaction is anaphylactic in nature, and its incidence is 1 in 20 treatments. Ethylene oxide (ETO) has been incriminated in the majority of these cases. In patients taking angiotensin-converting enzyme (ACE) inhibitors and using AN69 membranes concomitantly, similar events have been observed. Allergy to heparin is another cause. Using ETO-free dialyzers and avoiding AN69 membranes in patients taking ACE inhibitors are recommended. Type A reaction manifests in the first 20 to 30 minutes. Stopping dialysis immediately without blood return is of paramount importance, and steroids, epinephrine, and H1 blockers may be needed. Type B reactions, uncommon now with synthetic membranes, are unspecific (with a poorly defined etiology). They are less severe, occur later in treatment, and manifest themselves with back and chest pain. Their treatment is supportive.

Pruritus occurring exclusively during dialysis is most likely caused by an allergy to one or more materials of the extracellular circuit. Chronic itching is often found in the presence of an elevated Ca x P product. Changing the membrane and the bloodline may be helpful. In addition, H1 blockers are used as a nonspecific treatment. In patients with febrile reactions during dialysis, bacteremia from vascular catheters should be considered as a prime possibility.

Dialysis Disequilibrium Syndrome

Dialysis disequilibrium syndrome (DES) occurs most frequently within the first few dialyses. It is thought to be caused by an acute increase in brain water for osmotic reasons because at the beginning, blood urea nitrogen may be very high. Common symptoms are headache, nausea, and vomiting. In severe cases, seizures and coma may occur. The treatment is supportive, and elevating dialysate glucose concentration to 200 mg/dL (11 mmol/L) is of help. DES can be prevented by keeping dialysis efficiency low (e.g., with a urea reduction ratio below 40%) during the first couple of treatments (low blood and dialysate flow; small dialyzer) and increasing dialysis efficacy slowly over the next 2 to 4 weeks. A dialysate sodium concentration below the serum sodium concentration may worsen DES.

Air Embolism

Air embolism is a rare but potentially fatal complication of HD. The arterial site, improperly connected bloodlines, and disconnected central venous catheters are potential sources of venous air embolism. In a sitting patient, intravascular air is more likely to cause reduction of cerebral perfusion, resulting in focal neurologic symptoms. In the event of air embolism, the venous line has to be clamped immediately and the patient placed in a recumbent position on the left side. The head should be placed as the lowest point.

Falls

Early postdialysis falls occur frequently. Low blood pressure, orthostatic dysregulation, impaired balance, slippery floors, and unstable footwear are the leading causes. Patients at risk (older persons, previous IDH, patients with diabetes) should be accompanied when walking to the scale after treatment. Balance and muscle strength can be improved by specifically tailored physiotherapy programs.

CHAPTER 25

Arrhythmias in Hemodialysis Patients

Claudio Rigatto, MD • Patrick S. Parfrey, MD

Cardiac rhythm disturbances are common in dialysis. Multiple studies have shown a high prevalence of ventricular and atrial ectopy and conduction abnormalities in hemodialysis (HD) patients, reflecting both the proarrhythmic nature of the HD process itself and the high burden of structural heart disease in end-stage renal disease populations. The prevalence of chronic or recurrent rhythm disturbances, especially atrial fibrillation (AF), is 50% to 100% higher than in the general population. Treatment of arrhythmias in dialysis patients can be challenging, and, in many instances, the risk-to-benefit ratio of many therapies is altered or uncertain.

This chapter summarizes what is known about the etiology and management of rhythm disturbances in HD. The major emphasis is on chronic management of arrhythmias in dialyzed patients, especially AF. Because the acute management of life-threatening unstable arrhythmias deviates little from current advanced cardiac life support (ACLS) guidelines, only important differences are highlighted. The reader is encouraged to review the latest ACLS guidelines.

It should be remembered that most of the recommendations in this chapter are based on imperfect or evolving data mostly in nondialysis patients. In the future, direct evidence in HD populations may help refine the arguments presented here.

Etiology and Prognosis

Both patient factors and dialysis factors contribute to arrhythmic risk. Significant underlying cardiac disease, present in the majority of HD patients, is independently associated with conduction disturbances, atrial and ventricular ectopy, and death. Superimposed on this substrate, changes in volume and extracellular ion composition during dialysis enhance myocardial irritability (Table 25.1). Ventricular and atrial ectopy are more frequent during dialysis than in the interdialytic period. Both atrial (p-wave) and ventricular (t-wave) dispersion increase during dialysis, enhancing the likelihood of reentrant arrhythmias. Rapid extracellular fluid (ECF) volume fluxes are associated with catecholamine surges and subendocardial ischemia, which are, in turn, associated with ventricular ectopy. Rapid lowering of potassium, particularly in patients taking cardiac glycosides, is arrhythmogenic, and attenuation of these changes by stepwise ramping of dialysate potassium during dialysis seems to reduce ventricular ectopy. Many of the cardiac drugs commonly used in HD patients (e.g., digitalis preparations) exhibit arrhythmogenic toxicities because of altered pharmacokinetics, end-organ effects, or both.

The prognostic impact of arrhythmias in HD patients is incompletely defined. Frequent or complex ventricular ectopy is associated with decreased survival, but

Table 25.1

Factors That May Precipitate Arrhythmias During Hemodialysis

Digitalis
Acute volume shifts
Hypokalemia
Hypocalcemia
Hypomagnesemia
Myocardial ischemia

this effect is not independent of age, hypertension, and underlying heart disease and may simply be a marker of poor cardiac status.

Management

General Considerations

Unstable Rhythms

Acute unstable or life-threatening rhythms, defined as heart rhythms associated with chest pain or evidence of circulatory insufficiency (e.g., frank shock, hypotension, impaired mentation), should be managed as per current advanced cardiovascular life support (ACLS) guidelines. As a general rule, the dialysis procedure should be stopped unless a clear metabolic precipitant correctable by dialysis is present (e.g., hyperkalemia induced heart block). Intravenous access via the fistula or central line should be maintained. Because a thorough discussion of ACLS procedures is beyond the scope of this chapter, readers are encouraged to download the latest edition of the ACLS recommendations (see Recommended Reading). Any additional considerations in HD patients are discussed under specific rhythm disturbances.

Avoiding Arrhythmogenic Triggers

Avoidance of arrhythmogenic stimuli during dialysis may be helpful, particularly in patients in whom dialysis reliably precipitates arrhythmias. Measures such as strict control of interdialytic fluid gain and potassium intake may decrease the need for aggressive ultrafiltration and low potassium dialysate. Substitution of normal instead of the usual elevated calcium bath may be helpful. Discontinuation of arrhythmogenic drugs (e.g., cardiac glycosides) should be seriously considered. Conversion to an alternative dialysis modality, such as peritoneal dialysis, short daily HD, or long hours of nocturnal HD can be tried if other measures fail.

Treatment of Underlying Cardiac Disease

Aggressive medical and surgical therapy of underlying cardiac disease has been shown to prolong life and decrease morbidity in the general population. In contrast, with few exceptions, specific antiarrhythmic therapy does not prolong life and may increase mortality rates in patients with heart disease. In HD patients with arrhythmias, a search for and aggressive treatment of ischemic heart disease (IHD) and left ventricular dysfunction is probably more important than antiarrhythmic therapy.

Appropriate indications for established lifesaving therapies such as aspirin, beta-blockers, angiotensin-converting enzyme (ACE) inhibitors, and coronary revascularization are discussed elsewhere.

Specific Rhythm Disturbances

Ventricular Ectopy

Ventricular ectopic beats (also called ventricular premature contractions) are a common rhythm disturbance in dialysis. They may be precipitated or exacerbated by acute changes in volume and ECF composition. Minimizing these alterations may reduce or eliminate the ectopy (see Table 25.1). Medications should be reviewed to identify and stop medications associated with proarrhythmia (e.g., domperidone). Blood chemistry should be reviewed to identify and correct derangements in calcium, potassium, and magnesium.

Complex ventricular ectopy is usually associated with underlying structural heart disease. Underlying cardiac disease should be aggressively sought and treated. A cardiac history, electrocardiography, echocardiography, and cardiac perfusion scan are reasonable investigations to request in this regard. Referral to a cardiologist is indicated if significant cardiac disease is identified because treatment (e.g., coronary revascularization) will typically improve symptoms. In addition, cardiology referral is also indicated in patients with persistent ectopy despite review and optimization of the dialysis prescription and medications or if ectopy is complex or associated with persistent symptoms. Further therapeutic options for symptomatic patients or patients with frequent ectopic rhythms may include catheter ablation of an ectopic focus and consideration of an implantable cardioverter defibrillator (ICD) in patients meeting ICD criteria.

Ventricular Tachycardia

A wide QRS complex characterizes ventricular tachycardia (VT). The complexes may be identical (monomorphic) or variable (polymorphic). Polymorphic VT often oscillates between high and low amplitude as if the electrical axis were twisting (torsades de pointes).

Although a wide complex rhythm can be supraventricular (SVT) in origin, it is ventricular in more than 90% of patients who are older than 65 years of age or who have known structural heart disease. ECG-based criteria have been developed to help distinguish supraventricular from ventricular rhythms, but they are cumbersome to use and have poor predictive values for SVT given the low pretest probability of SVT in such patients. Wide complex tachycardia (WCT) in dialysis patients should be treated as VT unless the patient has known recurrent SVT with aberrancy.

Acute management of monomorphic and polymorphic VT is the same for dialysis patients as it is for nondialysis patients. These approaches are well summarized in the current ACLS guidelines and will not be elaborated on here because they require no modification. Polymorphic VT may be the result of hypomagnesemia, which should be corrected, or medications such as quinine, domperidone, metoclopramide, or antiarrhythmic drugs (e.g., sotalol, amiodarone), which should be discontinued. Long-term management depends on the underlying cause (e.g., coronary heart disease, cardiomyopathy), and some patients may require ICD implantation if indicated.

Paroxysmal Supraventricular Tachycardia

Paroxysmal supraventricular tachycardia (PSVT) is usually caused by an atrioventricular (AV) nodal reentrant circuit and rarely by an auxiliary AV bypass tract (Wolff-Parkinson-White [WPW] syndrome). Synchronized electrical cardioversion is the treatment of choice for patients with evidence of hemodynamic instability (e.g., systolic blood pressure <90 mm Hg, congestive heart failure [CHF], chest pain, or altered mental status). Termination of stable PSVT can be accomplished with vagal maneuvers (carotid sinus massage) or the use of AV nodal blocking agents, such as adenosine, diltiazem, or metoprolol, as described in the ACLS guidelines. Chronic therapy is rarely necessary for PSVT. In patients with recurrent symptomatic PSVT or WPW, catheter ablation of the reentrant pathway is the therapy of choice.

Atrial Fibrillation

Atrial fibrillation is the most common chronic arrhythmia in dialysis patients, having a prevalence of about 12% (range, 3%-27%) and an incidence of about 3 events (range, 1-6) per 100 patient years. These rates are about double the rates reported for older adults (age older than 55 years) in the United States general population.

Atrial fibrillation may be chronic (i.e., always present), persistent, or paroxysmal. Persistent AF is defined as AF that lasts for longer than 7 days or has required cardioversion for termination of the rhythm. Paroxysmal AF is self-terminating, usually within 24 to 48 hours, and is often recurrent. Valvular AF refers to AF occurring in the setting of valvular heart disease (e.g., rheumatic mitral valve disease) and has a much higher embolic risk than nonvalvular AF.

The significance of AF is twofold. First, it is a marker of probable underlying structural heart disease that should be investigated and treated. Second, it may be associated with a significantly elevated risk of embolic stroke in dialysis patients. This second point, and its corollary, whether anticoagulation with warfarin should be prescribed to all dialysis patients with nonvalvular AF, is the subject of significant current debate and uncertainty, as will be discussed below.

Approach to New-Onset Atrial Fibrillation in the Dialysis Unit

New onset of AF during the dialysis procedure is not a rare event. Some patients have significant symptoms (chest pain, heart failure [HF]) or hemodynamic instability and require immediate transfer to a monitored setting (e.g., emergency department, coronary care unit) for management by a cardiologist. However, many patients remain asymptomatic. In these cases, the diagnosis is typically made when the nurse notes a fast irregular pulse, and an ECG is ordered, which confirms AF. In our opinion, such stable cases can be managed in an outpatient setting (Fig. 25.1), provided that a low clinical probability of acute coronary syndrome (ACS), HF, pulmonary thromboembolism (PTE), or sepsis can be established.

Our approach therefore, is to obtain a focused cardiovascular history and physical examination, an ECG, cardiac enzymes, chest radiographs, a complete blood count,

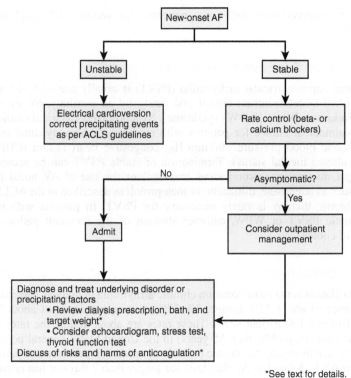

Figure 25.1

Overview of the treatment of acute atrial fibrillation (AF) in hemodialysis patients. ACLS, advanced cardiac life support.

and a transcutaneous O_2 saturation before the dialysis treatment is over. If the clinical suspicion of ACS, PTE, or sepsis is low; the ancillary tests above are negative or normal; the ventricular rate is less than 150 beats/min; and the patient is otherwise relatively high functioning, then outpatient management is selected. An oral rate control agent is prescribed, and the first dose is given in the unit (see section on rate control). We typically defer the decision to anticoagulate (see section on anticoagulation) pending a more thorough risk-to-benefit discussion in follow-up. The dialysis bath, ultrafiltration profile, and patient dry weight are reviewed and altered if possible to make them less arrhythmogenic (see general considerations provided earlier). The patient is then sent home at the end of the treatment, with instructions to return to the emergency department if symptoms or problems arise.

The rate of spontaneous termination of acute AF in nondialysis settings is high: 30% at 3 hours, 60% by 24 hours, and close to 80% by 48 hours. Although data are not available for dialysis, we have observed that many patients spontaneously convert to sinus rhythm (SR) by the time they present for their next dialysis treatment. In most cases, the rate control agent may be discontinued if there is spontaneous conversion to SR. At this time, an echocardiogram and an imaging cardiac stress test (e.g., adenosine sestamibi perfusion study) are requested to look for treatable structural heart disease, and thyroid function is assessed to exclude hypothyroidism. Finally, a careful weighing of the benefits and harms of anticoagulation for stroke prevention as described later is undertaken.

Readers are reminded that this approach is based on opinion and clinical experience and not on evidence from randomized controlled trials (RCTs).

Rate Control

Calcium blockers and beta-blockers are good first line agents for rate control in most patients. Beta-blockers should be avoided in patients with reactive airway disease. Although digoxin is effective at rest, it is less effective than either beta or calcium blockers in controlling the heart rate during exercise. Moreover, toxicity can be a problem in dialysis patients. For these reasons, it is considered a second line agent. Most guidelines recommend titration of the rate control agent to achieve a resting heart rate of 80 to 90 beats/min. Chronic heart rates above 130 beats/min have been associated with cardiomyopathy.

The approach to rate control paroxysmal AF is similar, although control of the rate during paroxysms may be more difficult. People with very rare paroxysms who tolerate a fast ventricular response well can probably forego chronic AV nodal-blocking drugs. Digoxin is poorly efficacious in paroxysmal AF and is not recommended. Beta-blockers and nondihydropyridine calcium channel blockers can successfully control ventricular rates during paroxysmal AF.

Stroke Prevention

Nonvalvular atrial fibrillation. In the general population, there is strong, concordant RCT evidence that anticoagulation with warfarin is superior to antiplatelet therapy for prevention of stroke and all-cause death in patients with nonvalvular AF. The evidence is much less clear in dialysis patients, however (extensively reviewed in Clase et al). Although the risk of stroke is higher, the risk of bleeding is also much higher, especially for catastrophic bleeding; for example, intracranial hemorrhage risk is 2.6%/year in dialysis patients on warfarin versus 0.4% per year in nondialysis cohorts. This increased risk of catastrophic bleeding may well nullify any net clinical benefit of anticoagulation. The efficacy of warfarin may also be lower in dialysis patients, further diminishing the benefit-to-risk ratio of treatment. Several recent, large, observational studies have noted a disturbing trend toward net harm in dialysis patients with AF treated with warfarin (reviewed in Clase et al). In the absence of direct RCT evidence in dialysis patients, it is unknown whether warfarin reduces the risk of stroke or death in dialysis patients with AF. This uncertainty is reflected in highly variable practice patterns worldwide. For example, fewer than 3% of dialysis patients with AF are anticoagulated with warfarin in Germany compared with 30% to 40% of AF patients on dialysis in the United States and Canada.

In the face of this knowledge gap, the practitioner has three possible, equally valid, options: (1) no anticoagulation, (2) anticoagulation as per recommendations in the general population ($CHA_2DS_2VASc > 1$, absent contraindication to warfarin), or (3) individualized care based on individual patient risks and preference. Of these options, we prefer the third (individualization). First, we formally calculate the CHA_2DS_2VASc (stroke risk) and HASBLED (bleeding risk) scores, mainly to see if either clotting (CHADS2DS2VASc) or bleeding (HASBLED) risk is dominant.

In most cases, both will be moderate-high. In these cases, we heavily weigh patient preference. Most patients are much more stroke averse than bleed averse, and unless there is a huge estimated risk of bleeding, most elect a trial of anticoagulation. If the consensus of patient and team is not to anticoagulate, we typically recommend continuing or starting antiplatelet therapy with aspirin.

Valvular atrial fibrillation. The risk of embolic stroke from valvular AF is much higher than from nonvalvular AF. Anticoagulation is probably reasonable for all patients with valvular heart disease (especially mitral).

New non–vitamin K antagonist anticoagulants. Several new direct thrombin inhibitors have been approved for anticoagulation in AF. The main advantages of these new agents over warfarin are a fixed dose administration and absent need for international normalized ratio monitoring. The major disadvantages are the long half-life and lack of reversibility in cases of bleeding or overdose. Of these agents, all of them except apixaban are contraindicated in kidney failure. The approval by the Food and Drug Administration for apixaban use in kidney failure was based solely on pharmacokinetic data and not on efficacy and safety data in this population. In the absence of such data, the concerns described above regarding warfarin therapy in dialysis patients also apply to apixaban.

Rhythm Control Versus Rate Control

Physicians have debated for years whether attempts should be made to achieve and maintain SR using drugs, cardioversion, catheter ablation, or various combinations of these, in nonvalvular AF. A recent meta-analysis of seven RCTs concluded that rate control and rhythm control are equivalent in terms of major clinical outcomes (all-cause death, cardiovascular death, and stroke). There was insufficient evidence to conclude whether catheter ablation was better than pharmacologic interventions. Thus, given equivalent efficacy, we generally recommend a rate control approach because it is simpler, it is associated with lower health care costs, and there is less concern about the risks of antiarrhythmic drug therapy (e.g., torsades de pointes) or invasive procedures (radiofrequency catheter ablation).

Rhythm control strategies should be considered in individuals who remain symptomatic despite rate control (e.g., difficult to control rate, frequent heart failure episodes, frequent symptomatic palpitations). Given the added complexity and different risks of a rhythm control approach, we recommend such strategies be prescribed and supervised by a cardiologist.

Bradyarrhythmias

Bradycardia is defined as a heart rate less than 60 beats/min. Immediate treatment is indicated for cardiovascular instability (hypotension systolic blood pressure <90 mm Hg, CHF, acute myocardial infarction, or chest pain). Early transthoracic pacing, if available, is preferable to repeated doses of atropine. Reversible causes of bradycardia such as SA or AV node depression with drugs (digoxin, calcium channel blockers, beta-blockers) should be sought. Hyperkalemia may manifest as SA arrest or AV block with a junctional or ventricular escape rhythm in the absence of classical QRST changes. Temporization with intravenous calcium gluconate and insulin–glucose are useful until the patient is dialyzed. Many patients on dialysis may have chronic SA or AV nodal disease secondary to age, CAD, or calcification of the AV valve annuli. In these cases, a permanent pacemaker is required if a superimposed reversible cause is not identified or if there is either third-degree or type 2 second-degree AV block.

Cardiac Arrest in the Dialysis Unit

Cardiac arrest during a dialysis run is, fortunately, a rare event, occurring three or four times per 100,000 treatments. The usual rhythms associated with a pulseless state are ventricular fibrillation (VF), VT, asystole, and pulseless electrical activity (PEA). The ACLS guidelines for management of these rhythms are published elsewhere and require little modification. Only special considerations in dialysis patients are discussed below.

Asystole in the adult general population is most often an agonal rhythm. However, asystolic arrest in a HD patient may reflect profound bradyarrhythmia secondary to hyperkalemia. As discussed earlier, this phenomenon may occur in the absence of antecedent, classical QRST changes, particularly in patients with underlying SA and AV conduction problems who may not exhibit a junctional or ventricular escape rhythm. It should be suspected in patients arresting with asystole immediately before dialysis. Treatment with calcium gluconate and insulin–glucose may be lifesaving.

Cardiac tamponade in patients with uremic pericarditis is a correctable cause of PEA in HD patients. Immediate volume infusion to improve cardiac filling and pericardiocentesis to decompress the pericardial sac are necessary for survival.

The long-term prognosis of witnessed cardiac arrest in the HD unit is abysmal. Only 15% to 19% survive to 30 days, and only 7% to 9% make it to 1 year after the event.

Sudden Cardiac Death

Sudden cardiac death (SCD) is defined as death from an unexpected circulatory arrest, occurring within 1 hour of symptom onset, or an unwitnessed, unexpected death without obvious noncardiac cause in patients known to have been well within the previous 24 hours. The mechanism is thought to be arrhythmic in most cases. SCD accounts for about 25% of deaths among patients with kidney failure. As described earlier, very few of these events occur during dialysis, the majority occurring at home.

The optimal strategies to prevent SCD are not yet known (reviewed in Pun 2014). Because SCD is thought to result from arrhythmogenic triggers (e.g., ECF changes, hypokalemia) acting on an arrhythmogenic substrate (underlying uremic and coronary heart disease), a sensible approach emphasizes optimizing treatment of underlying cardiac disease and minimizing dialysis-related arrhythmia triggers (Table 25.2). The role of ICDs in the prevention of SCD in kidney failure patients is at present unclear. It seems reasonable to consider an ICD in dialysis patients who otherwise meet ICD criteria.

Digoxin Toxicity

Digoxin toxicity may manifest as atrial or ventricular ectopy, AF or atrial flutter, high-grade AV block, VT, or VF. Atrial flutter with 4 : 1 AV block is a classic presentation. Toxicity may result from an inappropriate dosage schedule in light of severely impaired excretion or concomitant use of drugs that increase digoxin levels

Table 25.2

Strategies for Managing Sudden Cardiac Death Risk in Kidney Failure Patients.

Strategy	Possible Intervention
Manage Underlying Cardiomyopathy	
Systolic heart dysfunction	Assess left ventricular systolic and diastolic function within 3 months of dialysis initiation and every 3 years thereafter. Use carvedilol in patients with dilated cardiomyopathy.
Diastolic heart dysfunction (LVH)	Consider frequent hemodialysis to reduce left ventricular mass; consider the use of ACE inhibitors or ARBs.
Minimize Arrhythmic Triggers	
Potassium shifts	Monitor potassium more frequently, especially after hospitalization, and change dialysis prescription accordingly. Avoid low-potassium (<2 mEq/L) baths.
Calcium shifts	Avoid low calcium baths, especially in the context of concurrent use of QT-prolonging medications.
Metabolic alkalosis	Account for acetate in dialysis acid concentrate to determine total buffer; avoid high-dialysate bicarbonate concentrations in patients who are alkalotic.
Rapid ultrafiltration	Encourage patient compliance with fluid restriction between treatments. Avoid sodium ramping and large dialysate/serum sodium gradients. Extend dialysis time to reduce ultrafiltration rate.
Dialysis-induced myocardial ischemia	Cool dialysate temperature
Weigh Benefits and Risks of Implantable Cardioverter Defibrillators	
	Consider secondary prevention ICDs after cardiac arrest

ACE, angiotensin-converting enzyme; ARB, angiotensin receptor blocker; ICD, implantable cardioverter defibrillator; LVH, left ventricular hypertrophy.
Adapted from Pun PH. The interplay between CKD, sudden cardiac death, and ventricular arrhythmias. *Adv Chronic Kidney Dis* 2014;21(6):480-488.

(e.g., erythromycin, quinidine, verapamil, amiodarone). Acute lowering of serum potassium concentration during dialysis may further exacerbate toxicity. If suspected, digoxin should be stopped. Unstable rhythms need to be electrically cardioverted (VT) or defibrillated (VF). Stable ventricular arrhythmias can be treated with lidocaine or procainamide. Cardioversion should be avoided because of the risk of precipitating VF in this setting. In severe cases, consideration should be given to antidigoxin Fab therapy. Often, superior alternatives to digoxin exist for chronic therapy of heart failure or arrhythmias (e.g., ACE inhibitors for CHF), and consideration should be given to switching to these alternative drugs.

Summary

Arrhythmias are frequent in dialysis patients. They are often a reflection of underlying structural heart disease, which should be aggressively sought and treated. Mitigation of large or rapid swings in ECF volume and electrolyte composition may minimize triggering of arrhythmias during dialysis, and the dialysis prescription should be modified accordingly. The role of ICDs in prevention of fatal ventricular arrhythmias and SCD is not yet clear.

CHAPTER 26

Prevention and Therapeutic Management of Bleeding in Dialysis Patients

Federica Mescia, MD • Paola Boccardo, BiolSciD • Miriam Galbusera, BiolSciD • Giuseppe Remuzzi, MD, FRCP

The association between uremia and a bleeding tendency has been well established since its first appearance in the literature in 1764 in Morgagni's *Opera Omnia*. Most of the landmark studies on the pathogenesis and treatment of uremic bleeding were carried out in the 1970 and 1980s, when the key role of platelet dysfunction was clearly demonstrated. Modern dialysis techniques and the use of recombinant erythropoietin have markedly reduced hemorrhagic risk in end-stage renal disease (ESRD) patients; nonetheless, bleeding remains a frequent complication in this setting. For example, among the control group of a clinical trial, 24% of hemodialysis (HD) patients experienced clinically significant bleeding over less than 1 year. The clinical manifestations vary from minor events, such as ecchymoses, epistaxis, mucosal bleeds, or bleeding from venipuncture sites to life-threatening hemorrhages. Compared with the general population, patients with ESRD have a 10-fold greater risk of cerebral hemorrhage, a 10- to 20-fold higher risk of subdural hematomas, and a 100-fold increase in the risk of gastrointestinal (GI) bleeding. Hemorrhagic pericarditis is a well-known serious complication of uremia, which is still rarely seen in patients with advanced renal failure or inadequate dialysis. Bleeding events carry a significant burden of morbidity and mortality. Prevention is fundamental to minimize bleeding risk in dialysis patients and, in the case of hemorrhages, issues specific to ESRD patients need to be addressed in order to offer optimal treatment.

Pathogenesis of Uremic Bleeding

The pathogenesis of uremic bleeding is multifactorial but most important is a defect in primary hemostasis, involving platelet–platelet and platelet–vessel wall interactions. Of note, prothrombotic abnormalities in coagulation and fibrinolysis pathways often coexist with platelet defects in uremic patients, who represent a unique population at simultaneously increased risk of both bleeding and thrombosis.

Platelet Dysfunction and Uremic Toxins

Thrombocytopenia, caused by inadequate production or platelet overconsumption, is commonly found in ESRD patients but is usually mild or moderate and only rarely severe enough to cause bleeding. Numerous platelet biochemical changes and functional abnormalities have been documented in uremic patients, together leading to defective primary hemostasis. Platelet dense granules from patients with advanced chronic kidney disease (CKD) present reduced levels of the aggregation agonists serotonin and adenosine diphosphate (ADP) and an increase in the ratio of adenosine triphosphate (ATP) to ADP. Arachidonic acid and prostaglandin metabolism is deregulated in uremia; synthesis or release of thromboxane A2 is impaired, resulting in reduced platelet adhesion and aggregation, and plasma levels of prostacyclin, a platelet inhibitor and vasodilator, are increased. Elevation in prostacyclin and pathologic hyperactivity of platelet adenylate cyclase cooperate in increasing intracellular levels of cyclic adenosine monophosphate (cAMP), which in turn contributes to impaired platelet aggregation.

Platelets from uremic patients also undergo enhanced proteolysis of glycoprotein Ib (GPIb), resulting in reduced availability of GPIb on the cell surface. GPIb is a key component of the GPIb/V/IX complex, an adhesion receptor that binds von Willebrand factor (VWF) and collagen and is responsible for platelet capture to the subendothelium at sites of vascular damage. Platelet adhesion to subendothelial surfaces leads to activation of the glycoprotein IIb–IIIa receptor complex (GPIIb-IIIa), another platelet receptor that binds VWF and fibrinogen. Defective function of IIb-IIIa is an additional constant finding in uremic patients that has been ascribed to competitive binding of the receptor by fibrinogen fragments and possibly other dialyzable toxic substances that accumulate in uremic plasma.

Release of platelet α-granule proteins, including β-thromboglobulin, and thrombin-induced secretion of ATP are impaired in uremia. Intracellular calcium content is increased in platelets from uremic patients, and mobilization of these calcium stores after different stimuli is abnormal, which can result in functional platelet defects. The platelet cytoskeletal contraction system is dysfunctional in the uremic milieu, hindering platelet motility and secretory function.

Soluble plasma factors play a key role in determining platelet defects, consistent with the observation that, after mixing with plasma from healthy subjects, uremic platelets show improvement of many functional parameters, but mixing of uremic plasma with normal platelets leads to platelet dysfunction. The already cited elevation in prostacyclin and fibrinogen fragments, together with reduced thromboxane A2 in uremia, partially account for these findings. The metabolites phenol, phenolic acid, and guanidinosuccinic acid rise in CKD and impair platelet aggregation to ADP in vitro. On the other hand, several uremic solutes such as urea, creatinine, and guanidoacetic acid do not significantly interfere with platelet function when added to normal plasma. Parathyroid hormone (PTH) has been consistently shown to impair platelet aggregation in vitro, but its clinical relevance in influencing hemostasis has been questioned because of the lack of correlation between skin bleeding time and serum concentrations of intact PTH or PTH fragments in dialysis patients.

Higher than normal plasma concentrations of the stable nitric oxide (NO) metabolites, nitrites and nitrates, have been well documented in uremic animals. NO, produced by endothelial cells and platelets, may interfere with hemostasis by inhibiting platelet aggregation and by preventing the vasoconstriction that normally follows vessel injury. Plasma from HD patients, unlike normal plasma, strongly induces NO synthesis in cultured human microvascular endothelial cells. Increased NO synthesis is likely the main mechanism by which the uremic toxins guanidinosuccinic acid and methylguanidine interfere with platelet function. Cytokines such as tumor necrosis factor-α (TNF-α) and interleukin-1β (IL-1β), which increase in the setting of CKD, are also potent activators of the inducible isoform of NO synthase.

Chronic volume overload in dialysis patients has been proposed to be an additional factor predisposing to bleeding and, in particular, to increase the risk of spontaneous subdural hematomas. The putative pathogenic mechanism entails venous hypertension, predisposing to small venous tears of dural bridging veins.

Anemia

Anemia is a common finding in ESRD patients and has a multifactorial origin, encompassing shortened survival of red blood cells (RBCs) in the uremic milieu; reduced responsiveness of the erythroid marrow; repeated blood loss during dialysis; and, most important, defective secretion of erythropoietin. Anemia plays a key role in uremic bleeding, mainly through rheologic factors. At a low hematocrit, platelets tend to be dispersed along the blood vessels, which impairs their interaction with the vascular walls. At a hematocrit above 30%, erythrocytes mainly localize at the center of the vessels, and platelets are displaced more peripherally, closer to the endothelial surface, where their efficiency in forming a plug, when exposed to the subendothelium, is optimized. RBCs also stimulate the release of platelet aggregation agonists ADP and thromboxane A2, inactivate prostacyclin, and scavenge NO by hemoglobin. In the setting of anemia, all of these effects of RBCs are significantly impaired, further contributing to the bleeding diathesis.

Effects of Dialysis

Dialysis can have opposing effects on hemostasis. On the one hand, it allows removal of the uremic toxins that induce platelet dysfunction and hemostatic derangements. As a proof of concept, for example, skin bleeding time is significantly shortened, albeit rarely normalized, in uremic patients after the initial dialysis sessions. However, dialysis cannot effectively remove all uremic retention solutes, especially those with high molecular weight or protein bound, and thus only partially corrects uremia.

Importantly, dialysis itself can increase bleeding risk, especially in the case of HD, in which blood comes in contact with the extracorporeal circuit and systemic anticoagulation is usually required. In patients on chronic HD, skin bleeding time is often longer right after the dialysis session than before, an effect independent on heparin use. Despite significant advances in biocompatibility with current HD technology, exposure of blood to the dialyzer membrane, to circuit tubing, and to microbubbles in the circuit and to shear stress, particularly in the roller pump segment, inevitably leads to a certain degree of activation of platelets, inflammatory cells, coagulation, and the complement system. As well documented also in the setting of cardiopulmonary bypass, continual platelet activation can bring about mild thrombocytopenia and transient functional platelet exhaustion caused by reiterated degranulation and loss of glycoprotein receptors. The platelet count is typically around 180,000/mmc in HD patients, below the average of 250,000/mmc in the general population. Various studies have consistently shown that the platelet count slightly falls (typically 5%–15%) during the first 15 to 30 minutes of HD and then returns to the predialysis level or overshoots it slightly by the end of the treatment. Platelets taken from the dialyzer outlet blood display surface markers of activation and degranulation and form spontaneous platelet–platelet and platelet–leukocyte aggregates, the clinical significance of which is unknown. In vitro platelet aggregation, assayed through different tests, has been found either to be unaffected or, more frequently, to decrease during HD, consistent with functional exhaustion.

In the course of the HD session, hemostasis is modulated also by oscillations in the plasma levels of NO, which are the result of two opposing processes. HD removes uremic toxins that stimulate NO synthesis and, at the same time, activates inflammation pathways in the extracorporeal circuit, raising the levels of potent NO inducers such as the cytokines TNF-α and IL-1β. In particular, NO induction has been attributed to complement-activating dialyzer membranes, acetate-containing dialysate, and dialysate contamination by intact endotoxin, endotoxin fragments, and other bacterial toxins that may cross the dialysis membrane. The current use of synthetic, more biocompatible membranes; the widespread availability of bicarbonate dialysis; and the adoption of more and more stringent standards of dialysate purity could hopefully tip the balance toward a net reduction in NO during HD, thus improving hemostasis.

Administration of anticoagulants to avoid circuit clotting during HD is an additional factor that can raise bleeding risk. In particular, heparin, the drug most widely used for this purpose, is known to promote platelet self-aggregation and activation through nonimmunogenic mechanisms, which can exacerbate the functional alterations generated by the extracorporeal circulation. These effects of heparin are distinct from the rare idiosyncratic heparin-induced thrombocytopenia, a serious immuno-mediated thrombophilic condition.

From the standpoint of bleeding risk, peritoneal dialysis (PD) presents clear theoretical advantages over HD, by avoiding the need of intradialytic anticoagulation and the exposure of blood to the extracorporeal circuit. Compared with patients on HD, those on PD often have a shorter skin bleeding time and display fewer derangements in platelet functional in vitro studies. Along the same line, epidemiologic studies have documented a lower incidence of GI and intracranial bleeding in PD patients compared to HD patients. For example, in a large cohort study in Taiwan, the risk of bleeding from peptic ulcers was significantly higher in HD patients compared with patients on PD. Nonetheless, the hemorrhagic risk in patients on PD remained elevated compared with that seen in the general population and was comparable to that of patients with stage 4 to 5 CKD: Relative to subjects with normal renal function, hazard ratios for peptic ulcer bleeding were 3 to 4 in CKD patients and those on PD and were almost 12 in HD patients.

Medications

Because of their comorbidities, ESRD patients are often treated with anticoagulant and antiplatelet agents. Compared with the general population, these drugs increase bleeding risk more markedly in uremic patients, likely through both pharmacokinetic and pharmacodynamic mechanisms. For example, some medications, such as low-molecular-weight heparins (LMWHs) and fondaparinux, rely on a primarily renal metabolism and tend to accumulate in ESRD patients. Bleeding risk caused by bioaccumulation is significantly raised also with the new oral anticoagulants, targeting either thrombin (e.g., dabigatran) or factor Xa (e.g., apixaban), which are contraindicated in ESRD. Furthermore, β-lactam antibiotics accumulate in advanced renal failure and may perturb platelet membrane, interfering with the adenosine diphosphate receptor and therefore inhibiting platelet aggregation. These effects are dose and duration dependent and resolve after discontinuation of the drugs. Among the β-lactam antibiotics, third-generation cephalosporins may affect hemostasis the most because of concomitant interference with the coagulation cascade, in addition to platelet inhibition.

On the other hand, the uremic milieu might also alter pharmacologic activity; this has been demonstrated for aspirin, which causes a transient, cyclooxygenase-independent marked prolongation of the bleeding time in uremic patients but not in normal subjects.

Nonsteroidal antiinflammatory drugs (NSAIDs) increase hemorrhagic risk by both reversibly inhibiting platelet cyclooxygenase and directly disrupting the integrity of the GI mucosa.

Clinical and Laboratory Findings

The most common bleeding complications in uremia are minor skin and mucosal hemorrhages, such as petechiae, blood blisters, ecchymoses at venipuncture sites, and trivial bleeds from the oral and nasal mucosa. Moreover, women on dialysis frequently present with abnormal uterine bleeding, for which as many as 10% of patients may require gynecologic intervention.

Most major bleeding events originate from the GI tract. The sources of upper GI hemorrhage in uremic patients are similar to those in patients with normal renal function and include gastric and duodenal ulcers, vascular ectasias, gastric erosions, esophagitis, Mallory-Weiss tears, and gastric cancer. Hemorrhoids, colonic diverticular disease, and polyps are common sources of lower GI hemorrhages both in dialysis patients and people with normal renal function. Angiodysplasias (telangiectasias, arteriovenous malformations) are small vascular lesions of the GI mucosa and submucosa that may cause acute or subacute hemorrhage. They have been observed in any tract of the GI system and have been reported as a cause of bleeding more frequently in dialysis patients than in the general population. It is not clear whether this finding reflects a higher incidence of angiodysplasias in the setting of CKD or an increased risk for these lesions to bleed and thus to be diagnosed in dialysis patients. Ischemic colitis is another important differential diagnosis in dialysis patients with lower GI bleeding, especially in those with widespread vascular disease and prone to intradialytic hypotension. Alternative rare causes of digestive hemorrhage, such as Kaposi sarcoma, cytomegalovirus colitis, and non-Hodgkin lymphoma, need to be considered in dialysis patients with concomitant severe immunodepression, such as those with HIV nephropathy or a history of long-term exposure to immunosuppressant drugs for kidney transplantation or immunomediated systemic diseases.

Other severe, albeit less common, hemorrhagic events are intracranial bleedings, including subdural hematomas, intracerebral hemorrhages, and subarachnoid hemorrhages. ESRD patients are more prone to intracranial bleedings than the general population, and such events are often spontaneous, without apparent trauma. Brain magnetic resonance imaging studies have also shown that small hemosiderin deposits, indicative of prior microscopic cerebral hemorrhage, are highly prevalent among HD patients. These alterations, known as cerebral microbleeds, are closely associated with other cerebral small-vessel diseases and likely contribute to cognitive dysfunction; age and high blood pressure are significant risk factors.

Limited, fibrinous pericardial and pleural effusions are common findings in patients with advanced renal failure. Without adequate dialysis, serous effusion can undergo hemorrhagic transformation, leading to life-threatening uremic pericarditis, with possible tamponade, or pleuritis. These presentations used to be frequent in the predialysis era and are now rarely encountered, but they remain medical emergencies that require prompt recognition and treatment, the core of management being intensive, anticoagulant-free dialysis.

Renal cysts frequently occur in dialysis-associated renal cystic disease and can occasionally give rise to unprovoked bleeding, ranging from asymptomatic, trivial intracystic hemorrhage to massive retroperitoneal hematomas. Spontaneous severe intraocular bleedings have been occasionally reported in dialysis patients; minor subconjunctival hemorrhages or self-limited bleeds after cataract surgery are by far more common. Subcapsular liver hematoma is another serious hemorrhagic complication that has been rarely observed in uremic patients.

Notably, patients with CKD from autosomal dominant polycystic kidney disease may be at higher than average bleeding risk, caused by predisposing anatomic abnormalities such as kidney and liver cysts, an elevated frequency of colon diverticulosis, and susceptibility to develop intracranial aneurysms.

Finally, despite the current improvements in standards of care, major surgery and invasive procedures, including kidney or liver biopsy, still entail perioperative hemorrhagic risks that are elevated to a greater extent in dialysis patients than in the general population, with subsequent higher morbidity and mortality.

Extensive efforts have been made to find out which abnormal laboratory findings in uremia can best predict clinically significant bleeding. Urea or creatinine levels alone do not correlate well with hemorrhagic risk. Coagulation assays (prothrombin time and activated partial thromboplastin time) are usually within limits, and plasma levels of coagulation factors are normal (or clotting factors elevated) in ESRD patients, unless there is concomitant coagulopathy. Thrombocytopenia is rarely severe enough (<50,000/mmc) to significantly raise bleeding risk, but low hematocrit (<30%) is significantly associated with hemorrhagic diathesis in uremic patients.

The single assay that best correlates with uremic bleeding is skin bleeding time, an in vivo test measuring the primary phase of hemostasis. The skin bleeding time is most commonly determined using the Ivy method. A blood pressure cuff is applied above the cubital fossa and inflated at 40 mm Hg to elevate venous pressure and increase test sensitivity. A small cut is made on the ventral side of the subject's forearm in an area where there are no hairs or visible veins. The cut is done quickly by an automatic device, which provides a standardized width and depth. The blood is blotted away every 30 seconds by filter paper until the platelet plug forms and the bleeding terminates. The time it takes for the bleeding to stop is measured and represents the skin bleeding time. Normal values are below 7 minutes; prolongation above 10 minutes correlates with a significantly increased risk of bleeding in uremic patients. The skin bleeding time was established as a predictor of hemorrhagic events in CKD patients in the 1970s and suffers from poor reproducibility and accuracy; nonetheless, it remains the best available test at present.

Several in vitro assays of platelet function have been developed, such as closure time test (also known as platelet function analyzer or PFA-100, which measures platelet aggregation in response to ADP and epinephrine), whole blood platelet aggregation (WBPA), thromboelastography (TEG), and cone platelet analyzer (CPA). However, none of these tests has been validated in clinical practice in the setting of uremic bleeding, and their use remains investigational.

Prevention of Bleeding in Dialysis Patients

Guidelines for the management of hemorrhagic complications of uremia are outlined in Table 26.1.

Dialysis Prescription

The incidence and severity of hemorrhagic complications in ESRD patients decreased significantly after dialysis became available for widespread use. Adequate dialysis is the mainstay in the prevention of uremic bleeding. However, as already discussed, current dialysis technologies allow only partial correction of the bleeding diathesis associated with uremia, and HD in particular interferes with hemostasis.

For these reasons, in the absence of other contraindications, PD is a reasonable choice for patients with clinical conditions that put them at particularly high bleeding risk.

As part of the HD prescription, intradialytic anticoagulation needs to be personalized, balancing individual thrombotic and hemorrhagic risks. The minimum dose of heparin effective in preventing circuit clotting should be determined for each patient. Reduced intensity intradialytic anticoagulation is a sensible option in patients treated with oral anticoagulants: In many such cases, even complete avoidance of intradialytic anticoagulation is feasible, provided that the INR is within the target range, there is minimal inflammation, an autologous vascular access with adequate blood flow rate is available, and synthetic high-flux membranes are used.

As detailed elsewhere in this textbook, use of minimum-dose heparin or no-heparin HD is possible in patients at high bleeding risk at the cost of increasing the possibility of circuit clotting. Regional citrate anticoagulation, if locally implemented, is a useful alternative.

Table 26.1

Guidelines for the Management of Hemorrhagic Complications of Uremia

- For patients with hemorrhagic complications or undergoing major surgery, the dialysis prescription should be carefully reviewed, ensuring adequacy and personalizing intradialytic anticoagulation.
- Correction of anemia by red blood cell transfusion or erythropoiesis-stimulating agents (or both) is the first key step in the prevention and treatment of uremic bleeding. The hematocrit should be kept above 30% to improve hemostasis.
- Desmopressin acetate can be useful to improve hemostasis during acute bleeding episodes. It can be administered intravenously ($0.3\,\mu g/kg$ added to 50 mL of saline over 30 minutes), subcutaneously ($0.3\,\mu g/kg$), or intranasally ($3\,\mu g/kg$). The effect of desmopressin acetate has a fast onset but lasts only a few hours. Desmopressin loses efficacy after repeated administrations.
- Conjugated estrogens, given by intravenous infusion in a cumulative dose of 3 mg/kg as a daily divided dose (i.e., 0.6 mg/kg for 5 consecutive days), can be a useful adjunct to achieving long-lasting hemostasis in cases of persistent chronic bleeding.
- Because the favorable effect of cryoprecipitate on bleeding time has not been uniformly observed, we do not recommend its use.

When a central venous catheter is used as HD access, a heparin lock is an often underrecognized factor possibly contributing to bleeding risk. In fact, a certain degree of spillage of lock solution into the systemic circulation is practically inevitable and, if high-concentration heparin (5000–10,000 units/mL) is used, this can occasionally contribute to clinical bleeding. Low-dose heparin (1000 units/mL) or 4% citrate are safe and effective alternatives as lock solutions.

Anemia Treatment

Adequate treatment of kidney disease–related anemia is a cornerstone in the prevention of uremic bleeding. Use of recombinant human erythropoietin has largely replaced transfusions and significantly lowered hemorrhagic risk, after its widespread introduction into clinical practice in the late 1980s. Partial correction of anemia, increasing the hematocrit above 30%, consistently shortens bleeding time, likely by displacing platelets from a midstream position toward the vessel wall, thus encouraging platelet–endothelium interactions. In addition, recombinant human erythropoietin impacts hemostasis independently of anemia correction. For instance, it increases the number of reticulated platelets, which are more metabolically active, raises the density of GPIIb/IIIa receptors on the platelet surface, improves platelet calcium signaling, and enhances thrombin-induced phosphorylation of platelet proteins.

Appropriate Prescription of Antiplatelet and Anticoagulant Medications

Dialysis patients often take antiplatelet and anticoagulant medications for primary or secondary cardiovascular prevention. These drugs often result in a relatively higher increase in bleeding risk in ESRD patients than in those with preserved renal function, which should be considered in the risk-to-benefit assessment. For instance, in a systematic review, warfarin use in HD patients doubled the rate of major bleeding events compared with HD patients not taking warfarin. The absolute risk of major bleeding in ESRD patients on warfarin ranged from 0.10 to 0.54 events per patient-year, which was 10 times higher than rates for the general population. Studies looking at treatment with single antiplatelet agents in dialysis patients have yielded mixed results and have not consistently demonstrated a significant increase in hemorrhagic events. On the other hand, combination antiplatelet therapy appears to invariably raise bleeding risk in patients on HD. For example, major hemorrhage was noted in 7.6% of HD patients on a trial of aspirin and clopidogrel compared with 3.7% of nonuremic patients enrolled in the Clopidogrel in Unstable Angina to Prevent Recurrent Events (CURE) Trial, despite the use of the same two antiplatelet agents.

To further complicate decision making, we must consider that the indications for antiplatelet and anticoagulant medications derive from clinical trials that mostly excluded patients with advanced CKD. It is therefore unknown whether the risk-to-benefit profile demonstrated for these therapies in the general population can be reliably extrapolated to dialysis patients. For instance, several investigators have cast doubts on the overall clinical benefits of warfarin anticoagulation for prevention of thromboembolism in dialysis patients with atrial fibrillation. Based on retrospective case series, the efficacy of warfarin has not been consistently demonstrated in this setting, but clear potential for harm has emerged because of increased hemorrhagic risk. In addition, animal studies have highlighted an enhanced predisposition to vascular calcifications by warfarin, which could be of particular relevance in CKD patients.

Anticoagulant and antiplatelet agents are frequently prescribed also for preservation of HD access patency, despite the lack of clinical studies demonstrating clear-cut evidence of benefit for this indication. The excess in bleeding risk secondary to these therapies has been well documented instead, which should encourage critical revision of prescription appropriateness on a case-by-case basis.

Particular attention should be paid while prescribing LMWHs, which are primarily renally excreted and are therefore at risk of accumulation in dialysis patients. For this reason, many physicians prefer unfractionated heparin, that is administered intravenously or through multiple daily subcutaneous injections and can be easily monitored by activated partial thromboplastin time measurements. The convenience of less frequent dosing by the subcutaneous route still makes LMWHs an attractive alternative. In case LMWHs are chosen, the dose needs to be empirically reduced, for example, by 50%, and the effects should be monitored through the anti-Xa activity assay. Of note, anti-Xa monitoring may not be promptly available in all settings, and its use has not been validated in large trials.

New oral anticoagulants have not been studied in ESRD patients. They are eliminated through the kidneys and, in the absence of clinical data on putative dose adjustments, their use is contraindicated in dialysis patients. Nonetheless, a recent report has documented that as many as 5.9% of anticoagulated dialysis patients in the United States are currently started on dabigatran or rivaroxaban, which carry a higher risk of hospitalization or death from bleeding when compared with warfarin.

Proton Pump Inhibitors

Preliminary reports, based on limited case series or small randomized clinical trials, suggest that preventive use of low-dose proton pump inhibitors (PPIs) reduces the risk of upper bleeding in dialysis patients. Further data are needed before universal use of PPIs can be recommended, also in light of the emerging risks of long-term treatment with PPIs, such as predisposition to reduced bone density, to hypomagnesemia, or to *Clostridium difficile* infection. We commonly prescribe PPIs for primary prevention in dialysis patients treated with anticoagulants, antiplatelet agents, or NAIDs.

Preparation for Invasive Procedures

In comparison with the general population, ESRD patients run increased risks of morbidity and mortality after invasive procedures. This situation is multifactorial, and reduced hemostatic efficiency plays a key role. In case of elective interventions, patients can be prepared in advance. Anemia should be adequately corrected, raising the hematocrit above 30%, and medications interfering with hemostasis should be, if possible, temporarily suspended. Although there are no clinical data supporting this approach, it seems reasonable to schedule procedures at least some hours after HD, even if no intradialytic anticoagulant is used, because of transitory platelet dysfunction after contact with the extracorporeal circuit.

Preventive administration of medical treatments that ameliorate uremic bleeding, as detailed in the following section, can be advantageous in selected cases. For example, desmopressin has been shown to shorten bleeding time and reduce the risk of complications in uremic patients undergoing kidney biopsy.

Treatment of Dialysis Patients With Active Bleeding

Clinical management of hemorrhagic complications in dialysis patients includes diagnostic and therapeutic measures similar to those used in the general population and measures peculiar to ESRD patients.

The first approach to active bleeding is not specific for dialysis patients and includes hemodynamic support whenever necessary; identification of the hemorrhagic source; and, possibly, subsequent treatment by surgical, endovascular, or endoscopic techniques. Correction of concomitant factors predisposing to bleeding, if present, is another key intervention. This includes transfusion of platelets or plasma (or both); withdrawal of medications that interfere with hemostasis; or, if appropriate, reversal of anticoagulant treatments, for instance, by protamine for heparin or by vitamin K, alone or in association with prothrombin complex concentrates, in patients on warfarin. ESRD should be carefully accounted for in the risk assessment of patients with active bleeding and in the subsequent planning of therapeutic interventions. For example, markedly higher rebleeding rates from endoscopically treated peptic ulcers have been observed in ESRD patients, even when these patients had low-risk ulcer stigmata on endoscopy. While awaiting more comprehensive data, it would thus be reasonable to manage all dialysis patients with peptic ulcer bleeding, and maybe other bleeding disorders as well, as high-risk patients.

In addition to these general measures, the issues discussed in the previous section on prevention need to be specifically addressed in dialysis patients with ongoing bleeding disorders. Because of its well-characterized hemostatic effects in ESRD patients, correction of anemia should be prompt and more aggressive than what is normally done in nonuremic patients with hemorrhages, aiming at keeping the hematocrit above 30%. Transfusions are necessary to quickly correct anemia during active bleeding because recombinant erythropoietin requires at least 7 days to significantly increase the RBC mass. Nonetheless, it may be reasonable to administer erythropoietin also in the acute setting because of its direct effects on platelet activation and to limit the need for future transfusions. Prescription of intradialytic anticoagulation needs to be reviewed in HD patients. In case of life-threatening bleeding, such as intracranial hemorrhages, complete avoidance of anticoagulants is advised, usually for a period of at least 2 weeks. Dialytic adequacy must be carefully considered, especially in patients presenting with uremic or dialysis-associated pericarditis. In this setting, it is mandatory to initiate a trial of intensive dialysis, usually defined, in the case of HD, as daily sessions for 10 to 15 days, preferably without heparin to minimize the risk of hemopericardium and cardiac tamponade.

In particular cases, it is possible also to use medications that directly affect the hemostatic system and have been shown to be of benefit in uremic bleeding, such as desmopressin acetate, cryoprecipitate, estrogens, or tranexamic acid (TXA).

Desmopressin Acetate and Cryoprecipitate

Even if quantitative or qualitative defects in VWF have not been consistently demonstrated in uremic patients, therapies that increase VWF plasma levels, such as desmopressin acetate and cryoprecipitate, improve platelet–VWF interaction and significantly shorten bleeding time in patients with advanced CKD.

Desmopressin acetate or 1-deamino-8-d-arginine-vasopressin (dDAVP) is a synthetic derivative of antidiuretic hormone, with fewer vasopressor effects. dDAVP induces the release of high-molecular-weight multimers of VWF from endothelial storage sites into the plasma. It may also increase platelet membrane glycoprotein expression. dDAVP was initially used successfully in patients with von Willebrand disease and later proposed for control of uremic bleeding in the early 1980s; other indications include bleeding associated with hemophilia A and diabetes insipidus. In two randomized double-blind crossover trials in uremic patients, dDAVP was effective in shortening bleeding time at a dose of 0.3 µg/kg, administered either intravenously (added to 50 mL of saline over 30 minutes) or subcutaneously. Peak responses are achieved 1 hour after intravenous administration or 1.5 to 2 hours when the subcutaneous route is used. The effect lasts 6 to 8 hours, and bleeding time subsequently returns to basal values. dDAVP can also be given intranasally, using 10 to 20 times the intravenous dose (3–6 µg/kg). Tachyphylaxis typically develops after the second dose and is probably caused by progressive depletion of the VWF from storage sites. Adverse effects include mild to moderate decrease in platelet count, facial flushing, transient headache, nausea, abdominal cramps, and tachycardia. Thrombotic events after dDAVP administration have been rarely reported, particularly in patients with underlying advanced cardiovascular disease. Contraction of urinary volume and hyponatremia may also seldom occur if residual diuresis is present. Thanks to its rapid onset of action, dDAVP is commonly used as the first-line hemostatic agent in patients with active bleeding or those who are about to undergo surgery.

Cryoprecipitate is a transfusional product obtained when plasma is frozen and thawed, enriched with factor VIII : VWF multimers and fibrinogen. It has been found to shorten bleeding time, enhance resolution of bleeding in uremic patients, and reduce blood losses in uremic patients undergoing major surgery. The effect of cryoprecipitate on bleeding time is detectable by 1 hour after infusion, maximal after 4 to 12 hours (on average, 8 hours), and vanishes by 24 to 36 hours. The usual dose is 10 units given intravenously over 30 minutes. Cryoprecipitate has important drawbacks: As many as 50% of patients fail to respond to it and, being a blood product, it carries a minimum, yet not negligible, risk of transmission of infectious agents. Rare but severe reactions are possible, including anaphylaxis, pulmonary edema, and intravascular hemolysis. For these reasons, the use of cryoprecipitate is usually limited to patients with life-threatening bleeding who are resistant to blood transfusions and dDAVP.

Conjugated Estrogens

Estrogens were first proposed to mitigate uremic bleeding based on the observation that pregnancy ameliorates the hemorrhagic diathesis of women affected by von Willebrand disease. Several studies have established estrogens as a useful adjunct to the treatment of bleeding in ESRD patients, especially when a slow-onset but long-lasting effect is favorable.

Estrogens do not significantly affect the multimeric structure of VWF, platelet aggregation, or platelet thromboxane production. Their main effect on hemostasis is instead decreasing the production of l-arginine, which is a precursor of NO.

Accordingly, administration of estrogens to uremic rats almost normalizes plasma levels of nitrates and shortens bleeding time, which is abrogated by giving the animals l-arginine. Although none of the studies on uremic bleeding has looked into the effects of estrogens on coagulation, it is plausible that the well-documented capacity of these hormones to decrease the levels of antithrombin III and protein S and to increase factor VII concentrations play a role as well.

The minimum dose of conjugated estrogens to reduce bleeding time is 0.6 mg/kg, administered intravenously over 30 to 40 minutes. Dosing is the same in women and men. Four or five daily infusions are needed to shorten the bleeding time by at least 50%. The effect is manifest only after several hours, becomes maximum over 5 to 7 days, and lasts up to 14 to 21 days. More data exist to support the use of intravenous estrogens, but the oral and transdermal routes have been shown to be effective as well. One oral dose of 25 mg of conjugated estrogens (Premarin) normalizes bleeding time for 3 to 10 days. Courses of 25 to 50 mg/day, for an average of 5 to 7 days, have been demonstrated to be efficacious in clinical studies. Low-dose transdermal estrogens (estradiol 50–100 µg/24 hours), applied as a patch twice a week, effectively reduced bleeding time and lowered the risk of recurrent GI bleeding. In all of the clinical trials on estrogens in uremic bleeding, the hormones were administered only for a few days. With such short courses of treatment, no significant adverse effects were reported other than hot flashes. The clinical use of estrogens in uremic bleeding is mainly reserved for selected cases where long-lasting amelioration of hemostasis is needed, for example, in the preparation for elective surgery at high hemorrhagic risk.

Tranexamic Acid

Tranexamic acid is a potent inhibitor of the fibrinolytic system that stabilizes clots by preventing the binding of plasminogen to fibrin and the activation of plasminogen to plasmin. TXA rapidly decreases bleeding time in uremia. Case reports showed that TXA was effective in controlling chronic bleeding from colonic angiodysplasias and spontaneous subdural and cerebral hematomas in dialysis patients. In a pilot study, adjunctive therapy with TXA effectively reduced rates of rebleeding in dialysis patients with major upper GI hemorrhage. The dosage used was 20 mg intravenously followed by 10 mg/kg/48 hours orally for the next 4 weeks. Because of accumulation in renal failure, use of TXA is contraindicated in the long term in dialysis patients, and it should be limited to the treatment of acute episodes. Severe side effects, such as seizures and visual impairment, have been linked to TXA overdose.

SECTION X

Alternative Hemodialytic Techniques

C H A P T E R   2 7

Hemofiltration and Hemodiafiltration

Martin K. Kuhlmann, MD

Conventional hemodialysis (HD) is based on diffusive transport of solutes across a semipermeable membrane and is effective in removing water-soluble small-molecular-weight solutes and electrolytes. The removal of solutes with larger molecular sizes, such as phosphate and β_2-microglobulin, however, is limited by diffusive resistance. Because insufficient removal of these larger uremic toxins may contribute to the high cardiovascular mortality risk observed in the chronic HD population, the need for alternative therapies that provide better removal of those solutes has become evident. It has long been known that larger molecules can be removed across membranes more efficiently by convective transport, which is less size limited than diffusive transport.

In the 1970s, hemofiltration was developed as a pure convective therapy, which was later followed by the introduction of the concept of hemodiafiltration (HDF), which combines the advantages of diffusion and convection into one therapy. In both HF and HDF, plasma water is filtered across the dialyzer membrane in excess of the ultrafiltration volume (UFV) required to control hydration status. To maintain hemodynamic stability, the volume of excessively filtered fluid needs to be substituted to the blood in the form of a sterile, nonpyrogenic substitution fluid.

In the early days, sterile replacement fluid was produced independently from the dialysis procedure and, similar to peritoneal dialysis solution, was provided in plastic bags. For reasons of cost and practicability, the total fluid replacement volume per session was therefore limited. The understanding that sufficient removal of uremic middle-molecular-weight substances may only be achieved by enhanced convective transport led to the development of online production of sterile, nonpyrogenic dialysis fluid, which at the same time can be safely used as dialysate as well as replacement fluid. Today modern online HDF (ol-HDF) equipment allows the production of nearly unlimited volumes of dialysate and substitution fluid during treatment and therefore allows much higher convection and substitution volumes than traditional fluid bag-based HDF. Among all intermittent extracorporeal treatment strategies ol-HDF has the potential to provide the largest removal of the widest range of solutes.

Currently, ol-HDF is used in routine clinical practice for more than 10% of the European dialysis population with an increasing trend. In northern European countries, more than a quarter of patients and in Switzerland more than 60% of dialysis patients are treated with this modern form of convective therapy. In the United States, the use of ol-HDF lacks behind because only until recently, the necessary technology was not approved for use in chronic dialysis patients by the Food and Drug Administration.

Definitions

Hemofiltration is a technique in which water and solutes are driven by positive hydrostatic pressure across a semipermeable membrane from the blood compartment into the filtrate compartment, from where it is drained. With the flow of water, both small and large solutes get dragged through the membrane at a similar rate (solvent drag effect). Dialysate is not used in hemofiltration.

Hemodiafiltration combines diffusive and convective solute transport using a high-flux membrane with a dialysate flow rate that is similar to that of conventional HD (400–800 mL/min). Fluid is removed by ultrafiltration (UF), and the volume of filtered fluid exceeding the target weight loss is replaced by ultrapure, nonpyrogenic infusion solution. ol-HDF refers to the online production by the dialysis equipment of nearly unlimited amounts of ultrapure, nonpyrogenic dialysate, which is also used as infusion solution. *High-volume* HDF refers to an effective convection volume of at least 20% of the total blood volume processed.

Preparation of Ultrapure Replacement Fluid: Technical Issues

Water used for convection-based therapies needs to fulfill very stringent criteria of purity. Such high refinement in water purity has led to the concept of "ultrapure water," which means virtually sterile and nonpyrogenic. This concept aims to ensure both the chemical and microbial purity of all fluids used during treatment. The basic technical setup includes pretreatment of water by microfiltration, activated charcoal, and downstream microfiltration that is followed by two reverse-osmosis modules in series. Such ultrapurified water is delivered to dialysis machines via a distribution loop that ensures continuous recirculation of water. Ultrapure dialysate is then produced by "cold sterilization" of freshly prepared regular dialysis solution using additional sterilizing ultrafilters. Finally, replacement fluid is generated online by filtering dialysis fluid through bacteria- and endotoxin-retentive filters to prepare a sterile and nonpyrogenic solution that can be immediately infused into the patient. A double-filtered substitution fluid is thus generated from ultrapure dialysate (Fig. 27.1). All filters need to be replaced periodically.

Modes of Hemodiafiltration

Modes of HDF are differentiated depending on the site, in relation to the dialyzer, where replacement fluid is infused to the patient's blood.

Postdilution Hemodiafiltration

This is the most common form of HDF worldwide and so far the only HDF mode studied in several large prospective trials. In the postdilution mode, the replacement fluid is infused downstream of the dialyzer, usually into the venous bubble trap (Fig. 27.2, *A*). The concentration of filtered substances in the ultrafiltrate depends on the sieving coefficient for each compound. For solutes with a sieving coefficient of 1, which can pass the membrane unimpeded, the concentration in the ultrafiltrate will be identical to the plasma water concentration. Because UF is enforced on the undiluted blood, hemoconcentration occurs within the blood compartment of the dialyzer. Postdilution HDF is the most efficient mode in terms of increasing solute removal.

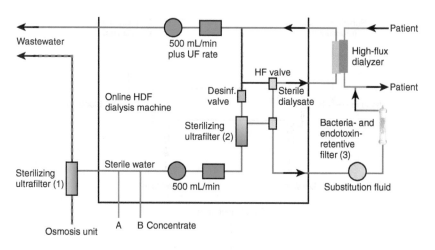

Figure 27.1

Hemodiafiltration (HDF) dialysis and substitution fluid circuit. Ultrapurified water is delivered from the osmosis unit and is sterile filtered through sterilizing ultrafilter *(1)*. Freshly prepared regular dialysis solution is then "cold sterilized" using the additional sterilizing ultrafilter *(2)*, thus generating ultrapure dialysate. "Sterile" replacement fluid is generated online by filtering ultrapure dialysis fluid through a bacteria- and endotoxin-retentive filter *(3)* to prepare a sterile and nonpyrogenic solution, which in postdilution HDF is infused to the patient downstream to the dialyzer. HF, hemofiltration; UF, ultrafiltration.

Predilution Hemodiafiltration

In the predilution mode, the replacement fluid is added upstream of the dialyzer, which results in dilution of the patient's blood (Fig. 27.2, *B*). In contrast to the postdilution mode, filtration rates up to 100% of blood flow rate are possible with predilution HDF. However, predilution reduces the efficiency of both the diffusive and convective components by reducing the solute blood concentration and thus the solute gradient. For equivalent clearance, the ultrafiltration rate (UFR) in predilution mode needs to be about two times greater than in postdilution HDF.

Mixed-Dilution Hemodiafiltration

In the mixed-dilution mode, the replacement fluid is infused both upstream as well as downstream of the dialyzer. The ratio of upstream and downstream infusion rates can be varied to achieve the optimal compromise between maximizing clearance and avoiding the consequences of a high transmembrane pressure and hemoconcentration.

Mid-Dilution Hemodiafiltration

Here, the replacement fluid is infused within specifically designed dialyzers partway down the blood pathway. Thus, the first part of the blood circuit is operated in post-dilution mode and the second part in predilution mode.

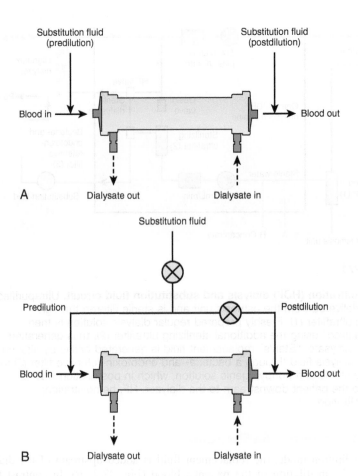

Figure 27.2

Hemodiafiltration modes. A, In the predilution mode, the substitution fluid is infused upstream; in postdilution mode, it is infused downstream of the dialyzer. **B,** In the mixed-dilution mode, the substitution fluid is infused upstream as well as downstream of the dialyzer. In the mixed-dilution mode, the relation of predilution to postdilution volume depends on various factors affecting blood side hemoconcentration.

Principles of Hemodiafiltration Dosing

Quantifier of Hemodiafiltration Dose

Traditionally, dialysis dose is defined by mass removal of uremic toxins; in conventional HD, an index of urea removal (Kt/V or urea removal ratio [URR]) is used as a surrogate marker for the elimination of small-molecular-weight toxins. However, diffusive urea clearance during standard HD treatment is already high and does not increase by more than 10% when convective clearance is added. Therefore, urea removal is not an adequate marker of middle molecule clearance in HDF. Overall, diffusive clearance of higher-molecular-weight solutes is considerably lower than convective clearance across dialysis membranes. For any solute, the convective clearance is dependent on its sieving coefficient and UFR; therefore, mass removal during HDF treatment is directly related to total UFV, which is also referred to as the convection volume. Effective convection volume in addition to standard adequacy measures, such as Kt/V, is currently used as the key quantifier for HDF dosing. In this regard, the "effective convection volume" relates to the undiluted UFV, which is identical to total convection volume in postdilution mode but is considerably lower in the predilution or mixed-dilution modes.

A measure of serum β_2-microglobulin clearance would also be a logical quantifier of the effect of HDF, but as long as the membrane β_2-microglobulin sieving coefficient is greater than 0.6, the β_2-microglobulin clearance will be proportional to the effective UFR.

Target Dose

Three randomized controlled studies (RCTs) (CONTRAST, ESHOL, and the Turkish HDF Study) have failed to demonstrate convincingly that survival times with postdilution HDF are superior to survival times with conventional low- or high-flux HD. However, there were major differences in mean delivered HDF dose among these three trials, and each of them, either in primary or secondary analysis, showed a dose-effect relationship between achieved convection volume and mortality. Those patients receiving the highest convection volume had a significantly lower mortality risk compared with control patients and with patients receiving a lower HDF dose. These data may be interpreted to suggest that convection volumes greater than 20 to 23 L per treatment may result in improved outcome.

Current treatment recommendations conclude that independent of patient body size, a total convection volume of 20 to 24 L per session should be targeted and achieved in *high-volume postdilution* HDF. Whether these target volumes need to be adjusted for some measure of body size, such as body weight or body surface area, still remains to be established. The fact that both generation rate as well as distribution volume of uremic toxins are related to body mass makes this consideration appear reasonable.

Prescription of Hemodiafiltration Dose

Membrane Selection

To guarantee unimpeded filtration of fluid and higher-molecular-weight solutes throughout the treatment session, selection of an adequate dialysis membrane is essential. High-flux membranes offering both a high hydraulic permeability *and* a high middle-molecule clearance are required for adequate HDF. Whereas hydraulic permeability is reflected by the membrane UF coefficient, membrane permeability is defined by the sieving coefficients (S) for selected middle molecules. For high-volume, high-efficiency ol-HDF, a high-flux membrane with an UF coefficient greater than 20 mL/h/mm Hg/m^2 and a sieving coefficient for β_2-microglobulin greater than 0.6 is recommended.

Blood Flow Rate, Filtration Fraction, and Treatment Time

The two major aims governing the prescription of HDF dose are (1) adequate delivery of the target effective convection volume and (2) prevention of excess hemoconcentration. The major determinants for the prescription of target convective volume are blood flow rate, filtration fraction, treatment time, and HDF mode.

In *postdilution* HDF, UF occurs in undiluted blood and necessarily leads to hemoconcentration and lowering of blood flow rate within the dialyzer. Both effects may contribute to the deposition of plasma proteins on the membrane surface, clogging of the membrane pores and occlusion of the blood channels within the dialyzer. These effects can raise transmembrane pressure, cause safety alarms, reduce clearance, or result in filter clotting. The hemoconcentration effects are on the one hand dependent on blood viscosity, which is determined by hematocrit and concentration of blood proteins, and on the other hand on the rate of UF.

The **blood flow rate (Qb)** needs to be optimized in high-volume postdilution HDF to minimize the effects of hemoconcentration. As explained later, extracorporeal Qb is directly related to the treatment time required to achieve the target convection volume. Extracorporeal Qb should be individualized for each patient, taking into account vascular access characteristics and the potential presence of conditions that increase blood viscosity, such as high hematocrit, cryoglobulinemia, and gammopathies. Ideally, a Qb of 300 mL/min or higher is recommended, but a lower Qb does not preclude successful high-volume postdilution HDF. It is essential to repeatedly measure recirculation when optimizing Qb.

Filtration fraction (FF) describes the relationship between the UFR and blood flow rate and is defined as the fraction of plasma water that is filtered during passage of blood through the dialyzer. To avoid excessive hemoconcentration in *postdilution* HDF, it is recommended to limit filtration fraction to 20% to 25% of blood flow rate. Higher filtration fractions up to 30% can only be safely achieved with modern dialysis systems designed to optimize filtration rate, based on automatic adjustment of transmembrane pressure.

Treatment time (TT) has to be recognized as an important prescription variable to achieve the target effective convection volume. Total treatment time required to reach the prescribed convection volume can be calculated from prescribed Qb, FF, and UFR:

$$UFR = Prescribed\ blood\ flow\ rate \times Prescribed\ filtration\ fraction \qquad (1)$$

$$Treatment\ time = Prescribed\ convection\ volume/UFR \qquad (2)$$

Complete and regular delivery of the prescribed target convection volume should become the priority in high-volume ol-HDF, with treatment time being an important variable in cases in which inadequate vascular access limits blood flow rates. When achievement of target HDF dose is regarded as the highest priority, then the treatment time will vary from treatment to treatment depending on individual blood flow rate and filtration fraction.

Anticoagulation

Adequate anticoagulation is a prerequisite for successful high-volume HDF treatment. It is important to realize that a loss of anticoagulant may occur during high-volume postdilution HDF because of high first-pass removal rates for nonprotein-bound low-molecular-weight (≤80%) or unfractionated heparin (≤50%) when infused upstream of the dialyzer. Therefore, the initial heparin bolus should be infused via the venous needle or blood line and allowed to mix with patient blood for at least 3 to 5 minutes before initiating extracorporeal blood flow.

Selection of Hemodiafiltration Mode

As demonstrated by the CONTRAST trial and the Turkish HDF trial, convection volumes longer than 20 L/session may be difficult to achieve in the postdilution mode when treatment time is fixed to a maximum of 4 hours. In cases of limited treatment time, other dilution modes may be applied to achieve treatment targets. However, in predilution and mixed-dilution modes, the convection volume required to remove a given mass of solutes is significantly higher than in postdilution mode because of the dilution of blood solutes by upstream infusion of the replacement fluid. In these cases, the target convection volume will be the effective convection volume (target convection volume in postdilution mode) multiplied by a dilution factor, which is 2.0 for predilution mode and approximately 1.3 for mixed-dilution mode.

So far no large trials have examined the effects of predilution or mixed-dilution HDF modes on patient outcome. In the future, mixed-dilution HDF with feedback control of transmembrane pressure may become the method of choice to achieve target effective convection volumes in a reasonable treatment time.

Safety of Hemodiafiltration

Online HDF is characterized by the intravenous infusion of large volumes of replacement fluid to maintain fluid balance. Because of the large volumes of fluid added to blood, patients are exposed to risks beyond those associated with routine HD. These additional risks relate to the systems used to prepare the replacement fluid, including the water treatment system, and to control fluid balance. Therefore, equipment used for online convective therapies needs to be subject to more stringent safety standards and regulatory oversight than those generally adopted for equipment used for conventional HD.

In general, high-volume ol-HDF can be considered a safe treatment modality. The RCTs mentioned earlier did not provide any indication that HDF is an unsafe treatment modality and demonstrated that substitution fluid of adequate quality can be produced online over a prolonged period of time without increasing the risk for infection or resulting in a significant increase in inflammatory markers. In fact, in some of these studies, mortality risk from infectious causes was significantly lower among patients randomized to ol-HDF compared with conventional HD.

The potential long-term risks of high-volume HDF are related to the induction of deficiency syndromes caused by the increased removal of proteins, vitamins, and nutrients as well as other solutes. Supplementation of vitamins B_{12} and folate, trace elements such as zinc and selenium, and other micronutrients, as well as regular monitoring of vitamin C and serum albumin levels is recommended in patients on long-term HDF treatment.

C H A P T E R 2 8

Continuous Renal Replacement Therapies for Acute Kidney Injury

Celina Denise Cepeda, MD • Piyush Mathur, MD •
Ravindra L. Mehta, MD, FACP

Acute kidney injury (AKI) is a clinical syndrome characterized by an abrupt decrease in kidney function. It leads to the inability of the kidney to excrete waste products, manage electrolytes, regulate fluid balance, and maintain acid–base status. AKI complicates 21% of hospital admissions with 2% of hospital admissions and 11% of all AKI patients requiring dialysis. AKI itself is associated with mortality greater than 50%, but when renal replacement therapy (RRT) is required, the mortality rate is as high as 80%. In the past 20 years, significant advances have been made in RRT, which now represents an important treatment for AKI. After its introduction in the early 1980s, continuous renal replacement therapy (CRRT) has been increasingly used, especially in critically ill AKI patients. Findings from accumulating research on this treatment modality suggest that continuous therapies will continue to be used increasingly for patients with AKI. This chapter reviews the basic techniques of CRRT and its applications, timing of initiation of therapy, dosing, and outcomes in AKI.

Basic Principles and Operational Characteristics

Continuous renal replacement therapy is actually an umbrella term for the four different continuous modalities: slow continuous ultrafiltration (SCUF), continuous venovenous hemofiltration (CVVH), continuous venovenous hemodialysis (CVVHD), and continuous venovenous hemodiafiltration (CVVHDF). The type of modality chosen depends on the goal of therapy; treatment may be used for solute removal, fluid removal, or both. Solute clearance through a dialysis filter occurs by diffusion, convection, or combination, called hemodiafiltration (Tables 28.1 to 28.3 and Fig. 28.1).

Convective techniques (ultrafiltration and hemofiltration) rely on solvent drag, whereby dissolved molecules are dragged along with ultrafiltered plasma water across a semipermeable membrane in response to a hydrostatic or osmotic force. The process of forcing a liquid against a membrane is called ultrafiltration (UF); the fluid collected after it passes through a membrane is the ultrafiltrate. UF does not require replacement of the fluid removed. Hemofiltration requires fluid replacement, either before or after the filter (or both before and after), so as to prevent hemodynamic instability from the loss of large amounts of fluid; the composition of the replacement fluid can vary. No dialysate solution is used. Solute removal depends on the size of the pores in the membrane, the size and weight of the molecule, the

Table 28.1

The Four Principle Modalities Used for Continuous Renal Replacement Therapy

Modality	Urea Clearance (g/d)	Replacement Fluid	Dialysate	Solute Transport	UF Flow (mL/hr)	Dialysate Flow (mL/hr)
SCUF	1–4	No	No	Convection	100–400	0
CVVH	22–24	Yes	No	Convection	500–4000	0
CVVHD	24–30	No	Yes	Diffusion	0–350	500–4000
CVVHDF	36–38	Yes	Yes	Convection + diffusion	500–4000	500–4000

CVVH, continuous venovenous hemofiltration; CVVHD, continuous venovenous hemodialysis; CVVHDF, continuous venovenous hemodiafiltration; SCUF, slow continuous ultrafiltration.

From Galvagno SM Jr, Hong CM, Lissauer ME, et al. Practical considerations for the dosing and adjustment of continuous renal replacement therapy in the intensive care unit. *J Crit Care* 2013;28(6):1019-1026.

Table 28.2

Mechanisms of Clearance for Various Solutes and Molecules in Continuous Renal Replacement Therapy

Molecular Size	Small Solutes (<300 Da)	Middle Molecules (500–50,000 Da)	Low-Molecular-Weight Proteins (50,000–50,000 Da)	Large Proteins (<50,000 Da)
Substances	Urea, creatinine, amino acids	Myoglobin, B_{12}, vancomycin	Inflammatory mediators	Albumin
Clearance mechanism	Convection/diffusion	Convection	Convection ± absorption	Convection

From Galvagno SM Jr, Hong CM, Lissauer ME, et al. Practical considerations for the dosing and adjustment of continuous renal replacement therapy in the intensive care unit. *J Crit Care* 2013;28(6):1019-1026.

transmembrane pressure, and the ultrafiltration rate (UFR; Q_{uf}). Middle- and large-molecular-weight solutes are more effectively cleared by convection. SCUF and CVVH only use convective transport for removal of solutes.

Diffusive techniques (dialysis) rely on a solute concentration gradient between the blood and the dialysate for clearance across a semipermeable membrane. Solute removal depends on the size of the pores in the membrane, the size and weight of the molecule, and the magnitude of the concentration gradient; the gradient is affected by the dialysate, dialysate infusion rate (Q_d), and blood flow rate (Q_b). The dialysate can be customized to promote diffusion of specific molecules. It runs countercurrent to the blood, so faster Q_b allows for a greater gradient. This is the same technique used in intermittent hemodialysis (IHD), but Q_d is much slower than Q_b, so there is complete saturation of the dialysate. Therefore, the Q_d is the rate-limiting factor for solute removal, but it allows for enhanced clearance. The

Table 28.3

Continuous Renal Replacement Therapy Terminology

Term	Definition
Ultrafiltrate (UF)	Fluid collected in bag distal to hemofilter
Dialysate	Fluid instilled into filter countercurrent to flow of blood
Effluent	UF (+ dialysate)(+ replacement fluid) (depending on which modality of CRRT is used)
Replacement fluid	Fluid instilled pre- or postfilter to replace UF volume
Sieving coefficient (SC)	Ability of substance to pass through filter Ratio of solute concentration in filtrate to solute concentration in plasma
Solvent drag	Free circulating, unbound solute carried with water during UF
Filter permeability/efficacy	Ratio of effluent FUN to BUN <1, decreased efficacy
Concentration polarization	Accumulation of rejected solutes on the blood compartment side of the ultrafiltration membrane
Q_b	Blood flow rate
Q_d	Dialysate flow rate
Q_r	Replacement flow rate
Q_{uf}	UF rate
Q_{net}	Net fluid removal rate
Q_{bw}	Blood-water flow rate $= (1 - \text{Hematocrit}) \times Q_b$

BUN, blood urea nitrogen; CRRT, continuous renal replacement therapy; FUN, fluid urea nitrogen.
Adapted from Galvagno SM Jr, Hong CM, Lissauer ME, et al. Practical considerations for the dosing and adjustment of continuous renal replacement therapy in the intensive care unit. *J Crit Care* 2013;28(6):1019-1026.

smaller the size and weight of the solute and the greater the gradient, the more efficiently solute clearance occurs. CVVHD uses diffusion to remove solutes. The amount of effluent is equal to the amount of the dialysate.

Hemodiafiltration (CVVHDF) combines both of these techniques to clear solutes. Dialysate and replacement fluids are needed. This modality allows for removal of small- and middle-sized molecules. Solute clearance for this combination technique is equal to the sum of the convective and diffusive clearances. The clearance is the product of a solute's sieving coefficient (SC; ratio of solute concentration in filtrate to solute concentration in plasma) and effluent flow rate. A solute with a SC of 1 means that it can pass freely through a filter; if the SC is 0, then a solute cannot pass through the filter at all. The amount of effluent in this case is equal to the amount of fluid removed from the patient by UF plus the dialysate and replacement fluid.

Technical Issues

Vascular Access

The location and size of the vascular access are important for ensuring successful CRRT. The preferred catheter for CRRT use is a double-lumen uncuffed central venous catheter. Although tunneled cuffed catheters are associated with significantly

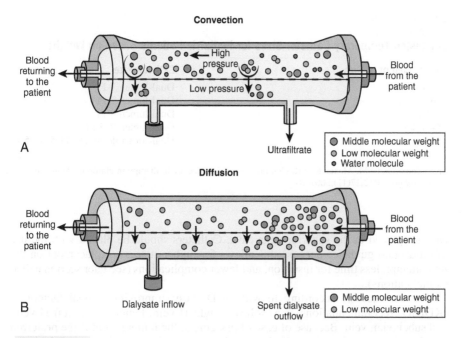

Figure 28.1

A, Convection occurs when solutes are transported across a semipermeable membrane with plasma water in response to a hydrostatic pressure gradient that is created on the blood side of the hemofilter. Convection enhances the removal of low- and middle-molecular-weight molecules. As shown in **B,** in diffusion, movement of solute across a semipermeable membrane is driven by a concentration gradient between the blood and the dialysate. Solutes move from the side with the higher concentration of particles to the side with the lower concentration. Diffusion is best for clearing low-molecular-weight solutes, such as urea and creatinine. (From Tolwani A. Continuous renal-replacement therapy for acute kidney injury. *N Engl J Med* 2012;367(26):2505-2514.)

better catheter survival and fewer infectious and thrombotic complications, they are not regularly placed in the acute setting; they require more time for insertion and have an increased risk of hematoma formation, so their placement is reserved for patients who will need prolonged RRT. CRRT circuit survival is improved when a larger bore catheter is used because it allows for higher Q_b rates. The diameter of the catheter has more influence on flow resistance than the length of the catheter. For adults, diameters range from 11 to 14 Fr. See Table 28.4 for suggested catheter sizes in pediatric patients. A longer catheter does allow placement into a larger vessel, such as the femoral vein. A single center, randomized trial by Morgan et al found that placement of a longer (20–24 cm) soft silicone short-term catheter into the right atrium, from the internal jugular (IJ) or subclavian vein, improved dialyzer life span and daily dialysis dose compared with a shorter (15–20 cm)

Table 28.4

Suggested Temporary Catheter Sizes for Pediatric Patients Based on Weight

Patient Weight or Size	Catheter size
Neonate	Dual-lumen 7 Fr
3–6 kg	Dual-lumen 7 Fr
6–15 kg	Dual-lumen 8 Fr
15–30 kg	Dual-lumen 9–10 Fr
>30 kg	Dual- or triple-lumen 11.5–12.5 Fr

From Sutherland SM, Alexander SR. Continuous renal replacement therapy in children. *Pediatric nephrology.* 2012;27(11):2007-16.

catheter placed in the superior vena cava. Catheters should be placed with the use of ultrasound guidance because this allows for higher success of placement on the first attempt, less time for insertion, and fewer complications (see later section called Complications).

The best access, according to Kidney Disease: Improving Global Outcomes (KDIGO) recommendations, is as follows: right IJ vein, femoral vein, left IJ vein, and subclavian vein. Because of ease of placement, the femoral vein is the preferred site for placement for some physicians. However, patient sedation or paralysis for placement is usually needed. Also, the catheter is often sensitive to patient movement, therefore restricting patient movement. Previous studies also showed a higher incidence of complications, including infection, when the femoral vein is used. In 2008, however, Parienti et al found in adult intensive care unit (ICU) patients that jugular access does not appear to reduce the risk of catheter-related infections compared with femoral access, except in patients with a high body mass index. The subclavian vein is avoided because if it becomes thrombosed or stenosed, it cannot be used in case permanent access is eventually needed. In children, a catheter in the IJ has been associated with better circuit survival compared with catheters placed in the femoral or subclavian vessels. Arteriovenous fistulas and grafts are not recommended for use in CRRT because accessing them continuously leads to trauma; there is also the risk of the needle dislodging leading to bleeding. If a fistula or graft is used, plastic needles should be used and taped securely to prevent tears in the access site.

Dialyzer Membranes

Semipermeable hollow-fiber dialyzers are standard of care for use during CRRT. All membranes lead to some degree of bioincompatibility or activation of blood products. Older membranes made of cuprophane or unmodified cellulose led to reactions, including complement activation, proinflammatory marker release, and oxidative stress, which in turn led to hypotension and vasodilation, hypoxia, fever, and leukopenia. The newer membranes are modified cellulosic and synthetic membranes made of polyacylnitrile, polysulfone, or polymethylmethacrylate, which are rarely associated with such reactions. There are also low- and high-flux membranes. The high-flux or high-permeability hemofilters have larger pores that can clear larger solutes (filter cut points of 60 kDa as opposed to 20–30 kDa) and allow for higher rates of fluid removal. KDIGO recommends the use of a biocompatible membrane or modified cellulose acetate membrane.

Of note, one of the biocompatible membranes, the AN-69 membrane, is often associated with the bradykinin release syndrome when blood priming of the extra-corporeal circuit is needed (e.g., in small children when the extracorporeal volume is >10%–15% of their blood volume). The syndrome is self-limited and pH depen-dent; it manifests more prominently in patients with severe acidosis, when banked blood is used, and in patients receiving angiotensin-converting enzyme (ACE) inhib-itors. When the membrane is exposed to blood, bradykinin is released and leads to vasodilation, which can cause extreme hypotension within 5–10 minutes after start-ing CRRT; ACE inhibitors prevent the breakdown of bradykinin, leading to pro-longed hypotension. Because of the potential for this serious complication, use of this membrane is usually avoided. However, other measures, such as normalizing banked blood pH or giving the patient (rather than the circuit) the blood prime, can prevent or decrease the reaction if no other membrane options are available.

Dialysate and Replacement Solutions

There are many commercially available solutions for use in CRRT. The composition of dialysate and replacement fluids is very similar, and many of the dialysates are used off-label for replacement. When choosing a fluid, it should restore acid–base balance and physiologic electrolyte concentrations. The solutions have varying amounts of sodium, potassium, chloride, glucose, phosphate, calcium, and magne-sium (Table 28.5). Electrolyte adjustments may be needed depending on specific circumstances (e.g., hyperkalemic patients will initially need a solution with 0–2 mmol/L concentration of potassium). The pharmacy can also add electrolytes to make different electrolyte compositions, but there is the chance for error. Calcium is not included in solutions that contain phosphate because an insoluble precipitate may form. A buffer anion is also necessary in solutions because bicarbonate is lost through the hemofilter. Bicarbonate, acetate, lactate, and citrate are available, but bicarbonate is the preferred buffer (see later section Correction of Acid–Base Abnormalities).

Anticoagulation

When blood comes into contact with the surface of the extracorporeal circuit, the intrinsic and extrinsic coagulation pathways and platelets become activated. Some form of continuous anticoagulation is therefore needed to prevent dialyzer or hemo-filter clotting. Anticoagulation is recommended for AKI patients if they do not have increased risk of bleeding or impaired coagulation or are not already being given systemic anticoagulation. If there are no contraindications to regional citrate, its use is recommended rather than heparin. When there are contraindications to citrate, unfractionated or low-molecular-weight heparin should be used. If heparin-induced thrombocytopenia (HIT) occurs, heparin should be stopped, and a direct thrombin inhibitor (argatroban) or factor Xa inhibitor (danaparoid or fondaparinux) should be used instead. Prefilter replacement fluid can be used to prevent filter clotting when anticoagulation is not or cannot be used. More details on anticoagulation can be found in Chapter 29 on anticoagulation for CRRT.

Table 28.5

Composition of Commercial Replacement and Dialysate Solutions

	PrismaSate		PrismaSol		PrismOcal	Accusol		Baxter Premixed	Normocarb HF	
	Ca	No Ca	Ca	No Ca		Ca	No Ca			
Intended use	D	D	RF	RF	D/RF	D	D	D for HDF	RF	D
Sodium (mEq/L)	140	140	140	140	140	140	140	140	140	140
Chloride (mEq/L)	109.5–113	108–120.5	109–113	106.5–110.5	106	109.5–116.3	113.5	117	106.5–116.5	105
Bicarbonate (mEq/L)	32	22–32	32	32	32	30–35	30	0	25–35	35
Lactate (mEq/L)	3	3	3	3	3	0	0	30	0	0
Potassium (mEq/L)	0–4	2–4	0–4	0–4	0	0–4	2	2	0	0
Calcium (mEq/L)	2.5–3.5	0	2.5–3.5	0	0	2.8–3.5	0	3.5	0	0
Magnesium (mEq/L)	1–1.5	1–1.5	1–1.5	1–1.5	1	1–1.5	1.5	1.5	1.5	1.5
Dextrose (mmol/L)	0–6.1	0–6.1	0–5.6	0–5.6	0	0–5.6	5.6	5.6	0	0
SID	35	25–35	35	35	32	30–35	30	29	25–35	36.5
Number of compartments	2	2	2	2	2	2	2	1	—	—
Base in small compartment	N/A	N/A	Yes	Yes	Yes	N/A	N/A	—	—	—

Ca, calcium; D, dialysate; K, potassium; N/A, not available; RF, replacement fluid; SID, strong ion difference, assuming that lactate is transformed into bicarbonate.
From Claure-Del Granado R, Bouchard J. Acid-base and electrolyte abnormalities during renal support for acute kidney injury: recognition and management. *Blood Purif* 2012;34(2):186-193.

Treatment Dosing

The clearance of solutes is related to the effluent flow, which is why the latter is commonly referred to as the dose of CRRT. Based on randomized controlled trials (RCTs), KDIGO guidelines recommend delivering an effluent dose of 20 to 25 mL/kg/hr for patients with AKI; other references recommend a dose of 25 to 30 mL/kg/hr. In 2000, Ronco and colleagues performed a prospective, randomized trial of CRRT UF dosing that compared doses of 20 mL/kg/hr, 35 mL/kg/hr, and 45 mL/kg/hr AKI ICU patients. They demonstrated that a dose of at least 35 mL/kg/hr improved survival at 15 days after stopping CRRT compared with the lower dose; there was no significant difference in survival between patients receiving 35 mL/kg/hr and 45 mL/kg/hr. After this study, a dose of 35 mL/kg/hr became the standard dose widely used.

These concepts changed after two large studies were published. The Veterans Affairs/National Institutes of Health Acute Renal Failure Trial Network (ARFTN) performed a large, multicenter study comparing standard-dose CVVHDF of 20 mL/kg/hr with high-intensity CVVHDF of 35 mL/kg/hr in critically ill AKI patients; it demonstrated no significant difference in 60-day all-cause mortality, rate of recovery of renal function, and duration of RRT. The Randomized Evaluation of Normal vs. Augmented Level (RENAL) Renal Replacement Therapy Study was another large, multicenter study comparing CVVHDF effluent flow of 40 mL/kg/hr to 25 mL/kg/hr to see if there was a difference in 90-day mortality and continued need for RRT in ICU patients with AKI; there was no significant difference in either outcome between the two groups.

Duosol Bicarbonate 35 Dialysate 0K/3Ca	Duosol Bicarbonate 35 Dialysate 2K/3Ca	Duosol Bicarbonate 25 Dialysate 2K/0Ca	Duosol Bicarbonate 32 Dialysate 2K/0Ca	Duosol Bicarbonate 35 Dialysate 4K/3Ca	Duosol Bicarbonate 25 Dialysate 4K/0Ca	multiBic			
D	D	D	D	D	D	D	D	D	D
140	140	136	136	140	136	140	140	140	140
109	111	115	107.5	113	117	109	111	112	113
35	35	25	32	35	25	35	35	35	35
0	0	0	0	0	0	0	0	0	0
0	2	2	2	4	4	0	2	3	4
3	3	0	0	3	0	1.5	1.5	1.5	1.5
1	1	1.5	1.5	1	1.5	0.5	0.5	0.5	0.5
1	1	0	0	0	0	1	1	1	1
—	—	—	—	—	—	—	—	—	—
2	2	2	2	2	2	2	2	2	2
Yes	Yes	Yes	Yes	Yes	Yes	Yes	Yes	Yes	Yes

Table 28.6

Factors Affecting Continuous Renal Replacement Therapy Dose Delivery

Filter clotting or type of anticoagulation
Decreased sieving coefficient
Secondary membrane formation
Concentration polarization
Changing catabolic rate/urea generation in AKI and critically ill patients
Catheter-related problems (type of catheter, site of placement, hygiene, etc.)
Circuit down-time (routine filter changes)
Time off for diagnostic procedures and therapeutic interventions

AKI, acute kidney injury.

An international survey of intensivists reported that use of CRRT hemofiltration doses of at least 45 mL/kg/hr were prescribed for septic AKI patients despite little recent evidence supporting this. As stated earlier, there is no difference in outcomes when using HVHF versus standard-volume hemofiltration in these patients.

In most of these studies, greater than or equal to 85% of the prescribed dose was delivered to AKI patients. This is usually much more than what is delivered in clinical practice (see Table 28.6 for factors that affect dose delivery). Therefore, when prescribing a treatment dose, clinicians should have about a 25% safety margin; prescribing a dose of 30 to 35 mL/kg/hr may then deliver an adequate dose.

Factors That Impact Dialysis Dose

As noted earlier, effluent volume (derived from blood-based kinetics) is thought to represent clearance and is used to prescribe and measure the dose in CRRT. This assumes that filter permeability stays the same over time; filter permeability is equal to the ratio of effluent fluid urea nitrogen (FUN) to blood urea nitrogen (BUN), which should be equal to 1. This is not actually seen in practice, however, and effluent volume may overestimate delivered dialysis dose, as noted by Claure-Del Granado et al in 2011 and Lyndon et al in 2012. The delivered dose can be decreased by several factors. Secondary membrane formation and concentration polarization affect water and solute permeability of an UF membrane. Exposure of the membrane to plasma leads to adsorption and deposition of proteins on the membrane. Concentration polarization results from accumulation of solute rejected by the UF membrane. Both phenomena result in a concentrated layer along the membrane, causing resistance to mass transfer. To overcome this, transmembrane pressure needs to be increased to maintain an adequate Q_{uf} and to lower the concentration of important solutes in the effluent. A second factor is progressive filter clotting, which decreases the SC and filter permeability. The CRRT machine measures effluent volume but cannot take into account changes in filter permeability (Fig. 28.2). The use of predilution is a third factor, which may decrease urea clearance by as much as 15%. Using replacement fluid prefilter reduces the concentration of solutes in the plasma and decreases solute clearance. Table 28.6 lists other factors impacting dose delivery.

To assess the dose in CRRT, the FUN-to-BUN ratio should be measured at least daily. Table 28.7 shows the calculations to assess dialysis dose in CRRT. These calculations help correct dialysis prescriptions with regards to small solute clearance, but changes in filter permeability also affect middle molecule clearance. It has been

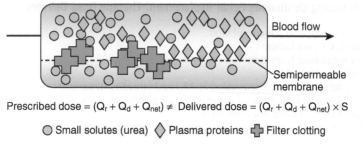

Prescribed dose = $(Q_r + Q_d + Q_{net}) \neq$ Delivered dose = $(Q_r + Q_d + Q_{net}) \times S$

○ Small solutes (urea)   ◇ Plasma proteins   ✚ Filter clotting

Figure 28.2

The effect of concentration polarization and clotting on delivered dialysis dose. Filter efficacy declines over time; protein fouling and filter clotting occur on the membrane and decrease the surface available for diffusion or convection, which reduces the amount of dose being delivered. These important factors must be frequently monitored during continuous renal replacement therapies. BUN, blood urea nitrogen; FUN, effluent fluid urea nitrogen; Q_d, dialysate fluid rate; Q_{net}, net fluid removal rate; Q_r, replacement fluid rate; S, FUN/BUN ratio. (From Macedo E, Claure-Del Granado R, Mehta RL. Effluent volume and dialysis dose in CRRT: time for reappraisal. *Nat Rev Nephrol.* 2012;8(1):57-60.)

Table 28.7
Continuous Renal Replacement Therapy Dose Assessment

CVVH

Prescribed dose = $Q_r + Q_{net}$

Delivered dose = $(Q_r + Q_{net}) \times (FUN/BUN)$

CVVHDF

Prescribed dose = $Q_r + Q_d + Q_{net}$

Delivered dose = $(Q_r + Q_d + Q_{net}) \times (FUN/BUN)$

Correcting for predilution effect

Delivered dose = $Q_{net} \times ([Q_{bw}/\{Q_{bw} + Q_r\}] + Q_d \times [Q_{bw}/\{Q_{bw} + Q_r\}]) \times (FUN/BUN)$

$Qbw = (1 - hematocrit) \times Qb.$

BUN, blood urea nitrogen; *CRRT*, continuous renal replacement therapy; *CVVH*, continuous venovenous hemofiltration; *CVVHDF*, continuous venovenous hemodiafiltration; *FUN*, effluent fluid urea nitrogen; Q_{bw}, blood-water flow rate; Q_d, dialysate fluid rate; Q_{net}, net fluid removal rate; Q_r, replacement fluid rate.

Adapted from Macedo E, Claure-Del Granado R, Mehta RL. Effluent volume and dialysis dose in CRRT: time for reappraisal. *Nat Rev Nephrol.* 2012;8(1):57-60.

suggested that future studies include measured clearances of small and middle molecules to determine the actual delivered dose.

Because the effluent rate only provides an inaccurate estimate of delivered dose, in 2012, Claure-Del Granado et al actually recommend measuring and expressing delivered dose as urea clearance (K_D or K_{urea}), derived from dialysate-side kinetics. This is the ratio of mass removal rate to blood concentration and is calculated using the formula: K delivered = (FUN × EV)/BUN, where FUN is urea nitrogen in the effluent (mg/dL), BUN in urea nitrogen in the plasma (mg/dL), and EV is effluent volume (mL/min). K_D takes into account filter function and duration and effective time of treatment. They also suggest that the equivalent renal urea clearance (EKR), based on urea kinetic modeling, provides a good estimate of delivered dialysis dose (please see reference for calculating EKR) and can be used as a tool to compare different types of therapies. These recommendations are based on findings evaluating six different methods of assessing and expressing CRRT delivered dose (three equations from blood-side kinetics and three equations from dialysate-side kinetics) in critically ill AKI patients treated with predilution CVVHDF and regional citrate anticoagulation. The dialysate-side measurement ensures delivery of dose, and the blood-side measurement helps determine if changes need to be made in the prescription.

Fluid Management

Patients with AKI often develop oliguria or anuria and fluid overload. Many publications have described the negative influence of fluid overload on morbidity and mortality in adult and pediatric patients. Therefore, optimizing fluid status in these patients is essential.

Continuous renal replacement therapy is highly effective for fluid control. Fluid balance can be maintained without compromising metabolic–solute balance because they can be dissociated from each other. Ultrafiltration allows fluid removal to be achieved. Bouchard and Mehta describe three techniques for achieving fluid balance with CRRT (Table 28.8). The level 1 technique is to vary the net UFR (Q_{uf}) to meet the anticipated fluid balance needs over 8 to 24 hours; the net ultrafiltrate is the difference between the total ultrafiltrate (the plasma water removed) and the total replacement (the fluid given to the patient). For example, a patient may have a total anticipated fluid intake of 3 L with a desired 1-L net loss over 24 hours; the Q_{uf} would be set at −170 mL/hr (3 L + 1 L/24 hr). This may not be the best technique to use because there may be unanticipated changes in clinical status and fluid needs, leading to a different net ultrafiltrate that is different from the desired fluid balance. In addition, effluent volume and treatment dose will vary because net Q_{uf} are not constant with this method.

The level 2 method of maintaining fluid balance is to vary the amount of postdilution replacement fluid administered; the net ultrafiltrate stays the same and exceeds the anticipated hourly intake. With this technique, the postdilution fluid is not given through the CRRT pump but through a separate pump. A patient can be maintained in negative fluid balance by decreasing the amount of postdilution fluid received to be less than the total output, in positive fluid balance by increasing postdilution replacement to be greater than all output, or in even balance by having equal postdilution replacement and total output. This method allows for variation in intake and a predetermined convective clearance because net ultrafiltrate does not vary as in the first technique.

The level 3 technique is similar to the second, but fluid balance is tailored to achieve a targeted hemodynamic parameter every hour. Predefined targets are set for parameters, such as central venous pressure (CVP), mean arterial pressure (MAP), or pulmonary arterial wedge pressure, and algorithms are used to achieve these targets. For example, if the CVP is to be maintained between 8 and 12 mm Hg, when this is achieved, the algorithm would determine that net fluid balance be set to zero. If the CVP is above target, the algorithm would call for fluid removal; if CVP is below target, then fluid would be added. This technique allows for greater flexibility and maximally uses CRRT as a fluid regulatory device.

Applications

When RRT is needed, AKI can be managed with IHD, CRRT, and peritoneal dialysis (PD). The specific role of CRRT versus IHD is not well defined, but transitions between the two are common. The use of PD for AKI is not well established, but it is used more often in the pediatric setting. The choice of which modality to use is based largely on available resources and experience with a specific modality. The 2012 KDIGO Clinical Practice Guideline for AKI recommends using continuous and intermittent RRT as complementary therapies. Nephrologists have traditionally managed AKI with IHD as it allows for rapid removal of solutes by diffusion and volume by UF. However, critically ill patients with hemodynamic instability would likely not tolerate this without serious drawbacks; for these patients, KDIGO suggests using CRRT. It offers the advantages of slower fluid removal for better hemodynamic stability and control of fluid balance; slower changes in solute concentrations to prevent large fluctuations and fluid shifts; ability to remove fluid restrictions which allows for proper nutrition, medications, and blood product administration; and the flexibility to adapt to a patient's changing treatment needs.

Table 28.8

Continuous Renal Replacement Therapy Fluid Balance Techniques

Variable	Level 1	Level 2	Level 3
Intake	Variable	Variable	Variable
Non-CRRT output	Variable	Variable	Variable
Ultrafiltration rate	Variable to achieve fluid balance	Fixed to achieve target effluent volume	Fixed to achieve target effluent volume
Substitution fluid rate	Fixed = or < Q_{uf}	Postdilution replacement varies to achieve −, zero, or + fluid balance	Postdilution replacement varies to achieve −, zero, or + fluid balance
Fluid balance	Achieved by varying Q_{uf}	Achieved by adjusting amount of substitution fluid	Targets the hourly fluid balance to achieve a predefined hemodynamic parameter
Key difference	Output varies to accommodate changes in intake and fluid balance goals	Output is fixed to achieve desired solute clearance and allow flexibility in accommodating varying intake	Output is fixed to achieve desired solute clearance and allow flexibility in accommodating varying intake
Examples	SCUF, CVVHD	CVVH, CVVHDF	CVVH, CVVHDF
Advantages			
Patient factors	Strategy similar to fluid removal in intermittent dialysis	Solute clearance is constant. Allows variation in intake. Individualizes prescription.	Solute clearance is constant. Allows variation in intake. Individualizes prescription.
CRRT factors	Fluid balance calculations can be deferred to longer intervals (every 8–12 hours)	Clearance requirements dissociated from fluid balance. Decreases interactions with CRRT pump to adjust UFR. Regimen simplified for caregiver.	Clearance requirements dissociated from fluid balance. Decreases interactions with CRRT pump to adjust UFR. Regimen simplified for caregiver.
Disadvantages			
Patient factors	Patient assumed to be in static state. Similar to ESRD prescription. Intake may fluctuate. Fluid boluses not accounted for. Commonly over- or undershoot. Fluctuations in solute clearance, especially when dependent on convection.	Requires hourly calculations for amount of fluid replacement to be given. Potential for fluid imbalances if balance sheet not used.	Requires hourly calculations for amount of fluid replacement to be given. Potential for fluid imbalances if balance sheet not used. Requires scale be made for hemodynamic parameter targets.

Continued

Table 28.8

Continuous Renal Replacement Therapy Fluid Balance Techniques—cont'd

Variable	Level 1	Level 2	Level 3
CRRT factors	Requires frequent interactions with CRRT pump to adjust UFR. Underutilizes CRRT for fluid removal only.	Requires use of external pump to achieve fluid regulation.	Requires use of external pump to achieve fluid regulation.

CRRT, continuous renal replacement therapy; *CVVH*, continuous venovenous hemofiltration; *CVVHD*, continuous venovenous hemodialysis; *CVVHDF*, continuous venovenous hemodiafiltration; Q_{uf}, ultrafiltration rate; *SCUF*, slow continuous ultrafiltration.
Adapted from Bouchard J, Mehta RL. Volume management in continuous renal replacement therapy. *Semin Dial* 2009;22(2):146-150.

Table 28.9

Potential Applications for Continuous Renal Replacement Therapy in Patients With Acute Kidney Injury

Renal Replacement	Renal Support
Acute kidney injury	Fluid management
Chronic renal failure	Solute and electrolyte management
	Acid–base management
	Nutrition
	Sepsis, cytokine removal, or multiple organ failure

When managing AKI patients with any form of RRT, the goals of therapy must be defined. In patients with end-stage renal disease (ESRD), the aim is to postpone starting dialysis until a substantial amount of renal function is lost. This should not be the strategy used for patients with AKI, however. RRT for these patients should be thought of as a way to prevent or halt the rapid decline in renal function and to support other organs to allow time for recovery. In this way, RRT is more like renal support rather than renal replacement. Table 28.9 lists potential applications for CRRT.

Traditional and Special Indications for Treatment

There is no question that starting CRRT is appropriate when patients meet standard criteria for IHD but are hemodynamically unstable: hyperkalemia, severe acidosis, volume overload, severe uremia leading to complications, pronounced azotemia, severe oliguria or anuria, and drug intoxications. Other indications for which CRRT may be started include sepsis, increased intracranial pressure (ICP), heart failure, correction of severe electrolyte and acid–base abnormalities, and removal of poisons. Table 28.10 also includes contraindications to starting CRRT.

Table 28.10

Indications and Contraindications for Continuous Renal Replacement Therapy in Critically Ill Acute Kidney Injury Patients

Indications

Classic indications
  Hyperkalemia
  Severe metabolic acidosis
  Diuretic-resistant volume overload
  Oliguria or anuria
  Uremic complications
  Some drug intoxications
Potential indications
  Hemodynamic instability
  Disrupted fluid balance (caused by cardiac failure or multiorgan failure)
  Increased ICP
  Electrolyte abnormalities

Contraindications

Advance directives indicating that the patient does not want dialysis
The patient or his or her health care proxy declines continuous RRT
Inability to establish vascular access
Lack of appropriate infrastructure and trained personnel for continuous RRT

ICP, intracranial pressure; *RRT*, renal replacement therapy.
From Tolwani A. Continuous renal-replacement therapy for acute kidney injury. *N Engl J Med* 2012;367(26):2505-2514.

Septic Acute Kidney Injury

Sepsis is the main cause of AKI in the ICU. About 30% to 50% of septic AKI patients need some form of RRT. Sepsis-associated AKI (SAKI) is preferably treated with continuous therapies for the reasons stated earlier. In addition, CRRT allows for temperature and acid–base status control. It could also be thought of as organ support for SAKI, such as in patients with acute respiratory distress syndrome (ARDS); CRRT has been shown to improve and stabilize oxygenation, decrease duration of mechanical ventilation, and decrease cytokine levels in the blood.

Newer, high-flux membranes have the ability to remove inflammatory mediators, such as cytokines and chemokines, by convection. Using conventional CRRT techniques, however, may not be of clinical significance because these mediators have high turnover rates. De Vriese et al failed to show an effect on serum cytokine levels using CVVH. In 2012, Atan et al performed a systematic review of ex vivo studies on cytokine removal using extracorporeal circulation modalities. They found standard hemofiltration led to insignificant removal of most cytokines. Studies involving the use of high-volume hemofiltration (HVHF) have been conducted to see if clinically significant removal of inflammatory mediators can be achieved. The systematic review and meta-analysis by Clark et al aimed to evaluate the effects of HVHF versus standard-volume hemofiltration in septic AKI; this included the IVOIRE (hIgh VOlume in Intensive caRE) study (high-volume vs. standard-volume hemofiltration for septic shock patients with AKI); no significant difference in mortality, hemodynamics, or organ improvement between the two groups of patients was found. High cutoff membranes, which have larger pore sizes, have better cytokine removal compared with standard high-flux membranes; this has been noted in ex vivo studies, animal experiments, and preliminary clinical studies. They also have favorable effects on immune cell function and increase survival in animal models of sepsis. More studies of the use of these membranes for septic shock patients are needed, however.

Increased Intracranial Pressure

About 8% to 23% of acute brain injury (ABI) patients develop AKI; this is an independent predictor of poor outcome. Between 30% and 75% of liver failure patients develop AKI, making it more difficult to medically manage hepatic encephalopathy and increased ICP. For patients with ABI or increased ICP, KDIGO suggests using CRRT rather than IHD. IHD may lead to decreased cerebral perfusion pressure (CPP) and worsening neurologic status. The goal for ABI and increased ICP patients is to maintain CPP above 60 mm Hg; this is done by ensuring MAP stays up because CPP = MAP − ICP. With IHD, intradialytic hypotension is common, leading to decreased MAP and CPP and increased ICP by compensatory cerebral vasodilation. This may result in infarction or secondary brain injury.

In addition, dialysis disequilibrium results when solutes are removed quickly, causing shifts in intracellular fluid; worsening cerebral edema and further increases in ICP ensue. Decreased CPP and dialysis disequilibrium can be avoided with CRRT's slow, steady fluid and solute removal. This was demonstrated in a report by Ronco et al in which there was increased brain density or water content on CT scans in all patients after IHD but no change in density in patients who had CVVH.

To attenuate the problem of dialysis dysequilibrium, hypertonic saline infusions have been used. It has been associated with improvements in hepatic encephalopathy, cerebral edema, and ICP because it produces an osmotic force to draw fluid from the brain parenchyma to the intravascular compartment. However, it can lead to volume overload and decreased oxygenation. CVVH or CVVHDF can be used to maintain hypernatremia while keeping the patient euvolemic or in negative fluid balance. High-dialysate sodium concentrations or addition of sodium to replacement solutions is the key. It is recommended that a sodium concentration of at least 140 mEq/L be used during treatment, although a target of about 150 to 160 mEq/L is the usual. There is also a case report on the use of trisodium citrate to aid in sustaining hypernatremia and providing regional anticoagulation; changes in the composition of the replacement fluid can be made to compensate for alkalosis or hypocalcemia that may occur because of the trisodium citrate.

Heart Failure and Cardiorenal Syndrome

Acute decompensated heart failure (ADHF) accounts for more than 1 million hospitalizations yearly. Patients often develop hypotension and diuretic resistance, requiring higher doses of diuretics. These factors often lead to progressive AKI and the cardiorenal syndrome. AKI occurs in up to 40% of patients with ADHF. UF with or without RRT (depending on degree of AKI) is used to relieve congestion. The Ultrafiltration Versus Intravenous Diuretics for Patients Hospitalized for Acute Decompensated Heart Failure trial (UNLOAD) study compared outcomes between patients who received standard diuretic treatment versus slow intermittent UF, although patients with serum creatinine of 3 mg/dL or greater were excluded. UF patients had greater weight loss at 48 hours and lower hospital readmission and emergency department visit rates at 90 days. However, the Cardiorenal Rescue Study in Acute Decompensated Heart Failure trial (CARESS-HF), which compared the effect of UF versus stepped pharmacologic therapy on renal function and weight (also excluded patients with serum creatinine ≥3.5 mg/dL), revealed different results. There was no difference in weight loss or readmission rates between the two groups; there was also an increased risk of AKI in the UF group.

In 2015, Prins et al studied in-hospital mortality in patients with ADHF requiring inotropes or vasopressors (or both) and CRRT for severe AKI (cardiorenal syndrome 1). CRRT was performed with CVVHDF and effluent rate of 25 to 30 mL/kg/hr. They found that CRRT in this setting was associated with high in-hospital mortality; most patients did not recover renal function (even with volume removal), and long-term prognosis was poor. This study, the CARESS-HF study, and a few other studies looking at UF with or without RRT for cardiorenal syndrome suggest these treatments may not be effective for this group of patients.

Correction of Severe Electrolyte Abnormalities

Patients with AKI who have severe electrolyte abnormalities often need RRT. IHD is the usual treatment of choice, but certain abnormalities are best corrected slowly to prevent neurologic sequelae.

Hypo- and Hypernatremia

The above is especially true for sodium disturbances that are chronic. Correction of sodium should not be above 8 mEq/L in 24 hours. With CRRT, lower volumes of replacement and/or dialysate fluid per hour can be used and sodium levels can be customized. Sodium content in replacement fluid is 140 mEq/L, so to correct hyponatremia, 5% dextrose in water (D5W) can be infused separately to slowly increase sodium levels. As an example:

$$\text{Target sodium concentration} = 123 \text{ mEq/L}$$

$$\text{Replacement fluid sodium content} = 140 \text{ mEq/L}$$

$$\text{D5W sodium content, peripheral} = 0 \text{ mEq/L}$$

$$\text{Desired clearance} = 2.5 \text{ L/hr}$$

$$\text{Replacement fluid rate} = \frac{\text{Target sodium concentration}}{140} \times \text{Desired clearance}$$

$$= \frac{123}{140} \times 2.5 \text{ L/hr} = 2.2 \text{ L/hr}$$

$$\text{D5W rate} = \frac{(140 - \text{Target sodium concentration})}{140} \times \text{Desired clearance}$$

$$= \frac{(140 - 123)}{140} \times 2.5 \text{ L/hr} = 0.3 \text{ L/hr} = 300 \text{ mL/h}$$

As stated earlier, some neurologic problems may require a patient to be hypernatremic. In these cases, infusing NaCl 3% separately or adding NaCl or $NaHCO_3$ directly to replacement fluid can be done. As an example:

$$\text{Target sodium concentration} = 150 \text{ mEq/L}$$

$$\text{Replacement fluid sodium content} = 140 \text{ mEq/L}$$

$$\text{NaCl 3\% sodium content, peripheral} = 513 \text{ mEq/L}$$

$$\text{Desired clearance} = 2.5 \text{ L/hr}$$

$$\text{NaCl 3\% rate} = \frac{(\text{Target sodium concentration} - 140)}{513} \times \text{Desired clearance}$$

$$= \frac{(150 - 140)}{513} \times 2.5 \text{ L/hr} = 0.05 \text{ L/hr}$$

$$\text{Replacement fluid rate} = \text{Desired clearance} - \text{NaCl 3\% rate}$$
$$= 2.5 \text{ L/hr} - 0.05 \text{ L/hr} = 2.45 \text{ L/hr}$$

In both situations, serum sodium levels should be checked every 2 hours to ensure correction is not too rapid.

Hypo- and Hyperkalemia

Hypokalemia is a much less frequent complication of AKI than hyperkalemia. To prevent hypokalemia, CRRT replacement fluid should contain 3 to 4 mEq/L of potassium. Correction of hypokalemia is the same as in patients not on RRT–potassium boluses.

Hyperkalemia is common in AKI. Because it can lead to changes in cardiac conduction, emergent treatment with IHD may be needed. However, if a patient cannot tolerate IHD or if the hyperkalemia is not life threatening, CRRT is an option. This is performed by increasing the volume of replacement or dialysate solution and using solution with zero or low (2 mEq/L) potassium concentration. Serum potassium levels should be monitored every 2 to 4 hours, especially if zero potassium solutions are used, and should continue after CRRT is discontinued; this allows identification of rebound hyperkalemia or hypokalemia.

Other Electrolytes

Hypocalcemia, hyperphosphatemia, and mild hypermagnesemia are also commonly seen in AKI. CRRT dialysate and replacement fluids come with (usually 2.5–3.5 mEq/L) and without calcium so the concentration in the fluids can be increased. These fluids do not contain phosphate so calcium-based phosphate binder or other phosphate binders can be used if hyperphosphatemia occurs. Hypermagnesemia does not usually cause clinical issues, but the amount of magnesium in the solutions can be decreased (range, 1–1.5 mEq/L).

Correction of Acid–Base Abnormalities

Metabolic Acidosis

In AKI patients, this is the most common acid–base disorder. It results from the inability to regenerate bicarbonate and excrete ammonium ions. Calculating the anion gap is important to help identify metabolic acidosis because bicarbonate and pH levels may be normal in some patients. When acidosis is severe and pH is below 7.1 to 7.15, RRT is indicated. Bicarbonate, lactate, citrate, and acetate are the four buffers in dialysis and replacement solutions used to treat acidosis. Acetate, however, is no longer used because it negatively affects hemodynamics and does not correct acidosis as well as the other buffers.

Bicarbonate concentrations range from 25 to 35 mEq/L. Despite its lower concentration compared with IHD bicarbonate (31–39 mEq/L), CVVHDF more often normalizes bicarbonate levels than IHD. Bicarbonate and lactate are equivalent in their ability to correct acidosis. Lactate is less expensive and more stable, though. Caveats to its use include liver failure, lactic acidosis, and shock because it can accumulate and not be converted to bicarbonate. Citrate is an anticoagulant and a buffer. Its use can lead to metabolic alkalosis, especially in higher doses because 1 mmol of citrate is converted to 3 mmol of bicarbonate. Again, caution should be used in patients with liver failure because its conversion to bicarbonate may be decreased.

Bicarbonate is the most frequently used buffer. To control acidosis, the highest concentration of bicarbonate should be used to stabilize levels; then the dose can be titrated based on the patient's needs. To prevent fluid overload, it can be delivered prefilter concurrently with UF.

Metabolic Alkalosis

Metabolic alkalosis occurs very rarely in AKI, but it can be caused by diuretic use, posthypercapnia in ventilated patients, in those receiving blood products, and when citrate anticoagulation is used. It should be managed by decreasing the bicarbonate concentration in solutions to the lowest concentration available. Custom-made bicarbonate solutions may be made by the pharmacy. Chloride concentration in solutions should also be increased, and if sodium levels are high, sodium concentration should be decreased.

Respiratory Acidosis and Alkalosis

Acute kidney injury can be seen concurrently in patients with ARDS. These patients are often treated with permissive hypercapnia, which leads to respiratory acidosis. CRRT permits adjustment of bicarbonate and pH levels in conjunction with a patient's pCO_2. Respiratory alkalosis is treated like metabolic alkalosis, by decreasing the bicarbonate concentration in solutions to maintain normal pH.

Removal of Poisons

The removal of drugs and toxins by CRRT can be done, but IHD is the usual treatment of choice. As stated previously, the clearance of a solute depends on blood and/or dialysis flow rate(s) and membrane characteristics, as well as molecular weight (MW) of solute, proportion of solute bound to plasma protein, and volume of distribution (VD) of solute. For example, a molecule that is large or highly protein bound and has a large VD is not cleared as well as a low-MW solute that is not bound to protein and has a small VD.

The advantage to using CRRT is that it can be used in hemodynamically unstable patients. Molecules as large as 20,000 to 40,000 Da can be cleared through CRRT membranes, but the clearance rate is lower compared with IHD. There is no rebound of compounds removed from the blood when CRRT is used, though this could be because of lower clearance; the lack of rebound may not be beneficial because the compounds stay in the intracellular space, where they likely have toxic effect rather than move to the extracellular space where they could be removed with treatment.

Lithium is a mood stabilizer with a low MW (<7 Da) that is not protein bound and has a VD of 0.6 to 0.9 L/kg. Altered mental status, clonus, and muscle fasciculations are signs of poisoning. The mainstay of treatment is administration of normal saline to enhance elimination. The Extracorporeal Treatments in Poisoning (EXTRIP) Workgroup performed a systematic review of extracorporeal treatments (ECTRs) in lithium poisoning. ECTR is recommended when there is AKI and the lithium concentration is greater than 4 mEq/L or if decreased level of consciousness, seizures, or life-threatening dysrhythmias occur irrespective of the concentration; it is suggested if the concentration is greater than 5 mEq/L, significant confusion is present, or it is expected to take more than 36 hours to achieve a concentration of less than 1 mEq/L. The workgroup states IHD is the preferred method of treatment, but CRRT is an alternative. CRRT can also be used after a session of IHD. Leblanc et al found lithium could be cleared at 48 to 62 mL/min with CVVHDF; clearance with IHD is 70 to 170 mL/min. They also noted that rebound did not occur and concluded that it could be used when chronic poisoning occurred. Treatment should be continued until there is clinical improvement or the concentration is less than 1 mEq/L.

Acetylsalicylic acid (aspirin) has a MW of 138 Da, is 90% protein bound at therapeutic levels, and has a VD of 0.17 L/kg. Toxicity can lead to multiorgan dysfunction, especially metabolic acidosis and neurotoxicity. It is metabolized by the liver and excreted by the kidneys. Overdose is treated with activated charcoal and urinary alkalization. A systematic review of ECTR for salicylate poisoning by the EXTRIP Workgroup recommends ECTR if its concentration is greater than 100 mg/dL, if there is AKI and concentration greater than 90 mg/dL, if there are mental status changes, and if oxygen therapy is needed for hypoxemia. When standard therapy fails, ECTR is suggested if concentration is greater than 90 mg/dL, if there is AKI and concentration is greater than 80 mg/dL, or if blood pH is 7.2 or less. IHD is the treatment modality of choice, but CRRT is an option if this is not available or the patient is unstable. Treatment cessation is indicated if there is clinical improvement, if concentration is less than 19 mg/dL, or if treatment has lasted at least 4 to 6 hours when salicylate levels are not available.

Carbamazepine, an anticonvulsant, is moderately dialyzable. It has a MW of 236 Da, is 75% to 78% protein bound, and has a VD of 0.8 to 1.8 L/kg. Toxicity may present with ataxia, seizures, tremors, drowsiness, slurred speech, or oliguria. It is remediated with activated charcoal. The EXTRIP Workgroup also performed a systematic review of ECTR for carbamazepine poisoning and suggests IHD as the preferred choice in severe poisoning; if this is not available, CRRT can be performed. One case report used albumin-enhanced CVVHDF to successfully remove carbamazepine; 25% albumin was added to the dialysate to adsorb the drug and maintain a concentration gradient; conventional CVVHDF would not be expected to clear the drug as well. ECTR is recommended if multiple seizures refractory to treatment or life-threatening dysrhythmias occur; it is suggested if prolonged coma or respiratory depression requires mechanical ventilation or if concentrations rise or stay elevated after use of multiple-dose charcoal and support measures. Treatment can be stopped after clinical improvement is noted or when the concentration is less than 10 mg/dL.

Initiation of Treatment

Currently, minimal data are available regarding the optimal time to initiate RRT in general. The question of whether to start CRRT "early" versus "late" is controversial, especially because there is no consensus on what constitutes early and late. Determining a patient's likelihood of recovering renal function may be difficult. There is the risk that patients may be placed on CRRT too early when they could have recovered renal function with conservative treatment or that starting may hinder recovery of function. Often markers of kidney function, such as serum creatinine, BUN, or urine production, are used to decide when to start CRRT. These markers may be misleading because their levels can be influenced by patient factors such as nutritional status, fluid accumulation, and medication usage. Neutrophil gelatinase–associated lipocalin, kidney injury molecule 1, cystatin C, and interleukin-18 are some of the plasma and urine biomarkers that may be useful in detecting AKI earlier than the current markers used. These in turn may facilitate the decision of when to start CRRT. Other factors that influence initiation of treatment can be seen in Table 28.11.

To date, there are few RCTs and some observational studies looking at timing of RRT initiation and outcomes. In 2011, Karvellas et al performed a systemic review and meta-analysis of 15 studies, two of which were RCTs, comparing early versus late initiation of RRT in critically ill AKI patients. The other studies were prospective and retrospective observational studies. Eight studies, including the two RCTs, used CRRT as the main RRT modality; the other had a combination of CRRT and IHD. Serum urea; serum creatinine; urine output; and Risk, Injury, Failure, Loss, End-stage (RIFLE) criteria were used to determine early and late initiation of RRT. Findings suggested there might be some benefit in survival at 28 days to initiating RRT early; however, studies were of low quality, and there was much heterogeneity with no standard definition for what constitutes "early" initiation of RRT.

Table 28.11

Factors Influencing Initiation of Renal Replacement Therapy in Acute Kidney Injury

Patient safety
Unnecessary procedure
Possibility of patient recovering renal function
Risk associated with RRT procedure
Complications associated with catheter placement
Hypotension and cardiac events during procedure
Fear of prolonging renal injury after initiation of RRT
Factors affecting implementation
Logistics
Vascular access availability
Availability of equipment and personnel
Time of decision to initiation (Sundays, late night)
Treating physician decision

RRT, renal replacement therapy.
From Macedo E, Mehta RL. Tailored therapy: matching the method to the patient. *Blood: Purif* 2012;34(2):124-131.

The Beginning and Ending Supportive Therapy for the Kidney (BEST Kidney) study was a large multicenter prospective, observational study comparing septic and nonseptic ICU patients with AKI. It showed that a higher proportion of septic AKI patients received CRRT rather than IHD. Investigators also noted that these patients were in the ICU longer before being placed on RRT. Overall this study showed that early initiation of RRT (based on time from admission to ICU) led to better outcomes with a decrease in mortality and length of hospital stay and shorter RRT duration.

The degree of fluid overload at CRRT initiation has also been shown to impact outcomes in both adult and pediatric patients. Several studies have shown that more than 10% to 20% of fluid accumulation in the ICU when starting CRRT is associated with increased mortality. In their analysis of the prospective pediatric continuous RRT registry, Sutherland et al found a 3% increase in mortality for each 1% increase in severity of fluid overload. Heung et al showed that in adults, a higher degree of fluid overload at RRT initiation predicts worse renal recovery at 1 year.

Thus, available data seem to show an association between better clinical outcomes and initiation of CRRT early in the course of AKI and at lower degrees of fluid accumulation. It is also known that delaying or avoiding RRT is associated with higher mortality rates, longer hospital and ICU stays, and decreased renal function in septic AKI patients. Two ongoing trials—STARRT-AKI (Standard versus accelerated initiation of RRT in AKI) trial and the IDEAL-ICU (Initiation of dialysis early versus late in intensive care unit) study—will hopefully better delineate the optimal time to initiate RRT.

Monitoring and Complications

Vascular access–related problems, such as vascular injury and infection, are common, occurring in up to 20% of patients, depending on access site. Uncuffed, nontunneled catheters are semirigid. Common complications after placement include hematoma, hemothorax, and pneumothorax, thrombus formation, pericardial tamponade, air embolism, and retroperitoneal hemorrhage. Therefore, ultrasound guidance should be used for line placement, and before using an IJ or subclavian line, a chest radiograph should be obtained to check for correct positioning. Catheter-line infections are also a concern and should be avoided by placement under sterile technique and appropriate dressing and catheter care. The use of topical antibiotics at the skin insertion site and use of antibiotic locks are not suggested because they may promote fungal infections and antimicrobial resistance.

Hypothermia is common with CRRT. This occurs because replacement fluids and dialysate are not warmed, leading to cooling of core body temperature. Newer CRRT machines have warming devices to prevent heat loss. Body temperature cooling can mask fevers, delaying infection recognition and treatment. In some instances, however, such as hyperthermia, after cardiac arrest, or with brain injury, this cooling effect may be advantageous. The extracorporeal circuit or filter membrane may activate inflammatory immune mediators, including various cytokines, which may increase protein breakdown and energy expenditure. As mentioned earlier, rarely, anaphylactoid reactions caused by bradykinin activation do occur.

Complications of anticoagulation include the risk of bleeding, especially if systemic anticoagulation, such as with heparin, is used. Heparin should be titrated to a postfilter partial thromboplastin time of 1.5 to 2 times normal or an activated clotting time of 180 to 220 seconds. The use of heparin can also lead to HIT, which may cause repeated premature filter clotting. Regional anticoagulation with citrate has less bleeding risk but has its own set of possible complications: hypocalcemia (citrate binds calcium), metabolic alkalosis (citrate is metabolized to bicarbonate), and hypernatremia (when sodium citrate is used). Citrate toxicity is noted by an increase in the total serum calcium, decrease in ionized calcium concentration, metabolic acidosis, and increased anion gap; if the ratio of total serum calcium to ionized calcium is greater than 2.5 (when both measured in mmol/L) or greater than 10 (when total calcium measured in mg/dL), toxicity is likely. To correct this, the citrate infusion should be decreased or stopped, the dialysate flow rate should be increased, and the calcium infusion should be increased. Careful monitoring should be carried out with the circuit-ionized calcium kept between 0.2 and 0.4 mmol/L and patient-ionized calcium in the physiologic range of 1.1 to 1.3 mmol/L, although sometimes a lower target of 0.9 to 1.0 mmol/L is acceptable. Monitoring of electrolytes, circuit- and patient-ionized calcium, and blood gases should occur at least every 6 hours, and total calcium levels should be measured at least once daily.

Electrolyte complications result from their removal by dialysis or hemofiltration and insufficient replacement occurs, as well as from the use of citrate anticoagulation, as noted earlier. Table 28.12 lists the potential electrolyte complications of CRRT. If severe derangements are present, laboratory measurements should be done frequently, about every 2 to 4 hours. Otherwise, electrolytes can be monitored at least every 6 hours, but this can be decreased to every 12 hours when they are stable.

When managing fluid issues, the potential for volume depletion needs to be kept in mind. This can occur if there is inadequate monitoring or inaccurate calculations are performed. Vigilant monitoring is important because there is the potential to remove large volumes of fluid quickly. Drops in blood pressure, tachycardia, or change in invasive monitoring (e.g., a decrease in CVP) are signs that this is occurring. To prevent this, flow sheets for recording and monitoring fluid balance should be used. Also, a nurse-to-patient ratio of at least one to one is needed to ensure appropriate management.

Nutritional losses in critically ill patients on CRRT are common. These patients are hypercatabolic and need extra nutrition. Amino acid loss ranges from 10 to 20 g/day. Severe protein-energy wasting ensues, leading to loss of lean body mass,

Table 28.12	

Electrolyte Derangements With Continuous Renal Replacement Therapy

Derangement	Cause
Hypophosphatemia	Removal and inadequate replacement
Hypokalemia	Removal and inadequate replacement
Hypernatremia	Sodium citrate anticoagulation without lowering dialysate or replacement fluid sodium concentration
Hypocalcemia	Citrate anticoagulation and inadequate replacement
	Excessive citrate in hepatic failure patients
Hypercalcemia	Citrate anticoagulation and excessive calcium replacement
Hypomagnesemia	Removal and inadequate replacement

Adapted from Fall P, Szerlip HM. Continuous renal replacement therapy: cause and treatment of electrolyte complications. *Semin Dial* 2010;23(6):581-585.

reduction of fat mass, and low urea concentrations; all of these worsen in-hospital mortality rates, extend hospital stays, and increase the likelihood of infectious complications. Patients should receive increased daily protein or amino acid intake to about 1.5 to 2.5 g/kg/day. Glucose loss also occurs but is not well documented. Dialysate and replacement solutions contribute up to 40 to 80 g/day, although they do not usually lead to hyperglycemia. If glucose-free solutions are used, there is a risk of hypoglycemia or inadequate nutrition. For adequate intake, carbohydrates should be given at 5 to 7 g/kg/day. CRRT readily removes vitamins and minerals. Their supplementation has not shown benefit on survival, but they are still replaced, especially because water-soluble vitamins and active vitamin D are easily depleted. Of note, vitamin A supplementation is not recommended because its accumulation can be toxic. In addition, vitamin C intake should not exceed the recommended daily dose because it can lead to oxalosis.

Finally, drug clearance may be significantly impacted by CRRT. High CRRT doses influence the pharmacokinetics and pharmacodynamics of medications. Therefore, patients may be underdosed, especially with regard to antimicrobials, vasoactive medications, sedatives and paralytics, or antiseizure medications. Medications should be titrated based on effect, or when available, medication levels in the blood should be followed to adjust doses.

Outcomes

Patient outcomes after starting CRRT are influenced greatly by underlying disease states, comorbidities, and indication for initiation, among other clinical criteria. In 2013, Schneider et al conducted a systematic review and meta-analysis of the literature at the time to analyze data on dialysis dependence among critically ill survivors of an episode of AKI that required acute RRT; patients who initially received intermittent RRT (IRRT) were compared with those who initially received CRRT. Seven RCTs and 16 observational studies were identified. Pooling all studies together demonstrated that IRRT was associated with 1.7 times the increased risk of dialysis dependence compared with CRRT. This increased risk was present even when subgroups were analyzed (RCTs pooled and observational studies pooled separately); however, the increased risk was not statistically significant among RCTs.

Allegretti and colleagues analyzed a prospective cohort of ICU patients started on CRRT with AKI at a single center to examine renal recovery and in-hospital and postdischarge mortality rates. They found only 25% of AKI patients were dialysis free at the end of the follow-up period (4 years of rolling postdischarge data). While in the hospital, the mortality rate was about 61%; after discharge, about 28% of patients died. The total rate of renal recovery was 93% by the end of the study period.

More recently, Wald et al performed a retrospective cohort study matching 1 : 1 CRRT and IRRT patients in the ICU with AKI. Only patients who survived past 90 days after RRT initiation were followed for a median duration of 3 years. It was found that chronic dialysis risk was lower in those patients who received CRRT versus IRRT (hazard ratio, 0.75; 95% confidence interval, 0.65–0.87). These results confirmed the findings of Schneider et al's review and meta-analysis.

Data for children regarding mortality have been gathered from the Prospective Pediatric Continuous Renal Replacement Therapy (ppCRRT). The overall mortality rate was 42%. Survival was lowest for patients who had fluid overload and electrolyte imbalances at CRRT initiation. Children weighing more than 10 kg and those older than 1 year of age had better overall survival rates. Other reviews and observational studies that have shown worse outcomes seem to be associated with greater burden of illness, multiple organ involvement, and hemodynamic instability. In addition, infant survival has been consistent between about 35% to 45%, and infants weighing less than 3 kg have worse survival, around 24% compared with infants over 3 kg (41%) as reported by Symons et al in 2003.

Cost

Publications in the past 15 years have looked at costs for different forms of RRT for AKI. Many of these studies look at short-term costs of RRT in the hospital and compare IRRT with CRRT. These studies have shown that CRRT is more costly than IRRT, even when IRRT was used more intensively (e.g., daily IHD). These studies, however, did not consider short- and long-term costs of the different RRT modalities in patients with AKI. They mostly focused on in-hospital or ICU costs and costs related to specific resources, such as dialysate or replacement fluids, anticoagulation, and circuit requirements. In 2015, Ethgen and colleagues performed a cost-effectiveness analysis comparing IRRT and CRRT in ICU patients with AKI. Despite finding higher up-front costs for CRRT, the total cost over 5 years (including dialysis dependence costs) was lower when CRRT was used as initial treatment compared with IRRT.

Conclusion

Continuous renal replacement therapy is being used more as an alternative to IRRT in the management of AKI, especially in critically ill patients. It has many applications, and its use can be adapted to fit different situations. Further research is needed, however, to see which patient populations are most likely to benefit from CRRT, to provide definitive criteria for appropriate initiation of treatment, and to determine long-term outcomes related to its use.

CHAPTER 29

Anticoagulation for Continuous Renal Replacement Therapy

Vinay Narasimha Krishna, MD • Keith Wille, MD, MSPH •
Ashita Tolwani, MD, MSc

Continuous renal replacement therapy (CRRT) has evolved as the preferred form of dialysis in hemodynamically unstable critically ill patients with acute kidney injury (AKI). It is applied continuously and achieves solute clearance and fluid removal by convection as in continuous venovenous hemofiltration (CVVH), diffusion as in continuous venovenous hemodialysis (CVVHD), or a combination of both as in continuous venovenous hemodiafiltration (CVVHDF). CRRT requires anticoagulation for the prevention of clotting of the extracorporeal circuit. Clotting of the hemofilter reduces total therapy time and leads to decreased dialysis efficacy, blood loss in the extracorporeal circuit, and increased cost because of frequent hemofilter replacements. Although observational studies have demonstrated that CRRT without anticoagulation is feasible in patients with coagulopathy, most critically ill patients require some form of anticoagulation to achieve adequate dialysis. The ideal anticoagulant for CRRT should have a short half-life and provide optimal antithrombotic activity with low bleeding risk and minimal systemic adverse effects. It should be inexpensive and readily available with simple monitoring methods and have an antidote for easy reversal. This chapter discusses the anticoagulation options available for CRRT with their advantages and disadvantages.

Selecting Anticoagulation Approaches for Continuous Renal Replacement Therapy

The most common anticoagulant options for CRRT include unfractionated heparin (UFH), regional citrate anticoagulation (RCA), and no anticoagulation. Less common anticoagulation options include UFH with protamine reversal, low-molecular weight heparin (LMWH), thrombin antagonists, and platelet-inhibiting agents. The anticoagulant choice should be determined by the bleeding risk of the patient and the presence of liver failure or heparin-induced thrombocytopenia (HIT) (Table 29.1). The Kidney Disease: Improving Global Outcomes (KDIGO) AKI guidelines recommend using RCA rather than UFH in patients who do not have contraindications to citrate and are with or without increased risk of bleeding. In patients who have contraindications to citrate and are without an increased bleeding risk, they recommend using UFH or LMWH rather than other anticoagulants. KDIGO also recommends avoiding regional heparinization during CRRT in patients at increased risk of bleeding. They recommend no anticoagulation in patients with contraindications to citrate use and who are at increased risk of bleeding.

Table 29.1

	Choice of Agent	
Clinical Characteristics	**No Liver Failure**	**Severe Liver Failure**
Low risk of bleeding	UFH, citrate	UFH
High risk of bleeding	Citrate	No anticoagulation
Heparin-induced thrombocytopenia	Citrate, argatroban	Bivalirudin

UFH, unfractionated heparin

Specific Agents and Anticoagulation Techniques (Table 29.2)

Unfractionated Heparin

In patients at low risk of bleeding, minimal-dose UFH is preferred because it is easy to use, inexpensive, and readily accessible, and it has an antidote (protamine). UFH is a mixture of glycosaminoglycans with molecular weights between 3000 to 30,000 daltons. It acts by binding to antithrombin III and inhibiting factors IIa and Xa. A single optimal regimen for UFH administration during CRRT has not been identified. Typical heparin protocols administer UFH into the arterial limb of the dialysis circuit as a bolus of 1000 to 5000 IU (30 IU/kg) followed by a continuous infusion of 5 to 15 IU/kg/hr. Anticoagulation is monitored by maintaining an activated plasma prothrombin time (aPTT) goal between 45 and 60 seconds or 1.5 to 2.0 times normal. However, the optimal target aPTT is not known with certainty, and the therapeutic benefit of preventing clotting in the extracorporeal circuit must be balanced with the risk of systemic bleeding. Disadvantages of UFH include dosing variability arising from complex and unpredictable pharmacokinetics, risk of heparin resistance caused by low patient antithrombin levels, the development of HIT, and the risk of hemorrhage. UFH is contraindicated in patients at high risk of bleeding (e.g., recent surgery, coagulopathy, thrombocytopenia).

Citrate

Regional citrate anticoagulation is a widely used alternative to UFH as an anticoagulant for CRRT and limits anticoagulation to the extracorporeal circuit. Advantages of RCA include the avoidance of both systemic anticoagulation and HIT. Furthermore, multiple randomized controlled trials (RCTs) have demonstrated RCA to have a lower risk of bleeding compared with UFH, reduced requirement for transfusion of blood products, and improved hemofilter survival.

Citrate is infused into the blood at the beginning of the CRRT extracorporeal circuit, where it chelates ionized calcium (iCa^{++}) and prevents clotting by making free calcium unavailable to the coagulation cascade (Fig. 29.1). Optimal regional anticoagulation is attained when the postfilter iCa^{++} concentration in the extracorporeal circuit reaches less than 0.35 mmol/L, correlating with a citrate blood concentration of 3 to 6 mmol/L. The majority of the formed calcium–citrate complex is freely filtered across the hemofilter and lost in the effluent. Intravenous calcium chloride or calcium gluconate is infused at an initial rate of 2 to 3 mmol/hr to replace the calcium lost in the effluent and titrated to maintain a normal serum iCa^{++}

Table 29.2

Agent	Dosing	Monitoring	Comments
Heparin	Bolus: 2000–5000 IU (30 IU/kg) Maintenance: 5–15 IU/kg/hr	aPTT goal: 45–60 sec or 1.5 to 2 times normal	Contraindicated in high bleeding risk patients Increased risk of HIT
Citrate	Depends on the CRRT operating characteristics and citrate solution composition Infused to achieve a postfilter ionized calcium <0.35 mmol/L or citrate blood concentration of 3–6 mmol/L	Postfilter ionized calcium, blood electrolytes, and calcium ratio (total calcium to ionized calcium)	Requires IV calcium and frequent electrolyte monitoring Contraindicated in severe liver failure
Argatroban	Bolus 100 mcg/kg followed by infusion to achieve a target aPTT of 1.5–3.0 Doses range between 0.7 and 1.7 µg/kg/min	aPTT	No antidote Dose reduction in liver failure
Regional UFH with protamine	UFH is infused prefilter at 1000–1500 U/hr Protamine is infused at 10–12 mg/hr postfilter to neutralize heparin	Circuit and systemic aPTT	Regional anticoagulation reduces risk of systemic bleeding Technically complicated HIT risk
Nadroparin Dalteparin	Loading dose of 15–25 IU/kg followed by a maintenance dose of 5 IU/kg/hr	Anti-Xa levels with target levels between 0.25 and 0.35 units/mL	High risk of bleeding Expensive Less reversal with protamine

aPTT, activated partial thromboplastin time; CRRT, continuous renal replacement therapy; HIT, heparin-induced thrombocytopenia; IV, intravenous; UFH, unfractionated heparin.

concentration. The remaining calcium–citrate complex that is not filtered is then returned to the patient and metabolized by the liver, kidneys, and skeletal muscles to bicarbonate. Each citrate molecule potentially yields three bicarbonate molecules. Calcium released from the calcium–citrate complex helps restore the serum iCa^{++} levels back to normal.

Because of the lack of universally available commercial citrate formulations specific for CRRT, the citrate solutions used for RCA are either custom made by a pharmacy or available in a concentrated formulation with high sodium content that are not intended for CRRT use. These hypertonic citrate formulations often require compensatory hyponatremic replacement or dialysate solutions with either no or reduced bicarbonate concentrations to prevent the development of metabolic alkalosis. The most commonly used hypertonic citrate formulations in the United States include: 2.2% Anticoagulant Citrate Dextrose Solution (ACD-A), which contains 224 mmol/L sodium, 74.8 mmol/L citrate, and 38 mmol/L citric acid, and 4%

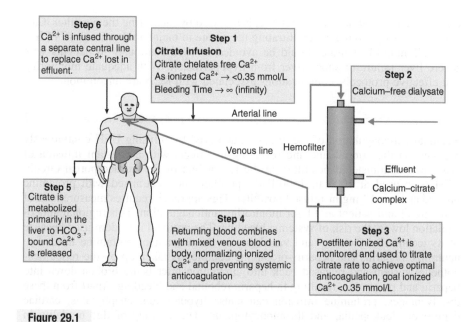

Figure 29.1

Schematic representation of regional citrate anticoagulation for continuous renal replacement therapy.

trisodium citrate solution (TSC), which contains 420 mmol/L sodium and 136 mmol/L citrate. Two isotonic dilute citrate formulations specific for CRRT have become commercially available in Europe: Prismocitrate 10/2, which contains 10 mmol/L citrate, 2 mmol/L citric acid, and 136 mmol/L sodium, and Prismocitrate 18/0, which contains 18 mmol/L citrate. These isotonic solutions are meant to function as a combined anticoagulant and replacement fluid for convective clearance in CVVH and CVVHDF. Neither of these solutions is available in the United States. Citrate is not currently a Food and Drug Administration–approved anticoagulant for CRRT and therefore is used off label as an anticoagulant for CRRT in the United States.

Electrolyte abnormalities specific to citrate anticoagulation include hypernatremia from the use of hypertonic citrate formulations, metabolic alkalosis, metabolic acidosis, hypomagnesemia, and hypo- or hypercalcemia. Metabolic alkalosis can occur with an excessive citrate load or the administration of exogenous bicarbonate with citrate anticoagulation. Metabolic acidosis can occur when citrate accumulates in patients who cannot metabolize citrate, such as those with liver failure or severe lactic acidosis, resulting in negative buffer balance. Hallmarks of citrate accumulation include worsening metabolic acidosis, ionized hypocalcemia from unmetabolized calcium–citrate complexes, rising total calcium levels caused by a progressively higher calcium infusion rate, and a disproportional rise in total systemic calcium to iCa^{++} ratio of greater than 2.5. Severe ionized hypocalcemia can cause hypotension, arrhythmias, and eventual cardiac arrest. Protocol driven care with frequent monitoring (every 4–6 hours) of acid–base status and other electrolytes, including ionized calcium, total calcium, phosphorous, and magnesium, is necessary for preventing errors. Adequate citrate anticoagulation is assessed by measuring the postfilter iCa^{++} concentrations periodically and titrating the citrate to maintain the circuit iCa^{++} less than 0.35 mmol/L. Citrate should be avoided or used cautiously in patients with severe liver failure or shock liver from hypoperfusion. With adequate monitoring and effective protocols, complications associated with RCA are uncommon.

Regional Unfractionated Heparin With Protamine Reversal

Regional anticoagulation of the circuit is achieved by infusing UFH continuously prefilter via the arterial line and reversing its effects with a constant infusion of protamine administered postfilter on the return line of the extracorporeal circuit. UFH is infused at 1000 to 1500 IU/hr prefilter and neutralized with protamine infused at 10 to 12 mg/hr infused postfilter. This approach requires measurement of both circuit and patient aPTT for monitoring anticoagulation. This regional anticoagulation lowers the risk of systemic bleeding. The protocol is seldom used because of its technical difficulties and variability in the amount of protamine needed to neutralize heparin. The heparin–protamine complex is taken up by the reticuloendothelial system and released back into circulation after being broken down into heparin and protamine, resulting in heparin rebound and bleeding. Apart from these disadvantages, protamine infusion can cause hypotension, anaphylaxis, cardiac depression, leukopenia, and thrombocytopenia. The efficacy of this modality in prolonging filter lifespan has been variable, although studies have demonstrated its feasibility and safety. Given the risks of HIT from heparin and side effects of protamine, this modality of anticoagulation is not recommended over UFH.

Low-Molecular-Weight Heparin

Low-molecular-weight heparin acts by inhibiting factor Xa and has a higher anti-Xa/anti IIa activity than UFH because of the lower molecular weight. The pharmacokinetics for LMWH is more predictable with a reliable anticoagulant response. LMWH is associated with a lower incidence of HIT. Dalteparin, enoxaparin, and nadroparin have been studied among patients receiving CRRT and differ in size, half-life, and activity. Nadroparin and dalteparin are administered at a loading dose of 15 to 25 IU/kg followed by a maintenance dose of 5 IU/kg/hr. Anticoagulation is monitored using anti-Xa levels with target levels between 0.25 to 0.35 units/mL. Higher anti-Xa levels between 0.45 and 0.8 units/mL have been associated with bleeding complications. The disadvantages associated with LMWH include prolonged anticoagulation effect in patients with renal failure, less effective reversal with protamine because of a stronger anti-Xa effect, requirement of special assays to measure anti-Xa activity, and increased cost compared with UFH. RCTs have shown that fixed-dose LMWHs are as effective as but not superior to standard heparin in prolonging circuit life.

Thrombin Antagonists

The most common thrombin antagonists used for anticoagulation of the CRRT circuit in the setting of HIT are argatroban and bivalirudin. Argatroban is metabolized in the liver and has a short half-life of 35 minutes even in patients on chronic dialysis. Anticoagulation is monitored by measuring aPTT levels. Argatroban is administered as a loading dose of 100 mcg/kg followed by an infusion to achieve a target aPTT of 1.5 to 3.0. Dosing can range between 0.7 and 1.7 μg/kg/min. A dose reduction is needed in patients with hepatic failure. Disadvantages include bleeding risks and the absence of an antidote. Bivalirudin is used as an alternative to argatroban in patients who have both liver and renal failure because it has both extrarenal and extrahepatic clearance. It has a short half-life with reversible thrombin binding. One study comparing bivalirudin anticoagulation with heparin anticoagulation in CVVH found longer filter survival times associated with bivalirudin use, which was well tolerated.

Platelet-Inhibiting Agents

Prostacyclin (PGI$_2$) and its synthetic derivative epoprostenol act by inhibiting platelet aggregation and adhesion. Prostacyclin is infused prefilter at 2 to 8 ng/kg/min. It can be used individually or in combination with low-dose UFH at a rate of 5 to 6 IU/kg/hr. Its main disadvantages are its high cost and potential to cause hypotension. There is only limited clinical experience with prostacyclin use with few published reports about its safety and efficacy.

Nafamostat mesylate is another prostacyclin analog that does not cause hypotension and is currently not available in the United States. It is a synthetic serine protease inhibitor that is administered at a dosage of 0.1 mg/kg/hr. Anaphylaxis, agranulocytosis, hyperkalemia, and circuit clotting because of decreased protein C activity resulting from increased levels of thrombin–antithrombin III complex and prothrombin activation fragment 1+2 are some of the disadvantages limiting its use.

Conclusions

There is no consensus on which anticoagulant should be the first choice for all CRRT patients. The choice of anticoagulation primarily depends on patient characteristics such as the risk of bleeding or the presence of other contraindications such as HIT or the presence of liver failure. This choice is also influenced by local expertise, nursing comfort, ease of monitoring, and issues related to pharmacy. Although UFH is most commonly used, citrate anticoagulation is gaining wider acceptance as an alternative anticoagulation approach with the evolution of simplified and safer protocols.

CHAPTER 30

Wearable and Implantable Renal Replacement Therapy

William Henry Fissell IV, MD

Dialysis is the semiselective removal of solutes from a solution by diffusion across a semipermeable membrane. It was first used in vitro by Thomas Graham in 1861 to separate ions from macromolecules in a colloidal solution. Early in the 20th century, John Jacob Abel isolated epinephrine, insulin, and other hormones from the blood of living dogs using dialysis, which he termed "vividiffusion." Kolff is generally credited with the first successful dialytic treatment of renal failure in a human patient in 1944. Alwall independently developed a hard-shell dialyzer, allowing for pressure-driven ultrafiltration (UF) to control extracellular fluid volume in addition to solute clearance. In 1960, Scribner, Quinton, and Dillard developed a reliable make-and-break connection to the circulation, the Scribner Shunt, and maintenance hemodialysis (HD) became possible. The technology and medical, economic, and social infrastructures of dialysis have evolved so that by 2010, more than 400,000 American patients with end-stage renal failure (ESRD) are able to survive for months and years after kidney failure. Dialysis is thus the first engineered replacement for a failed organ and has been successful in that a procedure that 40 years ago was rationed because of scarcity is now the standard of care. Recent literature has suggested that overenthusiastic prescription of dialysis to inappropriate patients is a concern rather than scarcity. However, a patient dependent on HD is medically distinct from a patient with normal kidneys or with advanced chronic renal insufficiency. Some of the most compelling data in this regard are the vastly prolonged survival times of renal failure patients who receive a transplant compared with those remaining on the waitlist for an organ. Time to first appropriate shock from an implantable defibrillator is much sooner in dialysis than in chronic kidney disease (CKD), and epicardial atherosclerosis appears much more resistant to therapy in dialysis patients compared with subjects without renal failure. Patients dependent on dialysis have impaired vaccine responses and die of pulmonary infection at a rate 20 times the rate in the general population. Young women with renal failure on dialysis often do not menstruate and rarely conceive or carry a pregnancy to term. The clinical presentation of a dialysis patient who is "well dialyzed" by present standards may be disappointingly similar to the presentation of a patient with renal failure who has not been dialyzed at all.

Limits of Conventional Hemodialysis

Maintenance HD is an episodic extracorporeal membrane blood purification procedure, and in the United States, it is generally performed three times each week for between 3 and 5 hours at a session. The dialysis dose is in practice adjusted by setting the duration of the treatment. The treatment time is chosen to clear approximately one volume of distribution of urea per patient per treatment using a membrane that has an area approximately equivalent to the patient's body surface area. Urea is in many ways a sensible choice for a biomarker of dialytic adequacy because the nitrogenous wastes of protein metabolism are clearly linked to acute uremia, and diets that are sparing in protein can delay the onset of uremic symptoms when dialysis is not feasible. This episodic treatment pattern is essentially unlike the continuous around-the-clock solute removal of healthy kidneys. In this section, we describe how the episodic treatment schedule of dialysis contributes to the morbid phenotype of dialyzed renal failure.

Solute Removal

Urea

Urea is the end product of protein metabolism. Typical dietary protein intake in adults results in about 10 to 13 mg/min of urea nitrogen production. In the course of a dialysis session, small solutes are removed in proportion to their concentration. In the case of urea, a two-compartment first-order kinetic model describes urea removal well, and a single-compartment model is sufficient for most urea kinetic modeling.

$$U_{final} = U_{initial} \times e^{-\frac{Kt}{V}}$$

where K is the instantaneous clearance, V is the volume of distribution of urea, and t is treatment time. Net urea removal per session is generally targeted to a single-pool Kt/V value of about 1.2 to 1.4. A Kt/V of 1.0 is approximately equivalent to a dialysis session clearance of one urea volume of distribution. In practice, there is some urea rebound from the (not modeled) peripheral compartment, so the single-pool Kt/V target is 20% to 40% higher than 1.0. From this, we can estimate net urea removal in a single session:

$$U_{removed} = K \times \int_0^{\tau} U_{initial} \times e^{-\frac{Kt}{V}}$$

Over 2 days between dialysis sessions, somewhere between 28 and 43 g of urea will be generated and need to be removed. Because removal is concentration dependent, one might ask, how high must the predialysis urea nitrogen rise to achieve this removal? HD urea clearance is usually limited by blood flow rather than dialysate flow or membrane efficiency. If we assume K is around 300 to 350 mL/min, we can evaluate the integral in the second equation and learn that the predialysis urea nitrogen must rise to around 70 mg/dL or greater to remove urea generated at a rate of 10 mg/min. The time-averaged urea concentration is likely close to 40 mg/dL. The lesson is that in maintenance dialysis on a thrice-weekly schedule, azotemia is the price of nutrition. The dialysis patient with a low predialysis BUN either has significant residual renal function or is not eating enough protein.

In contrast, the time-averaged concentration of any solute that is continuously cleared by a first-order mechanism tends toward the ratio of the generation rate to the clearance (G/K). If urea is being generated at 10 mg/min and being cleared at

15 mL/min, the long-term concentration will be about 0.66 mg/mL or 66 mg/dL. If we double the clearance to 30 mL/min, the time averaged concentration will still be elevated: 33 mg/dL.

Phosphorus

Phosphorus is an unusual molecule in dialysis. Inorganic phosphate is a small molecule with molecular weight (100 Da) less than that of creatinine (113 Da); it is negatively charged and passes through modern dialyzer membranes slightly less freely than creatinine. However, dialytic removal of phosphorus is inadequate to balance dietary intake, so dietary restriction and oral phosphorus binders are required to keep phosphorus levels low. Very few dialysis patients are able to attain target phosphorus levels through dialysis, binders, and diet. The basis for limited dialytic removal of phosphorus is that phosphorus is best described by a multicompartment kinetic model with nonlinear kinetics. Extracellular phosphate falls rapidly during treatment, decreasing the concentration gradient that drives removal, but refilling of the extracellular space from intracellular stores is slow. Thus HD can extract phosphorus from blood but not from all body tissues. Interestingly, phosphorus concentrations in blood decrease precipitously but then plateau as incompletely understood regulatory mechanisms mobilize phosphorus from reservoirs, possibly bone, to prevent more severe hypophosphatemia. The role of intradialytic hypotension in decreasing blood flow to phosphorus-rich tissues such as striated muscle remains uncertain but a plausible factor complicating dialytic phosphorus removal. In contrast, continuous renal replacement therapies (CRRTs) as are practiced in some critical care units have instantaneous clearances an order of magnitude lower than HD but can remove so much phosphorus over 1 to 2 days that supplementation is often needed. This is not surprising when one recalls that long-term steady-state serum concentrations will tend towards G/K. To balance dietary absorption of 800 mg/day or 0.5 to 0.6 mg/min, an instantaneous clearance of only 15 mL/min can maintain phosphorus levels of about 3 mg/dL. More than that, as in CRRT, will always drop levels lower.

β_2-Microglobulin

A significant difference between glomerular filtration and HD is the clearance of so-called middle molecules between 2 and 25 to 40 kDa, although definitions vary. β_2-Microglobulin is an approximately 12-kDa protein member of the immunoglobulin superfamily of proteins. It is expressed on the surface of all nucleated cells as a component of the type I major histocompatibility complex. β_2-Microglobulin passes through the glomerular capillary wall almost unimpeded. In contrast, β_2-microglobulin is not well cleared by conventional HD membranes. Even high-flux and high-cutoff dialyzers have β_2-microglobulin clearances 10% to 20% of the urea clearance. Although β_2-microglobulin levels in serum may fall by half during a treatment, postdialytic rebound from peripheral compartments is considerable. β_2-Microglobulin is not merely a benign marker of middle molecule clearance but is mechanistically pathological in ESRD. β_2-Microglobulin polymerizes to form amyloid, and, over time, this affects nearly every organ system, from nerve entrapment in the carpal tunnel to immune response to cardiovascular disease. So, in part, the barrier confronting dialytic management of β_2-microglobulin in the setting of thrice-weekly in-center dialysis is twofold: The dialyzer membranes do not allow much β_2-microglobulin to pass through them, and β_2-microglobulin is somewhat sequestered in a peripheral compartment.

The disappointing middle-molecule clearance of hollow-fiber dialyzers is likely related to the underlying technology used to manufacture polymer membranes. Although membranes are loosely described as having a "cutoff," even idealized membranes such as track-etch membranes or microfabricated membranes do not show an abrupt transition from unhindered passage to complete retention at some particular solute size or weight. Instead there is a transition range of molecular weights that are partially and incompletely retained. The pores in polymer membranes are formed using a solvent-demixing process. A polymer is dissolved in a mix of incompletely miscible solvents; typically, the polymer partitions more strongly into one solvent than the other. Some condition, such as temperature, is changed, and the solvents separate into individual phases, one with and one without the polymer. Micro- or nano-sized droplets of one solvent form the pores within the mix of the other solvent and polymer. These droplets have a dispersion of sizes: They are not all uniform in radius, and consequently, the membrane has a thermodynamic distribution of pore sizes, most small but many large. Fluid flow will disproportionately channel through the large pores as resistance to flow varies as the fourth power of the pore radius. If passage of a large solute, such as albumin, is to be blocked, there must be diminishingly few large pores. There are two ways to achieve this. First, the pore size distribution must be very narrow, with the droplets that form the pores being very uniform in size. Thus, there are few large pores. Second, the pore distribution must be based on a very small average pore size so that the distribution will have tailed off so that there are few large pores. In practice, both paths are followed, but the mean pore size of most polymer dialyzers is much smaller than albumin and smaller even than the middle molecules we describe. For example, it is common to see myoglobin (a 15-kDa monomer) in urine, but even in cases of severe rhabdomyolysis, one rarely or never sees pigmented in spent dialysate. Some of the difference between HD and native kidney function is also due to the difference in pore size between the glomerulus and the dialyzer.

Salt and Water Removal

The kidney, guided by redundant neuroendocrine feedback loops, maintains extracellular fluid volume to within a few kilograms despite widely varying salt and water intake. In the setting of CKD, renal sodium handling gradually adapts to decreased glomerular filtration rates at the cost of a greatly narrowed range of sodium intake that can be managed. Patients who depend on HD gradually lose residual renal function. Diuretic use can limit interdialytic weight gain (IDWG) and appears to delay loss of residual renal function. Again, as in the discussion of urea, the episodic nature of dialysis can explain some of the challenges in dialytic management of patients with ESRD. Typical fluid intake in adults is around 1500 mL/day, and stool losses are usually only 100 to 200 mL/day; 1300 mL/day is a little over 9 L per week, although insensible losses may blunt that slightly. Nine liters per week translates to 3 L of fluid removal per dialysis session. Patients with diabetes or who do not carefully restrict their salt intake will experience osmolality-driven thirst and will drink more. Despite similar urea reductions, patients with IDWGs in excess of 3 kg had worse mortality rates than those with IDWGs less than 3 kg. Rapid removal of fluid during dialysis is associated with cardiovascular mortality. Acute decreases in intravascular volume that occur with UF can cause myocardial ischemia through several mechanisms. Dialysis patients with left ventricular hypertrophy, atrial fibrillation, or both have an exaggerated hypotensive response to hypovolemia compared with healthy subjects. Catecholamine-mediated tachycardia in response to hypovolemia decreases the duration of diastole and thus the filling of epicardial coronary arteries. At the same time, systemic vascular resistance increases, increasing myocardial workload. Thus, demand ischemia is an understandable consequence of UF, and echocardiography shows intradialytic myocardial stunning related to UF. In contrast, prolonged or frequent dialysis sessions decrease IDWG, UF rates, and myocardial stunning, suggesting that transient myocardial dysfunction is not intrinsic to the patient or the dialytic removal of solutes but instead directly related to the hemodynamic stresses of cyclic severe hypovolemia.

Wearable Systems

Very quickly after maintenance dialysis became feasible and reimbursed by Medicare in the United States, technology development for convenient dialysis emerged. It is worth considering that in the early 1970s, self-care HD at home was usual practice. The network of in-center dialysis clinics that provide the vast majority of HD in the United States had not yet emerged. Patients were essentially homebound during treatments. In the context of widespread self-care, the drive even then to facilitate portable, personalized systems is understandable. Kolff, Friedman, and others published theoretical and clinical data regarding portable and wearable systems in the 1970s. However, as in-center dialysis became more widely available, patients were relieved of the burden of bringing their equipment with them because they could be reasonably assured of locating a unit that could accommodate them as they traveled. Dialysis accommodations for leisure travel became available as well. Thus, the need for portable or wearable systems for dialysis appeared less pressing, and efforts were directed elsewhere.

The episodic and intermittent nature of conventional dialysis poses barriers to health, and several groups have examined the role of intensive maintenance dialysis prescriptions with increases in treatment time, frequency, or both. The apparent benefits of these therapies and the growing recognition that less expensive and less burdensome treatment paradigms have stimulated a resurgence in wearable or even implantable devices for the treatment of renal failure. The most burdensome aspects of wearable systems for renal replacement are broadly similar to key features of conventional dialysis. Vascular access, the Achilles heel of all dialysis procedures, is an especially thorny problem for wearable HD systems. The concept of conducting activities of daily living with one or more needles in a fistula or graft is anxiety provoking. An accidental disconnect or venous needle dislodgement might not be immediately detected, and normal movement might allow the needle tip to traumatize the access. Catheter use is associated with inferior survival compared with a fistula or graft. It may be that patients who dialyze through catheters are substantially different from patients with fistulas and grafts in vascular health, wound healing, and access to care. Requiring catheter access as a precondition for wearable HD may create a therapeutic quandary for physicians counseling patients regarding modality choice.

If we somewhat arbitrarily choose a minimum delivered dialysis dose equal to 10 mL/min, a device needs to supply at least 14 L of dialysate per day and in general much more. Typical dialysate requirements for conventional HD are on the order of

200 L; hybrid therapies such as NxStage in which dialysate flow need not be in great excess of blood flow may require 40 to 50 L per session. Peritoneal dialysis (PD), which is the original "wearable" dialysis system, typically requires 10 to 15 L of dialysate. All of these volumes and their attendant weights are prohibitively cumbersome for a true wearable or implantable system. The cumbersome requirements for tens to hundreds of pounds of dialysate water has been recognized for decades. A longstanding and remarkably successful strategy to minimize water requirements has been the use of sorbents to regenerate fresh dialysate from waste dialysate.

The most widely used dialysate regeneration paradigm is clever and worthy of description. Spent dialysate bearing urea, potassium, phosphorus, and other organic uremic solutes is regenerated in a four-step process corresponding to each of these solutes. Dialysate is passed over a column bearing an enzyme, urease, that cleaves urea into ammonia and carbon dioxide gas. The pKa of the ammonia-ammonium (NH_3/NH_4+) system is around 9, so the newly generated ammonia rapidly binds all free protons in the dialysate, raising the pH of the spent dialysate. The spent dialysate then passes through a cation exchange resin that absorbs NH_4+, potassium, and other cations. Next, an anion-exchange column absorbs phosphate, sulfate, and other anions. Finally, a layer of activated charcoal absorbs creatinine and other organic solutes, as well as serves as a safety layer if the cation-exchange column becomes saturated and ammonia breaks through. The regenerated dialysate generally requires supplementation with calcium and magnesium to replace cations that bind to the cation exchange column, as well as supplementation with bicarbonate. Nevertheless, this approach was highly effective when implemented as the REDY system.

There are three commercial efforts at wearable systems for dialysis as of the date of writing. Public information about the state of development of technologies remains somewhat limited, which is understandable because entities protect trade secrets and corporate strategy, as well as navigating the regulatory environments in their potential markets. The descriptions of the four technologies is based on published literature as well as personal communication with the clinical engineering leaders of each effort.

Peritoneal Dialysis

Peritoneal dialysis was the first "wearable" dialysis. Despite the much smaller dialysate volumes involved in PD compared with HD, patients on PD have enviable survival statistics and autonomy in fitting their treatment to their lives and not the reverse. Recycling PD with the REDY system was reported as early as 1976. AWAK Technologies in Singapore is developing a PD-based automated wearable artificial kidney (AWAK) for around-the-clock therapy. The device is described as being about the size of a paperback book, weighing 2 lb, and consisting of a small control module containing a pump and the electronics, an infusion reservoir containing electrolyte concentrates, and a larger disposable container of sorbents. The sorbent system appears to be very similar to the REDY system, using urease, zirconium oxide, and zirconium phosphate in tandem with activated carbon.

As with the REDY system, an infusion of divalent cations is essential to replace calcium and magnesium bound to the ion exchange columns. Unlike the REDY system, peritoneal systems rely on an osmotic gradient between blood and dialysate to shift salt and water from the vasculature to the dialysate to be discarded. The standard osmotic agent in peritoneal dialysate is glucose, which is absorbed by the patient to varying degrees depending on the characteristics of the peritoneal membrane. As a result, the AWAK system infuses glucose as well as calcium and magnesium. The key innovation of the AWAK device is its combination of *tidal PD* with sorbents. In tidal PD, small volumes and short dwells are substituted for large volumes and long dwells. The AWAK device has a total fluid volume of 750 mL divided into a tidal volume of 250 mL and a reserve volume of 500 mL. The 250-mL tidal volume is exchanged almost continuously to attain a flow rate of 4 L/hr. In simulations with a commercial PD cycler operating in tidal mode, creatinine clearances of 10 to 11 mL/min, phosphate clearances of around 6 mL/min, and β_2-microglobulin clearances just under 2 mL/min were observed in human subjects. Whether the use of tidal PD results in greater clearance is unclear; the technique may be selected for patient comfort and practical issues with catheter drainage. For the AWAK device, the primary benefit of a tidal prescription seems to be that less fluid—and thus less weight—is required. The ability of a recycling system to match the clearance of a conventional single-pass system is strongly dependent on avoiding saturation of the sorbents. In particular, if there is breakthrough of the cation exchange layer, ammonia generated by the urease layer could be transported to the patient with potentially devastating consequences. If the AWAK can deliver 10 mL/min creatinine clearance around the clock in a small portable package, this would be remarkable. Whether selection of AWAK by a patient results in improved long-term modality or patient survival remains to be tested.

Hemodialysis

There are two systems, both sorbent based, being developed for continuous ambulatory HD. The Wearable Artificial Kidney, or WAK, is presently in United States–based clinical trials following pilot studies in Vincenza, Italy. The large package size and high blood flow rates of conventional HD are not intrinsic to extracorporeal therapy but are instead a consequence of the short treatment times used in conventional dialysis. Continuous therapy does not require dialyzer urea mass transfer coefficients in the thousands in order to remove urea and creatinine at high enough rates to balance endogenous production. Gura and colleagues combined a small rocker pump that alternately propels blood and dialysate through a small off-the shelf dialyzer. The dialysate is sequentially recirculated through a series of reactors containing the components of the REDY system. Syringe pumps supply calcium, magnesium, and heparin for anticoagulation. The apparatus can be worn similar to a utility belt, with a package weight of about 5 kg. Extensive effort was devoted to optimizing efficiency of the reactors because improved efficiency results in decreased package size and weight.

Two clinical studies have been published describing the use of this technology. The combination of the pump system with a central venous catheter was first tested as an isolated UF device in patients with symptomatic volume overload in the context of ESRD. In 2006, six patients were treated for an average of 5.7 hours with no obvious adverse reaction, other than one patient experiencing a thrombosis of his or her central venous catheter. Mean UF volume was slightly over 1 L. In 2007, Davenport and colleagues tested the WAK in eight patients with ESRD. At a relatively modest blood flow rate ($\approx$50 mL/min), they attained urea clearance of 22 mL/min. The maxim that access is the Achilles heel of dialysis was reaffirmed in that two vascular accesses clotted, and one venous needle dislodgement occurred in eight treatment sessions. A follow-up study reported phosphate and β_2-microglobulin clearances in the eight patients. Phosphate clearance was similar to urea clearance (21.7 mL/min), and β_2-microglobulin clearance was 11.3 mL/min. These data reinforce the earlier comments: The rate-limiting step in solute removal may not be the dialyzer but rather intercompartmental clearances within the patient. As of this writing, a 10-patient open-label safety and efficacy trial is enrolling (ClinicalTrials. gov identifier: NCT02280005), and results are eagerly awaited.

A different approach is adopted by a Netherlands-based company, Nanodialysis. Their sorbent-based approach has two fundamental differences from the REDY system and similar urease–zirconium–carbon regeneration schemes. First, the Nanodialysis system uses a FeOOH anion exchanger and a sodium polystyrene sulfonate cation resin with the intent that the resin be regenerated by the user. The principle is similar to the home water softener that removes minerals from well water. The solution of interest, such as spent dialysate, is circulated through the column. The cations and anions (e.g., potassium and phosphate) to be removed from solution displace the cations and anions on the column because of their higher affinity. When the column becomes saturated, it is switched out of the circuit and is bathed in a regeneration solution in which bound cations and anions are driven off and washed away. In a dialysis device for home use, the total volume of electrolyte solutions could be decreased significantly, and the disposables cost of daily or twice-daily replacement of saturated sorbent cartridges is reduced as well.

The second innovation of Nanodialysis is that it dispenses with the immobilized urease enzyme and instead uses an electrical current to oxidize urea to gaseous nitrogen, gaseous hydrogen, and carbon dioxide. This approach trades one set of challenges for another: The system does not have to manage ammonia generated by urease but will need to address gas generation by the recirculating system. The gas that is generated is removed from the dialysate by a degasser. The electrodes themselves are graphite-based, avoiding possible leaching of heavy metals into the dialysate. Data from preclinical testing of the Nanodialysis device are anticipated soon.

Fully Implantable Systems

A fully implantable device for treatment of renal failure is the holy grail of tissue engineering. The Achilles heels of dialysis are access and infections, and a permanent internal connection to the vasculature could ameliorate both problems. There are challenges to the design engineering of implantable therapy. Present hollow-fiber dialyzers require superphysiologic pressures to circulate blood and have very limited service lifetimes before fouling and thrombosis reduce membrane clearances. Therapeutic strategies that involve replacement of saturated sorbent cartridges or supply of dialysate will continue to require periodic or chronic percutaneous access, with the risk of infection that repeated cannulation or a chronic catheter entails. Successful long-term implanted solutions for ESRD care will likely be based on strategies that avoid the need for dialysate or sorbents.

Recellularization Approaches

Several investigators have examined whether stem cells, engineered cells, or kidney-derived cells can be manipulated to rejuvenate an injured kidney or establish functioning nephrons within an engineered construct. Here we discuss two approaches that have received widespread attention in the popular press: somatic cell nuclear transfer and "reanimation" of decellularized organs. We consider these approaches together because they appear to share common challenges that threaten to delay clinical success for some time. Lanza and colleagues describe a strategy for cloning syngeneic donor tissue. Bovine oocyte nuclei were replaced with nuclei from allogeneic fibroblasts from a donor cow. These cloned oocytes underwent implantation and embryogenesis in a surrogate mother cow. Fetal calves were harvested at 5 to 6 weeks of gestation, and cells from specific embryonic organs were cultured and then implanted into the individual animal from which the fibroblast nuclei had been originally isolated. Tissues from noncloned embryos were rejected by the host, but tissues from cloned embryos were not rejected by the syngeneic host. A small device made from hollow fibers, a collection pouch, and a cluster of embryonic renal tissue formed clear fluid and was implanted in the animals' flanks. At explant, tissue that had histologic features of renal cortex was identified, and a small amount of straw-colored fluid was present in the collection pouch. The authors argued on the basis of slightly elevated urea and creatinine levels as well as low glucose levels that the cloned tissue had produced urine. However, the authors did not report albumin or protein concentrations in the fluid, which might have been a more convincing demonstration that their cloned tissue had formed functional nephrons.

The kidney has a highly elaborate spatial organization of blood vessels and epithelial cells that is essential to healthy function. This intricacy is challenging to design into an artificial construct. Investigators considered using the existing structures in an animal kidney as the scaffold onto which human kidney cells might be grown. Building on early successes with heart tissue, Ott and colleagues published an early result with rodent tissue in 2013. A decellularized rat kidney was seeded with human umbilical vein endothelial cells via the renal artery and a slurry of neonatal rat kidney cells via retrograde infusion into the ureter. After perfusion culture, the recellularized kidney was fixed, sectioned, and stained. Structures similar to glomeruli and tubules were identified. In vitro testing of recellularized implants showed creatinine clearances much less than matched cadaveric kidneys. Albumin retention was poor (47%), and glucosuria persisted, suggesting that differentiated function of engrafted cells was incomplete.

Both approaches are highly exciting because they are innovative strategies to expand the limited the donor pool with organs for transplant. However, both approaches as published require the destruction of a fetus to obtain cells, which is ethically challenging for human applications. Both approaches rely to some extent on the idea that parenchymal cells retain their full differentiated identities despite extensive laboratory manipulation. If allowed to attach to a particular ecologic niche consisting of extracellular matrix epitopes, paracrine signals from surrounding cells, and endocrine signals from the host, it is expected that the parenchymal cells will assume a phenotype with quantitative fidelity to some cell in a natural organ. Data supporting this idea are scarce; indeed, cell culture stress is common in vivo as in vitro. Kidney podocytes, the glomerular cell most closely associated with filtration, have a fragile phenotype in vivo and do not assume the same phenotype in cell culture as they do in vivo. Growing replacement kidneys from isolated cells is likely to prove more complex than initially hoped.

Implantable Renal Assist Device

Fissell and Roy have pursued a biomimetic hybrid approach to build an implantable renal assist device (iRAD) as a permanent solution to ESRD. Healthy kidneys are composed of 1 million or more nephrons. Each nephron is composed of two modules in tandem. First, a glomerulus separates water and small molecules from the protein and cellular constituents of blood at a high enough rate to deplete the blood of wastes and toxins. In aggregate, the nephrons in a healthy adult kidney filter about 140 L/day of salt water and toxins from blood. Second, a long glandular structure lined with metabolically active epithelial cells reabsorbs 99% of the salt, water, glucose, and amino acids produced by the filter, progressively concentrating the filtered wastes into the 1 to 2 L of liquid urine we excrete every day. The Renal Assist Device (RAD) is a large-scale extracorporeal bioartificial kidney that recapitulates the tandem filtration and reabsorption architecture of the kidney. The Kidney Project is a multidisciplinary effort to miniaturize the large-scale RAD to a compact and durable package for implantation: the iRAD.

Implantable Filters

Conventional dialyzer membranes are bulky, have short service lives, and are unsuitable for implantation. The idea of using kidney cells to grow glomeruli in the laboratory is an attractive alternative to artificial membranes. As of this writing, the cells that make up the kidney's filters appear to be terminally differentiated with limited regenerative potential and fragile phenotype. The specific cues needed to coax these cells into functioning filters remain unknown. A tissue-cultured glomerulus remains in the far future, so the iRAD requires an alternative to conventional polymer membranes and tissue-engineered filters. Roy and Fissell pioneered an entirely new membrane for renal replacement. A new technology, silicon micromachining, allows precise control of pore size and shape. Roy developed thin-film membranes that copy the highly regimented and orderly structures of the glomerular slit diaphragm of the kidney. These silicon nanopore membranes optimize the permeability–selectivity tradeoff inherent to all membrane separation processes. Although silicon has been seen as a challenging biomaterial, especially for blood-contacting devices, highly hydrated polymer films effectively block the protein adsorption that initiates the coagulation cascade. Silicon membranes show promise in preclinical implant studies.

Bioreactor

The renal tubule has a remarkable ability to discriminate between metabolically valuable substrates and toxic wastes. The molecular mediators of uremia remain incompletely defined. In clinical practice, patients with prerenal azotemia may have extreme perturbations of urea and creatinine yet be cognitively intact, yet patients with tubular injury may have overt uremia despite less impressive laboratory measurements. The uncertainty regarding the mediators of uremia is a barrier to the design of passive devices. Humes et al pioneered the harvest, isolation, expansion, and packaging of renal tubule cells into a therapeutic device. The choice of scaffold in the large-scale RAD, a hollow-fiber dialyzer, is a good one, because in addition to mechanical support, the dialyzer membrane is a barrier between the patient and the cultured cells. The molecular and cellular effectors of the innate and acquired immune response could not engage the allogeneic tubule cells, thus obviating the need for immunologic immune suppression. Thus, the best membrane for a hemofilter may also be repurposed as an excellent scaffold for the tubule cell bioreactor. The innovative silicon nanopore membranes that form the hemofilter of the iRAD also serve as substrate for tubule cell growth. Cultured renal tubule cells display metabolic features of the healthy tubule and respond to fluid shear stress in vitro.

A patient facing impending renal failure has a wide variety of modality choices today: in-center conventional HD, in-center nocturnal dialysis, self-care home conventional, short daily, and nocturnal dialysis, or PD. In the near future, the range of treatment possibilities will expand further to encompass a variety of wearable and implanted therapies. Each of the technologies discussed here would lower barriers to self-care of renal failure and relocate ESRD care away from the dialysis clinic. If these options emerge into the market, they could significantly reduce the cost of the $32 billion Medicare ESRD program. In fiscal year 2015, the National Institute of Health's budget allocation for the Division of Kidney, Urologic and Hematologic diseases was $419.8 million, less than 2% of the annual cost of the Medicare ESRD program. All of us who care for patients with kidney disease hope that federal support for research on treatment of ESRD will come to match the immense burden of suffering and the immense financial cost of dialysis.

Peritoneal Dialysis:
Clinical Practice

C H A P T E R   3 1

Determination of Continuous Ambulatory Peritoneal Dialysis and Automated Peritoneal Dialysis Prescriptions

Scott G. Satko, MD • John M. Burkart, MD

According to the United States Renal Data System (USRDS) 2014 Annual Report, 9% of the prevalent end-stage renal disease (ESRD) patients in the United States without a functioning kidney transplant are currently performing peritoneal dialysis (PD). This percentage has been slowly increasing and is expected to continue to do so in the near future. In several South and Central American countries, this prevalence rate is considerably higher, exceeding 50% of all dialysis patients. PD can be performed manually (continuous ambulatory peritoneal dialysis [CAPD]) or with the assistance of a cycler machine (automated peritoneal dialysis [APD]). Selection of appropriate patients for either of these two modalities is mainly based on lifestyle considerations but also on the patients' physical characteristics and transporter status of the peritoneal membrane.

Rationale for Current Clearance Guidelines

When a patient initiates PD, it is important for the clinician to take into account the amount of residual renal function that is still present. The most recent set of National Kidney Foundation–Kidney Disease Outcomes Quality Initiative (NKF-KDOQI) Clinical Practice Guidelines from 2006 recommends that initiation of renal replacement therapy should be considered when a patient's estimated glomerular filtration rate (eGFR) declines to less than 15 mL/min, a level corresponding to CKD stage 5.

After PD has been initiated, it is recommended that one prescribe dialysis so that the total (peritoneal plus residual renal) weekly Kt/V_{urea} is above the minimum small solute clearance goal of 1.7/wk. This recommendation is based on the following data.

Historical univariate and multivariate analyses of retrospective data obtained on prevalent PD patients suggested that those patients with weekly Kt/V less than 1.89 to 1.96 were more likely to have lower 5-year survival rates. However, because of limited sample size, limited patient follow-up, and retrospective study designs, the true effect of small-solute clearance on morbidity and mortality was still not entirely certain from the conclusions of these studies. The CANUSA (Canada–U.S.A.) Study, a prospective, multicenter cohort study of 680 incident PD patients, suggested that total small-solute clearance *did* predict outcome. The investigators in this study followed 78 patients for 2 years. In this population, every 0.1-unit/wk increase in total Kt/V was associated with a 6% decrease in the relative risk of death over 2 years of follow-up. Every 5-L/1.73 m^2/wk increase in total creatinine clearance (Ccr) was also associated with a 7% decrease in the relative risk of death. The total weekly Kt/V and total weekly Ccr values that were associated with a 78% 2-year survival rate were 2.1 and 70 L/1.73 m^2, respectively. These data were analyzed using two assumptions: (1) total solute clearance did not change over time (an assumption that turned out to be incorrect), and (2) the predicted benefit from 1 unit of residual renal Kt/V was equal to that of 1 unit of peritoneal Kt/V (an assumption that has not been proven). In fact, reexamination of the CANUSA data has suggested that much of the change in the mortality rate may be more related to the level of residual renal function than to actual changes in peritoneal clearance.

Two randomized controlled trials from the previous decade have suggested that peritoneal clearance may play much less of a role in affecting overall mortality rate than other factors such as residual kidney clearance. The first such trial to show this was adequacy of PD in Mexico (ADEMEX), in which Mexican CAPD patients were randomized to a standard dialysis prescription (four daily exchanges of 2 L) or a modified prescription (adjusted to maintain a target peritoneal clearance of 60 L/wk/1.73 m^2). As expected, the mean total weekly Kt/V was lower in the control arm (1.80 vs 2.27 in the intervention arm). Surprisingly, the two groups had identical survival after 2 years of follow-up (69.3% in the standard group vs 68.3% in the modified prescription group). In these patients, the level of peritoneal small-solute (urea or creatinine) clearance had very little impact on the mortality rate, suggesting that the level of residual renal function may be a more important prognostic factor. In a subgroup analysis of anuric patients, there was also no difference in survival between the groups.

Similar findings were noted in a trial in Hong Kong, in which CAPD patients were randomized to three treatment arms with varied solute clearance goals (target total weekly Kt/V of 1.5–1.7, 1.7–2.0, or >2.0). Patients in all three arms of this study had minimal residual renal function, with mean residual renal Kt/V approximately 0.4 to 0.5/wk and mean GFR of approximately 2.4 to 2.6 mL/min. As in the ADEMEX trial, all three groups had similar survival rates. These data suggest that to optimize 2-year survival, a minimal total small solute clearance goal for CAPD should be a Kt/V of more than 1.7/wk. The recent KDOQI adequacy guidelines also recommended the same minimal total solute clearance goals (Kt/V urea of >1.7/wk) for both APD and CAPD. Extrapolation of these data should be taken with the following two caveats: First, these were patients on dialysis in Mexico and Hong Kong, where total protein intake may be different from that in patients from other countries or in patients of different ethnicities. Second, these patients were on 24 hours per day of PD dwell.

Discrepancy Between Kt/V and Creatinine Clearance

In a relatively high percentage of patients, total weekly Kt/V and Ccr are positively correlated (based on observational data and the original KDOQI targets of either a weekly Kt/V urea of >2.0 or a weekly Ccr of >60 L/wk/1.73 m^2). In others, these two measurements of small-solute clearance are discordant. There are multiple reasons for this discrepancy, including the amount of residual renal function, peritoneal membrane transport type, body size, and dialysis prescription. Kt/V and Ccr values also differ significantly when calculations of V (urea volume of distribution) and body surface area (BSA) are normalized using *desired* rather than *actual* body weights. Total small-solute clearance has been shown to be an important predictor of morbidity and mortality in PD patients. Detailed examination of this data has suggested that this relationship is mainly related to the residual renal component of small-solute clearance. There are no data to definitively determine which of the two major indicators of adequacy (Kt/V or Ccr) is better. The randomized trials listed earlier suggest that one can use Kt/V as the "dose" surrogate measurement and that there is no additional benefit to using Ccr. In actual clinical practice, nephrologists historically were frequently faced with a situation in which only one of these values (Kt/V or Ccr) was above target. Unfortunately, there are no rigorous outcomes data to help guide clinical decisions in this situation. In our experience, this discrepancy between Kt/V and Ccr occurs from 23% to 25% of the time, depending on whether actual or ideal body weight is used in the calculation of V and BSA for normalization of these parameters. An additional issue is the fact that at times one could change the dialysis prescription in a way that Kt/V increased while Ccr decreased. The current KDOQI guidelines recommend targeting dose using Kt/V.

To understand why the two clearance measurements are often discordant, it is important to remember how creatinine and urea are handled by both the nephron and the peritoneum. Renal clearance of creatinine occurs by both glomerular filtration and tubular secretion. With advanced degrees of renal insufficiency, the renal Ccr overestimates the true GFR. Renal clearance of urea also occurs by glomerular filtration, but urea can be reabsorbed by the renal tubules. For this reason, renal urea clearance usually represents an underestimation of the true GFR. When calculating total weekly Ccr for PD patients, it is recommended that an estimation of GFR be used for the residual renal clearance. This is most commonly estimated as the mean of the residual renal urea and Ccr. Even when the estimated GFR is used for Ccr, the residual renal Ccr tends to be relatively higher than the residual renal urea clearance. For this reason, residual renal function tends to contribute relatively more to Ccr/1.73 m^2 than to Kt/V for total weekly solute clearance. On the other hand, small-solute clearance by the peritoneum is mainly dependent on diffusion. Urea undergoes more rapid diffusion through the peritoneal membrane than does creatinine because of its smaller molecular weight. The typical CAPD dwell time for a patient using dextrose-containing peritoneal dialysate is 4 to 6 hours. During this time, dialysate urea usually becomes equilibrated with blood in patients of all transport types. On the other hand, because creatinine is transported relatively more slowly, equilibration of creatinine between blood and dialysate is likely to occur only in rapid transporters during the typical dwell times used for CAPD. Given these diffusive characteristics of the peritoneal membrane, anuric patients typically have a relatively higher Kt/V than Ccr. This finding becomes most apparent in low transporters, especially patients using either APD or CAPD with unusually short dwell times.

Previous guidelines have suggested that one should attempt to change the dialysis prescription so that both Kt/V and Ccr are at target. If only one of these values can be at or above target, the nephrologist should aim to have that parameter be the weekly Kt/V. As mentioned, the current KDOQI guidelines recommend only measuring solute clearance in terms of Kt/V and not measuring peritoneal Ccr to avoid the inconsistencies previously discussed. Additionally, measuring Ccr in addition to urea clearance provides little additional data that are useful in predicting short-term (2-year) clinical outcome.

It is acknowledged that small solutes are not the only uremic toxins. "Adequacy" of dialysis entails more than just removal of small solutes. It is known that to optimize outcomes, one must control blood pressure, blood volume, acid–base status, and other metabolic issues related to kidney failure. It is also acknowledged that recent randomized trials only evaluated short-term risk of death related to small-solute clearance. They did not evaluate long-term outcomes or risk of death related to middle-molecular-weight solute clearance or dose of dialysis related to metabolic control of other solutes such as phosphate, for example.

Epidemiologic data suggest that the relative risk of death is related to serum phosphate levels and calcium and phosphate metabolism. Phosphate control may be predictive of long-term outcome. In terms of diffusive transport across the peritoneal membrane, phosphorus acts as a larger molecule than suggested by its molecular weight, and therefore its rate of diffusive clearance across the peritoneal membrane is more like that of creatinine than urea. If a patient's dialysis prescription is adjusted in such a manner to raise or lower the total weekly Kt/V, the degree of phosphate removal will usually change in a similar fashion. However, similar to that of creatinine, if a low transporter is changed from CAPD to APD, it is possible that despite an increase in Kt/V, there will be little increase in phosphorus removal. Because of transport kinetics such as already discussed, if one wanted to increase phosphorus removal by PD in a patient on APD, one might consider adding a midday exchange, especially in a low transporter. Further studies are needed to see if the lower total small-solute clearance targets for PD have an adverse effect on long-term outcomes in PD patients with a higher protein and phosphate intake than patients in Mexico and Hong Kong.

Peritoneal Transport Characteristics

When an initial PD prescription is selected, the transporter characteristics of the peritoneal membrane are not known. For this reason, the initial prescription empirically assumes that the patient is an "average" transporter. Peritoneal equilibration testing (PET) should be performed within 1 month of initiation of PD. In the initial KDOQI guidelines, it was recommended that PET testing be repeated at least semiannually to monitor the patient's transporter status. However, it has now been recognized that transport status is generally stable, and therefore PET testing is now recommended only at the start of dialysis and then subsequently when problem solving such as during an evaluation of a volume-overloaded patient (Fig. 31.1).

Patients who are high, or "rapid," peritoneal transporters (4-hour dialysate/plasma [D/P] creatinine >0.81) usually have adequate peritoneal clearance while on a

4-Hour Dialysate/Plasma (D/P) Creatinine Ratio	Transporter Status
≤0.50	Low
0.51–0.65	Low-average
0.66–0.81	High-average
>0.81	High

Figure 31.1

Peritoneal transport characteristics.

standard CAPD regimen but frequently encounter difficulty with ultrafiltration (UF). This is because of excessive reabsorption of glucose, which diminishes the osmotic gradient necessary for UF to occur. In these cases, if the dwell time is too long, they may absorb enough fluid so that the net UF for that dwell is minimal or negative. Because total solute removal is a function of drain volume and the concentration of the solute in question in that drain volume (usually most dependent on diffusive characteristics of membrane), rapid transporters may not be adequately dialyzed on long dwell therapies such as CAPD. These patients often do better when given a dialysis prescription with short dwell times. APD is often the optimal modality for these patients. With APD, one could prescribe multiple short dwells overnight and at times a "dry" day, avoiding the long nighttime dwell of CAPD. In these patients (high and high-average transporters), if a daytime dwell is used, the daytime dwell should be appropriately shortened either by the performance of a midday manual exchange or midday drainage of fluid with the remainder of the day "dry." On the other hand, patients who are low, or "slow," peritoneal transporters (4-hour D/P creatinine <0.50) may experience underdialysis when given short dwell times. For these patients, the long dwells used in CAPD (e.g., three 5-hour daytime dwells and a single long, 9-hour nighttime dwell) are optimal. To reach clearance targets, anuric patients who are low transporters usually need to perform a continuous modality of dialysis, with each 24-hour day divided evenly into dwell periods. When performing CAPD, this is most effectively done by using a nighttime exchange device to divide the long nighttime dwell. Similarly, when performing APD, this is most effectively done by performing a midday manual exchange. Finally, remember that solute removal is the product of drain volume and the concentration of the solute in question in that drain volume. As such, another way to increase solute removal is to increase the instilled volume (and thus the drain volume) per exchange.

Many patients, especially those who are rapid transporters or have diabetes with suboptimal glycemic control, may have difficulty achieving adequate UF. This problem is often associated with rapid uptake of dextrose-containing peritoneal dialysate through the peritoneal membrane with associated diminution of the osmotic gradient for UF. These patients often respond better to the use of 7.5% icodextrin during the longest daily dwell in place of dextrose-containing dialysate. Icodextrin is a glucose polymer produced via hydrolysis of starch, which is not significantly metabolized or transported through the peritoneal membrane. Icodextrin solution uses a colloid osmotic gradient (7.5% icodextrin vs the typical serum albumin concentration) for UF, resulting in slow but sustained UF rates not influenced by peritoneal transport characteristics. The UF profile for a 15-hour icodextrin dwell would typically exceed that of a 2.5% dextrose dwell and equal or exceed that of a 4.25% dextrose dwell in most patients. Compared with dextrose-containing dialysate, icodextrin appears to be more biocompatible and is associated with a lower rate of formation of advanced glycation end products. Although, in theory, icodextrin should be associated with a lower long-term risk of peritoneal damage, it is important to note that no long-term mortality data yet exist proving better outcomes in patients using icodextrin.

Other Uremic Toxins

It is well recognized that urea and creatinine are not the only retained solutes in uremia. Rather, they are surrogates for all solutes with similar molecular weights.

There are other identified "uremic toxins" such as β_2-microglobulin, a surrogate for middle molecules, and p-cresol, a surrogate for protein-bound solutes that are retained in uremia. In cross-sectional observational cohort studies, the levels of these substances have been associated with increased morbidity or mortality. Obtaining the minimal Kt/V target should be the start of the thinking about adequacy, and concern for control of bone mineral metabolism, acidosis, volume status, and optimal removal of solutes other than urea and creatinine should follow. For now, there is no prospective randomized trial in PD patients to guide one in targeting middle-molecule solute removal. It should be remembered that in the randomized trials of adequacy in terms of Kt/V urea discussed earlier, the patients were on 24 hours/day of PD dwell, which optimizes middle-molecule removal. Therefore, the most recent KDOQI guidelines recommended that if the patient was anuric, one should consider 24 hours/day of PD dwell.

Blood Pressure and Volume Control

When managing any dialysis patient, one should not forget that along with solute removal, one should also adequately remove excess salt and water to normalize blood volume and blood pressure. There is an observed association in anuric PD patients between UF volume and probability of survival. This makes sense physiologically given the risks of volume overload and its association with left ventricular hypertrophy, increased sympathetic tone, and congestive heart failure. As a result, as one prescribes PD, one also needs to optimize the removal of sodium and water. There are differences in potential UF volumes during a dextrose dwell that are related to dwell time and transport type. These differences vary by modality (CAPD vs APD), and the prescriber must be aware of them as the individual patient is managed. If using dextrose solutions, rapid transporters rapidly absorb the dialysate glucose. As a result, the hypertonic gradient that favors fluid movement from the blood side to the dialysate side rapidly dissipates, and when peritoneal tonicity is equal to blood, UF ceases, and absorption of intraperitoneal fluid predominates. For these reasons, rapid transporters usually do better with short dwell therapies such as APD. In these cases, one must remember that during the daytime dwells with a dextrose solution, UF will be problematic, and unless the most hypertonic dextrose dwell (4.25% dextrose) or an alternative osmotic agent that tends not to be absorbed (icodextrin) is used, the patient may actually gain fluid during the daytime dwell of APD. In contrast, slow transporters tend not to absorb solutes as quickly, so that during a dextrose dwell, the UF profile lasts longer, and therefore slow transporters tend to do better with longer dwell therapies such as CAPD.

Calculation of Prescribed Kt/V for Peritoneal Dialysis

In a patient who is an average transporter (i.e., with 4-hour D/P creatinine 0.50–0.81), dialysate and plasma are nearly 100% equilibrated with urea during the typical dwell time used in CAPD. Four-hour D/P urea values are usually 80% to 100% in this population. For this reason, it can be assumed that K (urea clearance in L/day) is roughly equivalent to the 24-hour dialysate drain volume. Estimated weekly Kt would then be equal to (24-hour drain volume in L/d) × (7 days). V (volume of distribution of urea in liters) is equivalent to the volume of total body water. This value can be estimated using the Watson formulae:

For men, V (L) $= 2.447 + (0.3362 \times$ Body weight [kg]) $+ (0.1074 \times$ Height [cm])
$- (0.09516 \times$ Age [yr])

For women, V (L) $= -2.097 + (0.2466 \times$ Body weight [kg]) $+ (0.1069 \times$ Height [cm])

Alternatively, V can be more roughly approximated by multiplying body weight (in kilograms) by a factor of 0.55 for women and 0.60 for men. Estimations using equations such as the Watson formulae are recommended, however.

For example, consider the situation in which an anuric 75-kg man is performing CAPD using four exchanges of 2 L/day. Assume he is 100% saturated for urea during each exchange and that his drain volume is 2.3 L/exchange, giving him a daily ultrafiltration volume (UFV) of 1.2 L. It then follows that:

$$Kt = (2.3 \text{ L} \times 4/\text{day}) \times (7 \text{ days/wk}) = 64.4 \text{ L/wk}$$

$$V = (75 \text{ kg}) \times (0.60 \text{ L/kg}) = 45 \text{ L}$$

$$Kt/V = (64.4 \text{ L/wk}) \div (45 \text{ L}) = 1.43/\text{wk}$$

This calculation illustrates that a "typical" CAPD regimen of 4×2.0 L would not provide acceptable small solute clearance for an anuric 75-kg male.

Suppose the patient above increased the number of exchanges per day to 6×2.0 L in an attempt to provide better clearance. If he is an average transporter and is performing 3-hour dwells during the daytime to accommodate six daily exchanges, it is likely that urea may not become fully equilibrated between dialysate and plasma during the short dwells. During these short dwells, let us assume that urea is only 80% equilibrated between dialysate and plasma (see the PET curve for urea in Fig. 28.1). Assuming the daily UFV is unchanged, the patient's clearance is now as follows:

$$Kt = (2.2 \text{ L} \times 6/\text{day}) \times (7 \text{ days/wk}) \times (3\text{-hour D/P urea } 80\%) = 73.9 \text{ L/wk}$$

$$V = (75 \text{ kg}) \times (0.60 \text{ L/kg}) = 45 \text{ L}$$

$$Kt/V = (73.9 \text{ L/wk}) \div (45 \text{ L}) = 1.64/\text{wk}$$

Although this patient's clearance has now improved, he still does not meet recommended guidelines for dialysis adequacy.

Suppose, however, that instead of increasing the number of daily exchanges, this patient increases his exchange volume from 2 to 3 L. If he performs four daily exchanges, his total daily exchange volume will be 12 L, the same as in the previous scenario. However, with the longer dwell time, urea will again become more fully equilibrated between dialysate and plasma, leading to an increase in clearance. Assuming his daily UFV is the same as before, his clearance is now as follows:

$$Kt = (3.3 \text{ L} \times 4/\text{day}) \times (7 \text{ days/wk}) = 92.4 \text{ L/wk}$$

$$V = (75 \text{ kg}) \times (0.60 \text{ L/kg}) = 45 \text{ L}$$

$$Kt/V = (92.4 \text{ L/wk}) \div (45 \text{ L}) = 2.05/\text{wk}$$

This case illustrates the point clearly that, for the average CAPD patient, increasing exchange volume has a substantially greater effect on improving peritoneal small-solute clearance than does increasing the number of exchanges. Although the effect of changing exchange volume and dwell time can be predicted using kinetic modeling, in clinical practice, it is necessary to perform a 24-hour dialysate collection after each change in prescription to verify the actual effect of these changes in any individual patient.

A recent study by Perez et al examined the effect of increasing the number of nightly APD exchanges upon urea and Ccr, net UF, and monetary cost. Using 9 × 2 L nightly exchanges compared with 5 × 2 L nightly exchanges provided peritoneal urea and Ccrs 21% and 25% higher, respectively, and 47% more UFV. These increases, however, were obtained at the expense of using 80% more dialysate fluid (18 L vs 10 L) and a 54% greater monetary cost. As the number of nightly exchanges increases, a proportionally greater amount of time is spent filling and draining compared with dwelling. This leads to less efficient use of dialysate because much less small solute clearance occurs during the filling and draining periods than during the dwelling periods.

To perform PD most efficiently, it is important to optimize dialysate dwell time. As illustrated in the case above, if it is necessary to adjust a patient's prescription to improve clearance, the first step should be to attempt to increase the exchange volume. In situations in which the exchange volume is already maximized (i.e., 3 L) or the patient is unable to tolerate such an increase, the next step should be to increase the number of daily exchanges. From a practical standpoint, it is rather difficult for a CAPD patient to perform more than four manual exchanges a day. If these patients require more than four daily exchanges and wish to continue CAPD, the best solution is to add an extra automated exchange with a nighttime exchange device, or cycler. Similarly, APD patients who require extra exchanges often benefit from performing one or two daytime manual exchanges to optimize clearance.

By optimizing dwell times through the manipulations described earlier, it is possible to use the patient's time and peritoneal dialysate most efficiently. In this era when cost-containment issues are of paramount importance, it is especially prudent to prescribe PD in the most efficient way possible.

Patient Preference for Continuous Ambulatory Peritoneal Dialysis Versus Automated Peritoneal Dialysis

Although we have spent the majority of this chapter discussing "clinical" reasons for choosing one treatment regimen over another and using those clinical characteristics to help guide our decision making, it is important to understand that the majority of patients will do well on *either* CAPD or APD. In most cases, the determination of whether CAPD or APD will be the most appropriate modality for the patient will be made by the patient him- or herself, with input from family and other caregivers, as well as from the clinical team (nephrologist, nephrology nurses, renal social worker, renal dietitian, and so on). In our experience, most patients initially indicate a preference for APD because it gives them more free time during the day when they do not have to spend time performing manual exchanges. Other patients (e.g., those who live in areas with frequent power outages, those who sleep less than 6 hours per night) prefer to perform manual exchanges so as to avoid dependence on a mechanical device for a long span of the nighttime. A recent prospective cohort study from The Netherlands Cooperative Study on the Adequacy of Dialysis (NECOSAD) Study Group in the Netherlands reported equivalent mortality and technique failure rates from either CAPD or APD when patients are given the option to make their own choice of modality.

Conclusion

A number of different factors must be taken into consideration when selecting an appropriate PD prescription for a patient. These include a patient's lifestyle, body size and habitus, transporter status, and level of residual renal function, as well as specific indications or contraindications for selecting one modality over another. For patients with significant amounts of residual renal function, it is important to measure residual renal function periodically so that the dialysis prescription can be adjusted appropriately.

CHAPTER 32

Peritoneal Dialysis Solutions

Anand Vardhan, MBBS, MD, DNB, FRCP, MD •
Alastair J. Hutchison, MBChB, FRCP, MD

The basis of peritoneal dialysis (PD) is the removal of various metabolic products and excess fluid from the patient across the peritoneal membrane by instilling a suitable dialysis solution into the peritoneal cavity. This process can be altered by variations to the composition and volume of dialysis solution used and the duration of "dwell" in the peritoneum. Solute removal is achieved by diffusion (down a concentration gradient) and convection, which allows movement of solutes across the membrane along with the ultrafiltrate by virtue of "solvent drag." The electrolyte composition of the dialysis solution can be modified such that certain solutes are either not removed or diffuse into the patient. Fluid balance can be altered by varying the concentration of an osmotic agent, resulting in net fluid absorption or removal as required. Thus, the ability to appropriately prescribe differing PD solutions is a key factor in achieving electrolyte homeostasis, acid–base neutrality, an even fluid balance and a nonuremic state.

Historical solutions used included 0.8% saline, 5% dextrose and Ringer's lactate, but were associated with pulmonary edema and electrolyte and acid-base disturbances. Subsequent research led to the realization that the composition of dialysate needed to be similar to interstitial fluid and hypertonic to plasma in order to achieve fluid removal by ultrafiltration (UF). Several osmotic agents were evaluated and glucose was found to be effective, safe, and inexpensive. It became the standard osmotic agent for PD solutions, and little has changed since the 1950s. However, a better understanding of peritoneal anatomy and physiology led to the development of newer PD solutions that are more biocompatible and some of which are glucose free. This has paved the way for improved management of PD patients, with preservation of residual renal function and peritoneal membrane integrity, and will hopefully translate into improved survival times and fewer complications in the future.

There are numerous PD solutions in use today, and these include the "conventional" lactate-based solutions as well as newer "biocompatible" multichamber bicarbonate-based solutions. Unequivocal evidence for the superiority of biocompatible over conventional solutions has never materialized, and coupled with their higher cost, this has resulted in variable usage across the world. The composition of these solutions varies little among manufacturers and comprise three essential components, namely:

- Electrolytes
- Osmotic agents
- Acid–base buffers

The general composition of currently available PD solutions is shown in Table 32.1.

Electrolytes

Electrolyte disturbance is a common feature of end-stage renal disease (ESRD). To maintain homeostasis, solutions must contain sodium, potassium, calcium, and magnesium as major cations along with anions lactate–bicarbonate and chloride to maintain electrical neutrality.

Sodium

The concentration of sodium in currently available PD solutions is between 131 and 134 mmol/L. Clinical studies have not reported any specific side effects related to these concentrations, but nomograms are available to predict net sodium removal adjusted for the glucose concentration of the solution. Interestingly, studies in continuous ambulatory peritoneal dialysis (CAPD) patients have shown that varying the sodium concentration from 132 to 141 mmol/L has little effect on the serum sodium concentration.

The net removal of sodium per liter of ultrafiltrate ($\approx$70 mmol) is much less than one would expect from the extracellular fluid concentration. This is due to sodium sieving at the peritoneal membrane and the Donnan equilibrium whereby charged particles across a semipermeable membrane fail to distribute equally because the large anionic plasma proteins attract the smaller cations and drive the small anions out. However, in symptomatic hypotensive patients, higher sodium concentrations in PD fluids (137–142 mmol/L) have been used with benefit. Conversely, "very-low-sodium" concentrations (100–120 mmol/L) have been tried in a limited way (with some success) in managing hypertension and fluid overload. These solutions are not currently commercially available.

Residual renal function (when present) plays a significant role in sodium homeostasis and may account for the limited effects of small variations in PD fluid sodium concentration. Hypernatremia may occasionally occur, especially in rapid-cycling APD because of sodium sieving, which results in disproportionate water loss compared with sodium removal in the ultrafiltrate.

Potassium

Hyperkalemia is a common and life-threatening problem in ESRD patients. Potassium homeostasis in PD patients is dependent on numerous factors, including the amount of dietary potassium intake, variable intestinal excretion, residual renal function, serum potassium levels, insulin bioavailability, cell membrane Na/K ATPase activity, dialysate potassium concentration, and acid–base balance.

The current commercially available PD solutions do not contain any potassium. This ensures maximal potassium removal, which occurs predominantly by diffusion rather than solvent drag because of the low concentration of potassium in extracellular fluid. Hypokalemia is reported in 10% to 36% of patients but can be corrected easily by relaxing dietary restrictions, prescribing oral potassium supplementation, or (less easily) by adding 1 to 4 mmol/L of potassium to the dialysate as required. Again, nomograms are available to predict potassium removal.

Table 32.1

Composition of Peritoneal Dialysis Solutions

Type	Conventional	Low GDP		Glucose Free		Bicarbonate Based	
Name	Dineal	Balance	Gabrosol Trio	Nutrineal	Extraneal	Physioneal	Bicavera
Solute	Glucose	Glucose	Glucose	Amino acids	Icodextrin	Glucose	Glucose
Solute concentrate (%)	1.36/2.27/3.86%	1.5/2.3/4.25%	1.5/2.5/3.9%	1.1	7.5	1.36/2.27/3.86%	1.5/2.3/4.25%
pH	4–6.5	7	5.5–6.5	5.7–6.8	5.0–6.0	7.4	7.4
Osmolarity (mOsmol/L)	345/395/485	345/395/509	357/409/483	365	284	344/395/483	358/401/511
Na (mmol/L)	132	132	131–133	132	133	134	134
Ca (mmol/L)	1.25–1.75	1.25–1.75	1.7–1.79	1.25	1.75	1.25–1.75	1.75
Mg (mmol/L)	0.25	.025	0.24–0.26	0.25	0.25	0.25	0.5
Cl (mmol/L)	95–96	95–96	96	105	96	95–101	104.5
Lactate (mmol/L)	40	40	39–41	40	40	10–15	0
Bicarbonate (mmol/L)	0	0	0	0	0	25–30	34

GDP, glucose degradation product.

Calcium

Calcium homeostasis is dependent on the direction of the diffusive gradient and the UF rate. Transfer from dialysate to patient is negatively correlated with the degree of UF. Calcium homeostasis is also related to oral calcium intake, vitamin D prescription, parathyroid hormone levels, and phosphate levels. Whereas the normal serum ionized calcium level varies from 1.15 to 1.29 mmol/L, the calcium concentration of dialysate (in which all of the calcium is ionized) usually ranges from 1.25 to 1.79 mmol/L. In the 1980s, solutions using 1.75 mmol/L were commonly used but were found to be associated with an increased incidence of hypercalcemia.

The optimal dialysate calcium concentration is not known and depends on oral intake and the individual's serum calcium level. The majority of physicians now prescribe a more physiologic calcium concentration (1.25–1.55 mmol/L) because of concern relating to calcium "overload" and vascular mineralization. However, the current controversy regarding the maximum advisable calcium intake has tended to focus on oral intake from calcium-containing phosphate binders and dialysate calcium has been to some extent neglected.

Several studies have shown that a PD solution calcium level of 1.0 to 1.25 mmol/L can lead to adequate calcium balance and phosphate control with oral calcium binders and reduces the risk of hypercalcemia. However, hypocalcemia may occur, especially if compliance with vitamin D analogs or calcium-containing phosphate binders is incomplete. Lower dialysate calcium levels are available (0.6–1.0 mmol/L) and are used by some centers in PD patients with severe hyperparathyroidism who need increasingly high doses of calcitriol. The introduction of cinacalcet in the recent past has largely obviated the need for high-dose vitamin D therapy, although low-dose supplementation is still required to prevent significant hypocalcemia. The earlier formulations containing 1.75 mmol/L are still used in hypocalcemic patients and in patients who are nonadherent to prescribed calcium or calcitriol supplements.

Better understanding of calcium homeostasis should allow the dialysate calcium prescription to be tailored in accordance with the serum calcium level and phosphate binder prescription. However, little is known of peritoneal calcium balance in automated PD, and this undoubtedly needs further study.

Magnesium

The normal serum value for magnesium is between 0.60 and 1.00 mmol/L, depending on the laboratory reference range. In PD patients, the serum level is largely dependent on both dietary intake and gastrointestinal and urinary losses in those with residual renal function and the concentration of magnesium in the dialysate. In addition, the duration of the dwell, degree of UF, and peritoneal permeability can affect peritoneal transport. However, as with calcium, little is known of magnesium balance in APD.

Currently available PD solutions contain ionized magnesium at concentrations between 0.25 and 0.5 mmol/L. In most studies, the use of 0.75 mmol/L has resulted in elevated serum magnesium levels in many patients. However, there are no reported side effects from this. Some authors have suggested that hypermagnesemia may inhibit bone remodeling, but others believe it may have a preventive effect on soft tissue calcification but no sizeable prospective studies exist. Experience with a dialysate magnesium concentration of 0.25 mmol/L has shown a normalization of serum magnesium with no hypomagnesemia. A zero-dialysate magnesium concentration has also been tested to allow the use of oral magnesium as an additional phosphate binder, but this approach is limited because of the laxative effect of magnesium and the need to monitor serum levels at regular intervals.

Osmotic Agents

Glucose

Until the late 1990s, glucose was the only osmotic agent available for PD. It has the advantages of being effective, inexpensive, readily available, and not immediately toxic. Three standard concentrations are available, namely, 1.5%, 2.3%, and 4.25% dextrose monohydrate (or 1.36%, 2.27%, and 3.86% of anhydrous dextrose, respectively). High concentrations of glucose allow effective UF to be achieved.

Ultrafiltration is greatest at the beginning of an exchange but dissipates as the glucose in dialysate is absorbed systemically across the peritoneal membrane. In patients who have a "fast" transporter status, rapid absorption of glucose can result in UF failure and net fluid gain even with the use of high-glucose dialysate. This absorption of glucose can contribute up to 20% of the patient's caloric intake per day. Hyperglycemia and hyperinsulinemia have been observed in nondiabetic patients undergoing PD because of the large amount of glucose absorbed. This may therefore precipitate or exacerbate diabetes mellitus. Weight gain caused by the caloric load has also been observed, as well as hypertriglyceridemia and abnormal serum lipoprotein levels. All of these metabolic abnormalities can increase the cardiovascular burden associated with ESRD.

It is perhaps not surprising that glucose has been associated with peritoneal membrane changes in long-term PD patients. Therefore, although glucose is non-toxic in the immediate sense, it is clearly not devoid of longer term side effects. With long-term PD, morphologic changes occur in the peritoneum, resulting in derangement of membrane function. There are several mechanisms by which these progressive changes in the peritoneal membrane occur. Constant exposure of the mesothelium to glucose in such high concentrations—way beyond the diabetic range—has been shown in vitro and in vivo to be detrimental to membrane structure and function. Diabetiform changes are observed with glycation of membrane proteins and increased production of proinflammatory growth factors, particularly vascular endothelial growth factor (VEGF), which is implicated in peritoneal neoangiogenesis. This results in increased effective peritoneal vasculature surface area, resulting in more rapid dissipation of the osmotic gradient generated by this low-molecular-weight osmotic agent.

Glucose also activates the polyol pathway (also called the sorbitol–aldose reductase pathway), causing the secretion of transforming growth factor $\beta 1$ (TGF-$\beta 1$), monocyte chemoattractant protein-1 (MCP-1), and fibronectin in cultured mesothelial cells. Excessive activation of the polyol pathway leads to increased levels of sorbitol and reactive oxygen molecules and decreased levels of nitric oxide and glutathione. This also places osmotic stresses on the cell membrane. Any one of these elements alone can promote cell damage within the peritoneum.

Glucose has the potential to bind nonenzymatically to free amino groups on proteins or to lipids, resulting in the formation of advanced glycation end products (AGE). AGE formation is accelerated when ambient glucose levels are elevated or when the prevailing oxidant stress is high, as in uremia. The peritoneal cavities of PD patients thus provide good conditions for accelerated AGE formation and accumulation. AGE have been detected immunocytochemically in the mesothelium, submesothelial stroma, and the vascular wall of PD patients. AGE can induce VEGF expression in diverse cell types and therefore may have the potential to promote peritoneal neoangiogenesis.

The presence of glucose degradation products (GDPs) generated during steam sterilization and storage of dialysis solutions is associated with direct cytotoxicity and acceleration of the process of AGE formation. The formation of GDPs can be reduced by sterilizing glucose solutions separately at a low pH and dispensing dialysis solutions in multichambered bags to separate the glucose and buffer solutions.

Although glucose-based PD fluids have enabled PD to become an established therapy for thousands of patients who might otherwise not have received dialysis, it is clear that important goals for the clinician today are to reduce peritoneal exposure to glucose, minimize the total amount of glucose absorbed, and avoid hyperosmolar stress and GDP exposure. Non–glucose-based PD solutions and lower GDP-containing solutions are now available and offer a positive way forward.

Icodextrin

Icodextrin is a glucose polymer preparation used as a primary osmotic agent at a concentration of 7.5%. It uses colloidal oncotic, rather than crystalline osmotic, pressure to produce a sustained UF profile that is beneficial for long dwells. Because of its colloidal properties, a 7.5% icodextrin solution exerts a modest osmotic pressure of only 282 mOsmol/L compared with glucose 1.36%, 2.27%, and 3.86% PD solutions (which exert osmotic pressures of 345, 395, and 485 mOsmol/L, respectively). However, it is three to five times more efficacious than 1.36% glucose in terms of UF generation and equivalent to a 3.86% glucose solution over long dwells. Furthermore, the GDP content of icodextrin is very low compared with that of glucose-containing solutions. Its beneficial effects on fluid removal are explained by its large molecular size and consequent slow absorption from the peritoneum, sustaining the UF effect and resulting in an almost linear increase in UF during a long dwell. Increased UF also results in improved solute clearances.

Other potential benefits include a reduction in glucose-induced lipid abnormalities and improved phagocytosis by polymorphonuclear lymphocytes and monocytes. It is recommended as a once-daily replacement for a single glucose exchange during the long nocturnal dwell in CAPD or the long daytime dwell in APD, although regimens using two bag exchanges are gaining popularity based on reports on small groups of patients. The indications for use and characteristics of icodextrin are summarized in Tables 32.2 and 32.3.

The European Automated Peritoneal Dialysis Outcomes Study (EAPOS) examined how peritoneal function was affected by exposure to glucose and by the use of icodextrin for long dwells. At baseline, patients using icodextrin had significantly higher solute transport and lower UF capacity (poorer membrane function) than those using glucose only. Despite this, UF capacity remained unchanged in the icodextrin group but decreased significantly in the patients not using icodextrin. In addition, solute transport remained unchanged at 12 months and decreased significantly at 24 months compared with the non-icodextrin group (in which it increased

Table 32.2

Indications for Using Extraneal (7.5% Icodextrin)

For Sustained UF in:
Long overnight dwell in CAPD
Long daytime dwell in APD

For Effective UF in:
UF failure caused by aquaporin loss
UF failure in peritonitis
Fast transporters

For Reduced Glucose Exposure:
In all patients and
Particularly in patients with diabetes

For Ultrafiltration Alone in:
Severe diuretic-resistant heart failure

APD, assisted peritoneal dialysis; CAPD, continuous ambulatory peritoneal dialysis; UF, ultrafiltration.

Table 32.3

Summary Characteristics of Newer Peritoneal Dialysis Solutions

7.5% Icodextrin Solution
Reduced overall glucose exposure
No GDP exposure
Better and longer UF
Suitable for long dwells
Effective in peritonitis and UF failure caused by aquaporin loss
May interfere with CBS monitoring

1.1% Amino Acid Solution
Reduced overall glucose exposure
Similar UF profile as 1.36% glucose
No GDP exposure
May prevent or help manage malnutrition
May increase urea and acidosis

Bicarbonate–Lactate Buffered Solutions
Standard glucose exposure
Standard ultrafiltration profiles
Low GDP levels
Physiologic pH
Less inflow pain
Biocompatible, so better tolerated
Possibly less peritonitis and longer technique survival
Possibly preservation of residual renal function

CBS, capillary blood sugar; GDP, glucose degradation product; UF, ultrafiltration.

significantly at 12 and 24 months). These differences were independent of age, time on dialysis, and peritonitis episodes.

Icodextrin use is associated with nonphysiologic plasma levels of maltose (the end product of icodextrin metabolism by amylase). These appear to have no associated toxicity but can interfere with the glucose dehydrogenase pyrrolquinoline quinone (GDH-PQQ) method of capillary glucose measurement on finger prick glucose monitors, potentially resulting in falsely high results even in hypoglycemic PD patients. This is obviously dangerous in the context of a hypoglycemic event, when capillary blood glucose levels might be reported as normal or even high due to the presence of maltose. In patients on icodextrin, CBS monitors using GDH-PQQ should be avoided.

Amino Acids

Amino acid–based solutions can be used as a substitute for glucose-based solutions and as a nutritional supplement. Albumin losses in PD constitute up to 63% of the total protein lost in the dialysate. Amino acid–based solutions have been shown to replace amino acids lost during PD and may help to correct protein malnutrition. A 1.1% amino acid–based solution containing 87 mmol/L amino acids is available as Nutrineal (Baxter Healthcare Corporation) with an osmolarity of 365 mOsmol/L. With an absorption rate of 70% to 80% over 4 to 6 hours, a single exchange coinciding with a major meal can contribute up to 25% of the target daily protein intake in an average adult. This is achieved without the phosphate loading associated with dietary protein supplementation. This may be beneficial in severely malnourished patients, but the clinical results of treatment with amino acid PD fluids are disappointing.

Although amino acid–based solutions are effective osmotic agents, their use is associated with increased acidosis and urea generation, leading to increased alkali and dialysis needs. Thus, they can replace a single glucose exchange and serve as a nutritional supplementation in severe malnutrition or in hypercatabolic states such as peritonitis and to reduce membrane exposure to glucose and GDP. There is no evidence that they prevent malnutrition.

Glycerol

Glycerol, a low-molecular-weight sugar alcohol, has been the subject of trials primarily in PD patients with diabetes. It produces more UF initially than equivalent glucose concentrations, but because of its low molecular weight, it is absorbed rapidly, resulting in a lower total net UF overall. A higher pH makes it more biocompatible, and despite higher calorie loads, glucose homeostasis and insulin requirements are better than in PD patients with diabetes treated with a standard glucose dialysate. The risk of hyperosmolar symptoms and raised triglycerides has limited its use and it is not commercially available.

Fructose, Xylitol, and Sorbitol

These have been the subject of trials in patients with diabetes on PD but have failed to show any advantage over glucose-based solutions (or were limited by their side effect profile).

Acid–Base Buffers

Metabolic acidosis is a common complication of ESRD. Patients on PD tend to have better control of metabolic acidosis, as reflected by normal mean bicarbonate levels. This correction is predominantly achieved by continuous supplementation with alkali from PD solutions. The buffer composition of available PD solutions can be divided into three categories:

- Nonbicarbonate buffers
- Bicarbonate–lactate combination buffers
- Bicarbonate buffers

Nonbicarbonate Buffers

Nonbicarbonate buffers (including lactate, acetate, and pyruvate) are naturally occurring compounds with established metabolic fates, such as the glycolytic pathway. Acetate is no longer used because of an association with peritoneal membrane injury. Pyruvate buffers are not commercially available. Lactate is used either alone or in combination with bicarbonate. It is a naturally occurring molecule that is produced during anaerobic glycolysis and has a long safety history of intravenous administration as Ringer's lactate solution. In the liver, it is either metabolized back to pyruvate, which is then converted to acetyl CoA and with full oxidation to CO_2 and H_2O (80%) or to glucose (20%) via neoglucogenic pathways. In mitochondria-rich tissues, lactate is converted to pyruvate by the "ox-phos" shuttle with eventual conversion to acetyl CoA and finally CO_2 and H_2O. Either of the processes results in the generation of bicarbonate (Fig. 32.1). The load of lactate absorbed from PD solutions is small compared to the rate of lactate production in vivo, with no elevations in serum lactate occurring as a result. Problems with lactate solutions include pain upon infusion, peritoneal macrophage and mesothelial cell toxicity, enhanced glucose-mediated peritoneal toxicity and peritoneal fibrosis through TGF-β1 and MCP-1 production.

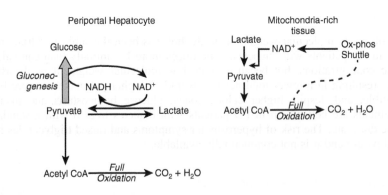

Figure 32.1

Modes of lactate removal from plasma.

Bicarbonate–Lactate Combination Buffers

In an attempt to improve biocompatibility, a glucose-based solution buffered with a combination of lactate (15 mmol/L) and bicarbonate (25 mmol/L) has been produced (Physioneal, Baxter Healthcare Corporation). This solution has an osmolality similar to that of a standard glucose-based solution, with a pH of 7.4 as opposed to the standard pH of 5.5. The bag is double chambered, with the glucose separate from the sodium bicarbonate and sodium lactate.

The development of novel gas-tight plastic bag materials has made it possible to store bicarbonate-based solutions for extended periods. This allows the glucose portion to be heat sterilized at a lower pH, resulting in less GDP production and thus improving its biocompatibility. Compared with lactate-buffered solutions, this solution is associated with lower peritonitis rates, improved function of macrophages and neutrophils, and less peritoneal membrane damage as measured by lower effluent interleukin-6, hyaluronan, and VEGF levels and higher CA 125 levels. The long-term outcome of this biocompatible solution compared with conventional solutions remains unclear, but there seems to be a general consensus on the superiority of biocompatible solutions.

Bicarbonate Buffers

Recent advances in manufacturing technology have provided the option of separate alkaline and acidic fluid compartments. This permits the sterilization of glucose at very low pH, with greatly reduced glucose-degradation product formation. With the use of lactate or bicarbonate (or both) as a buffer, this sterilization produces neutral-pH final dialysis solutions. A pure bicarbonate-buffered CAPD solution with 34 mmol/L of bicarbonate buffer is commercially available (see Table 32.1).

Advantages suggested for such solutions include better patient acceptance (because of reduced pain during the fluid infusion) and a significant increase in serum bicarbonate concentration. A higher bicarbonate concentration of 39 mmol/L has also been examined and may provide additional acid–base correction in patients who remain mildly acidotic with 34 mmol/L solution. Whether bicarbonate fluids or bicarbonate–lactate fluids have specific advantages over each other under long-term use conditions in clinical practice remains unknown. Despite a lack of hard clinical evidence of superiority of the newer more "biocompatible" solutions over "conventional" solutions, there is general consensus that they are the preferred solutions. Clinical use is often guided by affordability of therapy and varies across the globe. In many parts of Europe and the United States, the newer biocompatible solutions are now used as standard, but conventional solutions are still the first choice in much of the developing world.

C H A P T E R 3 3

Lymphatics, Peritoneal Fluid Losses, and Peritoneal Dialysis

Ramesh Khanna, MD

The role of lymphatics in the peritoneal cavity is to absorb materials presented to it. The range of material it can absorb includes fluid, electrolytes, proteins, colloid materials, cells, and inert particles. Studies in continuous ambulatory peritoneal dialysis (CAPD) patients using tagged colloid fluids from the peritoneal cavity have showed absorption rates of 1.0 to 1.5 mL/min. Similarly, a continuous absorption of fluid (regardless of the tonicity of the dialysis solution) significantly reduces the measured net ultrafiltration (UF) during a dwell time in CAPD patients. Indeed, a century ago, intraperitoneal blood transfusions were used to correct anemia in neonates and fetuses.

Pathways of Fluid Absorption

There are two pathways through which fluid absorption may occur from the peritoneal cavity: Fluids and electrolytes and small solutes are absorbed across the mesothelium in response to concentration, osmotic, or hydrostatic pressure gradients, and macromolecules from the interstitium are likely absorbed through the lymphatics slowly or by convective absorption into the lymphatics located both in the subdiaphragmatic area and the interstitium of the abdominal wall. Researchers in the mid-1900s assumed that all fluid absorbed from the peritoneal cavity along with proteins passed through lymphatics and that the rate of absorption was directly proportional to intraperitoneal hydrostatic pressure. It has not been possible to directly measure lymph flow from the peritoneal cavity. There is a marked discrepancy between the observed rate of fluid absorption from the peritoneal cavity and the appearance in the plasma of the protein equivalent fluid. It is estimated that the plasma appearance rate of fluid is less than 25% of the total fluid absorbed from the peritoneal cavity.

The specialized end lymphatics (stomata) were first observed in 1862 and were recently reconfirmed as allowing entry of intraperitoneal fluid, solutes, particles, and cells by extracellular pathways. A negative pressure created by diaphragmatic movement during inspiration aided by the intraperitoneal positive hydrostatic pressure causes absorption of fluid through lymphatics. Nearly 80% of the peritoneal lymphatic drainage enters the venous circulation via the right lymph duct. Estimations of peritoneal lymphatic absorption of ascitic fluid in patients with hepatic cirrhosis have ranged from 24 to 225 mL/hr; in patients with malignant ascites, the range is from 1 to 63 mL/hr.

Rate of Fluid Loss From the Peritoneal Cavity During Peritoneal Dialysis Exchanges

In hypertonic peritoneal dialysis (PD), the net transcapillary UF rate is highest during the exchange at time zero and decreases exponentially as the dialysate glucose concentration is dissipated by a combination of dilution by the ultrafiltrate and transperitoneal glucose absorption. The peak intraperitoneal fluid volume is observed much before the cessation of UF and osmotic equilibration. After the peak, the intraperitoneal volume begins to decrease indicating that the net fluid absorption occurs much before net transcapillary UF is complete. In addition, osmolar equilibrium is reached before osmotic pressure and glucose equilibrium. The dialysis solution becomes isoosmolar with the plasma before glucose equilibrium because of solute sieving. That the dialysis solution becomes hypoosmolar to the plasma toward the end of the dwell time further suggests that net transcapillary UF continues after osmolar equilibrium. Consequently, the reduction in intraperitoneal volume after attaining the peak volume really represents absorption through lymphatics and not into the microcirculatory capillaries. Direct measurements of drain volumes after sequential dwell times suggest that the rate of decrease in the intraperitoneal volume averages 39 mL/hr. The net absorption rate is not significantly different irrespective of whether 2-L volumes of 1.5%, 2.5%, or 4.25% dextrose dialysis solution are instilled. Irrespective of the initial solution tonicity and infusion volumes, a near constancy of absorption rate reflects a nonosmotic or non–hydrostatic-driven absorption of isosmotic fluid, presumably through lymphatic channels.

Direct measurement of lymphatic drainage (thoracic duct and caudal mediastinal lymph duct) of the peritoneal cavity in anesthetized sheep after administration of 50-mL/kg volumes of 1.5% dialysis solution estimated a total rate of lymph flow of 0.454 mL/hr/kg over a 6-hour period. The direct estimation of lymph flow rate in this study is likely a gross underestimation of the true rate because of the use of anesthesia. Anesthetic agents may depress active lymphatic pumping. The estimation of lymph flow response to excess intraperitoneal fluid in five awake sheep after cannulation of the caudal mediastinal node efferent lymphatic vessel showed a sevenfold increase in the flow rate from that of the baseline. In the caudal mediastinal lymph vessel alone, the rate of lymph flow was 0.5 mL/min.

In conclusion, by extrapolation from previous studies of drain volumes after infusion of isotonic and hypertonic solutions (by analogy with ascites and by direct estimation of lymph flow rates in response to dialysis solution in awake sheep), the average fluid loss from the peritoneal cavity is about four- to fivefold larger than plasma appearance of fluid, measured directly or indirectly.

Clinical Implications

Net UF volumes (UFVs) are significantly decreased by cumulative intraperitoneal reabsorption of fluid after long dwell exchanges in CAPD patients. Nevertheless, such reductions of total UF generated during an exchange causes a relatively greater reduction in net UF in children or adults with fast or high peritoneal solute transport characteristics. Reduction in such fluid volumes during an exchange also contributes to reduced solute clearances because clearances depend on net UFVs and solute mass removal. Accordingly, it is not surprising that the efficiency of the peritoneum as a dialyzing membrane is greater than observed and appreciated. Appreciation of true UF capacity of the peritoneum in response to an osmotic agent during a dialysis exchange and its eventual reduction of net UFV and solute clearances due to major reabsorption of generated UFV provide an opportunity for alternative means of increasing net UF and solute clearance without increasing the osmotic load. Preliminary studies in animal models and human subjects suggest the potential exists for decreasing such reabsorption of generated UFV through pharmacologic action of certain drugs or through measures that reduce intraperitoneal hydrostatic pressure. None of the studies reported so far has provided a clinically effective way to enhance net UF and solute clearances in human subjects.

Summary

Reduction in generated UFV caused by back reabsorption of nearly 80% to 90% of fluid from the peritoneal cavity during a PD exchange causes PD to be a very inefficient dialysis system. Such reductions have a major impact on the kinetics of UF and solute clearances during an exchange. Lower net UF reduces both effective UFV and solute clearances. Nevertheless, currently available osmotic agents allow sufficient net UFV to be achieved such that adequate fluid balance and small-solute clearance in the majority of CAPD patients are obtained. However, such reductions in volumes impact greatly on patients with fast or high peritoneal transport characteristic. Many such patients are unable to maintain adequate fluid balance such that they either have to use higher osmotic loads of glucose or are unable to continue on PD. Attempts to manipulate back reabsorption of fluid has not been clinically successful. Future research should attempt focus on reducing such fluid back reabsorption through pharmaceutical or physical methods.

SECTION XII

Peritoneal Dialysis:
Infectious Complications

Peritoneal Dialysis: Infectious Complications

CHAPTER 34

Abnormalities of Host Defense Mechanisms During Peritoneal Dialysis

Clifford Holmes, PhD

The prevention of peritoneal microbial contamination is the primary consideration in the prevention of peritonitis related to peritoneal dialysis (PD). The widespread use of PD solution delivery systems designed to minimize the probability of touch contamination in both continuous ambulatory peritoneal dialysis (CAPD) and automated peritoneal dialysis (APD)—combined with overall improvements in catheter placement and exit-site care protocols and continuous quality improvement programs and patient training—has continuously reduced the incidence of peritonitis over the past 3 decades. The 2011 International Society for Peritoneal Dialysis position statement on reducing the risk of PD-related infections identifies the achievement of selected centers around the world in attaining peritonitis rates as low as one episode in every 70 patient-months or less. Therefore, what, if any, is the role of the peritoneal cavity and its cellular and tissue architecture in the prevention of peritonitis after contamination occurs, and how does the process of PD therapy affect the host defense of the peritoneal cavity?

Evidence exists from longitudinal studies in the 1980s, using repeated effluent culture techniques, that recovery of viable microorganisms from drained peritoneal effluent did not always result in clinical peritonitis. A first line of peritoneal host defense mechanisms must therefore be operative in PD patients, as in normal healthy subjects, that prevents microbial contamination of the peritoneal cavity from progressing to overt clinical peritonitis despite the process of infusion and drainage of large volumes of dialysis fluid afforded by modern PD techniques. Animal models, in the 1980s, established that peritoneal macrophages account for the majority of early phagocytosis of bacteria injected into the peritoneum and combined with direct translymphatic absorption of bacteria account for the first line of host defense. Overwhelming of these first-line defense mechanisms, in an inoculum dependent manner, results in the amplification of the immune response involving a rapid influx of polymorphonuclear neutrophils, as typically seen in the clinical presentation of PD-related peritonitis.

Peritoneal macrophages and opsonins were first characterized in the dialysis effluent of CAPD patients in 1983. Since then, much research has led to the understanding of many cellular and soluble factors of numerous tissue and cell types involved in the immune response to peritonitis in PD patients. This chapter provides a brief review of peritoneal host defense mechanisms in PD patients followed by a description of therapeutic interventional strategies aimed at augmenting identified deficiencies.

Host Defense Mechanisms of the Peritoneal Cavity

Relative to the normal peritoneum, the chronically dialyzed peritoneal cavity is considered an immunocompromised site. Factors that are likely important in this respect include inefficient lymphatic removal of contaminating microorganisms; critically reduced levels of antibody, complement, and leukocytes; the presence of granulocyte inhibitors; and possibly the use of bioincompatible dialysis solutions. Lymphatic removal, particularly via the subdiaphragmatic lacunae, is believed to play a diminished role in the prevention of PD-related peritonitis compared with that of normal subjects. It is proposed that the large volume of dialysate required for dialysis impairs efficient convection of bacteria and phagocytosed cells to the lymphatics. Furthermore, the infusion of large solution volumes into the peritoneum reduces the concentration of two important opsonins (immunoglobulin G and complement C3) to approximately 1/30 to 1/70 that of normal peritoneal fluid—and the leukocyte count is reduced to 10^3 to 10^4 cells/mL from a normal range of 10^6 to 10^7/mL.

As described earlier, the peritoneal macrophage is the predominant cell type in uninfected peritoneal dialysate effluent and is considered the first line of cellular defense. Peritoneal macrophages recovered from PD effluent appear as phenotypically activated or immature cells putatively believed to derive from bone marrow via omental and parietal tissue milky spots and other peritoneal tissue routes. Effective functioning of the peritoneal macrophage within the peritoneum is assumed to be initially dependent on effective opsonization of the invading pathogen by IgG, by C3b, and perhaps to a lesser extent by fibronectin.

Microorganisms are engulfed by macrophages by a process termed *receptor-mediated phagocytosis*. Intracellular killing of the microbe by macrophages then ensues via oxidative and non-oxidative mechanisms. Generation of chemotactic factors such as leukotriene B_4 may attract more phagocytes to the site of microbial invasion, thereby assisting in the immune response. Neutrophils will be recruited, potentially in very large numbers, to the site of inflammation in a classic amplification manner. In this respect, mesothelial cells play a pivotal role. Human peritoneal mesothelial cells have now been reported to secrete cytokines, chemokines, and growth factors and to express several important adhesion molecules, suggesting that these cells are critically involved in the orchestration of the inflammatory response to injury.

Ongoing research into peritoneal host defense continues to illustrate its complexity (Fig. 34.1). To exemplify this, consider the following collection of recent mechanistic insights into peritoneal host defense mechanisms in dialysis patients:

- Elevated levels of interferon-γ, tumor necrosis factor-α (TNF-α), interleukin-12 (IL-12), and IL-18 during peritonitis in PD patients represent a bias toward a Th1-type immune response, that is, a response that activates cell-mediated immunity rather than humoral (antibody) immunity.
- Within the pool of peritoneal CD14+ cells that differentiate into macrophages or dendritic cells, there is an additional subset of cells (described as myeloid dendritic precursor cells) that is likely pivotal to the Th1 response in peritonitis.
- Lymphocyte-derived IL-17 is now recognized as playing an important role in neutrophil recruitment via the release of the chemokine Growth Regulated alpha protein (GRO-α) from mesothelial cells, and high levels of IL-7 during the early phase of peritonitis may be associated with a favorable outcome.

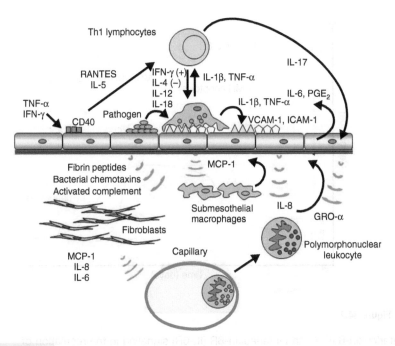

Figure 34.1

Cells and mediators involved in the host defense of peritoneal dialysis (PD) patients. This diagram represents some of the described cells and mediators putatively involved in peritoneal host defense in PD patients. GRO-α, Growth Regulated alpha protein; ICAM, intercellular adhesion molecule; IFN-γ, interferon-γ; IL, interleukin; MCP-1, monocyte chemotactic protein-1; PGE$_2$, prostaglandin E$_2$; RANTES, regulated on activation, normal T-cell expressed and secreted; TNF-α, tumor necrosis factor-α.

- Human peritoneal mesothelial cells respond to bacterial ligands through a specific subset of Toll-like receptors.
- IL-6 signaling via its soluble IL-6 receptor coordinates the transition from neutrophil to mononuclear cell infiltration during the amplification and resolution of the peritoneal immune response to infection and as such plays a critical role in the clearance of infection (Fig. 34.2).

Is Opsonic Activity of Peritoneal Dialysate Important?

The most compelling evidence that effective intraperitoneal opsonization of potential pathogens is important in the prevention of peritonitis is the finding that there is an inverse relationship between the opsonic activity or IgG concentration of effluent and the frequency of peritonitis. Several groups have reported this finding. However, an almost equal number of studies have found no such correlation within their patient populations. Reasons for disagreement among studies are unclear but may include inadequate sample sizes and differences in methodologies, such as dwell times used or the assays used for determination of opsonic activity.

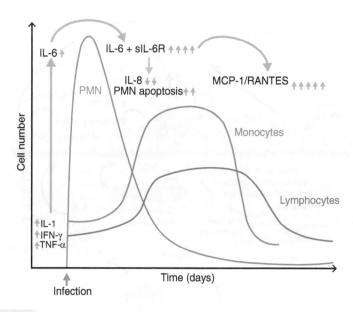

Figure 34.2

Interleukin-6 (IL-6) and interleukin-6R (IL-6R) signaling in the regulation of leukocyte trafficking in the peritoneal cavity. IFN-γ, Interferon-γ; MCP-1, monocyte chemotactic protein-1; PMN, polymorphonuclear neutrophil; RANTES, regulated on activation, normal T-cell expressed and secreted; sIL-6R, soluble IL-6 receptor; TNF-α, tumor necrosis factor-α. (Modified from: Devuyst O, Margetts P, Topley N. The pathophysiology of the peritoneal membrane. *J Am Soc Nephrol* 2010;21:1077-1085.)

Serum IgG levels have been reported to be low in pediatric CAPD patients, with no selective absence of any subclass. In contrast, total serum IgG levels were reported to be normal in a Dutch adult CAPD population, with a selective decrease in IgG_2 and IgG_4 caused by decreased synthesis. In neither study was a correlation with peritonitis identified.

Phagocytosis and Intracellular Killing

The in vitro phagocytic capability of peritoneal macrophages of most CAPD patients appears to be comparable to that of peritoneal macrophages obtained from women undergoing laparoscopy and of peripheral blood monocytes. In fact, not only is phagocytic function unhindered in most patients, but such dialysate-elicited macrophages appear to resemble stimulated or activated cells as described by a variety of functional and phenotypic characteristics. Studies that have included peritoneal macrophages from laparoscopy patients for comparison have found that peritoneal macrophages from CAPD patients also exhibit some characteristics of immature cells. Together, these observations suggest that the peritoneal macrophage population of PD patients consists of young inflammatory cells.

Some reports have identified specific functional defects or changes in peritoneal macrophage function associated with PD. In patients with frequent episodes of peritonitis (e.g., two per patient-year), there appears to be impairment in intracellular killing of bacteria by macrophages associated with enhanced prostaglandin E_2 production and decreased IL-1 production, Fc receptor expression, and respiratory burst activity. Because of the cross-sectional design of these latter studies, it is impossible to determine cause or effect. A single-center longitudinal study of PD patients has identified a transient decrease in the phagocytic capacity of macrophages in the few days before peritonitis. To date, two reports have identified changes in macrophage-receptor expression and in cytokine synthesis that occur with time in patients on PD, although no specific relationship to peritonitis was reported.

Impaired phagocytosis and intracellular killing by both peripheral blood and peritoneal polymorphonuclear leukocytes have been reported in CAPD patients. In a follow-up clinical study, a trend toward higher peritonitis rates and more catheter removals in patients with proven defective intracellular killing by peripheral blood polymorphonuclear neutrophils (PMNs) was reported, which did not, however, reach statistical significance.

Therapeutic Approaches

Immunologically based therapeutic interventions designed to prevent peritonitis in PD patients have focused on enhancing opsonic activity of effluent or on correcting leukocyte defects in patients at high risk for peritonitis. Unfortunately, neither of these strategies was originally derived from prospective studies, and immunoprophylaxis for PD patients has not yet been proven either safe or effective in the long term. In the following sections, both historical and current approaches to the therapeutic enhancement of peritoneal host defenses of PD patients are discussed.

Immunization Strategies

Passive immunization by chronic intraperitoneal instillation of intravenous-quality IgG and active immunization with commercially available staphylococcal vaccines have been used to enhance opsonization. Clinically, several uncontrolled studies have reported some benefit of intraperitoneal IgG therapy in patients with a high incidence of peritonitis. However, because of the inability to accurately identify patients at high risk for peritonitis by measurement of effluent IgG in a prospective manner and in the absence of controlled randomized studies, contemporary experience with intraperitoneal instillation of IgG appears to be restricted to the treatment of refractory peritonitis in conjunction with antibiotic therapy in a small number of selected centers.

The development of an effective *Staphylococcus aureus* vaccine has been a desired goal for many years, and several attempts using various vaccine development strategies have been attempted with little success. For instance, a decade ago, an experimental vaccine consisting of a conjugate between *S. aureus* capsular polysaccharides 5 and 8 (conferring specificity) and detoxified *Pseudomonas aeruginosa* exotoxin (conferring T cell–dependent memory) failed to confer protection against *S. aureus* peritonitis and exit-site infection. More recently, a candidate vaccine containing the highly conserved *S. aureus* 0657nI iron surface determinant B failed in phase III trials to prevent *S. aureus* infections in either patients undergoing cardiothoracic surgery or patients with end-stage renal disease undergoing hemodialysis.

Strategies to Enhance Cell Function

Until recently, experience in enhancing cell function was limited to a few uncontrolled studies of either intraperitoneal α-interferon or calcitriol (1,25-dihydroxy vitamin D_3). The rationale for exogenous α-interferon was simply to supply this mediator of immune function to correct for decreased production of lymphocyte interferon. Calcitriol enhances the antimicrobial function of macrophages by improving superoxide production and intracellular killing. However, reports describing a significant reduction in peritonitis rates using these agents are limited and small in study size.

Several groups have suggested that granulocyte colony-stimulating factor (G-CSF) or granulocyte-macrophage colony-stimulating factor (GM-CSF) may be of use in patients presenting with recurrent peritonitis or who have proven impaired PMN killing. The colony-stimulating factors have shown clinical benefit in many studies of patients with pathologic states associated with abnormal phagocytic cell function and increased risk of infection (e.g., HIV, hematopoietic malignancy, and cirrhosis). Despite the demonstration of transient changes in peritoneal cell numbers, phagocytic index, cell-receptor expression, and dialysate cytokine levels observed after a 3-day course of intraperitoneal GM-CSF, the usefulness of GM-CSF as an adjunctive treatment of recurrent or refractory peritonitis has not been established.

Peritoneal Membrane Resting

The practice of "resting" the peritoneum during treatment for recurring or relapsing peritonitis by temporarily discontinuing PD with continuation of antibiotic therapy is occasionally used by some clinicians, although its role appears to be limited to uncomplicated and clinically mild cases. This approach is based on the logic that enhanced opsonic activity, leukocyte function, and possibly lymphatic removal will ensue, thereby allowing either less aggressive antibiotic therapy or reduced potential for relapse. Unfortunately, no controlled studies have been published on such approaches.

Peritoneal Dialysis Solution Biocompatibility

In addition to the previously described immunologic alterations within the population with a high peritonitis incidence, it is now well established that several aspects of conventional PD solution formulations can impair in vitro peritoneal leukocyte, mesothelial, and fibroblast function. The acidic pH of commercially available dialysis fluids, in combination with their high lactate concentration, can inhibit phagocytosis and oxidative metabolism of peritoneal phagocytes, as well as the ability of mesothelial cells to secrete cytokines. Hypertonicity, especially of the highest glucose concentrations used (e.g., 4.25% glucose monohydrate), can diminish phagocytic function and respiratory burst activity. Similarly, the concentrations of glucose degradation products (again, especially in the highest glucose levels) can suppress cell function in vitro. Several animal models have also shown an improvement in peritoneal membrane function with more biocompatible solutions. In recent years, a total of 13 randomized controlled trials (RCTs) have compared biocompatible solutions with standard PD solutions with PD-related infection being a secondary outcome for most of these studies. Only two of these RCTs showed a significant benefit. In contrast, a recent observational study of the Australia and New Zealand Dialysis and Transplant registry of all incident PD patients between 2007 and 2010 reported a significantly greater overall rate of peritonitis and a shorter time to first peritonitis with the use of biocompatible solutions even in propensity score-matched cohorts.

Summary

Today a relatively large body of published research characterizing the host defense system of PD patients exists. Abnormalities of local peritoneal immunity include the dilution and bioincompatible effects of the dialysis solution itself, specific leukocyte functional defects, and the presence of functional leukocyte inhibitory uremic molecules. Despite growing insight into the pathobiology of PD-related peritonitis, there has been limited translation of this knowledge as yet into practical clinical measures for enhancing peritoneal host defense. The promise of biocompatible PD solutions enhancing peritoneal host defense leading to more favorable peritonitis related outcomes remains to be confirmed.

C H A P T E R   3 5

Peritoneal Catheter Exit Site and Tunnel Infections

Sharon J. Nessim, MD

Peritoneal dialysis (PD)–related infections, including peritonitis, exit-site infections (ESIs), and tunnel infections (TIs), remain important causes of morbidity and technique failure. Although peritonitis is usually the most frequent and morbid event among the infectious complications, ESIs and TIs are relevant and concerning complications of PD. This chapter focuses on the risk factors for their occurrence, as well as optimal strategies for their prevention and management.

Definitions

The definition of an ESI has evolved over time, and there have been several classifications created to try to improve the consistency in the diagnosis and reporting of ESI. In the simplest terms, based on the International Society for Peritoneal Dialysis (ISPD) guidelines, an ESI is defined by purulent drainage from the site at which the PD catheter emerges through the skin. Although erythema is often present during an ESI, the presence of erythema alone in the absence of purulent drainage may reflect inflammation of the skin rather than infection. Furthermore, a positive culture from an exit site in the absence of purulent drainage should be interpreted with caution because it may simply reflect colonization of the skin.

The PD catheter tunnel is the soft tissue space that the catheter passes through between the exit site and the peritoneal cavity. A tunnel infection is defined by the presence of tenderness, edema or induration, or erythema over the PD catheter tunnel or by the presence of a fluid collection along the catheter tunnel on ultrasonography. Because a TI usually results from migration of organisms from an infected exit site into the adjacent tunnel tract, most TIs occur in the presence of an associated ESI with the same organism.

Frequency

Data on the frequency of ESIs and TIs are not as readily available as those for peritonitis. In addition to the paucity of reported data on the frequency of their occurrence, the existing studies suggest an extremely wide variation in the rates of catheter infections. Some of this variability may relate to differences in the patient populations being studied, but part of it also likely relates to the relative subjectivity in diagnosing an ESI or TI as compared with a peritonitis episode. Based on one large U.S. observational data set of patients on PD between 1998 and 2004, 21% of patients developed an ESI, with an annual rate of 0.184 infections per patient-year at risk (or 1 infection every 65.2 patient months at risk). A similar ESI rate was reported in a randomized trial of exit site care among 203 Canadian PD patients (0.19 episodes per patient-year), while another randomized trial of 371 PD patients from Australia and New Zealand reported an ESI rate was 0.35 episodes per patient-year.

Causative Organisms

Several large observational databases have informed our understanding of the spectrum of organisms causing ESI. Approximately three quarters of ESIs are caused by gram-positive organisms, with the remainder mostly accounted for by gram-negative organisms. Among the gram-positive bacteria, the most common organism is *Staphylococcus aureus*, which is known to colonize some PD patients. Other gram-positive organisms that can cause ESI include coagulase-negative *Staphylococcus*, *Corynebacterium*, and *Streptococcus* spp. Among the gram-negative organisms, the most common cause of ESIs by far is *Pseudomonas* spp. Fungal ESI is usually rare but may occur with greater frequency when broad-spectrum topical antibacterial agents are used at the exit site. Because most TIs occur in association with an ESI, the causative organisms for TIs mirror those for ESIs.

Risk Factors

Because *S. aureus* is an important and frequent cause of ESI, one of the major risk factors is colonization with *S. aureus*. Nasal carriage of *S. aureus* has been reported to be present in approximately half of PD patients overall, with an almost twofold increased frequency of nasal carriage among patients with diabetes. Because *S. aureus* nasal carriage can be intermittent, repeating nasal swabs over time is prudent to ensure identification of patients who are colonized. It has been shown that *S. aureus* nasal carriage is associated with a dramatic increase in the risk of *S. aureus* ESIs and peritonitis and that strategies to eradicate *S. aureus* nasal colonization can reduce the incidence of *S. aureus* ESIs.

In addition, factors pertaining to the catheter position and orientation could augment the risk of ESIs and TIs. The location of the exit site is critically important to minimizing the risk of ESIs. For example, an exit site that is located under the pannus of an obese patient may lead to poor visualization of the exit site by the patient and a reduced likelihood of the area remaining dry and clean. Similarly, having an exit site in close proximity to a colostomy or ileostomy may increase the risk of ESIs. Furthermore, it is important to ensure that the exit site is not located at the level of the patient's belt line because this could contribute to chronic irritation and subsequent infection. Another important consideration is the direction of the catheter as it emerges from the skin. Based on observational data, a downward-directed tunnel has been associated with a reduced risk of infection, presumably by minimizing the risk of debris and organisms getting into the exit site.

Treatment and Outcomes

If a patient is diagnosed with an ESI, a Gram stain and culture of the discharge from the exit site should be obtained. Depending on the severity of the infection, the introduction of antibiotics can be deferred until the results of the Gram stain or culture are available, or one may elect to initiate empiric antibiotics pending the results. If the latter strategy is adopted, the initial choice of antibiotics should cover *S. aureus*, and consideration should be given to covering *Pseudomonas* spp. as well in patients with a history of *Pseudomonas* infections. After the causative organism is known, the antibiotics should be adjusted accordingly. Oral antibiotics are recommended as the preferred route of administration because topical antibiotics may be insufficient to overcome the bacterial burden of an ESI, and there is no evidence to suggest superiority of intraperitoneal administration over oral administration for ESI. The optimal duration of therapy is unknown, but the ISPD recommends continuation of antibiotics until the exit site appears normal, with a minimum treatment time of 2 weeks and a more lengthy course recommended for *S. aureus* and *Pseudomonas* infections.

Because TI typically represents the extension of an ESI into the PD catheter tunnel tract, a longer duration of therapy may be required when treating TIs, and consideration may be given to using intraperitoneal antibiotics. Tunnel sonography can be a useful adjunct for both diagnostic purposes as well as for identifying response to therapy.

If an ESI or TI does not resolve despite appropriate antibiotic therapy, or if a patient develops peritonitis with the same organism as that causing the catheter infection, the PD catheter should be removed. Such severe or nonresolving ESIs and TIs are most typical of *S. aureus* and *Pseudomonas* spp., which are very difficult to eradicate. For example, in one study, it was shown that complete resolution of a concomitant *Pseudomonas* ESI and peritonitis with antibiotic therapy occurred in only 11% of patients. One possible alternative to catheter removal for chronic, refractory ESI and TI is unroofing of the infected PD catheter tunnel. In the few reports of its use by experienced surgeons, there is a high rate of catheter salvage, but the data on this strategy remain quite limited.

The relationship between ESI and the risk of subsequent peritonitis has been investigated in several studies. In 2013, a qualitative review of nine such studies was performed, with eight of the nine studies suggesting that a history of ESI increased the risk of subsequent peritonitis, although evidence for a causal link was not present. In the most recent of these studies, it was found that having an ESI was associated with a sixfold higher risk of developing peritonitis within 30 days, even if the ESI was appropriately treated. The highest risk was early on, and it diminished with time. Interestingly, the subsequent peritonitis was only rarely caused by the same organism as the previous ESI, suggesting that high-risk patient characteristics, the immune response to the ESI, or the use of antibiotics to treat it may have contributed to the subsequent increased risk of peritonitis.

Prevention

Because some ESIs and TIs can be hard to eradicate, the best strategy is prevention. Preventive strategies that can reduce the frequency of PD-associated ESIs and TIs can be divided into appropriate early peri-implantation care and proper long-term exit site care.

At the time of PD catheter insertion, there are several important considerations. First, the selection of the exit site location is critical. Although most exit sites are located in the lower abdomen, consideration should be given to upper abdominal or presternal exit sites in the presence of a stoma or obesity with a large pannus. Furthermore, special attention should be paid to avoid placement of the exit site at the level of the patient's belt line. In all cases, the exit site should be visible to the patient so as to optimize chronic catheter care and early identification of changes in the appearance of the exit site. The superficial catheter cuff should be located approximately 2 to 3 cm deep to the exit site in order to avoid extrusion of the cuff, which can irritate the exit site and augment the risk of infection. The placement of an anchoring stitch or sutures at the exit site should be avoided because it may serve as an unnecessary nidus for infection. After the catheter is placed, a semiocclusive dressing should be used, and this dressing should not be removed or manipulated for the first week after catheter placement unless the dressing becomes soaked. Avoidance of frequent early dressing changes can help to prevent the introduction of organisms at the exit site (even if aseptic technique is used). In addition, this will minimize trauma and catheter movement, such that healing and epithelialization of the tunnel tract will be optimized. The catheter should be properly stabilized on the skin to minimize the mechanical stress transmitted to the exit site and tunnel, particularly during the healing period. If a PD catheter is being implanted well in advance of the expected date of use, embedding the catheter below the surface of the skin with exteriorization only at the time of PD initiation is another strategy that may minimize the risk of infection, although the evidence to support this strategy for infection prevention is inconclusive. It is unclear whether preoperative antibiotics reduce the risk of ESIs and TIs after catheter implantation, but they have been shown to reduce the risk of peritonitis in the postimplantation period and are therefore recommended.

After the exit site is healed, the dressing can be changed every day or every other day using aseptic technique. At the time of each dressing change, cleansing of the exit site should be performed. Several cleansing strategies have been used, including use of antibacterial soap and water, povidone-iodine, chlorhexidine, and sodium hypochlorite. No studies to date have definitively shown one strategy to be superior to another.

Based on the finding that *S. aureus* nasal carriage increases the risk of *S. aureus* ESI and peritonitis, one of the most studied strategies to prevent ESI involves the eradication of *S. aureus* colonization. The first agent used for eradication of *S. aureus* nasal carriage was oral rifampin for 5 days of every month, and although this strategy was effective, the routine use of this drug was limited by side effects, drug interactions, and the risk of developing resistance to rifampin over time. A more favorable strategy was identified in the form of mupirocin, a topical agent known to have excellent antibacterial activity against gram-positive organisms, including *S. aureus*. Several studies have reported on the use of topical mupirocin, either intranasally in *S. aureus* carriers or at the exit site in all PD patients, and have shown a significant reduction in the risk of *S. aureus* ESI and peritonitis. Despite some reports of the development of mupirocin resistance over time, the widespread adoption of mupirocin prophylaxis has led to a dramatic decrease in the frequency of *S. aureus* ESIs over the past 2 decades.

Although the risk of *S. aureus* ESIs and peritonitis declined significantly with the advent of strategies targeting *S. aureus* colonization, the risk of *Pseudomonas* ESIs over the same time period did not change. This led to the idea that topical gentamicin, an agent with antibacterial activity against both gram-positive and gram-negative organisms, might provide further benefit over mupirocin. In a single-center, randomized trial, exit-site application of topical mupirocin and gentamicin was compared, and it was found that although both were very effective at reducing gram-positive

ESIs, topical gentamicin was superior in the prevention of gram-negative ESIs and peritonitis. However, three subsequent observational studies have not been able to confirm the superiority of gentamicin over mupirocin, and some have raised questions about the possibility of gentamicin resistance over time with routine and prolonged use. Two subsequent randomized trials of other exit site strategies have been performed. In one trial in which Polysporin triple ointment was compared with mupirocin, the Polysporin triple ointment was not shown to be superior, and there was a higher risk of fungal ESIs. In the second trial, exit-site application of antibacterial honey in all patients was compared with intranasal mupirocin in *S. aureus* carriers, but there was an increased risk of infection among patients with diabetes in the antibacterial honey group.

Based on these findings, the 2011 ISPD position statement on prevention of PD-related infections recommends that all PD patients should use topical antibiotic either at the catheter exit site or intranasally or both. Because the choice of the topical agent is left to the discretion of the clinician, it should ideally be based on local patterns of infection (including the frequency of *Pseudomonas* catheter infections) and local antibiotic resistance. For patients colonized with methicillin-resistant *S. aureus*, mupirocin should be the topical agent of choice. A final point is that topical mupirocin ointment (as opposed to mupirocin cream) should not be used at the exit sites of polyurethane catheters because of the potential for structural damage to the catheter over time.

Summary

Although ESIs and TIs tend to be less common than peritonitis in most PD programs, they remain important complications of PD. Early diagnosis and appropriate treatment are critical in order to improve the likelihood of resolution of the infection. Despite optimal care, some severe catheter infections require removal of the PD catheter. Several preventive strategies have been shown to reduce the risk of ESIs and TIs.

C H A P T E R 3 6

Peritonitis in Peritoneal Dialysis Patients

Cheuk-Chun Szeto, MD, FRCP

Peritoneal dialysis (PD) is now a standard therapeutic modality for end-stage renal disease (ESRD) and is used in about 15% of the dialysis population worldwide. In some parts of the world, the use of PD is considerably higher, reaching about 80% of ESRD patients in Hong Kong. Nonetheless, peritonitis in PD remains a major cause of technique failure and morbidity. Although fewer than 4% of peritonitis episodes result in death, peritonitis is a "contributing factor" to death in 16% of deaths in patients on PD. Furthermore, peritonitis accounts for 30% of the cases of treatment failure and 15% to 35% of hospital admissions.

Peritonitis Rate in PD Patients

Peritonitis rates can be calculated using months of PD at risk, divided by number of episodes, and expressed as the interval in months between episodes or episodes per year. Alternatively, it can be expressed as percentage of patients per period of time who are peritonitis free or as median peritonitis rate for the program.

With improved patient training, PD delivery systems, and prophylactic measures, the rate of peritonitis has fallen over the past 2 decades. Many centers now report a peritonitis rate of 0.2 to 0.6 episodes per year at risk, or one episode per 20 to 60 patient-months of PD. In some centers, overall rates as low as 1 episode every 41 to 52 months (0.29–0.23/year) have been reported. The International Society for Peritoneal Dialysis (ISPD) 2010 updated guidelines for PD-related infections suggested that every program should regularly monitor infection rates, at a minimum, on a yearly basis. The center's peritonitis rate should be no more than 1 episode every 18 months (0.67 per year at risk), although the rate achieved will depend to some extent on the patient population.

Risk Factors for Peritonitis

The risk factors for peritonitis include patient related, technique related, and environment related (Table 36.1).

Patient age has been found to be a risk factor. Although older patients are commonly considered to be at risk, patients younger than 20 years of age also have a much higher risk compared with middle-aged ones. The socioeconomic status of patients has also been shown to be associated with peritonitis risk. Education level significantly influences the peritonitis rate. Previous studies suggest that patients with fewer than 9 years of education have almost double the peritonitis rate compared with those with more than 12 years of education. Depression (e.g., as indicated by a Beck Depression Inventory score) has been shown previously to be associated with the development of peritonitis.

Table 36.1

Risk Factors for Peritonitis

	Nonmodifiable	Modifiable
Patient related	• Older age • Female • Black ethnicity • Lower socioeconomic status • Diabetes mellitus • Coronary artery disease • Chronic lung disease • Hypertension • Poor residual kidney function	• Obesity • Smoking • Depression • Hypoalbuminemia • Hypokalemia • Medical procedures • No vitamin D supplement • Bioincompatible fluids • Nasal *Staphylococcus aureus* carrier • Previous ESI
Technique related	• Center effect	• Method of patient training • Connecting system • Prophylactic antibiotics for nasal carriage • Prophylactic antibiotics for exit site care
Environment related	• Hot and humid climate	• Living distantly from PD unit • Pets

ESI, exit-site infection; PD, peritoneal dialysis.

Peritoneal dialysis patients with diabetes mellitus are at particular high risk for peritonitis. This can possibly be attributed to the adverse effect of diabetes on peritoneal defense mechanisms by interfering with the migration of phagocytic cells into the peritoneum. Formation of advanced glycation end products might further suppress the phagocytic activity of resident peritoneal macrophages in patients with diabetes. In addition to an increased risk of touch contamination, a decrease in intestinal motility or slower colonic transit time among patients with diabetes also favors bacterial overgrowth with the increased risk of peritonitis secondary to enteric organisms.

Patients with *Staphylococcus aureus* nasal carriage are at a higher risk for *S. aureus* peritonitis. The rate of such infections may be reduced with prophylactic antibiotics such as mupirocin nasal ointment; the addition of chlorhexidine bath seems to have no extra benefit. A previous study shows that intermittent nasal mupirocin application is effective in preventing redevelopment of *Staphylococcus aureus*-carriage in PD patients, and the risk of antibiotic resistance is not increased.

Climate may play a role in predisposing to peritonitis. A number of studies have shown that there is a substantial seasonal variation in the incidence of dialysis-related peritonitis, with peak incidence in the months that are hot and humid. Keeping a cool and dry living environment may help to reduce peritonitis in PD patients, particularly in tropical countries.

It is important to note, however, that although a number of the risk factors for PD peritonitis listed in Table 36.1 are modifiable, there is currently little published evidence that modifying these risk factors will lead to reduced peritonitis rates, with the exception of topical exit-site antimicrobial prophylaxis and nasal eradication of *S. aureus*.

Pathogenesis and Causative Organisms

Several routes leading to peritonitis in PD are known: intraluminal (mainly through touch contamination), periluminal (through exit-site infections [ESIs] or tunnel infections [TIs]), intestinal, systemic (through bloodstream), and rarely ascending (through the vagina).

Using appropriate culture techniques, an organism can be isolated from the peritoneal fluid in more than 90% of cases in which clinical features of peritonitis are present. The responsible pathogen is most commonly a bacterium. With the extensive use of the "flush before fill" technology and double-bag disconnect systems, our recent data showed that gram-positive and gram-negative organisms accounted for about 40% and 32% of all the peritonitis episodes, respectively (Table 36.2). Among all gram-negative organisms, *Pseudomonas* and those from the family Enterobacteriaceae were the most common. Enterobacteriaceae often are labeled as "enteric bacteria" with a number of major human intestinal pathogens (e.g., *Shigella* spp., *Salmonella* spp.) and several others being normal colonizers of the human gastrointestinal tract (e.g., *Escherichia* spp,. *Klebsiella* spp.). Peritonitis caused by Enterobacteriaceae may be due to touch contamination; ESI; or possibly a bowel source, such as constipation, colitis, or transmural migration, but the etiology is often unclear.

Table 36.2

Causative Organisms of Peritoneal-Dialysis Related Peritonitis in Prince of Wales Hospital From 2005 to 2014

Causative Organisms	Percentage
Gram-Positive Organisms	40.4
Coagulase-negative staphylococcus	11.6
Staphylococcus aureus	10.4
Streptococcus spp.	11.0
Enterococci	0.8
Diphtheroid species	1.9
Corynebacterium species	1.7
Miscellaneous	2.9
Gram-Negative Organisms	27.5
Escherichia coli	8.0
Pseudomonas spp.	6.7
Klebsiella spp.	3.9
Acinetobacter spp.	1.9
Miscellaneous	7.0
Polymicrobial	15.3
Culture-Negative Peritonitis	13.2
Fungi	1.5
Mycobacterium spp.	2.1

Diagnosis of Peritonitis in Peritoneal Dialysis Patients

The diagnosis of PD-related peritonitis can be confirmed when at least two of the following conditions are present: (1) symptoms and signs of peritoneal inflammation, (2) cloudy peritoneal fluid with an elevated peritoneal fluid cell count (>100/µL) due predominantly (<50%) to neutrophils, and (3) demonstration of bacteria in the peritoneal effluent by Gram stain or culture. However, PD patients presenting with cloudy effluent should be presumed to have peritonitis. It is important to initiate empiric antibiotic therapy for PD-associated peritonitis as soon as possible. In theory, there are other causes of cloudy peritoneal effluent, including chemical peritonitis, eosinophilia of the effluent, hemoperitoneum, and rarely malignancy and chylous effluent. Nonetheless, there are potentially serious consequences of peritonitis (relapse, catheter removal, permanent transfer to hemodialysis, and death), which are more likely to occur if treatment is not promptly initiated. Although a number of novel diagnostic techniques (e.g., leukocyte esterase, broad-spectrum polymerase chain reaction [PCR], quantitative bacterial DNA PCR) have been explored, there is as yet not enough evidence for recommending them for the routine diagnosis of peritonitis.

Clinical Assessment

Assessment of the patient should include history taking for possible touch contamination, compliance with sterile dialysis technique, recent procedures that may have led to peritonitis, and changes in bowel habits (either diarrhea or constipation). Careful physical examination including vital signs should be performed, especially to look for septicemia resulted from the peritonitis as this may affect the route of administration of the antibiotics. One must also carefully assess the exit site and tunnel for edema, erythema, tenderness, and discharge to look for evidence of associated ESI, which may be the cause of the peritonitis.

Collection of Peritoneal Dialysis Effluent for Cell Count and Culture

After the initial clinical assessment, PD effluent should be obtained for cell count, differential, and culture. The diagnosis of peritonitis and the subsequent management depend on good specimen collection. A sample of peritoneal fluid (preferably the first bag of PD fluid) should be collected before the addition of antibiotics, and the specimen should be sent immediately to the laboratory for absolute cell count and differential counts as well as culture. If the collection is done after flush out cycles, the clinician should use the percentage of neutrophils rather than the absolute number of white blood cells (WBCs) to diagnose peritonitis.

Cell count is important because it can differentiate cellular element of the peritonitis from those without cells (e.g., fibrin, chyle). The WBC count should exceed 100/mm^3 before the diagnosis of peritonitis is made. The majority of the cell count in an untreated effluent sample of suspected infective peritonitis should be composed of neutrophils or lymphocytes. An abundance of eosinophils should alert the clinician to the diagnosis of chemical peritonitis, in which chemicals causing irritation to the peritoneum render an eosinophilic response. A predominance of lymphocytes or macrophages should raise the suspicion of tuberculous peritonitis. Most laboratories will make a smear with a direct differential cell counting after staining, with or without dilution. One caution is that cell lysis can occur after 24 to 48 hours of specimen collection, and then the cell morphology cannot be identified.

Traditionally, the specimen for culture is collected in universal sterile bottles; the fluid is centrifuged, and the sediment is used for Gram stain and plate culture. However, the yield of this method is often low. The standard culture technique recommended by the latest ISPD guideline is the use of blood-culture bottles. This method gives a good yield of microbiologic data because factors and nutrients inside this system will enhance growth of the organism. Furthermore, a large-volume culture (e.g., culturing the sediment after centrifuging 50 mL of effluent) could further improve the recovery of microorganisms. Peritoneal fluid should be cultured promptly. If immediate delivery to the laboratory is not possible, the inoculated culture bottles should ideally be incubated at 37°C. Routine blood cultures are not necessary unless a patient appears septic or if an acute surgical abdominal condition is suspected.

Management of Peritonitis

Peritoneal dialysis patients presenting with cloudy effluent should be presumed to have peritonitis. It is important to initiate empiric antibiotic therapy for PD-associated peritonitis as soon as possible, without waiting for confirmation from the laboratory of the cell count so as to prevent delay in treatment. Empiric antibiotics must cover both gram-positive and gram-negative organisms. The ISPD 2010 updated guidelines recommend center-specific selection of empiric therapy depending on the history of sensitivities of organisms causing peritonitis in that center. In addition, it suggests that gram-positive organisms may be covered by vancomycin or a cephalosporin, and gram-negative organisms by a third-generation cephalosporin or aminoglycoside.

Fig. 36.1 shows the initial management of PD-related peritonitis. The authors favor cefazolin rather than vancomycin because of the potential of the emergence of vancomycin-resistant organisms. Although aminoglycosides are theoretically associated with a more rapid loss of residual renal function, this problem was not observed in recent randomized studies. The ISPD 2010 updated guideline states that short-term aminoglycoside use appears to be safe and inexpensive and provides good gram-negative coverage. Nonetheless, an extended course of aminoglycoside therapy should be avoided because it may increase the risk for both vestibular toxicity and ototoxicity.

Antibiotic Administration

In general, intraperitoneal administration of antibiotics is superior to intravenous (IV) dosing for treating peritonitis. If the patient has septicemia or appears toxic as a result of the peritonitis, antibiotics should be administered intravenously in addition to other resuscitative measures. The ISPD 2010 updated guideline on intraperitoneal antibiotic dosing recommendations for patients receiving continuous ambulatory peritoneal dialysis (CAPD) is summarized in Table 36.3. For patients with substantial residual renal function (e.g., residual glomerular filtration rate ≥ 5 mL/min/1.73m^2), the dose of antibiotics that have renal excretion may need to be adjusted accordingly

Intraperitoneal antibiotics can be given in each exchange as continuous dosing or once daily as intermittent dosing, and both are equally efficacious. In intermittent

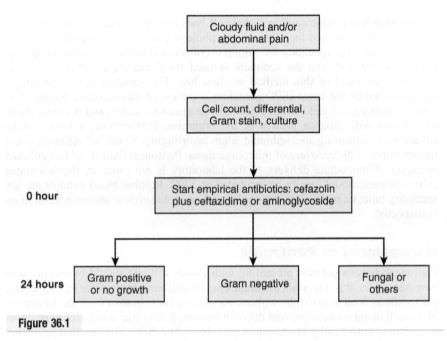

Figure 36.1

Initial management of peritoneal dialysis–related peritonitis.

dosing, the antibiotic containing dialysis solution must be allowed to dwell for at least 6 hours to allow adequate absorption of the antibiotic into the systemic circulation. Once-daily therapy has the advantage of ease of use by patient and staff, both in the hospital and at home. In addition, once-daily dosing may result in less ototoxicity and nephrotoxicity. Evidence supports good efficacy of intermittent dosing of aminoglycosides and vancomycin. For example, once-daily dosing of gentamicin (40 mg IP in 2 L) is as effective as dosing in each exchange (10 mg/2 L intraperitoneal in four exchanges per day) for CAPD peritonitis. Intraperitoneal vancomycin is well absorbed when given in a long dwell and subsequently crosses again from the blood into the dialysate with fresh exchanges. On the other hand, data in support of intermittent dosage of cephalosporin are less complete, and we recommend continuous administration.

With effective treatment, the patient should begin to improve clinically within 12 to 48 hours, and the total cell count and percentage of neutrophils in the peritoneal fluid should begin to decrease. When culture results and sensitivities are known, antibiotic therapy should be adjusted to narrow spectrum agents as appropriate.

Adjunctive Treatment

Fibrinous clots are commonly found in PD effluent during peritonitis, and there is a risk of catheter obstruction. Heparin (500–1000 units/L) is often added to the dialysis solution until the dialysis effluent clears up and fibrinous clots are no longer visible. Because the majority of fungal peritonitis episodes are preceded by courses of antibiotics, fungal prophylaxis during antibiotic therapy may prevent some cases

Table 36.3

Intraperitoneal Antibiotic Dosing Recommendations

	Intermittent (Per Exchange, Once Daily)	Continuous (mg/L, All Exchanges)
Aminoglycosides		
Amikacin	2 mg/kg	LD 25, MD 12
Gentamicin	0.6 mg/kg	LD 8, MD 4
Netilmicin	0.6 mg/kg	LD 8, MD 4
Tobramycin	0.6 mg/kg	LD 8, MD 4
Cephalosporins		
Cefazolin	15 mg/kg	LD 500, MD 125
Cefepime	1000 mg	LD 500, MD 125
Cephalothin	15 mg/kg	LD 500, MD 125
Ceftazidime	1000–1500 mg	LD 500, MD 125
Penicillins		
Ampicillin	ND	MD 125
Oxacillin	ND	MD 125
Nafcillin	ND	MD 125
Amoxicillin	ND	LD 250–500, MD 50
Penicillin G	ND	LD 50,000 units, MD 25,000 units
Quinolones		
Ciprofloxacin	ND	LD 50, MD 25
Others		
Vancomycin	15–30 mg/kg q 5–7 days	LD 1000, MD 25
Daptomycin	ND	LD 100 mg/L, MD 20 mg/L
Linezolid	PO 200–300 mg qd	
Aztreonam	ND	LD 1000, MD 250
Antifungals		
Fluconazole	200 mg IP q 24–48 hr	
Amphotericin	NA	1.5
Combinations		
Ampicillin–sulbactam	2 g q 12 hr	LD 1000, MD 100
Trimethoprim–sulfamethoxazole	160 mg/800 mg PO twice daily	
Imipenem–cilastin	ND	LD 250, MD 50

LD, loading dose in milligrams; MD, maintenance dose in milligrams; ND, no data; NA, not applicable; PO, oral; q, every; qd, every day.
Adapted from Li PK, Szeto CC, Piraino B, et al; International Society for Peritoneal Dialysis. Peritoneal dialysis-related infections recommendations: 2010 update. *Perit Dial Int* 2010;30: 393-423.

of *Candida* peritonitis in programs that have high rates of fungal peritonitis. Nystatin prophylaxis should be considered in programs with high baseline rates of fungal peritonitis.

Urokinase has been used by some investigators in the treatment of refractory or relapsing peritonitis. In theory, fibrinolytic treatment could release bacteria entrapped in fibrin within the peritoneum or along the catheter, thus making it possible to eradicate the infection. However, studies of intraperitoneal urokinase show conflicting results, and this treatment is not routinely recommended.

Treatment of Specific Organisms

Gram-Positive Organism Cultured (Fig. 36.2)

If *S. aureus*, *Staphylococcus epidermidis*, or a *Streptococcus* spp. are identified, then continued therapy with cefazolin or vancomycin is recommended. Many *S. epidermidis*–like organisms reported to be resistant to first-generation cephalosporins are sensitive to the levels achieved in the peritoneal cavity. As a result, if the patient is clinically responding to treatment, there is usually no need to change the

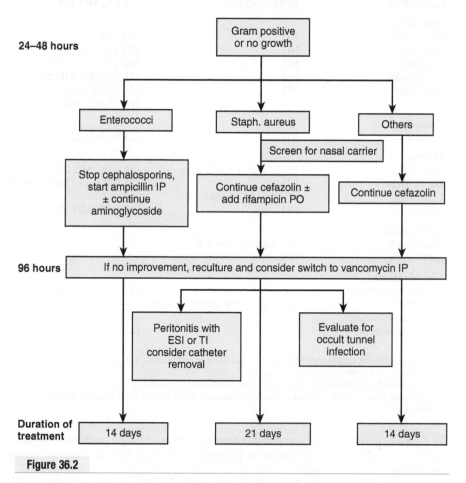

Figure 36.2

Management of peritonitis caused by gram-positive organisms. ESI, Exit-site infection; IP, intraperitoneal; PO, oral; TI, tunnel infection.

antibiotic regimen. Enterococcal peritonitis tends to be severe and is best treated with IP ampicillin, with or without an aminoglycoside, when the organism is susceptible. If the improvement is prompt, antimicrobial therapy should be continued for a total of 14 days, but *S. aureus* peritonitis requires antimicrobials for 3 weeks. Peritonitis caused by *S. aureus* with concurrent ESI or TI is unlikely to respond to antibiotic therapy without catheter removal. These patients also require screening for possible nasal carrier state. Rifampicin could be considered as an adjunct for the prevention of relapse or repeat *S. aureus* peritonitis, but the enzyme inducer effect of rifampicin should be considered in patients taking other medications.

Gram-Negative Organism Cultured (Fig. 36.3)

If a single, non-*Pseudomonas* species is recovered, the peritonitis can usually be treated by continuation of the initial intraperitoneal third-generation cephalosporin or aminoglycoside alone, or by another single appropriate antibiotic. Treatment should be continued for 14 days. If a *Pseudomonas* spp. or *Stenotrophomonas maltophilia* is recovered, then two anti-*Pseudomonas* antibiotics are needed. Suitable choices include aminoglycoside, third-generation cephalosporin, semisynthetic penicillin with anti-*Pseudomonas* activity (e.g., piperacillin), fluoroquinolone,

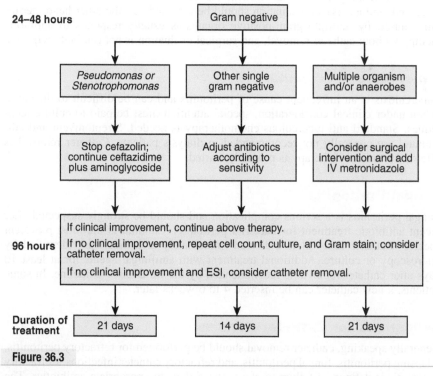

Figure 36.3

Management of peritonitis caused by gram-negative organisms. ESI, Exit-site infection; IV, intravenous.

aztreonam, imipenem, and trimethoprim–sulfamethoxazole. It should be noted that semisynthetic penicillins can inactivate aminoglycosides in vitro and thus should not be coadministered intraperitoneally. The duration of therapy should be 21 days. *Pseudomonas* peritonitis is often related to a catheter infection; in such cases, catheter removal is required. If the peritoneal catheter is removed, appropriate antipseudomonal antibiotics should be continued for another 2 weeks.

Culture-Negative Peritonitis

If the culture results are negative at 24 hours, then the most likely explanation is that a bacterial infection was present but that the responsible organisms failed to grow in the culture sample. However, if a program has a rate of culture-negative peritonitis greater than 20%, then the culture methods should be reviewed and improved. Management depends on whether the patient is improving clinically. Most authorities recommend continuing cefazolin alone for 2 weeks if the patient is improving. On the other hand, patients with culture-negative peritonitis who do not improve should be recultured to look for unusual organisms such as fungus and mycobacteria.

Polymicrobial Peritonitis

Management should be individualized. In general, if multiple enteric organisms are grown, particularly in association with anaerobic bacteria, the risk of death is increased, and a surgical evaluation should be obtained. On the other hand, peritonitis caused by multiple gram-positive organisms usually responds to antibiotic therapy without catheter removal, and surgical evaluation is not routinely required.

Tuberculous Peritonitis

Tuberculosis is an infrequent cause of peritonitis and can be difficult to diagnose. When under clinical consideration, special attention must be paid to culture techniques. Standard anti-tuberculous chemotherapy is needed. Streptomycin and ethambutol are generally not recommended in dialysis patients. Catheter removal is often not required if therapy is promptly started.

Fungal Peritonitis

Fungal peritonitis is a serious complication and should be strongly suspected after recent antibiotic treatment for bacterial peritonitis. *Candida* is the most prevalent species. Catheter removal is indicated immediately after fungi are identified by microscopy or culture. Additional treatment with antifungal agents for at least 10 days after catheter removal is recommended by the ISPD 2010 guideline. In some patients, a new catheter can be inserted 4 to 6 weeks later.

Indications for Catheter Removal

Generally speaking, catheter removal should be performed for refractory peritonitis, relapsing peritonitis, fungal peritonitis, and refractory catheter infections. Refractory peritonitis is defined as failure to clear after 5 days of appropriate antibiotics. The focus should always be on preservation of the peritoneum rather than saving the peritoneal catheter. After catheter removal, systemic antibiotics should be continued for another 2 weeks, and reinsertion of a new catheter can be considered after 4 weeks. Resumption of PD is possible in approximately half of the patients, but problems with ultrafiltration (UF) are common.

Relapsing, Recurrent, and Repeat Peritonitis

Under the current terminology stated by the ISPD 2010 guideline, relapsing peritonitis is defined as an episode that occurs within 4 weeks of completion of therapy of a prior episode with the same organism or one sterile episode, recurrent peritonitis is an episode that occurs within 4 weeks of completion of therapy of a prior episode but with a different organism, and a repeat episode is one that occurs more than 4 weeks after completion of therapy of a prior episode with the same organism. Pathogenically and clinically, relapsing, recurrent, or repeat peritonitis episodes represent distinct entities, which portend a worse outcome (particularly for recurrent peritonitis). Timely catheter removal should be seriously considered. With less serious infections, it may be possible to insert a new catheter simultaneously with removal of the old catheter after the infection is cleared.

Special Considerations in Automated Peritoneal Dialysis

The choice of first-line antibiotics in CAPD applies also to automated peritoneal dialysis (APD). Nonetheless, the recommendations for antibiotic treatment are based mainly on data obtained in CAPD patients and experience in patients on APD is limited. From a practical point of view, it is often more convenient to administer the loading dose intravenously for APD patients. For APD patients with a daytime dwell, antibiotics can be administered conveniently just in the daytime dwell. For patients with no daytime dwell, temporary conversion to a CAPD regimen may be considered because of the ease of antibiotic administration, although this may require additional patient training and sometimes result in fluid retention in rapid transporters. Alternatively, a daytime dwell could be added, and antibiotics can be administered just in the daytime dwell. There are few data concerning the efficacy of first generation cephalosporins given intermittently for peritonitis, particularly for the patient on APD. In contrast, it would be a safe approach to add a first-generation cephalosporin to each exchange. Doses of selected antimicrobials in patients who remain on APD during treatment of peritonitis are given in Table 36.4.

Predictors for Treatment Failure in Peritonitis

Recent studies have shown that the number of years on PD, the presence of diabetes mellitus, and peritonitis with gram-negative organisms, *Pseudomonas*, fungal or *Mycobacterium* species are independent risk factors predictive of treatment failure. In addition, the peritoneal dialysate total WBC count on day 3 of peritonitis predicts treatment failure independent of standard risk factors. Using a peritoneal dialysate WBC count cut point of $1090/mm^3$ or greater on day 3, the sensitivity is 75% and the specificity is 74% for the prediction of treatment failure (defined as catheter loss or peritonitis-related death).

Table 36.4

Intermittent Dosing of Antibiotics in Automated Peritoneal Dialysis

Drug	IP Dose
Vancomycin	Loading dose 30 mg/kg IP in long dwell; repeat dosing 15 mg/kg IP in long dwell q 3–5 days (aim to keep serum trough levels >15 µg/mL)
Cefazolin	20 mg/kg IP qd in long day dwell
Tobramycin	Loading dose, 1.5 mg/kg IP in long dwell; then 0.5 mg/kg IP each day in long dwell
Fluconazole	200 mg IP in one exchange per day q 24–48 hours
Cefepime	1 g IP in one exchange per day

IP, intraperitoneal; q, every; qd, every day.
Adapted from Li PK, Szeto CC, Piraino B, et al; International Society for Peritoneal Dialysis.
   Peritoneal dialysis-related infections recommendations: 2010 update. *Perit Dial Int* 2010;30:
   393-423.

Impact of Peritonitis

The permeability of the peritoneum to water, glucose, and proteins is increased during peritonitis. Rapid absorption of glucose from the dialysis solution reduces the amount of UF and often results in fluid overload. Higher dialysis solution glucose levels and shorter dwell times may be needed to maintain adequate UF. Partly as a result of rapid glucose absorption, glycemic control may worsen in patients with diabetes during peritonitis. Blood glucose monitoring with appropriate adjustments of insulin dosage is needed. In addition, protein loss during peritonitis is also increased, and the nutritional status of patients may worsen rapidly. In the long run, an episode of severe peritonitis often results in lasting effects, including a rise in peritoneal permeability and loss of UF. As discussed previously, among patients with refractory peritonitis and catheter removal, about half of the patients could resume treatment with PD. However, there is usually a substantial decline in the UF capacity of these patients, and nearly 90% of them require additional dialysis exchanges or hypertonic cycles to compensate for the loss of solute clearance or UF.

The risk of dying during an episode of peritonitis is 0.8% to 2.5%. Looking from another angle, peritonitis is the direct cause of death in more than 15% of all PD patients. Our previous study showed that the 2-year technique survival of PD patients was 88% without peritonitis but 70% when the patient had peritonitis. Peritoneal permeability characteristics have prognostic implications for patient and technique survival.

Prevention of Peritonitis

Strategies to prevent peritonitis include better patient selection, better patient training, improved exit-site care, treatment of *S. aureus* nasal carriage, antibiotic prophylaxis, better systems of PD, and possibly improving peritoneal defense by using biocompatible PD solutions.

Careful selection of patients could diminish the rate of peritonitis secondary to contamination. The method of training has a substantial influence on the risk of peritonitis. A nurse should provide the training whenever possible according to standard guidelines. Each PD program should consult the standard ISPD guidelines to prepare the trainer and develop a specific curriculum for PD training. Although there are few published data, retraining should be considered after peritonitis or catheter infection and after change in dexterity, vision, or mental acuity. After each peritonitis episode, it is prudent to perform a root cause analysis to determine the etiology so that interventions can be planned to prevent future episodes. Continued monitoring of the peritonitis rate is necessary in all dialysis programs. A high rate of peritonitis in a dialysis center should be followed by a critical appraisal of the pathogenic organisms as well as the training program with appropriate interventions taken.

For the choice of catheter placement, double-cuff catheters are preferred because they are less likely to require catheter removal for ESI compared with single-cuff catheters. The standard silicon Tenckhoff catheter remains a good choice, and there is no evidence that other catheter designs are superior in preventing peritonitis. The downward-pointing exit-site locations, suggested as a method of reducing ESIs, may decrease the risk of catheter-related peritonitis.

Good exit-site care also helps to prevent catheter infections and thus peritonitis. Catheter immobilization, proper location of the exit site, sterile wound care immediately after placement of the catheter, and avoidance of trauma are useful preventive measures. For routine exit-site care, there are sufficient data to support the use of PD catheter exit-site antibiotic creams (either mupirocin or gentamicin). Previous trials showed that mupirocin ointment applied daily to the exit site decreased the rate of both ESIs and peritonitis compared with a historical control group, and gentamicin cream was as effective as mupirocin in preventing *S. aureus* infections and reduced *P. aeruginosa* and other gram-negative catheter infections. Peritonitis, particularly that caused by gram-negative organisms, was reduced by 35%. However, the risk of antibiotic resistance after prolonged usage has not been assessed.

Improved connection systems have the benefit of reducing the incidence of peritonitis. With the technique of "flush-before-fill," Y-set disconnect systems consistently give a lower peritonitis rates than standard spike set in several clinical trials, and the double-bag system, which is a completely sterilized disposable integrated system that contains an empty bag and a fresh dialysate-containing bag, is superior to the Y-set disconnect systems.

Nasal carriage of *S. aureus* has been associated with an increased risk of ESIs, TIs, peritonitis, and possibly catheter loss. The rate of such infections may be reduced with eradication therapy. Both oral rifampin and topical mupirocin applied at the exit site or intranasally could reduce the risk of *S. aureus* catheter infection. In general, topical application is preferred to oral antibiotics. To prevent relapse after eradication and at the same time reduce the risk of developing resistance, one option is to use intranasal mupirocin intermittently (e.g., twice per day for 5–7 days every month). Another option is to treat only in response to documented relapses by a positive culture result.

Short-term prophylactic antibiotics are beneficial in the following settings: (1) before catheter placement; (2) before invasive procedures, such as dental procedures, colonoscopy, hysteroscopy, or cholecystectomy; and (3) after wet contamination. For prophylactic antibiotics administered at the time of catheter insertion, the usual recommendation is a single IV dose of first-generation cephalosporin. IV vancomycin is also an effective alternative, but the potential risk of hastening resistant organisms has to be considered.

SECTION XIII

Peritoneal Dialysis: Noninfectious Complications

CHAPTER 37

Peritoneal Membrane Dysfunction: Inadequate Solute Removal, Ultrafiltration Failure, and Encapsulating Peritoneal Sclerosis

Mark Lambie, MD, PhD • Simon J. Davies, MD

Solute Removal

Physiology of Solute Transport

Solute transport occurs between peritoneal capillaries and intraperitoneal dialysate. The barrier between blood and dialysate is therefore composed of the following parts of the peritoneal membrane: capillary endothelium, loose connective tissue, submesothelial compact zone, basement membrane, and mesothelium. The main barrier to peritoneal transport, according to animal model work, seems to be the endothelium. Several models describe peritoneal membrane function, the first of which, and most commonly used, is the three-pore model.

Described in 1990, this model predicted that peritoneal transport through the peritoneal capillaries occurs through large, small, and ultra-small pores (Fig. 37.1). The large pores are relatively rare and are large enough to let large proteins through by solute drag, with transport dominated by hydrostatic pressure gradients driving convective flow of water. Small pores, the anatomic equivalent of which are uncertain but thought to be interendothelial clefts, are numerous, and ultrafiltration (UF) across them is dictated by both osmotic and hydrostatic pressures. Ultra-small pores are water-specific channels, confirmed to be aquaporins by knock-out models, and UF across them is dictated by osmotic pressure only.

There are a variety of methods for measuring membrane function, with the most widely used being the peritoneal equilibration test (PET) (Fig. 37.2), but frequently used in a modified form, with alternatives including the personal dialysis (PD) capacity test, the standard peritoneal permeability analysis, and the double mini-PET. For a summary of these tests, see Table 37.1. In essence, they are based on timed measures of the level of UF for a given concentration of glucose and of the diffusion of small water-soluble solutes into dialysate. Creatinine is usually chosen to measure differences in solute transport because it is larger than urea and diffuses more slowly, but urea tends to reach equilibrium quickly in all patients.

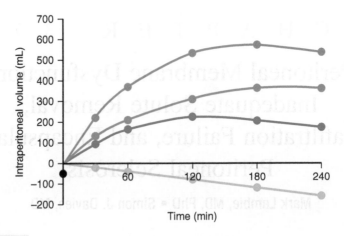

Figure 37.1

The main pathways of fluid transport across the peritoneal membrane as described by the three-pore model in response to a hypertonic (4.25%) glucose exchange. The net ultrafiltration (UF; *top*) is mostly made up of two components, the ultra-small pore aquaporin pathway *(second from top)* and the small pore pathway *(third from top)*. A small amount of fluid (too small to show here) leaks via a third large pore pathway. Throughout the exchange, there is fluid reabsorbed *(bottom)*, either directly or indirectly via lymphatics. Net UF peaks at around 180 minutes, the point when glucose absorption results in loss of the osmotic gradient, causing fluid to be reabsorbed via the small pore pathway because of Starling forces (hydrostatic and oncotic pressure gradients). Fast transporters have an earlier and lower peak in the net UF and more rapid small pore pathway reabsorption, which explains their worse fluid removal. UF failure is defined as less than 400 mL net fluid removal at 4 hours.

Measurement of Dialysis Adequacy

Measures of solute removal have primarily focused on small water-soluble molecule clearance, assessed for urea by Kt/V and for creatinine by clearance (or combined urea–creatinine clearance for residual renal function). Because peritoneal dialysis (PD) is a steady state, the calculations are simple but not comparable with hemodialysis (HD). For Kt/V, this equates to total weekly urea removed/plasma urea concentration corrected for the volume of distribution (e.g., using the Watson estimation of volume). For creatinine clearance the calculation is total weekly creatinine removed/plasma creatinine concentration corrected to a body surface area of $1.73m^2$ (e.g., using the DuBois formula). Although it is now clear that peritoneal and renal clearances are not equivalent, for simplicity, targets are often set for a combined clearance.

There are only two randomized controlled trials of adequacy. Of 965 patients in the Adequacy of PD in Mexico (ADEMEX) study, the intervention group received a peritoneal creatinine clearance of more than 60 L/wk per 1.73 m², and the control group received four daily 2-L exchanges, providing an average of 46 L/wk per 1.73 m². Over a follow-up of 2 years, there was no difference in outcomes. In the Hong Kong study, 320 patients received a total Kt/V of 1.5 to 1.7, 1.7 to 2.0, or

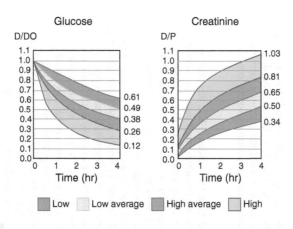

Figure 37.2

D/DO, Ratio of dialysate glucose after time of dwell to initial dialysate glucose. Four categories of the rate of peritoneal transport as originally described for the peritoneal equilibration test, ranging from low (slow) to high (fast) rates according to glucose disappearance *(left panel)* or the dialysate/plasma (D/P) creatinine ratio at 4 hours *(right panel)*. The categories of transport described here will differ among centers because the methods of measuring plasma and dialysate creatinine or glucose are affected by local factors. When monitoring longitudinal change, it should be remembered that the solute transport rate is a continuous, not categorical, measurement.

greater than 2.0. The 1.5 to 1.7 group had a higher dropout rate and worse anemia, but there was no difference in outcomes between the groups otherwise.

The interpretation of creatinine clearances and Kt/V is not identical, although there is no evidence to support use of one over the other. Peritoneal solute transport rates affect larger molecules more than smaller ones such that fast transporters achieve higher creatinine clearances without differences in Kt/V. There are also caveats for patients at extremes of body size in whom the estimates of total body water, and to a lesser extent, body surface area may be inaccurate. Because of this, malnourished patients may have deceptively high Kt/Vs, and conversely, obese patients may have low values.

On the basis of these trials and the caveats in interpretation, most guidelines recommend minimum targets for total Kt/V of 1.6 or 1.7 or total clearance of 50 L/wk per $1.73m^2$. Some guidelines suggest a higher clearance target for fast transporters, such as 60 L/wk per $1.73m^2$. Because the numeric targets focus exclusively on small water-soluble molecule clearance and use potentially inaccurate methods of correcting for body size or metabolic load, other markers, such as phosphate levels, acid–base balance, and symptom burden, should be used in the overall assessment of adequacy. Most guidelines recommend that changes to the dialysis regimen are only made after considering all these issues

Management of Underdialysis

The simplest solution to underdialysis is to increase the volume of dialysate used. How best to achieve this depends on the current regimen. Extra exchanges can be

Table 37.1

Summary of the Different Approaches for Testing Peritoneal Membrane Function*

	Component of Membrane Function				
Test	Solute Transport	Ultrafiltration Capacity	Sodium Sieving	Osmotic Conductance	Notes
Standard 4-hr PET	4-hr dialysate/plasma creatinine (or glucose) ratio	Net fluid removal at 4 hr (taking account of overfill)	Not assessed	Not assessed	Initially described using a midstrength (2.5%) glucose, but now hypertonic (4.25%) is recommended, and <400 mL UF capacity indicates potential membrane failure. For categories of solute transport, see Fig. 37.2.**
SPA: uses 4.25% glucose over 4 hr	As above	As above	Dialysate sodium dip at 1 hr; because of net excess water transport via the aquaporins, should be <125 mmol/L	Not assessed	Basic components as for standard PET; this also assesses fluid transport via the ultra-small pathway (sodium dip), which is likely a more sensitive measure of membrane injury by whatever mechanism. It also estimates large pore protein leak and "lymphatic" absorption as a research tool.
Double mini-PET: two back-to-back 1-hr dwells using 1.5% and 4.25% exchanges in turn	Measured from dialysate/plasma ratios for creatinine and glucose in both dwells, which should agree, providing internal quality control	Net UF measured from both dwells	As above for both dwells; there will be minimal change in dialysate sodium concentration for the 1.5% exchange (132 mmol/L)	Calculated from the difference in UF capacity between the two dwells	This test helps to discriminate among the three main causes of UF failure. Typically, a <400-mL difference in net UF between exchanges indicates a poorly functioning membrane, especially if the difference in sodium dip is also small. If these measures are preserved, then the problem is either fast solute transport or a leak causing fluid loss from the peritoneal cavity; this usually manifests as marked negative UF capacity in the 1.5% exchange but preserved osmotic conductance and sodium dip.***

*The peritoneal equilibration test (PET) and standardized permeability analysis (SPA) are useful screening tests; the double mini-PET provides more detailed information and can be reserved for more complex cases.

**For more information, see La Milia V, Limardo M, Virga G, Crepaldi M, Locatelli F. Simultaneous measurement of peritoneal glucose and free water osmotic conductances. Kidney Int. 2007;72(5):643-50.

***For more information, see Pannekeet MM, Imholz AL, Struijk DG, Koomen GC, Langedijk MJ, Schouten N, et al. The standard peritoneal permeability analysis: a tool for the assessment of peritoneal permeability characteristics in CAPD patients. Kidney Int. 1995;48(3):866-75.

UF, ultrafiltration.

added, either through switching continuous ambulatory PD to automated PD, or the long dwell can be split into two dwells (see Chapter 31).

Clearances of small molecules depend more on dialysate volume so increase with number of exchanges, but larger molecules such as phosphate or β_2-microglobulin depend on the length of contact with dialysate. Any days off or periods with no exchanges should therefore be stopped, particularly for patients with little residual renal function, even if urea or creatinine targets are met.

Caution needs to be taken with increases in dwell volume because the intraperitoneal pressure rises linearly with this. Although most case control studies have not found any evidence of dwell volume increasing the risk of leaks or hernias, this remains a concern, as does splinting of the diaphragm.

If these simple measures have been tried but a significant problem persists, then consideration should be given to switching to HD. This is not a common problem; for example, in the ANZDATA 2013 report, only 9.6% of reasons for stopping PD were caused by inadequate solute clearance.

Ultrafiltration Failure and Peritoneal Fibrosis

Clinical Significance of Ultrafiltration

Low UF rates have independently predicted mortality rates in PD patients generally, although this has been most clearly shown for anuric patients. In the European APD Outcome Study (EAPOS) study of anuric PD patients, the baseline UF volume of less than 750 mL/day independently predicted patient survival, although this was not significant when analyzed time dependently (relative risk [RR], 0.57 per L/day; P 0.088). However, the Netherlands Co-operative Study on the Adequacy of Dialysis (NECOSAD) study found the RR for time-dependent UF to be both significant and similar (RR, 0.48 per L/day; 95% confidence interval 0.23–0.97).

This evidence has driven attempts to measure fluid overload more accurately, primarily using bioimpedance. This technique provides information on the total body water, as well as the body cell mass, which in the limbs mainly reflects muscle mass, and from these two pieces of information, a measure of relative overhydration is derived. Overhydration has been associated with patient survival, both in HD and PD, but this association may be confounded by the role of inflammation, which affects both body cell mass and endothelial function. Evidence from comparative studies of HD and PD also suggest that PD patients may be more fluid loaded. Interventional studies demonstrating the true effect of clinical management based on bioimpedance measures are awaited.

A further problem with UF may affect patients through forcing a switch to HD (i.e., technique failure caused by UF failure). This is usually defined clinically (i.e., inability to maintain adequate fluid status), but the consensus membrane definition is less than 400 mL at 4 hours using a hypertonic (4.25%) glucose exchange (see Fig. 37.1). Clear data on the incidence of this as a problem are generally limited, with a notable exception being the ANZDATA report. UF failure was responsible for 6.3% of all causes of technique failure in the 2013 report, with technique failure affecting 19.6% of all PD patients in that year. UF failure appears to be time dependent, with data from the NECOSAD study finding rates of underdialysis or UF failure (which are likely predominantly UF failure) vary with the duration of PD, from 5 per 1000 patient years between 0 and 3 months of PD to 25 per 1000 patient years between 2 and 3 years of PD.

Aside from effects on mortality and technique failure, the other significant impact of UF failure is on the risk of encapsulating peritoneal sclerosis, discussed later.

Principles of Ultrafiltration

Convection across capillaries is governed by the following equation, devised by Ernest Starling in 1896:

$$J_v = K_f([P_c - P_i] - \sigma[\pi_c - \pi_i])$$

where J_v is the net fluid flux across the capillary, K_f is a proportionality constant (a function of the liquid permeability of the membrane and its area), P is the hydrostatic pressure and π is the capillary and colloid osmotic pressure in capillary or interstitium, and σ is the reflection coefficient (i.e., proportion of the osmolyte reflected back from membrane rather than passing through the pores). UF in PD is therefore driven by a crystalloid or colloid osmotic pressure exerted by solutes in the dialysate (glucose, amino acids, or icodextrin).

Causes of Ultrafiltration Failure

Impaired Ultrafiltration Caused by Fast (High) Solute Transport

Solute transport is a key determinant of UF because faster solute transport leads to increased absorption of either glucose or amino acids and faster loss of the osmotic pressure (see Fig. 37.1). After the dialytic osmotic pressure has disappeared, not only is there no further UF, but fluid reabsorption occurs through the small pores driven by intravascular oncotic pressure. Solute transport is recognized to increase with time on PD, likely mainly driven by peritoneal inflammation with subsequent angiogenesis creating more peritoneal capillaries. Drivers of this change may include the level of glucose exposure, solution type, diabetes, and catheter exposure. Other associations of a faster solute transport include male gender (likely because of an association with body size), plasma albumin levels (faster solute transport correlates with increased protein losses in dialysate, although inflammation may also be a confounder in this relationship), and the residual urine volume (the mechanism for which is unclear but may represent an effect of intravascular filling), although it seems unlikely that these are the drivers of the long-term changes.

Because of this rise in solute transport, UF failure commonly occurs after several years on PD because of an increase in solute transport, but there are now two important strategies to manage this. First, because of its large size, icodextrin does not get absorbed to the same extent as glucose, so it provides ongoing UF for 8 to 12 hours or even more. At least four randomized trials have examined the UF effects of icodextrin, and a meta-analysis of these found a mean difference of 448 mL/day; this is particularly true in patients with fast solute transport.

Second, automated PD uses short dwells such that the osmotic gradient cannot dissipate in time to cause a problem and can prevent UF problems. This is thought to be the reason why the use of APD appears to have a survival benefit in faster transporters. The combination of icodextrin and APD usage generally solves the problem of low UF in fast transporters.

Alongside the use of these two strategies, the entire prescription should be reviewed and dwells adjusted to avoid fluid reabsorption. Excess time spent draining fluid can be minimized with tidal APD. The urine volume should be maximized by diuretics, such as 250 mg of furosemide daily, and salt intake and fluid restriction should be reviewed.

Impaired Ultrafiltration Caused by Reduced Membrane Efficiency and Fibrosis

The increase in vascularity that drives faster solute transport is not the only pathologic change that occurs in the peritoneal membrane with time on PD. There is also a large increase in the submesothelial compact zone caused by fibrosis. A tight fibrotic mesh is thought to act as a resistance to the convective flow of water such that for a given osmotic gradient, less UF is achieved. This result has been predicted through modeling, the physiologic effect has been demonstrated, and now a study has demonstrated a correlation between more fibrosis (both depth and density) and less UF.

This is usually assessed through the osmotic conductance to glucose, literally a reduced amount of UF for a given osmotic gradient (K_f in Starling's equation), measurable through investigations such as the double mini-PET, with lower values indicating more fibrosis and worse UF. However, another surrogate for a fibrotic membrane has been described recently—sodium sieving. Sodium sieving is a phenomenon whereby the water-selective ultra-small pores (i.e., aquaporins) allow the transfer of pure water without sodium across the capillary membrane driven by a crystalloid osmotic pressure. Through dilution of any solutes within the dialysate, this causes a measurable drop in dialysate sodium concentration during the first hour or two of a dwell; then as the osmotic driving force dissipates, sodium diffusion will increase the dialysate sodium back toward the plasma value. The extent of sodium dipping can be used to calculate ultra-small pore water transport, but accumulating evidence suggests that the sodium dip is affected by fibrosis, too.

The sodium dip, or the free water transport calculated from it, often decreases with time on PD, but it particularly appears to decrease in patients developing UF failure due to fibrosis. One possible explanation for the association between changes in sodium sieving and osmotic conductance or fibrosis is a selective decrease in aquaporins with increased fibrosis or inflammation. However, a recent study found that aquaporin expression was maintained in the presence of severe fibrosis and UF failure. It is possible that fibrosis impedes the penetration of glucose into the interstitium, leaving a lower glucose concentration around the capillary, as suggested by the distributed model, although the reduction in sodium dipping is also predicted by the fiber matrix or three-pore model. The true explanation of this phenomenon remains unclear.

Because of the difficulty in measuring the osmotic conductance to glucose, there have been no large studies capable of defining predictors of a deteriorating membrane. The determinants are likely to be similar to those affecting solute transport, with increasing glucose concentrations as well as dialysate exposure playing a significant role. Whether biocompatible solutions mitigate membrane fibrosis is not clear from clinical studies yet, although animal studies suggest they should. In Japan, a national policy of using biocompatible solutions has been associated with a reduction in encapsulating peritoneal sclerosis (EPS), but this was confounded by other changes. Recurrent and severe peritonitis has been shown to have long-term effects on membrane function, although the effect of single episodes was uncertain.

The management of this form of UF failure is more problematic because there is no simple solution to the problem. Because a decreased osmotic conductance tends to occur with faster solute transport, the same general strategies described should be used to mitigate the impact of solute transport, but these will not overcome a low osmotic conductance to glucose. An increasing need for stronger concentrations of glucose in the dialysate may be noticed as a marker for this. When fluid overload is developing or the need for high concentrations of glucose is problematic, consideration must be given to switching to HD. Furthermore, as discussed later, increased fibrosis predisposes to encapsulating peritoneal sclerosis.

Other Factors Determining Ultrafiltration

Because UF is driven by the balance of hydrostatic and osmotic pressures, other factors might have a role in determining UF, although clinical evidence to support this is not strong. During dialysis with glucose-based solutions, the intraperitoneal pressure may drive greater lymphatic absorption; this is discussed in Chapter 33.

It is now clear that there is variability in UF achieved with icodextrin, with some of this variability correlating with dwell length, although the reasons for this are not yet well understood. From theoretical modeling, the oncotic gradient is of greater importance for icodextrin than glucose dwells, so UF with icodextrin could be preferentially affected by plasma albumin or by dilution from the residual volume. Because of the latter possibility, in cases of poor UF with icodextrin, it is reasonable to check the drainage of the dwell immediately preceding the icodextrin fill.

Encapsulating Peritoneal Sclerosis

Encapsulating peritoneal sclerosis is an uncommon but severe disease with significant mortality and morbidity. In PD patients, it was initially recognized in Japan and Europe, but it is now widely recognized as occurring elsewhere. EPS is defined by the combination of symptoms of gastrointestinal (GI) function, especially obstructive, with radiologic or surgical evidence of encapsulation in the absence of another cause for the symptoms. There is a clear association with PD, although it is not specific to this, with reported associations including postsurgical cirrhosis, with ascites, generalized peritonitis, and beta-blocker treatment. Initial reports used terms such as *sclerosing peritonitis, calcific peritonitis, sclerotic obstructive peritonitis,* and *abdominal cocoon,* but there is now consensus on *encapsulating peritoneal sclerosis.*

Pathologic Features

The hallmark of this condition is an exuberant proliferation of the peritoneum, with subsequent cocooning of the GI tract, and the symptomatology is of gastrointestinal dysfunction. Macroscopic appearances can vary, with three different types suggested varying from a sticky fibrinous coating of the membrane to a sclerotic cocoon, and the extent can also vary, from a global problem to a very focal issue. The biggest difficulty in identifying histologic changes specific for EPS is differentiating it from simple peritoneal sclerosis associated with UF failure. Changes in EPS include a relative increase in fibroblast-like cells, mesothelial denudation, calcification, vasculopathy, and acute and chronic inflammatory changes. Podoplanin, a cell surface marker usually found on mesothelial and lymphatic endothelial cells, has been found more specifically in EPS on a diffuse infiltration of cells with fibroblastic appearance. Of note, the changes of EPS and simple peritoneal sclerosis may differ between the visceral and parietal peritoneum, with greater parietal fibrosis in simple sclerosis and vice versa for EPS.

Clinical Features

Symptoms are mainly those of GI dysfunction but can vary from complete obstruction to a milder phenotype, with some nausea and vomiting, and these symptoms usually cause some degree of malnutrition. Some reports have identified cases with radiologic or macroscopic evidence of EPS but with no symptoms, although this highlights the variation in how the diagnostic criteria have been applied.

There is inconsistency among different authors over the role of peritonitis in EPS: Some authors include persistent peritonitis as a feature, others have explicitly excluded this from groups considered to have EPS, and most authors do not comment. This may be partly because of the complexity of the potential relationships between peritonitis and EPS. There is often evidence of increased systemic inflammation during EPS, which can compound the severe malnutrition that patients often develop.

Epidemiology of Encapsulating Peritoneal Sclerosis

The prevalence of EPS varies in reports, from 0.4% in Australia and New Zealand up to 2.5% in Japan, although diagnostic variability, clinical awareness, and differences in data collection at least partly explain this variability. The risk of EPS rises with time on PD, with rates after 5 years of PD rising to 2.1% in Japan, 6.4% in Australia, and up to 8.1% in Scotland, so the differences among countries also depends on rates of transplantation, death, and technique failure within those countries.

This finding suggests that prolonged PD predisposes to EPS by driving progressive membrane damage. This can only be examined by using functional surrogates for membrane damage. Solute transport, a surrogate for vascularity, is known to rise with time on PD and is faster in patients with EPS, who have generally been on PD longer. Three studies have used UF data to infer changes in osmotic conductance to glucose and have consistently shown that, for a given time on PD, patients with subsequent EPS have a worse osmotic conductance and therefore likely increased fibrosis. As discussed earlier, sodium sieving may be a clinical measure of fibrosis that is easier to measure.

The other main risk factor for EPS appears to be stopping PD, although again reported rates vary widely, from 74% to 21% of cases diagnosed after stopping PD, with the low rates possibly due to ascertainment bias. In the largest case series, the median time to diagnosis after stopping PD was 5.5 months, and most cases were within 6 months with some exceptions diagnosed up to 3 years after stopping PD. The most likely pathophysiologic explanation for this slightly counterintuitive finding is an accumulation of profibrotic or inflammatory cytokines after the lavage effect of PD has stopped.

Some reports have suggested that transplantation may be a distinct form of EPS, but this has been limited to reports from one country; other reports have not shown a transplant to be a particular risk, and a comparison of cases after HD and after transplant has found no apparent differences in clinical or pathologic features.

Peritonitis has often been cited as a risk factor for EPS, although almost all recent studies have found no evidence for this. The most likely reason for the surprising lack of association is the association between peritonitis and technique failure. Recurrent peritonitis is therefore likely to prevent prolonged periods of time on PD and therefore minimize the strongest risk factor for EPS even though it may damage the membrane.

There are other possible roles that peritonitis could play in precipitating EPS, but there is little evidence for or against them (e.g., peritonitis could act as an acute precipitant on an already chronically damaged membrane, or peritonitis necessitating catheter removal stops PD and thereby precipitates EPS). Other risk factors have been identified that are no longer available or used, notably the beta-blocker practolol and the use of chlorhexidine to sterilize tubing connections.

Treatment of Encapsulating Peritoneal Sclerosis

Management principles of EPS consist of supportive treatment, medication, and surgical interventions. Supportive therapy consists primarily of total parenteral nutrition, a necessity for a large number of patients, particularly when seeking to optimize patients before surgical therapy. Stopping PD is also necessary because PD exposure is the primary driver of the condition, but because stopping PD appears to act as a precipitant for EPS, it could theoretically make diagnosed EPS worse in the short term.

The medications that have been tried most commonly are steroids and tamoxifen, although the evidence for either is weak. Tamoxifen, a selective estrogen receptor modulator, is known to affect transforming growth factor-β and has been used in fibrotic conditions such as retroperitoneal fibrosis and Riedel thyroiditis. The best evidence for its use in EPS comes from a Dutch retrospective nonrandomized case series with limited information on confounders reporting an advantage, although a series from London found no benefit.

Steroids have been associated with marked clinical improvements in some case reports and case series, although indication bias and reporting bias are likely to affect both of these. The most obvious presentation in which steroids might be beneficial is a significantly systemically inflamed patient, a common feature of this condition.

Surgery usually involves peritonectomy and enterolysis and is generally considered a mainstay of therapy, certainly for the more severe cases. In Japan some degree of improvement has been reported in 81 of 86 cases undergoing surgery. Unfortunately, recurrence postsurgery necessitating further surgery is also common with one report finding 11 of 47 patients followed for 2 years afterward developing a problem. With a large inflamed area, patients are often very unwell postoperatively, frequently requiring intensive care. Because of difficulties like this and the rarity of the condition, treatment is usually limited to a few specialist centers.

CHAPTER 38

Abdominal Catastrophes, Peritoneal Eosinophilia, and Other Unusual Events in Peritoneal Dialysis

Rajnish Mehrotra, MD, MS • Pranay Kathuria, MD

Repeated instillation and drainage of dialysate during the course of peritoneal dialysis (PD) is a unique clinical situation, which infrequently draws attention to primary intraabdominal events. These events are often unrelated to the PD treatment itself but are brought to attention because of an abnormal appearance of drained dialysate, with or without abdominal pain. They are important for two reasons. First, some conditions such as visceral perforation present with peritonitis. Thus, unless a nephrologist considers the diagnosis of a primary intraabdominal event, definitive intervention may be delayed. Second, some conditions such as hemoperitoneum are alarming but often require only reassurance of the patient. This chapter discusses several such primary intraabdominal events; complications of PD such as encapsulating peritoneal sclerosis are discussed in other chapters.

Abdominal Catastrophe

In patients undergoing PD, the term *abdominal catastrophe* refers to the signs and symptoms associated with either severe visceral inflammation or perforation. This disorder is also called *secondary peritonitis, intrinsic peritonitis*, or *peritonitis due to bowel perforation*. Peritonitis secondary to visceral injury represents between 3.5% and 25% of published series of PD-associated peritonitis, with a mortality rate of approximately 50%.

Enteric peritoneal contamination may occur as a result of perforated diverticulitis, appendicitis, incarcerated hernia, ischemic colitis or nonocclusive mesenteric ischemia, gangrenous cholecystitis, or perforated gastric or duodenal ulcer. It has been suggested that patients undergoing PD present with abdominal catastrophes more frequently than those undergoing hemodialysis (HD) or in the general population. However, these data are based on small, single-center studies, and no definitive conclusions can be made in this regard. Rarely, erosion of the Tenckhoff catheter into the ileum or colon may be the primary event leading to visceral perforation; this often is limited to patients with a dormant, indwelling access not being used for PD.

Notwithstanding the early reports, patients with autosomal dominant polycystic kidney disease do not appear to be at a higher risk for either diverticular disease or enteric peritonitis. Furthermore, the relationship of the presence of colonic diverticula to the occurrence of enteric peritonitis or abdominal catastrophe remains unclear. It appears that a large number (≥10) or size (≥10 mm) of diverticuli or a nonsigmoid location may predispose patients to a higher incidence of enteric peritonitis. Yet most patients with diverticular disease never develop enteric peritonitis or visceral perforation; thus, the presence of diverticulosis should not be considered as a contraindication to PD.

The initial clinical presentation of peritonitis associated with abdominal catastrophes is indistinguishable from PD-associated peritonitis from other causes. An occasional patient will present with abdominal pain with clear dialysate effluent or with septic shock. The presence of fecal or biliary material in the effluent, although highly suggestive, is rarely observed. The peritoneal white blood cell (WBC) count is usually higher than with other causes of peritonitis; however, the data are not sufficiently clear to recommend a reliable cut-off value for the peritoneal cell count. Pneumoperitoneum can be present in patients undergoing PD (see later discussion) and does not help in diagnosing visceral perforation. Other imaging studies, such as computed tomography (CT), are often unrevealing as well.

There is an increasing body of data that allows one to challenge the conventional wisdom associating polymicrobial peritonitis with abdominal catastrophes. Fewer than 20% of patients with abdominal catastrophes have polymicrobial peritonitis; cultures of peritoneal effluents usually demonstrate a single gram-negative or rarely, an anaerobic organism. Conversely, fewer than 10% of patients with polymicrobial peritonitis have an underlying surgical cause (Table 38.1); thus, routine use of laparotomy in patients with more than one organism on peritoneal fluid culture is probably inappropriate. The concentration of amylase in the peritoneal effluent appears to be promising—levels that exceed 500 IU/L seem to be highly suggestive of visceral perforation.

Given the above, the diagnosis of abdominal catastrophes in patients undergoing PD is often delayed and this, in turn, leads to a greater probability of an adverse outcome. Thus, a high index of clinical suspicion is needed to diagnose episodes of peritonitis associated with abdominal catastrophes and should be considered in patients with enteric peritonitis who respond inadequately or incompletely to conventional therapy. Early evaluation by a surgeon is recommended in patients suspected of having an abdominal catastrophe. Large perforations, such as those associated with gastric or duodenal ulcers or ischemic colitis, are often fatal, but

---

Table 38.1

Relationship of Polymicrobial Peritonitis and Surgical Causes: Fact or Fiction?

	Episodes of Polymicrobial Peritonitis (*n*)	Catheter Removal (*n*)	Death (*n*)	Surgical Causes (*n*)
Pittsburgh	39	17	1	3
New Haven	80	12	4	6
Chicago	43	14	1	3
Hong Kong	140	45	9	4
Total	302	88 (29%)	15 (5%)	16 (5%)

Adapted from Szeto CC, Chow KM, Wong TYH, et al. Conservative management of polymicrobial peritonitis complicating peritoneal dialysis—a series of 140 consecutive cases. *Am J Med* 2002;113:728-733.

smaller, such as those associated with appendicitis or diverticulitis have a somewhat better prognosis.

Pneumoperitoneum

In the general population, the presence of air under the diaphragm is considered to be diagnostic of visceral perforation and a trigger for surgical intervention. The PD catheter provides an additional port of air entry into the peritoneal cavity, and patients undergoing PD may have demonstrable air under the diaphragm on plain radiography or CT.

Pneumoperitoneum is particularly common after the placement of a PD catheter or manipulation or intervention involving the peritoneal access or after gastrointestinal (GI) endoscopic procedures. Pneumoperitoneum has been reported to occur in settings such as the use of a cycler or if the patient eliminates the step of flushing the line before filling the peritoneal cavity.

Inadvertent introduction of air into the peritoneal cavity may result in patients' presenting with sharp abdominal pain that radiates to the shoulder. However, most cases are diagnosed incidentally, and in an asymptomatic patient with an unremarkable abdominal examination, pneumoperitoneum is generally of little consequence. In the setting of peritonitis, the presence of pneumoperitoneum has a somewhat higher probability of being associated with underlying visceral perforation and requires aggressive radiologic workup. Contrary to earlier reports, the size of pneumoperitoneum has little predictive value for the diagnosis of visceral perforation. Furthermore, diagnostic laparotomy should still be used only when the clinical suspicion is high and other corroborative evidence (e.g., high peritoneal effluent amylase levels or other suggestive radiologic studies) presents a strong possibility for visceral perforation.

Iatrogenic Complications of Gastrointestinal or Gynecologic Procedures

There have been several case reports that have documented episodes of peritonitis after sigmoidoscopy or colonoscopy (particularly if accompanied with polypectomy or argon photocoagulation), gastroscopy (particularly if it involves sclerotherapy or heat coagulation), hysteroscopy, endometrial biopsy, or the placement of intrauterine devices. The nature of published reports does not allow one to estimate the incidence of peritonitis after endoscopic procedures or interventions. Furthermore, it is unlikely that a randomized controlled trial will be conducted to test the benefit of routine antibiotic prophylaxis when patients treated with PD undergo GI or gynecologic procedures. In light of these considerations, it is recommended that prophylactic antibiotics that provide coverage against enteric gram-negative and anaerobic bacteria be routinely administered before such procedures in patients treated with PD. It is also recommended that patients drain dialysate from their abdomens before such procedures.

Percutaneous endoscopic gastrostomy (PEG) tubes are used to provide enteral nutrition. The presence of a well-healed PEG tube is not a contraindication to treat a patient with end-stage renal disease (ESRD) with PD. However, the PEG tube and the PD catheter should be clearly marked because inadvertent administration of enteral nutrition feeds into the peritoneal cavity can lead to severe, and often fatal, chemical peritonitis. On the other hand, placement of a new PEG tube in a patient undergoing PD carries a high risk of infection, particularly fungal peritonitis. Thus, if a patient requires the placement of a PEG tube, PD should be interrupted for 2 to 6 weeks, and the patient should undergo temporary HD, if needed.

Pancreatitis

Several single-center studies have suggested that the incidence of pancreatitis may be up to threefold higher in patients undergoing PD compared with patients undergoing maintenance HD. The pathophysiologic basis for the increased incidence is unclear, but systemic abnormalities such as hypertriglyceridemia or hypercalcemia or local events such as irritation of the pancreas from the retroperitoneal diffusion of peritoneal dialysate have been proposed as possible culprits.

The clinical presentation of acute pancreatitis in patients undergoing PD is often the same as that observed among patients without ESRD. The peritoneal dialysate is often clear, but it may demonstrate increased total WBC count with or without positive effluent cultures. Hemoperitoneum or chyloperitoneum may be seen occasionally; rarely, the dialysate may be brownish-black because of the presence of methemalbumin in patients with hemorrhagic pancreatitis. Although serum amylase levels may be helpful, dialysate amylase (>100 IU/L) provides greater diagnostic information. However, serum and dialysate amylase are up to sixfold lower among PD patients treated with icodextrin-based dialysate; serum and dialysate lipase levels are more reliable under these circumstances. If radiologic testing is pursued to either diagnose pancreatitis or any of the complications, it is prudent to completely drain all the intraperitoneal dialysate before imaging is performed to provide a better and more complete visualization of the pancreas.

The data on the prognosis of PD patients with pancreatitis are inconsistent, and some centers have reported a higher morbidity and mortality compared with patients without ESRD. Thus, early diagnosis and careful management are critical to ensure optimal outcomes.

Peritoneal Eosinophilia

Among the differential diagnosis of cloudy effluent in patients on PD is peritoneal eosinophilia, a condition with eosinophils constituting greater than 10% of the total peritoneal WBC count and the eosinophil count exceeding 100 cells/mL^3 of peritoneal effluent.

Peritoneal eosinophilia can be seen in the presence of PD-associated peritonitis; however, many cases occur in the absence of peritonitis. In the past, the leading cause was hypersensitivity to the PD catheter material, possibly the plasticizers or sterilants. Introduction of air or blood into the peritoneum has also been associated with peritoneal fluid eosinophilia. A rare cause is encapsulating peritoneal sclerosis.

Most episodes of peritoneal eosinophilia develop in the first 3 months after initiating PD with an occasional patient presenting years after starting the therapy. Prior reports put the incidence between 5% to 61%, but the incidence has significantly decreased in recent years because of improvement in the quality of materials used to make PD catheters. Patients typically present with cloudy effluent, and some may have abdominal pain or fever. An elevated blood eosinophil count and elevated IgE levels are found in fewer than half the patients. While awaiting cell counts and cultures, it is common to initiate antimicrobial therapy for presumed bacterial peritonitis. With a confirmed diagnosis of noninfective peritoneal eosinophilia, it is appropriate to follow a course of watchful expectancy because most cases resolve spontaneously. Steroids (intraperitoneal or orally) may be used for patients with a protracted course or frequent recurrences. Steroids may also be used in patients with severe abdominal pain or very turbid fluid to maintain catheter patency. Other successful treatment options reported in the literature include antihistamines, ketotifen (a mast cell stabilizer), and glycyrrhizin (an extract of licorice with antiinflammatory properties).

Hepatic Subcapsular Steatosis

Subcapsular steatosis or fat accumulation in the liver appears to occur exclusively among patients with diabetes undergoing PD who are receiving intraperitoneal insulin. This condition is clinically asymptomatic, is not associated with any liver function test abnormalities, and appears to be without clinical consequence. However, the recognition of this entity by a nephrologist is important to avoid misinterpreting hepatic subcapsular steatosis as more serious lesions such as metastatic malignancy.

Increasing body weight, higher intraperitoneal insulin dose or serum triglycerides, and higher peritoneal transport rate appear to increase the likelihood for the development of hepatic subcapsular steatosis. Recent studies also suggest that the intraperitoneal administration of insulin rather than the glucose load leads to the steatosis. It has been proposed that insulin gets absorbed from the liver surface into the subcapsular hepatocytes, where it suppresses the oxidation of fatty acids; this leads to the esterification of the fatty acids to form triglycerides, which accumulate and result in hepatic subcapsular steatosis.

On ultrasonography, the steatosis appears as a bright echogenic rim or discrete, echogenic, subcapsular nodules, best seen in the subdiaphragmatic segments of the liver. On CT, it is seen as discrete, nodular, low-attenuation subcapsular nodular or thin rindlike lesions. On magnetic resonance imaging (MRI), hepatic subcapsular steatosis is identified as hyperintense lesions and chemical shift imaging demonstrates the presence of fat in the liver. Serial imaging has shown the lesions to be reversible upon discontinuation of intraperitoneal insulin. However, it may take several months for complete resolution.

Hemoperitoneum

Hemoperitoneum is a common complication associated with PD. The presence of even minimal amounts of blood can color the peritoneal fluid pink or red. Performance of the dialysis procedure by PD patients often brings cases to light, which would have been otherwise clinically silent.

The various causes of hemoperitoneum are categorized in Table 38.2. Hemoperitoneum is more common among premenopausal women with causes related to gynecologic conditions such as retrograde menstruation, ovulation, cyst rupture, and endometriosis. Hemoperitoneum with retrograde menstruation or endometriosis usually presents before the onset of vaginal bleeding. These patients are most likely to have recurrent hemoperitoneum. In a number of patients, no definite etiology can be determined; it has been suggested that hemoperitoneum may have been a result

Table 38.2

Causes of Hemoperitoneum

Gynecologic Disorders
Ovulation (midcycle)
Retrograde menstruation (with periods)
Ruptured ovarian cyst
Endometriosis (with periods)
Ectopic pregnancy

Associated With Acute Abdomen
Acute hemorrhagic pancreatitis
Acute cholecystitis
Splenic rupture or infarction
Peritonitis

Peritoneal Membrane Abnormalities
Encapsulating peritoneal sclerosis
Peritoneal carcinomatosis
Peritoneal calcification
Radiation injury

Miscellaneous
Trauma
Exercise
Postcolonoscopy
Bleeding disorders
Rupture of hepatic or renal cysts
Kidney or liver tumors
Retroperitoneal hematoma
IgA nephropathy
Idiopathic

of minor tears of the omental vessels. Occasionally, the peritoneal catheter has been reported to erode into the major mesenteric vessels, leading to hemoperitoneum.

Most cases of hemoperitoneum are benign. Uncommonly, hemoperitoneum is a sign of underlying intraperitoneal pathology; in these patients, bleeding often persists beyond 36 hours. Major hemorrhage is uncommon, and it is highly unusual for patients to require blood transfusions or surgical intervention. An initial assessment includes a thorough history, including details of menstruation, recent trauma, and use of anticoagulant or antiplatelet drugs. The patient should undergo assessment of the hemodynamic status and be examined for signs of an abdominal catastrophe. Subsequent evaluation is often dictated by this initial assessment.

The management of hemoperitoneum is often expectant and, if necessary, directed at the primary cause. To prevent occlusion of the PD catheter, the addition of 500 to 1000 units of heparin to each bag of dialysate is often recommended. Instillation of unwarmed dialysate, at room temperature, has also been proposed to induce vasoconstriction of the peritoneal circulation by the cooler dialysate to slow the bleeding. However, care should be exercised to avoid hypothermia during the winter months in cold locales. Desmopressin and unconjugated estrogens can ameliorate uremic bleeding.

Chyloperitoneum

Chyloperitoneum results from the leakage of chyle into the peritoneal cavity. Patients present with turbid or typical milky dialysate. The diagnosis is confirmed if chylomicrons are detected or dialysate triglyceride levels are higher than the plasma level. Patients undergoing PD can lose substantial amounts of protein and lymphocytes with repeated exchanges leading to protein-energy wasting and immunosuppression. Excessive fluid loss causing dehydration can also be an issue.

The underlying causes are related to either interruption or obstruction of the lymphatic system. Malignancies, especially lymphomas, are reported as the most common cause of chyloperitoneum. Trauma, either at the time of insertion of the peritoneal catheter, or from repeated catheter movement, acute and chronic pancreatitis, cirrhosis, amyloidosis, superior vena cava syndrome, and tuberculous peritonitis are other causes of chyloperitoneum. Elevations of peritoneal triglycerides have also been associated with the use of dihydropyridine calcium channel blockers.

Evaluation of patients should include a detailed history and physical examination along with CT scans, MRI, or lymphoscintigraphy, as indicated. Strategies on the treatment of chylous ascites focus on decreasing production of chyle and treatment of the underlying cause. Long-chain fatty acids are absorbed from the bowel directly into the lymphatic system and contribute to chyle flow, and medium-chain triglycerides are absorbed directly into the bloodstream and decrease chyle flow. Thus, high-protein, low-fat diets containing medium-chain triglycerides can be used and over several months have been shown to be effective. Bowel rest with total parenteral nutrition is an alternative. Octreotide, a somatostatin analog, has been reported to be effective in anecdotal reports.

C H A P T E R   3 9

Metabolic Effects of Peritoneal Dialysis

Rajnish Mehrotra, MD

The removal of solute and water for the management of end-stage renal disease (ESRD) with peritoneal dialysis (PD) is achieved by exposing the naturally occurring peritoneal lining of the abdomen to 6 to 20 L of dialysate every day. It is widely believed that the exposure of the peritoneum to large volumes of dialysate has significant and wide-ranging deleterious systemic effects. This chapter reviews the evidence for and the clinical implications for the purported systemic metabolic effects of PD.

Weight Gain

Every patient treated with PD either uses glucose-based solutions exclusively or for most of the treatment through the day, with the remaining time with either icodextrin- or amino acid–based solutions. Treatment with glucose- or icodextrin-based solutions is associated with an obligatory absorption of 50 to 150 g of carbohydrates daily. As a result, it is widely believed that patients treated with PD are significantly more likely to gain weight than those undergoing hemodialysis (HD). This is an important consideration in the selection of dialysis modality for some patients either because of effects on body image or future eligibility for transplantation.

Caution must be exercised in interpreting data on changes in weight over time because they may result from alterations in volume status, fat mass, or fat-free edema-free body mass. Initiation of dialysis is associated with two competing events—improvement in volume status with fluid removal with dialysis as well as improvement in appetite from the amelioration of anorexia, a cardinal manifestation of the uremic state. This results in a net decrease in weight in the first few months of initiation of dialysis followed by weight gain in most patients irrespective of dialysis modality. Three large multicenter studies have compared the magnitude of the subsequent weight gain and demonstrated either no significant difference in the trajectory of change in weight over time for patients treated with HD or PD or a higher probability of significant weight gain for patients treated with HD. Hence, the notion that patients are more likely to gain significant weight with PD is not supported by the available evidence. Limited evidence suggests that the magnitude of weight gain with PD may at least in part be determined genetically. Small single-center studies also seem to indicate that patients treated with PD may be more likely to gain visceral fat mass than those undergoing HD. These findings need to be validated in larger studies, and their clinical implications are unclear.

The data to date seem to imply that after the first few months of treatment, patients gain weight upon initiation of dialysis irrespective of modality, and concerns about a higher probability of weight gain with PD are not supported by the available evidence. It follows then that concerns about weight gain should not figure in the selection of dialysis modality.

Metabolic Syndrome

Metabolic syndrome is defined as the presence of a cluster of risk factors that are associated with a significantly higher risk for cardiovascular disease in the general population. The definitions for metabolic syndrome from different expert groups are somewhat different but generally include measures of adiposity, dyslipidemia, hypertension, and abnormal fasting blood glucose levels. Insulin resistance is the dominant but not the only condition underlying the pathogenesis of metabolic syndrome. The different components of the metabolic syndrome are independent risk factors for the development and progression of chronic kidney disease (CKD); hence, patients with metabolic syndrome are significantly more likely to have CKD. Conversely, metabolic syndrome is highly prevalent in patients with ESRD, including among those undergoing maintenance dialysis.

Similarly, several studies have demonstrated that up to half or more of patients undergoing PD have metabolic syndrome, and at least one study has demonstrated a significant increase in the prevalence with initiation of PD therapy. The only study that made a head-to-head comparison concluded that metabolic syndrome was significantly more prevalent in patients undergoing PD compared with in-center HD. These observations have raised concerns that PD therapy itself may contribute to the development of metabolic syndrome. However, the prevalence of metabolic syndrome in patients undergoing in-center HD in the only study with head-to-head comparison was substantially lower than in other studies. Moreover, there are two challenges with the diagnosis of metabolic syndrome in patients undergoing PD. First, the intraperitoneal instillation of dialysate with PD results in an increase in waist circumference, an important component for the diagnosis of metabolic syndrome. Second, there is continuous systemic absorption of glucose from intraperitoneal dialysate, and hence, patients undergoing PD are never in a postabsorptive state. This results in overestimation of fasting glucose and lipid parameters. Finally, the results from studies examining the association of metabolic syndrome with cardiovascular events or all-cause mortality have been inconsistent. This is not surprising because the individual components of metabolic syndrome themselves do not portend a higher risk for death or cardiovascular events in patients with ESRD, including among those undergoing PD.

For these reasons, the contribution of PD to the development of metabolic syndrome and its clinical relevance for these patients is at best uncertain.

New-Onset Diabetes Mellitus in Nondiabetic Patients

It is common for patients undergoing maintenance dialysis to be diagnosed with new-onset diabetes mellitus. There are several possible reasons for the occurrence of new-onset diabetes mellitus, including an increase in insulin resistance over time with loss of residual kidney function or weight gain with amelioration of uremic anorexia. It is also possible that some patients may have had previously undiagnosed diabetes mellitus that becomes apparent with improvement in the uremic state or increase in dietary intake with initiation of dialysis. Concern has been raised that systemic glucose absorption with PD may also contribute to new-onset diabetes mellitus, but as discussed earlier, caution must be exercised in interpreting fasting blood glucose concentrations given the continuous systemic carbohydrate absorption with PD. To determine the contribution of PD therapy to the occurrence of new-onset diabetes mellitus, two studies from Taiwan have made a head-to-head comparison of the incidence of the condition in patients treated with PD and HD. Although one study demonstrated no difference by the modality, the second showed a significantly higher risk among patients undergoing in-center HD. Hence, evidence to date does not support the notion for a higher risk for new-onset diabetes mellitus in patients undergoing PD. Nevertheless, the condition is common enough that nondiabetic patients undergoing maintenance dialysis should have periodic measurement of blood glucose with further workup with measurement of fasting levels or glycosylated hemoglobin as appropriate.

Hyperglycemia in Patients With Diabetes Mellitus

In patients with diabetes mellitus, initiation of PD is associated with worsening of glycemic control both because of increased dietary intake and obligatory systemic carbohydrate absorption with the therapy. The magnitude of increase in blood glucose levels is associated with the concentration of glucose in the dialysate. Given these observations, it is imperative patients with diabetes mellitus monitor home blood glucose levels closely in the first few months of initiation of PD. Furthermore, most patients with diabetes treated with PD require an escalation of glucose-lowering therapy or need to initiate treatment for diabetes mellitus in patients who had previously been diet controlled.

It is important to take into account the PD prescription when adjusting glucose-lowering therapy. As discussed earlier, patients undergoing PD are invariably absorbing glucose through the 24-hour period, and in patients undergoing automated PD, a substantial proportion of this absorption occurs overnight when most other patients are in the postabsorptive state. It is also important to adjust glucose-lowering therapy when patients adjust the tonicity of the dialysate. In that context, at least two multicenter clinical trials have demonstrated that glucose-sparing PD regimens that variably use icodextrin and/or amino acid solutions throughout the day are associated with an improvement in glycemic control.

The data on health benefits of improved glycemic control in patients undergoing PD, however, are substantially limited. Like in the general population, improved glycemic control should be expected to prevent or slow the progression of microvascular disease (e.g., retinopathy or neuropathy). However, there are no data to date for patients undergoing PD. Furthermore, it is not clear if improved glycemic control would reduce the progression of macrovascular disease or lower all-cause mortality. As for the general population, observational studies have demonstrated an association between measures of glycemic control (blood glucose, glycosylated hemoglobin, or glycosylated albumin) with risk for death in patients undergoing PD. In contrast, none of the clinical trials to date has been able to demonstrate reduction in risk for death with improvement in glycemic control in patients with diabetes mellitus in the 3 to 5 years span of life expectancy of patients with PD. It would then be unreasonable to expect reduction in cardiovascular risk or increased life expectancy with aggressive glycemic control in individuals with diabetes mellitus undergoing PD. Given this uncertainty and potential risks with hypoglycemia, it is currently not possible to recommend a target range for various indices for glycemic control in patients undergoing PD.

Lipid Abnormalities

It is often said that patients undergoing PD have a more atherogenic lipid profile than patients undergoing HD and by extension that the PD therapy itself contributes to the dyslipidemia. Lipid abnormalities in patients undergoing PD have been attributed to obligatory glucose absorption and peritoneal protein loss with consequent hypoalbuminemia as with patients with nephrotic syndrome. Although conceivable, there are few head-to-head comparisons of lipid profiles of patients treated with different dialysis modalities that preclude a definitive conclusion about the relative prevalence of dyslipidemia and contribution of PD to the same. Moreover, as discussed earlier, patients undergoing PD are never in the postabsorptive state, so lipid parameters in these patients cannot be considered to be "fasting" values.

Statin drug therapy remains the mainstay for the management of hyperlipidemia in patients undergoing PD and are safe and similarly effective as in the general population. Clinical trials have demonstrated that substituting glucose-based dialysate in one or more exchanges with icodextrin- and/or amino acid–based solutions are associated with a modest reduction in total or low-density cholesterol or triglycerides. However, the magnitude of reduction and the lipid parameters that improve have been inconsistent among studies. Nevertheless, adjusting the PD prescription is a reasonable approach for patients for whom drug therapy is not effective in achieving the desired goal or who develop unacceptable adverse effects of treatment.

There are limited clinical trial data on the health benefits of lipid lowering in patients undergoing PD. The Study of Heart and Renal Protection (SHARP) enrolled a large population of patients treated with PD, and many more patients initiated treatment with PD during the course of the trial. The clinical trial demonstrated that treatment with simvastatin-ezetimibe was associated with a significant reduction in risk for cardiovascular events, and there was no effect modification with dialysis status. Put differently, the same nature and magnitude of benefit could be expected for patients undergoing maintenance dialysis as observed in the study at large. Yet there was no significant reduction in all-cause or cardiovascular mortality with such treatment. Hence, the magnitude of health benefit with lipid lowering in patients with kidney disease, including those undergoing PD, is significantly lower than in the general population.

Hypokalemia

Unlike virtually any other population of patients with kidney disease, hypokalemia is common in patients undergoing PD. There are likely several factors contributing to the high prevalence of hypokalemia, including dialysate potassium loss particularly in the face of low intake, transcellular shift induced by endogenous insulin release in response to systemic glucose absorption, renal losses with use of diuretics, or intestinal losses with use of laxatives. Observational studies have also demonstrated a consistent association of low serum potassium levels with a higher risk for gram-negative peritonitis, and all-cause, cardiovascular, and infection-related mortality.

Not only are there no clinical trials that have demonstrated the health benefits of treatment of hypokalemia in patients undergoing PD, but none is likely to be done in the near future. Given the frequency of occurrence of hypokalemia and the associated health risks, it is important to routinely monitor and correct serum potassium levels in patients undergoing PD. As a first step, dietary restrictions on potassium intake should be removed and the intake liberalized. In patients with persistent hypokalemia, inhibitors of the renin–angiotensin–aldosterone axis should be considered (e.g., angiotensin-converting enzyme inhibitors, angiotensin receptor blockers, or spironolactone). Most patients, however, are likely to require oral potassium supplements.

SECTION XIV

Peritoneal Dialysis: Intra-Abdominal Pressure-Related Complications

Peritoneal Dialysis:
Intra-Abdominal Pressure-
Related Complications

C H A P T E R   4 0

Abdominal Hernias in Continuous Ambulatory Peritoneal Dialysis

Farhanah Yousaf, MBBS • Chaim Charytan, MD •
Bruce S. Spinowitz, MD, FACP

Complications related to peritoneal dialysis (PD) can be categorized as infectious or noninfectious. Non-infectious complications, including abdominal hernias, catheter malfunction, and exit site leaks occur in continuous ambulatory peritoneal dialysis (CAPD), continuous cycling peritoneal dialysis/automated peritoneal dialysis (CCPD/APD), and intermittent peritoneal dialysis (IPD), although some of these complications are more common in the CAPD population. More serious complications such as catheter erosion into the bowel, bladder, or vagina are rare and related to the presence of a catheter irrespective of the form of PD used.

Abdominal hernias are the most common of the anatomic complications of PD (Van Dijk et al 2005) and contribute significantly to morbidity, increased medical costs, and withdrawal from PD.

Incidence and Prevalence

The prevalence of PD-related hernias ranges from 9% to 32%. However, the incidence of hernias has dropped from 0.21 hernias per PD-year at risk since the early 1980s (Khanna et al 1981) to about 0.06 hernias per PD-year at risk in late 1990s (Hussain 1998). This finding may be attributable to the discontinuation of midline catheter insertions and resorbable suture material. Emerging evidence demonstrates a further decline in the incidence of hernias with 0.04 hernias per PD-year at risk being reported in 2014 (Yang et al 2014).

Types of Abdominal Wall Hernias

Several locations of hernia formation have been described in patients undergoing PD, including inguinal, catheter exit site, umbilical, incisional, ventral, epigastric, pelvic, femoral, and obturator. Although the prevalence rates vary in the literature, the most commonly occurring hernias are umbilical, inguinal, ventral, and incisional. Hernial sacs may contain subcutaneous fat, bowel, or peritoneal fluid (or a combination). Unusual hernias such as spigelian, Ritchers, foramen of Morgagni or diaphragmatic, rectocele, cystocele, and uterine prolapse have also been reported in the PD population.

Risk Factors

Normal intraabdominal pressure in an empty peritoneal cavity is about 0.5 to 2.2 cm H_2O, which increases to nearly 2 to 10 cm H_2O with instillation of dialysate volumes commonly used in clinical practice. The increase in intraabdominal pressure is linearly correlated to the volume of dialysate instilled. Therefore, a theoretical association between increased dialysate volumes and intraabdominal pressure and risk of hernia exists, but supportive evidence in the literature is lacking (Durand et al 1992; Bleyer et al 1998; Hussain et al 1998; Del Peso et al 2003). Factors that may contribute to increased intraabdominal pressure include coughing or straining, which can transiently elevate abdominal pressure to as high as 120 to 150 cm H_2O, with varying volumes of intraperitoneal dialysate (Twardowski et al 1986).

The PD modality plays a role in hernia formation based on the presumptive principle that intraabdominal pressures are lower during recumbency compared with the ambulatory state. In IPD, the patient remains supine throughout the treatment, which attenuates the rise in intraabdominal pressure. In CCPD, patients maintain a full volume in their abdominal cavity throughout the day, but the bulk of their treatment occurs during the night while the patient is in the recumbent position. In contrast, patients undergoing CAPD perform dwells and drains during the day. A mean intraabdominal pressure increase of 2.0, 2.7, and 2.8 cm H_2O per liter of instilled dialysate volume has been demonstrated in supine, upright, and sitting positions, respectively (Twardowski et al 1983). However, evidence in the literature is inconclusive. A survey of 75 randomly selected dialysis units in the United States and Canada involving 1864 PD patients found no difference in hernia incidence among the various PD modalities (CAPD, APD, and nocturnal IPD). The association of PD modality and hernia risk was lacking in a study of 47 automated PD and 14 CAPD patients (Dejardin et al 2007). However, the rate of hernia was higher but not statistically significant, among CAPD patients versus CCPD patients in a 5-year retrospective review from Spain (Del Peso et al 2003).

Each year on CAPD increases the risk of hernia formation by 20% (O'Connor et al 1986). PD duration is therefore an important risk factor for hernia formation (Yang et al 2014). Additional risk factors associated with hernia include acquired focal abdominal wall weakening caused by previous abdominal surgery or multiparous status (Digenis et al 1982) and increasing age (Digenis et al 1982). However, the rate of hernia formation was not statistically significant between those who had previously undergone abdominal surgery versus those who did not (Del Peso et al 2003). The role of gender in the development of hernia in PD population is controversial; some studies indicate female gender increases the risk, but more recent data suggest that female gender reduces this risk (Van Dijk et al 2005; Yang et al 2014). The suggestion that small body size (Tokgoz et al 2003; Afthentopoulos et al 1998) is associated with increased risk for hernia formation has not been confirmed in recent studies (Van Dijk et al 2005; Dejardin et al 2007). Hernias appear to be more common among PD patients weighing less than 90 kg versus those weighing more than 90 kg (Ananthakrishan et al 2014). A lower rate of hernia formation was evident with a weekly Kt/V greater than 2 compared with a weekly Kt/V less than 2 (Van Dijk et al 2005). Although constipation is common and could significantly increase intraabdominal pressure during straining, its contribution to risk of hernia formation in PD population has not been defined.

There is no correlation between the etiology of renal disease and development of hernia, with the exception of polycystic kidney disease (PKD). The large size of polycystic kidneys may contribute to increased intraabdominal pressure by limiting peritoneal space. Alternatively, a PKD-associated generalized collagen disorder may predispose to hernia formation. The collagen defect has been postulated to explain the renal and liver cysts that develop in PKD, as well as the increased incidence of diverticulosis, valvular defects, and aneurysms. Although the risk for hernia formation is higher in PKD population undergoing PD, the overall survival rate and peritonitis risk remain comparable to that of nondiabetic PD patients (Li et al 2011). PKD is not an absolute contraindication for PD therapy.

No correlation has been identified with the type of catheter used (Van Dijk et al 2005) or with type of incision (midline vs paramedian transrectus), although a paramedian transrectus incision has been suggested as a means of decreasing the incidence of incisional hernias (Spence et al 1985; Stegmayr et al 1990). Moreover, paramedian incisions are associated with fewer early postoperative complications and longer PD catheter survival (Kanokkantapong et al 2011). Similar incidences of hernia development have been associated with open versus laparoscopic PD catheter insertion approaches (Xie et al 2012).

Complications

Untreated hernias may cause cosmetic concerns, discomfort, or loss of ultrafiltration or lead to bowel incarceration and strangulation. Umbilical hernias have a high likelihood of incarceration, strangulation, and recurrence (Cherney et al 2004; Afthentopoulos et al 1998). Strangulated hernial sacs predispose to peritonitis. Early detection of hernias may be difficult; therefore, it is common for patients to present with acute incarceration requiring emergent surgery. Even when a hernia is recognized early, its correction requires hospitalization and interruption of CAPD therapy, contributing to morbidity, cost, and patient inconvenience. The development of hernias, particularly recurrent hernias, is therefore a significant factor influencing a permanent switch to hemodialysis (HD).

In addition, the dialysate may leak into the soft tissues if there is a break in the supporting structures of the abdominal wall with hernia formation.

Diagnosis and Management

Most hernias are asymptomatic but may be appreciated on a thorough physical examination. The standard diagnostic procedure for locating subclinical hernia, hernial sac tear, or patent processus vaginalis, is computed tomography peritoneography. Other procedures such as peritoneal scintigraphy and magnetic resonance imaging have also demonstrated diagnostic usefulness.

Because of complications associated with hernia development, timely surgical repair of hernia is recommended despite some increased 30-day mortality, morbidity, and requirement for reoperation that have been observed in dialysis patients undergoing elective ventral hernia repair (Tam et al 2014). Conventional hernia repair consists of suture closure of the abdominal wall defect and is associated with a recurrence rate of 22% to 29% (Wetherington et al 1985; Afthentopoulos et al 1998; Suh et al 1994). Nowadays, hernioplasty is performed using a prosthetic mesh as a low-tension or tension-free repair to reduce the risk of recurrence. It comprises an underlay patch which provides reinforcement from inside of the abdominal wall, a connector, and an onlay patch that lies over the abdominal wall. In addition, low tension mesh repair of hernia allows rapid resumption of CAPD (Lewis et al 1998).

Continuation of Continuous Ambulatory Peritoneal Dialysis After Hernioplasty

The temporary interruption of CAPD and use of HD in the interim period after hernia repair or other intraabdominal surgery may decrease the likelihood of hernia recurrence. If HD cannot be performed, low-volume PD or nighttime continuous cycling PD should be used for at least 2 to 4 weeks after abdominal surgery for hernia repair to allow sufficient time for incisional wounds to heal, which is often slow in the presence of uremia. Emerging literature suggests that interim HD and its associated complications can be avoided in most patients. In one series, early postoperative dialysis was not necessary in 26 of 49 PD patients who underwent hernia repair, and only 7 patients required temporary HD (Balda et al 2013). In other reported series, the immediate resumption of CAPD after hernia repair has been successful without giving rise to early hernia recurrence or leakage (Lewis et al 1998; Crabtree et al 2006; Shah et al 2006; Gianetta et al 2004).

Prophylactic Measures

Prophylactic measures to prevent hernia formation in the CAPD population have been suggested but have not been established. The simultaneous repair of preexisting hernias during PD catheter placement is highly recommended (Wetherington et al 1985; Nicholson et al 1989; Afthentopoulos et al 1998). A paramedian transrectus incision may decrease the incidence of incisional hernias at the site of catheter insertion (Spence et al 1985; Stegmayr et al 1990). Administration of antitussives and laxatives when indicated may be useful. It is advisable to refrain from vigorous physical activities with a full peritoneal cavity.

The incidence of hernia recurrence is approximately 25% after surgical repair (Wetherington et al 1985; Suh et al 1994; Afthentopoulos et al 1998). A reinforcing prosthetic polypropylene mesh may prevent local recurrence by guarding against increased abdominal wall tension. Indeed, prosthetic mesh reinforcement overlying the abdominal wall has been effective in preventing hernia recurrence during a follow up of 2 to 45 months (Martínez-Mier et al 2008). In a small retrospective analysis of CAPD patients with large or multiple abdominal hernias who were not candidates for HD, placement of a polypropylene mesh at the time of hernia repair was reported to prevent hernia recurrence (Imvrios et al 1994). In addition, there was a lower incidence of peritonitis after mesh placement compared with before mesh placement. Extraperitoneal placement or neoperitonealization of the mesh may reduce the risk of secondary mesh infection (Lewis 1998; Schoenmaeckers et al 2011). Failure of mesh hernia repair is rare but has been reported in the setting of unusual comorbidities (Abraham et al 1997).

There is no evidence that abdominal binding or the wearing of a corset will in any way decrease the incidence of hernia development. APD with low daytime dialysate volume may be recommended for patients at risk of recurrent hernia based on the principle of lower intraabdominal pressures during recumbency and relative lower rate of hernia formation in APD patients compared with the CAPD population (Bargman et al 2008; Del Peso et al 2003).

C H A P T E R 4 1

Peritoneal Dialysate Leaks

Sassan Ghazan-Shahi, MD, FRCPC • Joanne M. Bargman, MD, FRCPC

Leak of dialysis fluid out of the peritoneal cavity is a significant and common mechanical complication of peritoneal dialysis (PD) therapy. It results from the loss of integrity somewhere in the peritoneal compartment, leading to egress of the dialysate to adjacent anatomic spaces.

The reported incidence of PD leaks varies, but it is described in the literature to happen in up to 5% of patients.

The leaks that happen within 4 weeks of PD initiation are considered "early," and the "late" leaks occur after this time. Early leaks usually present shortly after PD catheter insertion and mostly manifest as movement of PD fluid along the catheter tract, or at the median or paramedian surgical incision site. Late leaks are mainly due to passage of the dialysate into the adjacent anatomic spaces outside of the peritoneum. These internal leakages can move into the abdominal wall, pleural space, and external genitalia in both males and females. (Movement of PD fluid into the pleural cavity is referred to as PD hydrothorax; see Chapter 42.)

Herniation of bowel or even mesentery represents another break in the integrity of the peritoneal compartment, and leak of PD fluid commonly accompanies these hernias. Both leaks and hernias are the result of increased intraabdominal pressure (IAP) that is a result of instillation of a significant volume of dialysis fluid into the peritoneal cavity. Intraabdominal pressure increases with the volume of dialysate infused; the typical value is 12 ± 2 cm of water (cm H_2O) with an intraperitoneal volume (IPV) of 2 L, with linear increases of 2.2 cm H_2O for each additional liter infused. IAP is highest when the patient is sitting, compared with the supine position with the same IPV; factors such as obesity, coughing, or Valsalva, such as in straining with bowel movements, all increase the intraperitoneal pressure as well and hence make the patient prone to develop abdominal wall hernias and leaks.

The technique used for PD catheter insertion is thought to influence the incidence of leakage, especially early leaks. The paramedian incision is associated with a lower incidence of early leak compared to a midline incision through the linea alba. In addition, early initiation of PD therapy after catheter insertion, prescribing large dialysate volumes during the early break-in period, and regimens that involve patients carrying dialysate in the nonsupine position all increase the risk of early leaks. Abdominal wall characteristics also affect the probability of developing leaks. Previous abdominal surgeries, polycystic kidney disease, chronic corticosteroid use, and multiple pregnancies are all factors that compromise abdominal wall strength and increase the chance of leaks.

Leaks into the pleural space and consequent development of hydrothorax may occur because of passage of the fluid through the preexisting defects in the diaphragm, or defects that may develop following trauma, pregnancy, or surgeries (discussed in Chapter 42). Leaks into the scrotal sac are the result of a patent processus vaginalis (see below) or palpable or nonpalpable inguinal hernias with defects in the hernia sac. Vaginal leaks are rare but may occur as a result of tracking of the dialysate through the fallopian tubes or due to fascial defects.

Depending on the location and amount of peritoneal leak, the clinical manifestations can be subtle or dramatic. External leaks that usually happen early in the course of PD therapy often manifest as visible wetness around the exit site, or soaking of the dressing used to cover the surgical site. In cases where the leaks track into subcutaneous tissues, the abdominal wall appears edematous upon exam, with changes in the appearance of the skin in the affected areas and deep impressions made by waist bands, dialysis tubing, etc. (Fig. 41.1). The leaks into the abdominal wall may go on for a relatively long time before they are recognized.

The processus vaginalis is a connecting pathway between the peritoneal cavity and the scrotum or labia that usually obliterates during fetal development. However, a significant minority of patients continue to have patency of this structure. The presence of the spermatic cord in males leads to a greater prevalence of patency and risk for hydrocele in that gender. Patients with leaks into the patent processus vaginalis usually present with an uncomfortable and enlarged scrotum (i.e. hydrocele). The fluid also may track across the tunica vaginalis into the overlying scrotal wall, causing edema there as well. In most cases of PD leaks, especially the ones with large fluid shifts, inadequate ultrafiltration, or continuous failure to drain the expected amount of effluent dialysate after a dwell, in the setting of weight gain and absence of generalized edema, should clue the clinician to consider possibility of PD fluid leak into other potential spaces. The leaks into the abdominal wall subcutaneous tissues, new appearance of hernias, or leak through a patent processus vaginalis become more prominent or appear de novo after the patient's PD prescription has typically been advanced to larger dwell volumes and initiation of dwells in the nonsupine position. In many of these cases, a temporal association between changing the prescription and start of the leak can be discerned.

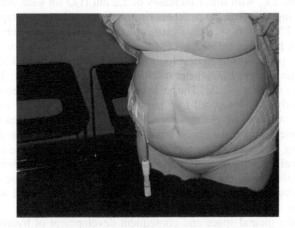

Figure 41.1

Protuberant Abdomen Resulting From Leak of Dialysis Fluid.

In the approach to most PD leaks, clinical history and physical exam are the mainstay of establishing the diagnosis. Exit site leaks usually can be confirmed with testing the fluid around the exit site for glucose using urinary dipsticks. For abdominal wall leaks, leaks into hernias, and leaks through the patent processus vaginalis, computed tomography (CT), with intraperitoneal contrast dye, and following the track of the instilled dye, can aid the diagnosis. For this purpose, 100 mL of Omnipaque 300 (iohexol preparation) is added to a 2-L bag of dialysis solution and instilled into the peritoneal cavity. Following the instillation, the patient should be ambulatory and walk for about 2 hours, in order to increase the IAP and facilitate the movement of the contrast fluid along the leakage track so that it can be easily seen in the images (Figs. 41.2 and 41.3). If magnetic resonance imaging (MRI) is to be used for this purpose, the dialysis solution itself acts as the MRI contrast and gadolinium is not necessary.

Treatment of the PD leaks depends on the type and location. Pericatheter leaks usually can be dealt with by leaving the peritoneal cavity empty and discontinuing the PD for a few days. The longer the PD therapy can be held, the greater the chance the leak will seal off. If necessary, the patient can be supported by hemodialysis while the PD is on hold. In most cases the leak stops after the trial of withholding PD, and it can be restarted. Modifying the prescription to a low-IAP regimen by avoiding large dialysate volumes and excluding the day dwell in the beginning while restarting the PD may help to prevent the leak from recurring. Indeed, in patients at greater risk for leak, such as those with known or previous hernias, malnourished patients, those with PKD or chronic corticosteroid therapy, a low-pressure regimen should be prescribed from the start. Patients with failing renal transplants who are

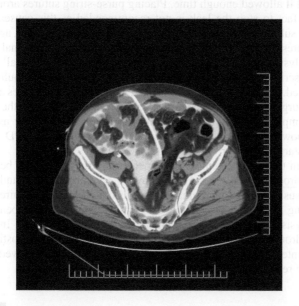

Figure 41.2

Computed Tomography With Intraperitoneal Contrast Dye Demonstrating a Pericatheter Leak of Dialysis Fluid.

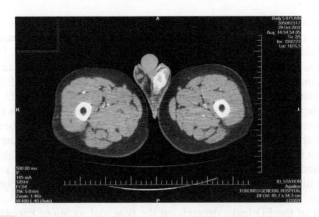

Figure 41.3

**Computed Tomography With Intraperitoneal Contrast Dye Demonstrating
Herniated Bowel and Dialysis Fluid in the Left Scrotal Sac.**

receiving mTor inhibitor immunosuppression, such as sirolimus, should stop this drug before the PD catheter is implanted.

In recurrent and protracted exit-site leaks, the catheter may have to be removed and placed at a different site. This maneuver should be a rare occurrence as most leaks will seal if allowed enough time. Placing purse-string sutures around the catheter after the fact to stop the leak is not recommended as this causes the fluid to divert into the subcutaneous tissues. In cases of abdominal wall leaks, again, modifying the PD prescription to supine position cycles (NIPD: nocturnal intermittent peritoneal dialysis) usually results in resolution of the abdominal wall edema. This change in prescription often allows the wall defect to heal, and ambulatory PD can then be restarted. In recurrent cases, or in cases where the leak involves an abdominal wall hernia, surgical repair is needed. Depending on the situation, the patient may need to be temporarily placed on hemodialysis. However, as long as there is no evidence of bowel incarceration or strangulation, a low-pressure PD regimen can usually be restarted a day or two after hernia repair.

Similarly, in the case of genital leaks, peritoneal dialysis should be temporarily withheld. Hydrocele usually resolves following scrotal elevation and bed rest. A patent processus vaginalis, after imaging confirmation, can be repaired surgically. While awaiting surgery and in the weeks following surgery, depending on the patient's dialysis needs, NIPD using small volumes may be used. In the case of suspected hydrothorax, PD should be stopped immediately. Diagnostic and therapeutic thoracentesis may be needed depending on the situation followed by different diaphragmatic repair options (see Chapter 42).

CHAPTER 42

Hydrothorax and Peritoneal Dialysis

Ali Al-Lawati, MD • Joanne Bargman MD, FRCPC

Introduction

PD hydrothorax is a well-described, albeit uncommon, complication of peritoneal dialysis. It was first reported in 1967 by Edwards and Unger in a 69-year-old patient who developed acute severe respiratory distress with radiographic evidence of right-sided hydrothorax soon after the commencement of peritoneal dialysis.

It is reported in 1.6%–10% of peritoneal dialysis patients. Observational studies have documented it to occur almost exclusively on the right side (Fig. 42.1). Several risk factors have been associated with the development of hydrothorax, including female sex, polycystic kidney disease (PKD), previous surgery, and peritonitis.

Pathophysiology

Pleural effusions develop when fluid accumulates in the pleural space in excess of the rate at which it can be reabsorbed. This can happen as a result of increased production of the fluid, such as in congestive heart failure, or through fluid entering from the peritoneal cavity, which is what happens in the case of ascites from portal hypertension, or PD hydrothorax.

Normally, the diaphragm functions as a wall that separates the thoracic and abdominal cavity. Although the normal diaphragm has both large and small openings (stomata) that allow the passage of structures such as the aorta, inferior vena cava, and the esophagus, none of these anatomic stomata allows for transit of intraperitoneal dialysate into the pleural cavity. This is thought to be due to the interface of muscle fibers with serous membranes and other connective tissues.

Several mechanisms have been described to explain how fluid could migrate from the peritoneal cavity to the pleural cavity. Gagnon and Daniels proposed that an embryonic remnant, namely, the persisting pneumatoenteric recess and the infracardiac bursa, provides a passage connecting the peritoneal cavity to the right pleural space. It remains unclear why in the majority of patients the fluid accumulates on the right side of the chest, a phenomenon that is also seen in several other conditions such as hepatic hydrothorax, and Meig syndrome (ovarian fibroma in association with ascites and right-sided pleural effusion). In liver cirrhosis, it has been proposed that pleural effusion is due to increased transport by lymphatics, which are more numerous on the right side. Another potential explanation is the presence of the heart and pericardium in the left hemithorax, which could block some of these diaphragmatic defects and prevent fluid from entering into the left side of the chest.

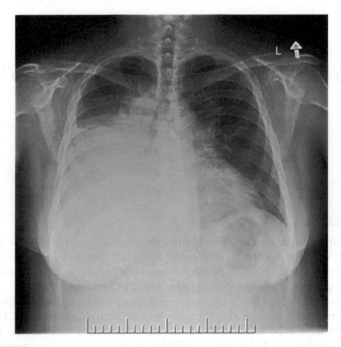

Figure 42.1.

Twenty-Five-Year-Old Woman With Acute Shortness of Breath Days After Starting PD. Note the large right pleural effusion.

Symptoms and Presentation

PD-related hydrothorax most commonly presents with shortness of breath, which can be sudden in onset. Physical examination may show signs of pleural effusion, with no other features to suggest volume overload as a cause of the dyspnea, such as peripheral edema. Another clue to the presence of a peritoneo-thoracic leak is a persistent decrease in effluent fluid volume. About 25% of patients may remain asymptomatic, and the pleural effusion is discovered incidentally. Hydrothorax classically develops shortly after initiation of peritoneal dialysis, but has been reported to occur as late as 8 years after being on PD. The difference in onset may represent two distinct mechanisms, where early fluid migration happens due to preexisting congenital communications, and later ones through acquired defects due to an increase in intra-abdominal pressure. In the case of hydrothorax occurring coincident with PD peritonitis, it has been suggested that the inflammation associated with the infection leads to sloughing of a fragile cellular layer overlying a diaphragmatic defect.

Diagnosis

Early diagnosis of PD hydrothorax is essential, as failure to recognize pleuroperitoneal communication as a cause of shortness of breath could result in inappropriate prescription of hypertonic dialysis exchanges, which would increase intraperitoneal volumes and pressure and worsen the hydrothorax.

Thoracentesis is of both diagnostic and therapeutic value. Many of these patients present with shortness of breath secondary to the presence of a significant amount of fluid in the pleural cavity, which can be promptly relieved by thoracentesis. In addition, fluid analysis can confirm the diagnosis. The fluid in this case should be a sterile transudate, ruling out infectious or malignant etiologies. Although the higher the absolute pleural fluid glucose concentration, the more likely there is a communication, there is no cut-off value that can reliably distinguish pleuroperitoneal communication from other causes of hydrothorax. Comparison with a simultaneous plasma glucose has been advocated by some. In a study by Chow et al, a pleural fluid to serum glucose concentration gradient of greater than 50 mg/dL may be used to differentiate pleuroperitoneal communication from other causes of transudative pleural effusion in PD patients. However, if the dialysis has dwelled in the pleural cavity for a long time before thoracentesis, it is possible that the glucose has had time to diffuse out of the pleural space into the systemic circulation. In that situation, the pleural fluid glucose concentration may not be elevated compared to blood glucose. In addition, if the patient's most recent dwell was with a glucose-free solution, such as icodextrin or amino acids, the pleural fluid glucose concentration would not be expected to be increased.

After an initial chest radiograph, other imaging modalities are available to document a pleuroperitoneal leak.

Peritoneal scintigraphy using technetium-99m tagged macro-aggregated albumin or Tc-99m sulfur colloid infused into the peritoneal dialysis fluid can confirm pleuroperitoneal communication in a noninvasive fashion, by demonstrating radioactive tracer leakage into the thoracic cavity. Because the rate of movement of dialysis fluid from the peritoneal to the pleural cavity can be slow, late images may be needed to show the presence of tracer above the hemidiaphragm.

Leaks can also be diagnosed using CT technology. Twardowski proposed the addition of contrast to PD fluid to improve detection. This has the advantage of diagnosing small leaks, adhesions, and loculated fluid collections. Its preparation is similar to that for scintigraphy.

Magnetic resonance imaging (MRI) can also be used to diagnose peritoneal defects with similar accuracy to that of CT scans. Previously, gadodiamide, a gadolinium-based contrast, was used in these studies. However, MRIs can be used without the need for additional contrast media administration, where the dialysate, because of its electrolyte content, is used as the contrast medium, which appears bright on T2-weighted images and can therefore detect leaks. This is particularly important given the risk of development of nephrogenic systemic fibrosis with the administration of gadolinium-based contrast media in patients with low GFR. The main advantage of using MR images is lack of radiation, which is an important consideration in younger patients.

Methylene blue has been suggested where the dye is added to the dialysis fluid, the fluid instilled in the peritoneal cavity, and then thoracentesis is done to look for blue discoloration of the pleural fluid. However, methylene blue has been reported to cause chemical peritonitis and is therefore not recommended.

Management

Conservative management has been reported to be successful in up to 50% of patients. The hypothesis is that the presence of the acidic, hypertonic peritoneal dialysis fluid in the pleural cavity leads to pleural inflammation sufficient to lead to pleurodesis in the healing phase. The patient should be left empty of PD fluid for several weeks. If dialysis is necessary, a temporary dialysis catheter will have to be inserted for hemodialysis. The patient could be rechallenged with PD after these 4–8 weeks to see if there is recurrence of the hydrothorax.

The movement of fluid from the peritoneal to the pleural cavity is pressure-driven secondary to the increased intraabdominal pressure incumbent in PD. Hydrothorax is sometimes improved or even eliminated by using a "low pressure" PD regimen. This regimen involves using smaller volumes of PD fluid and having the patient assume the supine position. There is a general impression that the supine position may allow fluid to move into the pleural cavity more easily, but insofar as it is pressure-driven the supine position would be advantageous in reducing the occurrence of hydrothorax.

Because the diaphragmatic defects only become manifest when there is sufficient intraperitoneal fluid, it should be explained to the patient that if they transition to hemodialysis they will not need any further intervention for the hydrothorax. However, if they want to persevere with peritoneal dialysis, pleurodesis will be necessary if the defects do not heal during the resting phase.

Pleurodesis, by instilling a sclerosing agent into the pleural cavity, works by irritating the epithelial surface, leading to inflammation and fibrosis, resulting in obliteration of the trans-diaphragmatic route of dialysate leakage. This procedure can be done blindly through a chest tube, or under direct visualization of the pleural cavity using video-assisted thoracoscopy (VATS). The latter has the advantage of being able to evenly distribute the sclerosing agent and potentially achieve better success rates. Different agents have been used in the pleurodesis procedure, including talc and tetracycline, with similar response rates. Autologous blood has also been used with variable success rates. A 10-day waiting period is the minimum time recommended before PD can be restarted, based on follow-up data using scintigraphy that showed pleuroperitoneal communication healing 10 days after pleurodesis.

In addition to the above, VATS has the advantage of being able to directly inspect the diaphragm for communications between the pleural and peritoneal cavities, which can then be repaired. Di Bisceglie and colleagues first described this procedure in 1996, and it has become the surgical intervention of choice. Prior to that, patients who failed closed pleurodesis had to undergo open thoracotomy, where the diaphragm was visualized and defects directly sutured. Although open thoracotomy carried a high success rate, given the perioperative risks, not all dialysis patients were eligible. Fortunately, this is not a major concern with VATS. Through VATS, the defects can be surgically repaired. An automatic stapler with glue or absorbable polyglycolic acid felt can be used to seal the leakage areas. Lastly, VATS allows immediate intraoperative evaluation for air leakage to confirm successful closure of a pleuroperitoneal communication. In the case of microscopic defects in the hemidiaphragm with slow leaks, VATS may not confer any advantage over simple pleurodesis.

Efficacy of thoracoscopic treatment has been confirmed by several case series from various centers with a more than 90% success rate reported.

SECTION XV

Acid-Base Homeostasis

CHAPTER 43

Acid–Base Homeostasis in Dialysis

F. John Gennari, MD

When renal replacement therapy is initiated, regulation of acid–base balance by the kidneys is replaced by a new homeostatic process responding to the physical principles of diffusion and convection rather than to the pH of the body fluids. Balance is achieved by bicarbonate addition during dialysis, not by regulated acid excretion. Consequently, serum [HCO_3^-] in the steady state is dependent in large part on the kinetics of HCO_3^- diffusion across the dialysis membrane—which in turn is highly dependent on the characteristics of the dialysis treatment used. Despite the lack of a pH-dependent regulatory system, a new equilibrium is achieved during dialysis therapy in which HCO_3^- consumption by endogenous acid production (including any alkali lost in the stool) is matched by HCO_3^- addition during dialysis.

Although dialysis therapy creates a new equilibrium, it is much less able to adapt to day-to-day changes in acid production or to superimposed disorders of acid–base equilibrium. This chapter reviews the nature of this unique regulatory process and the tools for identifying disturbances of acid–base homeostasis in dialysis-dependent patients. Throughout the chapter, the term *serum [total CO_2]* refers to the routinely measured variable that correlates closely with serum [HCO_3^-], and the term *[HCO_3^-]* itself refers to the value calculated from measurements of Pco_2 and pH in blood or to the concentration of bicarbonate in the dialysate solution.

Determinants of Serum [Total CO₂] in Dialysis Patients

The amount of alkali added during hemodialysis or peritoneal dialysis is related to the dialysance of the alkali source used (HCO_3^- or lactate) and to the transmembrane concentration gradient (Fig. 43.1). Because dialysance (a function of membrane permeability and surface area) and bath [HCO_3^-] or [lactate] are fixed by the dialysis prescription, serum [HCO_3^-] is the variable that determines the amount of alkali added. The lower the serum value, the more alkali is added. Consequently, a new equilibrium is achieved in which the alkali consumed in buffering endogenous acid production (a process that reduces serum [HCO_3^-]) is matched by the alkali added during treatment.

Hemodialysis

In patients receiving hemodialysis, predialysis serum [total CO_2] is determined by the dialysis and patient characteristics outlined in Table 43.1. The dialysis prescription is fixed and unless blood flow rate is compromised should not be a source of great variation in predialysis serum [total CO_2]. Hemodialysis bath solutions typically contain 32 mEq/L of bicarbonate, and the concentration can be adjusted (see later). In addition, the bath contains an organic anion, either acetate or citrate, in

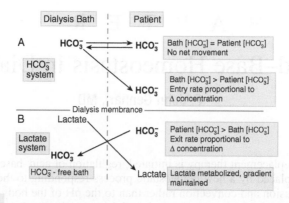

Figure 43.1

(A) Role of Patient's Serum [HCO₃⁻] in Determining Rate of [HCO₃⁻] Movement Across the Dialysis Membrane. (B) Dynamics of Lactate Entry and [HCO₃⁻] Loss Across a Dialysis Membrane Using a Lactate-Based Bath. Note that the same principles (although in the opposite direction) govern HCO_3^- movement across the membrane.

Table 43.1

Determinants of Predialysis or Steady-State Serum [Total CO₂] in Patients Receiving Dialysis Therapy

Hemodialysis prescription
    Bath [HCO₃⁻] (or [lactate] used in some forms of daily hemodialysis)
    Permeability and surface area of dialysis membrane
    Blood and dialysate flow rates
    Duration and frequency of dialysis treatments
Peritoneal dialysis prescription
    Bath [lactate] (or [HCO₃⁻] used in some cases)
    Volume and dwell time of exchanges
    Permeability and surface area of peritoneal membrane
Patient characteristics
    Endogenous acid production
    Fluid retention[a]
    Renal HCO₃⁻ generation or loss (in patients with residual renal function)
    Organic acid production during dialysis treatments

---

[a]Fluid retention affects the space of distribution and therefore the concentration of HCO₃⁻ in the extracellular fluid.

---

low concentration. While metabolism of these organic anions also adds new bicarbonate, this added bicarbonate simply reduces the transmembrane gradient for entry from the bath and therefore does not have a notable influence on serum [total CO₂].

    Of the patient characteristics outlined in the table, the first two, endogenous acid production and fluid retention between treatments, have the major impact on predialysis serum [total CO₂]. Renal generation and loss of HCO₃⁻ are usually trivial, and

Table 43.2

Effect of Endogenous Acid Production and Fluid Retention on Predialysis Serum [Total CO$_2$] in Patients Receiving Hemodialysis With a Bath [HCO$_3^-$] = 35 mEq/L

Endogenous Acid Production, mEq/day[a]	Predialysis Serum [Total CO$_2$], mEq/L[b]
30	24.2
60	21.9
90	19.6
120	17.3
Fluid Retention (L)[c]	
0	23.1
2	21.9
4	20.8
6	19.8

[a]Assuming 2 L fluid retention between treatments.
[b]After long interval between treatments (68 hours).
[c]Total fluid gain between treatments, assuming 60 mEq/day endogenous acid production.
Other assumptions: Weight 70 kg, postdialysis serum [total CO$_2$] = 28 mEq/L, HCO$_3^-$ buffer space = 0.5 × body weight.

organic acid production (which influences the net retention of alkali during dialysis) has little impact unless it is unusually large (see discussion of metabolic acidosis later in the chapter). The estimated effects of variations in endogenous acid production and fluid retention between treatments are outlined in Table 43.2. In this table, predialysis serum [total CO$_2$] has been calculated using some simple assumptions to illustrate the magnitude of these effects. These estimates have been substantiated by experimental and clinical observations.

As shown in Table 43.2, variations in acid production over a reasonable range can change predialysis serum [total CO$_2$] from normal to frankly acidotic values. Endogenous acid production varies directly with dietary intake of sulfur-containing proteins. Thus, patients with limited intake of animal protein and grains will have a higher predialysis serum [total CO$_2$] than will patients eating a diet high in these foods. Variations in fluid retention have a smaller, but still significant, effect.

Dialysis against a bath with a [HCO$_3^-$] of 35 mEq/L three times weekly does not restore predialysis serum [total CO$_2$] to 24 mEq/L unless endogenous acid production is quite low. The usual values range from 19 to 23 mEq/L in stable hemodialysis patients. It is important to emphasize that predialysis [total CO$_2$] is a nadir value. Serum [total CO$_2$] rises to 28–30 mEq/L just after each hemodialysis treatment and then gradually falls to the predialysis level over the interval between treatments.

Two large cohort studies have demonstrated an increased mortality risk both in patients with low (<19 mEq/L) and high (>24 mEq/L) predialysis values. In the former group, the increased risk is attributable to the presence of acidosis. By contrast, in the latter group, the increased risk appears to be unrelated to alkalosis and is largely due to nutritional and inflammatory factors. Predialysis serum [total CO$_2$] can easily be varied by adjusting bath [HCO$_3^-$], and short-term studies have shown that in patients with low values, increasing bath [HCO$_3^-$] sufficiently to increase serum [total CO$_2$] to 24 mEq/L has beneficial effects on both muscle and bone metabolism. Although this practice has been adopted by many dialysis units in the

United States, a recent large cohort study suggests that increasing bath $[HCO_3^-]$ is an independent risk factor for death, raising the likelihood by 8% for every 4-mEq/L increase. Thus both the optimal predialysis [total CO_2] and the optimal bath $[HCO_3^-]$ remain uncertain, but at this point the data suggest that the latter should not be increased above 37 mEq/L. Patients receiving daily hemodialysis have higher serum [total CO_2] values without any change in bath $[HCO_3^-]$, and bath $[HCO_3^-]$ usually must be decreased to avoid sustained alkalemia.

Peritoneal Dialysis

In patients receiving peritoneal dialysis, steady-state serum [total CO_2] is also determined by the dialysis and patient characteristics outlined in Table 43.1. Bath lactate concentration has empirically been set at 40 mEq/L, a value that maintains serum [total CO_2] in the normal range in most patients. In some centers in Europe, peritoneal dialysis with a HCO_3^--containing bath solution (mixed just before instillation) has improved acid–base status further, but this technique is technically difficult and has not gained wide acceptance. The higher exchange volumes and shorter dwell times now routinely used in continuous cycling peritoneal dialysis have had little impact on serum [total CO_2].

Normal Values

The ranges of "normal" values for predialysis serum [total CO_2] and for arterial blood pH, P_{CO_2}, and $[HCO_3^-]$ in patients receiving conventional hemodialysis or peritoneal dialysis are shown in Table 43.3. In patients receiving hemodialysis, average serum [total CO_2] has risen by 1–2 mEq/L in the last decade without any change in dialysis prescription, possibly reflecting a lower protein intake in the older population now receiving this treatment. Blood P_{CO_2} and pH measurements indicate

Table 43.3		

Steady-State Acid–Base Values in Stable Dialysis Patients

	Conventional Hemodialysis	Peritoneal Dialysis
[Total CO_2] mEq/L	23.9 ± 2.1 (175)[a]	26.4 ± 3.0 (109)[b]
$[HCO_3^-]$ mEq/L	21.6 ± 2.4 (30)[c]	21.5 ± 2.4 (33)[d]
pH	7.39 ± 0.04 (30)	7.38 ± 0.04 (33)
P_{CO_2} mm Hg	37 ± 4.5 (30)	37 ± 5.1 (33)

Means ± SD, numbers in parentheses are the numbers of patients.

[a]Gennari FJ, 2015. Personal observations measured either in graft or fistula blood samples predialysis after long interval between treatments. Hemodialysis bath $[HCO_3^-]$ = 35 mEq/L.

[b]Venous blood measurements. Data from Gennari FJ, Feriani M. Acid base problems in hemodialysis and peritoneal dialysis. In N Lameire, RL Mehta, eds. *Complications of Dialysis*. New York: Marcel Dekker 2000:361–376.

[c]$[HCO_3^-]$, pH, and P_{CO_2} values in hemodialysis patients obtained predialysis from arterial blood. Hemodialysis bath $[HCO_3^-]$ = 35 mEq/L. Data from Marano et al, *Int Urol Nephrol* 2015;47(4):691–694.

[d]$[HCO_3^-]$, pH, and P_{CO_2} values in peritoneal dialysis patients obtained from arterial blood. Peritoneal bath [Lactate] = 40 mM. Data from Feriani M. Use of different buffers in peritoneal dialysis. Semin Dial 2000;13:256–260.

a mild acidosis with an appropriate secondary respiratory response. Patients receiving peritoneal dialysis have average values for serum [total CO_2] in the normal range, but arterial acid–base measurements in these patients also show a very mild acidosis.

Diagnosis and Management of Acid–Base Disorders

The nephrologist caring for patients receiving dialysis therapy has two tasks with regard to their acid–base status. The first task is to identify patients with either persistently low values for serum [total CO_2] (less than 20 mEq/L) or persistently high values for serum [total CO_2] (greater than 26 mEq/L) and to determine whether treatment modification can improve this situation. The second task is to uncover superimposed acid–base disturbances. In making either assessment, serum samples for total CO_2 must be processed and run in a timely fashion. Shipment of blood samples to a distant laboratory and delay in analysis may spuriously reduce the value by as much as 5 mEq/L.

The Patient With a Persistently Low Serum [Total CO₂] Level

Dialysis patients with predialysis or steady-state serum [total CO_2] values less than 20 mEq/L are at increased risk for muscle catabolism and for worsening renal osteodystrophy. Those with predialysis values less than 19 mEq/L have a higher mortality risk. In patients receiving intermittent hemodialysis with a low predialysis serum [total CO_2], one should first assess whether the treatment is effectively increasing serum [total CO_2] by measuring a post-dialysis level. In a small minority of patients, typically those with severe hypotension during the procedure, organic acid (presumably lactic acid) production can consume virtually all of the added HCO_3^-.

If the treatment is effective, assessment of protein and fluid intake should be undertaken (patient characteristics in Table 43.1), and appropriate modifications instituted. If these measures fail, increasing bath [HCO_3^-] by 1 to 4 mEq/L will increase predialysis serum [total CO_2] in most patients, with the caveat that higher bath [HCO_3^-] may by itself increase mortality risk. Management is more difficult in patients receiving peritoneal dialysis. If nutritional measures fail, the only option is to switch back to hemodialysis or to a bicarbonate-containing peritoneal dialysis solution.

The Patient With a Persistently High Serum [Total CO₂] Level

Predialysis serum [total CO_2] values >26 mEq/L are associated with an increased mortality risk, but this risk appears to be correlated with nutritional and inflammatory factors rather than the prescribed dialysis treatment. There is no evidence to suggest that lowering bath [HCO_3^-] will influence this risk. Instead, attention should be focused on the patient's nutrition and causes of inflammation.

Identifying Superimposed Acid–Base Disorders

The presence of a superimposed metabolic acid–base disorder in a patient receiving dialysis therapy can be brought to one's attention by a change or new abnormality

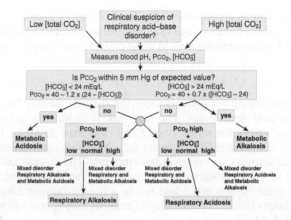

Figure 43.2

Approach to the Diagnosis and Characterization of Acid–Base Disorders in Dialysis Patients. See text for definitions of high and low serum [total CO₂]. (Adapted from Gennari FJ. Acid-base considerations in end-stage renal disease. In WL Henrich, ed. Principles and Practice of Dialysis. Baltimore: Lippincott, Williams, & Wilkins 2003:402.)

in serum [total CO_2] (Fig. 43.2). By contrast, respiratory disorders can only be suspected from clinical signs and symptoms. Serum [total CO_2] varies widely among dialysis patients. Fortunately, this parameter is usually measured on a regular basis, allowing a baseline for comparison. Assessment of a suspected new acid–base disorder involves the same three steps as in patients with functioning kidneys:

1. Identification of the primary disorder (i.e., metabolic acidosis or alkalosis, respiratory acidosis or alkalosis).
2. Assessment of the secondary response, in order to determine whether the disorder is simple or mixed (simultaneous presence of two or more acid–base disorders).
3. Determination of the cause. For this last step, assessment of whether the anion gap has changed is useful.

Steps 1 and 2 require measurement of arterial P_{CO_2} and pH and calculation of $[HCO_3^-]$. In patients with functioning fistulas or synthetic grafts, a separate arterial puncture is not required for this measurement. Blood from fistulas or grafts is equivalent to arterial blood.

Rules for Identification of the Primary Disturbance in Dialysis Patients

- Metabolic acidosis: Serum [total CO_2] lower than the usual value by 3 mEq/L or more.
- Metabolic alkalosis: Serum [total CO_2] higher than the usual value by 3 mEq/L or more.
- Respiratory acidosis: Arterial P_{CO_2} higher than predicted for the prevailing serum $[HCO_3^-]$ by 5 mm Hg or more (see equations following).
- Respiratory alkalosis: Arterial P_{CO_2} lower than predicted for the prevailing serum $[HCO_3^-]$ by 5 mm Hg or more (see equations following).

Evaluation of the Secondary Response

Arterial P_{CO_2} responds to changes in serum [HCO_3^-] in dialysis patients in the same fashion as in individuals with normal renal function. Thus, the rules of thumb are the same.

- For serum [HCO_3^-] <24 mEq/L: Arterial P_{CO_2} (mm Hg) = 40 – 1.2 × (24 – serum [HCO_3^-])
- For serum [HCO_3^-] >24 mEq/L: Arterial P_{CO_2} (mm Hg) = 40 + 0.7 × (serum [HCO_3^-] – 24)

In contrast to patients with functioning kidneys, serum [HCO_3^-] does not change in response to changes in P_{CO_2}. As discussed previously, it is fixed primarily by the dialysis prescription and by endogenous acid production. Thus, there is no secondary change in serum [HCO_3^-] in response to hypocapnia or hypercapnia.

Causes of Acid–Base Disorders

Metabolic Acidosis

Although many patients receiving dialysis therapy have a chronic stable mild metabolic acidosis, a key management issue is to recognize the development of a new and more severe metabolic acidosis; that is, a further reduction in serum [total CO_2] (see previous rules for recognition). Assessment in these patients should include measurement of the anion gap, $[Na^+] – ([Cl^-] + [HCO_3^-])$, to determine whether it is increased. For this assessment, one should compare the value obtained with the most recent value prior to development of acidosis. If serum albumin has also changed significantly, one must adjust the anion gap for this change. The causes of metabolic acidosis are outlined in Table 43.4.

Virtually all of the causes of a superimposed metabolic acidosis in patients receiving dialysis therapy produce an increase in the anion gap. The most common cause is diabetic ketoacidosis. In contrast to patients with functioning kidneys, fluid and alkali replacement are unnecessary for treatment. In the absence of kidney function,

---

Table 43.4

Causes of Metabolic Acidosis in Dialysis Patients

Increased Anion Gap
Endogenous causes
    Diabetic ketoacidosis
    Lactic acidosis
    Alcoholic ketoacidosis
    Increased endogenous acid production (high protein intake or catabolic state)
Toxin ingestions
    Methyl alcohol
    Ethylene glycol
    Salicylates
    Paraldehyde

No Increase in Anion Gap
Gastrointestinal alkali loss
    Expansion acidosis

no fluid or ketoanion losses occur. Insulin therapy rapidly leads to metabolism of the retained ketoanions, regenerating the HCO_3^- consumed, and quickly restores serum $[HCO_3^-]$ to the premorbid level. With other organic acidoses, dialysis removes the offending toxins and replenishes alkali stores quickly.

If the anion gap is not increased, only two causes need to be considered. The first cause is gastrointestinal alkali loss. Such losses are straightforward to diagnose and can be replaced rapidly by dialysis at the same time losses are curtailed by therapeutic intervention. The second cause is excessive fluid volume expansion with salt and water. As outlined in Table 43.2, predialysis serum [total CO_2] is inversely related to fluid retention between treatments. The effect is usually only a mild reduction in serum [total CO_2]. Iatrogenic volume expansion with isotonic saline in these patients will produce the same effect.

Metabolic Alkalosis

A new metabolic alkalosis may be missed in patients receiving dialysis treatment because serum [total CO_2] may still be in the normal range for patients with functioning kidneys. For example, in a dialysis patient with a steady-state serum [total CO_2] of 21 mEq/L, a sudden increase to 26 mEq/L indicates the development of a metabolic alkalosis. Hypokalemia, a characteristic feature of metabolic alkalosis in patients with functioning kidneys, does not occur. Moreover, dialysis patients have no way to excrete excess alkali added to the body. Once metabolic alkalosis is induced, it is sustained by the dialysis procedure itself, which does not remove HCO_3^- unless serum [total CO_2] is greater than 35–40 mEq/L.

None of the renal causes of metabolic alkalosis (e.g., aldosterone adenoma, Bartter syndrome) can produce this disorder in patients without kidney function. Metabolic alkalosis has only two causes in dialysis patients: gastrointestinal HCl loss and excess alkali administration. The most common cause of metabolic alkalosis is vomiting or nasogastric suction. In patients without kidney function such losses can lead to severe and sustained alkalosis. An increase in serum [total CO_2] may be the key to identifying the presence of bulimia in a dialysis patient.

A sometimes-overlooked cause is exogenous alkali administration. In addition to sodium bicarbonate ingestion (e.g., Alka-Seltzer, baking soda), a common source is organic anion administration. Citrate, lactate, acetate, and other organic anions given in various parenteral solutions can all increase serum [total CO_2]. Discontinuation or a reduction in the amount given will correct or ameliorate the disorder. Metabolic alkalosis in the intensive care unit is often caused by daily hemodialysis in patients with low rates of endogenous acid production, or by excess HCO_3^- or lactate replacement in patients receiving continuous renal replacement therapy. The combination of sodium polystyrene sulfonate (Kayexalate, Sterling Drug) and aluminum hydroxide can cause metabolic alkalosis by acting together to bind H^+ in the stomach.

Rapid reduction in serum [total CO_2] is rarely required for the treatment of metabolic alkalosis. Hemodialysis limits the increase to about 35 mEq/L unless H^+ losses are very large. If rapid removal is necessary, bath $[HCO_3^-]$ can be reduced to facilitate alkali loss during hemodialysis. Alternatively, one can institute continuous venovenous hemofiltration and use only saline for replacement fluid.

Respiratory Acidosis

Detection of respiratory acidosis requires clinical suspicion and measurement of arterial pH and P_{CO_2} is necessary to confirm the diagnosis (Fig. 43.2). Serum [total

CO_2] does not increase in response to hypercapnia in patients receiving dialysis therapy. Even the small increase normally engendered by the buffer response to hypercapnia may be modified by the dialysis treatment. With the exception of the patient on a ventilator with fixed minute ventilation in whom an increase in CO_2 generation can increase arterial Pco_2, respiratory acidosis is caused by pulmonary insufficiency. Thus, the first approach to management should always be an attempt to improve ventilation. If ventilation cannot be improved, increasing serum $[HCO_3^-]$ can mitigate the acidemia. To achieve this goal, bath $[HCO_3^-]$ can be increased or the patient switched to peritoneal dialysis.

Respiratory Alkalosis

Hypocapnia induces severe alkalemia in patients receiving dialysis therapy because there is no secondary renal response, and the body buffer response is reversed by alkali addition during treatment. Diagnosis requires clinical suspicion and measurement of arterial pH and Pco_2. Respiratory alkalosis has multiple causes, including hypoxemia, anxiety, central nervous system disease, pulmonary disease, and hepatic failure. Correction of the cause of the hypocapnia, if possible, is the first approach to treatment. If the alkalemia is severe (pH >7.65), arterial Pco_2 should be increased acutely using a rebreathing device. Sustained hypocapnia is more difficult to manage. The only option is to dialyze the patient against a bath with a low $[HCO_3^-]$, but chronic hyperventilation is a very poor prognostic indicator and no therapy is very effective.

Mixed Acid–Base Disorders

Two or more acid–base disorders can coexist in patients receiving dialysis therapy, but the occurrence of such mixed disorders is rare. Mixed disorders are diagnosed by demonstrating that the secondary response to a given acid–base disorder is either less than or greater than that predicted by the rules presented previously (Fig. 43.2). Table 43.5 lists the possible mixed disorders in dialysis patients. The importance of detecting the presence of more than one disorder lies in the approach to management. For example, the presence of metabolic acidosis (low serum $[HCO_3^-]$) and respiratory acidosis (arterial Pco_2 not appropriately reduced) requires that attention be directed to the patient's ventilatory status as well as correcting the metabolic acidosis.

Table 43.5

Mixed Acid–Base Disorders in Dialysis Patients

Mixed Metabolic and Respiratory Acid–Base Disorders

Metabolic acidosis $[HCO_3^-]$ ↓
    + respiratory acidosis Pco_2 ≥ 5 mm Hg or more above expected value[a]
    + respiratory alkalosis Pco_2 ≤ 5 mm Hg or more below expected value
Metabolic alkalosis $[HCO_3^-]$ ↑
    + respiratory acidosis Pco_2 ≥ 5 mm Hg or more above expected value
    + respiratory alkalosis Pco_2 ≤ 5 mm Hg or more below expected value
Mixed metabolic acidosis and alkalosis
    Anion gap ↓ without equivalent ↑ in serum $[HCO_3^-]$

---

[a]See Fig. 43.2 for formulas defining appropriate Pco_2 for any given serum $[HCO_3^-]$.

Nutritional Management of Dialysis Patients

SECTION XVI

Nutritional Management of Dialysis Patients

C H A P T E R 4 4

Nutritional Management of Hemodialysis Patients

T. Alp Ikizler, MD • Serpil Muge Deger, MD

Introduction

One of the most commonly encountered complications of end-stage renal disease (ESRD), especially for patients undergoing maintenance hemodialysis (MHD), is the subtle but clinically important progressive deterioration of nutritional status. Advanced chronic kidney disease (CKD) leads to a unique state of metabolic and nutritional derangements, more aptly called protein–energy wasting (PEW). PEW is closely associated with major adverse clinical outcomes such as increased rates of hospitalization and death in MHD patients. PEW is complicated and includes a number of clinically relevant aspects that require special attention. These include, but are not limited to, how to appropriately screen and assess nutritional status, implement preventive measures, and prescribe effective interventions.

Screening and Assessment of Nutritional Status in MHD

A clinically meaningful assessment of nutrition and metabolic status should be able to identify and risk-stratify patients with PEW, distinguishing the causes and consequences of both PEW and the underlying disease states, and determine whether there is potential benefit from nutritional or metabolic interventions. Therefore, no single nutritional marker is likely to adequately phenotype this highly complicated comorbid state requiring several concurrent or consecutive measurements (Table 44.1). It is recommended that MHD patients should undergo routine screening tests that are easy to perform, readily available, and inexpensive. Screening parameters should be collected routinely in clinical practice by any health professional and mostly provide a trigger to conduct more extensive assessment, to confirm or establish the diagnosis and determine the best course of treatment, if needed. The most commonly used screening tests in MHD patients are serum albumin concentration and assessment of body weight especially immediately following hemodialysis (i.e., estimated dry weight). Any clinically meaningful change in these metrics is adequate to initiate a more thorough workup. On the other hand, nutritional assessment generally requires extensive training, provides comprehensive information to make a nutritional diagnosis, to aid in intervention and monitoring planning, and should be performed by qualified individuals, preferably dietitians. Most commonly used tests in MHD patients include serum prealbumin concentration, assessment of dietary nutrient intake, anthropometric measures, and subjective global assessment. These tests should also be used for guiding nutritional therapies once the patient is deemed to be at risk or has overt PEW. A diagnosis of PEW necessitates confirmation by several tools and can be as strict as requirement of multiple findings as suggested by the

Table 44.1	

Suggested Strategies to Screen and Assess Nutritional Status in Advanced CKD

Screening	Threshold for Detailed Assessment
Body weight	Continuous decline or <85% IBW
Dietary nutrient intake	DEI <25 kcal/kg IBW/d
	DPI <0.8 g/kg IBW/d
Serum albumin	<4.0 g/dL
Serum creatinine	Relatively low value
MST	>2

Assessment	Threshold for Intervention
Serum prealbumin	<28 mg/dL
hsCRP	>10 mg/dL
Anthropometrics	Deviation from norms
SGA	B or C (moderately or severely malnourished)
MIS	>5

Diagnosis (2 of the 4)[a]	Threshold for Intervention
Serum chemistry	
Albumin	<3.8 g/dL
Prealbumin	<28 mg/dL*
Cholesterol	<100 mg/dL
Body mass	
BMI	<23
Weight loss	>5% over 3 months or 10% over 6 months
Total body fat %	<10%
Muscle mass	
Muscle wasting	>5% over 3 months or 10% over 6 months
Reduced MAMC	>10% reduction compared to norms
Creatinine appearance	<1 g/kg/IBW
Dietary intake	
Low DPI	DPI <0.8 g/kg IBW/d
Low DEI	DEI <25 kcal/kg IBW/d

DEI, dietary energy intake; DPI, dietary protein intake; hsCRP, high sensitivity C-reactive protein; IBW, ideal body weight; MIS, malnutrition–inflammation score; MST, Malnutrition Screening Tool; SGA, subjective global assessment.
[a]Based on International Society of Nutrition and Metabolism Criteria, Fouque et al, 2008; *influenced by kidney function.
Adapted from Ikizler, T.A. A patient with CKD and poor nutritional status. Clin J Am Soc Nephrol 2013;8:2174-2182.

International Society of Renal Nutrition and Metabolism (ISRNM) criteria or could be less specific as suggested by others. It is also important that a number of considerations must be made on the unique situation of CKD patients for appropriate screening and assessment of their nutritional status. Some of these include the fluid status of the patient, which could alter body composition and biochemical markers, presence of systemic inflammation that could change serum concentrations of acute phase proteins, presence and the extent of proteinuria, a major determinant of serum albumin concentrations and the level of residual renal function, which could influence serum concentration of some biochemical markers such as prealbumin that are cleared by the kidneys.

Epidemiology of PEW in MHD Patients

Virtually every study evaluating the nutritional status of MHD patients reports some degree of protein and energy depletion. The clinical relevance of these observations is that practically every nutritional marker used in this patient population has been associated with hospitalization and death risk. Of note, most of the epidemiologic reports on nutrition in MHD patients have been mainly based on serum albumin concentrations, especially studies in large cohorts. Smaller studies using other nutritional markers such as serum prealbumin and SGA also are suggestive of increased risk associated with poor nutritional status in MHD patients. These observations are reproducible irrespective of patient demographics and geographic area. Because of the many different diagnostic tools utilized in separate studies, the prevalence of PEW in this patient population varies widely among different reports, ranging from 20% to 60%. Although there is evidence of improvement in nutritional parameters within 3 to 6 months following initiation of maintenance hemodialysis, PEW is still present in up to 40% or more of those patients and the prevalence seems to increase as the time on dialysis extends. Recent epidemiologic data also indicate a survival benefit with improvement in these markers over time.

Results from large cohort studies suggest a higher prevalence of hypoalbuminemia in the United States compared with other countries. Whereas the lowest mean serum albumin level was observed in the United Kingdom for Europe, the U.S. value was significantly lower than in all European countries (3.60 vs 3.72 g/dL [36 vs 37 g/L]). Overall, Japan had significantly higher serum albumin concentrations compared with other countries. More recent data showed that 20.5% of U.S. patients had a serum albumin level less than 3.5 g/dL (35 g/L). Results from the DOPPS also showed a prevalence ranging from 7.6% (United States) to 18% (France) for moderately malnourished and 2.3% (Italy) to 11% (United States) for severely malnourished MHD patients as diagnosed by subjective global assessment (SGA).

Etiology and Prevention of PEW in MHD Patients

A large number of factors affect nutritional and metabolic status in CKD patients leading to multiple adverse consequences (Fig. 44.1). Accordingly, prevention and treatment of PEW in CKD should involve an integrated approach to reduce protein and energy depletion, in addition to therapies that will avoid further losses and replenish already wasted stores.

Dietary Nutrient Intake

A frequent and important cause of PEW in MHD patients is inadequate dietary protein and energy intake relative to the needs, primarily due to uremic anorexia. The spontaneous decrease in dietary protein and energy intake seen in nondialysis CKD patients usually improves once maintenance dialysis is commenced. Nevertheless, a significant portion of MHD patients could still suffer from anorexia as a result of inadequate dialysis and retention of uremic toxins, intercurrent illnesses, chronic systemic inflammation, and depression. Of note, some of the dietary restrictions are

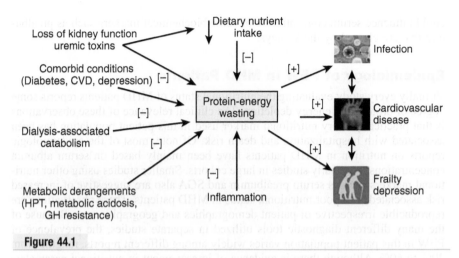

Figure 44.1

The Etiology and Consequences of Protein Energy Wasting in Kidney Disease. GH, growth hormone, HPT, hyperparathyroidism.

continued in an attempt to prevent hyperphosphatemia, hyperkalemia, or metabolic acidosis even if the CKD patients are initiated on maintenance dialysis. It is therefore imperative to identify these potential factors and treat the root cause before prescribing aggressive nutritional supplementation.

Increased Catabolism Due to Renal Replacement Therapy

Provision of an adequate dialysis dose has long been considered as a cornerstone among measures to prevent and treat PEW in maintenance dialysis patients and a minimum dose of dialysis has been recommended to avoid uremic anorexia and maintain optimal dietary nutrient intake. Data from RCTs in MHD (HEMO study) and PD (ADEMEX Trial) patients indicate that what is currently considered adequate dialysis in various guidelines is sufficient to preserve the nutritional status although the HEMO study showed that MHD patients lose weight over time regardless of "adequate" dialysis dose. Increasing dialysis dose beyond the targets studied in these trials has not been shown to improve the nutritional status any further. In addition, in the HEMO and MPO trials most nutritional parameters studied did not differ among patients exposed to different dialysis membranes (i.e., high-flux vs low-flux) although there was a nominally significant survival benefit in patients with baseline serum albumin levels <40 g/dL (prespecified analysis) and with diabetes mellitus (DM) (post hoc analysis) randomized to high-flux dialysis in the latter. The results of the Frequent Hemodialysis Network Trial indicate no appreciable difference in nutritional markers between subjects randomized to 6×/week in-center HD versus standard 3×/week in-center HD.

Nutrient losses through hemodialysis membranes (6–8 g per HD session), loss of renal residual function due to long-term dialysis treatment, increased inflammation due to indwelling catheters, bioincompatible hemodialysis membranes, and peritoneal dialysis solutions could also lead to an overly catabolic milieu and increase the minimal amount of nutrient intake needed to maintain a neutral nitrogen balance. In patients who cannot compensate for this increased need, a state of semistarvation ensues leading to the development or worsening of PEW. One potential strategy to prevent the immediate protein catabolic effects of hemodialysis is to allow stable patients to consume a reasonable amount of regular meals during hemodialysis. This practice has shown to be safe in multiple settings and is a routine process except in a few countries such as the United States and Canada.

Chronic Inflammation

Systemic inflammation is a major contributor to PEW in MHD patients (Fig. 44.2). Increased levels of inflammatory cytokines such as interleukin-1 (IL-1), interleukin-6 (IL-6), and tumor necrosis factor-alpha (TNF-α) play a crucial role in the exaggerated protein and energy catabolism, resulting in sarcopenia and frailty in chronic disease states. Despite convincing data in animals, there are very limited studies examining the mechanisms and nature of inflammation-induced catabolism in MHD patients. In addition to increasing protein breakdown, the chronic inflammatory state is associated with reduced physical activity, impaired insulin, and growth hormone actions and may also contribute to anorexia because of its central effects.

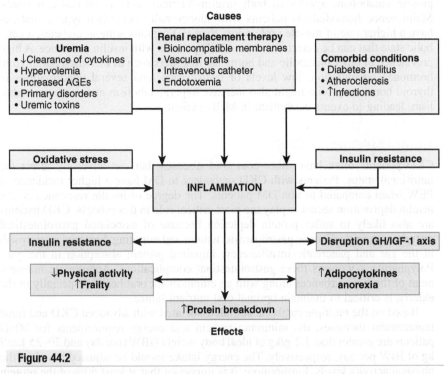

Figure 44.2

Proposed Etiology of Systemic Inflammation in Kidney Disease and Its Adverse Effects Leading to Protein Energy Wasting.

The initial step for treatment of persistent inflammation should be elimination of etiologic factors such as the use of central hemodialysis catheters in MHD patients. As the dialysis procedure per se might stimulate the immune system, proinflammatory effects of dialysis membranes and fluids should also be taken into account in maintenance dialysis patients. Many uremic toxins are also known to be proinflammatory. Current dialytic strategies are inadequate for their removal, and alternative removal techniques, such as strategies to modify intestinal generation or absorption, are necessary. Appropriate management of fluid status might improve systemic inflammation in ESRD patients as well. Volume overload leads to immunoactivation and increased cytokine production via bacterial or endotoxin translocation.

Metabolic Acidosis and Hormonal Derangements

Metabolic acidosis is associated with increased muscle protein catabolism and promotes PEW in patients with advanced CKD. There are a number of studies indicating improvement in nutritional status with oral bicarbonate supplementation in CKD patients. Recent epidemiologic data indicate adverse outcomes with high predialysis serum bicarbonate levels, requiring a target of 22–24 mmol/L in MHD patients in order to avoid alkalosis after hemodialysis.

Resistance to insulin and to the growth hormone (GH)/IGF-1 axis are two key endocrine abnormalities implicated in loss of muscle mass in CKD patients. Enhanced protein catabolism applies to both insulin-deficient and insulin-resistant states. Maintenance hemodialysis patients with suboptimally controlled type 2 diabetes have a higher rate of muscle protein loss than HD patients without diabetes, a catabolic state that can be detected even in MHD patients with insulin resistance. A high prevalence of other metabolic and hormonal disorders such as increased parathyroid hormone concentration, low levels of testosterone, and several abnormalities in thyroid hormone profile might also increase hypermetabolism and decrease anabolism, leading to excess catabolism in MHD patients.

Comorbidities in CKD

CKD patients often have other comorbid diseases that can adversely affect the nutritional status. Patients with CKD secondary to DM have a higher incidence of PEW when compared to non-DM patients. The degree of insulin resistance and/or insulin deprivation seems to play the most critical role in this process. CKD patients are also likely to suffer protein depletion because of associated gastrointestinal disturbances (e.g., diabetic gastroparesis, nausea and vomiting, bacterial overgrowth in the gut and pancreatic insufficiency, impaired protein absorption in the gut). Polypharmacy worsens these gastrointestinal complications. Appropriate management of these disturbances along with an emphasis on oral health, especially in the elderly, is critical to maintain optimal oral nutrient intake.

Based on the multiple catabolic stimuli associated with advanced CKD and renal replacement therapies, the minimum protein and energy requirements for MHD patients are greater than 1.2 g/kg of ideal body weight (IBW) per day and 30–35 kcal/kg of IBW per day, respectively. The energy intake should be adjusted based on the physical activity levels. Furthermore, it is important that at least 50% of the protein intake should be of high biologic value. An important consideration regarding strategies to improve dietary protein intake in MHD patients is the potential increase in the intake of several potentially harmful elements, especially phosphorus. Dietary recommendations to improve protein intake should take into account the phosphorus content of the specific protein sources (i.e., vegetarian diet leading to lower serum phosphorus levels) and other phosphorus-containing nutrients especially ones with additives/preservatives in processed food.

Treatment of PEW in MHD Patients

Oral and Enteral Nutritional Supplementation

In certain MHD patients, the aforementioned standard preventive measures are unable to diminish loss of protein and energy stores. In these circumstances, nutritional supplementation is a suitable next step with appropriate indications (Fig. 44.3). Oral supplementation should be given two to three times a day, preferably 1 hour after main meals and/or during dialysis for MHD patients. Oral supplementation can provide an additional 7–10 kcal/kg per day of energy and 0.3–0.4 g/kg per day of protein. This requires a minimum spontaneous dietary intake of 20 kcal/kg per day of energy and 0.4–0.8 g/kg per day of protein in order to meet the recommended dietary energy intake (DEI) and dietary protein intake (DPI) targets.

The efficacy of oral supplementation has been studied in multiple settings. The beneficial nutritional effects of these supplements ranged from improvements in serum biomarkers such as albumin, prealbumin, and transferrin to gains in different body compartments such as weight and lean body mass. The effects were evident as early as within a month and were sustained in most if not all studies. There were also improvements in quality of life and physical functioning. In several of these studies, improvements in hospitalizations and death were reported but none of the studies had the statistical power to appropriately assess the efficacy of these interventions. For patients who are unable to tolerate nutritional supplementation by mouth, nasogastric tubes, percutaneous endoscopic gastroscopy or jejunostomy tubes can be considered. Tube feeding is most often used in conditions such as severe anorexia, swallowing troubles secondary to neurologic or head and neck diseases, perioperative periods, and stress.

Two recent large-scale observational studies reported significant survival benefit in favor of hypoalbuminemic MHD patients receiving nutritional supplementation versus similarly matched controls. Specifically, in a retrospective cohort study of 4289 matched pairs, death rates were 30.9% versus 37.3% in treated versus historically matched untreated groups, respectively. In a prospective observational study, the effects of an oral nutritional supplementation (ONS) program performed as part of a disease management plan were reported in 276 MHD patients who received supplements versus 194 MHD patients who did not receive ONS because they were deemed inappropriate or refused. ONS use was associated with higher serum albumin and lower hospitalization at 1 year, but there was no significant reduction in mortality risk in this study. The limitations of these studies include their retrospective design, convenience sampling, and residual confounding from unmeasured variables. Parenteral provision of nutrients, especially during the HD procedure (i.e., IDPN), has been shown to be a safe and convenient approach for individuals who cannot tolerate oral or enteral administration of nutrients (see Chapter 46).

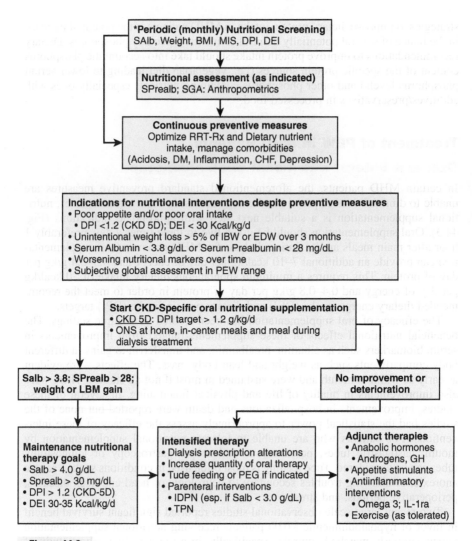

Figure 44.3

Algorithm for Nutritional Management and Support in Patients With Chronic Kidney Disease. *Minimum every 3 months, monthly screening recommended. ^Only for ESRD patients without residual renal function. BMI, body mass index; CHF, congestive heart failure; CKD, chronic kidney disease; DEI, dietary energy intake; DM, diabetes mellitus; DPI, dietary protein intake; GH, growth hormone; IDPN, intradialytic parenteral nutrition; IL-1ra, interleukin-1 receptor antagonist; LBM, lean body mass; MIS, malnutrition–inflammation score; ONS, oral nutritional supplement; PEG, percutaneous endoscopic gastrostomy; PEW, protein energy wasting; RRT-Rx, renal replacement therapy prescription; SAlb, serum albumin (measured by bromocresol green); SGA, subjective global assessment; SPrealb, serum prealbumin; TPN, total parenteral nutrition. (Used with permission from Ikizler TA, et al, Prevention and treatment of protein energy wasting in chronic kidney disease patients: a consensus statement by the International Society of Renal Nutrition and Metabolism. Kidney Int 2013;84(6):1096-107.)

Anabolic Hormones

Recombinant human growth hormone (rhGH), an approved treatment for short stature in pediatric CKD patients, leads to improved growth, confirming that rhGH could overcome the GH resistance associated with CKD. In adults with CKD, resistance to native GH may be responsible for the premature decline in body composition. In a large multicenter RCT, significant decreases were observed in C-reactive protein (CRP) and homocysteine levels along with increases in serum high-density lipoprotein (HDL) cholesterol and transferrin levels in hypoalbuminemic MHD patients in the rhGH group. Unfortunately, this large RCT was prematurely terminated due to slow recruitment, without the ability to assess the effects rhGH has on hospitalization or death.

Testosterone deficiency is also very common in male MHD patients and is associated with increased mortality risk. Several RCTs performed in MHD patients showed significant benefits of nandrolone decanoate (ND) treatment on both anthropometric and biochemical parameters, including body weight, body mass index, skinfold, MAMC, and serum levels of total protein, prealbumin, and transferrin. No consistent effect of ND was demonstrated on physical functioning in several studies, and high-dose ND (100 mg/week) was poorly tolerated in females because of its virilizing effects. In clinical practice, anabolic steroids could be used for preventing sarcopenia, albeit under close supervision, and such use should be limited to 6 months.

Exercise

Abnormalities in muscle function, exercise performance, and physical activity begin in the early stages of CKD and progress dramatically as ESRD develops. In MHD patients, there are metabolic and structural muscle abnormalities, with reductions in oxidative capacity and type 1 fibers with associated decrease in muscular endurance. Although a number of studies have examined the effects of cardiopulmonary fitness training in MHD patients, relatively few studies have examined the role of exercise training on stimulating muscle growth. Collectively, the available data indicate that the presumed beneficial effects of exercise such as improvements in muscle quality and quantity, strength, and physical functioning are not consistently observed in ESRD patients. The possible explanations for the limited efficacy of exercise in CKD patients include the limitations of methods to assess body composition, inadequate intensity and/or duration of exercise, and the lack of understanding of the actual metabolic and morphologic abnormalities related to PEW in the setting of advanced CKD.

Emerging Therapies

Antiinflammatory Agents

The fact that systemic inflammation leads to an exaggerated protein catabolic response has suggested that treatment with specific and nonspecific antiinflammatory agents as a novel strategy to prevent development or worsening of PEW in kidney disease patients might be effective. Although a limited number of studies have shown the beneficial effects of these approaches on markers of systemic inflammation, only a few have extended these to nutritional outcomes. Biolo et al investigated the effect of pentoxifylline on whole body protein turnover and reported a significant decrease in protein breakdown and also net positive anabolic effect when pentoxifylline was combined along with amino acid administration. Tietze et al documented that the administration of supplemental fish oil (8 g daily) up to 6 months somewhat improved nutritional status. A recent pilot study of 3 g daily of omega-3 administration showed significant improvements in protein breakdown rates in MHD patients. Although current data are intriguing, further long-term studies are warranted to determine the reproducible effects of antiinflammatory strategies on prevention or treatment of PEW in advanced CKD patients.

Appetite Stimulants

Ghrelin is a stomach-derived growth hormone–releasing hormone that stimulates appetite via the central nervous system. Administration of ghrelin has been shown to increase muscle mass in experimental animal studies. Longer-term ghrelin administration resulted in net positive energy balance in an elderly population demonstrating that it may be an alternative agent for treatment of PEW in CKD patients. In animal models of CKD, ghrelin administration resulted in increased appetite and decreased muscle protein degradation. In a pilot study, administration of subcutaneous ghrelin administration resulted in increased appetite in 9 PD patients with PEW, suggesting that future clinical trials of longer-term administration of ghrelin could reveal intriguing results in advanced CKD patients at risk for PEW. Appetite stimulants such as megestrol acetate, melatonin, cyproheptadine, and dronabinol have long been used for improving appetite in MHD patients although their efficacy has not been systematically examined.

Summary and Recommendations

Because of its metabolic and functional importance in whole-body homeostasis, preservation of muscle mass is the ultimate goal in the management of PEW in MHD patients. In MHD patients, in whom a number of catabolic signals dominate, it is critical to maintain a dietary protein and energy intake relative to needs. Preemptive treatment of concurrent conditions that contribute to catabolism, such as metabolic acidosis, insulin resistance, and systemic inflammation is of paramount importance for the prevention of PEW. When supplemental nutrition is indicated, it is crucial to take into account all the determinants of body and muscle mass: protein and energy content, exercise, anabolizing hormones, antioxidants and antiinflammatory nutrients or drugs, and other specific nutrients. Finally, it is important to assess the impact of nutritional supplements not only in terms of changes in nutritional parameters but to translate these observations into potential improvements in hospitalization, mortality, and cost-effectiveness. It should be noted that although numerous epidemiologic data suggest that an improvement in biomarkers of nutritional status is associated with improved clinical outcomes such as hospitalization and mortality, there are no large adequately powered randomized clinical trials that have tested the effectiveness of nutritional interventions on morbidity and mortality.

CHAPTER 45

Intradialytic Parenteral Nutrition and Intraperitoneal Nutrition

Ramanath Dukkipati, MD • Kamyar Kalantar-Zadeh, MD, MPH, PhD

Introduction

Protein–energy wasting (PEW) is common in patients undergoing dialysis and is one of the strongest risk factors for death. The prevalence of PEW in observational studies ranges from 18% to 75%. The presence of PEW is indicated by a number of signs, symptoms, and biomarkers, including decreased body mass index (BMI) and muscle mass and reduced serum levels of albumin and transthyretin (prealbumin), increased markers of inflammation and decreased food intake and appetite.

Inadequate protein and energy intake and inflammatory disorders are the most common and dominant causes of PEW in maintenance dialysis patients. This led to the hypothesis that nutritional support can potentially prevent or minimize PEW and can also improve quality of life along with reduction of morbidity and mortality. Indeed it is argued that even if inadequate nutritional intake is not the primary cause of PEW in CKD, enteral and parenteral nutritional support can still provide an important corrective and supportive intervention, similar to the nutritional support in cancer cachexia that is per se due to inflammation and oxidative stress and not inadequate dietary intake. Unintentional weight loss harbors increased mortality over time, but increasing nutritional intake has not been shown to reduce mortality risk in randomized prospective clinical trials. Nevertheless, the search for interventions to reduce high mortality in dialysis patients is of utmost importance in changing the natural history of survival in these patients.

Intradialytic Parenteral Nutrition (IDPN)

IDPN solutions are commonly prepared from base solutions. The base solutions for amino acids, carbohydrates, and lipids can vary in concentrations. Up to 10% of essential and nonessential amino acids, 50% or 70% D-glucose and 10%–20% lipids, or IDPN can also be prepared lipid free. Trace elements, vitamins, and selected minerals can be included. IDPN solutions can be tailored to individual patient needs. When IDPN is given, it is initiated at the beginning of hemodialysis and is infused into the venous line distal to the dialyzer. The infusion is usually planned to be completed about 25–30 minutes before the end of the hemodialysis session.

Components of commonly prescribed oral nutritional supplements are presented in Table 45.1, and typical components of IDPN solution are presented in Table 45.2.

Table 45.1

Typical IDPN Formulations

Dextrose Infusion Rates	Lipids	Protein Infusion Rates

Moderate to high
  Carbohydrate controlled
    4–6 mg/kg/minute
  Non–carbohydrate controlled
    6–8 mg/kg/minute
	4 mg/kg/minute
	or
	12–12.5 g/hour
		1.2%–1.6%

Low ≤3 mg/kg/minute	4 mg/kg/minute or 12–12.5 g/hour	1.2%–1.6%
Low ≤3 mg/kg/minute	No lipids	1.2%–1.6%

Table 45.2

Currently Available Oral Nutritional Formulations

	Total Carbohydrates (g)	Total Protein (g)	Total Fat (g)	Total Calories (kcal)	kcal/mL
Nepro (240 mL)	39.4	19.1	22.7	425	1.8
Nepro (1000 mL)	166.8	81	96	1800	1.8
Boost glucose control (237 mL)	20	14	12	250	1.06
Boost glucose control (1000 mL)	84	58.2	49.4	1060	1.06
Boost (240 mL)	41	10	4	240	1.0

Limitations of Clinical Trials of IDPN therapy

The experimental design of nearly all published studies conducted on IDPN has limitations. These include inadequate statistical power due to limited sample size, absence of a control group, and lack of rigorous description and use of inclusion and exclusion criteria to select patients with PEW. The dose of dialysis that patients received in the studies was not standardized and also was not clearly described. The length of IDPN therapy was not of adequate duration to draw firm conclusions regarding the effectiveness of IDPN. Follow-up periods were often brief. The intake of oral nutritional supplements or the intake of food was not standardized and was not well described. Because of these limitations, definitive conclusions regarding the effectiveness of IDPN cannot be drawn. Selected nonrandomized studies are summarized in Table 45.3, and randomized studies are summarized in Table 45.4.

Nonrandomized Studies of IDPN

Heidland and Kult in 1975 published the first report describing the use of IDPN therapy during a 60-week study period in 18 patients receiving maintenance hemo-dialysis three times a week. Patients were given 16.7 g of essential amino acids,

Table 45.3

Nonrandomized Studies in IDPN

Study	Design	Treatment Duration	No. With PEW	Parameters Measured	Outcome
Heidland and Kult 1975	18 pts; 16.75 g EAA, 100 kcal; no control	60 weeks	Most did not	Alb, total protein, complement levels, transferrin	Increase in Alb, total protein, transferrin, complement levels after 16 weeks' therapy in 13 pts. When therapy was discontinued for 6 weeks, decrease in complement levels, transferrin
Piriano 1981	16 pts: 16.5 g EAA + 1 NEAA, 200 g glucose; 5 pts: 10.2 g glucose/EAA only	20 weeks	5 (in EAA group lost >15% of usual BW)	BW	In EAA + NEAA group, 8 pts gained >10% BW; the other 8 lost weight. Pts in EAA group gained weight if did not have acute illness.
Powers 1989	18 pts; 250 mL 50% glucose, 250 mL RenAmin[a]	46–165 infusions	All	Weight gain, Alb, TSF, MAMC	Weight gain (12.6 ± 4.9 lb) in 11 of 18 pts. No change in Alb. Only MAMC improved
Bilbrey 1989	20 pts; 50 g EAA + NEAA, 50 g lipids, 125 g glucose	90 days minimum	All	BW, MAMC	BW, MAMC improved
Matthys 1991	10 pts; 16.75 g EAA	3 months	All	Quality of life, Hct, BW, degree of edema	BW increased starting from first month of therapy (p <.01). Scoring index of general condition increased (p <.01).
Bilbrey 1993	47 pts; 400 mL 15% AA, 150 mL 70% glucose, 250 mL 20% lipids	90 days minimum	All	Alb, transferrin, mortality	29 survived, 18 died. Survivors had increase in Alb, transferrin. No data on cause of death, dialysis dose

Continued

Table 45.3

Nonrandomized Studies in IDPN—cont'd

Study	Design	Treatment Duration	No. With PEW	Parameters Measured	Outcome
Chertow 1994	1679 pts: 1.2 g protein/kg, 15 kcal/kg 22,517 pts: no IDPN	12 months or until death		Alb, URR, odds of death	Decrease in mortality in IDPN-treated pts who had Alb ≤3.3 g/dL
Capelli 1994	50 pts: 50 g EAA, 50 g lipids,125 g glucose, dietary supplement (discontinued once IDPN started) 31 pts: dietary supplement	9 months	All had Alb <3.5 g/dL, BW < 90% of desirable BW or BW loss >10% over 2 months	Alb, BW, mortality	32 of 50 treated pts and 16 of 31 untreated pts survived Weight gain in treated survivors, no weight gain in survivors who were untreated No weight gain in nonsurvivors in either group 6 months of IDPN before change in weight or Alb
Foulks 1994	72 pts; 0.64 g N/kg, 3.78 kcal/kg as lipids, glucose	Mean of 159 days in responders, 222 days in nonresponders		Mortality, hosp rate	Decreased mortality and hosp rate in responders
Smolle 1995	16 pts; 0.8 g/kg EAA + NEAA	16 weeks		Alb, skin test reactivity, WBC, SCr	NA[b]
Cranford 1998	43 pts; 63 g EAA + NEAA, 18.4 g lipids, 92.5 g carbohydrates	6 months		Alb, BUN, hospitalizations	NA[b]

Study	Treatment	Duration	Patients	Measurements	Results
Hiroshige 1998	10 pts: 200 mL 50% glucose, 200 mL 7% EAA, 200 mL 20% lipids; 18 pts: dietary counseling	12 months	All	BW, BMI, TSF, MAMC, Alb, transferrin, plasma AA profile, mortality	All IDPN-treated pts survived, 5 pts without IDPN therapy died (3 due to sepsis, 1 due to GI bleeding) during study period
Mortelmans 1999	26 pts (16 pts completed study, 10 pts withdrew); 250 mL 50% glucose, 250 mL 20% lipids, 250 mL 7% AA	9 months	All	BW, MAMC, lean body mass, transferrin, serum pre-Alb levels	BW increased ($p < .05$); transferrin, PA increased; TSF increased ($p < .05$); No such change in patients who withdrew
Blondin 1999	45 pts[c]	6 months	All had mean Alb <3.2 g/dL ±0.4	Alb, BUN, morbidity, URR, hosp. rate	Decrease in hosp rate ($p < .05$), increase in Alb ($p < .05$)
Cherry 2002	24 pts; 250 or 500 mL 10% AA, 250 mL 50% glucose, 250 mL 20% fat emulsion	4.3 months (mean)	All	Alb, dry BW	Increase in dry BW, Alb
Dezfuli 2009	196 pts IDPN No control group	3–12 months	All	Serum albumin	72% of patients had increase in serum albumin with a mean increase of 0.4 g/dL

AA, amino acids; Alb, albumin; BUN, blood urea nitrogen; BW, body weight; EAA, essential amino acids; GI, gastrointestinal; IDPN, intradialytic parenteral nutrition; pts, patients; hosp, hospitalization; NEAA, nonessential amino acids; MAMC, mid-arm muscle circumference; NA, not applicable; SCr, serum creatinine; TSF, triceps skinfold thickness; URR, urea reduction ratio; WBC, white blood cells.

[a]RenAmin, a solution of essential and nonessential amino acids, is manufactured by Baxter (www.baxter.com).
[b]Publication not accessible to authors.
[c]Incomplete data provided.

Table 45.4

Randomized Studies in IDPN

Study	Design	Treatment Duration	No. With PEW	Parameters Measured	Outcome
Wolfson 1982	8 pts: EAA + NEAA + glucose solution vs normal saline	NA	NA	Plasma amino acid levels	Unclear if plasma amino acid levels increased
Toigo 1989	11 pts: 26.5 g modified EAA 10 pts: 24 g EAA + NEAA	6 months	None	Nerve conduction velocity, Alb	Decrease in Alb in the EAA + NEAA group
Cano 1990	12 pts: 0.08 g N/kg (per HD session) from EAA + NEAA, 1.6 g/kg (per HD session) lipids 14 pts: no intervention	3 months	All	BW, appetite, MAMC	Increase in calorie (9 kcal/kg/day) and protein intake (0.25 g/kg/day) in IDPN-treated pts
McCann 1999	19 pts: 70% glucose, 15% amino acids, 20% lipids	11 weeks	NA	Delivered Kt/V, URR	Reduction in delivered Kt/V in pts who received amino acid–containing IDPN
Navarro 2000	17 pts	3 months	NA		Positive net balance of amino acids
Cano 2006	17 pts: olive oil–based IV lipid emulsion 18 pts: soybean oil–based IV lipid emulsion	5 weeks	NA		Increase in PCR, Alb, transferrin Both groups showed similar improvement in nutritional status, plasma lipid, oxidative and inflammatory parameters
Cano 2007	89 pts: IDPN 93 pts: control	12 months	All	Primary endpoint, all-cause mortality; secondary endpoints, hosp rate, BW, Karnofsky score, BMI	No difference in hosp rate or mortality between 2 groups

Alb, albumin; BMI, body mass index; BW, body weight; EAA, essential amino acid; IV, intravenous; pts, patients; hosp, hospitalization; IDPN, intradialytic parenteral nutrition; NA, not available; NEAA, nonessential amino acid; PCR, protein catabolic rate.

including histidine and 250 mL of a mixture of D/L-malic acid, xylitol, and sorbitol during the last 30 minutes of hemodialysis. During the first 3 months, some nonessential amino acids were added to the IDPN. After 16 weeks of IDPN therapy, 13 of the 18 patients were discontinued. With every hemodialysis session, about 100 g of protein was also included. The food intake was not constant. After 30 weeks of IDPN therapy, serum albumin and serum total protein levels were reported to increase significantly. Serum transferrin and complement levels and the hemoglobin level decreased. In a study of 21 MHD patients by Piriano who had lost at least 10% of their dry weight, 16 were treated with one type of IDPN mixture for 20 weeks. IDPN that was given to these 16 patients had 400 mL of 50% glucose, 400 mL of 8.5% essential amino acids, and nonessential amino acids. Five of 21 patients who had lost at least 15% of their dry weight were treated with a solution mix of 50% glucose and essential amino acids. The dialysis dose, the volume of IDPN, and the comorbid conditions of these MHD patients were not well described. Neither of these groups gained weight, and neither of these groups had any significant increase in serum albumin level. The only exception is those patients who received essential and nonessential amino acids who did not have hyperparathyroidism who gained weight.

Bilbrey et al reported that in 47 MHD patients with severe PEW who for 3 months received IDPN there was a significant increase in serum albumin level (from 3.30 ± 0.38 SD to 3.71 ± 0.30 g/dL, $p <.001$) and serum transferrin level (165 ± 37 to 200 ± 62 mg/dL, $p <.001$) in survivors. There was no increase in serum albumin or serum transferrin level in the nonsurvivors. The dialysis dose, comorbid conditions, and duration of therapy of IDPN was not reported. Capelli et al reported a survival difference between 50 patients who received IDPN and 31 patients who did not receive IDPN in their retrospective study of 81 MHD patients. All patients in the study had reduced serum albumin levels. In the 31 control patients, a history of recent weight loss or low body weight was not consistently present. All of the patients in the study group received oral nutritional supplements and/or nutritional counseling at the initiation of the study. In those patients who did not respond to this supplementation, IDPN was started. This IDPN solution had a 10%–20% lipid emulsion (20–500 kcal/dialysis session), variable amounts of D-glucose based on the presence or absence of diabetes, and 50 g of essential amino acids. The mortality rate was 36% in the IDPN-treated patients ($p >.05$) and 48% in the control group. The time to death was significantly greater (16.9 ± 7.9 [SD] vs 7.5 ± 4.2 months, $p <.001$) in the nonsurvivors in the IDPN-treated patients. A nonrandomized study reported by Foulks et al reported on 72 patients with PEW who failed to respond to dietary counseling and who received IDPN. If there was a 10% increase in dry body weight or an increase in serum albumin of ≥0.5 g/dL these patients were stratified as responders while they received IDPN. In these responders mortality was significantly lower. The responders had a significantly lower serum albumin level compared to nonresponders (2.2 ± 0.7 vs 3.0 ± 0.8 g/dL, $p <.0001$). Both the responders and nonresponders had similar body weights both before and after treatment with IDPN. Responders had higher hospitalization rates during the 6 months prior to the initiation of IDPN ($p <.0001$) but during IDPN therapy only 52% of responders were hospitalized as compared to 76% of nonresponders ($p <.0001$). It is a plausible hypothesis that the nonresponders' increased morbidity reduced their ability to respond to IDPN therapy. It is also conceivable that the improved clinical course of the responders was due to the IDPN.

A retrospective study compared 22,517 control MHD patients with 1679 MHD patients who received IDPN. In the 1679 patients who received IDPN, the composition of IDPN was not identical. There was a significant decline in the odds ratio of death at 1 year in those patients with serum albumin level of ≤3.3 g/dL treated with IDPN after correction for case mix and predialysis serum creatinine level compared to patients who had comparable serum albumin level who did not receive IDPN therapy. In patients who were treated with IDPN who had a serum albumin level of ≥3.5 g/dL at 1 year, the mortality was higher. In the MHD patients who had a predialysis serum creatinine level of 8.0 mg/dL or lower, the survival effect of IDPN was greater.

Hiroshige et al in a nonrandomized study published results of IDPN therapy in 10 MHD patients. The control group were 18 MHD patients who refused IDPN therapy and were given dietary counseling. The treated group received IDPN for 12 months consisting of 200 mL of 50% glucose, 200 mL of 20% lipid emulsion, and 200 mL of 7.1% essential amino acids per dialysis session. The baseline nutritional measures between the two groups did not differ significantly. In the treated group, there was a significant rise in serum albumin and transferrin, triceps skinfold thickness, body weight, and mid arm muscle circumference during the IDPN therapy. A reduction in the plasma essential amino acids was seen in the control group for the duration of the study.

In a prospective cohort of 196 MHD patients with reduced serum albumin levels, Dezfuli et al examined predictors of response to IDPN in a multivariate logistic regression model (Fig. 45.1). One hundred thirty-four patients had severe hypoalbuminemia, defined as a baseline serum albumin level of less than 3.0 g/dL. The average period of IDPN therapy was 5.8 months. The baseline level of serum

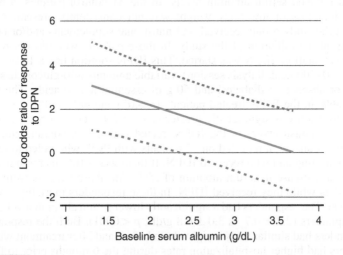

Figure 45.1

Association of serum albumin at baseline to odds ratio of response to intradialytic parenteral nutrition (IDPN) adjusted for patient demographics and length of treatment based on cubic spline analysis: solid line is odds ratio, and dotted line is 95% confidence interval.

albumin was lower in MHD patients who responded to IDPN. A multivariate logistic regression analysis adjusted the associations for age, gender, diabetes, and IDPN time. The presence of severe hypoalbuminemia (serum albumin <3.0 g/dL) at baseline was associated with a 2.5 times higher chance of responding to IDPN. The same severe hypoalbuminemia was associated with a 3.5 times increased likelihood of serum albumin correction by at least 0.5 g/dL. The authors concluded that the degree of response to IDPN correlated with the severity of hypoalbuminemia. This study also led to advancing the funnel hypothesis of hypoalbuminemia response to IDPN in that the lower the serum albumin, the more likely one is to see faster and more incremental response (Fig. 45.2).

Randomized Prospective Controlled Trials of IDPN

Key randomized trials in IDPN have been presented in Table 45.4. Over 12 weeks, Cano et al studied 26 MHD patients with PEW. The treated group exhibited a significant rise in body weight, serum transthyretin (prealbumin), and serum albumin

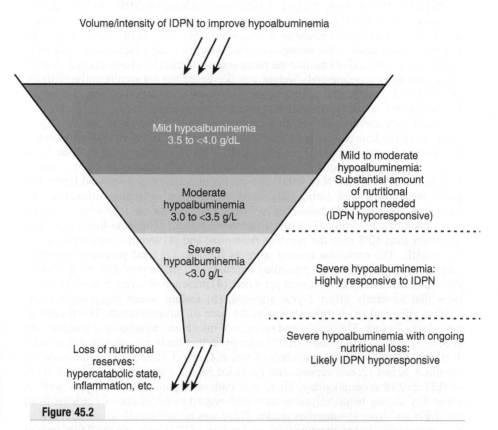

Figure 45.2

Hypothetical model to explain the association between the degree of response to intradialytic parenteral nutrition (IDPN) with severity of hypoalbuminemia.

levels. There were also increases in mid-arm muscle circumference, skin test reactivity, and in plasma Apo lipoprotein A-1 and plasma leucine levels. None of the control patients experienced a rise in any of these parameters. Of note, the IDPN-treated group had a statistically nonsignificant lower baseline value of many of these measures. This may or may not have predisposed them to increases of these measures during therapy with IDPN. The plasma lipid levels did not change but the plasma Apo lipoprotein A-1 levels increased. The IDPN therapy provided an estimated 1.6 g/kg body weight of fat and 0.08 g/kg of nitrogen from essential and nonessential amino acids.

In a study of 18 MHD patients by Guarnieri et al, patients were assigned in a random fashion to three IDPN treatment regimens. These regimens differed according to the amino acid content of the solutions. In these 18 patients, most had PEW. Patients received either only essential amino acids or a combination of nonessential and essential amino acids or amino acid–free solution with an isocaloric infusion of 5% glucose. All three IDPN regimens contained vitamins, minerals, and trace elements. IDPN was given three times weekly for 2 months. The only change experienced in the three groups was that the patients who received only essential amino acids had a gain of body weight. Twenty-one patients on MHD were randomly assigned to receive IDPN therapy for 6 months. Ten patients were given a combination of nonessential and essential amino acids, and 11 patients were given only essential amino acids as the nitrogen source. Baseline energy input before initiation of IDPN was low, and at baseline the mean serum albumin level was normal. Protein intake and mean baseline body weight was decreased but not significantly. With the essential and nonessential amino acids, there was a reduction in serum albumin levels and an increase in normalized protein nitrogen appearance.

The French Interdialytic Nutrition Evaluation Study (FineS) is to date the largest prospective randomized study to examine the benefit of IDPN in dialysis patients. One hundred eighty-six MHD patients aged 18–80 years undergoing dialysis for at least 6 months were randomly assigned to receive IDPN therapy (n = 93) or not to receive therapy with IDPN (n = 93). The treatment period was 1 year and IDPN was given three times a week during dialysis. All patients received oral nutritional supplementation and had PEW defined as having at least two of the following: (1) body mass index of <20 kg/m^2; (2) serum albumin <3.5 g/dL; (3) edema-free weight loss of greater than 10% over the previous 6 months; and (4) serum transthyretin levels <30 mg/dL. The exclusion criteria were as follows: (1) total parenteral nutrition received within the 3 months preceding the study; (2) single-pool Kt/V <1.2; (3) less than 12 hours of dialysis treatment per week; (4) presence of severe comorbid conditions that adversely affect 1-year survival; (5) fasting serum triglyceride levels >300 mg/dL; and (6) hospitalization at the time of randomization. The follow-up period was 2 years. The energy and nutritional intake was monitored at baseline and at 3, 6, 12, 18, and 24 months. IDPN therapy in this study was provided at months 3, 6, and 12 and was the equivalent of 6.6, 6.4, or 6.1 kcal/kg of amino acids. At months 3, 6, and 12, oral supplements provided 5.9 ± 2.7 kcal/kg/day and 0.39, 0.38, or 0.37 ± 0.18 protein/kg/day. There was patient to patient variability as well as variability among hemodialysis centers with regard to the intake of nutrients from the IDPN and from spontaneous intake. There was no statistically significant difference in mortality, hospitalization rates, and indices of PEW between the IDPN-treated group and the control group. The Karnofsky scores did not change from baseline in either the control group or in the groups that received IDPN. Both the groups received oral nutritional supplements, and this may have played a role in the failure to demonstrate any difference in outcomes between the groups. Of note, the patients in the IDPN-treated groups who had a rise in serum transthyretin of greater than 30 mg/L within the first 3 months of the study showed an approximately 50% reduction in mortality at 2 years. The authors note that although this is the largest prospective randomized trial to date, it was still underpowered.

Indications for Initiation of IDPN

The first step in the management of a patient with PEW is to explore reversible causes, and if none is found oral or enteral feeding (nasogastric tube or percutaneous gastrostomy PEG tube) should be attempted. Many patients will not choose a PEG tube, and a nasogastric tube is a very temporary solution. When sustained use of oral nutritional supplements fails to improve nutritional status, an initial trial of IDPN can be attempted. One needs to encourage the patient to have a spontaneous protein intake of at least 0.8 g/kg/ideal body weight and at least a calorie intake of 20 kcal/kg/ideal body weight before IDPN can be initiated.

Administration of IDPN

Care should be taken to keep the IDPN infusion rate to less than a maximum infusion rate of 250 mL/hour. The serum lipid clearance rate may reach its maximum limit at an infusion exceeding 250 mL/hour. Symptoms such as nausea and vomiting associated with hypertriglyceridemia can be reduced if the infusion rate is less than 250 mL/hour. Reducing the infusion rate to 50% (125 mL/hour) in the FineS study resulted in resolution of nausea and vomiting. After a 2-week period, the infusion rate was increased to 250 mL/hour with no recurrence of symptoms.

Monitoring of IDPN Therapy

In patients with diabetes mellitus, particularly in patients with a history of uncontrolled hyperglycemia, the blood glucose should be checked at the beginning and at the end of IDPN administration during the first week of dialysis and once a week thereafter. Endogenous insulin released in response to IDPN can induce postinfusion reactive hypoglycemia due to a delay in the action of endogenous insulin. At 30–45 minutes before the end of a dialysis session, IDPN can be completed, which allows time to monitor for reactive hypoglycemia. A low-carbohydrate IDPN formulation is available from commercial IDPN companies. In the FineS study, 15%–25% of patients experienced nausea and vomiting. This side effect can be mitigated with reduction of the infusion rate or by reduction of the total amount of IDPN. Hypertriglyceridemia can occur with IDPN therapy. Lipid-free formulations are available to be prescribed in patients who experience hypertriglyceridemia. Reduction of the infusion rate can partially correct development of hypertriglyceridemia. It is prudent to measure serum lipids and liver function tests at least once a month though development of fatty liver associated with IDPN is rare.

Advantages and Disadvantages of IDPN

Nutrition is provided with IDPN independent of the patient's appetite, gastrointestinal motility (e.g., patients with diabetes mellitus may suffer from gastroparesis), or anorexia. Compliance of the patient or the patient's ability to consume a diet does not influence the nutritional intake as IDPN is given intravenously. Because this is given using the patient's vascular access that is used for hemodialysis, there is no need for an additional intravenous access. IDPN can be tailored to a patient's individual needs such as lipid-free or low glucose for example. Fluid that is administered with IDPN can be removed during the same hemodialysis session. The labor involved with administration of IDPN is not onerous and does not add a significant amount of burden to the dialysis care team.

IDPN is more expensive than any of the available enteral or oral nutrition therapies. The limited nature of the supplementation that is provided by IDPN is usually not adequate if the spontaneous oral intake of the patient is not substantial enough to meet a large portion of the patient's nutrition demands. Spontaneous intake of the patient should be greater than 20 kcal and at least 0.8 g protein/kg of the ideal body weight per day. IDPN is of limited value if the patient's spontaneous intake is less than the aforementioned calorie and protein intake. IDPN cannot be used as the sole source of nutrition. The time that a given patient is exposed to intravenous nutrition is only about 9–15 hours per week as it is given only during dialysis. Because IDPN bypasses the gut interaction of nutrients, it is not physiologic and lacks the trophic effects of nutrition on the gastrointestinal tract. In the United States, reimbursement for IDPN is controversial and therefore many patients are not covered.

Intraperitoneal Nutrition

In peritoneal dialysis patients with PEW, peritoneal dialysis–specific etiologies should be looked for such as extraperitoneal sclerosis, delayed gastric emptying, and excessive protein loss due to high transport status.

Intraperitoneal nutrition can be provided by a mixture of nine essential and six nonessential amino acids that are added to a peritoneal dialysate solution. This is

---

Table 45.5

Composition of 1.1% Nutrineal

Essential Amino Acids		Nonessential Amino Acids	
L-Valine	1.39 g/L	Arginine	1.07 g/L
L-Leucine	1.02 g/L	Alanine	0.95 g/L
L-Isoleucine	0.85 g/L	Proline	0.59 g/L
L-Methionine	0.85 g/L	Glycine	0.51 g/L
L-Lysine	0.76 g/L	Serine	0.51 g/L
L-Histidine	0.71 g/L	Tyrosine	0.30 g/L
L-Threonine	0.65 g/L		
L-Phenylalanine	0.57 g/L		
L-Tryptophan	0.27 g/L		
Sodium	132 mEq/L	Chloride	105 mEq/L
Calcium	5 mg/L	Lactate	40 mEq/L
Magnesium	0.50 mEq/L		
Total amino acids	1.1%		
Osmolarity	365		
Ph	6.7		

usually a 1.1% amino acid solution along with a reduction in glucose concentration. Typical components of a 1.1% Nutrineal solution are shown in Table 45.5. This peritoneal dialysate is used for one or two peritoneal dialysate exchanges every day. The dwell times are increased to typically 4–6 hours to enhance uptake of about 80% of the amino acid content in the peritoneal dialysate. The addition of amino acids to the peritoneal dialysate increases protein synthesis and the plasma levels of several proteins and amino acids. To avoid high serum urea nitrogen levels and metabolic acidosis, it is prudent to prevent an excessive load of amino acids and protein from the combined intake of intraperitoneal and oral intake. The effects of intraperitoneal amino acid supplementation on the long-term function of the peritoneal membrane and on peritoneal protein loss and cytokine production have not been rigorously studied in long-term clinical trials.

CHAPTER 46

Nutritional Management in Peritoneal Dialysis

Joline L.T. Chen, MD, MS • Kamyar Kalantar-Zadeh, MD, MPH, PhD

Protein–Energy Wasting and Its Impact in Peritoneal Dialysis Patients

Patients with chronic kidney disease (CKD) are at risk for development of protein–energy malnutrition. The factors associated with protein–energy wasting (PEW) include uremia, suppression of appetite, inadequate diet, overly restrictive diet prescription, frequent hospitalizations, loss of protein during dialysis, and inflammatory states associated with the kidney disease and its complications. The expert panels from the International Society of Renal Nutrition and Metabolism (ISRNM) have previously used the term PEW to describe malnutrition often seen among patients with CKD. PEW is specifically defined as the syndrome of depletion of protein mass and/or energy fuel supplies with specific diagnostic criteria. In this chapter, we will use PEW as an inclusive syndrome that also includes the protein and energy malnutrition and the complications associated with insufficient intake and increased catabolism seen in kidney disease patients.

By the time patients with CKD progress to end-stage renal disease (ESRD) that requires dialysis initiation, the prevalence of PEW is particularly high. Almost half of patients treated with maintenance dialysis have mild to moderate PEW, and this is even more prevalent in peritoneal dialysis (PD). Recent investigations have assessed the incidence of protein–energy malnutrition and have found that approximately 40% of PD patients were at least mild to moderately malnourished and that 4%–8% were severely malnourished.

Although the prevalence of PEW is high in dialysis patients, few studies have compared the severity of PEW between hemodialysis (HD) and PD patients. A Korean study evaluated PD and HD patients using five different measures incorporating albumin, body weight loss, and symptoms. A higher percentage of PD patients are found to have a more severe degree of PEW than HD patients. However, long-term comparative analyses have shown that the trend does not necessarily persist as patients continue to perform PD in comparison with those treated with HD. Thus, decisions regarding modality selection should not be based on patient nutritional status alone.

Why do we need to assess nutritional status in PD patients? PEW is a particularly important risk factor for mortality and morbidity in the CKD population in general including in ESRD. Many studies have repeatedly shown that PEW is the strongest predictor of patient outcomes in ESRD. Among patients treated with PD, the prognostic role of nutrition in patient outcome has been demonstrated in clinical trials and observational studies. The ADEMEX trial noted that patients with better nutritional status, represented by higher normalized protein of nitrogen appearance (nPNA) had better survival. Lower albumin level was also associated with worse outcomes. The largest study of the association of serum albumin and mortality in PD patients was performed by Mehrotra et al in 12,850 PD patients who were examined from 2001 and 2007 in the United States. Comparison with more than 100,000 HD patients showed that in both PD and HD patients serum albumin has by far the strongest association with mortality, so that even a 0.1–0.2 g/dL higher or lower serum albumin or any such minor change in serum albumin over time in PD patients is associated with greater and worse survival, respectively (see Fig. 46.1). In the prospective cohort study of 14 clinical centers in the CANUSA study, patients with lower albumin and lower subjective global assessment (SGA) scores had a higher risk for mortality. In fact, with every unit decrease in the SGA score, the risk of mortality increased by 25%.

Importantly, one needs to recognize that the association of poor nutritional state and worse outcome may not be a cause-and-effect relationship in these studies. Malnutrition and low albumin may be a result or surrogate marker of other complications of dialysis or intercurrent illnesses. Nevertheless, PEW per se may be contributing to the overall poor outcomes. Independent of the cause of PEW it is

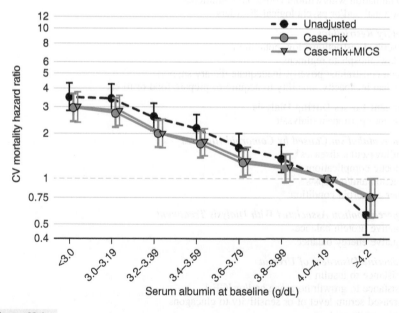

Figure 46.1

Association of Baseline Serum Albumin Concentration With Cardiovascular Outcomes in Patients Undergoing Peritoneal Dialysis (n = 12,171). Reference Group: Peritoneal Dialysis Patients With Serum Albumin Between 4.00 and 4.19 g/dL. (Adapted from Mehrotra R, Duong U, Jiwakanon S, et al. Serum albumin as a predictor of mortality in peritoneal dialysis: comparisons with hemodialysis. Am J Kidney Dis. 2011;58(3):418-428.)

believed that nutritional support can improve PEW and outcomes. In this chapter, we will explore the potential risk factors for PEW in PD patients and measures to evaluate nutritional status and provide recommendations for nutritional management in PD.

Risk Factors for PEW in PD

The causes of PEW in dialysis including PD patients are multifactorial, and a summary of potential risk factors are listed in Table 46.1. Main causes may include inadequate food and nutrient intake as well as increased catabolism seen in kidney disease. Protein loss via PD treatment is another important factor as discussed below.

Table 46.1

Causes of Wasting and PEM in Dialysis Patients

Inadequate Nutrient Intake
Anorexia* Caused by
Uremic toxicity
Impaired gastric emptying
Inflammation with/without comorbid conditions*
Emotional and/or psychological disorders

Dietary Restrictions
Prescribed restrictions: low-potassium
    low-phosphate regimens
Social constraints: poverty, inadequate dietary support
Physical incapacity: inability to acquire or prepare food or to eat

Nutrient Losses During Dialysis
Loss into peritoneal dialysate

Hypercatabolism Caused by Comorbid Illnesses
Cardiovascular diseases*
Diabetic complications
Infection and/or sepsis*
Other comorbid conditions*

Hypercatabolism Associated With Dialysis Treatment
Negative protein balance
Negative energy balance

Endocrine Disorders of Uremia
Resistance to insulin
Resistance to growth hormone and/or IGF-1
Increased serum level of or sensitivity to glucagons
Hyperparathyroidism
Other endocrine disorders

Acidemia With Metabolic Acidosis

---

*The given factor may also be associated with inflammation.
Adapted from Kalantar-Zadeh K, Ikizler TA, Block G, Avram MM, Kopple JD. Malnutrition-
   inflammation complex syndrome in dialysis patients: causes and consequences. Am J Kidney Dis.
   Nov 2003;42(5):864-881.

Kidney disease and dialysis-associated factors, such as uremia, metabolic acidosis, volume overload, or loss of residual renal function, also contribute to decreased energy and protein intake. Additionally, increased comorbidities and hospitalization may also increase inflammation and catabolism, subsequently leading to PEW. PD patients may have lower peak hunger, less change in fullness rating, and lower nutrient intakes compared with controls. These findings may be related to the following modality-associated characteristics (Fig. 46.2).

Protein Loss

A substantial amount of protein is lost through the peritoneal membrane during each exchange. This may range between 5 and 15 g per day. Patients with high peritoneal membrane transport properties are particularly at risk with more albumin loss with each exchange. However, the high membrane transport status alone has not been consistently linked with poor nutritional status. This complicated relationship

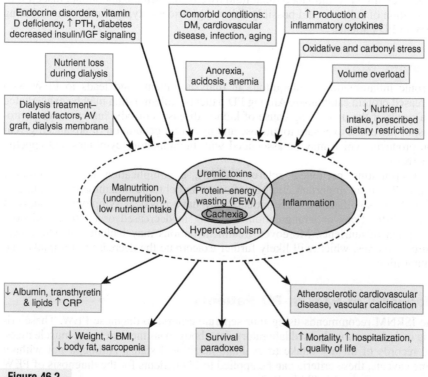

Figure 46.2

Schematic Representation of the Causes and Manifestations of the Protein–Energy Wasting Syndrome in Kidney Disease. (Adapted from Fouque D et al, A proposed nomenclature and diagnostic criteria for protein–energy wasting in acute and chronic kidney disease. Kidney International 2008;73:391-398).

between membrane status and nutritional status is likely due to the use of albumin as a surrogate marker for nutrition status. Whereas a higher amount of albumin may be lost in the effluent, the low serum albumin may not necessarily represent malnutrition. During episodes of peritonitis, the inflammatory changes to the membrane also result in high amounts of protein losses in the effluent. This will directly lead to lower serum albumin levels, especially if patients do not increase protein intake. The inflammation and decreased oral intake associated with an infectious episode will directly contribute to PEW.

Early Satiety/Fullness

Absorption of dialysate carbohydrate from dextrose-based exchanges can contribute to a large proportion of total daily energy intake. The amount of glucose absorbed can be calculated based during a peritoneal equilibrium test or a 24-hour dialysate collection. Up to 60% of daily dialysate glucose load may be absorbed, resulting in glucose absorption of 100–200 g of glucose per day. This significant amount of caloric intake may contribute to decreased appetite and subsequently poor oral intake. Additionally, intraabdominal fluid dwells may lead to abdominal discomfort, a sensation of fullness, and possibly delayed gastric emptying, further exacerbating PEW in PD patients.

Inflammatory States

Chronic inflammation is ubiquitous in dialysis patients and leads to PEW with increased protein catabolism. Among PD patients, inflammation may be exacerbated as a result of the underlying cause of kidney disease, episodic infections or peritonitis, or increased exposure to glucose and increased generation of advanced glycation products, which may be associated with inflammatory cytokines and appetite suppression.

Encapsulating peritoneal sclerosis (EPS), a complication not uncommonly seen in PD, is an important etiology of acute and chronic inflammation, leading to PEW. More significantly, EPS patients may have physical symptoms or signs of bowel obstructions or strangulation, resulting in decreased oral intake and poor absorption of nutrients. Moreover, treatment options may include episodic bowel rest or surgeries, which will likely further exacerbate the decreased oral intake and malnutrition.

Diagnosis of PEW in PD Patients

The ISRNM recommends using four separate criteria to diagnose PEW. These criteria include commonly used laboratory data, body mass measurement, muscle mass, and records of dietary intake to evaluate nutritional status. Although not without some caveats, these criteria can be applied to PD patients for the diagnosis of PEW and are summarized in Table 46.2.

Serum Chemistry

Serum albumin is the most essential diagnostic criterion for PEW in CKD. Among PD patients, albumin per se is negatively and linearly associated with mortality and poor outcome. Although low serum albumin levels in PD patients is not specific for

Table 46.2

Readily Utilizable Criteria for the Clinical Diagnosis of PEW in AKI or CKD

Serum Chemistry
Serum albumin <3.8 g per 100 mL (Bromcresol Green)[a]
Serum prealbumin (transthyretin) <30 mg per 100 mL (for maintenance dialysis patients only; levels may vary according to GFR level for patients with CKD stages 2–5)[a]
Serum cholesterol <100 mg per 100 mL[a]

Body Mass
BMI <23[b]
Unintentional weight loss over time: 5% over 3 months or 10% over 6 months
Total body fat percentage <10%

Muscle Mass
Muscle wasting: reduced muscle mass 5% over 3 months or 10% over 6 months
Reduced mid-arm muscle circumference area[c] (reduction >10% in relation to 50th percentile of reference population)
Creatinine appearance[d]

Dietary Intake
Unintentional low DPI <0.80 g/kg/day for at least 2 months[e] for dialysis patients or <0.6 g/kg/day for patients with CKD stages 2–5
Unintentional low DEI <25 kcal/kg/day for at least 2 months[e]

AKI, acute kidney injury; BMI, body mass index; CKD, chronic kidney disease; DEI, dietary energy intake; DPI, dietary protein intake; GFR, glomerular filtration rate; nPCR, normalized protein catabolic rate; nPNA, normalized protein nitrogen appearance; PEW, protein–energy wasting.
At least three of the four listed categories (and at least one test in each of the selected category) must be satisfied for the diagnosis of kidney disease–related PEW. Optimally, each criterion should be documented on at least three occasions, preferably 2–4 weeks apart.
[a]Not valid if low concentrations are due to abnormally great urinary or gastrointestinal protein losses, liver disease, or cholesterol-lowering medicines.
[b]A lower BMI might be desirable for certain Asian populations; weight must be edema-free mass, e.g., postdialysis dry weight. See text for the discussion about the BMI of the healthy population.
[c]Measurement must be performed by a trained anthropometrist.
[d]Creatinine appearance is influenced by both muscle mass and meat intake.
[e]Can be assessed by dietary diaries and interviews, or for protein intake by calculation of normalized protein equivalent of total nitrogen appearance (nPNA or nPCR) as determined by urea kinetic measurements.
Adapted from Fouque D, Kalantar-Zadeh K, Kopple J, et al. A proposed nomenclature and diagnostic criteria for protein-energy wasting in acute and chronic kidney disease. Kidney Int. 2008;73(4):391-398.

PEW and is often associated with fluctuating volume status, it is most commonly due to protein loss in dialysis effluent and may occur without obvious signs of inflammation. Nevertheless, it remains a powerful indicator of PEW and a significant prognosticator of long-term outcome. Because of its limitations, the National Kidney Foundation–Kidney Disease Outcomes and Quality Initiative (NKF-KDOQI) nutrition guideline recommends the use of additional markers to evaluate PEW. Other useful laboratory measures to evaluate malnutrition and inflammation often include C reactive protein, leptin, adiponectin, and prealbumin (also known as transthyretin). However, many of these laboratory markers are also prone to fluctuations in the setting of inflammatory or infectious episodes. Hence, to properly assess nutritional status, one should always evaluate the presence of any active inflammation because it will likely lead to anorexia and PEW. Although low cholesterol level may be another surrogate marker for low oral intake, one needs to be cognizant of the abnormal lipid metabolism in renal disease as well as the ubiquitous use and effect of lipid-lowering agents.

Body Mass

The diagnostic criteria for PEW included an absolute body mass index (BMI) <23 or unintentional weight loss or low body fat. As in other CKD patients and those treated with HD, the paradoxical relationship between high BMI and mortality, known as obesity paradox or reverse epidemiology, is similarly observed among PD patients. PD patients with low BMI have the highest risk for mortality whereas higher BMI tends to confer protective effects. It is important to know that in the general population, BMI between 18.5 and 25 may be considered the normal range, whereas ISRNM has suggested that a BMI <23 is in the lower range for dialysis patients. East Asian dialysis patients, however, may be within lower BMI ranges as their desirable BMI.

Muscle Mass

Muscle mass is an important criterion for the diagnosis of PEW. Surrogates for muscle mass may be extrapolated from anthropometric measurements of midarm muscle circumference, waist circumference, or validated equations using serum creatinine. Serum creatinine is a useful surrogate of muscle mass in ESRD patients when there is no residual renal function and it is not affected by inflammation. Noori et al has created a creatinine-based equation to estimate lean body mass in mainte-nance HD patients; however, the validity of this equation has not been studied in the PD population. Among PD patients, lean body mass has been found to correlate with creatinine kinetics, anthropometry, and bioelectrical impedance, but there are conflicting results on whether it may represent steady-state nutritional status or if it can prognosticate long-term outcomes.

Dietary Intake

PD patients with persistently low protein intake <0.8 g/kg/day or daily energy intake <25 kcal/kg/day are at particularly high risk for PEW. The estimation of caloric or protein intake is best estimated by a food intake diary or by normalized protein of nitrogen appearance (nPNA), also known as normalized protein catabolic rate (nPCR), as discussed below.

Other tools for PEW assessment recommended by the ISRNM are used com-monly among clinicians and researchers during the care of PD patients. The follow-ing are examples of nutrition screening tools.

nPNA (Also Known as nPCR)

Among patients in a steady state, urea nitrogen appearance is calculated to estimate daily protein intake, and nPNA can be used to estimate protein intake. In PD patients, PNA can be calculated by estimating the generation of urea nitrogen in the dialysate and then normalized based on body weight. However, it is important to note that nPNA has many potential limitations when used in PD. For example, its accuracy is questionable among patients not in a steady state and may lead to overestimation of daily protein intake in catabolic states. Among patients receiving intraperitoneal amino acids for 1 exchange per day, the nPNA may be falsely elevated, giving an incorrect impression of improved nutritional state. Therefore, nPNA should be used in collaboration with other criteria to provide an accurate reflection of nutritional status.

Body Composition

Dual-energy x-ray absorptiometry or bioelectrical impedance analysis are useful tools that inform clinicians of patients' volume status and anthropometry. However, they are not often readily available for clinical use in most dialysis clinics. Importantly, intraabdominal dwells of dialysate solutions will also change the accuracy of the bioimpedance measurement and patients need to have the peritoneal dialysate drained prior to this measurement.

Nutritional Assessment Scores

Subjective global assessment (SGA), a nutritional status assessment based on history and physical examination, has been validated in PD patients and found to be a strong predictor of mortality risk. The malnutrition–inflammation score (MIS), a newer tool that incorporates components of the SGA, laboratory measurements including albumin and transferrin, and BMI, has been found to be well correlated with mortality and morbidity risk among HD patients. The use of MIS in PD patients is less common, but it is also significantly associated with other measures of PEW in small studies. Thus, it may be an important patient care tool as well as a prognosticating instrument for PD patients.

Management of Protein Energy Malnutrition in PD Patients

Daily Energy Intake Goal

The 2000 KDOQI guideline recommends a total daily energy intake of 35 kcal/kg/day for patients 60 years of age or younger and 30–35 kcal/kg/day for those who are older. The European Best Practice Guideline also recommends a similar energy intake. This recommendation includes both oral intake and the absorbed glucose from dialysate. As discussed above, the high proportion of absorbed glucose may adversely affect patient appetite, resulting in patient difficulty in attaining the goal. Importantly, there are no interventional trials evaluating the recommended calorie intake and correlating this with outcomes. Guideline recommendations were made based on the observations of the association of poor outcome and low body weight/PEW.

Daily Protein Intake

The 2000 KDOQI guideline has recommended a daily protein intake of 1.2–1.3 g/kg/day for stable PD patients. However, this recommendation remains a matter of debate, especially because it will lead to a higher dietary phosphorus load, a higher risk of metabolic acidosis, and a higher probability of increased fluid intake. Others argue that a daily protein intake of approximately 0.7–1 g/kg/day may be adequate for the patient to remain in nitrogen balance especially on incremental transition to PD from non–dialysis dependent CKD status, where many patients were already on a low protein diet of 0.6–0.8 g/kg/day. Nevertheless, recent data examining the impact of dietary phosphorus counseling efforts on dialysis patients noted that restriction of dietary phosphorus intake can lead to lower dietary protein intake and worse nutritional status. Thus, we would recommend high dietary protein intake to PD patients because of the increased risk for PEW and subsequent adverse outcomes.

Dialysis Prescription and Metabolic Acidosis

Although most randomized controlled trials have not shown a direct benefit of high PD dosage on nutritional status or outcomes, the ADEMEX study did find that those who achieved a higher *Kt/V* target had a higher nPNA level. Notably, *Kt/V* and nPNA are mathematically linked, and the improvement of nPNA may not implicitly represent better food intake or nutritional status. Thus, it remains unclear whether a change of PD prescription to improve adequacy would result in less PEW. Importantly, patients who have maintained residual kidney function had better nutritional status. Therefore, an effort to maintain residual kidney function is paramount. The assessment of dialysis adequacy and residual renal function should be performed regularly.

Although mild metabolic acidosis may be observed among patients with excellent protein intake, more severe degrees of metabolic acidosis with serum bicarbonate level less than 19 mmol/L is likely a complication of kidney failure and possibly a sign of inadequate dialysis. As acidosis may further worsen protein catabolism, it is a potentially reversible and treatable factor. A change in the prescribed dialysate buffer level may be beneficial. Treatment with oral sodium bicarbonate has been evaluated in a randomized controlled study and has been shown to result in improved bicarbonate levels, nutritional status, and shorter hospitalizations. Thus, oral sodium bicarbonate supplementation may serve as an important therapeutic tool to improve nutritional status.

Intraperitoneal Nutrition

This nutritional support option can be recommended to PD patients with more severe PEW, including those with lower serum albumin levels (e.g., albumin <3.0 g/dL or <30 g/L). Intraperitoneal nutrition (IPN) is provided in different combinations; a more commonly used mixture includes 15 amino acids (9 essential and 6 nonessential amino acids) that are added to a peritoneal dialysate solution, resulting in a 1.1% amino acid solution with reduced glucose concentration. The impact of using one exchange with 1.1% amino acid PD to treat malnutrition in PD remains controversial. Although many studies examining the safety as well as protein synthesis and membrane characteristics showed a potential benefit, data on long-term nutritional status or anthropometric measurements are not available and there are currently no well-designed multicenter controlled studies to examine the effects and outcomes of IPN or to compare it with other types of nutritional support. It is also unclear if patients in significant inflammatory and catabolic states will be able incorporate the additional amino acids into protein synthesis. Although intraperitoneal amino acid dialysate may be a potentially useful method to treat PEW in PD patients, the clinician must remain cognizant of potential side effects including metabolic acidosis, worsening uremia, and further reduction of oral intake. More details on IPN can be found in Chapter 45.

Appetite and Hormonal Stimulants

The use of appetite stimulants including megestrol acetate, cannabinoids, pentoxyphylline, and certain appetite-stimulating antidepressants such as mirtazapine has not been systematically evaluated in large interventional trials in PD. However, in small studies, 160 mg of oral megesterol daily increased weight gain and serum albumin after 3 months.

Other agents such as recombinant human growth hormone (rhGH) and insulinlike growth factor-1 have been studied in a small number of PD patients. The short-term studies suggested potential anabolic effects. However, no long-term studies are available to further evaluate the effect to prevent or to treat PEW.

Oral Nutritional Supplementation

The effectiveness of oral nutritional supplement has not been well established in large randomized controlled trials among PD patients. Whereas the supplementation may increase the protein and caloric intake of PD patients and may increase the nutritional parameters, the long-term effect on patient outcomes has not been studied. In one interventional trial, patients had difficulty tolerating the taste of protein supplementation, which is not uncommon in clinical practice.

The use of tube feeding including intermittent nasogastric tube or percutaneous endoscopic gastrostomy (PEG) tube feeding in PD is rarely recommended. In studies where adult and pediatric patients received PEG tube feedings for supplemental nutrition, the risk of complications was exceedingly high, including development of bleeding and fungal and bacterial peritonitis. Thus, PEG tube feeding should be considered as a last resort in PD patients with severe PEW.

Impact of Nutritional Support on Outcome of PD Patients

In a hypothetical model, it was shown that if an intervention can increase serum albumin to >3.8 g/dL in dialysis patients and by doing so can improve survival in PD and HD patients, at least one-third of all deaths among dialysis patients can be hypothetically prevented. Because among the more than 400,000 dialysis patients in the United States, approximately 80,000 die every year, hypoalbuminemia-correcting intervention can theoretically prevent 20,000 to 25,000 deaths every year. If this is correct, effective nutritional interventions are urgently needed to correct hypoalbuminemia (albumin <3.8 g/dL) and PEW in PD patients irrespective of the cause of PEW. As an analogous argument, the entire field of nutritional support that is devoted to cancer cachexia is based on the premise that irrespective of the cause of cancer cachexia (which is often inflammation and oxidative stress and not inadequate food intake), provision of nutritional support still helps many such patients.

Dietary Counseling

The 2000 NKF-KDOQI guideline recommended nutritional counseling for all patients with ESRD. Every PD patient should receive nutritional education and interventions by a dietitian, who can provide assessment and monitoring of the PD patient's dietary intake. Many PD patients have difficulty increasing protein intake to achieve recommended goals, especially if they are transitioning from a recommended low protein diet prior to dialysis initiation. An individualized diet plan for a PD patient should take into consideration the PD prescription, membrane characteristics, evaluation of glucose absorption, and protein loss in the effluent, not to mention the social, cultural, and dietary preferences of the PD patient. As physicians and dietitians may impose dietary restrictions on their patients regarding dietary phosphorus, sodium, and fluid intake, patients may find it quite challenging to find suitable food choices and may exacerbate PEW. Hence, nutritional education and patient empowerment on the choice of food with higher protein to phosphorus ratio, required carbohydrate intake, and weight management, are also paramount.

Conclusion

PEW is a common phenomenon in ESRD patients treated with PD and is associated with poor long-term prognosis. Development of PEW may be associated with kidney disease itself, chronic or acute inflammatory states, and modality-associated factors. A comprehensive nutritional assessment should include the use of laboratory measures, dietary record, and validated instruments. Clinicians need to be aware of the caveats of these tools when they are used to diagnose and monitor the treatment of PEW. Frequent assessment of nutritional status is important. Treatment options should include intensive and individualized dietary counseling with specific dietary protein and energy intake goals. Dialysis adequacy and metabolic acidosis may be corrected, as these conditions will likely exacerbate PEW. More interventional trials that include multimodal therapy to include nutritional support, intraperitoneal amino acid, or additional anabolic agents are needed to evaluate long term effects in PD patients with severe PEW.

SECTION XVII

Gastrointestinal Disease

C H A P T E R 4 7

Liver Disease and Gastrointestinal Disorders in Dialysis Patients

Fabrizio Fabrizi, MD • Alessio Aghemo, MD • Paul Martin, MD

Introduction

Patients with end-stage renal disease on maintenance dialysis show a variety of acute and chronic diseases of the liver (Table 47.1). Viral hepatitis continues to be the most frequently recognized cause of liver damage in patients on regular dialysis; the most important causes of hepatitis in this population remain chronic hepatitis B and C infection. The majority of the literature on liver disorders in the dialysis population refers to patients on hemodialysis. Patients receiving peritoneal dialysis are at lower risk for acquisition of blood-borne infections for several reasons: the absence of extracorporeal blood manipulation; it is performed in the patient's home, where there is no exposure to pathogens from other patients; and there is a decreased likelihood of blood transfusions among patients undergoing peritoneal dialysis.

The most important causes of death in patients on maintenance dialysis remain cardiovascular diseases and infections; cirrhosis and hepatocellular carcinoma (HCC), two major complications related to chronic viral hepatitis, are uncommon among patients on intermittent dialysis. A large Asian registry based on patients with HCC does not frequently list end-stage renal disease on maintenance dialysis (1.2%) as a comorbid condition. Although there was no significant difference in the comparison of long-term survival between HCC patients receiving dialysis or not, hepatitis B and C infections were much more prevalent in dialysis patients with HCC than the entire HCC population.

Hepatitis B

Hepatitis B virus (HBV) is a partially double-stranded compact DNA virus that is spread by intimate and nonintimate contact as well as parenterally. The most common modes of transmission of HBV in the adult population of the developed world are sexual contact and intravenous drug use; maternal-to-infant transmission is an important mode of transmission in endemic areas such as Asia and sub-Saharan Africa.

Interpretation of Diagnostic Tests

Hepatitis B surface antigen (HBsAg) is the first marker of HBV detectable in serum in acute infection. By the time clinical and biochemical hepatitis is present after an incubation period of up to 140 days, other serologic markers of HBV infection appear—including antibody to HBV core antigen (anti-HBc). Hepatitis B core

---

Table 47.1

Liver Disease in Dialysis Patients

Acute viral hepatitis: hepatitis A virus (HAV), hepatitis B virus (HBV), hepatitis C virus (HCV), hepatitis E virus (HEV)
Chronic viral hepatitis: hepatitis B virus (HBV), hepatitis C virus (HCV)
NASH: nonalcoholic steatohepatitis
Drug hepatotoxicity
Iron overload
Congestive heart failure

---

antigen, a marker of viral replication found in infected hepatocytes, does not circulate in serum. However, its corresponding antibody (anti-HBc) does. Documented HBsAg positivity in serum for 6 or more months suggests chronic HBV with a low likelihood of subsequent spontaneous resolution. Chronic HBV is diagnosed by the absence of IgM anti-HBc antibody. IgM anti-HBc antibody is a marker of acute or recent acute hepatitis B and is detectable for 6 months after infection, whereas IgG anti-HBc is lifelong. If acute HBV resolves, neutralizing antibody against HBsAg (anti-HBs) develops. If HBV infection becomes chronic, other HBV markers—including HBV viremia (HBV DNA) and hepatitis e antigen (HBeAg)—should be sought. Both of these markers imply viral replication and thus greater infectivity, although any patient who is HBsAg positive is potentially infectious.

Natural History of HBV in the Dialysis Population

The course of HBV infection is frequently asymptomatic and indolent among patients on maintenance dialysis; some symptoms that typically occur in nondialysis patients with HBV (ie, asthenia, fatigue, and cognitive impairment) are common in the dialysis population irrespective their HBsAg serologic status. Evaluation of the seriousness of HBV infection in patients on long-term dialysis is hampered by the observation that serum aminotransferase levels are commonly lower in patients on dialysis or with predialysis chronic renal failure than among individuals with intact kidney function. No marked elevations of liver enzymes have been observed but serum aminotransferase and gamma-glutamyl transpeptidase are frequently greater in HBsAg-positive than HBsAg-negative individuals on long-term dialysis. In contrast to renal transplant recipients with chronic HBV infection, there is no evidence of accelerated progression to decompensated cirrhosis or HCC.

Mortality is an unequivocal endpoint in the natural history of HBV, but data concerning the relationship between HBV infection and risk for death among HBV-infected patients on long-term dialysis are not abundant. One survey from financially constrained dialysis facilities has shown that the death rate was greater among HBsAg-seropositive than HBsAg-seronegative patients undergoing long-term dialysis. Liver failure was more common in HBsAg-seropositive than HBsAg-seronegative patients. These investigators concluded that clinical outcomes of renal replacement therapy are apt to be adversely affected by inadequate dialysis or infections due to limited financial resources.

Epidemiology of Hepatitis B Virus in Dialysis Units

Soon after the discovery of HBV (late 1960s), hepatitis B was recognized as an important threat for staff and patients within dialysis units. In 1977, the Centers for Disease Control and Prevention (CDC) issued isolation guidelines to prevent transmission of HBV within dialysis centers. In addition to the CDC recommendations, the screening of blood products for HBsAg and antiHBc antibody and a lower need for blood products resulted in a fall of incidence and prevalence of HBV among patients and staff within dialysis units from North America and western Europe during the period 1974 to 1995. The most recent and large (n=263,820) survey on the epidemiology of HBV among patients undergoing long-term dialysis in the developed world remains the 2002 survey by the CDC. It reported a 1.0% mean prevalence of HBsAg-seropositive patients; the incidence of HBV infection was 0.12%. HBV appears more frequent in many low-income countries where the rate of patients on maintenance dialysis who are chronic HBsAg carriers ranges between 1% and 15%.

The delivery of health care in the developed world has changed over recent years, leading to an increased number of patients treated outside of acute care hospitals. Thus, numerous outbreaks of HBV infection in nonhospital health care settings, including dialysis units, have been reported. An incomplete compliance to standard and dialysis-specific infection control precautions is likely the most important cause of patient-to-patient transmission of HBV in dialysis units, according to a recent systematic review of reports on outbreaks.

Strategies to Control HBV Transmission in Dialysis Units

To prevent transmission of blood-borne pathogen agents in general health care settings, "universal precautions" have been recommended by the CDC. These procedures are now referred to as "standard precautions" and include (1) hand washing after touching blood and other potentially infectious material, (2) wearing of gloves when touching blood or other potentially infectious material, and (3) use of gowns and face shields when exposure to blood or body fluids has been anticipated.

In addition to these "standard precautions," there are routine hemodialysis unit precautions that are unique to the hemodialysis setting and are more stringent than the "universal precautions." The infection control practices specific to the hemodialysis environment recommend that glove use is necessary whenever patients or hemodialysis equipment is touched, and that there should be no sharing of supplies, instruments, or medications between HD patients, including ancillary supply equipment (trays, blood pressure cuffs, clamps, scissors, and other nondisposable items). Further, the hemodialysis center precautions specify the separation of clean areas (used for handwashing and handling and storage of medications) from contaminated areas (handling blood samples and hemodialysis equipment after use), cleaning and disinfection of nondisposable items, machines and environmental surface between uses. In addition, other precautions to prevent HBV acquisition in the hemodialysis environment are needed: monthly serologic testing for hepatitis B surface antigen (HBsAg) of all susceptible patients, prompt review of results, physical separation of HBsAg-positive from susceptible patients and cohorting of separate dialysis staff, instruments, supplies, and hemodialysis machines to patients with HBsAg positivity.

Treatment of HBV-Related Liver Disease

Several drugs have received approval for the treatment of chronic HBV infection including conventional or pegylated interferons, the nucleoside analogs lamivudine and telbivudine, and the nucleotide analogs entecavir, adefovir, and tenofovir. Antiviral therapy is recommended in HBsAg-positive patients with active viral replication, HBeAg-positive status, and elevated ALT levels. Clearance of HBsAg with anti-HBs seroconversion is an important aim of treatment for all HBV antiviral therapies. However, this goal can only be reached in a small proportion of immunocompetent patients, and reaching this goal is likely to be even less frequent in immunocompromised patients such as those on HD. Clearance of HBeAg and loss of HBsAg, indicating complete resolution of HBV infection, are more commonly obtained with interferons than with nucleos(t)ide analogs. The ultimate goal for treatment of chronic HBV is to prevent the development of irreversible complications such as cirrhosis, liver failure, and hepatic cancer.

The evidence in the literature on antiviral therapy of chronic HBV in dialysis patients is very limited; the low rate of HBsAg-positive patients undergoing intermittent dialysis in the developed world clearly hampers the implementation of randomized or cohort clinical trials in this area. The information available on this point mostly relies on lamivudine. Small and uncontrolled prospective clinical studies have shown that lamivudine is effective and safe for HBV in many dialysis patients: treatment results in normalization of ALT values and persistent clearance of HBV DNA. A major limitation of lamivudine is a high rate of viral resistance. The data on the use of other nucleos(t)ide analogs for HBV in the dialysis population remain anecdotal.

Hepatitis B Vaccination

Hepatitis B vaccination has been recommended for all seronegative dialysis patients and staff members since the early 1980s. Safe and effective vaccines that contain HBsAg, either plasma derived or manufactured by recombinant DNA technology, are currently available. However, the fall of the incidence of HBV infection within dialysis units of developed countries (between 1976 and 1980) antedated the availability of the HBV vaccine. Patients on maintenance dialysis show cellular immunodeficiency that impairs not only the clearance of HBV but also the immunoresponsiveness to HBV vaccine—the frequency of responders (i.e., patients developing anti-HBs titers with protective concentration) is lower than in the general population. Moreover, after completion of the vaccination schedule, antibody titers of responder dialysis patients are low and fall rapidly. Different approaches have been used to overcome the nonresponsiveness of chronic uremic patients—the intramuscular administration of multiple or double doses, the coadministration of zinc or immune modulators such as levamisole, thymopentin, interleukin-2, γ-interferon, and the intradermal administration of HBV vaccine. Despite these attempts, the proportion of nonresponders (patients who are not able to develop anti-HBs concentrations above the protective level of 10 mIU/mL, after HBV vaccine) remains higher among dialysis patients. Currently a 0-, 1-, 2-, and 6-month schedule with double doses of hepatitis B surface antigen (2×20 µg HBsAg) of recombinant HB vaccine by the intramuscular route (deltoid muscle) is recommended in dialysis patients, with regular monitoring of antibody levels and administration of one booster dose whenever antibody titers decline below the protective concentration. In order to improve the immunogenicity of recombinant HB vaccines, various adjuvant systems have been recently developed, and one of them (AS04) appears to give encouraging results in terms of efficacy and safety, according to some randomized controlled trials. Studies in unselected cohorts of patients on maintenance dialysis are under way to confirm these findings.

Hepatitis C

Hepatitis C virus (HCV) is a single-stranded RNA virus. The route of contamination by HCV is almost entirely parenteral, making HCV significantly less infectious than HBV. Prior to the 1990s, the main routes of transmission were blood product transfusion, intravenous drug use, or unsafe injection procedures. Since the systematic screening of blood products, the residual risk of transfusion-related HCV infection is extremely low (around 1/2,000,000). In industrialized countries, important routes of transmission remain intravenous or nasal drug use, mother to child transmission, and unsafe medical or surgical procedures. The risk of heterosexual transmission is currently low but high in HIV-positive men who have sex with other men. It has been calculated that around 30% of cases of HCV infection are still unexplained, and occasional transmission has been observed with acupuncture or tattoos. The risk related to dialysis is 1%–2%/year, and it varies in different countries.

Interpretation of Diagnostic Tests

The diagnosis of HCV infection is based on the detection of anti-HCV antibody by third-generation enzyme-linked immunosorbent assay (ELISA). Anti-HCV–positive patients need to be tested for HCV viremia (HCV RNA) in serum by polymerase chain reaction (PCR) techniques; patients with active HCV infection are anti-HCV–positive, HCV RNA–positive whereas HCV RNA–negative patients have inactive HCV infection. A small but significant minority of anti-HCV–negative patients on regular dialysis show detectable HCV RNA in serum; this implies that PCR testing should be done if there is concern about HCV infection despite negative serologies. A variety of PCR tests for HCV are available; quantitative tests measure HCV viral load (HCV RNA), whereas qualitative tests are more sensitive and can detect even low-level viremia. Improper collection, handling, and storage of samples may also impact test results.

Natural History of HCV in Dialysis Population

The long-term consequences of HCV infection are difficult to assess among patients on long-term dialysis for several reasons. HCV infection is usually asymptomatic with an apparently indolent course, the natural history of HCV extends over decades rather than years, and adverse consequences of chronic HCV infection may not be obvious in individuals followed for short periods of time such as dialysis patients. Patients undergoing maintenance dialysis have a shortened life expectancy because their average age is high and they have a large number of comorbidities. The recent implementation of guidelines recommending antiviral therapy for HCV infection in the dialysis population makes it difficult to the conduct of longitudinal clinical trials on the natural history of HCV infection in patients on long-term dialysis. Clinicians are usually reluctant to perform liver biopsy in dialysis patients because of platelet dysfunction due to uremia.

An updated meta-analysis of fifteen observational studies (n = 195,370 unique patients) about the effect of anti-HCV serologic status on survival in dialysis patients demonstrated an independent and significant impact of HCV on mortality among individuals receiving long-term dialysis. The adjusted relative risk (all-cause mortality) was 32% higher in anti-HCV positive patients on maintenance dialysis. Various mechanisms support the excess death risk of HCV-infected patients, in addition to liver-related mortality. There was an increased risk of cardiovascular mortality among HCV-infected patients, and this has been associated in part to malnutrition and chronic inflammation. An impairment of health-related quality of life has been also documented.

Epidemiology of Hepatitis C Virus in Dialysis Units

A high prevalence of HCV among patients receiving long-term dialysis has been observed in the early 1990s but the universal introduction of sensitive tests for screening blood products, as well as the widespread availability of erythropoiesis-stimulating agents and the compliance with infection control procedures, have helped to reduce the prevalence of HCV among patients on maintenance dialysis in the developed world. The prevalence of HCV in dialysis populations currently ranges from below 5% in northern Europe, around 10% in southern Europe and the United States, and between 10% and 70% in developing countries (including North Africa, Asia, and South America). The prevalence of HCV is highly variable from unit to unit within the same country, with recent reports from some dialysis units in the United States still reporting prevalences of 25%–30%. Nosocomial transmission is now the most likely source when patients on regular hemodialysis in industrialized countries develop anti-HCV antibodies. The nosocomial spread of HCV among patients on long-term dialysis has been supported by several epidemiologic findings and confirmed in studies based on molecular virology. In fact, portions of the HCV genome are greatly variable and lend themselves to fingerprinting of each strain using nucleic acid testing (NAT) and sequencing. This strategy is analogous to the sequencing of the V3 region used in studies on human immunodeficiency virus (HIV) transmission.

Strategies to Control HCV Transmission in Dialysis Units

The most important mechanism in nosocomial transmission of HCV among patients receiving long-term hemodialysis is currently suboptimal adherence to infection control procedures against blood-borne pathogens. These include "universal precautions," and other precautions specific to the hemodialysis setting, as reported above. Unlike the procedures for HBV, additional hemodialysis precautions (physical separation of HCV-positive from HCV-negative patients) and the cohorting of separate dialysis machines, instruments, supplies, and staff to HCV-infected patients are not recommended in various clinical guidelines (CDC and KDIGO). In fact, large prospective studies have not identified isolation of HCV-infected hemodialysis patients as an effective measure to reduce nosocomial HCV transmission. The use of dedicated dialysis machines for HCV-infected patients also is not indicated. It has been suggested that monthly monitoring of serum aminotransferase levels, and periodic retesting for anti-HCV antibody in patients on HD who test negative for HCV be done routinely. Quarterly monitoring of serum aminotransferase levels in patients on peritoneal dialysis is also recommended.

Therapy of HCV in the Dialysis Population

The treatment of HCV in patients on chronic dialysis is predicated on the premise that HCV is associated with decreased patient survival. However, recent evidence supports the view that HCV-infected patients on intermittent dialysis very rarely receive antiviral therapy; this is probably related to several factors, including concerns about side effects with pegylated interferon and ribavirin, the need of experienced clinicians to give antiviral therapy, among others. The KDIGO HCV study group recommends the antiviral treatment of all HCV-infected patients on the waiting list for a renal transplant, irrespective of whether they are dialysis-dependent or not. Monotherapy with standard interferon has been considered over the past decades the mainstay of antiviral therapy of chronic hepatitis C in patients receiving long-term dialysis. Tolerance to initial monotherapy with recombinant interferon appears to be lower in dialysis than nonuremic patients with chronic HCV infection. However, more than one-third of dialysis patients with HCV have been successfully treated with sustained clearance of circulating HCV RNA.

More recent data have been accumulated on pegylated interferon monotherapy in patients with end-stage renal disease and HCV; pegylated interferon does not provide an added benefit in terms of virologic response in comparison with standard interferon monotherapy in the hemodialysis population, treatment discontinuation due to adverse events was also similar. A novel meta-analysis (254 unique patients on regular hemodialysis with chronic hepatitis C) found that the summary estimate for SVR and drop-out rate was 33% (95% CI, 24-43) and 23% (95% CI, 14-33), respectively. The most frequent side effects requiring interruption of treatment were hematologic (18%) and gastrointestinal (14%).

Nephrologists have been reluctant to use combined therapy in dialysis patients with HCV as ribavirin in this setting had been contraindicated. Impaired excretion of ribavirin occurs in patients with chronic kidney disease, as ribavirin is mostly eliminated by kidneys. Very little ribavirin is removed by dialysis, so there is a propensity for the drug to accumulate, exacerbating hemolysis in the dialysis population already at significant risk for anemia as well as other comorbidities (e.g., cardiac ischemia) at baseline. Recent studies suggest that with marked dose reduction and careful monitoring of the hematocrit it may be feasible to use ribavirin in dialysis patients to enhance response rates to interferon-based regimens. The gold standard for treating HCV-positive hemodialysis patients is based on the combined use of pegylated interferon plus low-dose ribavirin (200 mg daily). According to some randomized clinical trials that have been recently published, pegylated interferon plus low-dose ribavirin gave a sustained viral response up to 64% and a drop-out rate ranging between 7% and 23% among patients on hemodialysis; no data are available in patients on peritoneal dialysis.

A better understanding of the viral cycle of HCV, and the characterization of viral enzymes that are potential targets, has resulted in the development of new molecules, direct-acting antiviral drugs targeted against HCV, either specific of genotype 1 (NS3/NS4A protease inhibitors and NS5 polymerase inhibitors) or with a wider spectrum (NS5A or entry inhibitors), and nonspecific antivirals (new interferons,

Table 47.2

New Hepatitis C Antiviral Drugs: Direct-Acting Antivirals (DAAs) and Host-Targeting Antivirals (HTAs)

Protease Inhibitors	NS5A Inhibitors	Polymerase Inhibitors (Nucs)	Polymerase Inhibitors (Non-Nucs)	HTAs
Telaprevir	Daclatasvir	Sofosbuvir	Deleobuvir	Alisporivir
Boceprevir	Ledispavir	VX-135	ABT-333	Miravirsen
Simeprevir	Samatasvir	ACH-3422	PPI-383	NIM811
Faldaprevir	ABT-267			SCY-635
Asunaprevir				
ACH-2684				

Nucs, nucleos(t)ide analogs.

cyclophilin inhibitors; Table 47.2). Thus, treatment of chronic hepatitis C has evolved considerably; at the moment, for HCV-positive patients with intact kidney function, as well as liver transplant recipients who are HCV-positive, HCV infection treatment no longer relies on pegylated interferon but instead on a combination of new drugs, such as sofosbuvir, daclatasvir, simeprevir, and ledispavir. It is also not clear yet whether ribavirin is still valuable in addition to these new drugs, and little is known about treatment in groups different from the general population, including patients on maintenance dialysis. Affordability of these innovative regimens will also be an issue, particularly in resource-constrained countries.

Nephrogenic Ascites and Other Gastrointestinal Disorders in the Dialysis Population

Gastrointestinal (GI) disorders are common among patients on regular dialysis with almost 80% of dialysis patients reporting dyspepsia or other symptoms of GI distress. Some nonspecific GI symptoms including nausea, vomiting, anorexia, metallic taste, or loss of taste were encountered commonly in the past as they mirror advanced uremia. These symptoms can still be seen in patients where dialysis is delayed or not available. Their presence can be useful in order to evaluate dialysis adequacy or the time to start renal replacement therapy.

Dyspepsia is characterized by nausea, vomiting, upper abdominal pain or bloating, and early satiety; it has been frequently associated with delayed gastric emptying. Early satiety or poor appetite could be caused by gastroparesis even in the absence of overt problems such as nausea and vomiting. Gastroparesis is better recognized in diabetics; however, it is common in all-cause end-stage renal disease, varying between 36% and 62% among patients on chronic dialysis. Various mechanisms have been suggested in the pathogenesis of delayed gastric emptying, including peritoneal dialysate volume, prolonged postprandial suppression of ghrelin secretion, and uremic autonomic neuropathy despite seemingly adequate dialytic therapy. The symptoms of gastroparesis may negatively impact on nutritional status and decrease quality of life among patients on maintenance dialysis. Pharmacologic interventions such as prokinetics and antiemetic drugs or nonpharmacologic interventions (i.e., gastric surgery and gastric electrical stimulation) have not been conclusively proved to be effective and safe.

It is well known that an increased rate of upper (such as gastritis and gastroparesis) and lower (diverticular disease and colonic perforation) GI disorders occurs in the dialysis population compared with the nonuremic population. Chronic renal failure has been previously associated with an increased frequency of peptic ulcer disease among patients receiving long-term dialysis but endoscopic studies have shown that peptic ulcer disease is no more common in dialysis than nondialysis patients. *Helicobacter pylori* has a close association with development of peptic ulcer, gastric cancer, and gastric lymphoma; it had been considered one of the major risk factors for gastrointestinal symptoms among patients on intermittent dialysis. Recent consensus shows that the prevalence of *H. pylori* in dialysis patients is significantly lower than in subjects with intact kidney function.

Hemodialysis patients carry a higher risk of peptic ulcer bleeding, and recent data have shown a higher risk of nonpeptic, nonvariceal gastrointestinal bleeding in hemodialysis patients after adjustments for age, gender, underlying comorbidities, and ulcerogenic medications.

A number of studies have addressed the prevalence of biliary lithiasis in the hemodialysis population with inconsistent results. Some investigators have found prevalence rates similar to those observed in the local general population; others have found a greater prevalence among patients receiving long-term dialysis. According to a large and recent survey from southern America, the prevalence of cholelithiasis among end-stage renal disease patients awaiting kidney transplant was 12%, with half of them being symptomatic.

Nephrogenic ascites is another GI disorder that affects dialysis patients; it is uncommon (probably <5%) and appears to be declining. Nephrogenic ascites is a clinical diagnosis defined as refractory ascites in patients with end-stage renal disease where infection, portal hypertension, heart failure, and malignant processes are excluded. Most of these patients are undergoing hemodialysis. The exact cause of ascites formation is unclear, and patients frequently present with moderate to massive ascites and cachexia. The ascitic fluid has a high protein content, low serum–ascites albumin gradient, and low leukocyte count. Hypoalbuminemia may predispose uremic patients to ascites development. The diagnosis is made by ruling out other causes, and it has been suggested that the pathogenesis of the ascites is an alteration in peritoneal membrane permeability or impaired resorption due to peritoneal lymphatic channel obstruction. Daily hemodialysis should be the initial therapy and is successful in up to three-fourths of patients within 3 weeks. Alternative approaches include continuous ambulatory peritoneal dialysis, with renal transplantation being the most effective form of therapy, with the success rate approaching 100%.

Conclusions

Liver disease is currently a significant cause of morbidity and mortality among patients receiving long-term dialysis. Hepatitis B and C infections are important agents of dialysis-associated liver disease. Combined antiviral therapy (pegylated interferon plus low-dose ribavirin) has improved the efficacy and safety of chronic hepatitis C in dialysis population and the advent of direct-acting antiviral agents will change shortly the natural history of chronic hepatitis C in these patients. Compliance to infection control procedures against blood-borne pathogens is recommended to control HCV and HBV infections within dialysis units; isolation of HBsAg-positive patients is also needed to limit HBV spread. Gastrointestinal disorders are frequently encountered among patients on chronic dialysis even if the prevalence of *H. pylori* is not higher than that observed in patients with intact kidney function.

The HIV-Infected Patient

SECTION XVIII

The HIV-Infected Patient

C H A P T E R   4 8

Care of the HIV-Infected Dialysis Patient

Andrew Brookens, MD • Rudolph A. Rodriguez, MD

The incidence and prevalence of end-stage renal disease (ESRD) among patients with AIDS increased until 2000, and according to USRDS data, between 2000 and 2008, the incidence of ESRD has plateaued but the prevalence has continued to increase. The increase in prevalence is due to the increase in survival among ESRD patients with HIV infection. African Americans continue to comprise more than 80% of patients with ESRD and HIV infection.

Prior to 2000, HIV-associated nephropathy (HIVAN) became the fourth leading cause of ESRD among African Americans aged 20–64 years, a condition felt to develop largely in patients with uncontrolled viremia. Much of the subsequent improvement in the incidence of ESRD is attributed to improvements in antiretroviral therapy (ART) and access to care and occurs at a time when other known comorbid risk factors for ESRD among the general population are rising. Although HIVAN burden has decreased with increasing ART, the strongest predictor of progression to ESRD is the CD4 count, and as the HIV population ages, the traditional renal risk factors like diabetes and hypertension are now important risk factors among the HIV population. Recent research is exploring immune activation in HIV-infected individuals. In HIV-infected patients, hepatitis C and hepatitis B coinfections, *APOL1* high-risk allele carriers in patients of African descent, and socioeconomic status are risk factors leading to faster progression to ESRD that continue to attract attention.

The HIV-infected ESRD patient provides specific medical and logistic challenges to dialysis care providers. Hemodialysis, peritoneal dialysis, and transplantation are options for these patients—and each modality has advantages and disadvantages, with no treatment showing a survival advantage in HIV-infected patients. Over the past 10 years, many dialysis facilities have both developed familiarity with HIV-infected ESRD patients and standardized protocols for treating patients and protecting dialysis personnel. Updated guidelines for the management of chronic kidney disease in HIV-infected patients and recommendations of the HIV Medicine Association of the Infectious Diseases Society of America were published in *Clinical Infectious Diseases* to help with the management of these complicated patients (see Recommended Reading section).

Improved Survival of the HIV-Infected ESRD Patient

Early data from the 1980s showed that newly diagnosed patients with ESRD and AIDS were dying on average 1–3 months after starting hemodialysis, but predominantly included AIDS patients late in the course of the HIV disease. Present-day early detection, treatment, and prophylaxis of HIV infection and opportunistic infections have led to dramatic improvements in the survival of HIV patients. Data from the United States Renal Data System have shown a steady increase in survival among ESRD patients with HIV infection since the advent of antiretroviral therapy in the mid- to late 1990s. CD4 count, serum albumin, older age, and lack of adherence on chronic dialysis seem to be strong determinants of survival in these patients.

Hemodialysis and Vascular Access

The most common renal replacement modality used in HIV-infected patients is hemodialysis. There appear to be no technical difficulties associated with placement of arteriovenous fistulas in HIV-infected patients. Patency rates for prosthetic grafts are lower in HIV-infected ESRD patients compared with the general ESRD population. Not surprisingly, infection rates are seen at a higher rate in HIV-infected patients with prosthetic grafts than with native arteriovenous fistulas. HIV-infected patients appear to have an increased risk of infection with tunneled dialysis catheters including gram-negative sepsis, associated more frequently with low serum albumin, intravenous drug use, and low CD4 counts. Therefore, HIV-infected patients with chronic kidney disease should be referred to a nephrologist early—and all possible efforts should be made for early surgical placement of a native arteriovenous fistula.

Infection Control in Hemodialysis

Unlike hepatitis B virus–infected ESRD patients, HIV-infected ESRD patients do not require special isolation procedures during dialysis, and routine testing for HIV infection for infection control purposes is not necessary or recommended. Of note, there is an increased incidence of false-positive EIA and intermediate Western blot testing when screening ESRD versus other low-risk patient populations. Dialyzer-reuse programs may include HIV-infected patients, although a policy of non-reuse among HIV-infected patients could eliminate the remote possibility of mistaken transmission to any HIV-uninfected patient through dialyzer reuse. In 1993, a tragic incident occurred in Colombia, South America, where nine hemodialysis patients were infected with HIV. Improperly reprocessed patient care equipment was the likely mode of transmission. This incident highlights the fact that strict guidelines emphasizing universal precautions and common sense must be enforced in all dialysis units because of HIV and other blood-borne pathogens. Routine infection-control precautions such as blood precautions, routine sodium hypochlorite cleaning of dialysis equipment and surfaces that are frequently touched, and restriction of non-disposable supplies to individual patients are sufficient in HIV-infected patients on hemodialysis.

Providing hemodialysis to HIV-infected patients carries the potential risk of exposure to contaminated blood or needles for dialysis personnel and other patients. All dialysis care personnel should take precautions against needle-stick injuries, including barrier precautions such as wearing gloves. Such injuries constitute the major potential risk for HIV transmission to personnel, although the risk of infection from needle stick is far lower than with hepatitis. The current regulations of the Division of Occupational Safety and Health (OSHA) state that needleless systems should be in place. This regulation requires needleless systems for withdrawal of blood once venous access is established and for administration of medications and fluids. If needleless systems are not used, needles with injury-protection devices should be used.

Dialysis staff that receive a needle stick or are exposed to HIV-contaminated blood or other body fluids should be immediately referred to a hotline or a medical provider experienced in dealing with blood-borne pathogen exposure and postexposure prophylaxis. The size of the HIV particle is much larger than most dialyzer membrane pore sizes, making it unlikely to cross the dialyzer membrane into the dialysate or ultrafiltrate. Despite noting a small decrease in plasma HIV RNA levels pre- versus posthemodialysis, one study could not measure HIV RNA in the ultrafiltrate of 10 HIV-infected hemodialysis patients. However, there are few data on the presence of HIV in dialysate—especially with regard to reused dialyzers. Despite this lack of evidence, dialysate should be treated as potentially contaminated body fluid.

Peritoneal Dialysis

There are advantages and disadvantages to offering peritoneal dialysis to HIV-infected patients. Peritoneal dialysis compares favorably with hemodialysis in HIV-infected patients, with comparable patient survival and very few reports of peritoneal dialysis technique failure. From a public health standpoint, the potential exposure by contaminated blood or needles to dialysis personnel is not present with peritoneal dialysis. On the other hand, peritoneal protein losses in malnourished HIV patients and severe peritonitis are potential concerns in this population. The incidence and spectrum of peritonitis have been reported in several small series of HIV-infected patients.

One study of 39 HIV-infected ESRD patients on continuous ambulatory peritoneal dialysis (CAPD) confirmed that HIV-infected patients have a higher overall risk of peritonitis and are more likely to have peritonitis attributed to *Pseudomonas* spp. and fungi compared to other ESRD patients, although *Staphylococcus aureus* is a similarly predominant pathogen. Interestingly, the higher peritonitis rate may not be due to HIV infection itself but to confounding variables such as low socioeconomic status and intravenous drug use.

HIV has been identified in peritoneal dialysate tubing and fluid bags for up to 7 days, and it should be handled as contaminated body fluid. Peritoneal dialysis patients should be instructed to pour dialysate into the home toilet and to dispose of dialysate bags and lines by placing and tying them in plastic bags and disposing of the plastic bags into conventional home trash systems.

Medical Management

Dialysis Care

The Kidney Disease Improving Global Outcomes (KDIGO) recommendations should be followed for HIV-infected patients with ESRD. As noted previously, native arteriovenous fistulas are preferred in these patients in order to reduce the incidence of catheter and graft infections. The goals for Kt/V, renal osteodystrophy and anemia management, and vascular access monitoring should be followed as outlined in KDIGO. Anemia targets are as in KDIGO, and different studies have demonstrated that HIV patients respond similarly to dosing of erythropoietic stimulating agents (ESAs).

Nutrition and Diet

Already a problem in many ESRD patients, malnutrition can be a life-threatening condition in HIV-infected ESRD patients—and hypoalbuminemia at the initiation of dialysis therapy is as strong a predictor of mortality as a low CD4 count. The prevalence and treatment of malnutrition or wasting among HIV-infected ESRD patients are not well understood. Successful initiation of antiretroviral therapy may increase weight and should be the first step in addressing malnutrition in these patients. Aggressive dietary interventions with the assistance of a dietitian should also be initiated in any HIV-infected patient with ESRD and significant weight loss.

Other therapies that have been studied in HIV patients with wasting include exercise, caloric supplements, the administration of hormones, and the administration of hormonelike drugs. The hormonal agents are reserved for HIV patients with documented endocrine deficiencies. Most studies using these agents have not included patients with chronic kidney disease and have only demonstrated short-term benefits. In addition, the risks of these agents are significant.

Hepatitis C and Hepatitis B Coinfection

Coinfection with hepatitis C virus (HCV) is very common in HIV-infected ESRD patients. More than 50% of patients with HIVAN are intravenous drug users, and 40%–90% of intravenous drug users are infected with HCV. Non-ESRD patients coinfected with HIV and HCV may progress more rapidly to end-stage liver disease compared with non–HIV-infected patients. In non–HIV-infected patients, novel antiviral therapies for HCV lead to unprecedented cure rates, are being studied in renal failure, and suggest promise for changing outcomes in HIV-infected and ESRD patients. At a minimum, patients coinfected with HIV and HCV should be discouraged from alcohol use and should be vaccinated against hepatitis A and B viruses. HIV-infected patients have an 88% antibody response rate to hepatitis A virus vaccine but only a 50% response to hepatitis B virus vaccine.

Transplantation

Kidney transplantation for HIV-infected ESRD patients, once thought to be risky in this population because of the potential risks of immunosuppression in the context of HIV infection, occurs routinely at transplant centers in the United States and globally. The results of a 2011 prospective nonrandomized trial found that HIV patient survival rates at 1 and 3 years were 94.6% ± 2.0% and 88.2% ± 3.8% (± standard deviation), respectively, and mean kidney graft-survival rates were 90.4% and 73.7% at 1 and 3 years, respectively. These rates fall between those reported nationally for elderly (>65 years old) patients and all kidney transplant recipients. Immunosuppression has not led to rapid progression of HIV infection or to unexpected reductions in CD4 counts. Despite the encouraging patient and graft survival rates, a consistent finding among HIV kidney transplant patients is a substantially higher acute graft rejection rate. The potential mechanisms explaining the increase in acute graft rejection remain unclear.

HIV Care

Recent improvements in the survival of HIV-infected patients are due not only to ART but to improved prophylaxis and treatment of opportunistic infections.

Table 48.1

Dosing of Antiretroviral Drugs in Adults With Renal Insufficiency and Hemodialysis

All Dosing Information Updated May 1, 2014, Reference, or Per Package Insert

All Agents Should Be Used With Caution and Monitored Carefully

Drug	Standard Dosage	Dosing in Renal Insufficiency and Hemodialysis		References
Nucleotide Reverse Transcriptase Inhibitors				
Abacavir (ABC)	300 mg PO bid or 600 mg PO daily	No dosage adjustment necessary, hemodialysis		Ziagen package insert, 9/13
Didanosine (ddI) (enteric-coated capsules)	250 mg PO daily, <60 kg 400 mg PO daily, ≥60 kg	**CrCl (mL/min)** 30–59 10–29 <10, HD, PD	**Wt ≥60 kg** 200 mg DAILY 125 mg DAILY 125 mg DAILY **Wt <60 kg** 125 mg daily 125 mg daily Use 75 mg (pediatric powder for suspension) daily	Videx EC package insert, 11/14
Emtricitabine (FTC)	200 mg PO daily or 240 mg oral solution daily	**CrCl (mL/min)** 30–49 15–29 <15 or HD	**Capsule** 200 mg Q 48H 200 mg Q 72H 200 mg Q 96H give dose after dialysis **Solution** 120 mg Q 24H 80 mg Q 24H 60 mg Q 24H	Emtriva package insert, 11/12
Lamivudine (3TC)	150 mg PO BID or 300 mg PO daily	**CrCl (mL/min)** 30–49 15–29 5–14 <5 or HD	**Dosage** 150 mg daily 150 mg first dose, then 100 mg daily 150 mg first dose, then 50 mg daily 50 mg first dose, then 25 mg daily	Epivir package insert, 1/2013
Stavudine (d4T)	30 mg PO BID, <60 kg 40 mg PO BID, ≥60 kg	**CrCl (mL/min)** 26–50 10–25 or HD	**Wt ≥60 kg** 20 mg bid 20 mg daily **Wt <60 kg** 15 mg bid 15 mg daily	Zerit package insert, 12/12

Continued

Table 48.1

Dosing of Antiretroviral Drugs in Adults With Renal Insufficiency and Hemodialysis—cont'd

All Dosing Information Updated May 1, 2014, Reference, or Per Package Insert

All Agents Should Be Used With Caution and Monitored Carefully

Drug	Standard Dosage	Dosing in Renal Insufficiency and Hemodialysis	References
Tenofovir disoproxil fumarate (TDF)	300 mg PO daily	**CrCl (mL/min)** **Dosage** 30–49 150 mg daily 10–29 150 mg daily <10, not on HD No recommendation HD 300 mg weekly, 12H post dialysis	Viread package insert, 2/16
Zidovudine (AZT, ZDV)	300 mg PO bid	**CrCl (mL/min)** **Dosage** <15 or HD 300 mg daily	Retrovir package insert, 9/08
Fixed-Dose Combinations			
Combivir (zidovudine/lamivudine)	1 tab PO bid	Substitute component drugs, dose adjusting each drug for CrCl	Combivir package insert, 1/13
Descovy (tenofovir alafenamide/emtricitabine)	1 tab PO DAILY	Not recommended for CrCL <30 or hemodialysis	Descovy package insert 4/16
Epzicom or Kivexa (abacavir/lamivudine)	1 tab PO daily	Substitute component drugs, dose adjusting each drug for CrCl	Epzicom package insert, 3/12
Trizivir (zidovudine/lamivudine/abacavir)	1 tab PO bid	Substitute component drugs, dose adjusting each drug for CrCl	Trizivir package insert, 5/13
Truvada (emtricitabine/tenofovir)	1 tab PO daily	**CrCl (mL/min)** **Dosage** 30–49 1 tab Q 48H <30 or HD Not recommended	Truvada package insert, 4/16

Non-Nucleotide Reverse Transcriptase Inhibitors

Drug	Dose	Adjustment	Reference
Delavirdine (DLV)	400 mg PO tid	No dosage adjustment necessary	Rescriptor package insert, 8/12
Efavirenz (EFV)	600 mg PO QHS	No dosage adjustment necessary	Sustiva package insert, 3/15
Etravirine (ETR)	200 mg PO bid	No dosage adjustment necessary	Intelence package insert, 8/14
Nevirapine (NVP)	200 mg PO bid or 400 mg PO daily	Patients on dialysis should receive an additional dose of 200 mg following each dialysis treatment; otherwise no dosage adjustment necessary	Viramune package insert, 1/14
Rilpivirine (RPV)	25 mg PO daily	No dosage adjustment necessary	

Fixed-Dose Combinations

Drug	Dose	Adjustment	Reference
Atripla (efavirenz/ tenofovir/emtricitabine)	1 tab PO daily	Substitute component drugs, dose adjusting each drug for CrCl	Atripla package insert, 1/15
Complera (rilpivirine/ tenofovir/disoproxil fumarate/emtricitabine)	1 tab PO daily	Substitute component drugs, dose adjusting each drug for CrCl	Complera package insert, 5/15
Odefsey (rilpivirine/ tenofovir alafenamide/ emtricitabine)	1 tab PO DAILY	Not recommended for CrCL <30	Odefsey package insert, 3/16

Protease Inhibitors

Drug	Dose	Adjustment	Reference
Atazanavir (ATV)	400 mg PO daily, or 300 mg PO daily + ritonavir (RTV) 100 mg PO daily For ART-naïve patients on HD, 300 mg + RTV 100 mg PO daily For ART-experienced patients, not recommended	No dosage adjustment necessary off HD	Reyataz package insert, 9/15

Continued

Table 48.1

Dosing of Antiretroviral Drugs in Adults With Renal Insufficiency and Hemodialysis—cont'd

All Dosing Information Updated May 1, 2014, Reference, or Per Package Insert

All Agents Should Be Used With Caution and Monitored Carefully

Drug	Standard Dosage	Dosing in Renal Insufficiency and Hemodialysis	References
Darunavir (DRV)	ART-naïve and ART-experienced with DRV resistance mutation: 800 mg + RTV 100 mg PO daily ART-experienced with >1 DRV resistance mutation: 600 mg + RTV 100 mg PO bid	No dosage adjustment necessary	Prezista package insert, 6/16
Fosamprenavir (FPV)	1400 mg PO bid, or 1400 mg + 200 mg RTV PO daily, or 700 mg + RTV 100 mg PO bid	No dosage adjustment necessary	Lexiva package insert, 9/09
Indinavir (IDV)	800 mg PO q8H	No dosage adjustment necessary, though not studied in renal failure, per package	Crixivan package insert, 3/15
Lopinavir (LPV)/Ritonavir (Kaletra)	400 mg + RTV 100 mg PO bid, or 800 mg + RTV 200 mg PO daily	Avoid once-daily dosing on patients on HD	Kaletra package insert, 3/15
Nelfinavir	1250 mg PO bid	No dosage adjustment necessary	Viracept package insert, 5/13
Ritonavir (RTV)	As a PI-boosting agent: 100–400 mg daily	No dosage adjustment necessary	Norvir package insert, 11/15

Saquinavir (SQV, hard-gel capsules or tablets)	1000 mg + RTV 100 mg PO bid	No dosage adjustment necessary	Invirase package insert, 3/16
Tipranavir (TPV)	500 mg + RTV 200 mg PO bid	No dosage adjustment necessary	Aptivus package insert, 3/15
Fixed-Dose Combinations			
Prezcobix (darunavir/cobicistat)	1 tab PO daily	Not recommended if CrCl <70 mL/min if used with TDF No dosage adjustment necessary if not used with TDF	Prezcobix package insert, 1/15
Integrase Inhibitors (INSTI)			
Dolutegravir (DTG)	50 mg PO daily or 50 mg PO bid	No dosage adjustment necessary, though caution warranted in INSTI-experienced patients as higher risk for loss of therapeutic effect and development of resistance.	Tivicay package insert 12/14
Elvitegravir (EVG)	50 mg PO daily	No dosage adjustment necessary	Vitekta package insert, 9/14
Raltegravir (RAL)	400 mg PO bid	No dosage adjustment necessary	Isentress package insert, 2/15
Fixed-Dose Combinations			
Genvoya (elvitegravir/ tenofovir alafenamide/ cobicistat/emtricitabine)	1 tab PO DAILY	Not recommended if CrCl <30	Genvoya package insert, 11/15
Stribild (elvitegravir/ tenofovir/disoproxil fumarate/cobicistat/ emtricitabine)	1 tab PO daily	Substitute component drugs, dose adjusting each drug. Not recommended if CrCl <70 mL/min	Stribild package insert, 2/16

Continued

Table 48.1

Dosing of Antiretroviral Drugs in Adults With Renal Insufficiency and Hemodialysis—cont'd

All Dosing Information Updated May 1, 2014, Reference,
or Per Package Insert
All Agents Should Be Used With Caution and Monitored Carefully

Drug	Standard Dosage	Dosing in Renal Insufficiency and Hemodialysis	References
Triumeq (dolutegravir/ lamivudine/abacavir)	1 tab PO daily	Substitute component drugs, dose adjusting each drug for CrCL	Triumeq package insert, 4/16
Fusion Inhibitors			
Enfuvirtide (T20)	90 mg SC bid	No dosage adjustment necessary	Fuzeon package insert, 6/14
CCR5 Antagonist			
Maraviroc (MVC)	Varies based upon concomitant medications and potential for drug–drug interactions	CrCl <30 or on HD, and without potent CYP3A inhibitors or inducers: 300 mg PO BID, reduce to 150 mg PO BID if postural hypotension occurs Not recommended with potent CYP3A inhibitors or inducers	Selzentry package insert, 8/07

BID, 2 times per day; CrCl, creatinine clearance; h, hour(s); HD, hemodialysis; PI, protease inhibitor; PO, orally; q, every; QHS, at bedtime; QW, once weekly; SC, subcutaneous (injection); TID, 3 times per day; Wt, body weight.

Table adapted from HIV InSite, http://hivinsite.ucsf.edu. Thank you to Jennifer Cocohoba, PharmD, for her assistance in adapting this table.

The following references support Table 1 dosing recommendations:

Armbruster C, Vorbach H, El Menyawi I, Meisl FT, Neumann I. Pharmacokinetics of nelfinavir during haemodialysis in a patient with HIV infection. *AIDS.* 2000;14:99-101.

Bohjanen PR, Johnson MD, Szczech LA, et al. Steady-state pharmacokinetics of lamivudine in human immunodeficiency virus-infected patients with end-stage renal disease receiving chronic dialysis. *Antimicrob Agents Chemother* 2002;46:2387-2392.

Grasela DM, Stoltz RR, Barry M, et al. Pharmacokinetics of single-dose oral stavudine in subjects with renal impairment and in subjects requiring hemodialysis. *Antimicrob Agents Chemother* 2000;44:2149-2153.

Personal communication with J. Flaherty, 2002.

Guardiola JM, Mangues MA, Domingo P, Martinez E, Barrio JL. Indinavir pharmacokinetics in haemodialysis-dependent end-stage renal failure. *AIDS.* 1998;12:1395.

Ian R. McNicholl, PhamD, University of California San Francisco.

Izzedine H, Aymard G, Hamani A, Launay-Vacher V, Deray G. Indinavir pharmacokinetics in haemodialysis. *Nephrol Dial Transplant* 2000;15:1102-1103.

Izzedine H, Launay-Vacher V, Aymard G, Legrand M, Deray G. Pharmacokinetics of abacavir in HIV-1-infected patients with impaired renal function. *Nephron* 2001;89:62-67.

Singlas E, Taburet AM, Borsa Lebas F, et al. Didanosine pharmacokinetics in patients with normal and impaired renal function: influence of hemodialysis. *Antimicrob Agents Chemother* 1992;36:1519-1524.

Izzedine H, Launay-Vacher V, Aymard G, Legrand M, Deray G. Pharmacokinetic of nevirapine in haemodialysis. *Nephrol Dial Transplant* 2001;16:192-193.

Izzedine H, Launay-Vacher V, Deray G. Dosage of lamivudine in a haemodialysis patient. *Nephron* 2000;86:553.

Izzedine H, Launay-Vacher V, Deray G. Pharmacokinetics of ritonavir and nevirapine in peritoneal dialysis. *Nephron Dial Transplant* 2001;16:643.

Izzedine H, Launay-Vacher V, Legrand M, Aymard G, Deray G. Pharmacokinetics of ritonavir and saquinavir in a haemodialysis patient. *Nephron* 2001;87:186-187.

Izzedine H, Launay-Vacher V, Legrand M, Lieberherr D, Caumes E, Deray G. ABT 378/r: a novel inhibitor of HIV-1 protease in haemodialysis. *AIDS.* 2001;15:662-664.

Johnson MA, Verpooten GA, Daniel MJ, et al. Single dose pharmacokinetics of lamivudine in subjects with impaired renal function and the effect of haemodialysis. *Br J Clin Pharmacol* 1998;46:21-27.

Kimmel PL, Lew SQ, Umana WO, Li PP, Gordon AM, Straw J. Pharmacokinetics of zidovudine in HIV-infected patients with end-stage renal disease. *Blood Purif* 1995;13:340-346.

Knupp CA, Hak LJ, Coakley DF, et al. Disposition of didanosine in HIV-seropositive patients with normal renal function or chronic renal failure: influence of hemodialysis and continuous ambulatory peritoneal dialysis. *Clin Pharmacol Ther* 1996;60:535-542.

Pachon J, Cisneros JM, Castillo JR, et al. Pharmacokinetics of zidovudine in end-stage renal disease: influence of haemodialysis. *AIDS.* 1992;6:827-830.

Paci-Bonaventure S, Hafi A, Vincent I, et al. Lack of removal of nelfinavir during a haemodialysis session in an HIV-1 infected patient with hepatic and renal insufficiency. *Nephrol Dial Transplant* 2001;16:642-643.

Taylor S, Little J, Halifax K, Drake S, Back D. Pharmacokinetics of nelfinavir and nevirapine in a patient with end-stage renal failure on continuous ambulatory peritoneal dialysis. *J Antimicrob Chemother* 2000;45:716-717.

Tartaglione TA, Holeman E, Opheim K, Smith T, Collier AC. Zidovudine disposition during hemodialysis in a patient with acquired immunodeficiency syndrome. *J Acquir Immune Defic Syndr* 1990;3:32-34.

It is beyond the scope of this chapter to review current guidelines for prophylaxis and treatment of opportunistic infections. All HIV-infected ESRD patients with advanced HIV disease and low CD4 cell counts should receive standard prophylaxis for *Pneumocystis carinii* pneumonia and *Mycobacterium avium*-complex infections. All patients should be vaccinated against pneumonia, influenza, and hepatitis A and B.

The current recommendations for initiation of ART are well outlined by the International Antiviral Society–USA Panel in a consensus statement published in the *Journal of the American Medical Association*. ART is now recommended regardless of CD4 cell count but the strength of the recommendation increases as the CD4 cell count decreases and in the presence of other conditions. For example, treatment is recommended for patients with HIVAN and CD4 cell counts of >500/μL.

Antiretroviral Therapy (ART)

In renal disease, several of the antiretroviral medications are excreted primarily through the kidney and must be dose adjusted accordingly (Table 48.1). There are limited data on the pharmacokinetic properties of the nonnucleotide reverse transcriptase inhibitors and protease inhibitors in patients with renal function impairment. Aside from those combination pills including tenofovir, the pharmacokinetic profile of these drugs suggests no dosage adjustment necessary in renal insufficiency. The nucleotide reverse transcriptase inhibitors require dose adjustments in patients with renal insufficiency (Table 48.1).

SECTION XIX

Anemia and Epoetin Use

C H A P T E R 4 9

Use of Erythropoiesis-Stimulating Agents in Hemodialysis Patients

Bonita A. Mohamed, MD • Jeffrey S. Berns, MD

Introduction

Erythropoietin is necessary for the survival, proliferation, and differentiation of bone marrow–derived erythroid cells that ultimately become mature circulating red blood cells. In the vast majority of patients on hemodialysis, erythropoietin synthesis is insufficient to stimulate adequate levels of erythrocyte production by the bone marrow, and anemia develops as a result. Although factors such as iron deficiency, inflammation, infection, and other comorbid conditions contribute to the anemia seen almost universally in hemodialysis patients, a relative deficiency of erythropoietin is the most important factor. Observational studies have shown that anemia in hemodialysis patients is associated with increased risk of death from noncardiac and cardiac causes, increased frequency and duration of hospitalizations, cardiac dysfunction, left ventricular hypertrophy, reduced quality of life, functional status, and exercise intolerance.

Replacement therapy with recombinant human erythropoietin (rHuEPO, epoetin alfa), first reported in hemodialysis patients in 1987 and approved by the US Food and Drug Administration (FDA) in 1989, markedly changed the management of anemia in these patients—as well as patients with chronic kidney disease (CKD) not on dialysis and those on peritoneal dialysis. Treatment with epoetin alfa raised hemoglobin levels and reduced transfusion requirements. Compared to the very low hemoglobin levels that were common before epoetin alfa became available, often in the range of 6–8 g/dL, moderately higher hemoglobin levels (>8–10 g/dL) were associated with improvement in symptoms related to anemia, left ventricular hypertrophy, quality of life, and functional status. What has become clear over the years, though, is that raising hemoglobin levels with erythropoiesis-stimulating agents (ESAs) to levels that approach normal does not reduce mortality risk, increases blood pressure, and increases the risk of stroke.

ESAs Available in the U.S.

There are three ESAs currently commercially available in the United States: epoetin alfa, darbepoetin alfa, and methoxy polyethylene glycol (pegylated)-epoetin beta. Optimal utilization of ESAs requires understanding of the pharmacology of these agents, their clinical effects and side effects, practical aspects of their use, and knowledge of clinical practice recommendations related to their use. To stimulate erythropoieses, ESAs interact with the same reactor on erythroid progenitor cells as the native erythropoietin, reducing apoptosis of these red blood cell precursors. Epoetin alfa is a 165-amino-acid glycoprotein with three N-linked and one O-linked carbohydrate chain produced using recombinant DNA technology using Chinese hamster ovary cells. The amino acid structure is identical to the native human erythropoietin hormone. Most other epoetin types, such as epoetin beta and epoetin omega, which are commercially available outside the United States, contain the same amino acid sequence as epoetin alfa but differ in their glycosylation and sialic acid content. For epoetin alfa, the terminal half-life following intravenous (IV) administration is approximately 4–13 hours, and following subcutaneous administration it is approximately 16–67 hours.

Darbepoetin alfa was approved by the FDA in 2001 for the treatment of anemia in patients with CKD, including dialysis patients. This ESA, also produced using recombinant DNA technology, differs in five amino acids compared to the native hormone and contains five N-linked carbohydrate chains rather than three as are present in epoetin alfa. As a result of its increased glycosylation, affinity of darbepoetin alfa for the erythropoietin receptor is less than that of epoetin alfa. However, because of an increase in serum half-life, clinical efficacy is enhanced. The darbepoetin alfa half-life is approximately 21 hours with IV administration and 46 hours with subcutaneous administration. Methoxy polyethylene glycol (pegylated)-epoetin beta was approved for use in the U.S. in 2007 but did not become commercially available until recently. It has been used for several years outside the U.S. and its use among U.S. hemodialysis patients has increased significantly since becoming available in this country. Methoxy polyethylene glycol-epoetin beta contains a chemical bond between either the N-terminal amino group of the ε-amino group of any lysine present in erythropoietin and methoxy polyethylene glycol (PEG) butanoic acid. Pegylated epoetin beta has a greated in vivo activity and longer half-life compared to epoetin alfa and darbepoetin alfa. The half-life is approximately 135–140 hours following IV or subcutaneous administration.

Subcutaneous administration of epoetin alfa tends to be more effective than IV administration. As a result, many patients can be treated with a lower epoetin dose when it is given subcutaneously rather than intravenously, with an overall average reduction in epoetin dose of 25%–30% while maintaining the same target hemoglobin level. The relatively short half-life of IV epoetin predicts the need for more frequent dosing than when it is administered subcutaneously and compared to darbepoetin alfa. In practice, whether administered intravenously or subcutaneously, epoetin is typically administered three times weekly for hemodialysis patients. Subcutaneous and IV darbepoetin alfa and pegylated epoetin beta administration appear to be of similar efficacy.

Dosing and Administration Guidelines

Epoetin use among hemodialysis patients has declined from greater than 95% to about 50% with increasing use of darbepoetin and peglyted epoetin beta. For reasons of convenience and patient preference, despite the reported superior efficacy of epoetin when administered by subcutaneous injection, most U.S. hemodialysis patients are treated with IV injections at each dialysis treatment. Specific dosing practices and goals of therapy with ESAs in hemodialysis patients have been influenced over the years by the package labeling, reimbursement policies, findings from various clinical studies, mostly in patients with CKD not on dialysis, and clinical practice guidelines. There is no evidence to support any specific ESA or ESA-dosing protocol over another, and each dialysis clinic or provider will generally have developed a protocol for use in their dialysis facility.

The approved prescribing information in the United States recommends an epoetin alfa starting dose of 50–100 IU/kg three times weekly IV or subcutaneously for adults on dialysis. The prescribing information recommends initiation of treatment when the hemoglobin level is <10 g/dL and stopping treatment or reducing the dose if the hemoglobin level approaches or exceeds 11 g/dL. The starting dose recommended in the U.S. prescribing information for darbepoetin alfa is 0.45 µg/kg intravenously or subcutaneously weekly or 0.75 µg/kg intravenously or subcutaneously every 2 weeks. The starting dose of pegylated epoetin beta recommended in the U.S. prescribing information is 0.6 mcg/kg every two weeks IV or subcutaneously. It is also recommended that once a stable maintenance dose is determined, that dose can be doubled for monthly administration. The IV route is recommended for patients on hemodialysis for all ESAs. The recommended hemoglobin levels for initiation and termination of treatment before darbepoetin and pegylated epoetin beta are the same as for epoetin therapy. For all ESAs, there is significant variability in responsiveness among patients. Prospective clinical trials in dialysis patients comparing once-weekly IV darbepoetin, twice-monthly pegylated epoetin beta and 2- to 3-times-weekly IV epoetin alfa have found that they have similar clinical efficacy with regard to endpoints such as absolute level of hemoglobin increase, time to achieve a hemoglobin response, ability to maintain target hemoglobin, and reduction in transfusion requirement.

Clinical use of ESAs has been largely guided by clinical practice guidelines ever since publication of the National Kidney Foundation Kidney Disease Outcomes Quality Initiative (NKF-K/DOQI) guideline on anemia in 1997. The most current clinical practice guideline in this arena is the 2012 Kidney Disease Improving Global Outcomes (KDIGO) Clinical Practice Guideline for Anemia in Chronic Kidney Disease. Specific recommendations concerning ESA use in dialysis patients from this report are listed in Table 49.1.

Initial interest in using ESAs to achieve normal or near-normal hemoglobin levels in patients on dialysis (as well as those with CKD not on dialysis) has been tempered by results of several prospective randomized controlled clinical trials (only one of which was conducted in hemodialysis patients). In sum, these studies failed to show significant clinical or quality of life benefit of attempting to maintain hemoglobin levels >11.5 g/dL or so and also demonstrated that risks of death and cardiovascular events including stroke were either not reduced or were increased. Individualization of therapy is recommended as it is recognized that some patients may have improvement in their quality of life with hemoglobin levels >11.5 g/dL and will be willing to accept some risks in return. It must also be recognized that virtually all patients in these studies were middle-age or older and most had diabetes, cardiovascular disease, and other significant comorbidities. As such, the extent to which the findings of these clinical trials should be applied to younger patients or those without diabetes and other comorbid conditions is not clear. Maintaining hemoglobin levels >13 g/dL is not recommended.

Approaches to ESA dosing and target hemoglobin levels in the United States have also been significantly impacted by reimbursement policies of the Centers for Medicare and Medicaid Services (CMS), which governs payment for patients receiving Medicare benefits. The ESRD Prospective Payment System (PPS) replaced the previous basic case-mixed adjusted composite payment system and the reimbursement of separately billable outpatient ESRD-related items and services. The Social Security Act was amended to require CMS to implement a fully bundled PPS for renal dialysis services furnished to Medicare beneficiaries for the treatment of ESRD, which went

Table 49.1

KDIGO Clinical Practice Guidelines for Treatment of Anemia in ESA-Treated Hemodialysis Patients

In initiating and maintaining ESA therapy, we recommend balancing the potential benefits of reducing blood transfusions and anemia-related symptoms against the risks of harm in individual patients (e.g., stroke, vascular access loss, hypertension). (1B)

We recommend using ESA therapy with great caution, if at all, in CKD patients with active malignancy—in particular when cure is the anticipated outcome (1B), a history of stroke (1B), or a history of malignancy (2C).

For adult CKD 5D patients, we suggest that ESA therapy be used to avoid having the Hb concentration fall below 9.0 g/dL by starting ESA therapy when the hemoglobin is between 9.0 and 10.0 g/dL. (2B)

Individualization of therapy is reasonable as some patients may have improvements in quality of life at higher Hb concentration and ESA therapy may be started above 10.0 g/dL. (Not Graded)

ESA Maintenance Therapy

In general, we suggest that ESAs not be used to maintain Hb concentration above 11.5 g/dL in adult patients with CKD. (2C)

Individualization of therapy will be necessary as some patients may have improvements in quality of life at Hb concentration above 11.5 g/dL and will be prepared to accept the risks. (Not Graded)

In all adult patients, we recommend that ESAs not be used to intentionally increase the Hb concentration above 13 g/dL. (1A)

ESA Administration

3.9.1: For CKD 5HD patients and those on hemofiltration or hemodiafiltration therapy, we suggest either intravenous or subcutaneous administration of ESA. (2C)

CKD, chronic kidney disease; ESA, erythropoiesis-stimulating agent.

Adapted from Kidney Disease: Improving Global Outcomes (KDIGO) Anemia Work Group. KDIGO Clinical Practice Guideline for Anemia in Chronic Kidney Disease. Kidney International, Suppl. 2012;2:279-335.

into effect January 2011; thus, ESAs are no longer separately billable items but instead their cost is now included in a global fee paid to dialysis facilities. Since the implementation of bundled reimbursement, mean hemoglobin levels among U.S. hemodialysis patients have declined from 11.5 g/dL to approximately 10.8 g/dL. Median weekly prescribed IV epoetin doses have declined from about 20,000 IU to just under 10,000 IU. Similar data is not available for the other ESAs.

Adequate iron availability is necessary for maintaining an optimal response to ESA therapy. Unfortunately, there is no single test that completely and accurately measures total body iron stores, the amount of iron readily available for erythropoiesis, or whether a patient's hemoglobin level or ESA dose will improve with additional iron supplementation. The two most commonly used tests are the serum ferritin and the percentage saturation of serum transferrin (TSAT). For adult hemodialysis patients on ESA therapy, a trial of IV iron is suggested if an increase in hemoglobin level or a decrease in ESA dose is desired and if TSAT is ≤30% and ferritin is ≤500 ng/mL. Most oral iron products are not well tolerated and are of limited efficacy in hemodialysis patients, and therefore are not recommended, although some newer oral agents may prove to be more useful in the future.

Clinical Outcomes Associated With ESA Treatment in Hemodialysis Patients

There have been remarkably few large prospective studies in ESA-treated hemodialysis patients. None have been published in the last decade. Observational studies have generally noted associations of higher hemoglobin levels, up to the range of 11–13 g/dL, with improved quality of life measures (less fatigue, depression, cognitive deficits, and exercise intolerance), and decreased mortality risk from cardiac and noncardiac causes. Only one large randomized controlled trial has been conducted in ESA-treated hemodialysis patients, in which a target hemoglobin level of 14 g/dL was compared to 10 g/dL. Patients assigned to the higher hemoglobin group had an increased rate of composite outcome of death or first nonfatal MI and the study was stopped early as a result. There were no differences between groups for all-cause hospitalization or other endpoints, with the exception of a higher thrombosis rate for AV (arteriovenous) fistulas and grafts in the higher target group.

In the most recent large randomized controlled clinical trial of ESA treatment in patients with CKD not on dialysis, more than 4000 patients with diabetes and anemia were randomly assigned to receive darbepoetin alfa to achieve a hemoglobin level of approximately 13 g/dL or placebo, with rescue darbepoetin alfa when the hemoglobin level was <9.0 g/dL. There was no reduction with darbepoetin in the primary endpoints of death or a cardiovascular event composite. Fatal or nonfatal stroke was nearly twice as likely in darbepoetin-treated patients. Red-cell transfusions were lower among darbepoetin-treated patients. There was only a modest improvement in patient-reported fatigue in the darbepoetin alfa group.

While some studies have shown improvement in some quality of life measures—such as physical symptoms, vitality, fatigue, exercise performance, and neurocognitive function—as hemoglobin levels are raised toward normal with ESA treatment in hemodialysis patients, this has not been a consistent finding. Higher hemoglobin levels do reduce the need for blood transfusions, which were once the mainstay of anemia treatment in hemodialysis patients. While transfusions in general are less common when the higher hemoglobin levels are chronically maintained in hemodialysis patients, transfusion rates increase substantially when baseline hemoglobin levels are <10 g/dL. Clinical studies, primarily retrospective in nature, have suggested an association between anemia and left ventricular hypertrophy (LVH) and dilation. Prospective studies in hemodialysis patients have generally failed, however, to demonstrate that treatment of anemia with ESA therapy to a hemoglobin level above 10 or 11 g/dL results in regression of LVH or amelioration of LV dilation.

Side Effects of ESA Therapy

Serious acute side effects directly related to use of ESAs are uncommon. All three agents have similar side-effect profiles in hemodialysis patients. Use of these agents is contraindicated in patients with uncontrolled hypertension or with prior hypersensitivity to the drug (including prior history of pure red cell aplasia, discussed below) or to its carrier components. The most common minor adverse effects are pain at the site of subcutaneous injection and rarely mild flulike symptoms. Allergic reactions such as urticaria and skin rash are uncommon and are rarely serious, but anaphylactic-like reactions have been very rarely described. More significant adverse effects include increased risks of vascular-access thrombosis, seizures, and hypertension. Vascular access thrombosis rates are greater in ESA-treated patients with higher hemoglobin levels and may be more of a problem for patients with synthetic arteriovenous grafts than with primary AV fistulas. Whether this increased vascular access thrombosis rate is due to a higher hemoglobin level itself or to other factors, including the higher ESA doses needed to achieve higher hemoglobin levels is not known.

The appearance of hypertension or worsening of existing hypertension is seen in as many as 30% of hemodialysis patients treated with an ESA. The specific mechanism for this is not defined but is thought to include direct effect of the ESA on endothelial cells, alterations in vascular reactivity with increased vasoconstriction and impaired vasodilation due to improvement in the anemia and effects on factors such as nitrous oxide and endothelin, increased blood viscosity and plasma volume related to higher red cell mass, and increased cardiac output. Seizures related to ESA therapy are very rare in hemodialysis patients but may be due to severe hypertension and very high hemoglobin levels—predisposing to cerebrovascular sludging and impaired cerebral blood flow. All ESAs are rated pregnancy category C (no teratogenicity or fetotoxicity in animal studies).

ESA-related pure red cell aplasia (PRCA) is a rare but potentially life-threatening condition characterized by severe anemia associated with a very low reticulocyte count, nearly complete absence of erythroid precursor cells in the bone marrow, and the development of neutralizing antierythropoietin IgG antibodies in the blood. These antibodies cross-react with the endogenous hormone as well as recombinant ESAs. An international outbreak of epoetin antibody-mediated PRCA began in 1998 in patients receiving primarily one particular epoetin alfa product made and used outside the United States (Eprex; Ortho-Biotech, Inc) by the subcutaneous route of administration. The specific product implicated was prefilled syringes with uncoated rubber stoppers with the stabilizer polysorbate-80 used instead of albumin as was used in other formulations. Subcutaneous ESA administration was subsequently considered contraindicated by regulatory authorities. The exact cause of this reaction is not known for certain, although it has been proposed that compounds leached from the uncoated rubber stoppers by polysorbate-80 led to the formation of anti-epoetin antibodies. Fortunately, with removal of this product from the worldwide market, the incidence of ESA-related PRCA has again become quite low (0.2–0.3/100,000 patient-years).

U.S. prescribing information includes a "black box warning" indicating that ESAs increase the risk of death, myocardial infarction, stroke, venous thromboembolism, thrombosis of vascular access, and tumor progression or recurrence. It also states that no trial has identified a hemoglobin target level, ESA dose, or dosing strategy that does not increase these risks. Hence, the recommendation is that the lowest ESA dose sufficient to reduce the need for red blood cell transfusions should be used.

ESA Hyporesponsiveness in Hemodialysis Patients

When the hemoglobin concentration does not increase as expected in response to ESA therapy, a correctable underlying disease state that limits the erythropoietic response should be suspected. Such conditions include iron deficiency, hemolysis, hemoglobinopathies, malignancy, infectious and inflammatory disorders, severe malnutrition, folic acid or vitamin B_{12} deficiency, severe hyperparathyroidism with marrow fibrosis, and infiltrative processes of the bone marrow such as leukemia and multiple myeloma. Although there is no single generally accepted definition of ESA hyporesponsiveness, the most recent KDIGO anemia clinical practice guidelines recommend classifying patients as having initial ESA hyporesponsiveness if there is no increase in hemoglobin concentration from baseline after 1 month on an appropriate weight-based dose. Acquired ESA hyporesponsiveness occurs when patients with stable ESA dosing require two increases in ESA dose up to 50% beyond their previous dose. In both circumstances, repeated ESA dose escalations beyond a doubling of the initial or subsequently stable dose are not recommended. The vast majority of hemodialysis patients are able to achieve currently recommended hemoglobin level with <30,000 IU epoetin alfa per week.

Iron deficiency is the primary cause for ESA hyporesponsiveness. Many hemodialysis patients are either iron deficient when ESA therapy is initiated or have inadequate iron stores to support the enhanced erythropoiesis that develops in response to ESA therapy. These patients quickly become iron deficient. Therefore, most ESA-treated hemodialysis patients require iron supplementation. KDIGO guidelines recommend iron treatment in hemodialysis patients receiving ESA therapy if TSAT is <30% and serum ferritin is <500 ng/mL if an increase in hemoglobin level is desired, especially if intended to avoid transfusions and anemia-related symptoms. The preferred route of iron administration in hemodialysis patients is intravenous. Oral iron has generally been found to be ineffective in dialysis patients, although newer agents may alter this.

Pharmacologic agents other than iron have been reported in some small studies to be effective for treating erythropoietin-resistant anemia. In the absence of documented folate or vitamin B_{12} deficiency, there is no role for routine supplementation of either of these compounds. Prior to the availability of ESAs, androgens were often administered by intramuscular injection to stimulate erythropoiesis. These agents are now not recommended because of their toxicity (including acne, virilization, liver disease, and injection site pain) and because of limited evidence that they enhance the response to ESA therapy. L-Carnitine is a carrier molecule involved in the transport of long-chain fatty acids into mitochondria, where they are oxidized to produce energy. An L-carnitine deficiency state has been described in hemodialysis patients, and anemia in hemodialysis patients has been attributed to this deficiency, although the pathogenetic mechanisms remain speculative. IV and oral L-carnitine have been studied for possible enhancement of ESA responsiveness, largely in case reports and small uncontrolled studies. Although some reports and consensus conference statements supported use of IV L-carnitine in ESA-hyporesponsive hemodialysis patients, the KDIGO guidelines recommend that it not be used in ESA-hyporesponsive hemodialysis patients. Vitamin C (ascorbic acid) may increase the release of iron from stores, improve iron utilization for red cell production, and modulate oxidative stress. Oral vitamin C can enhance absorption of iron from the gastrointestinal tract. However, there is no evidence that oral vitamin C is an effective adjuvant to ESA therapy. Studies of IV vitamin C have produced conflicting results and its use is currently not recommended. Other pharmacologic agents (including statins, pentoxifylline, and vitamin E) have not been studied sufficiently to recommend their use at this time.

Biosimilars and Other Future ESAs

As noted above, epoetin alfa remains the primarily used ESA in the U.S. hemodialysis population. Biosimilars are biologic products that are similar, but not identical to, a reference product. The passage of the Biologics Price Competition and Innovation (BPCI) Act provides a regulatory pathway for the development and approval of biosimilars by the FDA. The incorporation of biosimilar epoetins into the standard of care in European and other countries may be indicative of their potential success in the United States as well. It is likely that such biosimilar epoetins will become available in the United States also in the near future.

Considerable progress has been made in further understanding the regulation of EPO gene expression, which has led to the identification of certain cellular oxygen-sensing mechanisms. The transcription factor complex hypoxia-inducible factor (HIF)-1, a heterodimer of an alpha- and beta-subunit, is predominantly regulated by oxygen-dependent posttranslational hydroxylation of the alpha-subunit. Oral inhibitors of HIF-1 alpha, which lead to increased erythropoiesis, are undergoing clinical testing.

Summary

ESA treatment has dramatically altered the treatment of anemia in hemodialysis patients, but at substantial economic cost. Initially, ESA treatment was used successfully to rescue patients on hemodialysis from severe anemia, multiple transfusion, and iron overload. Currently available data and clinical practice recommendations support the use of ESA therapy to maintain hemoglobin levels of 10.0–11.5 g/dL in most hemodialysis patients, with the primary treatment goal of transfusion avoidance, although treatment goals should be individualized. Adequate amounts of iron, usually administered intravenously, should be provided to support erythropoiesis and efficient ESA therapy.

C H A P T E R 5 0

Anemia in Patients With End-Stage Kidney Disease

Hitesh H. Shah, MD • Steven Fishbane, MD

Anemia remains an important clinical complication of chronic kidney disease (CKD). It is defined by the World Health Organization as serum hemoglobin level <13 g/dL in adult men and postmenopausal women and <12 g/dL in premenopausal women. Similar to the anemia of chronic disease, anemia of CKD is generally normocytic and normochromic with bone marrow of normal cellularity. While several factors may play a contributing role in the development of anemia in CKD, inappropriately low secretion of erythropoietin from the diseased kidneys remains the most important cause. As the glomerular filtration rate (GFR) and renal function declines, there is a relative decline in the production of erythropoietin leading to an increased prevalence of anemia with progressive CKD. A recent data analysis from the National Health and Nutrition Examination Survey (NHANES) conducted in 2007–2008 and 2009–2010 showed the prevalence of anemia to be increased with the stage of CKD, from 8.4% at stage 1 (GFR ≥90 mL/min/1.73 m^2 plus evidence of kidney disease) to 53.4% at stage 5 (GFR <15 mL/min/1.73 m^2).

Several clinically relevant consequences result from the development of anemia in patients with CKD. Many of the symptoms that were formerly attributed to advanced renal failure and uremia were, in fact, at least in part from anemia. The most notable symptoms include fatigue, reduced exercise tolerance, and dyspnea. Other common complaints include insomnia, loss of appetite, cold intolerance, and reduced sexual and cognitive function. Anemia may lead to increased cardiac output and the development of left ventricular hypertrophy, angina, and congestive heart failure. Other problems as a result of anemia include impaired immune and hemostatic function. Anemia has also been associated with high morbidity and mortality in this population.

Treatment of anemia with erythropoietin-stimulating agents (ESAs) in patients with nondialysis CKD and end-stage kidney disease (ESKD) may not only decrease blood transfusion requirements, but may also improve the quality of life and symptoms related to anemia.

In this chapter, we will mainly review the causes of anemia seen in patients with ESKD. We will also briefly review the role of blood transfusion in the management of anemia of ESKD. Other treatment options including the use of ESAs and iron therapy will be reviewed elsewhere in this book.

Erythropoietin Deficiency

The erythropoietic system functions to ensure adequate delivery of oxygen to the body's organs and tissues. When anemia or hypoxia develops, cells recognize oxygen deprivation, and a group of genes are activated that protect the cells from damage due to hypoxia. The process is mediated by stabilization of hypoxia-inducible factors (HIFs) 1α and 2α. In the kidneys, activation of the HIF system plays a particularly important role by promoting quantities of erythropoietin production that result in a substantial increase in serum erythropoietin levels.

As the kidneys fail, erythropoietin deficiency develops. The deficiency is relative in that serum levels of erythropoietin are actually higher in CKD than among normal controls, however, lower than what the levels should be for the degree of anemia. In ESKD, levels become frankly deficient and most patients will require ESA therapy on a long-term basis.

Other factors, described below, contribute to the anemia of kidney disease, but erythropoietin deficiency is the most important cause. There are some patients on dialysis who maintain a relatively normal level of hemoglobin; in many of these cases, erythropoietin production remains sufficient. This is seen more commonly when polycystic kidney disease is the cause of ESKD. Interestingly, dialysis patients living at higher altitudes may maintain a greater ability to produce erythropoietin compared to patients living at sea level and tend to have higher hemoglobin levels.

Iron Deficiency

Most hemodialysis patients become iron deficient, which is multifactorial in origin. The most apparent problem is that blood (and iron) is lost during every hemodialysis treatment. There is blood retained in the dialysis filter and lines and occasional bleeding that occurs during and after the treatment. This has been estimated to result in 3–10 mg of iron lost per treatment. In addition, blood is frequently drawn for laboratory testing. Blood may also be lost during the surgical or interventional procedures that dialysis patients often undergo. In addition, gastrointestinal bleeding is more common among dialysis patients and may contribute to iron deficiency.

Dietary absorption of iron is probably decreased in dialysis patients compared to normal controls; however, data in this regard have been conflicting. Regardless of whether the inherent ability to absorb dietary iron is maintained, the use of phosphate binders and gastric acid–blocking drugs by dialysis patients probably does limit iron absorption. In addition, functional achlorhydria, often present in dialysis patients, also adversely affects iron absorption.

During the current era, where intravenous iron treatment has become almost universal in hemodialysis patients, true iron deficiency is probably far less common than previously observed. Recently, 60%–80% of hemodialysis patients in the United States have been treated regularly with intravenous iron, with mean serum ferritin in early 2014 nearing 800 ng/mL. Studies utilizing magnetic resonance imaging (MRI) have demonstrated iron overload in the liver of many hemodialysis patients, although the clinical relevance of this observation has been questioned. To be clear, intravenous iron therapy remains an important aspect of anemia management in dialysis patients, but some moderation of therapy may be justified to optimize the balance of benefits and risks.

Reduced Erythrocyte Survival

Red cell half-life is reduced among patients with advanced kidney disease. The exact magnitude of reduction has been difficult to characterize. While the normal red cell half-life is approximately 120 days, estimates in dialysis patients have been as low as 40–80 days. Mechanisms behind reduced erythrocyte life span in ESRD have not been fully elucidated. Uremic toxins, low-grade hemolysis due to shearing by dialysis needles, and other factors have all been implicated. Shortened half-life (eg, due to hemolysis) can be compensated for in nonuremic individuals through accelerated erythrocyte production. In patients on dialysis, erythropoietin deficiency limits this ability.

Inflammation

One of the most important contributing factors to the anemia of CKD is inflammation. Many patients with ESKD have a chronic occult inflammatory process, demonstrated by measurement of C-reactive protein, interleukin-6, and other markers. The etiology is unclear, perhaps because of atherosclerosis, infection, uremic toxins, or other factors yet to be identified. The presence of inflammation in these patients is associated with adverse outcomes and is linked to suboptimal nutrition as part of a broader malnutrition–inflammation complex.

Inflammation results in reduced hemoglobin concentrations and impaired responsiveness to ESA therapy. One of the important recent advances in science has been the identification of hepcidin, the key regulator of iron homeostasis. Serum hepcidin concentrations are very sensitive to inflammation. In the presence of inflammation, levels can rise sharply, up to 100-fold. The net effect is to block iron entry into the circulation both by limiting intestinal iron absorption and by greatly reducing movement into the circulation of iron held in storage tissue. In the classic anemia of chronic disease, better termed anemia of inflammation, hepcidin lowers iron in the circulation, thereby limiting iron availability for red cell production. The same occurs frequently in dialysis patients, where the chronic inflammatory state contributes to anemia. Iron is sequestered in storage tissues, raising serum ferritin, and reduced in the circulation, lowering transferrin saturation. This discordant combination of a relatively high serum ferritin in combination with normal or reduced transferrin saturation is a common finding in dialysis patients.

Infection

Infection also contributes to anemia in ESKD patients. Increases in serum hepcidin and reduced availability of iron for erythropoiesis play important roles. In addition, infection by itself may interfere with red cell production. Certain infections can cause hemolysis. Hemoglobin concentrations often decrease in chronic infections but may decline in acute infections as well. One interesting source of occult infection seen in dialysis patients could be their previously used but currently nonfunctioning arteriovenous grafts. These infections are hard to detect but may be an important cause of ESA hyporesponsiveness.

Hyperparathyroidism

Hyperparathyroidism is believed to contribute to the anemia of CKD, at least in part due to fibrosis of the bone marrow. The best proof of this relationship may be that after parathyroidectomy, anemia tends to improve whether hyperparathyroidism was primary or secondary to other factors. The decision on whether parathyroidectomy is necessary should not be based on anemia, but rather on more traditional mineral and bone parameters. Medical treatment of hyperparathyroidism does appear to have a beneficial effect on anemia. Goicoechea et al treated 28 patients with hyperparathyroidism with intravenous activated vitamin D therapy. The result of treatment was an improvement in hemoglobin concentration and reduction in ESA dose requirements.

Bleeding

Acute or chronic blood loss from either an occult or an obvious clinical source may contribute to the anemia of CKD. This is a particularly important cause, in that the usual response to worsening anemia in dialysis patients is to increase the ESA dose, often without a clinical evaluation. As a result, the diagnosis of occult blood loss may be substantially delayed. Whenever there is worsening of anemia or ESA hyporesponsiveness, there should be an evaluation for the possibility of blood loss, including, as appropriate, testing for gastrointestinal bleeding.

Other Hematologic Disorders

Because of the primacy of erythropoietin deficiency as a cause of anemia in ESKD and because of automated ESA dose adjustment protocols, the response to worsening anemia is usually repetitive increases in ESA dose. As discussed above, this may delay evaluation for occult bleeding. However, in addition, evaluation for other causes of anemia may also be delayed. Patients with ESKD may develop any of the large number of causes of anemia that individuals in the general population are subject to.

When a dialysis patient has reduced responsiveness to an ESA, then a basic anemia evaluation is called for. After ruling out iron deficiency and other issues discussed above, pathologic causes of reduced red cell production, sequestration, and hemolysis should be considered. Erythrocyte production defects can result from folic acid or vitamin B_{12} deficiency, among many other causes. Myelodysplasia is an important cause of anemia in older individuals and should be considered in ESKD patients resistant to ESA treatment. An epidemic of pure red cell aplasia due to anti-erythropoietin antibodies took place primarily in Europe in the late 1990s. Rare sporadic cases may still occur. Hemolytic conditions can be acute during hemodialysis, but chronic hemolytic conditions should be considered when unexplained anemia is present and suggestive clinical signs are present. In general, when response to ESA therapy is suboptimal and typical causes have been excluded, further evaluation with red cell indices, reticulocyte count, folic acid, vitamin B_{12} level, C-reactive protein, lactate dehydrogenase, and bilirubin should be completed. If the cause of ESA hyporesponse remains undetermined, hematologic consultation should be considered.

Role of Red Blood Cell Transfusion in Management of Anemia of ESKD

Although ESAs remain the main treatment option in the management of anemia of ESKD, the use of red blood cell transfusion in this population has recently increased in the Unites States. This increase in transfusion and decrease in ESA utilization among long-term dialysis patients in the U.S. may be a result of ESA-related safety concerns and major ESKD-related regulatory and reimbursement changes. In any case, transfusion of packed red blood cells should be considered in ESKD patients who are experiencing symptoms related to severe anemia and in patients with acute bleeding. Red blood cell transfusion also needs to be considered in chronically anemic ESKD patients in whom ESA therapy has been insufficiently effective (as a result of bone marrow failure, hemoglobinopathies, or ESA resistance) or when the risks of ESA therapy outweigh its benefits. The Kidney Disease: Improving Global Outcomes (KDIGO) Anemia Work Group suggests the use of red blood cell transfusions in patients in whom urgent correction of anemia is required to stabilize the clinical condition (eg, in cases of acute hemorrhage, unstable coronary artery disease) or when rapid preoperative hemoglobin correction is required.

Both benefits and risks of red blood cell transfusions should also be considered in this patient population. The clinical benefit of red cell transfusion primarily includes improvement in symptoms related to anemia. Although uncommon, several risks that are associated with red blood cell transfusions should be considered in a given ESKD patient. These include volume overload, hyperkalemia, citrate toxicity (causing metabolic acidosis and hypocalcemia), hypothermia, coagulopathy, and immunologic reactions, including transfusion-related acute lung injury (TRALI). Although rare, transmission of infections remains a concern with red blood transfusion. Another important concern, although disputed, is the risk of allosensitization and resulting diminished subsequent ability to receive a kidney transplantation. Hence, to minimize the risk of allosensitization, especially in patients who are candidates for kidney transplantation, the KDIGO guidelines suggest avoiding red blood cell transfusions in chronically anemic CKD patients, when possible. For the above-mentioned reasons, red blood cell transfusions should be used prudently in this population.

CHAPTER 51

Iron Use in End-Stage Renal Disease

Gopesh K. Modi, MD DM • Rajiv Agarwal, MD

Epidemiology of Iron Deficiency in CKD

Anemia is a common complication of chronic kidney disease (CKD). In the adult U.S. population, 1.2 million women and 390,000 men have anemia attributable to CKD. In population-based surveys of adults in the United States, CKD-attributable anemia occurs early in the course of kidney disease. Among men, a significant reduction in hemoglobin (Hgb) is seen when calculated creatinine clearance is <70 mL/min and among women when calculated creatinine clearance is <50 mL/min. The prevalence of anemia and its severity increase as GFR declines. Almost 50%–60% of patients with stage 4 CKD are anemic, and the vast majority (75%–92%) of patients with stage 5 CKD have anemia.

Although gender-based thresholds exist for the definition of anemia in the general population (<12 g/dL in women and <13.5 g/dL in men), in people with CKD Hgb cut-offs are similar. According to the 2012 Kidney Disease Improving Global Outcomes (KDIGO), anemia is defined as <13 g/dL for men and <12 g/dL for women. However, the threshold for treatment is independent of gender. In general, erythropoiesis-stimulating agents (ESA) are not administered until the Hgb declines to a level less than 10 g/dL. For unclear reasons, African Americans are more often anemic compared with other racial/ethnic groups.

The pathophysiology of anemia of CKD is complex. Although the relative deficiency of erythropoietin is important for the pathogenesis of anemia associated with CKD, there are multiple other factors involved. Iron deficiency or iron-restricted hematopoiesis is a common cause of anemia associated with CKD. Approximately 40% of women and 20% men have transferrin saturation of <20% irrespective of calculated creatinine clearance. For stage 4 CKD, between 40% and 50% of people have serum ferritin concentration of <100 ng/mL. Because most patients with advanced CKD will need replacement ESA to correct anemia, most patients will also need iron for effective erythropoiesis.

Pathophysiology

Systemic Iron Homeostasis

Iron is a micronutrient that is ubiquitous and indispensable for life. It can exist in several oxidation forms and thus has catalytic activity and potential for generation of free radicals that can damage biologically important molecules such as proteins, lipids, and DNA. In order to safeguard against its highly reactive forms, iron is distributed in three distinct pools: functional, storage, and transit. Of the total body iron content of 3000–4000 mg, the functional pool is the largest (2500 mg) and comprises hemoglobin, myoglobin, and various cellular enzymes. The storage pool in the liver and the reticuloendothelial system is the next largest (1500 mg) and is responsible for iron recycling recovered from senescent red blood cells (RBCs). Unlike most ions and minerals, the concentration of which are regulated by the kidney, the regulation of iron content in the body occurs in the small intestine and there is no significant excretion of iron by the kidneys. Dietary absorption of iron is only 1 mg per day but the formation of RBCs requires about 30 mg of iron daily, which is provided by the release of iron from the reticuloendothelial system.

The link between the functional and storage pool of iron is the transport or transit pool. In contrast to the other pools, the transit pool comprises only a tiny fraction of total body iron (3 mg or 0.1% of total body iron) but it is tightly regulated. The high turnover of this pool provides the much needed iron to the cells for hematopoiesis. This pool comprises iron bound to transferrin. Transferrin is the sole provider of iron for erythropoiesis. It also ensures that free iron, which is highly reactive and capable of damaging various molecules, does not circulate free in blood. The process of erythropoiesis has two phases: an EPO-dependent phase from stem cell to the erythroblast stage that does not require iron, and an EPO-independent stage of 3–4 days wherein erythroblasts develop into reticulocytes and mature erythrocytes and requires iron. The transferrin molecule saturated with iron is important for the delivery of iron to cells expressing transferrin receptors. Thus, this transport pool is crucial for the successful hemoglobinization of erythrocytes.

A normal diet contains 13–18 mg of iron per day, which is normally composed of heme and nonheme iron. The liberation of nonheme iron from food and its solubilization is aided by the acidic pH of the stomach. Iron absorption is maximal in the duodenum, less in the jejunum, and least in the ileum. Regulation of intestinal iron absorption is crucial for prevention of iron overload.

Nonheme iron is absorbed mainly in the duodenum, where a low pH (due to Na–H exchanger) in the unstirred layer at the brush border of the enterocyte favors solubility of iron. Iron is absorbed by the divalent metal transporter (DMT1) expressed on the surface of enterocytes in the upper small intestine (Fig. 51.1). DMT1 only transports ferrous iron, whereas dietary iron is mostly ferric; this conversion of ferric to the ferrous form is carried out by ferric reductases, and one such enzyme is duodenal cytochrome b (Dcytb). Ascorbic acid facilitates this reduction reaction. The expression of Dcytb enzyme is regulated by iron deficiency and follows the expected gradient from duodenum to ileum. Once inside the cell, iron can be either stored as ferritin and thus lost from the body when the enterocyte sheds from the mucosa or iron can be exported to the circulation. This export takes place on the basolateral aspect of enterocytes. Iron is released into the circulation via ferroportin (also known as IREG1 and MTP1) in combination with ferroxidases hephestin and ceruloplasmin, which convert ferrous iron to ferric ion, where it is captured by the butterfly-shaped transferrin. Ferroportin is the only known mammalian protein involved in export of intracellular iron to the circulation whether from enterocytes, macrophages (that have iron recycled from RBCs), or hepatocytes. The transferrin molecule can hold two atoms of iron—one in each wing. The diferric transferrin molecule preferentially binds to transferrin receptor-1 (TfR-1) expressed on tissues that requires iron for cellular function, including erythroblasts, and through clathrin-coated pits is internalized (Fig. 51.2). The resulting endosome is acidified to release iron in the cell and transferrin, devoid of iron, called apotransferrin, is recycled back to the circulation.

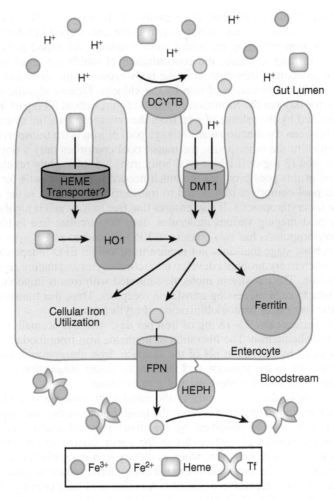

Figure 51.1

Iron is absorbed by the divalent metal transporter 1 (DMT1) expressed on the surface of enterocytes in the upper small intestine.

Heme iron, however, can be directly absorbed by enterocytes. The potential but not yet confirmed heme transporters are the heme-carrier protein 1 (HCP-1) and heme-responsive gene 1 (HRG-1) protein at the apical membrane of the enterocytes of the duodenum. Once inside, the enterocyte iron is released by heme oxygenase 1 (HO-1). Iron thus released can be either stored as ferritin in the cytoplasm or exported to be bound to transferrin. Additionally, there is some evidence that heme-iron could also be exported directly by the Bcrp/Abcg2 transporter. These heme-efflux proteins could potentially play a role in preventing toxicity due to heme overload.

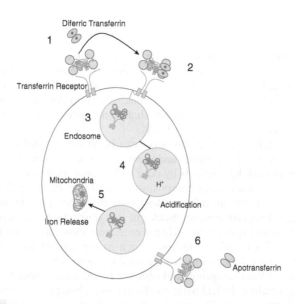

Figure 51.2

The diferric transferrin molecule preferentially binds to transferrin receptors expressed on tissues that require iron for cellular function, including erythroblasts, and through clathrin-coated pits is internalized.

The understanding of the iron cycle control has been enhanced by elucidation of the roles of its key control elements. At the center of this system is hepcidin, a *hep*atic bacteri*cidal* peptide. Ferroportin, the transporter of iron from cells to the bloodstream, is also the receptor for hepcidin. The binding of hepcidin to ferroportin leads to its internalization and subsequent degradation. This decreases the ability of the cell to export iron to be available for binding to transferrin. The hepcidin–ferroportin axis thus regulates systemic iron balance. Hepcidin production rises in inflammatory and iron overload states, and consequently the gut absorption of iron is suppressed. Furthermore, the release of iron from the reticuloendothelial system is also impaired when hepcidin concentrations are increased. These emerging data on the important role of hepcidin in iron biology shift the focus of regulation of iron absorption from the gut (and iron release from the reticuloendothelial system) to the liver.

Hepcidin production by the liver is influenced by many factors. Importantly, replete and/or overloaded iron stores and inflammation increase hepcidin levels. Increased intensity of erythropoiesis, hypoxia and certain endocrine factors, and steroids and growth factors suppress hepcidin expression. Hepcidin is also capable of influencing erythropoiesis by directly inhibiting erythropoietic cells, especially in states of low ambient EPO levels, such as that seen in CKD.

Besides relative EPO deficiency and iron-restricted erythropoiesis, resistance to the effect of EPO, largely because of manifest or occult inflammation, is important to the pathogenesis of anemia in CKD. Reduced RBC life span due to a uremic milieu or inflammation is another important cause of anemia in such patients.

Pathophysiology of Iron Deficiency in Renal Anemia

The use of parenteral iron in patients on dialysis is rising, as is the risk of iron overload. However, iron-restricted erythropoiesis remains an important cause of poor response to ESA. Iron-restricted erythropoiesis can be due to an absolute deficiency of iron or a functional deficiency. Functional iron deficiency broadly defines a state of adequate iron stores in the body that do not meet the requirement of erythropoiesis, especially when driven by ESAs.

Absolute iron deficiency is commonly seen in patients with CKD because of a mismatch between supply, demand, and increased losses of iron. The supply side is commonly affected in CKD patients by poor dietary iron intake or absorption, which in part may be due to the dietary composition, use of phosphate binders, and gastric pH changes. Furthermore, an inflammatory state that often goes hand in hand with CKD may trigger hepcidin release, block gut iron absorption, and sequester iron in the reticuloendothelial system. In CKD patients, iron losses are magnified 2–4 times normal because of a bleeding diathesis (such as through platelet dysfunction or aspirin use), high prevalence of gastrointestinal erosions, and arteriovenous malformations, frequent blood sampling, and obligate blood losses inherent to the hemodialysis (HD) procedure. In HD patients, dietary iron absorption is substantially less than losses and intravenous (IV) iron is often required. In fact, in the pre-EPO era, ferrokinetic studies demonstrated that gut iron absorption is sharply reduced when serum ferritin concentration exceeds 50–75 ng/mL. Whereas the ferritin is not causal in arresting gut iron absorption, ferritin likely reflects iron sufficiency which in turn arrests gut iron absorption.

Heme iron absorption may not be regulated in the same way as inorganic iron as inferred by its physiology. For example, in iron-deficient rats, nonheme iron absorption was increased several fold, but heme iron absorption was unaffected. However, other studies in iron-deficient rats demonstrated 3- to 10-fold increase in absorption of heme iron compared with controls. Whereas data in animals are conflicting, in subjects with serum ferritin concentration of >400 ng/mL heme iron absorption was >10 times greater than when iron was given as non-heme iron. Although these data are provocative, few head-to-head trials exist that help us in choosing between heme or non-heme iron supplements.

Diagnosis of Iron Deficiency in CKD Patients

Diagnosis of iron deficiency in CKD patients is often difficult because the commonly used tests in the general population do not have the same degree of sensitivity or specificity in the diagnosis of iron deficiency anemia in CKD patients. Two markers of iron status, transferrin saturation (the ratio of serum iron to serum transferrin iron-binding capacity (TSAT)) and serum ferritin concentration, help establish iron deficiency. Ferritin is a marker for evaluation of body iron stores and transferrin saturation is a marker that helps evaluate the ability to deliver iron to tissues that express a need for iron such as erythroblasts. Absolute iron deficiency is defined as TSAT <20% and ferritin <100 ng/mL. However, as we discuss below, these thresholds are prone to error. For example, inflammation may increase serum ferritin concentration and reduce transferrin levels, thus masking the presence of iron deficiency. These influences create the pathophysiologic state of functional iron deficiency a difficult diagnosis to confirm. Those patients who may have low transferrin saturation and high serum ferritin may still respond to parenteral iron with a rise in Hgb. Although response to IV iron is taken to justify a diagnosis of functional iron deficiency, this may not always be the case. This is because conditions that cause hyporesponsiveness to EPO such as inflammation, hyperparathyroidism, or infection may coincidentally resolve following administration of iron, and an erroneous diagnosis of functional iron deficiency may be made. Some have suggested that the distinction of absolute and relative iron deficiency can be made by bone marrow examination for iron stores. The prevalence of iron deficiency on bone marrow examination in CKD subjects has been reported to be between 23% and 74%. However, bone marrow examination cannot exclude functional iron deficiency. In fact, the performance of bone marrow examinations against the "gold standard" of Hgb response to IV iron therapy is modest at best. In one study, the positive and negative predictive values of bone marrow findings to predict a 1 g/dL Hgb response to IV iron ranged between 70% and 72%.

Because of these difficulties in accurate assessment of iron status, coupled with cautions regarding safety of overzealous use of ESA and IV iron, the current KDIGO guidelines suggest iron repletion for patients with TSAT <30% and serum ferritin concentration <500 ng/mL when an increase in Hgb with or without starting ESA treatment is desired.

Emerging Markers of Iron Status

Cellular hemoglobin in reticulocytes or reticulocyte Hgb content (CHr) reflects the Hgb content in the youngest of the erythrocytes—reticulocytes. Low levels of CHr suggest iron-deficient erythropoiesis. Although target CHr is not entirely clear, a level of >29 pg according to some and >32 pg according to others is considered consistent with adequate iron status.

Percent hypochromic RBCs measures the proportion of RBCs that have low Hgb concentration (hypochromic erythrocytes), that is, <28 g/dL. This measure is not to be confused with mean corpuscular hemoglobin concentration (MCHC). A value >6% of RBCs being hypochromic suggests iron-deficient erythropoiesis and thus predicts iron responsiveness of anemia.

Soluble Transferrin Receptor: Transferrin receptor 1 (TfR-1) is expressed on the surface of cells that require iron such as erythroblasts. Binding of the transferrin molecule to this receptor is responsible for the delivery of iron to these cells. The expression and release in plasma of soluble transferrin receptor (sTfR) are magnified in states of erythropoiesis and iron deficiency. It is not influenced by inflammation. However, expansion of the erythron by ESA can also cause an increase in sTfR, making it difficult to use this biomarker in those receiving ESAs.

Hepcidin: Measuring hepcidin level has been attempted but is technically complex and has large intraindividual variation. This coupled with the effects of inflammation, iron administration, and GFR on serum hepicidin concentration makes the use of this biomarker difficult to implement in clinical decision making.

Iron Use in CKD Patients

The treatment of anemia in CKD is complex and has undergone progressive evolution over the past few decades. The introduction of ESAs led to a reduction in blood transfusions and a subsequent enthusiasm to drive Hgb levels to normal to improve cardiovascular outcomes. Identification of adverse cardiovascular effects of Hgb normalization led to revision of guidelines to recommend cautious use of ESAs. The cut-off Hgb level for ESA initiation was lowered along with a moderation in the target Hgb level. The demonstration of a reduction in ESA dose and a better Hgb response with IV iron quickly catapulted IV iron into widespread use. It must be emphasized that the use of IV iron is the net result of observational studies and improvement in surrogate markers rather than hard outcomes. There have been only a few randomized controlled trials, and they have significant limitations; however, the financial pressures on ESA use have accelerated the adoption of IV iron use.

The main issues to be considered in iron therapy are the route of administration, available preparations, and their efficacy, safety, and cost. It has been shown in many studies that oral iron is particularly ineffective in patients on HD. Additionally, it has been observed that IV iron appears to be more efficacious in raising Hgb, TAST, and ferritin levels both in CKD patients who are not on dialysis (CKD-ND) and patients on HD. However, no studies have demonstrated definitive improvements in patient outcomes like mortality or QOL improvement between oral and IV iron. Even when oral iron was successful in iron repletion in short-term studies, there were associated falls in ferritin and TSAT levels raising questions on its efficacy over longer periods, especially with ESA use. Simultaneously, the safety issues with IV iron have not been resolved satisfactorily because of the short duration of most published studies.

Oral Iron Therapy in CKD

Oral iron therapy is still the preferred treatment for subjects with CKD-ND who are iron deficient. There have been a few studies that showed better results with IV iron on markers of iron status in this population, but the difference in Hgb level was small at least in the short term.

The usual dose of oral iron should be 200 mg elemental iron per day. The major limitations of oral iron are its low bioavailability and adverse gastrointestinal side effects. The treatment should continue for 4–6 months after correcting Hgb or may be needed indefinitely if the patient is on ESAs.

The various oral preparations are judged to be similar in safety and efficacy. These include ferrous forms (sulfate, fumarate, glutamate), carbonyl iron powder, and ferric polymaltose complex. Ferric polymaltose complex does not interact with food or drugs and hence can be taken with meals.

As stated earlier, oral heme iron absorption occurs independently of iron stores, and through a different pathway. It is possible that oral heme iron is superior in maintaining iron balance than nonheme iron. In a published study, 40 CKD-ND patients were randomized to receive heme iron polypeptide or IV iron sucrose. After 6 months of treatment, Hgb and TSAT were similar in both groups but serum ferritin was higher in the IV iron group. In patients on maintenance HD, an open-label study of orally administered heme iron polypeptide versus IV iron showed that the heme iron group was able to maintain the target Hgb without concomitant IV iron use. A significant reduction in serum ferritin was seen at months 4 through 6 in the heme iron group, whereas serum ferritin remained increased in the IV iron group. These data suggest a possible role for heme iron in both CKD-ND and HD patients on maintenance ESA therapy although the significance of falling ferritin is unknown and all studies are short term.

Oral liposomal iron preparations promise better absorption. In a short-term study in CKD-ND subjects, the Hgb increase with oral liposomal iron was similar to IV iron. However, after the withdrawal of iron, Hgb concentrations remained stable in the IV iron but not in the oral iron group. The replenishment of iron stores was greater in the IV group.

Ferric citrate is a new oral iron preparation available that has been used as a phosphate binder in CKD-ND and HD patients. Not only does it control phosphorus as well as conventional phosphate binders, it has salutary effects on iron stores and anemia. In a study involving 149 patients with CKD-ND and iron deficiency anemia, a 12-week trial of ferric citrate treatment increased mean TSAT from 22% to 32%, mean Hgb from 10.5 to 11 g/dL, and reduced serum phosphate levels whereas the placebo exerted no such effects. Similar findings were observed in another study that randomized 441 subjects on dialysis to ferric citrate or active phosphate-binding control drug over a 52-week period. The ferric citrate arm achieved phosphorus control equivalent to active control. It also achieved significantly higher levels of Hgb, TSAT, and ferritin with reduced ESA and IV iron use.

The status of oral iron in CKD-ND and dialysis patients has also been the subject of two meta-analyses. In the first meta-analysis comparing randomized trials of oral to IV iron on hemoglobin response among CKD-ND patients, Rozen-Zvi et al analyzed six studies. Five of these six trials were short term, 1–3 months', and compared with oral iron the mean increase in hemoglobin with IV iron was 0.31 (95% confidence interval [CI] 0.09–0.53) g/dL. However, one of the studies included in this meta-analysis was 6 months long and reported a mean decline in hemoglobin of 0.52 g/dL associated with IV iron administration. A Cochrane review of parenteral versus oral iron therapy in CKD in the year 2012 included 28 studies (2098 participants). Hgb, ferritin, and TSAT were significantly increased by IV iron compared with oral iron along with a significant reduction in ESA requirement. Mortality and cardiovascular morbidity did not differ significantly, but were reported in only a few studies. Gastrointestinal side effects were more common with oral iron, but hypotensive and allergic reactions were more common with IV iron.

In the largest randomized clinical trial comparing IV to oral iron in iron-deficient anemic patients with CKD, the Ferinject assessment in patients with Iron deficiency anemia and Non-Dialysis-dependent Chronic Kidney Disease (FIND-CKD) investigators randomized 626 patients in 193 centers in 1 : 1 : 2 ratio to IV ferric carboxymaltose targeting ferritin to high level (400–600 ng/mL), lower level (100–200 ng/mL), or oral iron. After a 52-week period, the mean increase in Hgb was 1.0 g/dL in the oral iron group, 0.9 g/dL when IV ferric carboxymaltose targeted ferritin to 100–200 ng/mL, and 1.4 g/dL when IV ferric carboxymaltose targeted ferritin to 400–600 ng/mL ($p = .014$). Although statistically significant, the difference in hemoglobin of 0.4 g/dL between oral iron and high-dose IV iron observed in that study should be viewed in light of the fact that oral ferrous sulfate administration was only 100 mg twice daily, which is much below the recommended intake of ferrous sulfate. It is possible that using 200 mg elemental oral iron may have increased the Hgb further in the oral iron group.

At this point, it would seem that oral iron in adequate doses has a definite place in CKD-ND and may also be used in an individualized manner in dialysis patients with close monitoring. IV iron will be needed for dialysis patients and those CKD-ND subjects who fail oral iron treatment.

Intravenous Iron

It has been shown that IV iron can to some extent bypass hepcidin-mediated iron blockade and treat iron-deficiency anemia even in the setting of inflammation. In the short term, randomized controlled trials lasting 1-3 months have consistently demonstrated that IV iron is superior to oral nonheme iron in patients on HD treated with ESAs. Most patients treated with ESAs will require iron to improve anemia and increase responsiveness to ESAs. Acute allergic and anaphylactic reactions are of major concern when dextran-containing irons are used and are rare with newer preparations. There are now many IV preparations available for use. The essential theme for designing IV iron molecules is the modification in the carbohydrate side chain (mitigating immunogenicity and allergic reactions) and iron binding (to reduce release of free iron/labile iron), thus reducing the harmful effects such as free radical generation, acute hypotension, back pain, and edema. The size and coating of the iron product affects its cellular uptake and disposition in the tissues. These attributes also affect the maximum one-time dose and the rapidity of injection in one sitting. The various nondextran IV iron preparations are iron sucrose, ferric gluconate, ferric carboxymaltose, ferumoxytol, and iron isomaltoside. The absolute rates of life-threatening adverse drug effects (ADEs) have been reported as 0.6, 0.9, and 3.3 per million for iron sucrose, sodium ferric gluconate complex, and low-molecular-weight iron dextran. There have been many studies comparing these IV preparations with oral iron. The IV preparations in general raise Hgb more than oral iron in the short term. Long-term safety data are notable by their absence.

The largest of these studies, REPAIR-IDA, randomized 2584 CKD-ND patients to two 750-mg IV doses of ferric carboxymaltose (FCM) in 1 week or up to 5 infusions of iron sucrose 200 mg in 14 days. In parallel with higher total delivered dose of FCM, at day 56 the TSAT and ferritin were higher in the FCM arm but the Hgb rise was not different. The side effect profile was also similar but these data do not ensure safety beyond 2 months.

Taken together, it seems that clinical trials on IV iron in HD have insufficient numbers of patients followed for an insufficient length of time to fully assess the long-term safety of IV iron treatment, particularly when used in individuals with serum ferritin >800 ng/mL.

Dialysate Iron Delivery

The US Food and Drug Administration (FDA) recently approved soluble ferric pyrophosphate (*Triferic*, Rockwell Medical) to replace iron and maintain hemoglobin in adults with chronic kidney disease who are undergoing dialysis. Ferric pyrophosphate is a water-soluble iron salt delivered through the dialysate. It is formulated to replace the 5–7 mg iron that is lost during every dialysis treatment.

Future Directions for Iron-Restricted Erythropoiesis

The recent knowledge about the iron cycle has kindled interest in therapies directed at the hepcidin–ferroportin axis. Several options are under study or development. One category of therapy is directed against hepcidin. These include antihepcidin antibodies, hepcidin-binding proteins (anticalins), hepcidin-binding spiegelmers, hepcidin siRNAs, and antisense oligonucleotides. Another strategy is to inhibit hepcidin production by targeting either the BMP–SMAD signaling pathway (e.g., anti-BMP6 antibodies) or the IL6-STAT3 pathway (e.g., anti-IL6 antibody Siltux-imab, anti-IL6 receptor antibody Tocilizumab, JAK2 inhibitors, and STAT3 inhibitors). A second category is to enhance ferroportin, and the strategies include anti-ferroportin antibodies and ligands that can interfere with hepcidin binding to ferroportin, as well as agents that block ferroportin internalization or potentiate ferroportin synthesis.

Independent Benefits of Iron Unrelated to Correction of Anemia

Several independent benefits of iron use traditionally thought to be due to improvement of anemia may be due to correction of the underlying iron deficiency. Several enzymatic hemoproteins such as catalase, peroxidase, cytochrome c, cytochrome p450, nitric oxide synthase, and nicotinamide adenine dinucleotide phosphate oxidase (NADPH) are ubiquitous and serve important functions. Thus, the benefits of iron repletion may extend beyond repair of anemia. Small studies have reported improvement in fatigue, cold intolerance, restless legs syndrome, and measures of quality of life. However, adequately powered randomized trials are needed to confirm these benefits. The best evidence for hemoglobin-independent benefits comes from studies in patients with congestive heart failure (CHF). Iron deficiency occurs in approximately one-third of CHF patients, even in the absence of anemia, and is independently associated with adverse outcomes. In the Ferinject Assessment in Patients With IRon Deficiency and Chronic Heart Failure (FAIR-HF) trial, 459 patients with CHF and iron deficiency were randomized to IV iron as ferric carboxy-maltose or placebo. The primary endpoints were the self-reported Patient Global Assessment and NYHA functional class, both at week 24. Irrespective of the presence or absence of anemia, the ferric carboxymaltose group experienced better outcomes. Further, in patients with anemia, ferric carboxymaltose therapy was associated with lower rates of death because of worsening heart failure and hospitalization for any cardiovascular reason.

Potential Long-Term Concerns of Harm With IV Iron Use

Iron, through the Haber–Weiss reaction, generates the highly reactive hydroxyl ion that is responsible for creating oxidative stress. Although oxidative stress can be quenched by normal individuals, in those with CKD, the mechanisms to combat oxidative stress are impaired. Thus, iron can be a particularly powerful prooxidant in these individuals. Intravenous iron induces oxidative stress, prooxidant cell signaling, tissue inflammation, cellular iron deposition, and cytotoxicity in cell culture models, animal models, and acutely in humans as well. Oxidative stress can generate endothelial dysfunction, promote atherosclerosis, and accelerate the progression of CKD.

In addition, iron is a growth factor for bacteria, even common ones such as *Staphylococcus epidermidis*. Iron is thought to limit absorption of zinc, whose deficiency can impair immune response to infection. Iron blocks the transcription of inducible nitric oxide synthase (iNOS), important in death of pathogens. Excess iron deposits in the liver are detrimental to response to interferon therapy in hepatitis C–infected patients, and iron load may promote the progression of hepatitis C. The inflammatory response to bacterial infections and even nonbacterial infections is enhanced with IV iron, which at least in animals is associated with increased morbidity and mortality. Direct evidence of harm exists in a randomized, placebo-controlled trial of oral iron and folic acid with or without zinc in 24,076 preschool children in Zanzibar, a country with a high malaria transfer setting. Those treated with active drug were 12% more likely to die or need treatment in a hospital for an adverse event and 11% more likely to be admitted to the hospital than the placebo group. Infection or malaria-related causes were the most likely reasons for admission to the hospital. Notably, those who were iron deficient and anemic had half the event rate when treated with active drug when compared to placebo. The evidence of harm was mainly seen in those children who were iron replete but received iron. Hoen et al followed 988 HD patients from 19 French centers for 6 months. There were 51 episodes of bacteremia, but there was no association with either IV iron dosing or serum ferritin concentration. A much larger study by Brookhart et al based on the DaVita dialysis data on 117,050 HD patients showed otherwise. Patients with higher IV iron doses had a slightly but significantly greater risk of infection-related hospitalization or death, which was most magnified in individuals with the combination of high serum ferritin and high iron saturation at baseline. It was also noted that compared with maintenance therapy, bolus treatment was associated with a greater risk of infection.

An important concern with iron administration is iron overload and/or hemosiderosis. The trends over the past two decades show that in 1993 the mean ferritin in HD patients was only 302 ng/mL. Subsequently mean ferritin has steadily increased to 526 ng/mL in 2001, 586 ng/mL in 2007 with 22% of patients having serum ferritin >800 ng/mL. This assumes significance with persisting concerns about safety of IV iron more so when iron is administered to dialysis patients who are already iron replete.

These cautionary remarks about iron overload are further supported by another study that examined liver iron stores in HD patients using MRI. The findings revealed that despite the use of iron and ESA as per standard guidelines, 80% of subjects had moderate hepatic iron overload and 30% had severe iron overload.

Observational data associating iron use with mortality in dialysis patients are conflicting. For example, Kalanter-Zadeh et al studied 58,058 DaVita Inc. dialysis patients. Among patients who received >400 mg IV iron per month, there was a significantly increased risk of death. On the other hand, Kshirsagar et al, reporting on 117,050 HD patients, found no association between the dose of IV iron and short-term risk of myocardial infarction, stroke, or death. A recent analysis of iron dose and clinical outcomes in 32,435 HD patients in 12 countries from 2002 to 2011 in the Dialysis Outcomes and Practice Patterns Study found that adjusted total and cardiovascular mortality and hospitalization risk was significantly higher in subjects receiving >300 mg/month IV iron.

In contrast to the observational data, the randomized trial to evaluate IV and oral iron in chronic kidney disease (REVOKE) reports harm associated with IV iron use. In order to determine whether in comparison to oral iron, IV iron accelerates decline in measured glomerular filtration rate among patients with stage 3 and 4 CKD and iron deficiency anemia, participants were randomly assigned to either open-label oral ferrous sulfate (n = 67) or IV iron sucrose (n = 69), each administered over 8 weeks. Ferrous sulfate was administered orally 325 mg three times daily for 8 weeks and iron sucrose 200 mg IV every 2 weeks for a total of 1 g. If further supplementation was needed, group assignment was adhered to. Hemoglobin was targeted to be between 10 and 12 g/dL; ESAs were used as needed. Plasma iothalamate clearance (12 samples over 5 hours) was used to measure glomerular filtration rate on 5 occasions over 2 years. The primary outcome variable was the between group difference in slope of GFR change.

An independent Data and Safety Monitoring Board recommended to stop the trial early based on little chance of discovering differences in GFR slopes over 2 years, but a higher risk of serious adverse events in the IV iron treatment group. There were 35 serious cardiovascular events among 19 participants assigned to the oral iron treatment group and 53 events among 15 participants of the IV iron group (adjusted incidence rate ratio [IRR] 2.57, 95% CI 1.59–4.17, p <.0001). There were 27 infectious events requiring hospitalization among 11 participants assigned to the oral iron treatment group and 37 events among 19 participants in the IV iron treatment group (adjusted IRR 2.12, 95% CI 1.24–3.64, p = .006). Serious adverse events from all causes (adjusted IRR 1.61, p <.0001) and hospitalizations for heart failure (adjusted IRR 2.08, p = .038) were also increased in the IV iron group. Over time, hemoglobin increased similarly between treatment groups. Iothalamate GFR declined similarly over 2 years in both treatment groups (oral iron, −3.6 mL/min/1.73 m^2; IV iron, −4.0 mL/min/1.73 m^2; between-group difference, −0.35 mL/min/1.73 m^2, 95% CI −2.9 to 2.3, p = .79).

Thus, among stage 3 and 4 CKD patients with iron deficiency anemia, compared with oral iron–based therapy, IV-based iron therapy was associated with an increased risk of all serious adverse events, including those from cardiovascular causes and infectious diseases. Accordingly, it is prudent to use oral iron therapy as first line among patients not on dialysis with CKD and iron deficiency anemia.

C H A P T E R   5 2

Resistance to Erythropoiesis-Stimulating Agent (ESA) Treatment

John C. Stivelman, MD

Historical Background and Current Definitions

The last nine years' experience with ESA treatment has seen a transformation of that therapy in chronic kidney disease (CKD)/end-stage renal disease (ESRD) and has also resulted in a change in the definition of and approach to hormone resistance. The findings of the major studies evaluating effects of increasing ESA doses and hemoglobin values on health outcomes, resulting changes in FDA labeling of ESAs, the institution of bundled payment in the Prospective Payment System for dialysis which includes intradialytic medications, the publication of the Kidney Disease Improving Global Outcomes (KDIGO) recommendations, and the elimination of the minimum hemoglobin performance measure by CMS in the Quality Incentive Program have all contributed to these developments, each in its own fashion.

First, publications of the Normal Hematocrit Cardiac Study (1998), followed by the CHOIR (Correction of Hemogloblin and Outcomes in Renal Insufficiency, 2006), CREATE (Cardiovascular Risk Reduction by Early Anemia Treatment with Epoetin Beta, 2006), and TREAT (Trial to Reduce Cardiovascular Events with Aranesp Therapy, 2009) trials raised the basic issue of what constitutes appropriate ESA dosing and hemoglobin goals. These randomized, controlled studies demonstrated either an increase or no improvement in cardiovascular/cerebrovascular morbidity with attempts at progressive ESA-driven increases in hemoglobin equal to or beyond 13.0 g/dL, compared to controls (control hemoglobin concentrations variably 9.0–11.5 g/dL). Second, in a series of increasingly restrictive black box labeling changes for ESAs appearing in 2007, 2009, and 2011, the Food and Drug Administration issued a series of warnings related to target hemoglobin and cardiovascular risk. The 2011 warning indicated that serious events occurred with ESA treatment when targeting a hemoglobin greater than 11 g/dL (the 2007 version indicated greater than 12.0 g/dL) and that no trial "has identified a hemoglobin, target level, ESA dose, or dosing strategy that does not increase these risks." Further, the FDA suggested (as it had in 2007 in analogous language) that "the lowest [ESA] dose sufficient to reduce the need for red blood cell transfusions" should be used. Third, the advent of bundled payment in 2011 for medications administered during dialysis compelled re-evaluation of many processes and economies of care, resulting in decreases in ESA utilization. Fourth, following the release by the National Kidney Foundation of Kidney Disease Outcomes Quality Initiative (K/DOQI) 2007 (which began to address concerns relating to hemoglobin target raised by some of these studies), the next anemia guideline to appear was from KDIGO in 2012: this document offered a more individualized spectrum of therapy for patients while giving heed to the concerns raised by both the studies and FDA warnings noted above. Last, at least partly in view of the FDA's labeling changes, CMS eliminated a floor value for hemoglobin as a quality measure in the Prospective Payment Program's Quality Incentive Program in 2013, thus removing a potential penalty to providers.

Taken together, many of these historical trends have contributed to the decline in both national mean ESA (EPO) dose per week (from 19,244 U/wk in January 2006 to 12,460 U/wk in December 2011), and mean monthly hemoglobin among hemodialysis patients (from 11.95 g/dL in January 2006 to 10.70 g/dL in December 2011) (Fig. 52.1). By virtue of the global change in the level of aggressiveness of ESA therapy as manifested by these trends, what is considered resistance to that therapy has changed, as well as how that resistance should be addressed by the clinician.

The definition of resistance to ESA treatment has a complex history evolving over the course of NKF-DOQI, K/DOQI, and KDIGO guidelines. In the first and second editions of NKF-DOQI/K/DOQI (1997, 2001), initial therapy was suggested to hemoglobin targets of 11–12 g/dL, using total starting doses of ESA (then, epoetin alfa) ranging from 120 to 180 U/kg/wk IV thrice weekly, and 80–120 U/kg/wk subcutaneously twice to thrice weekly in divided doses. Fifty percent increments in dose were suggested for negligible response after 2–4 weeks, as were downward adjustments of 25% in the weekly dose for overshooting of hemoglobin goals, or accelerated increases in hemoglobin. Resistance was defined as inability to reach target hemoglobin at 450 U/kg/wk IV (300 U/kg/wk subcutaneously) within 4–6 months in the presence of adequate iron stores, or failure to maintain target hemoglobin at that dose. For these first two editions of guidelines, refractory patients were recommended to receive therapies dating from the pre-ESA era. In 2006, however, hemoglobin thresholds were revised to ≥11.0, and <13, with guidelines for initial dosing, titration regimen, frequency, and route of administration now far less

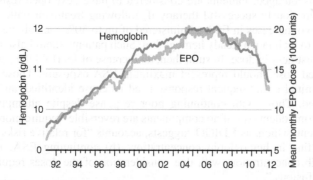

Figure 52.1

Temporal Trends in Both Mean ESA Dose per Week (in 1000s of Units) and Mean Monthly Hemoglobin (g/dL) Over the Interval Under Discussion Are Noted. (U.S. Renal Data System, USRDS 2013 Annual Data Report, Atlas of Chronic Kidney Disease and End-Stage Renal Disease in the United States, National Institutes of Health, National Institute of Diabetes and Digestive and Kidney Diseases, Bethesda, MD, 2013, vol 2, figure 2.3.) (The data reported here have been supplied by the United States Renal Data System [USRDS]. The interpretation and reporting of these data are the responsibility of the authors(s) and in no way should be seen as an official policy or interpretation of the U.S. government.)

prescriptive than previously. In this issue, resistance to ESA was now quantitatively defined as a failure to increase hemoglobin to beyond 11.0 g/dL with a dose of >500 U/kg/wk. Finally, in the last edition of K/DOQI in 2007—largely in response to CHOIR—the Anemia Workgroup limited the hemoglobin target to be "generally . . . in the range of 11–12 g/dL," and recommended it not be greater than 13.0 g/dL. Resistance was not addressed.

The 2012 KDIGO recommendations should be interpreted in light of this historical background, as well as the concern relating to ESA dose exposure and hemoglobin values. Its recommendation for hemoglobin threshold for starting therapy is now 9.0–10.0 g/dL (the lower value, the "rescue" level in TREAT), and for maximum hemoglobin, is, in general, no greater than 11.5 g/dL (the upper range of values for control groups in many of the randomized controlled trials cited previously). ESAs should not be used to raise the hemoglobin above 13.0 mg/dL intentionally. Epoetin alfa or beta doses for initiation are noted as usually from 60 to 150 U/kg/wk (20–50 u/kg TIW; with titration once a month of 60 U/kg/wk upward if required), and for darbepoetin at 0.45 µg/kg/wk. Downward titration of 25% as needed is recommended if the patient's hemoglobin is still increasing and nearing 11.5 g/dL, provided it does not continue to rise thereafter (temporary suspension of therapy is then appropriate, with resumption at a lower dose once it plateaus). Dose adjustments may occur every two weeks in the maintenance setting.

KDIGO defines resistance two ways: that noted at initiation of therapy, and that acquired in the setting of previously stable treatment. Patients are considered to have initial ESA resistance if, using a proper weight-adjusted dose, an increase in hemoglobin is absent during the first month of therapy. Repeated upward adjustment of ESA administered above doubling of the initial per kilogram/week dose in this setting is discouraged. Patients are considered to have developed resistance in the setting of previously successful therapy if, following treatment with stable doses, they need two increases in ESA administered of up to 50% each above the previous stable dose to maintain a steady hemoglobin. Such patients should also avoid further upward adjustment in dose. In sum, then, an increase of fourfold the patient's initial weight-based dose should represent maximum ESA exposure. Those who persist with poor initial or subsequent response need its cause identified, and where possible, treated. Those with continuing poor response despite attempts to address reversible components (or, if no components are reversible) require more individualized treatment, which, as KDIGO suggests, accounts "for relative risks and benefits of: (a) decline in hemoglobin concentration; (b) continuing ESA, if needed to maintain Hb concentration, with due consideration of the doses required, and (c) blood transfusions."

In addition to this changed landscape of care, it would also appear prudent to evaluate patients for sources of resistance to therapy (according to the following caveats from K/DOQI 2006) "whenever the hemoglobin is inappropriately low for the ESA dose administered. Such conditions include, but are not limited to: a significant increase in the ESA dose requirement to maintain a certain hemoglobin level or a significant decrease in hemoglobin level at a constant ESA dose."

Disorders Inducing Resistance to Treatment

Resistance to ESA therapy is a major clinical problem that has often been cited as entailing increased cardiovascular and mortality risk—whether due to increased ESA

Table 52.1

Etiologies of Resistance to ESA Treatment

Occurring Any Time During ESA Therapy	Occurring Commonly in the Setting of Successful Chronic ESA Therapy
• Iron deficiency	• Iron deficiency
• Inflammatory blockade	• Inflammatory blockade
• Hemoglobin "cycling"	• Hemoglobin "cycling"
• Aluminum intoxication	
• Secondary hyperparathyroidism	
• Hemoglobinopathy	
• Myelophthisic states and other malignancies	
• Hemolysis	
• ACEi treatment	
• Carnitine deficiency	
• Pure red-cell aplasia	

dose, presence of significant existing comorbidities, a combination of these issues, or other factors—and therefore should be approached in a thoughtful, physiologically rational fashion. A wide variety of clinical events and pathologic states engendering resistance, many of which are reversible, may occur at any time during treatment; those most commonly encountered during chronic, previously successful treatment—true and functional iron deficiency, and inflammatory blockade—pose particular problems in the maintenance of stable hemoglobin, which are detailed above (Table 52.1).

Iron and Other Cofactor Needs

Clinical experience with use of ESA has shown that most resistance to therapy likely has its origins in either iron deficiency (induced by effective ESA treatment, iron loss, or undetected functional iron deficiency) or inflammatory reticuloendothelial blockade. As hemoglobin synthesis increases following marrow stimulation with ESA, iron stores are consumed—a mark of successful treatment. With erosion of iron stores, loss of therapeutic response follows, which can be overcome initially by raising the ESA dose. This strategy ultimately fails, however, and response is diminished with those stores' further consumption. The rapidity with which this occurs depends on their adequacy pretreatment, as well as their chronic maintenance. Iron stores sufficient to attain the sought-after hemoglobin range are therefore desirable prior to or early in the course of ESA treatment. The need to guide therapy in both attaining and maintaining these stores has resulted in heavy reliance on values for percentage transferrin saturation (TSAT) and serum ferritin concentration.

Tools for Diagnosis

The most direct methods for ensuring adequacy of iron stores, whether beginning ESA treatment or maintaining stable hemoglobin levels, require measurement of transferrin saturation ([TSAT], Fe/TIBC × 100), and serum ferritin. Desirable adjuncts to these measurements may include either reticulocyte count, reticulocyte hemoglobin content (CHr), or percent hypochromic red cells. Reliability of both transferrin saturation and ferritin in diagnosing the need for iron supplementation has been subjected to close scrutiny in view of the lack of optimal sensitivity and specificity of both tests. Reliance on the serum ferritin values to assess iron stores, particularly without concurrent assessment of changes in transferrin saturation, ESA dose, serial hemoglobin values, and evaluation of prior clinical history, may also provide a misleading assessment of iron stores, since the serum ferritin is an "acute phase" protein. Thus fever, underlying inflammation, and liver disease affect its synthesis regardless of total body iron stores. In addition, rapid response to ESA may consume transferrin-bound iron (see Functional Iron Deficiency, below) before parenchymal stores and serum ferritin concentration decline, leading to an incorrect estimation of iron stores readily available for hemoglobin synthesis.

K/DOQI (2006) defined the appropriate range of iron sufficiency previously as a TSAT of >20% and ferritin of >200 ng/mL (hemodialysis) and >100 ng/mL (peritoneal dialysis [PD]), with an upper range of 500 ng/mL (there was insufficient evidence to recommend routinely higher ferritin values). KDIGO has indicated that appropriate ranges for iron therapy for adult CKD/ESRD patients receiving ESAs are TSATs ≤30% and ferritins ≤500 ng/mL. Routine use of iron supplementation at higher TSATs or ferritins is not recommended by KDIGO.

If the need for supplemental iron is found on the initial evaluation of anemic dialysis patients prior to beginning ESA treatment, its potential source needs identification and correction to ensure the sufficiency of substrate. Finally, the adequacy of cofactors essential for red cell synthesis, such as B_{12} and folate, should be ensured.

Differential Diagnosis

Iron deficiency as a source of evolving resistance to treatment should be excluded at the beginning or midcourse of treatment and suspected either in the patient requiring progressively higher ESA doses during treatment, the patient whose TSAT and ferritin are decreasing (see later), or whose hemoglobin and reticulocyte count actually fall despite stable ESA therapy. Exhaustion of iron available for erythropoiesis may simply reflect ESA-stimulated incorporation into new erythrocytes. Although intravenous iron administration has evolved as a therapy specifically to obviate this problem, other causes of iron deficiency, including gastrointestinal and dialysis-related losses still require exclusion. Isolating the source of iron loss may be difficult and obliges careful examination of technical components of the dialysis procedure for additional treatment-related losses (frequency and volume of routine phlebotomy; reuse procedures; adequacy of intradialytic heparinization; clotting frequency of dialyzer and tubing; postdialysis bleeding from sites, etc.) as well as losses unrelated to it. The magnitude of the latter should be inferred from medical history, physical findings, stool guaiacs, review of individual patient recent medical events, and recent hospitalization and surgical history (Table 52.2).

Functional Iron Deficiency

Functional iron deficiency evolves most often in the setting of effective treatment with ESAs, in which transferrin-bound iron is incorporated into red cell precursors more rapidly than tissue stores are mobilized to replace it (in contrast to true iron

---

Table 52.2

Potential Sources of Iron Loss

- Clotted dialyzers and tubing
- Poor reuse technique
- Slow clotting of access puncture sites post dialysis
- Occult GI blood loss
- Hospitalization, particularly with multiple caregivers/consultants
- Recent surgeries, particularly thrombectomies (especially if repetitive)
- Increased phlebotomy frequency at the dialysis unit

---

deficiency, which is characterized by both depleted tissue and circulating protein-bound stores). In the setting of continuous stimulation of erythropoiesis by ESAs, the ability to deliver iron to synthetic sites falls, transferrin is desaturated, and responsiveness to treatment—which can initially be sustained by increasing ESA dose—ultimately decreases. This clinical scenario, which is reversible by further iron administration, underscores the need for joint surveillance of transferrin saturation, serum ferritin, and hemoglobin, and an appreciation of their dynamic relationship to one another over time (see later). Functional iron deficiency may evolve in the setting of seemingly "appropriate" serum ferritin values and may occur manifesting only modest depressions of transferrin saturation (or even values within the normal range [Fig. 52.2]).

Treatment of Iron Deficiency

To provide proper surveillance of iron stores, KDIGO has recommended at least monthly or bimonthly follow-up of hemoglobin after initiation of ESAs, with routine values obtained at least monthly once stable hemoglobin is attained. Percent transferrin saturation and serum ferritin should be obtained at least quarterly or, as suggested by KDIGO, more frequently if the clinical situation suggests this may be of value (such as in the settings of blood loss, rising ESA dose, oversight of iron stores at risk for depletion, or assessing responses to a course of iron therapy).

KDIGO has outlined two strategies for preserving iron stores in dialysis patients: "repletion," and "maintenance" therapy. Initial and "repletion" courses of iron based on hemoglobin, TSAT, and ferritin usually comprise an approximately 1000-mg cumulative dose and are often administered on serial dialyses (or recurrent clinic visits for PD patients) in amounts based on the total dose infusion for the agent used. Transferrin saturation and ferritin values to verify adequate repletion thereafter should be drawn no less than 1 week after the last dose. An alternate strategy (also known as "maintenance therapy") for iron dosing in hemodialysis patients provides the patient smaller amounts of iron at more frequent, standardized intervals. This approach attempts to maintain sufficiency of TSAT and ferritin so that iron deficiency is averted. Use of oral iron therapy is not as effective in hemodialysis patients in either increasing hemoglobin production or decreasing ESA dose and often produces undesirable gastrointestinal side effects.

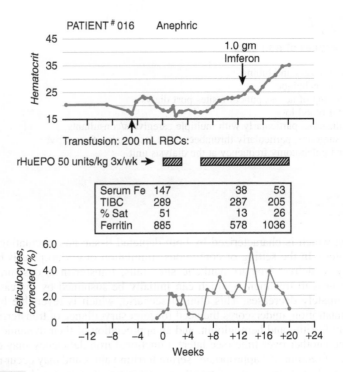

Figure 52.2

The Top Panel Illustrates One Patient's Response to Epoetin Alfa Treatment; the Bottom Panel, the Course of His Reticulocyte Count in Response to Therapy. The values in the hatched box reflect the change in his iron indices occurring with treatment. The patient's hematocrit rises, despite a brief hiatus in therapy, but reaches a plateau between weeks 8 and 12. At that time, the patient's protein-bound iron stores are depleted, manifested by a fall in transferrin saturation, and his reticulocyte response reaches a plateau, as well. The ferritin, though slightly decreased by week 12, remains robust. Following 1 g of further iron loading, transferrin saturation rises, and response is restored, demonstrating the presence of functional iron deficiency. (Eschbach, JW, Egrie, JC, Downing, MR, et al. Correction of the anemia of end-stage renal disease with recombinant human erythropoietin. N Engl J Med 1987;316(2):73-78.)

Identifying Clinical Problems in Iron Consumption and Bioavailability

Treatment of resistance resulting from iron deficiency, whether true or functional, is often avoidable with close surveillance of hemoglobin, serum ferritin, and transferrin saturation over periods of months. The availability of up to 12 months of these data, arranged chronologically, amplified by the physician's knowledge of the patient's recent clinical history, is invaluable in assessing whether a subtle change in one or more components of the patient's iron profile is occurring, and in evaluating the mechanics of poor response to treatment. Although examination of the TSAT and ferritin over time may aid in defining the patient's progressive iron status, this analysis may gain depth through scrutiny of TSAT and ferritin in relation to each other, to the patient's hemoglobin, the ESA dose, and the ongoing iron dose. TSAT and ferritin which decline in the same direction suggest iron consumption or possibly loss. Similarly, TSAT and ferritin, which fail to rise to some degree with iron repletion (or repetitive repletion), suggest rapid consumption or ongoing losses, as well. On the other hand, TSAT and ferritin, which over time appear to diverge from each other, suggest the advent of an inflammatory insult. It is thus through the longitudinal analysis of routinely obtained data that the most fruitful assessment of treatment resistance related to inflammation or iron deficiency ensues.

Underlying Inflammatory Disease

If iron or other substrate depletion is not detected in the patient with poor or absent initial response, or declining response, an inflammatory basis for treatment resistance should be sought and addressed where possible. Inflammatory sources of ESA resistance encompass infectious, neoplastic, or rheumatologic illnesses, as well as the postoperative state—the latter can include even minor procedures such as revision or replacement of vascular or peritoneal access, or central venous catheter placement. Extended investigation is often required to uncover sources of poor ESA response.

The pathophysiology of inflammatory reticuloendothelial blockade is multifaceted. Several mechanisms have been suggested for this problem, including roles for IL-1, IL-6, interferon gamma, and TNF-alpha in both inhibition of erythropoiesis and enhancement of apoptosis of early red cell elements; and hepcidin-mediated sequestration of iron within macrophages and the reticuloendothelial system, rendering it less available for red blood cell growth.

Many have also argued that ESRD per se is a chronic inflammatory state, and that poor response to ESA may reflect in certain patients the presence of a more global humoral disorder. Repetitive blood-membrane exposure, the catabolic effects of elevated parathyroid hormone (PTH) activity, waxing and waning degrees of metabolic acidosis, and the indirect effect of both vascular insufficiency and progressive atherosclerosis may all contribute to a chronic state of inflammation. The manifestations of this process, if severe, may include loss of visceral protein stores, hypoalbuminemia, anemia, and suboptimal ESA response. In support of this observation, a marked association of elevated CRP levels on increasing the ESA dose needed to maintain stable hemoglobin concentration has been previously noted, as has an inverse relationship between ESA dose and CRP levels with serum albumin and serum iron. By virtue of the diverse insults potentially responsible for this form of treatment resistance, the duration of diminished or nonresponse to treatment varies widely; resolution depends on the rapidity of identification of and ability to correct the presumed cause. Following assessment and, where possible, elimination of the inflammatory problem, effective ESA response often returns. Protracted resistance, however, should suggest incomplete resolution of the initial problem or a new, superposed insult. Given the experience of the last several years (particularly as outlined above), persistent escalation of ESA dose in the setting of poorly resolving resistance in the hope of enhancing response should no longer be relied on as an advisable treatment strategy, and the risks and benefits of therapy in such a setting should be reviewed.

Other Disorders Inducing Resistance to Treatment

The pathologic states detailed below may all impair the effectiveness of ESA treatment, but in the aggregate account for this phenomenon far less than do iron deficiency or inflammatory reticuloendothelial blockade.

Aluminum Intoxication

Aluminum intoxication may cause poor response by inducing modest resistance to ESA. This problem has dramatically diminished in frequency given regulatory requirements for uniform water quality, the negligible use of aluminum-containing phosphate binders, and use of selective vitamin D analogs with less phosphatemic effect. The mechanisms most frequently cited to explain this phenomenon have included aluminum-mediated impairment of iron uptake from transferrin into red cell precursors, and inhibition of iron's enzymatic incorporation into heme.

This now rare variety of ESA resistance may be considered in the poorly responding patient with adequate iron stores and microcytic anemia; low turnover bone disease and refractory normochromic normocytic anemia; abnormal unstimulated plasma aluminum concentration and anemia; or chronic aluminum exposure with otherwise unexplained anemia. In such patients, following exclusion of other causes of treatment resistance and anemia, assessment of body aluminum burden with deferoxamine stimulation test (if unstimulated level is elevated) and/or bone biopsy may be considered. If clinical suspicion of ESA resistance due to aluminum is high but evaluation inconclusive, empiric treatment may entail exclusion of exogenous aluminum (if not done already), and serial monitoring of blood levels. Presumptive treatment with deferoxamine without tissue documentation of aluminum excess must be weighed against the risks of opportunistic infection, neurotoxicity, and (possibly) iron deficiency, potentially complicating its chronic administration. Treatment endpoints could include diminishing ESA requirements and stable hemoglobin with either deferoxamine treatment (persisting after its discontinuation) or aluminum exclusion, or tissue verification of aluminum removal.

Secondary Hyperparathyroidism

Given exclusion of more common causes of resistance discussed previously, poor response in the presence of significant secondary hyperparathyroidism should prompt suspicion that PTH may be causally implicated. Two pathophysiologic mechanisms have been postulated in the contribution of hyperparathyroidism to both anemia and ESA resistance. One centers on a toxic effect of PTH on red cell precursor proliferation in the marrow and antagonism of the effect of endogenous erythropoietin (several observations of some reversal of anemia following parathyroidectomy have supported this consideration). A second focuses on the physical effects of high turnover bone disease and marrow fibrosis in diminishing the size of the erythron responsive to ESAs. Of interest in both regards is a recent study that has shown a potentiation of ESA effect with cinecalcet in the setting of effective treatment of secondary hyperparathyroidism. Bone biopsy was not performed. In patients with very elevated PTH levels and ESA resistance in whom other etiologies for poor response have been excluded, effective treatment of secondary hyperparathyroidism should be pursued. For those patients who continue to manifest significant resistance to ESA therapy in the face of effective medical management of this ailment, another etiology for ESA resistance should be entertained.

Hematologic Disorders

In patients with hemoglobinopathies, immunologically mediated hemolytic processes, and some myelophthisic states, initial response to ESA treatment may be poor. In patients with sickle cell anemia, initial expectations that aggressive ESA therapy would be beneficial in reducing transfusion requirements did not fully materialize. Alpha and beta thalassemia may respond poorly, as well. Resistance has also been reported among dialysis patients with hemolytic anemias resulting from chloramine exposure, reuse-related formaldehyde exposure (anti-N_{form} hemolysis), and prosthetic cardiac valves.

ESRD patients with myelodysplastic syndrome may also have less satisfactory response to ESA treatment, should such therapy be elected. Poor response in this setting as well as with hemoglobinopathies should prompt reassessment of the overall goals of ESA therapy, caution in escalation of dose, and consideration of transfusion as at least a partial therapeutic alternative.

Angiotensin-Converting Enzyme Inhibitors and Receptor Blockers

A relationship between activation of the renin-angiotensin system and erythropoietin production has been recognized for many years, but has not been well understood. Activation of the renin-angiotensin system as seen in renal artery stenosis is often accompanied by erythrocytosis, while polycythemia occurring post-renal transplant is often reversed by employment of angiotensin-converting enzyme inhibitors (ACEis). The physiologic basis for this latter relationship is unclear. One suggested mechanism for the role of ACEi in ESA resistance entails ACEi-mediated increases in levels of *N*-acetyl-seryl-aspartyl-lysyl proline, an inhibitor of stem cell recruitment. In the ESA era, however, hormone resistance has been inconsistently demonstrated, with many studies over recent years revealing divided opinions regarding the clinical impact of ACEi or ARB in this phenomenon. This suggests a potentially modest effect of ACEi/ARB in the etiology of this problem.

Carnitine Deficiency

Some have suggested a role for carnitine deficiency in impairing response to ESA treatment in ESRD, possibly by altering erythrocyte membrane stability, or marrow sensitivity to the hormone. It is difficult to draw a direct conclusion regarding the efficacy of carnitine therapy from many of the more recent studies in this area, as patients selected for some of those trials were not necessarily chosen on the basis of ESA resistance or carnitine deficiency. A meta-analysis in 2002 examining a variety of diverse studies revealed six randomized investigations evaluating whether ESA sparing could be accomplished with carnitine administration. Five of six showed ESA dose reducible with maintenance of hemoglobin in the desired target range. ESA resistance index (ERI, expressed as dose in units/g hemoglobin) in three of these trials decreased with therapy. On the other hand, a recent 1-year randomized controlled trial of 92 unselected incident dialysis patients, half receiving carnitine IV and the other placebo, found no improvement in the study patients' response to ESAs.

Two recent studies have suggested a potentially interesting role for non-acetyl acylcarnitine in the evolution of ESA resistance in ESRD. In one study that divided 87 unselected patients into high-ERI and low-ERI groupings, high ERI levels (in µg/kg/wk ESA/g hemoglobin) were significantly associated with low carnitine concentrations, whereas patients with normal carnitine values had low ERI levels. Of interest, ERI was positively correlated with the ratio of non-acetyl acylcarnitine to total carnitine. Another investigation examined the relationship of reduced physical activity (and several other parameters of health, including ESA dose in units) to dysfunctional fatty acid oxidation in ESRD patients with free carnitine levels <40 µmol/L. This study revealed a significant positive correlation between ESA dose and acylcarnitine's acyl chain length. These interesting findings would benefit from further investigation.

Adequacy of Dialysis

Enhanced erythropoiesis with more aggressive clearance has been noted as early as 1992 from experience in Tassin, France, in which a baseline dialysis prescription more robust than that of the United States at the time (mean delivered Kt/V of 1.67) yielded an average hematocrit of 28% unassisted by ESA therapy. Several studies over the past 20 years have shown improvement in ESA response with an increase in hemodialysis dose (whether these observations are related to dialysis dose, or dialyzer, however, is not always straightforward), whereas others have found it equivocal.

Of particular note in this regard has been the recent completion of the Frequent Hemodialysis Network study, a randomized, controlled trial assessing cardiac outcomes of patients receiving either short daily in-center dialysis, or frequent nocturnal hemodialysis compared to controls. In the nocturnal trial, 87 patients were randomized to either conventional dialysis 3×/wk (42), or 6×/wk nocturnal dialysis (45). These 45 patients had a 1.82-fold higher mean weekly stdKt/V than 3×/wk controls, and 2.45-fold higher average weekly treatment times. In the daily in-center trial, 125 patients were randomized to short daily dialysis 6×/wk, and 120 to conventional dialysis 3×/wk. In the short daily group, the 125 study patients had a 1.42-fold higher weekly stdKt/V than the 3×/wk patients. The effect of these two therapies combined on anemia management—specifically, ESA dose—was evaluated as a secondary study endpoint. Although the provision of this amount of dialysis might have been anticipated to improve the erythropoietic treatment efficiency and lower ESA dose (presumably by improving anti-uremia therapy and increasing erythrocyte survival), it had no significant effect on this component of anemia management in either daily or nocturnal trial as a whole. (There was, however, a nonsignificant trend toward ESA dose reduction in the daily frequent dialysis group and a significant reduction in dose among diabetics in the daily frequent dialysis group.) Possible reasons for this negative overall finding include the relatively small size of the trial (particularly the nocturnal trial), and observance of prior practice patterns in hemoglobin targeting and ESA dosing compared to those since the study was executed.

Hemoglobin Cycling and Variability

In previous years, considerable interest was generated by the phenomenon of hemoglobin cycling, characterized by sinusoidal fluctuation of hemoglobin concentration often resulting initially from the interaction of intercurrent clinical events with ESA dose (i.e., induction of transient resistance to treatment). As an example, hospitalized patients, depending on their diagnosis, may present with—or develop—substantial inflammatory insults during the course of their illness, resulting in resistance to ESA.

The patient's ESA dose is thereafter raised while hospitalized, resulting in an upward hemoglobin trajectory. "Cycling" ensues if the resulting hemoglobin concentrations ultimately exceed upper outpatient facility or protocol limits after discharge and require downward dose titration. Another previous contributor to this undesirable phenomenon included frequent dose change maneuvers born out of concerns relating to compliance of hemoglobin concentration with certain payment issues.

In more recent years, attention has been devoted to the relationship between hemoglobin variability (i.e., standard deviation: at facilities, among groups of patients, or individual patients) and a variety of outcomes, particularly mortality. This value serves as a surrogate for frequency and severity of patient illness (and by inference, ESA resistance), blood loss, or problematic hemoglobin management. Several studies that have examined this relationship from the perspectives of group, facility, or individual patient standard deviation have been divided in demonstrating clear relationships with mortality. It has been suggested, however, that enhanced measures to decrease facility intra- and interpatient variability (such as tightened anemia control, narrower hemoglobin targets, more frequent lab review, ESA adjustment based on hemoglobin trends, etc.) might not only be effective but could improve patient outcomes as well.

Pure Red Cell Aplasia

Casadevall et al reported 21 patients developing pure red cell aplasia in the setting of ESA (EPO) treatment between 1998 and 2001, traced to the presence of a neutralizing antibody which inhibited red cell proliferation from normal marrow. Nearly all patients developing this problem in that report were treated with Eprex via subcutaneous injection and, in most cases, responded either to discontinuation of the hormone or immunosuppressive treatment. Exhaustive evaluation by both manufacturers and investigators over several years has offered several possible mechanisms for the generation of anti-EPO antibodies: one suggestion is that compounds acting as adjuvants for an anti-EPO immune response were leached out of uncoated rubber stoppers from hormone-containing syringes by polysorbate 80 (at that time, an agent substituted for human serum albumin in the preparation). With new coating of the syringe rubber stoppers, this very serious problem was reduced to a rare occurrence. As suggested by MacDougall et al, other possible mechanisms for PRCA have appeared over ensuing years, including denaturation and aggregation of protein in the preparation related to tungsten contamination, or polysorbate 80–mediated decrease in compound stability, both generating an anti-EPO immune response.

PRCA is diagnosed by severe resistance to ESA therapy, rapidly declining hemoglobin, and accompanying falling reticulocyte count, without other cytopenias. In evaluation of PRCA, other sources of ESA resistance merit exclusion, and assays for neutralizing anti-EPO antibodies should be sent. Bone marrow examination, if done, should show absent erythroblasts. Treatment should entail discontinuation of ESA, support with transfusion, and immunosuppression, either alone or in conjunction with renal transplantation.

Future Developments

Given the dramatic change in the setting of ESA therapy over the last decade, forecasts of clinical developments in treatment of the patient with resistance to ESAs might now reasonably includ: first, sharper definition of the settings in which dose increases for the poorly responding patient are problematic (and either transfusion, a combination of ESA and transfusion, or total weekly weight-adjusted dose limitation are less so); second, whether newer agents can be developed to convert resistant states into nonresistant ones; and third, whether more effective hemoglobin management (i.e., protocol-driven tools such as trending hemoglobins to aid in dose adjustment, use of narrower target hemoglobin ranges, or employment of more sophisticated computerized dosing regimens, some now seeing use) can reproducibly improve response by limiting hemoglobin variability for both facilities and individual patients.

SECTION XX

Cardiovascular Disease

The Challenges of Blood Pressure Control in Dialysis Patients

Vito M. Campese, MD • Ravi S. Lakdawala, MD

Cardiovascular disease (CVD) is the leading cause of death in patients receiving maintenance hemodialysis (HD). Hypertension is extremely common in HD patients, occurring in upward of 82% of patients, and is considered the single most important predictor of coronary artery disease (CAD) and cardiovascular events. Thus, treatment of hypertension is considered crucial for long-term survival in these patients. Unfortunately, there is limited conclusive evidence on how to define, evaluate, and manage hypertension in the HD patient population. The approaches recommended by existing guidelines are largely based on opinions and not on hard evidence concerning efficacy and safety.

Challenges Defining Hypertension and in Establishing Goal Blood Pressure in Dialysis Patients

In the general population the definitions of optimal blood pressure (BP) (<120/80 mm Hg), normal BP (120–129/80–84 mm Hg), prehypertension (135–139/85–89 mm Hg), and hypertension (≥140/90 mm Hg) are well defined. For this population, there is a linear relationship between systolic BP (SBP) and CVD and events starting at levels of SBP above 115 mm Hg. According to the Eighth Joint National Committee (JNC 8) guidelines, the recommended goal BP is 140/90 mm Hg or less in patients with essential hypertension with and without diabetes and with or without CKD. In patients older than 60 years, the recommended goal BP is 150/90 mm Hg. It is not the scope of this review to critically analyze these recommendations.

The paradigms valid for the general population cannot be applied to patients with advanced chronic kidney disease (CKD) or end-stage renal disease (ESRD); therefore, the ideal goal BP in these patients has not been ascertained. The Kidney Disease Outcomes Quality Initiative (KDOQI) guidelines currently recommend a goal predialysis BP of less than 140/90 mm Hg. In hypertensive dialysis patients, each 10–mm Hg rise in mean arterial pressure (MAP) has been shown to increase the risk of left ventricular hypertrophy (LVH), increase the risk of de novo congestive heart failure (CHF), and increase the risk of de novo ischemic heart disease. However, a large body of evidence from observational studies indicates that low levels of BP may be associated with increased mortality compared with levels in the mild to moderate hypertension range. A "U-shaped" relationship exists between BP and mortality, with excess mortality risk in patients with the lowest and with the highest levels of BP. In patients with low estimated glomerular filtration rate (eGFR <30 mL/min per 1.73 m^2), the risk of all-cause mortality and death from CVD was higher in nonhypertensive participants (<120 mm Hg) than in hypertensive participants. Similar observations have been reported for dialysis patients.

Regardless of levels of BP, survival rate is better among those prescribed antihypertensive medication, primarily with renin–angiotensin–aldosterone (RAAS) inhibitors. However, uncertainty persists whether low levels of BP achieved with antihypertensive medications carrying the same adverse prognostic implications as low levels of BP achieved spontaneously. The reason for the controversies surrounding the relationship between hypertension and outcome may reflect the high prevalence of cardiomyopathy and autonomic dysfunction among patients with longstanding hypertension, particularly if associated with diabetes and CKD. Many of these patients develop cardiac failure with consequent reduction of BP values (so-called "reverse causality").

Challenges of Blood Pressure Measurements in Dialysis Patients

According to current guidelines, BP should be measured with patients seated in a chair with their backs supported and their arms bared and supported at heart level. Measurements should begin after at least 5 minutes of rest. Two or more readings separated by 2 minutes should be averaged. If the first two readings differ by more than 5 mm Hg, additional readings should be performed and averaged. BP measurements should be performed both before and after each dialysis or at every office visit and in the sitting position and after standing for 2 minutes. This is necessary to determine whether patients manifest orthostatic hypo- or hypertension. BP should be measured in both arms and, subsequently, the arm with the higher SBP should be used. Frequently, this practice cannot be implemented in dialysis patients because the arm with a fistula or a graft cannot be used for BP measurements. Often, BP cannot be measured in any of the two arms, and it is measured in the lower extremities. In this case, BP cannot be adequately assessed in the upright posture.

Importance of 24-Hour Blood Pressure Recording in Dialysis Patients

In the nondialysis population, the correlation between BP measured in the physician's office and CV endpoints is usually weak. A large body of evidence from subjects with essential hypertension has shown that average 24-hour ambulatory blood pressure monitoring (ABPM) correlates with the incidence of CVD better than office BP.

Among dialysis patients, BP measurements obtained in the peridialysis period lack precision in estimating ambulatory BP, and average interdialytic ambulatory BP levels predict mortality better than BP measured in the dialysis unit. Interdialytic BP measurement is best achieved with 24- or 44-hour ambulatory ABPM. This type of measurement has also allowed the study of the prevalence of white coat hypertension (an elevation of BP that occurs only in the office of the doctor and not outside) or masked hypertension (an elevation of BP that occurs outside of the office and that cannot be documented in the doctor's office). Both white coat and masked hypertension are common among ESRD patients and are relevant in the evaluation and management of these patients.

Unfortunately, ABPM is expensive and cannot be performed in most dialysis centers. As an alternative, inclusion of multiple intradialytic BP measurements, in addition to pre- and post-HD measurements, may be used to more accurately evaluate BP in these patients. Home self-measurements of BP correlate with CV outcomes better than pre- or postdialysis measurements, but they do not provide information pertaining to circadian variability of BP.

Normally, BP tends to be the highest during the morning, gradually decreasing during the course of the day to reach the lowest levels at night. Approximately 10% to 25% of patients with essential hypertension fail to manifest this normal nocturnal dipping of BP, defined as a nighttime BP fall of more than 10%. These patients are called "nondippers," and those with a normal circadian rhythm are called "dippers." The lack of diurnal BP variation and the loss of nocturnal dipping affect a significant number of ESRD patients. Sometimes in dialysis patients, nocturnal BP can be greater than BP measured during the day. Because BP is usually measured during the day, this may lead to the erroneous impression of good antihypertensive control. Using ABPM, it has been observed that in HD patients, BP decreases after dialysis and during the first night, but by the next morning, it reaches predialysis levels, and it does not decrease during the second night.

The mechanisms responsible for the abnormal circadian rhythm of BP in ESRD include autonomic dysfunction, reduced physical activity, sleep-disordered breathing, reduced arterial distensibility, and volume overload. One would predict that volume expansion plays a major role in the phenomenon of BP nondipping among HD patients. However, interdialytic weight gain (IDWG) does not correlate with the phenomenon of nondipping, and slow and short daily hemodialyses do not change nocturnal dipping despite reduced extracellular water and better BP control.

A relationship also seems to exist between the absence of the nocturnal dipping of BP and frequency and severity of CVD.

Pulse Pressure and Outcomes in Dialysis Patients

There is substantial evidence that pulse pressure (PP), particularly in middle-aged and older subjects, is an independent predictor of risk of coronary heart disease, cardiovascular mortality, and overall mortality. From age 30 to 50 years, SBP and diastolic BP (DBP) track together in a parallel manner. However, after the age of 60 years, DBP decreases while SBP continues to rise, accounting for the increase in PP after the age of 60 years.

One of the factors that may contribute to increasing PP in ESRD patients is aortic stiffness. Epidemiologic studies have shown that aortic stiffness is increased in ESRD patients and is an independent marker of CVD risk. Aortic stiffness is usually determined by the aortic pulse wave velocity (PWV), which frequently improves when BP is reduced, particularly when angiotensin-converting enzyme inhibitors (ACE) inhibitors or calcium channel blockers (CCBs) are used. In ESRD patients, failure of PWV to improve in response to decreased BP is associated with worse cardiovascular outcomes.

The ankle-to-arm blood pressure index (AABI) has also been found to be a strong predictor of cardiovascular and overall mortality.

Blood Pressure Variability and Cardiovascular Outcome in Dialysis Patients

Blood pressure is quite variable in dialysis patients before and after HD and in between visits. Increased intradialytic and interdialytic variability has been associated with an increase in all-cause, stroke, and cardiovascular mortality. Lower BP variability was associated with greater fluid removal, achievement of target weight postdialysis, and the absence of beta-blocker or renin–angiotensin system (RAS) blocking agent therapy. CCBs may have the greatest effect on visit-to-visit BP reduction compared with other antihypertensives, but this effect has not been studied in the dialysis population.

Pathogenesis of Hypertension in End-Stage Renal Disease Patients

See Table 53.1.

Management of Hypertension in Dialysis Patients

Because of the complexity of the factors that sustain hypertension in dialysis patients, the management is frequently challenging. Certainly, there is no one-size-fits-all solution, and the management of patients should be individualized based on certain factors, including whether the patient has frequent episodes of hypotension during dialysis, intradialytic hypertension, nocturnal hypertension, masked or white coat hypertension, or resistant hypertension. An adequate management cannot be accomplished without knowledge of the BP variability during and between dialysis and without knowledge of the circadian changes of BP. ABPM for 24 to 44 hours is essential for individually planning an adequate antihypertensive regimen. Treatment also requires knowledge of the pharmacokinetic and pharmacodynamic properties of the antihypertensive agents used.

Lifestyle modifications should be an integral part of the management of every patient with hypertension, including those with ESRD. In dialysis patients, achievement of dry weight is essential for BP control.

Lifestyle Modifications

Lifestyle modifications, such as dietary salt restriction, moderation of alcohol intake, and increased physical activity, can be used effectively as adjunct therapy in the management of hypertension in dialysis patients. Unlike in the general population

---

Table 53.1

Factors Implicated in the Pathogenesis of Hypertension in End-Stage Renal Disease

Sodium and volume excess
The renin–angiotensin–aldosterone system
The sympathetic nervous system
Reduced baroreceptors' sensitivity
Endothelium-derived vasodilators
Endothelium-derived vasoconstrictors
Erythropoietin
Divalent ions and PTH
Structural changes of the arteries
Miscellaneous: serotonin, vasopressin, calcineurin inhibitors, NSAID use, anticongestion
    agents

NSAID, nonsteroidal antiinflammatory drug; PTH, parathyroid hormone.

with essential hypertension, a high-potassium diet is not recommended for ESRD patients because of the risk of hyperkalemia.

Control of Fluid and Volume Status With Dialysis

Sodium retention and excessive extracellular volume are major pathogenic factors of hypertension in ESRD patients. In addition to sodium and fluid restrictions, an adequate dialysis strategy should be established to achieve and maintain dry weight, which is defined as that body weight at the end of dialysis below which further reduction results in hypotension.

The strongest evidence supporting a role of extracellular volume expansion derives from observations by the group in Tassin, France, who observed that when excessive body fluids are removed with long, slow dialysis and "dry weight" is achieved, BP normalized in more than 90% of HD patients, but fewer than 5% of them required antihypertensive drugs 3 months later. Other benefits of slow dialysis include hemodynamic stability with low incidences of hypotension and muscular cramps.

When initiating dialysis, optimum dry weight should be achieved gradually over 4 to 8 weeks, and the negative fluid balance should not exceed 1 to 2 kg per week. Overzealous ultrafiltration (UF) may result in hypotension, rapid reduction of the residual renal function, and cerebral or coronary ischemic events. Several methods have been proposed to estimate dry weight, but none of them is applicable to a large number of patients. The gold standard for evaluation of total body water is the use of tracer dilution techniques, but this is not clinically applicable. Some have proposed the use of postdialytic echocardiographic measurement of the diameter of the inferior vena cava, but this method is not without its critics. The most promising method to assess fluid status during dialysis is multifrequency electrical bioimpedance.

In a patient just beginning dialysis, if BP is only moderately elevated (stage 1), antihypertensive therapy should not be instituted until dry weight is achieved. In patients already taking antihypertensive agents, the dosage of medications should be gradually tapered as the BP progressively declines because of UF. When dry weight is achieved, BP becomes normal in more than half of these patients. During the interdialytic period, BP may rise again proportionally to the amount of sodium and fluid retention. If during the interdialytic periods, BP does not exceed 160/90 mm Hg, antihypertensive therapy may be withheld because administration of antihypertensive agents before dialysis may result in frequent and severe intradialytic hypotensive episodes. Antihypertensive therapy should be promptly instituted in patients with stage 2 hypertension; accelerated hypertension; or end-organ damage such as severe retinopathy, CHF, cerebrovascular accidents, or aortic aneurysm. Intensive UF should be instituted only in patients with signs of CHF, hypertensive emergencies, hypertensive encephalopathy, or pulmonary edema.

Dialysate Sodium Prescription and Blood Pressure Among Hemodialysis Patients

Dialysate concentration of sodium has been adjusted in numerous studies to assess effect on weight gain and hemodynamic stability. When high-dialysate sodium or sodium profiling—progressive adjustment of sodium from high concentration to low sodium concentration—is used, there may be increased fluid removal and hemodynamic stability; however, the consequences include increased IDWG as a result of increased thirst. Low-dialysate concentrations of sodium may reduce BP, IDWG, and intradialytic symptoms. However, an analysis from the International Dialysis Outcomes and Practices Patterns Study (DOPPS) has shown that patients assigned to higher dialysate sodium do not manifest higher predialysis BP than patients treated with lower sodium concentrations.

Therapy With Antihypertensive Drugs

An extensive number of effective antihypertensive agents are currently available. In choosing among antihypertensive agents, consideration should be given to the coexisting diseases as well as the patient's demographic characteristics, risk profile, and lifestyle, as well as the pharmacokinetic properties of the antihypertensive drugs used (Table 53.2). Diuretics should not commonly be used in dialysis patients unless they have an adequate residual urine output.

Patient Demographics

Patients who are less likely to comply with the antihypertensive regimen, either because of their lifestyle or poor intellectual capacity to adhere to a therapeutic regimen, should be treated with long-acting agents that can be administered once daily—or even better, once weekly—or postdialysis by nurses.

Certain antihypertensive agents, such as beta-blockers and centrally acting antiadrenergic agents, may affect mental acuity and physical strength and should be avoided in patients who perform activities requiring alertness, mental acuity, or strenuous physical feats. In these instances, drugs such as ACE inhibitors or CCBs, which have little impact on mental or physical performance, are preferred.

Antiadrenergic drugs are more likely to cause sexual dysfunction, an important consideration particularly when managing male dialysis patients, because 50% of them have significant impotence as a result of uremia.

Coexisting Disease

The presence of concomitant diseases should also guide the physician in the choice of antihypertensive drugs. For example, beta-blockers should not be used in patients with asthma or with peripheral vascular disease because these conditions can be aggravated by the administration of these drugs.

Patients with CAD, previous myocardial infarction, arrhythmias, hyperdynamic circulation, nervousness, or migraine headaches should be preferentially treated with beta-blockers or calcium antagonists. In patients with known CAD, direct vasodilators such as hydralazine or minoxidil should be avoided because they activate the sympathetic nervous system (SNS), thereby increasing heart rate, cardiac output, and myocardial oxygen consumption.

Patients with type 1 diabetes mellitus and autonomic dysfunction should not be treated with nonselective beta-blockers because they may aggravate the control of diabetes, cause or aggravate episodes of hypoglycemia, and mask the signs of hypoglycemia. Antiadrenergic agents that are more likely to cause or aggravate orthostatic hypotension should be avoided.

Table 53.2

Pharmacokinetic Properties of Antihypertensive Drugs in Patients With End-Stage Renal Disease

	Oral Bioavailability (%)	Protein Binding (%)	Half-life (hr)		Renal Excretion of Unchanged Drug (% Dose)	Dose Change With ESRD	Removal With Dialysis		Active Hemometabolites
			Normal	ESRD			Hemo	Peritoneal	
Antiadrenergic Agents									
Clonidine	75	20–40	5–13	17–40	50	↓ (50%–75%)	5%	NA	No
Guanabenz	40	40	50–100	83–323	Small	→ (Yes)	None	None	No
Guanethidine	5–60	0	48–72	Prolonged	30–50	→ (Yes)	None	None	Slight
Guanfacine	100	65	15–20	Slightly increased	30–50	→ (Yes, lowered dose)	None	None	No
Methyldopa	26–74	<20	1–2	1.7–3.6	50	12%–24%	60%	30–40	Yes
Moxonidine	90	7–9	1.7–3.5	3.2–10.6	55–65	50%	—	—	—
Rilmenidine	100	7–8	7–9	31–37	60–70	50%	—	—	—
α-Adrenergic Blocking Agents									
Doxazosin	60–70	98–99	10–15	10–15	9	None	None	NA	Yes/none
Guanadrel	70–80	20	3–5	10–30	40–50	→	NA	NA	—
Prazosin	48–68	97	2.5–4.0	2.5–4.0	<10	—	None	None	None
Terazosin	80–90	90–94	10–15	10–15	40	None	NA	NA	None
Urapidil	70–75	79–82	2–5	5–8	10–15	None	None	None	Yes
β-Adrenergic Blocking Agents									
Acebutolol	50	26	3.5	3.5	40	70%	50%	NA	Yes
Atenolol	50	10	6–9	<120	85–100	↓75%	53%	48%	No
Betaxolol	89 ± 5	50	14–22	28–44	15	50%	None	None	No
Bisoprolol	80–90	30	10–12	23–25	45–55	50%	25%–35%	None	No
Carteolol	80–85	20–30	5–7	30–40	55–65	25%	NA	NA	Yes
Carvedilol	25	95	4–7	4–7	2	None	None	None	Yes

Continued

Table 53.2

Pharmacokinetic Properties of Antihypertensive Drugs in Patients With End-Stage Renal Disease—Cont'd

	Oral Bioavailability (%)	Protein Binding (%)	Half-life (hr) Normal	Half-life (hr) ESRD	Renal Excretion of Unchanged Drug (% Dose)	Dose Change With ESRD	Removal With Dialysis Hemo	Removal With Dialysis Peritoneal	Active Hemometabolites
Cetamolol	—	—	6–8	10–12	30–40	33%	NA	NA	NA
Esmolol	—	55	7.2	7.1	2	None	None	None	Slight
Labetalol IV	NA	50	5.5	5.5	50–60	Smaller doses work	<1%	<1%	No
Labetalol PO	33	50	3–4	3–4	20–40	Slight →	<1%	<1%	No
La-propranolol	20	90	10	10	<1	Slight →	None	None	Yes
Metoprolol tartrate	40–50	12	3–4	3–4	13	None	High	NA	Slight
Metoprolol SA	50	12	3–7	—	10	None	—	—	Yes
Nadolol	30	30	14–24	45	70	50% ↓	High	NA	No
Pindolol	90	57	2–3	2–3	40	Slight →	Probable	NA	Yes
Propranolol	30	90	2–4	2–4	<1	Slight →	None	None	No
Timolol	75	10	4–6	4–6	20	Slight →	NA	NA	No
Nebivolol	—	98	12–19	—	38–67	—	—	—	—
Angiotensin-Converting Enzyme Inhibitors									
Alacepril	—	—	—	—	15–20	—	→	—	—
Benazepril	37	97	10–11	4–6	1	Yes ↓[b]	None	NA	—
Captopril	75	30	2–3	Prolonged	30–40	Yes[b]	Yes	—	No
Cilazapril	77	2–3	4–6	20–30	25	Yes	—	—	—
Delapril	55	0.5	—	65–85	?	—	—	—	Yes
Enalapril	60	High	11	2	70	Yes[b]	35%	NA	Yes
Fosinopril	36	95	12	Prolonged	Negligible	None	2	7	Yes
Lisinopril	25–30	3–10	12.7	54.3	29	↓75%	50%	NA	No
Moexipril	13	2–9	—	—	—	—	—	Yes	—

Pentopril	50	0.7–1.0	No change	20–25	—	—	—	—	—
Pentoprilat	—	2–3	10–14	35–45	→	—	—	—	—
Perindopril	66	—	—	78	Yes	NA	NA	NA	—
Quinapril	60	97	2–3	Prolonged	5–6	50%	Yes	NA	Yes
Ramipril	54–65	73	10.8	Prolonged	2	50%	NA	—	Yes
Trandolapril	10	80	6	12	33	50%	—	—	Yes
Zofenopril	96	80–85	5–6	10	5	—	—	—	—
Vasodilators									
Diazoxide	Low	85	20–36	Prolonged	50	None	Yes	Yes	?
Hydralazine	10–30	90	2–4	Prolonged	10	Yes, slight →	NA	None	No
Minoxidil	95	Minimal	2.8–4.2	4.2	10	None	Yes	Yes	No
Nitroprusside	0	?	3–4 min	Prolonged	High	None	Yes	Yes	No
Calcium Channel Blockers									
Amlodipine	60–70	97	30–50	10%	<1	None	NA	NA	?
Diltiazem	20	80	α: 20 hr (β: 4 hr)	Unchanged	35	None	NA	NA	No
Diltiazem ER									
Felodipine	15–20	97	10–20	<0.5%	<0.5	None	—	—	—
Isradipine	15–20	96	8–12	Unchanged	<5	—	—	—	—
Lercanidipine hydrochloride	6%	>98%	8–10	?	44%	NA	NA	NA	No
Nicardipine	6–30 (dose dependent)	98–99	3–6	Unchanged	<5	Decreased	—	—	No
Nifedipine	65	90	α: 2.5–3.0 hr (β: 5 hr)	Unchanged	70–80	None	Low	Low	No
Nilvadipine	15	85–90	10–13	<5	—	—	—	—	No
Nimodipine	6–10	98	1–1.5	<1	None	—	—	—	No
Nisoldipine	8–10	98–99	1.0–1.5	<1	None	—	—	—	No
Nitrendipine	10–30	98	1.0–1.5	<1	3–4	—	—	—	Yes
Verapamil	10–32	90	α: 15–30 hr (β: 3–7 hr[a])	α: 4.5 (β: 2.3 hr[a])	3	? (none)	None	Yes	

Continued

Table 53.2

Pharmacokinetic Properties of Antihypertensive Drugs in Patients With End-Stage Renal Disease—Cont'd

	Oral Bioavailability (%)	Protein Binding (%)	Half-life (hr) Normal	Half-life (hr) ESRD	Renal Excretion of Unchanged Drug (% Dose)	Dose Change With ESRD	Removal With Dialysis Hemo	Removal With Dialysis Peritoneal	Active Hemometabolites
Angiotensin II Receptor Blockers									
Azilsartan	60	>99	11	—	15	None	None	—	—
Candesartan	15	>99	9	?	26	Yes ↓	None	NA	No
Cilexetil	—	—	—	—	—	—	—	No	No
Eprosartan	13	98	5–9	NA	IV 37 PO 7	None	Poorly	No	No
Losartan	33	98.70	2	4	4	None	None	None	Yes
Olmesartan	26–28	NA	10–15	NA	35–50	NA	NA	NA	—
Medoxomil	—	—	—	—	—	—	—	—	—
Telmisartan	42–58	>99.5	24	NA	0.49–0.91	None	None	NA	No
Valsartan	10–35	95	6	NA	13	NA	None	None	No
Direct Renin Inhibitor									
Aliskiren	2.5	47–51	24	25	0–1	None	Low	—	—

a Maximum dose is same. Consider starting with lower dose (50% ↓).
b alpha (α) phase (initial fast decrease related to cell distribution); beta (β) phase (late, gradual decrease related to metabolism of drug).
ESRD, end-stage renal disease; IV, intravenous; PO, oral; NA, not applicable or not available.

Effects of Dialysis on Antihypertensive Drugs in End-Stage Renal Disease Patients

In ESRD patients, the metabolism and disposition of antihypertensive drugs may be abnormal, resulting in accumulation of the intact drug or of its metabolites and increased incidence of untoward effects. In general, drugs that are more water soluble and less protein bound are removed with dialysis more readily than lipid soluble and highly protein-bound agents. Postdialysis hypertension is more commonly observed in patients taking dialyzable drugs because the removal with dialysis may result in a sudden decrease in blood levels of drugs and result in rebound hypertension. For these reasons, the choice of antihypertensive drugs in dialysis patients requires knowledge of the pharmacodynamic and pharmacokinetic properties of these agents.

Antihypertensive Drugs in End-Stage Renal Disease Patients

We describe in this section some of the principal pharmacologic properties of the most commonly used antihypertensive agents in dialysis patients.

Inhibitors of the Renin–Angiotensin–Aldosterone System

Angiotensin-Converting Enzyme Inhibitors

The ACE inhibitor class of antihypertensive agents inhibits kininase II, thereby reducing the conversion of angiotensin I to angiotensin II. ACE inhibitors can be classified into three main chemical categories: sulfhydryl-, carboxyl-, and phosphoryl-containing compounds.

Sulfhydryl Agents

The sulfhydryl agents, such as alacepril, delapril, and moveltopril, are prodrugs and thus are converted to captopril in vivo. These sulfhydryl-containing compounds have a slower onset and longer duration of action than captopril. Zofenopril has greater potency and is partially eliminated by the liver.

Carboxyl Agents

The carboxyl-containing ACE inhibitors, such as enalapril and benazepril, are prodrugs converted in vivo to the active metabolite. The kidney principally excretes ACE inhibitors, with the exception of spirapril, which is totally eliminated by the liver. Benazepril has an earlier peak time and a slightly shorter terminal half-life than enalapril. Delapril, quinapril, trandolapril, and spirapril have earlier peak times and shorter half-lives, but perindopril has a peak time and half-life similar to enalapril. Lisinopril is an enalapril-like diacid, which is not a prodrug, and has poor oral bioavailability (30%).

Phosphoryl Agents

The last class of ACE inhibitors is the phosphoryl-containing group, which includes fosinopril, a drug that is partially eliminated by the liver and does not require dose adjustment in patients with renal failure.

The ACE inhibitors reduce BP by diminishing the circulating levels of angiotensin II and aldosterone. As a result of the negative feedback of angiotensin II on renin secretion, they result in increased levels of plasma renin activity (PRA). The ACE inhibitors are more effective antihypertensive agents in patients with increased PRA, but they are also effective, although to a lesser extent, in patients with low PRA. The reason for their efficacy in patients with low PRA is less clear, but this may be due to inhibition of intrarenal angiotensin II formation. Because kininase II blocks the degradation of kinin, the antihypertensive action of these drugs may depend in part on increased blood levels of bradykinin.

The ACE inhibitors decrease peripheral vascular resistance without increasing heart rate, cardiac output, or pulmonary wedge pressure and without reflex activation of the sympathetic nervous system. On the contrary, these agents may reduce BP in part via inhibition of SNS activity. The ACE inhibitors may reduce thirst, oral fluid intake, and possibly IDWG.

Side Effects of Angiotensin-Converting Enzyme Inhibitors
Captopril, the first ACE inhibitor to be introduced into the market, was initially associated with a high incidence of side effects in large part because of the high doses used at that time. Captopril contains a sulfhydryl group, which increases the frequency of some side effects. The most common side effects of ACE inhibitors are dry cough, skin rash, angioedema, and dysgeusia. Neutropenia and agranulocytosis may appear after 3 to 12 weeks of therapy, particularly in patients with autoimmune collagen vascular diseases.

Another notable side effect is worsening of anemia in dialysis patients. This is not associated with decreased levels of erythropoietin or increased hemolysis, but it appears to be related to a direct or indirect interference of angiotensin II with the signal transduction of erythropoietin at the cellular level.

Of particular interest is the report of anaphylactic reactions in dialysis patients treated with ACE inhibitors. Specifically, this phenomenon has been observed in the setting of patients treated with ACE inhibitors while undergoing dialysis with a high-flux (AN-69) capillary dialyzer. Symptoms may range from mild edema of the mucosa of the eyes to nausea and vomiting, bronchospasm, hypotension, and angioedema.

Angiotensin II Receptor Antagonists
Losartan, a derivative of imidazole, was the first orally active and highly specific antagonist of angiotensin II receptor with vasodilator and antihypertensive activity to be introduced into the market. Subsequently, several other angiotensin II receptor blockers have been introduced in the U.S. market, including valsartan, irbesartan, candesartan, telmisartan, eprosartan, and olmesartan.

The mechanism of antihypertensive action of these drugs is due to inhibition of the RAS, specifically blocking angiotensin II–induced responses. Because sartans do not affect the activity of kininase II, they do not appear to cause cough, a well-known adverse effect of ACE inhibitors. The effects of sartans and ACE inhibitors on BP and CVD outcome appear to be comparable.

Molecular techniques have identified at least two angiotensin II receptor subtypes, AT_1 and AT_2. AT_1 receptors mediate the vasoconstriction of resistance vessels; examples of selective AT_1 antagonists are losartan and valsartan. Stimulation of AT_2 receptors produces vasodilation, inhibits cell proliferation, increases apoptosis and cell differentiation, and regulates pressure natriuresis. Studies suggest AT_2 stimulation opposes the vasoconstrictor effect of angiotensin II.

Direct Renin Inhibitors

Renin, as part of the RAS, is an aspartic protease enzyme that is highly specific, only cleaving angiotensinogen. Pharmacologic blockade of ACE or angiotensin II receptors leads to upregulation of renin synthesis and activity. Renin itself may have deleterious cardiovascular and renal effects; thus, the blockade of renin at the top of the RAS cascade has been considered a target of therapy given the possible beneficial effects on BP and end-organ damage. Direct renin inhibitors decrease PRA and therefore inhibit the conversion of angiotensinogen to angiotensin I.

Aliskiren is a direct renin inhibitor and is a non–peptide-like compound that binds to several pockets in distinct regions around the active site of renin. Aliskiren is rapidly absorbed with maximal plasma concentrations reached between 1 and 3 hours after dosing; its elimination half-life is about 40 hours (range, 34–41 hours), which may account for slowness of maximum hypotensive effect. It is 47% to 51% bound in human plasma and has a substantial extravascular volume of distribution. Excretion occurs almost entirely by the biliary route, primarily as unchanged drug, with less than 1% renal excretion. Of the small amount that is metabolized, CYP 3A4 is the major enzyme responsible for metabolism. Direct renin inhibitors are likely to have sustained hypotensive effect and reduce PRA because of their long half-lives. In the initial studies of nondialysis-dependent healthy and hypertensive patients, aliskiren was shown to have similar BP-lowering effects as ARB monotherapy. Aliskiren may have a role in dialysis patients to lower BP and improve IDWGs, but more large-scale studies are needed to assess whether there is an overall benefit to using this medication on renal and cardiovascular outcomes in the long term.

Side Effects

The side effects of aliskiren include angioedema; periorbital edema; and edema of the face, hands, or whole body, which occasionally required discontinuation. Cough occurs but in much lower rates compared with ACE inhibitors. There is also an association with abdominal pain, reflux, dyspepsia, and diarrhea, which are dose dependent. Aliskiren should be avoided during pregnancy because of the concern for fetal and neonatal morbidity and mortality. There are also small risks of hyperkalemia, elevated creatine kinase levels, increase in uric acid levels, and tonic-clonic seizures.

Based on the results of the Aliskiren Trial in Type 2 Diabetes Using Cardiorenal Endpoints (ALTITUDE Trial) trial, in patients with type 2 diabetes mellitus, CKD, or both, the use of aliskiren with ACE inhibitors or ARBs is not recommended given the increased risk of hyperkalemia, renal dysfunction, hypotension, and, more significantly, cardiovascular events (death or stroke) compared with placebo plus ACE inhibitor or ARB.

Mineralocorticoid Receptor Antagonists

Spironolactone has been successfully used in dialysis patients to control refractory hypertension and to prevent cardiovascular events. Administration of spironolactone for 2 weeks decreased predialysis SBP without any significant effect on predialysis and postdialysis plasma potassium, aldosterone concentrations, or renin activity.

In dialysis patients, spironolactone may substantially reduce the risk of both cardiovascular morbidity and death among HD patients. In addition, some have observed an improvement in ejection fraction in patients with CHF on continuous ambulatory peritoneal dialysis treated with spironolactone 25 mg every other day. Side effects include gynecomastia or breast pain.

Potential Beneficial Effect of Drugs That Inhibit the Renin–Angiotensin–Aldosterone System on Cardiovascular Diseases Independent of Blood Pressure

Activation of the RAAS is considered to be an important contributor to hypertension in patients with ESRD; thus, RAAS inhibitors have been the drugs of choice in the management of hypertension in these patients. In addition to hypertension, the presence of CHF in this patient population supports the use of RAAS inhibitors. Unfortunately, there is no conclusive evidence that these agents are superior to other classes of antihypertensive agents in terms of BP control or in the prevention of cardiovascular events.

Anti-Adrenergic Drugs

β-Adrenergic Blocking Agents

In the past, beta-blockers in combination with vasodilators were extensively used in the management of hypertension in patients with CKD based on the notion that these agents would, at least in part, reduce BP by inhibiting renin secretion. Since the advent of ACE inhibitors and CCBs, the use of beta-blockers in the management of hypertensive patients with renal failure has decreased. In addition, based on the current recommendations of JNC 8, beta-blockers are to be used as second-line drugs. Some studies, however, have demonstrated that beta-blockers may improve survival in patients with CAD as well as in patients with CHF. Based on these studies and given the very high prevalence of coronary heart disease and CHF among dialysis patients, the use of these agents has received renewed interest.

Beta-blocking agents reduce morbidity and mortality in patients with ischemic heart disease and heart failure, and in patients with heart failure, they reduce the incidence of atrial fibrillation, ventricular arrhythmias, and sudden death. Because these comorbidities are very prevalent in patients with ESRD, beta-blockers have the potential to reduce cardiovascular morbidity and mortality in these patients. Thus, in dialysis patients with a history of CAD, beta-blockers are superior to other antihypertensive drug classes for secondary prevention.

An open-label study showed that atenolol-based antihypertensive therapy may be superior to lisinopril-based therapy in preventing cardiovascular morbidity and all-cause hospitalizations in dialysis patients with hypertension and left ventricular hypertrophy. Supervised administration of atenolol after HD produces a marked improvement in ABPM. In HD patients with drug-resistant hypertension, propranolol has also been shown to be very effective.

Although the mechanisms of action of beta-blockers are not well established, they reduce heart rate, myocardial contractility, atrioventricular (AV) conduction time, and automaticity. Thus, the antihypertensive action of beta-blockers may be partly due to reduction of cardiac output. Peripheral vascular resistances initially rise, presumably because of inhibition of β-receptors (which mediate vasodilatation) and unopposed stimulation of α-receptors or because of stimulation of the SNS as a secondary adaptive response to a decrease in cardiac output. After prolonged therapy, some studies found a persistent increase of peripheral vascular resistance, but others found a decrease in peripheral vascular resistance in patients in whom BP decreased. Nebivolol, a beta$_1$-blocker that also stimulates nitric oxide production, exerts vasodilatory actions that are unique for this class of agents.

Beta-blockers may reduce PRA, and some studies have shown a relationship between hypotensive action and pretreatment renin or degree of renin suppression. Other studies suggest that renin suppression is not a major mechanism of action because patients with low renin also respond to beta-blockers, and agents such as pindolol may effectively lower BP without decreasing PRA. Moreover, the hypotensive action of beta-blockers reaches its peak after several days of treatment, but the decrease in plasma renin occurs more rapidly.

A large number of β-adrenergic blocking agents with differing pharmacodynamic and pharmacokinetic properties are available (see Table 53.2). The most important pharmacologic differences among these agents are lipid solubility, intrinsic sympathomimetic activity (ISA), selectivity for $β_1$-adrenergic receptors (cardio-selectivity), and combined α- and β-antagonist actions.

Lipid Solubility
The degree of lipid solubility affects both central nervous system (CNS) penetration and the extent of hepatic metabolism. High lipid solubility results in both more CNS side effects, as well as more extensive hepatic metabolism. For example, propranolol, acebutolol, and metoprolol are well absorbed from the small intestine, but because of extensive first-pass metabolism by the liver, only 30% to 50% of these drugs reaches the systemic circulation. The concomitant use of drugs that affect hepatic blood flow may further reduce the bioavailability of these beta-blockers. By contrast, atenolol, acebutolol, and nadolol are agents with low degrees of lipid solubility that are primarily renally excreted. Accumulation of beta-blockers with low lipid solubility may result in excessive bradycardia. Consequently, the dose of most liposoluble agents do not need to be adjusted in patients with renal failure, but the dose of agents with low lipid solubility should be adjusted. Atenolol and nadolol are removed in significant amounts by HD and thus should be administered after dialysis. An observational study by Weir et al revealed a possible association between the use of highly dialyzable beta-blockers (e.g., metoprolol, atenolol, and acebutolol) and mortality compared with low dialyzability beta-blockers (e.g., bisoprolol and propranolol) when given to older patients on long-term HD.

Cardioselectivity
The second important characteristic distinguishing these agents is cardioselectivity, which is of limited clinical relevance with respect to the antihypertensive efficacy but is of considerable importance with respect to side effects. Cardioselective beta-blockers are less likely to cause bronchospasm, Raynaud phenomenon, or disturbances of lipid and carbohydrate metabolism. The $β_1$-selective beta-blockers include atenolol, metoprolol, bisoprolol, acebutolol, and nebivolol.

Intrinsic Sympathomimetic Activity
The third characteristic of beta-blockers worthy of note is the SA. Pindolol, and to a lesser degree acebutolol, has ISA and thus has a dual action of both blocking and directly stimulating β-adrenoreceptors. Hemodynamically, this results not only in decreased peripheral vascular resistance but also in less pronounced reductions in heart rate, cardiac output, and plasma renin secretion.

Some beta-blockers, such as labetalol and carvedilol, have combined β and α antagonistic properties. Labetalol is a nonselective beta-blocker with little ISA but with $α_1$-blocking properties. The ratio of α- to β-blocking activity is between 1:3

and 1 : 7. It lowers BP by decreasing both peripheral vascular resistance and cardiac output. After prolonged therapy, whereas the decrease in BP is sustained primarily by a fall in peripheral vascular resistance, cardiac output returns to pretreatment levels. Acutely, the drug may cause slight reflex tachycardia, but chronic administration may actually decrease heart rate. Labetalol is particular useful as adjunct therapy in patients with CKD and severe or refractory hypertension.

Labetalol can be used both orally and intravenously. The intravenous form has been used with some success in hypertensive emergencies even though its efficacy is not as predictable and immediate as that of sodium nitroprusside.

The most common side effect is orthostatic hypotension, which is related to the α-blocking properties. Labetalol is less likely to cause bronchospasm and has no deleterious effects on serum lipids. Occasionally, it can increase the titer of antinuclear and antimitochondrial antibodies.

Carvedilol is an antagonist of β_1-, β_2- and α_1-adrenergic receptors that has been used extensively in patients with heart failure, including patients with ESRD. Carvedilol is potentially a good beta-blocking agent for patients with ESRD because it is eliminated entirely by hepatic metabolism, is highly protein bound and not removed by HD, and has a favorable metabolic profile compared with other beta-blocking agents. In dialysis patients, carvedilol has been shown to improve endothelial function (monitored by changes in flow-mediated vasodilation and endothelial progenitor cells) as well as lower intradialytic and interdialytic BP and to cause fewer episodes of intradialytic hypertension.

Side Effects of Beta-Blockers

Simultaneous administration of beta-blockers and nondihydropyridine CCBs (particularly diltiazem and nifedipine) must be avoided in patients with chronic renal failure to avoid an increase of the negative inotropic effect each of these agents exerts on the heart. Similarly, administration of cyclooxygenase inhibitors should be avoided because they may antagonize the antihypertensive effect of beta-blockers. Hypotensive episodes during HD may occur more frequently with the use of beta-blockers as a result of a blunting of reflex tachycardia.

The most frequent side effects of beta-blockers are bradycardia, muscular fatigue, tiredness, AV blocks, sick sinus syndrome, heart failure, cold extremities, and Raynaud phenomenon. Bradycardia and heart failure are less likely to occur with beta-blockers with ISA.

Beta-blockers increase serum triglycerides and decrease high-density lipoproteins (HDLs), but they do not significantly affect serum levels of low-density lipoprotein (LDL) cholesterol. Beta-blockers with ISA, however, cause little or no increase in triglycerides. Carvedilol and nebivolol do not alter lipid profile in ESRD patients.

Beta-blockers can cause several CNS symptoms, including insomnia, nightmares, hallucinations, and depression. Because beta-blockers increase the number of receptor sites on vascular smooth muscle cells, caution must be exercised when these drugs are to be withdrawn because of the possibility of coronary artery spasm or arrhythmias.

Centrally Acting Antiadrenergic Agents

α-Methyldopa

The antihypertensive action of α-methyldopa is primarily caused by activation of α_2-adrenergic receptors in the brainstem and partially by biotransformation into a false neurotransmitter. The drug also lowers PRA, but this mechanism is not considered to be of primary importance for the drug's antihypertensive action.

α-Methyldopa is biotransformed into pharmacologically active metabolites, which may accumulate in patients with renal failure and subsequently may cause untoward side effects. The more common side effects of methyldopa involve the CNS such as drowsiness and lethargy. Orthostatic hypotension and impotence are also well-known side effects. Occasionally, the drug can cause hepatitis or Coombs-positive hemolytic anemia.

α-Methyldopa is easily removed by HD and should be administered after dialysis to avoid fluctuations in BP. The recommended initial dose is 250 mg twice daily. The dose for ESRD patients should not exceed 1000 mg daily. This drug has limited use in dialysis patients.

Clonidine

Clonidine is an imidazoline derivative that lowers BP primarily by activating presynaptic α_2-adrenergic receptors in the nucleus tractus solitarius and in the rostral ventrolateral medulla, thereby causing a decrease in sympathetic nervous system activity. Part of the antihypertensive effect of clonidine may be mediated by central I_1-imidazoline receptors localized in the rostral ventrolateral medulla. Inhibition of renin secretion contributes to the BP-lowering properties of clonidine but to a lesser extent. The drug is readily absorbed from the intestine and reaches peak plasma levels within 1 hour. The antihypertensive action appears within 30 minutes, and it peaks within 2 to 4 hours.

Because the kidneys excrete 40% to 50% of the drug, the dosage should be reduced in patients with ESRD. The mean HD clearance of clonidine is 59 ± 7.8 mL/min. The use of this drug has decreased substantially in recent years because of the high incidence of untoward CNS side effects, including drowsiness, lethargy, dry mouth, impotence, and orthostatic hypotension. In addition, hypertensive crisis may occur when the drug is discontinued abruptly. This rebound effect is more frequent and severe when the drug is given in dosages exceeding 0.6 mg daily or in combination with β-adrenergic blocking agents. In this instance, the surge of catecholamines that occurs after withdrawal of the drug binds preferentially to unoccupied α-receptors rather than to the drug-bound β-receptors, resulting in greater vasoconstriction and more severe hypertension.

The oral form of clonidine has limited use in dialysis patients. By contrast, the transdermal therapeutic system (TTS) allows for steady and continuous transdermal delivery of the drug over 1 week, which limits the fluctuations in BP that are commonly observed with oral dosing and reduces the incidence of side effects. The transdermal delivery system of clonidine is particularly useful for noncompliant dialysis patients; a dialysis nurse can apply the patient's patch once a week to ensure compliance. Despite some removal of clonidine with HD, the blood levels remained therapeutic beyond 1 week. The transdermal form of delivery can cause skin rash at the site of adherence of the patch. Clonidine may be useful in the management of restless legs syndrome in ESRD patients and in the treatment of gastroparesis in patients with diabetes.

Guanabenz and Guanfacine

Guanabenz and guanfacine are α_2-agonists similar in function to clonidine. The liver mainly excretes guanabenz, and no dose adjustment is necessary in patients with renal failure. The dosage is 4 to 16 mg given orally twice daily. Guanfacine has a more prolonged duration of action than clonidine and may be given twice daily. This drug likely causes less SNS side effects than clonidine.

Rilmenidine and Moxonidine

Rilmenidine and moxonidine are antihypertensive agents that lower BP by binding to central I_1-imidazolone adrenoceptors in the rostral ventrolateral medulla. These drugs cause sedation less frequently and less intensively than clonidine.

Peripherally Acting α_1-Adrenergic Receptor Blocking Agents

Prazosin

Prazosin is a quinazoline derivative with a dual mechanism of antihypertensive activity: direct smooth muscle relaxant effects and peripheral α_1-adrenergic receptor inhibition. Prazosin does not significantly affect presynaptic α_2 receptors and thus does not stimulate the heart rate or plasma renin release. Epinephrine and norepinephrine occupy the presynaptic inhibitory α_2 receptors, thereby reducing further release of catecholamines from the sympathetic end-terminals.

The efficacy of the drug is similar to that of hydralazine, but prazosin is less likely to cause tolerance. Prazosin has a short half-life (2–3 hours) and needs to be administered twice daily. Prazosin is primarily metabolized by the liver and no dose adjustment is necessary in ESRD patients.

The most troublesome side effect of prazosin is the "first-dose phenomenon," which is significant orthostatic hypotension occurring after administration of the first dose. This phenomenon is particularly common in patients receiving UF with dialysis and those on sodium restriction. Other side effects include syncope, dizziness, diarrhea, and nausea in addition to a postural hypotension that is independent of the first-dose effect. Prazosin has a favorable effect on the lipid profile in that it decreases LDL cholesterol and increases the cholesterol ratio.

Terazosin

Terazosin is a congener of prazosin with similar α_1-adrenergic inhibition. The oral absorption of this drug is more gradual than that of prazosin, resulting in higher blood levels 8, 12, and 16 hours after administration of an oral dose. The half-life of terazosin is approximately 12 hours and is not altered by renal failure, making it possible to administer the drug once daily. The side effects are similar to those of prazosin.

Doxazosin

Similar to terazosin, doxazosin is a quinazoline derivative with a long half-life, making it suitable for once-a-day administration. The main route of elimination is the gut, and it is poorly dialyzed. This drug (as well as other drugs of the same group) should not be used as first-line therapy because of an increased risk of heart failure Antihypertensive and Lipid-Lowering Treatment to Prevent Heart Attack Trial (ALLHAT).

Urapidil

Urapidil, a derivative of arylpiperazine uracil, is a peripheral α_1-adrenergic receptor-blocking agent with an additional central component that is different from that of clonidine as it does not involve stimulation of central α_2-adrenoceptors. This compound stimulates serotonergic receptors in the 5-hydroxytryptamine (5HT)-1A subtype located in the rostral ventrolateral medulla. Stimulation of these receptors lowers BP without causing sedation. The dose is not altered in renal failure, and it is poorly dialyzed.

Reserpine

Reserpine decreases BP by reducing norepinephrine storage at the adrenergic nerve terminals. The bioavailability of the drug is approximately 40%. Although the liver primarily metabolizes the drug, the dose is nonetheless reduced in cases of ESRD. The drug is not removed by dialysis.

This drug is of little use in patients with CKD and ESRD because of its side effects, which include a high incidence of depression, psychosis, Parkinson-like syndrome, impaired ejaculation, and peptic ulcer disease.

Guanethidine

Guanethidine decreases BP by inducing depletion of norepinephrine storage at the sympathetic nerve terminals. The oral bioavailability is variable, and the urinary excretion of the unchanged drug is 50%. In humans, guanethidine also undergoes extensive hepatic metabolism. The antihypertensive effects of the metabolites are one 10th that of the intact compound. Renal failure results in the accumulation of the drug and its metabolites, so the dosage must be reduced accordingly. The drug is not removed by dialysis.

Guanethidine has virtually no role in the management of patients with renal failure because of the high incidence of severe side effects. Orthostatic hypotension, impotence, and retardation of ejaculation are extremely common. Diarrhea, bradycardia, and nasal stuffiness are also common and are due to uninhibited parasympathetic activity.

Guanadrel

Guanadrel is an analog of guanethidine with a shorter half-life and a shorter duration of action. Disposition of this drug is significantly altered by renal insufficiency. The dose is substantially reduced in dialysis patients to 25 mg every 5 days.

Direct Vasodilators

Vasodilators exert their antihypertensive effect by a direct action on vascular smooth muscle cells. Relaxation of vascular smooth muscle cells occurs when there is reduced phosphorylation of myosin light chains. The mechanisms that cause reduced phosphorylation include reduced calcium entry into the cell (with CCBs), reduced release of calcium by the sarcoplasmic reticulum (antagonists of angiotensin II, norepinephrine, and vasopressin), inhibition of myosin light chain kinase by increased intracellular concentration of cyclic adenosine monophosphate (cAMP) (epinephrine), activation of a phosphatase that leads to dephosphorylation of myosin light chain (nitrates), and opening of K_{ATP} channels (prostaglandins, adenosine, isoproterenol, minoxidil, diazoxide).

Calcium Channel Antagonists

Intracellular calcium exerts critical functions in the regulation of vascular tone and BP. Calcium channel antagonists primarily inhibit the voltage-dependent calcium channels, leading to less movement of calcium across vascular smooth muscle and cardiac cells, inhibition of myosin light chain phosphorylation, and subsequent relaxation of smooth muscle cells.

These agents are classified as dihydropyridines and nondihydropyridines. The dihydropyridines include nifedipine, felodipine, amlodipine, nitrendipine, nimodipine, isradipine, nisoldipine, and nilvadipine. The nondihydropyridine agents include diltiazem, which is structurally related to the benzodiazepines, and verapamil, which is structurally similar to papaverine.

Calcium antagonists lower BP by reducing peripheral vascular resistance. As a result of their negative inotropic action, verapamil and diltiazem may lower BP in part by reducing cardiac output. The dihydropyridine derivatives have a more selective action on peripheral vascular smooth muscle cells and thereby are more likely to cause reflex stimulation of the SNS and tachycardia.

The N-type dihydropyridine CCBs, such as cilnidipine, may actually inhibit SNS activity. In pithed spontaneously hypertensive rats, cilnidipine inhibited the increase in BP and plasma norepinephrine levels in response to cold, stress, and electrical sympathetic neurotransmission. Cilnidipine also attenuated the decrease in renal blood flow and in urinary sodium excretion caused by renal nerve stimulation in anesthetized dogs.

The dihydropyridines have a significant hepatic first-pass effect, and their bioavailability is between 6% and 30%. Urinary excretion is less than 1% of felodipine, nisoldipine, nitrendipine, and nimodipine and approximately 10% in the other dihydropyridines. Because of their poor water solubility, high protein binding, and large volume of distribution, the dihydropyridines are not significantly cleared by HD, eliminating the need for adjustment or a supplementary postdialysis dose. The dihydropyridines form many inactive metabolites. Nondihydropyridine calcium channel antagonists are also poorly excreted by the kidneys and require no dose adjustment in ESRD patients.

Some calcium channel antagonists exert additional actions. For example, verapamil, and to a lesser extent diltiazem, may prolong AV conduction and is thereby useful in the treatment of supraventricular tachycardia. Verapamil is also useful for the prophylaxis of migraine headaches. Nicardipine and nimodipine appear to have more selective action on the cerebral circulation and to be useful in the setting of cerebrovascular accidents. Some studies have shown that these drugs may prevent ischemia-induced mitochondrial overload of calcium during reperfusion. As a result of peripheral vasodilation, dihydropyridines may reduce the incidence of Raynaud phenomena.

The calcium channel antagonists are usually well tolerated. The dihydropyridines are more likely to cause flushing, headache, tachycardia, ankle edema, and nausea. Verapamil is more likely to cause conduction disturbances, bradycardia, and constipation. Because verapamil and diltiazem have negative inotropic and chronotropic actions, they should not be combined with beta-blockers because CHF and severe, life-threatening conduction defects may occur.

Nifedipine capsules should not be used for the management of hypertensive crisis or severe hypertension because of increased risk of myocardial infarction and stroke. The practice of using this agent in patients with dialysis-induced hypertension has been abandoned.

Calcium channel blockers may increase blood levels of 25-hydroxy vitamin D but not the levels of 1,25-dihydroxy vitamin D.

Sodium Nitroprusside

Sodium nitroprusside is the most effective intravenous vasodilator available. It has the advantage of being both an arteriolar and venous vasodilator, thus reducing both preload and afterload of the heart so that no increase in cardiac output occurs. The antihypertensive activity ensues immediately, and it also terminates rapidly because the drug is quickly biotransformed into inactive metabolites such as thiocyanate and cyanogen. In patients with renal failure, these toxic metabolites can accumulate and cause delirium, seizures, coma, and hypothyroidism. To prevent these toxic effects, the drug should not be administered for more than 2 to 3 days. If more prolonged administration is required, serum thiocyanate and cyanate levels should be monitored closely, and, if needed, dialysis should be instituted to remove the toxic metabolites. Hydroxocobalamin may prevent cyanide transfer from red blood cells and plasma into tissue, thereby preventing cyanide toxicity from large intravenous doses of the drug.

Nitrates

Nitrates are effective antihypertensive drugs, but they cause a selective decrease in SBP and in PP. Because of these characteristics, nitrates are particularly useful in patients with isolated systolic hypertension and wide PP. This selective action of nitrates on PP without affecting DBP suggests that these drugs act primarily on large muscular arteries (from the medium-sized arteries to the origin of arterioles), but they have little effect on small resistance vessels.

Nitrates increase arterial compliance of elastic and muscular arteries. The increase in compliance is mainly due to an increase in arterial diameter, but distensibility and pulse-wave velocity do not change.

Diazoxide

Diazoxide is another vasodilator suitable for intravenous administration in hypertensive emergencies. Diazoxide is a benzothiadiazine derivative, chemically related to the thiazide diuretics. It primarily dilates arterioles and has little effect on capacitance vessels. This action results in decreased afterload with resultant increase in venous return, heart rate, and cardiac output. The drug has a rapid onset of action, and the antihypertensive activity may last from 4 to 24 hours. It has been customary to administer 100 to 150 mg of the drug by rapid intravenous bolus injection to achieve high concentrations of the unbound form at the level of the vascular smooth muscle cells, thus yielding a more rapid and effective antihypertensive response. More recently, it has been shown that slow intravenous infusion of diazoxide can cause a slower but equally effective reduction of BP. A slower reduction allows prevention of complications from sudden reductions in BP such as angina, myocardial infarction, and cerebral ischemia.

The most common adverse reactions are sodium and water retention, hyperglycemia, electrocardiographic ischemic changes, angina pectoris, hypotension, nausea and vomiting, and hyperuricemia.

Hydralazine

Hydralazine, like diazoxide, is predominantly an arteriolar vasodilator. The drug causes activation of the SNS and of the RAAS system, resulting in tachycardia, increased cardiac output, and sodium retention. Hydralazine, available in both oral and injectable forms, is of little therapeutic use as monotherapy, and it is more effective and tolerated when used in conjunction with a beta-blocker or an antiadrenergic agent. In patients with CHF, it is given in combination with nitrates. Hydralazine is metabolized primarily by the liver, but dose adjustment is required in dialysis patients. To prevent side effects, a daily dose of 200 mg should not be exceeded. The most frequent side effects are headache, tachycardia, nausea, vomiting, palpitations, dizziness, fatigue, angina pectoris, sleep disturbances, nasal congestion, and a lupus-like syndrome. Currently, there is very little place for hydralazine in the management of hypertension because of limited efficacy, the need of multiple daily doses, and the excessive number of adverse events. In patients with resistant hypertension, long-acting CCBs are more effective and better tolerated vasodilators. In patients with resistant hypertension, a trial with minoxidil, rather than hydralazine, is more likely to attain the desired BP goals.

Minoxidil

Minoxidil is an orally administered vasodilator more potent than hydralazine. It dilates primarily arterioles and has little effect on capacitance vessels. For patients with the most refractory forms of hypertension, it has been advocated as a valid alternative of bilateral nephrectomy. The liver primarily metabolizes minoxidil, so dose adjustments are not required in patients with renal failure. The drug induces reflex stimulation of the SNS as well as the RAAS system, producing tachycardia, increased cardiac output, and marked sodium and water retention. Minoxidil also exerts a direct sodium retaining action on renal tubular cells. Thus, minoxidil should be used in combination with a beta-blocker or ACE inhibitor and high doses of diuretics.

Patients receiving maintenance HD who are treated with minoxidil usually experience a greater increase in body weight during the interdialytic period. This is probably due to an increase in thirst and appetite for salt caused by reflex stimulation of the RAAS system. The most common adverse effects aside from fluid and sodium retention are tachycardia, angina pectoris, and ischemic electrocardiographic changes. Hypertrichosis is commonly seen, which may limit its use among women for cosmetic reasons. Pericardial effusion can develop in patients taking minoxidil, but its true incidence, particularly in patients with ESRD, is unknown.

The drug may be administered once or twice daily in doses of 5 to 20 mg.

Resistant Hypertension in Dialysis Patients

In the general population, hypertension is considered resistant if BP in an adherent patient remains above 140/90 mm Hg after treatment with full dose of three antihypertensive drugs, including a diuretic. In dialysis patients, there is no agreed-upon definition of resistant hypertension. We do not agree with the current definition of resistant hypertension and prefer the concept of refractory hypertension, which is a predialysis BP consistently above 150/90 mm Hg after achieving dry weight and after an adequate and appropriate antihypertensive drug regimen. The regimen should include nearly maximal doses of different pharmacologic agents selected from ACE inhibitors, calcium channel antagonists, beta-blockers, antiadrenergic agents, and direct vasodilators such as minoxidil and after a trial with spironolactone.

Several factors can cause resistant hypertension, including patient noncompliance, inadequate drug regimen, drug-to-drug interactions, pseudoresistance, secondary hypertension, and unrecognized pressor mechanisms. However, the inability to remove sodium and volume remains the most common cause of resistant hypertension in these patients.

In recent years, renal denervation has been used to treat resistant hypertension. The results so far have been mixed, and the trials involving the Symplicity renal denervation system, the only published randomized controlled trials, have demonstrated no benefit. There are no good data on the role of renal denervation in dialysis patients with refractory hypertension.

Effect of Frequent Hemodialysis on Blood Pressure Control in End-Stage Renal Disease Patients With Refractory Hypertension

Several observational and randomized trials have established that daily HD improves BP control and reduces the number of antihypertensive drugs needed and the rate of intradialytic hypotensive episodes.

Analysis of the Frequent Hemodialysis Network trials demonstrated frequent HD had sustained decreases in predialysis SBP and DBP, significantly fewer antihypertensive medications, and a lower risk of intradialytic hypotension. The reasons for the lower rates of intradialytic hypotensive episodes observed with more frequent dialyses treatment are not clear, but a lower UF rate seems to be responsible.

In other studies, frequent HD sessions were associated with significant benefits with respect to both left ventricular mass and self-reported physical health. A downside of more frequent HD is the increased likelihood of interventions related to vascular access. There were no significant effects of frequent HD on cognitive performance, self-reported depression, serum albumin concentration, or use of erythropoiesis-stimulating agents. In summary, frequent HD reduces BP and the number of prescribed antihypertensive medications.

Intradialytic Hypertension

Although most HD patients manifest a decrease in BP during HD, some patients experience an increase in BP, commonly referred to as intradialytic hypertension. Intradialytic hypertension is defined as an increase in SBP 10 mm Hg or greater

Table 53.3

Proposed Mechanisms of Intradialytic Hypertension

Extracellular volume expansion
Exaggerated cardiopulmonary receptor reflex leading to:
- Reflex activation of the renin–angiotensin–aldosterone system
- Reflex activation of the sympathetic nervous system
Endothelial cell dysfunction
Removal of dialyzable antihypertensive drugs during hemodialysis
Volume overload and ventricular dilation
Electrolyte changes (Na^+, K^+, Ca^{2+}) induced by the dialysate composition

from pre- to post-HD, and it has been associated with increased morbidity and mortality in prevalent and incident HD populations. Intradialytic hypertension occurs sporadically in most HD patients, but in 25% of patients, it occurs quite often. The mechanisms underlying intradialytic hypertension are complex, and this condition is not easy to manage (Table 53.3).

C H A P T E R   5 4

Management of Ischemic Heart Disease, Heart Failure, and Pericarditis in Hemodialysis Patients

Tara I. Chang, MD, MS

Introduction

Cardiovascular disease is exceedingly common in patients with end-stage renal disease (ESRD) on maintenance hemodialysis, and is the leading cause of death in this patient population. The rate of cardiovascular death in patients with ESRD is substantially higher than that of the general population at all ages, but the disparity is particularly prominent within younger age groups. Cardiovascular disease is also a major contributor to the total morbidity of hemodialysis patients.

This chapter discusses the diagnosis and management of ischemic heart disease (IHD), heart failure, and pericarditis in patients with ESRD on hemodialysis. Recommendations based on evidence taken directly from the ESRD population are discussed where possible. However, because the management of cardiovascular disease in patients with ESRD has been relatively understudied and evidence from randomized clinical trials is limited, data from observational studies are included where necessary.

Ischemic Heart Disease

The prevalence of IHD in patients on dialysis is estimated at 40%–50%. Also known as coronary artery disease, IHD in patients on dialysis tends to be diffuse, multivessel, and to have a high degree of calcification. Rates of acute myocardial infarction (AMI) in patients on dialysis increased between 1996 and 2002, reaching a peak of 80.8 events per 1000 patient-years, but then began to decline steadily to 73.1 per 1000 patient-years in 2011. Although the declining rate of AMI in patients on hemodialysis is encouraging, the absolute rates still far exceed the rate in the general population of approximately 2 per 1000 patient-years. The high rates of IHD in patients with ESRD stem from the high prevalence of traditional and nontraditional risk factors (Table 54.1).

Clinical Presentation

Patients with ESRD can have typical presentations of stable IHD (e.g., dyspnea or chest pain with exertion) or AMI (e.g., substernal chest pain and diaphoresis). However, they often present atypically, with symptoms such as epigastric pain, fatigue, or nausea, perhaps due in part to the high prevalence of concomitant diabetes

Table 54.1	
Risk Factors for Cardiac Disease in Dialysis Patients	
Traditional	**Nontraditional**
Hypertension	Anemia
Dyslipidemia	Chronic inflammation
Diabetes	Oxidative stress
Smoking	Disordered bone and mineral metabolism
Sedentary lifestyle	Accelerated vascular calcification
	Fluid overload
	Arteriovenous fistulae

mellitus or to uremia-related neuropathies. Moreover, symptoms and signs of acute coronary syndrome can be mistakenly attributed to complications of hemodialysis or ESRD, leading to its underrecognition. Therefore, a high index of suspicion is needed for accurate diagnosis of IHD and acute coronary syndromes.

Diagnosis

The hemodialysis procedure is a kind of "stress test" that can precipitate symptoms of IHD. A variety of factors contribute to this phenomenon, including tachycardia, dialysis-related hypoxemia, and intradialytic hypotension. The emergence of symptoms of IHD on dialysis is an indication for further evaluation (Fig. 54.1).

One-third to over one-half of patients with ESRD have significant IHD (>50% stenosis) by coronary angiography, despite having no symptoms. However, routine screening for IHD in asymptomatic patients with ESRD is generally not indicated, because randomized trials (albeit in non-ESRD populations) have shown that coronary revascularization in asymptomatic patients does not reduce cardiovascular morbidity or mortality, except possibly in patients with unprotected left main disease. Moreover, ESRD is considered an IHD risk equivalent with indications for maximal medical management and therefore not reliant on the results of screening tests.

One notable exception is potential kidney transplant recipients, who often do undergo noninvasive stress testing and subsequent revascularization. To date, there has been only one randomized trial of coronary revascularization in asymptomatic patients with ESRD awaiting kidney transplantation, all of whom also had diabetes mellitus. Manske et al randomized 26 patients with documented significant coronary lesions by angiography to medical management or revascularization. Ten of 13 patients in the medical treated group and 2 of 13 patients in the revascularization group experienced the composite cardiac endpoint of unstable angina, AMI, or cardiac death during a median of 8 months of follow-up ($P = .002$). However, this study was conducted more than 25 years ago, and the medical management group received only aspirin and calcium channel blockers, making it difficult to apply these results to contemporary clinical practice. Despite the weakness of the available evidence, most clinical practice guidelines support screening asymptomatic patients awaiting kidney transplant who have additional risk factors such as diabetes mellitus, known history of IHD, older age, or longer dialysis vintage for IHD with noninvasive testing followed by revascularization if warranted. However, there is little consensus

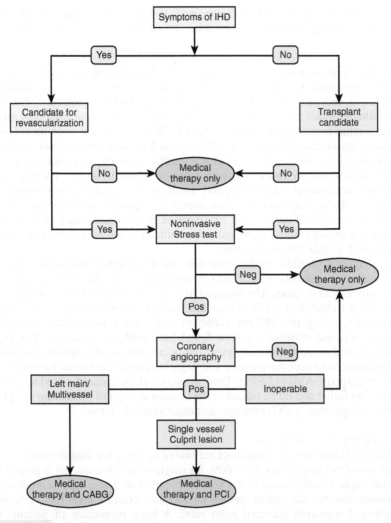

Figure 54.1

Evaluation and Management of Ischemic Heart Disease in Patients on Hemodialysis. Abbreviations: CABG, coronary artery bypass grafting; IHD, ischemic heart disease; PCI, percutaneous coronary intervention; Pos, positive; Neg, negative.

on the optimal timing for repeated screening tests, with some guidelines favoring annual testing, some recommending testing every 24 months, and others giving no specific interval for repeated testing. Some answers may be provided by the ongoing CADScreening (Coronary Artery Disease Screening in Kidney Transplant Candidates) trial. This pilot trial will randomize asymptomatic patients awaiting kidney transplant to annual noninvasive stress testing or not (NCT02082483). Being a pilot trial, the primary outcome of CADScreening is to assess the feasibility of a full-scale trial, but secondary outcomes will examine the occurrence of cardiac events.

Cardiac Troponins

Up to 70% of asymptomatic patients with ESRD have chronic elevations of cardiac troponins (troponin T and troponin I). These chronic elevations do not seem to be due solely to decreased renal clearance, as troponins are large molecules that would not be filtered intact by the kidney. Moreover, the elimination of troponins after an AMI is similar in patients with and without ESRD. Instead, the troponin elevations seen in asymptomatic patients with ESRD may reflect subacute ischemia, underlying cardiac structural disease, or recurrent myocardial stunning. Troponin elevations in patients on dialysis are associated with a two- to fourfold higher risk of all-cause mortality, cardiovascular mortality, and major adverse cardiovascular events, and the U.S. Food and Drug Administration approved troponin T testing in patients with ESRD for purposes of cardiac risk stratification over a decade ago. However, how best to use troponin values for clinical risk stratification and prognostication in stable patients with ESRD remains unclear.

For diagnosis of AMI, cardiac troponins are the standard biomarkers, but their interpretation in patients with ESRD is complicated by the high prevalence of chronically elevated values. The National Academy of Clinical Biochemistry recommends using a change of ≥20% in troponin values 6–9 hours after presentation with ≥1 value exceeding the 99th percentile, to define AMI in patients with ESRD. However, a recent systematic review found little evidence to support this recommendation, and could not identify clear cut-points that would maximize sensitivity and specificity and thus the positive and negative predictive values for cardiac troponins to diagnose AMI in ESRD. Thus, troponins alone cannot be used to diagnose an AMI, but rather should be placed in the broader context of presenting symptoms, electrocardiographic (ECG) findings, and other clinical factors.

Noninvasive Stress Testing

Exercise ECG has been the traditional method of noninvasive diagnosis of IHD. The sensitivity of this test is only 50%–60% for single-vessel disease, but is greater than 85% for triple-vessel disease in the general population. These figures are based on the assumption that the patient reaches an adequate exercise level (i.e., 85% of the age-adjusted predicted maximal heart rate). A large proportion of patients with ESRD are unable to achieve this target because of poor exercise tolerance or the use of beta-blockers, and many have abnormal baseline ECGs. Therefore, pharmacologic agents with imaging are therefore often used for noninvasive testing in these patients.

The sensitivity of radionuclide testing in ESRD patients ranges from 29% to 92%, with a specificity of 68%–88%. Dobutamine stress echocardiography may be the method of choice, as it avoids radiation exposure and has comparable sensitivity and specificity in patients with ESRD (35%–89% and 71%–94%, respectively). Patients with ESRD on dialysis have a much higher prevalence of coronary artery calcification compared to age-matched controls, which can be measured using electron beam computed tomography (EBCT). Studies of EBCT in patients with ESRD have shown that higher coronary artery calcification scores are associated with higher risks of death and cardiovascular events. However, patients with ESRD often have medial, rather than intimal, calcification, which may not have a causative role in IHD. Further study of EBCT and other tests such as coronary CT angiography, coronary flow reserve assessment using positron emission tomography, or hybrid imaging approaches require further study in patients with ESRD on dialysis before they can be routinely used to screen for IHD.

Coronary Angiography

Coronary angiography remains the gold standard for the diagnosis of IHD. The major side effects associated with this procedure in dialysis patients are the potential precipitation of pulmonary edema due to volume overload and possible nephrotoxicity in patients with residual renal function. The risk of both of these complications is minimized with the use of smaller volumes of contrast. In general, however, coronary angiography should be limited to those patients who have persistent symptoms of myocardial ischemia despite maximal medical therapy and in whom revascularization would be considered reasonable.

Medical Management

The treatment for acute coronary syndrome in patients with ESRD is similar to that of the general population and includes timely administration of aspirin, beta-blockers, angiotensin-converting enzyme (ACE) inhibitors or angiotensin receptor blockers (ARBs), and nitroglycerin, provided that there are no contraindications. Antithrombotic agents are often administered, particularly prior to percutaneous coronary interventions (PCIs), but special care to avoid renally cleared agents is required to reduce bleeding risks. A recent study showed that 22% of patients on dialysis undergoing PCI received a contraindicated antithrombotic agent (e.g., enoxaparin or eptifibatide), which was associated with a significantly higher risk of in-hospital major bleeding. Alternative antithrombotic agents are unfractionated heparin, abciximab, or bivalirudin.

For stable IHD, the National Kidney Foundation's Kidney Disease Outcomes Quality Initiative (NKF KDOQI) guidelines, published in 2005, recommend treating patients on dialysis in the same way as for the general population: aspirin, beta-blockers, ACE inhibitors or ARBs, and statins. However, the evidence on which these guidelines are based is weak (level C), as many studies are observational rather than randomized trials, and not all studies focused exclusively on secondary prevention. Consequently, whether to use these agents in patients with established stable IHD requires individual risk–benefit assessments by the physician and the patient.

Aspirin

Patients with ESRD on dialysis have a higher risk of bleeding complications due to uremic platelets, chronic inflammation, or repeated exposure to anticoagulation. In fact, two large observational studies, one using data from 41,425 patients in a large dialysis organization and the other a study of 28,320 patients from the DOPPS (Dialysis Outcomes and Practice Patters Study), showed higher risks of death and cardiac events in patients taking aspirin compared with patients not taking aspirin. However, given the nonrandomized nature of these studies, confounding by indication remains a concern.

Antihypertensive Medications

Optimal blood pressure targets have yet to be defined in hemodialysis. Current guidelines recommend targeting predialysis systolic blood pressure <140 mm Hg and postdialysis systolic blood pressure <130 mm Hg. However, these recommendations are based on extrapolation from the general population, as there have been no randomized trials of blood pressure targets in ESRD. In fact, observational studies show that the strongest associations with adverse cardiovascular outcomes and death are seen with lower rather than higher blood pressures. Despite the lack of evidence on blood pressure targets, several randomized trials and two recent meta-analyses have shown that treatment with medications that lower blood pressure is beneficial to patients on dialysis.

Treatment with beta-blockers in patients on dialysis with stable IHD to reduce cardiovascular morbidity and mortality remains uncertain. Results from observational studies have been mixed. One of the largest studies used data from 11,142 patients from the DMMS (Dialysis Morbidity and Mortality Studies) waves 3 and 4, and showed that beta-blocker use was associated with a 16% (confidence interval [CI] 7%–25%) lower risk of all-cause mortality. In contrast, several other observational studies showed no benefit associated with beta-blocker use in patients on hemodialysis. In the recent HDPAL (Hypertension in Hemodialysis Patients Treated with Atenolol or Lisinopril) study, patients on hemodialysis with left ventricular hypertrophy and hypertension randomized to an atenolol-based regimen had lower rates of heart failure and other cardiovascular events compared with patients receiving a lisinopril-based regimen. However, this was a relatively small study (200 patients) with predominately African American patients (86%), necessitating replication in larger, more diverse dialysis populations.

There have been several randomized clinical trials of ACE inhibitors or ARBs in patients on hemodialysis. A recent meta-analysis of these trials showed a definite benefit in terms of reduction in left ventricular mass (p <.001), but the association with reduction of cardiovascular events was not statistically significant (pooled rate ratio [RR] 0.66, CI 0.35–1.25). Given these data, along with reported benefit of ACE inhibitors or ARBs on preservation of residual renal function, ACE inhibitors and ARBs are recommended for patients with ESRD.

Use of aldosterone-receptor blockers has also been examined in ESRD. The DOHAS (Dialysis Outcomes Heart Failure Aldactone Study) randomized 300 oligo-anuric patients on hemodialysis to receive 25 mg/day of spironolactone or to control. After 3 years of follow-up, the spironolactone group had a significantly lower risk of death and cardiovascular and cerebrovascular events (hazard ratio [HR] 0.4, CI 0.2–0.7) compared to the controls. Serious hyperkalemia leading to discontinuation occurred in 3 patients (1.9%), all in the spironolactone group. However, the study was underpowered, open-label, and had no placebo control. The ongoing ALCHE-MIST (ALdosterone antagonist Chronic HEModialysis Interventional Survival Trial) may provide stronger evidence of the use (or not) of aldosterone, as this trial will randomize 825 patients on hemodialysis to spironolactone or placebo in a double-blinded fashion to examine cardiovascular endpoints (NCT01848639).

Lipid-Lowering Medications
The 2013 Kidney Disease: Improving Global Outcomes (KDIGO) lipid management guidelines recommended that adults with ESRD on dialysis not initiate treatment with statins or statin/ezetimibe combination, given the results of three large-scale randomized clinical trials that failed to show a benefit in this population. The 4D Study (Die Deutsche Diabetes Dialyse Studie) randomized 1255 patients on hemodialysis with

diabetes mellitus to receive atorvastatin 20 mg or placebo. Even though the impact on cholesterol reduction was similar to that observed in the general population, atorvastatin had no statistically significant effect on the primary composite endpoint of death from cardiac causes, fatal stroke, nonfatal myocardial infarction (MI), or nonfatal stroke (RR 0.92, CI 0.77–1.10). AURORA (A study to evaluate the Use of Rosuvastatin in subjects On Regular dialysis: An assessment of survival and cardio-vascular events) randomized 2776 patients on hemodialysis to rosuvastatin 10 mg or placebo. Again, despite a reduction in low-density lipoprotein of 43% in the interven-tion group, no benefit was seen in the primary combined endpoint of cardiovascular death, nonfatal MI, or nonfatal stroke (HR 0.96, CI 0.84–1.11). Finally, the SHARP (Study of Heart and Renal Protection) randomized 9270 patients with advanced CKD (3023 of whom were on dialysis) to receive simvastatin 20 mg + ezetimibe 10 mg or placebo. Although a significant reduction in the rate of the primary outcome of major atherosclerotic events was seen in the intervention group overall, no benefit of active treatment was seen for the subgroup of patients on dialysis.

In patients who are already using statins prior to initiation of dialysis, the 2013 KDIGO guidelines suggest that these medications can be continued, although the evidence on which these suggestions are based is graded as low quality. In a departure from previous guidelines, after an initial lipid panel measurement, repeated follow-up lipid measurements are not recommended for most patients.

Bone and Mineral Metabolism
There is considerable experimental and clinical evidence that the disordered calcium metabolism and hyperparathyroidism associated with uremia contribute to left ventricular (LV) dysfunction, atherosclerosis, myocardial ischemia, and vascular and cardiac calcification. Observational data indicate that hyperphosphatemia and raised calcium × phosphate product are independent predictors of mortality, especially death from IHD and sudden death. The appropriate use of vitamin D analogs and phosphate binders is recommended to achieve target levels for serum calcium and phosphate. Phosphate binders are generally divided into two categories: calcium-based (e.g., calcium acetate, calcium carbonate) or non-calcium-based (e.g., sevelamer and lanthanum). A recent meta-analysis of 11 randomized trials (4622 patients) comparing calcium-based versus non-calcium-based phosphate binders showed a significant reduction in all-cause mortality for patients on dialysis receiv-ing non-calcium-based phosphate binders (pooled RR 0.88, CI 0.79–0.99). However, none of the trials reported on fractures or vascular stiffness.

Calcimimetic agents like cinacalcet are quite effective in lowering serum para-thyroid hormone levels in patients with secondary hyperparathyroidism, but until recently their effects on cardiovascular outcomes had not been studied. In 2012, results of the EVOLVE (Evaluation of Cinacalcet Hydrochloride Therapy to Lower Cardiovascular Events) trial were published. In this multicenter, prospective study, 3883 patients with ESRD on hemodialysis with moderate to severe secondary hyperparathyroidism were randomized to receive cinacalcet or placebo, along with conventional therapy with phosphate binders, vitamin D sterols or both. In the intention-to-treat analysis, the cinacalcet group had a relative hazard for death or first nonfatal cardiovascular event (the primary composite endpoint) of 0.92 (CI 0.85–1.02). However, after accounting for the high rates of study-drug discontinu-ation in both arms with lag censoring at 6 months after study-drug discontinuation, cinacalcet use had a nominally significant effect on lowering the risk of the primary composite endpoint compared with placebo (HR 0.85, CI 0.76–0.95).

Anemia

Anemia has been associated with LV hypertrophy, development of de novo cardiac failure and death in patients on dialysis. Partial correction of severe anemia is associated with improvement in LVH and exercise-mediated cardiac ischemia. Complete normalization of hemoglobin is not recommended, based on several clinical trials in ESRD and in predialysis CKD cohorts demonstrating lack of significant clinical benefit but increasing risk of adverse cardiovascular outcomes and death. In 2012, KDIGO recommended evaluating iron status and supplementing with iron prior to initiation of an erythropoiesis-stimulating agent (ESA), which can be done when the hemoglobin falls below 9.0 g/dL. Targeting hemoglobin levels of 10.0–11.5 g/dL is generally appropriate for most patients on hemodialysis.

Coronary Revascularization

The indications for coronary revascularization in patients on dialysis are generally the same as those in the non-ESRD population (i.e., failure of medical therapy to control symptoms, left main disease, or triple-vessel coronary disease, particularly in patients with diabetes mellitus). There is very little information, even from observational studies, on how coronary revascularization compares with optimal medical management in the contemporary era. However, this important issue may be answered in the near future by the ongoing ISCHEMIA-CKD (International Study of Comparative Health Effectiveness with Medical and Invasive Approaches–Chronic Kidney Disease) Trial (NCT01985360). This study will randomize 1000 patients with advanced CKD (including patients on dialysis), all of whom will receive optimal medical therapy, to an invasive or conservative strategy group. All patients in the invasive strategy group will undergo cardiac catheterization followed by revascularization while patients in the conservative strategy group will receive cardiac catheterization only after failure of optimal medical therapy. Patients will be followed for up to 4 years with a primary composite endpoint of death or nonfatal MI.

There have been no randomized trials comparing coronary artery bypass grafting (CABG) with PCI in patients on dialysis, but observational studies have suggested a benefit in terms of lower risks of death and death or repeat MI in patients on hemodialysis undergoing multivessel coronary revascularization. However, the perioperative mortality of CABG in patients on dialysis is roughly three times the expected rate for non-ESRD patients, and overall survival following any kind of coronary revascularization is much lower than for the general population. For patients who opt for PCI, the type of stent (i.e., drug-eluting vs bare-metal) has not been adequately studied in patients with ESRD. Current guidelines recommend drug-eluting stents, based on observational studies and lower rates of restenosis observed in the general population. However, as drug-eluting stents require longer duration of dual antiplatelet therapy than bare-metal stents, for patients at high risk of bleeding or for patients with planned upcoming major surgery (e.g., kidney transplantation), bare-metal stents may be preferred. Therefore, patients should have careful counseling with a multidisciplinary team of nephrologists, cardiologists, and surgeons in order to make informed decisions about optimal methods of coronary revascularization.

Hemodialysis-Related Interventions

Whether more hemodialysis improves cardiovascular outcomes has been a topic of interest for several years, and there have been randomized clinical trials aimed at answering this question. One study was the landmark Hemodialysis (HEMO) Study. The HEMO study randomized 1846 patients on thrice-weekly hemodialysis to a standard dose (single-pool Kt/V urea = 1.3) or high dose (single-pool Kt/V urea = 1.67) of dialysis. There were no differences in the primary outcome of all-cause mortality or in any of the prespecified secondary outcomes, including cardiac hospitalization or cardiac death. The dialysis sessions in the high-dose group were approximately 30 minutes longer on average than in the standard dose group (219 minutes vs 190 minutes).

More recently, the FHN (Frequent Hemodialysis Network) Trial randomized 245 patients with ESRD to receive conventional, thrice-weekly hemodialysis, or frequent in-center hemodialysis (6 times/week) for 12 months. Patients in the conventional hemodialysis arm had an average session length of 213 minutes (10.4 hours/week), whereas patients in the frequent hemodialysis arm had an average session length of 154 minutes (12.7 hours/week). Results showed that patients in the frequent-hemodialysis group had lower risk of the primary composite outcome of death or increase in LV mass (HR 0.61, CI 0.46–0.82), as well as improved hypertension control (a prespecified secondary outcome).

The FHN Nocturnal Trial randomized 87 patients to conventional thrice weekly hemodialysis or to frequent nocturnal home hemodialysis (6 times/week). Patients in the conventional hemodialysis arm had an average session length of 256 minutes (12.6 hours/week), whereas patients in the frequent nocturnal hemodialysis arm had an average session length of 379 minutes (30.8 hours/week). No significant difference in death or LV mass was seen between the two groups, but patients in the frequent nocturnal hemodialysis arm had improved hypertension control (a prespecified secondary outcome). However, the study had difficulties with recruitment, resulting in a relatively small sample size and reduced power.

Lifestyle Modification

As with the general population, lifestyle modification for patients with ESRD also has a role in IHD management. Any patients with ESRD who smoke should be encouraged to quit. Although some data suggest that increased muscle mass confers a survival advantage over fat, weight loss in patients with ESRD is controversial, given the paradoxical survival advantage for heavier patients. Therefore, a gradual exercise program with the goal of increasing muscle mass and cardiovascular health can be encouraged in patients with ESRD on dialysis. Obese patients who are planning to undergo kidney transplant should be encouraged to lose weight.

Heart Failure

Heart failure is the most common cardiovascular diagnosis in patients with ESRD on hemodialysis, with rates of 655.5/1000 patient-years in 2011. The associated risk for death is high, with 2-year mortality rates estimated at 49% for patients on hemodialysis in 2013. Disorders of LV structure and function are highly prevalent in the dialysis population and begin long before dialysis therapy initiation. As with IHD, the etiology of cardiac dysfunction leading to heart failure in ESRD is partly attributable to the high prevalence of traditional cardiac risk factors, but also to the metabolic and hemodynamic changes associated with kidney failure (Table 54.1).

Approximately 80% of patients starting maintenance dialysis have LV hypertrophy or systolic dysfunction. In patients with diastolic dysfunction, heart failure results from impaired ventricular relaxation because of concentric or eccentric LV hypertrophy. This leads to an exaggerated increase in LV end diastolic pressure for a given increase in end diastolic volume. As a result, a small excess of salt and water can rapidly lead to a large increase in LV end diastolic pressure—culminating in pulmonary edema and symptomatic heart failure. In dilated cardiomyopathy, cardiac output is maintained at the expense of an increase in both end diastolic fiber length and end diastolic volume. As ventricular volume increases, inadequate hypertrophy leads to an increase in wall stress and an increase in end diastolic pressure, also leading ultimately to pulmonary edema.

Diagnosis

The clinical signs of heart failure are the same for patients on dialysis as for the general population: dyspnea, jugular venous distention, bilateral lung crackles, and a characteristic chest radiograph appearance. Although heart failure is often attributed to "volume overload" in the dialysis patient, the appearance of such symptoms suggests an underlying cardiac abnormality. Echocardiography remains the method of choice for assessment of LV geometry and function. In addition, echocardiography can diagnose valvular lesions that can contribute to cardiac dysfunction. NKF KDOQI guidelines recommend that all patients get an echocardiogram at initiation of dialysis after achieving their dry weight (because calculation of LV mass and volume are affected by volume status) and then routinely every 3 years or when there is a change in clinical status.

As with cardiac troponins, B-type natriuretic peptide (BNP) is often chronically elevated in patients with ESRD. In fact, some studies have shown that NT-proBNP (an inactive fragment of BNP) can be elevated in up to 99% of patients on hemodialysis and is therefore of limited diagnostic usefulness in this population. Elevated NT-proBNP levels are associated with the presence of LVH, reduced LV function, and higher risks of death and cardiovascular events. However, because the levels of NT-proBNP can vary within and between individuals, its precise role in providing additional prognostic information remains to be defined in future studies before its routine measurement can be recommended.

Management

For all patients with symptoms of heart failure, potentially reversible precipitating and aggravating factors (i.e., ischemia, tachycardia, arrhythmias, or hypertension) should be sought and managed appropriately.

Volume Control

Diuretics are an essential component of the symptomatic treatment of heart failure in non-ESRD populations, but are of more limited value for patients on maintenance dialysis. Loop diuretics should be continued as long as the patient continues to have residual renal function. For all patients on hemodialysis, but particularly in those patients with established heart failure, maintenance of an accurate dry weight is essential. Some patients may require more frequent or prolonged hemodialysis sessions to achieve adequate volume removal. Heart failure may be exacerbated by a high-flow arteriovenous fistula and banding or revision of the fistula may improve symptoms.

Sodium intake should also be monitored in order to reduce interdialytic weight gain, and patients should be counseled to consume no more than 2–3 g of sodium per day. Some guidelines suggest even lower daily sodium intake (<1500 mg/day), but this recommendation remains somewhat controversial. The use of lower dialysate sodium baths and discontinuation of sodium modeling have been advocated as ways to reduce the total sodium load experienced by patients after a hemodialysis session. However, optimal sodium dialysate prescriptions to minimize sodium exposure without precipitating intradialytic hypotension remains an area of active investigation.

Antihypertensive Medications

Beta-blockers are widely used in the management of heart failure with LV systolic dysfunction in the general population, as a result of studies showing improvement in mortality and morbidity. Current guidelines for the general population suggest the routine use of beta-blockers in clinically stable patients with an LV ejection fraction ≤40% and mild to moderate heart failure symptoms who are on standard therapy (i.e., diuretics, an ACE inhibitor, and digoxin). Such therapy should also be considered for asymptomatic patients with an LV ejection fraction >40%, but the evidence supporting its use in this setting is not as strong.

To date there has only been one randomized clinical trial of beta-blockers in patients on hemodialysis with heart failure. That study randomized 114 patients on hemodialysis with dilated cardiomyopathy to receive carvedilol or placebo in addition to standard therapy. After 2 years, treatment with carvedilol reduced the risk of death from any cause (52% vs 73%, p <.01) and cardiovascular death in particular (29% vs 68%, p < .00001). This, along with numerous observational data, supports the notion that beta-blockers may be safely used in the dialysis population in the same manner recommended for the general population. As in the nondialysis population, these agents should be started in low doses with careful clinical reevaluation during the titration phase.

In patients without ESRD, several studies have confirmed the utility of ACE inhibitors and ARBs to improve symptoms, reduce morbidity, and improve survival. The NKF KDOQI guidelines therefore recommend ACE inhibitors for treatment in patients with ESRD, despite the fact that there are no trials of ACE inhibition in patients with established heart failure on dialysis.

In 2010, Cice et al published results of a 3-year trial that randomized 351 patients on hemodialysis with LV ejection fraction ≤40% and heart failure (New York Heart Association functional class II to III) to receive telmisartan or placebo in addition to ACE inhibitor therapy. Results were impressive: the addition of telmisartan to standard therapy reduced death by 49% (CI 18%–68%), cardiovascular death by 59% (CI 49%–62%), and heart failure hospitalization by 62% (CI 49%–81%). However, there was a higher frequency of adverse events in the telmisartan group, which was predominantly hypotension. In contrast, a large observational study showed a significantly higher risk of cardiovascular mortality risk in patients on hemodialysis initiated on an ARB + ACE inhibitor, compared with patients initiated on an ARB + non-ACE inhibitor antihypertensive agent. Taken together, these data suggest that combined ACE inhibitor and ARB therapy can be considered in patients on hemodialysis with heart failure and systolic dysfunction, but with careful monitoring for possible adverse effects, including hypotension and hyperkalemia.

As noted above, the DOHAS trial showed benefit of spironolactone compared to standard therapy on lower risks of death and cardiovascular and cerebrovascular events in patients on hemodialysis. However, despite the words "heart failure" in the trial name, DOHAS did not focus on recruitment of patients with ESRD with established heart failure. Therefore, the use of aldosterone receptor blockers in ESRD is not currently recommended as part of standard heart failure treatment in these patients.

Digoxin

Current guidelines recommend use of digoxin in patients with ESRD primarily for ventricular rate control in patients with heart failure and atrial fibrillation. However, there are safety concerns given narrow therapeutic window and fluctuations in serum potassium levels that occur with hemodialysis. To date, there have been no randomized trials of digoxin in the ESRD population. An observational study of 120,864 incident patients on hemodialysis showed a 28% increased risk of death (CI 25%–31%) associated with digoxin use versus nonuse. These results were consistent in sensitivity analyses that limited the cohort only to patients with indications for digoxin (e.g., atrial fibrillation and/or heart failure). The increased mortality risk was highest among patients with the lowest predialysis serum potassium levels. The use of digoxin in patients on hemodialysis with heart failure can be considered with careful monitoring of drug levels and avoidance of hypokalemia. Digoxin should not be given to patients with primarily diastolic dysfunction, as the increased contractility could worsen diastolic impairment.

Uremic Pericarditis

Because of the earlier initiation of dialysis and higher delivered dialysis doses, clinically significant uremic pericarditis is now a relatively rare event. When it does occur, the symptoms may be sudden and have severe consequences if not recognized and treated promptly. A high index of suspicion is therefore required. Between 50% and 70% of patients with uremic pericarditis will respond to intensified dialysis, suggesting that uremia itself is responsible in some cases. Cases that do not improve with dialysis may be due to other etiologies, such as viral pericarditis.

Clinical Presentation and Diagnosis

The typical clinical presentation of pericarditis may include precordial pain, dyspnea, cough, or fever. The chest pain is not related to exertion, may be pleuritic in nature, and is often relieved by leaning forward. Most patients will have a pericardial friction rub. Those patients with a significant pericardial effusion may have jugular venous distention or a paradoxical pulse. Any of these symptoms in the presence of new-onset hypotension makes pericardial tamponade a likely diagnosis. Electrocardiograph findings (classically diffuse ST changes) are not sensitive or specific. Echocardiography should be performed in any patient suspected of having a pericardial effusion to estimate its size and guide further management.

Management

For patients who are hemodynamically stable and without impending tamponade, intensification of dialysis and analgesia are usually all that is required for management. Nonsteroidal anti-inflammatory drugs, used cautiously, are useful for reducing pain but do not appear to hasten resolution of the pericarditis. Prednisone is not recommended and may actually increase morbidity. Heparin should be avoided during dialysis therapy if at all possible to prevent hemorrhagic complications. Patients should be carefully monitored for clinical evidence of tamponade until all symptoms have resolved.

Hemodynamically unstable patients who have tamponade require immediate pericardiocentesis. Blind pericardiocentesis is associated with considerable risks and is therefore indicated only in the most urgent cases. Patients with a large pericardial effusion or those with unstable hemodynamics and/or echocardiographic evidence of cardiac-chamber compromise (even with a moderate pericardial effusion) should be referred for pericardiostomy, pericardial window, or pericardiectomy. The selection of the surgical procedure should be based on clinical and hemodynamic status, comorbid conditions, and the experience of the physician. Pericardial window is often the procedure of choice.

CHAPTER 5 5

Avoidance and Treatment of Cardiovascular Disease in Dialysis

Christopher W. McIntyre, MBBS, DM • Lisa E. Crowley, MBChB, MRCP (UK), PhD

Introduction

The prevalence and severity of cardiovascular disease in the dialysis population are well appreciated and represent one of the defining therapeutic challenges in nephrology. It is also one of the most difficult issues to approach as the unique pathophysiologic processes underpinning disease in the dialysis population mean there is inherent complexity in approaching the patient who is manifesting the symptoms and signs of vascular disease. There are a number of pitfalls in treating these patients. What may be a standard treatment recognized to be effective in the general population could potentially not only be ineffective but actually cause harm in the dialysis population. Furthermore, physicians from other specialties may not always be aware of the different set of "rules" that apply to our patients, making consulting with other specialties a not altogether straightforward process. It is therefore vital that nephrologists are fully informed of the hazards that can ensue in treating their patients according to a diagnostic and therapeutic context that has evolved from an understanding of cardiovascular disease in the non–chronic kidney disease (non-CKD) population, not receiving dialysis. Although many of the messages in this chapter may appear negative at first glance and serve to highlight the many uncertainties faced by a physician caring for a dialysis patient, an enhanced understanding of these uncertainties may well prevent patients from receiving inappropriate investigations and treatments. There are also areas where measures can be taken to improve symptoms and outcome, and although many of these measures are in the early stages of adaptation they provide potential ways forward in improving patient well-being, quality of life, and mortality outcomes.

Presentation and Diagnostic Tests for Coronary Arterial Disease

Despite the overwhelming prevalence of cardiovascular disease, the unique conflation of susceptibility and stressors experienced by dialysis patients results in prevention, identification, and treatment of vascular disease presenting a number of difficult challenges.

Diagnostics

Presentation of a cardiac event in dialysis patients is often atypical and may consist of shortness of breath, fatigue, or palpitations rather than classical chest pain. A high index of suspicion is warranted in all dialysis patients presenting with unexplained symptoms, and there should be a low threshold for hospital admission and investigation. However, the nephrologist must always be aware that there are considerable challenges involved in applying and interpreting standard diagnostic tests.

Cardiac Enzymes

There are well-evidenced cutoffs for values of cardiac enzymes that, combined with increased assay sensitivity, are the bedrock of diagnosing acute cardiac events in the general population. The issues with using cardiac enzymes such as troponin to identify a coronary event in patients with acute or chronic renal impairment are by now well known. These measurements are unreliable in end-stage renal disease patients. Most will have elevated troponins in the absence of a defined cardiac event, with elevated troponin levels being indicative of more general "ventricular distress"; these challenges are compounded by considerable variability between patients (and over time within a patient). They may have some utility in observing changes from baseline or in their evolution over a period of hours where the diagnosis of an acute coronary event may be uncertain. However, this depends on having a reliable baseline measurement in the first instance.

Electrocardiography

Interpretation of electrocardiograms (ECGs) in dialysis patients is not always straightforward. Studies have suggested that hemodialysis in particular induces repolarization abnormalities that may interfere with parameters such as the calculation of the QT interval, and indeed longstanding cardiac morphologic changes often leave highly abnormal patterns of repolarization that masquerade (especially to automated ECG reporting software) as acute changes. Having recent baseline ECGs to refer to is crucial in accurate interpretation in the setting of suspected acute cardiac events.

Exercise Stress Testing

Although exercise stress testing remains an integral part of the workup of transplantation candidates, its utility in the dialysis population is not proven. In terms of overall risk stratification, many patients, even those under consideration for transplantation, will be unable to complete an exercise test to the required heart rate because of physical frailty, mobility limitations, autonomic neuropathy, or medication preventing them from development of an appropriate stress response. Exercise stress testing is a poor predictor of posttransplant outcomes. Most physicians will accordingly proceed to alternative tests in order to assess the patient for reversible ischemia.

Isotope Stress Testing

In terms of risk stratification, in the general population isotope stress testing can be of use in patients unable to complete an exercise stress test to the required heart rate. There is evidence, however, that in dialysis patients the sensitivity of myocardial perfusion scans is reduced. In patients who have had a negative isotope stress test and then progressed to transplantation, a negative stress test is a poor predictor of which patients have gone on to have cardiovascular events. Although isotope testing again remains a standard tool in the transplantation workup, this poor predictive value should be borne in mind when counseling a patient for transplantation and the result of an isotope stress test should be interpreted in the context of the patient's other symptoms and overall health.

Coronary Angiography

This remains the gold-standard investigation in the general population, but one that again is more difficult to apply in the dialysis population. The decision to go ahead with diagnostic and therapeutic coronary angiography is not always clear-cut. Although percutaneous coronary intervention remains the treatment of choice in dialysis patients with an ongoing acute coronary syndrome such as an ST elevation myocardial infarction, many patients have cardiac events in the absence of significant stenotic lesions. Outside of an acute event, a significant proportion of symptomatic and high-risk (or higher risk as all patients regardless of age have a significantly elevated cardiovascular risk) individuals will have no treatable lesion identified (approximately 50% according to case series). Atheromatous coronary arterial disease is extremely common in dialysis patients, but the functional significance of individual lesions is much more difficult to determine. To determine the potential clinical significance of a lesion, further testing, such as the determination of fractional flow reserve, may be needed but as yet there is no evidence such a directed approach improves outcomes. Aside from the diagnostic accuracy of the test, the use of iodinated contrast and subsequent impact on residual renal function must also be considered. The decision to refer a patient for consideration of angiography should bear these realities in mind, and the potential benefits of this invasive procedure must be considered to outweigh the risks.

Treatment Challenges

It should be noted that there is a limited evidence base for all treatments, with dialysis patients being excluded from most previous studies, and what evidence there is has largely derived from underpowered substudies of much larger investigations. It is important to be aware that the potential harmful effects of many of the standard treatments used in the general population may have a disproportionate effect in the dialysis population, given their aggravated vulnerability, high comorbidity load, and commonly prescribed concomitant medications.

Antiplatelet Therapy

Platelet dysfunction and aggravated bleeding risk is a well-known complication of uremia. Use of antiplatelets in thrombotic disease must always be balanced against this increased risk. In CKD as a whole, the evidence of meta-analyses suggests that antiplatelet treatment reduces the incidence of myocardial infarction (MI) but has no effect on cardiovascular or all-cause mortality and increases the risk of hemorrhagic stroke. Given the increased risk of major bleeding, care must be taken in prescribing these drugs appropriately. This is particularly the case in end-stage renal disease (ESRD) where this bleeding risk is greatest and the effect on cardiovascular mortality is least. Combination therapy with multiple agents appears to be particularly associated with increased serious hemorrhagic risk.

Revascularization Therapy

Regardless of the method of revascularization, periprocedural mortality is higher than in the general population and long-term survival is lower. Coronary artery bypass grafting currently has the highest long-term survival of the revascularization therapies. However, it also carries with it the highest initial morbidity and mortality, much higher than the general population. These risks do not appear to be significantly modified by the use of more modern approaches avoiding cardiopulmonary bypass. Percutaneous interventions are associated with a lower initial mortality but also a lower long-term survival and it is clear that the efficacy of coronary artery stenting is attenuated in dialysis patients. Overall, there is little difference between the two interventions. The more limited efficacy of percutaneous coronary intervention is at least partly due to the type of lesions encountered in dialysis patients, the frequency of encountering multifocal lesions and the fact that the lesions are sited more proximally. It should be noted that the requirement for antiplatelet therapy also poses hazards in the form of the increased risk of major bleeding. Again a careful calculation of the relative risks and benefits must be performed before undertaking revascularization therapy. Intractable anginal chest pain resistant to reasonable conservative medical therapy remains the most consistent indication for percutaneous coronary intervention in this group.

Pharmacologic Management

All of the major cardiovascular trials establishing the efficacy of what we now consider to be standard treatment for cardiovascular disease excluded patients with severe CKD. In recent years as awareness of the increasing prevalence of CKD in the aging populations has increased, there have been attempts to redress this balance and perform robust clinical trials in the CKD population. So far success has been somewhat limited, particularly with regard to dialysis patients.

Statins

Following the failure of a number of smaller trials to show any effect on mortality from statin use in the dialysis population, the SHARP study (Study of Heart and Renal Protection, the largest trial of its type) was conducted in patients with CKD. A total of 1700 of these patients were receiving dialysis, and once again no mortality benefit was found in the ESRD population. At the time of writing, there is no convincing evidence that statins are of any benefit to dialysis patients in terms of primary or secondary prevention of cardiovascular disease.

Hypertension

Unlike the general population there is no accepted target blood pressure for ESRD patients. They are characteristically hypertensive, because of a combination of the extremely stiff nature of the vasculature causing increased peripheral resistance and fluid overload. They are commonly prescribed antihypertensive medications to reduce the risk of vascular events, often as extension of current prevailing hypertension guidelines. Although severe hypertension probably needs to be treated to lessen the risk of acute hemorrhagic stroke and risk of malignant hypertension transformation (with widespread failure of end organ autoregulation), the question of what to do about more moderate levels of hypertension is as yet unresolved. There is no solid evidence base that demonstrates an ability to reduce vascular events through blood pressure control, what level of blood pressure control is required to improve outcomes, and what the optimal antihypertensive regimen to achieve and target may be in this population.

Patients also commonly suffer from autonomic neuropathy with decreased baroreceptor sensitivity, and thus lack adequate compensatory mechanisms to help them adjust to changes in volume. Blood pressure control through management of fluid and salt intake is vital. The combination of autonomic neuropathy and aggressive treatment with antihypertensive medications leaves patients vulnerable to episodes of intradialytic hypotension during hemodialysis (HD) by further disabling what little is left of the vasoregulatory reserve. Recent evidence has suggested that the lower the blood pressure (BP) falls during HD, the so-called nadir BP, then the higher the mortality risk for the patient, with the number of such episodes that occur having a clear dose response association with mortality risk.

Any treatment of hypertension should therefore focus initially upon achieving adequate control of blood pressure through sodium and fluid management (the optimal level of hydration is also not clear at present but discussion of that is beyond the scope of this chapter). In addition to fluid and salt management, care should be taken with antihypertensive medications because of their potential negative contribution to isolated diastolic hypertension (IDH), potential arrhythmogenic, negative inotropic properties, and high incidence of side effects. A careful weighing of harm versus benefit must be carried out, especially with reference to the many drugs used in cardiovascular medicine that can increase the QT interval. The dialyzability of specific agents (e.g., beta-blockers and angiotensin-converting enzyme [ACE] inhibitors) needs also to be taken into account when trying to minimize the risk of cardiovascular events.

Treatment Interactions

As discussed above, a variety of pathologic processes leave the dialysis patient short of adequate mechanisms, allowing them to cope with physiologic challenge. This is most noticeable and acute in the setting of hemodialysis. It is increasingly recognized that the procedure often results in repetitive ischemic insults. It is now broadly accepted that a standard 4-hour HD session leads to a reduction in myocardial blood flow in a significant number of patients. This recurrent injury leads to a combination of recurrent acute ischemic episodes and maladaptive cardiac remodeling, which in turn leads to the high incidence of cardiac failure and sudden cardiac death (approximately 26% of dialysis patients). This remodeling begins early in a patient's time on HD and continues throughout the treatment lifetime. Some degree of recovery can occur posttransplantation, depending on how long the exposure to dialysis has been.

Optimization of the dialysis procedure, aimed at reducing the hemodynamic stress, has been the focus of much recent work. Interventions that have shown promise in small-scale trials include more frequent dialysis (takeup is limited by resources and patient acceptability) and cooling of the dialysate to improve vasoreactivity and potentially increase organ protection by inducing mild hypothermia during hemodialysis. The latter intervention is simple and inexpensive, but requires further evaluation in large-scale clinical trials. Simple alterations to the dialysis procedure and further clarification of optimum fluid status offer the best potential hope of attenuating the ischemic injury of HD in the short term. There may also be room for more novel therapies that add a cardioprotective element to these adjustments.

Peripheral Vasculature

The relatively unique properties of vascular disease in patients on dialysis are an important reason that an alternative approach and treatment are often required. One of the principal consequences of chronic kidney disease is that the cumulative effect on the vasculature alters arterial compliance. In turn, this increasing arterial stiffness leaves the patient particularly vulnerable to the consequences of demand ischemia in a variety of critical organ systems, such as the heart and brain. Later, we consider some of these factors in turn, and the influence of current accepted treatments upon each.

Vascular Calcification

Vascular calcification (VC) is highly prevalent in patients with chronic kidney disease, and studies using computed tomography (CT) have suggested a prevalence of greater than 80% in ESRD patients. The mechanisms are multifactorial and incompletely understood. Calcium can be deposited in the medial or intimal layers of the vessels although the hallmark of VC in renal patients is diffuse medial calcification as a result of direct ossification of the vessel. There has been understandable concern from physicians regarding the administration of calcium-containing phosphate binders; however, this phenomenon was already well recognized in the earlier era when aluminum-based salts were the predominant phosphate binder, exposure to calcium-containing binders alone certainly cannot explain the full extent of VC seen in ESRD.

Risk factors for VC include dialysis vintage, increasing age, hyperphosphatemia, high–calcium phosphate product, diabetes, vitamin D therapy, and inhibitors of vitamin K such as warfarin. Detection and quantification of VC have not gained traction in routine care, largely because of a lack of specific therapy to reverse it.

Inflammation and Oxidative Stress

As in VC, renal disease is associated with a progressive increase in markers of inflammation and oxidative stress reaching the highest levels in ESRD. Oxidative stress is an imbalance between the generation of oxidative compounds and their antioxidant regulatory mechanisms. Although the generation of oxidative compounds is important as a defense mechanism, and as a part of tissue repair and remodeling, an imbalance can result in vascular injury and in acceleration of the process of atherogenesis. The common phenotype of patients with CKD, that is, older, diabetic, and hypertensive, predisposes them to increased oxidative stress. This is compounded again by the hemodialysis procedure itself, where antioxidant vitamins are lost through the dialysis procedure, and reactive oxygen species (ROS) are generated on the dialysis membrane due to suboptimal biocompatibility. The elevated generation of ROS is a major cause of endothelial dysfunction and microcirculatory malfunction.

Inflammation is another important cause of increased oxidative stress. Renal patients exhibit a high degree of subclinical inflammation that is enhanced by multiple factors such as malnutrition and long-term volume overload as well as more specific processes. Poor oral health, including caries, tooth loss, and periodontitis, is ubiquitous worldwide and is potentially treatable and preventable. This set of problems is especially common in dialysis patients. Periodontitis is a prevalent and persistent peripheral infection that is associated with gram-negative anaerobic bacteria and is capable of promoting localized and systemic infections in the host.

There is well-recognized activation of polymorphs and elevated levels of numerous inflammatory markers and mediators in CKD patients. Along with this, dialysis patients have high circulating levels of endotoxin, which is linked to increased ultrafiltration volumes, suggesting that hemodynamic stress and gut ischemia may result in translocation of endotoxin from the gut into the bloodstream.

The endothelial dysfunction driven by increased inflammation and oxidative stress is of particular importance in our patient population. It is an independent predictor of myocardial infarction, heart failure, and death. Limiting inflammation and oxidative stress and thus attenuating or reversing endothelial dysfunction would be important.

Diagnostics

Pulse-Wave Velocity

Pulse-wave velocity (PWV) is a measurement of arterial stiffness that is an independent predictor of cardiovascular risk. It can be measured simply and noninvasively by measuring the carotid and femoral pulse pressures and the time delay between the two or by other methods relying on pulse-wave analysis. Direct measurement of aortic compliance is possible by magnetic resonance imaging (MRI). The value is affected by age, gender, and blood pressure and so should be adjusted for these factors. Studies in ESRD patients have shown that along with age, PWV is a potent predictor of cardiovascular and all-cause mortality.

Quantifying Vascular Calcification

The gold standard for measurement and quantification of vascular calcification is CT, which yields a calcification score that has been correlated with outcomes. Patients who score higher have a greatly elevated risk of mortality; this can be performed at a variety of sites. CT could also in standard clinical care theory be used to monitor progression of calcification and response to therapy; however, given the concerns about radiation exposure and the lack of an effective therapy that causes a regression of VC, routine quantification of VC by CT scanning is not currently recommended.

Treatment Approach

The most important therapeutic approach to the decreased arterial compliance of the vasculature is prevention.

Hypertension

Endothelial dysfunction is also seen in hypertensive patients in the general population. The majority of patients with ESRD will also have a long history of hypertension, either as the direct cause or secondary to their renal dysfunction. Controlling hypertension is key to limiting the progression of renal disease. Once the patient has reached ESRD the control of hypertension becomes more difficult due to the interaction between blood pressure, intravascular volume, hydration status, and the stiff vasculature. For patients on hemodialysis, treatment with antihypertensives can exacerbate intradialytic hypotension. Choice of drugs with antiarrhythmic actions may be inappropriate in some patients because of the risk of sudden cardiac death, that is, beta-blockers may be harmful in patients prone to bradyarrhythmias, an increasingly appreciated final cause of cardiac sudden death in hemodialysis patients (potentially the predominant cause).

Vascular Calcification

At present, the principal therapeutic approach to limiting the progression of vascular calcification has been careful attention to calcium and phosphate balance with restricted ranges of serum calcium and phosphate associated with a lower degree of progression. There has been concern that calcium-containing phosphate binders disrupt this aim, and therefore much interest has surrounded non-calcium-containing binders. To date, studies have suggested that there may be less progression of VC when these alternative agents are used, but the available evidence is not conclusive and as yet cannot be linked to any improvement in outcomes. Control of phosphate intake and vitamin D supplementation continue to play the primary role in preventing progression. There has been interest in the use of sodium thiosulfate and the possibility it may inhibit or regress VC. It is currently used as treatment in patients suffering from calciphylaxis, the most severe form of VC. Other therapeutic approaches have been suggested, but await robust clinical evidence before allowing their use to be recommended.

Oxidative Stress

Despite the fact that it is a broad target, a number of potential therapeutic options exist to reduce oxidative stress. ACE inhibitors are inhibitors of nicotinamide adenine dinucleotide phosphate (NADPH) oxidase activation and have been proposed as agents that could be effective in modifying endothelial dysfunction, although their utility in this context in ESRD patients is unproven. Another option that has been suggested is allopurinol, which studies have suggested can abolish oxidative stress in the vessels of patients with congestive heart failure (CHF) and slow progression of CKD and potentially reduce cardiovascular events. Again its efficacy in ESRD is unknown and a larger evaluation in clinical trials is awaited.

Inflammation

The recognition of end-stage renal failure as an inflammatory condition has led to much interest in potential therapeutic targets. In the first instance, factors that exacerbate the inflammatory state should be addressed. These include adequate nutrition and the prevention of excessive volume overload. Attention to the hemodynamic stresses of HD may also serve to limit translocation of endotoxin and thus reduce the inflammatory response. Other proposed interventions include statins that have antiinflammatory properties, which it has been suggested could be harnessed in CKD.

Peripheral Arterial Disease

It is important to consider not just coronary and cerebral vascular disease but also the very high incidence of peripheral arterial disease in dialysis patients, with high observed rates of amputation characteristic of dialysis patients, with and without diabetes. Amputations have a wide-ranging impact on quality of life as they are responsible for frequent hospitalizations and infections. Frequent infections exacerbate the preexisting inflammatory and metabolic stresses and contribute to the underlying microvascular pathology. It is plausible to suggest that hemodynamic stress further compromises peripheral blood supply and inhibits ulcer healing. Management of peripheral arterial disease requires a strong multidisciplinary approach and the active cooperation of vascular surgeons, multidisciplinary wound care specialists, and diabetologists.

Diagnostics

Similar challenges exist in the diagnosis of peripheral arterial disease as in coronary artery disease. The use of contrast potentially compromises residual renal function (although to a lesser extent than in coronary angiography, because of the volumes usually administered) and in symptomatic patients it can be difficult to find treatable occlusive lesions as microvascular disease may be the predominant pathophysiological process. It is not advisable to use magnetic resonance angiography to assess the vessels because of the risks associated with use of gadolinium-based contrast material.

Special Considerations

The occurrence of foot ulcers as a result of peripheral arterial disease has a particularly important impact upon patient quality of life. The risk of hospitalization due to infection or the need for amputation is higher than in the nondialysis diabetic population, also meaning that dialysis patients suffer a disproportionate impact on mobility and a resultant loss of physical conditioning and ability to live independently.

Much attention has focused on improving the multidisciplinary team approach to foot ulceration in order to improve outcomes. There has been increased training of dialysis nurses in surveillance and early referral to appropriate services. Continuing training of dialysis nurses and awareness from nephrologists are crucial to ensuring ulcers are not allowed to develop.

One overlooked aspect of chronic foot ulceration is the potential role in accelerating CKD progression to ESRD and worsening cardiovascular outcomes. Exacerbating the persistent subclinical inflammation of CKD will worsen microvascular disease. Thus the patient will progress more quickly to ESRD and, once there, will be trapped in a vicious cycle of chronic inflammation, poorly healing refractory ulceration, and susceptibility to demand ischemia, ultimately resulting in much poorer outcomes.

Other Critical Organ Systems Requiring Protection

As already discussed, the dialysis patient is uniquely exposed to cardiovascular risk as a result of structural and functional abnormalities of the cardiovascular system uniquely predisposing to demand ischemia in combination with treatment-specific stressors. This unfortunate conflation of vulnerability and stress is felt across the entire cardiovascular system.

There is strong emerging evidence that the HD procedure itself causes significant systemic circulatory stress. This circulatory stress interacts with complex hemodynamic factors causing perfusion anomalies that accelerate end organ damage in a wide range of vulnerable vascular beds. Initially this work focused on the heart, but emerging evidence strongly suggests that a much wider range of organs are affected. These include the gut, kidney, skin, and critically, the brain.

The Gut

Translocation of endotoxin across the gut wall is well described in severe heart failure, and occurs both in the setting of shock and portal hypertension and with severe decompensated hepatic impairment with portal hypertension. Endotoxin (without sepsis) was initially proposed as a stimulus for immune activation in the proinflammatory state in CHF. Endotoxin enters the circulation by translocation from the gut, with bowel edema and hypoperfusion being the two main factors thought to influence bowel wall permeability in CHF. A study of clinically stable CHF patients has shown structurally and functionally altered gut, with increased bowel wall thickness suggestive of edema, and increased intestinal mucosal permeability suggestive of inadequate bowel mucosal perfusion.

Patients on long-term maintenance hemodialysis have lower gastric mucosal pH compared with controls, at levels suggestive of mucosal ischemia. Acutely, HD with ultrafiltration causes a reduction in splanchnic blood volume. This associated reduction may occur with or without hypotension. This results in mesenteric ischemia leading to disrupted gut mucosal structure and function (with increased gut permeability). Grossly elevated levels in HD patients correlate with intradialytic instability, systemic inflammation, cardiac troponin T (cTnT) levels, ultrafiltration (UF) volumes, dialysis-induced myocardial stunning, and risk of subsequent mortality.

Vascular Brain Injury

Abnormalities of cognitive function and high levels of depression incidence are characteristic of hemodialysis patients. Although previously attributed to the humoral effects of uremia, it is becoming increasingly appreciated that many elements of the overall disease state in CKD patients contribute to functional disturbances and physical brain injury. These factors range from those associated with the underlying primary diseases (cardiovascular disease, diabetes, etc) to those specifically associated with the requirement for dialysis (including consequences of the hemodialysis process itself). They are however predominantly ischemic threats to the integrity of brain tissue.

There are multiple pathologies that have been described by brain MRI appearances in dialysis patients. These may be entirely asymptomatic or linked to more subtle defects in neurocognitive function, often only apparent on specific testing. Many of the same processes drive this entire spectrum and are often progressive. These abnormalities range from classic stroke to silent cerebral infarct (SCI) and more subtle changes both in the white matter (leukoaraiosis) and gray matter (cortical atrophy). In this way, the situation with cardiac injury on dialysis is mirrored—with more non–ST segment elevation myocardial elevation (NSTEMIs) than classical completed transmural myocardial infarctions.

Leukoaraiosis

Leukoaraiosis describes rarefaction of the brain white matter caused by loss of axons and myelin due to ischemic injury and appears to be of central importance in the neurocognitive defects associated with hemodialysis. The MRI appearance is that of high signal intensity on T2-weighted images. Leukoaraiosis has been described as a risk factor for developing dementia, mobility problems and strokes.

Recently more advanced brain imaging (brain diffusion tensor imaging [DTI]) has demonstrated it to be a universal finding in HD patients after only 3 months of dialysis. The severity of reduction in cognitive function was proportional to the distribution and amount of white matter injury and in turn this was proportional to the degree of cardiovascular instability during HD sessions. This further reinforces the central role that dialysis treatment might play in the development of functionally significant brain injury.

Direct evidence has recently been published relating to the direct link between hemodynamic tolerability of dialysis and brain injury as measured by brain DTI MRI to quantify and localized white matter ultrastructural injury. HD is associated with progressive further ultrastructural white matter injury and that this has the signal signature pathognomonic of vascular injury. The improvement of hemodynamic tolerability using individualized cooling of dialysate entirely abrogated this progressive injury in a recent pilot randomized controlled trial, strongly supporting the integral role that the HD process itself plays in the evolution of brain injury in HD patients.

Kidney and Residual Renal Function

Although data are currently lacking it is clearly possible that other vascular beds might also be damaged during conventional HD such as the kidney itself. Residual renal function (RRF) is an important factor contributing to better survival in dialysis patients. It has been observed that RRF declines more rapidly in HD patients than in those untreated by dialysis or maintained with peritoneal dialysis. In a preliminary study of a small cohort of patents new to dialysis, we combined HD and PD therapy; UF was confined to PD only. The use of HD in this context (extracorporeal blood—

membrane contact but with minimal perturbation of BP) resulted in unchanged RRF over a 12-month period.

Conclusion

Cardiovascular health in dialysis patients is clearly of prime importance. Because of the unique collection of processes that are at work, the therapeutic approach needs to be substantially different than that generated from study of patients with CKD and in particular not receiving dialysis. More specifically, addressing the negative consequences resulting from the current therapies we use (including dialysis itself) may be of central importance. Much of this appreciation is a matter of ongoing discovery. This combines therapeutic frustration for clinicians (given that robust evidence-based strategies are still to be largely developed and widely tested), with the exciting prospect that by increasing appreciation of the relative contributions made by the plethora of complex pathophysiological processes at play we may realistically expect real progress in addressing the most common cause of excess mortality for our patients.

Metabolic Abnormalities

C H A P T E R   5 6

Management of Dyslipidemia in Long-Term Dialysis Patients

Suetonia C. Palmer, MB, ChB, PhD •
Giovanni F.M. Strippoli, MD, MPH, MM, PhD

Dyslipidemia is commonly observed in adults treated with long-term hemodialysis (HD) and peritoneal dialysis (PD). The most prevalent pattern is increased plasma triglyceride concentrations (linked to an accumulation of triglyceride-enriched apolipoprotein-B particles) and decreased plasma concentrations of high-density lipoprotein (HDL). In addition, PD patients usually have increased low-density lipoprotein (LDL) concentrations. Atherogenic changes in the composition of lipo-proteins have also been documented in HD and PD patients. Dialysis patients experience grossly elevated risks of cardiovascular events and mortality. Accordingly, evidence of the benefits and harms of lipid management on cardiovascular risk in the setting of dialysis is of central importance to clinical practice.

In contrast to the general population and adults with cardiovascular disease, lipid abnormalities inversely correlate with cardiovascular disease (CVD) and all-cause mortality in observational studies among HD and PD patients. Notably, higher levels of serum total and LDL cholesterol are associated with lower risks of total and cardiovascular death, which may in part be explained by effect modification from systemic inflammation and/or malnutrition, which are independently associated with poor outcomes.

Uncertainty about the effects of lipid-lowering treatment in dialysis patients has occurred due to differing conclusions among large randomized trials of statin therapy with or without ezetimibe. Numerous randomized controlled trials evaluating lipid management in the dialysis setting are available. This chapter examines existing data for treatment effects of lipid management among dialysis patients.

Diet and Exercise

Trials evaluating the effects of dietary or lifestyle management of dyslipidemia among dialysis patients are sparse, and there can be very low confidence in the effectiveness of dietary and lifestyle modifications on clinical outcomes including serum cholesterol levels and cardiovascular events among HD and PD patients. Most existing randomized trials evaluate the effects of dietary management in predialysis patients. In observational studies, there is evidence that dietitian care for more than 12 months before dialysis therapy initiation has an independent association with lower cholesterol levels and lower mortality in the first year of dialysis treatment.

In a systematic review of randomized trials of regular exercise training (lasting 8 weeks or longer) among adults with chronic kidney disease, treatment effects on serum lipid levels were not known, although exercise training improved aerobic capacity, muscle and cardiovascular function, walking capacity, and health-related quality of life. In a small before–after study of exercise training over nine months among six HD patients, training lowered triglyceride levels and increased plasma HDL cholesterol levels, although other studies have shown little or no association between exercise and blood lipid composition. Until randomized trials of dietary interventions and exercise are conducted to examine treatment effects on patient-level outcomes such as cardiovascular risk, the benefits of exercise appear limited to improved quality of life and functional capacity and specific dietary management recommendations are not possible. This is despite dialysis patients, caregivers, and clinicians considering heart health promotion as a key treatment uncertainty in the setting of dialysis.

Lipid-Lowering Drugs

Several randomized controlled trials of lipid-lowering therapy in HD and PD patients are now available and provide moderate to high-quality evidence for the effects of treatment on mortality and cardiovascular events. Data for the effects of 3-hydroxy-3-methyl-glutaryl-coenzyme A (HMG-CoA) reductase inhibitors (statins) used with or without ezetimibe are available for 7982 HD and PD patients.

Despite clinically important reductions in serum levels of total cholesterol (–47.5 mg/dL [–1.2 mmol/L]), LDL cholesterol (–43.1 mg/dL [1.1 mmol/L]), and triglycerides (–21.9 mg/dL [–0.2 mmol/L]) during treatment lasting 6 months on average, statin therapy had little or no effect on all-cause mortality (relative risk 0.96, 95% confidence interval 0.88 to 1.04), cardiovascular mortality (relative risk 0.94, 95% confidence interval 0.82 to 1.07), and major cardiovascular events (relative risk 0.95, 95% confidence interval 0.87 to 1.03) (Fig. 56.1). Similarly, statin therapy had uncertain effects on risks of myocardial infarction (relative risk 0.87, 95% confidence interval 0.71 to 1.07) and stroke (relative risk 1.30, 95% confidence interval 0.79 to 2.11). The effects of treatment were predominantly examined in HD patients; information about treatment effects and safety of statins in PD patients is currently insufficient to make treatment recommendations. Overall, clinicians may reasonably choose not to initiate statin therapy in dialysis patients. In fact, the lack of clinical effect of lipid-lowering strategies on cardiovascular risk despite clinically important reductions in cholesterol and triglyceride levels in PD and HD patients suggests that pharmacologic treatment to target specific lipid levels is ineffective in long-term dialysis settings.

In a meta-analysis of randomized controlled trials of fibrate therapy among 16,869 adults with or at risk of chronic kidney disease, fibrates decreased total cholesterol (–12.4 mg/dL [–0.32 mmol/L]) and triglyceride (49.6 mg/dL [–0.56 mmol/L]) levels, increased HDL levels (2.31 mg/dL [0.06 mmol/L]), and had nonsignificant effects on LDL cholesterol. No information was available about fibrate treatment among HD or PD patients.

Other drugs with effects on lipid profiles in dialysis patients have not been shown to have effects on patient-level outcomes while safety data are sparse. These drugs include bile acid sequestrants, niacin, acipimox, pantetheine, and probucol and are not recommended for use in PD or HD patients.

Several possible explanations have been advanced to explain the smaller clinical effects of lipid-lowering treatment among dialysis patients compared with the consistent proportional reductions in cardiovascular events among people with or at risk

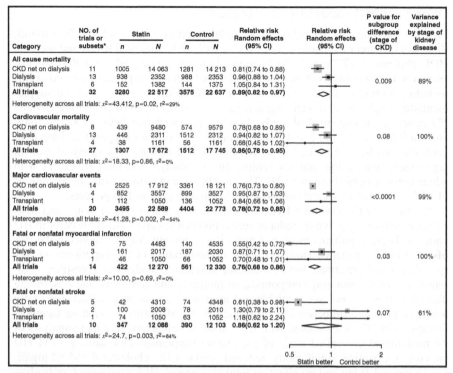

Category	NO. of trials or subsets*	Statin n	Statin N	Control n	Control N	Relative risk Random effects (95% CI)	Relative risk Random effects (95% CI)	P value for subgroup difference (stage of CKD)	Variance explained by stage of kidney disease
All cause mortality									
CKD net on dialysis	11	1005	14 063	1281	14 213	0.81(0.74 to 0.88)			
Dialysis	13	938	2352	988	2353	0.96(0.88 to 1.04)		0.009	89%
Transplant	6	152	1382	144	1375	1.05(0.84 to 1.31)			
All trials	32	3280	22 517	3575	22 637	0.89(0.82 to 0.97)			
Heterogeneity across all trials: x^2=43.412, p=0.02, r^2=29%									
Cardiovascular mortality									
CKD net on dialysis	8	439	9480	574	9579	0.78(0.68 to 0.89)			
Dialysis	13	446	2311	1512	2312	0.94(0.82 to 1.07)		0.08	100%
Transplant	4	38	1161	56	1161	0.68(0.45 to 1.02)			
All trials	27	1307	17 672	1512	17 745	0.86(0.78 to 0.95)			
Heterogeneity across all trials: x^2=18.33, p=0.86, r^2=0%									
Major cardiovascular events									
CKD net on dialysis	14	2525	17 912	3361	18 121	0.76(0.73 to 0.80)			
Dialysis	4	852	3557	899	3527	0.95(0.87 to 1.03)		<0.0001	99%
Transplant	1	112	1050	136	1052	0.84(0.66 to 1.06)			
All trials	20	3495	22 589	4404	22 773	0.78(0.72 to 0.85)			
Heterogeneity across all trials: x^2=41.28, p=0.002, r^2=54%									
Fatal or nonfatal myocardial infarction									
CKD net on dialysis	8	75	4483	140	4535	0.55(0.42 to 0.72)			
Dialysis	3	161	2017	187	2030	0.87(0.71 to 1.07)		0.03	100%
Transplant	1	46	1050	66	1052	0.70(0.48 to 1.01)			
All trials	14	422	12 270	561	12 330	0.76(0.68 to 0.86)			
Heterogeneity across all trials: x^2=10.00, p=0.69, r^2=0%									
Fatal or nonfatal stroke									
CKD net on dialysis	5	42	4310	74	4348	0.61(0.38 to 0.98)			
Dialysis	2	100	2008	78	2010	1.30(0.79 to 2.11)		0.07	61%
Transplant	1	74	1050	63	1052	1.18(0.62 to 2.24)			
All trials	10	347	12 088	390	12 103	0.86(0.62 to 1.20)			
Heterogeneity across all trials: x^2=24.7, p=0.003, r^2=64%									

0.5   1   2
Statin better   Control better

Effect of statin therapy versus placebo or no treatment control on total and cardiovascular mortality and major cardiovascular events grouped by stage of chronic kidney disease. 95% CI, 95% confidence interval; CKD, chronic kidney disease. *Subsets of trials refers to presence of data from subgroups with chronic kidney disease not on dialysis or cohorts on various types of dialysis (peritoneal dialysis or hemodialysis) within broader trials

Figure 56.1

Effect of Statin Therapy Versus Placebo or No Treatment on Total and Cardiovascular Mortality and Major Cardiovascular Events. (From Palmer SC, Craig JC, Navaneethan SD, Tonelli M, Pellegrini F, Strippoli GFM. Benefits and Harms of Statin Therapy for Persons with Chronic Kidney Disease. *Ann Intern Med* 2012;157:263-275 [figure on page 267].)

of cardiovascular disease and who have normal kidney function or mild to moderate kidney disease, in whom a proportional risk reduction in major cardiovascular events of 20% for every 40 mg/dL (1 mmol/L) reduction in LDL cholesterol is observed. The pathologic etiology of cardiovascular disease in HD and PD patients is dominated by vascular calcification, cardiac hypertrophy, and arterial stiffening, which are biologic processes that might be less amenable to the beneficial effects of lipid reduction with statin or fibrate therapy.

The existing evidence evaluating statin therapy in dialysis patients is high to moderate quality, indicating that additional trials of statin management in HD and PD patients are unlikely to change our confidence in the results. Based on existing evidence, there is little to support a recommendation for pharmacologic treatment of lipid abnormalities among HD and PD patients.

Other Lipid-Lowering Strategies

Fish oil supplements (0.9–3.0 g/day) reduce serum triglycerides (–20.4 mg/dL [0.23 mmol]) and total cholesterol (–4.63 mg/dL [0.12 mmol/L] levels and increase HDL cholesterol (7.7 mg/dL [0.20 mml/L]) levels among HD and PD patients. However, high-quality evidence for the effects of fish oils on patient-centered events including mortality are not available in randomized trials, whereas fish oil supplementation might increase bleeding and gastrointestinal side effects among HD and PD patients. An uncontrolled study showing an association between serum long-chain n-3 fatty acids and lower risk of sudden cardiac death suggest that long-term controlled studies are needed to assess the relative efficacy and safety of fish oil supplementation in the dialysis setting. In one study, short-term treatment with adrenocorticotrophic hormone (ACTH) was effective in reducing the concentrations of LDL cholesterol—as well as those of lipoprotein (a)—in HD patients.

Treatment with sevelamer hydrochloride, which is a non-aluminum- and non-calcium-containing polymer, reduces serum phosphorus and LDL cholesterol in HD patients. These simultaneous effects make it a candidate drug for reducing the risk of CVD in HD patients. However, clear demonstration of the superiority of any specific class of phosphate binder including sevelamer, lanthanum, colestilan, bixalomer, and iron-containing compounds, on mortality and cardiovascular risk among dialysis patients is not yet available. L-Carnitine is an essential cofactor for fatty acid transport into mitochondria for oxidation. Of all forms of renal replacement therapy, only HD is associated with free carnitine deficiency. In a meta-analysis of 49 randomized controlled trials of L-carnitine supplementation among 1734 HD patients, L-carnitine significantly reduced serum LDL cholesterol (–5.82 mg/dL [–0.15 mmol/L]) but had no effect on total cholesterol, HDL cholesterol, or triglycerides. Treatment effects of L-carnitine on mortality and cardiovascular events remain uncertain. Systemic heparinization that is used routinely in HD might adversely affect plasma lipids through the depletion of lipoprotein lipase, leading to the accumulation of triglyceride-enriched apolipoprotein-B particles. Low-molecular-weight heparin preparations are expected to have a favorable effect on lipid metabolism, because only fractions of high-molecular-weight account for lipolytic effects; however, a recent systematic review has reported conflicting effects of heparin formulations on lipid levels in HD patients. Reasons for these conflicting results potentially include differences among preparations and modes of administration of low-molecular-weight heparin preparations.

To date, attempts to improve lipid profiles by altering dialysate composition in HD have been largely unsuccessful. Moreover, studies examining the effects on serum lipids of different glucose-free dialysate fluids in PD patients are inconclusive. Modest reductions in total cholesterol have been observed after the substitution of glucose by amino acid fluids in PD patients. The use of high-molecular-weight glucose polymer-based solution led to a nonsignificant 6%–10% reduction in cholesterol and triglyceride levels over a 6-month period. Randomized trials have found that high-flux dialysis membranes have little or no effect on lipid profiles in HD patients.

Summary

Cardiovascular disease is a major complication of dialysis. The lipid abnormalities in dialysis patients are complex and are frequently manifest by multiple disturbances in this metabolic pathway of lipoprotein formation and clearance. In large dialysis population studies, cholesterol levels have been associated with a paradoxically reduced cardiovascular risk, potentially due to the lipid-lowering modification of systematic inflammation. Although treatment of LDL cholesterol abnormalities in the general population and among patients with mild to moderate chronic kidney disease has been shown to proportionally reduce the morbidity and mortality of CVD, there is little or no evidence of benefit with lipid-lowering therapy in dialysis patients. Information about treatment effects of statins in PD patients are sparse but unlikely to be different from the effects observed in HD patients. Treatment trials of lipid therapy are largely limited to statin therapy with or without additional ezetimibe; the benefits and harms of fibrates, fish oil supplementation, other pharmacologic lipid modification treatment, and diet and lifestyle interventions including exercise on mortality and cardiovascular events in the setting of end-stage kidney disease are unknown.

As the available evidence about statin treatment is moderate to high quality, a reasonable approach to patient management is to follow the current recommendations of the Kidney Disease Improving Global Outcomes (KDIGO) Clinical Practice Guideline for Lipid Management in Chronic Kidney Disease. These include consideration of not initiating statin or statin/ezetimibe combination in dialysis patients, although these treatments might reasonably be continued in patients who are receiving these agents when dialysis is commenced. Additional data are needed before widespread adoption of other lipid-lowering therapies can be considered safe and effective for PD and HD patients. Exercise provides quality of life and functional benefits for dialysis patients whereas dietary management has uncertain effects in the setting of HD and PD and more research is needed.

CHAPTER 57

Abnormalities of Thyroid Function in Chronic Dialysis Patients

Connie M. Rhee, MD, MSc

Introduction

Data spanning over three decades show that hypothyroidism, defined as an elevated thyrotropin (TSH) with normal or low free thyroxine (FT4) levels ("mild" subclinical and "severe" overt hypothyroidism, respectively), is highly prevalent in dialysis patients. However, there is likely underrecognition of disease in this population given its symptom overlap with uremia and coexisting comorbidities. Dialysis patients also frequently demonstrate other thyroid functional test abnormalities, such as low triiodothyronine (T3), low thyroxine (T4), and high reverse triiodothyronine (rT3) levels. Thyroid hormone receptors are present in most tissues, and in the general population hypothyroidism has been shown to have pervasive effects on multiple end-organs, and in particular the cardiovascular system. Although hypothyroidism was previously thought to be a physiologic adaptation in patients with end-stage renal disease (ESRD), a growing body of evidence suggests that hypothyroidism is associated with adverse cardiovascular sequelae and higher mortality risk. This chapter examines the epidemiology of hypothyroidism and other thyroid functional test alterations commonly observed in dialysis patients; the mechanistic pathways linking thyroid and kidney disease; and existing data on the prognostic implications and treatment of hypothyroidism in this population.

Prevalence of Hypothyroidism

Epidemiologic data have shown that there is an increasing prevalence of hypothyroidism with incrementally impaired kidney function. Data from 14,623 adults in the Third National Health and Nutritional Examination Survey (NHANES III) have demonstrated that the prevalence of hypothyroidism (defined as TSH >4.5 mIU/L or treatment with exogenous thyroid hormone) was 5%, 11%, 20%, 23%, and 23% among those with estimated glomerular filtration rates (eGFRs) of >90, 60–89, 45–59, 30–44, and <30 mL/min/1.73 m², respectively. After accounting for differences in age, sex, and race/ethnicity using multivariable logistic regression, there was still a twofold higher risk of hypothyroidism among participants with an eGFR of <30 versus those with an eGFR ≥90 mL/min/1.73 m². This study also showed that more than 50% of hypothyroid cases had subclinical disease (defined as TSH >4.5 mIU/L and total T4 ≥4.5 μg/dL). Although studies of hypothyroidism in ESRD have been conducted in comparatively smaller cohorts, a similarly high prevalence has been observed in a number of hemodialysis and peritoneal dialysis studies (Table 57.1). Varying prevalence estimates across these studies may be due to differences

Table 57.1

Studies of the Prevalence of Hypothyroidism and Thyrotropin (TSH) Elevation in Dialysis Patients

Study (Year)	Cohort (n)	Definition of Thyroid Functional Disease	Prevalence
TSH Elevation			
Lin et al (1998)	HD/PD (221)	TSH >3.1 mIU/L	14.9%
Kutlay et al (2005)	HD (87)	TSH >5.5 mIU/L	23.1%
Rhee et al (2013)	HD/PD (2715)	TSH >assay ULN	12.9%
Dreschler et al (2014)	HD (1000)	TSH 4.5–15.0 mIU/L	1.8%
Rhee et al (2015)	HD (8840)	TSH >5.0 mIU/L	22.0%
Subclinical Hypothyroidism			
Shantha et al (2011)	HD (137)	TSH 4.5–10 mIU/L + Normal FT4	24.8%
Ng et al (2012)	PD (122)	TSH >4 mIU/L + Normal FT4	15.6%
Meuwese et al (2012)	HD (218)	Diagnostic criteria not available	1.8%
Rhee et al (2013)	HD/PD (2715)	TSH: assay ULN to 10 mIU/L	8.9%
Dreschler et al (2014)	HD (1000)	TSH 4.5–15.0 mIU/L + Normal FT3/FT4	1.6%
Rhee et al (2015)	HD (8840)	TSH >5.0–10 mIU/L	12.9%
Overt Hypothyroidism			
Kaptein et al (1988)	HD[a] (306)	1. TSH ≥20 mIU/L, or 2. TSH 10–20 mIU/L + exaggerated TRH response + Low TT4 or FT4 index	2.6%
Lin et al (1998)	HD/PD (221)	TSH ≥20 mIU/L + Low TT4 or FT4	5.4%
Kutlay et al (2005)	HD (87)	TSH >5.5 mIU/L + Low FT4	3.4%
Meuwese et al (2012)	HD (218)	Diagnostic criteria not available	5.0%
Rhee et al (2013)	HD/PD (2715)	TSH >10 mIU/L	4.3%
Dreschler et al (2014)	HD (1000)	TSH 4.5–15.0 mIU/L + Normal FT3/FT4	0.2%
Rhee et al (2015)	HD (8840)	TSH >10 mIU/L	8.9%

FT4, free thyroxine; FT3, free triiodothyronine; HD, hemodialysis; PD, peritoneal dialysis; TRH, thyrotropin-releasing hormone; TSH, thyrotropin; TT4, total thyroxine; ULN, upper limit of normal.
[a]19% of patients had end-stage renal disease, but had not yet received HD.

in the criteria used to define hypothyroidism, age distribution, and iodine intake of the study populations.

Factors Contributing to Thyroid Functional Disease in Kidney Disease

Normal Thyroid Hormone Physiology

The production of thyroid hormone is stimulated by TSH from the pituitary, which in turn is regulated by thyrotropin-releasing hormone (TRH) from the hypothalamus. Although T4 is solely produced by the thyroid gland, 80% of T3 is generated from the deiodination of T4 to T3 by the types 1 and 2 5'-deiodinase enzymes (D1 and D2) in peripheral tissues. In humans, D2 is believed to be the principal enzyme responsible for peripheral T4 to T3 production. Consequently, both TSH and TRH are regulated by feedback inhibition from circulating T4, which is converted to T3 in the pituitary and hypothalamus by D2.

Thyroid Functional Disease Leading to Kidney Disease

The mechanistic link between thyroid and kidney disease has not been fully elucidated, but existing data suggest the relationship is bidirectional. Hypothyroidism adversely affects kidney size, weight, and structure both in development and adulthood. For example, in neonatal rats, hypothyroidism has been shown to result in decreased kidney size to body weight ratio, truncated tubular mass, and decreased glomerular basement membrane volume. Hypothyroidism has also led to diminished compensatory hypertrophy following unilateral nephrectomy in animal models, and histologic data have demonstrated that hypothyroidism is associated with glomerular basement membrane architectural changes.

Hypothyroidism may also lead to decreased kidney function, presumably due to reduced renal blood flow from (1) decreased cardiac output resulting from systolic dysfunction, diastolic impairment, and decreased blood volume; (2) increased peripheral vascular resistance; and (3) intrarenal vasoconstriction, as well as glomerular filtration rate reductions from impaired renin–angiotensin–aldosterone activity. For example, animal studies have shown that hypothyroidism leads to decreased single-nephron GFR, renal plasma flow, and glomerular transcapillary hydrostatic pressure (Table 57.2). Human case series have confirmed that severe hypothyroidism results in reversible plasma flow reductions, creatinine elevations, and decreased GFR as measured by indirect estimating equations and isotopic renal scans, confirming that changes in creatinine levels were due to actual changes in GFR as opposed to underlying myopathy or alterations in creatinine metabolism. Large population-based studies also corroborate an association between milder forms of hypothyroidism and kidney dysfunction. For example, in a cross-sectional study of 461,607 U.S. veterans with stages 3 to 5 chronic kidney disease (CKD), every 10 mL/min/1.73 m^2 decrement in eGFR was associated with an 18% higher risk of hypothyroidism (defined as TSH >5 mIU/L and/or receipt of thyroid hormone replacement therapy), independent of age, sex, race/ethnicity, and comorbidity burden (Fig. 57.1). In a longitudinal study of 104,633 patients with normal baseline kidney function who underwent annual to biennial TSH measurements, patients whose baseline TSH levels were in the highest quintile (TSH 2.85–5.00 mIU/L) had

Table 57.2

Risk Factors for Thyroid Functional Disease in Kidney Disease

Kidney Disease → Thyroid Functional Disease	Thyroid Functional Disease → Kidney Disease
• Metabolic acidosis	• Altered development and structure
• Selenium deficiency	• ↓ Kidney size–to–body weight ratio
• Iodine retention	• Truncated tubular mass
• Testosterone deficiency	• ↓ Glomerular basement membrane
• Protein losses	volume
• Nephrotic syndrome	• ↓ Compensatory hypertrophy after
• Peritoneal effluent losses	nephrectomy
• Nonthyroidal illness	• Altered function
• Medications	• ↓ Renal blood flow
	• ↓ Cardiac output
	• ↑ Peripheral vascular resistance
	• Intrarenal vasoconstriction
	• ↓ Glomerular filtration rate
	• Impaired renin–angiotensin–
	aldosterone activity

a 26% higher risk of incident CKD (defined as eGFR <60 mL/min/1.73 m^2) versus those in the lowest TSH quintile (TSH 0.25–1.18 mIU/L). It should be noted that cystatin C production may be affected by thyroid hormone independent of glomerular filtration rate and hence should not be used as a measure of kidney function in patients with thyroid functional disease.

Observational data also suggest that thyroid hormone replacement in subclinical hypothyroidism is associated with reduced CKD progression. Among 309 patients with stages 2 to 4 CKD and subclinical hypothyroidism, after a median follow-up of 35 months, patients who received thyroid hormone replacement therapy had a 36% lower likelihood of experiencing a halving of eGFR and had a 15% lower likelihood of developing ESRD compared with those who were untreated.

Kidney Disease Leading to Thyroid Functional Disease

Kidney disease may also lead to thyroid functional disease via several pathways (Table 57.2). First, metabolic acidosis has been associated with lower T3, lower T4, and higher TSH levels in nondialysis patients. In one study of hemodialysis patients, correction of metabolic acidosis with sodium citrate normalized FT3 concentrations but had no impact on FT4 or TSH levels. Second, selenium deficiency is common in hemodialysis patients and may impair peripheral T4 to T3 conversion, leading to lower T3. Third, iodine retention from iodinated contrast-enhanced imaging studies, fistulograms, angiograms, povidone–iodine solutions used to sterilize peritoneal dialysis catheter tips, and dietary sources may lead to hypothyroidism via the Wolff–Chaikoff effect. Fourth, testosterone deficiency is also common in dialysis patients and in animal studies has been associated with reduced peripheral deiodination of T4 to T3. Fifth, as the vast majority of circulating T3 and T4 (>99%) are bound to carrier proteins such as thyroid-binding globulin, transthyretin, albumin,

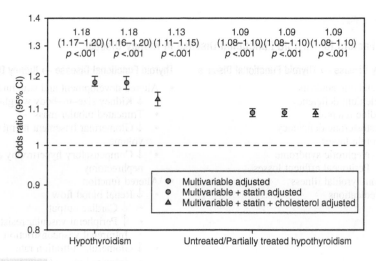

Figure 57.1

Association Between Kidney Dysfunction and Thyroid Functional Disease Among 461,607 U.S. Veterans With Stages 3–5 Chronic Kidney Disease (CKD). Association between estimated glomerular filtration rate (eGFR) and hypothyroidism (defined as serum TSH >5 mIU/L and/or receipt of thyroid hormone replacement therapy) estimated using multivariable random effects logistic regression. Multivariable analyses adjusted for age, sex, race/ethnicity, coronary heart disease, congestive heart failure, liver disease, malignancy, chronic lung disease, rheumatologic disease, peptic ulcer disease, and Charlson comorbidity index. Multivariable + statin adjusted analyses adjusted for covariates in multivariable model, plus statin use. Multivariable + statin + cholesterol adjusted analyses adjusted for covariates in multivariable + statin model, plus baseline cholesterol level. (Adapted from Rhee CM, Kalantar-Zadeh K, Streja E, et al. The relationship between thyroid function and estimated glomerular filtration rate in patients with chronic kidney disease. Nephrol Dial Transplant. 2015;30(2):282-287.)

and lipoproteins, heavy urinary losses of these proteins in nephrotic syndrome may lead to thyroid hormone deficiency. Sixth, malnutrition, inflammation, and underlying comorbidities prevalent in dialysis patients may lead to nonthyroidal illness (i.e., thyroid functional test alterations associated with underlying ill health in the absence of thyroid pathology [Table 57.3]). Lastly, various medications commonly prescribed in dialysis patients may lead to thyroid functional test alterations (Table 57.4).

Effects of Dialysis on Thyroid Functional Tests

Limited data suggest that dialysis therapy may contribute to alterations in thyroid hormone metabolism. Two case series of peritoneal dialysis patients demonstrated that 10%–30% of daily T4 production was lost in peritoneal dialysis effluent as free and protein-bound hormone; however, some have posited that the predominant etiology of hypothyroidism in peritoneal dialysis patients is iodine excess from

Table 57.3

Thyroid Functional Tests in Nonthyroidal Illness

Severity of Illness	Thyroid Functional Test		
	T3	**T4**	**TSH**[a]
Mild	↓	Normal	Normal
Moderate	↓↓	↓	Normal
Severe	↓↓	↓↓	↓

[a]TSH usually normal in nonthyroidal illness. In the recovery phase of severe illness, may see a transient rise in T3, T4, and TSH.

Table 57.4

Common Medications in Dialysis Patients That Alter Thyroid Functional Test Results

Mechanism	Medications
↓ Thyroid hormone synthesis/secretion	Thionamides
	Lithium
	Iodine-containing agents/medications
↓ Thyroxine absorption	Calcium carbonate
	Sevelamer
	Lanthanum carbonate
	Aluminum hydroxide
	Iron sulfate
	Proton pump inhibitors
	Cholestyramine
	Colestipol
↓ Thyrotropin	Dopamine
	Dobutamine
	Glucocorticoids
↑ Thyroid hormone synthesis/secretion	Amiodarone
	Iodine-containing agents/medications
Impaired thyroxine-hormone binding	Furosemide
	Heparin
	Salicylates
	Nonsteroidal antiinflammatory drugs
Impaired T4 to T3 conversion	Amiodarone
	Glucocorticoids
	Propranolol
	Nadolol
	Propylthiouracil

povidine–iodine cleaning agents as opposed to peritoneal effluent thyroid hormone losses. In hemodialysis patients, one study that measured thyroid functional tests pre- and postdialysis showed that TSH levels remained stable, whereas T3 and T4 demonstrated a significant rise postdialysis; these changes were thought to be due to medication effects and extravascular shifts in thyroid hormone.

Thyroid Functional Test Alterations in Dialysis Patients

The kidney bears an important role in the metabolism, degradation, and excretion of thyroid hormone and its metabolites. Uremic toxins may also alter the hypothalamic–pituitary–thyroid axis pathway and the results of thyroid hormone assays. As a consequence, various thyroid functional test alterations may be observed in euthyroid dialysis patients (Table 57.5).

Low Triiodothyronine (Low T3 Syndrome)

Low T3 levels are the most commonly observed thyroid functional test alteration in kidney disease patients. In a cross-sectional cohort of 2284 predialysis CKD patients with normal thyrotropin (TSH) levels, there was a graded association between the prevalence of low T3 with incrementally lower eGFRs: 8%, 11%, 21%, 61%, and 79% for eGFR levels ≥90, 60–<90, 30–<60, 15–<30, and <15 mL/min/1.73 m^2, respectively. In dialysis patients, a similarly high prevalence of low T3 has been observed.

The peripheral deiodination of T4 to T3 is highly sensitive to illness states, and low T3 levels are the most common thyroid functional test alteration observed in nonthyroidal illness (Table 57.3). Multiple factors may lead to reduced conversion of T4 to T3 in nonthyroidal illness, which include malnutrition; cytokines such as tumor necrosis factor, interferon-α, NF-κβ, and IL-6; high endogenous serum

---

Table 57.5

Common Thyroid Functional Disease Alterations in Dialysis Patients

Thyroid Function Test	Alterations
Triiodothyronine (T3)	Low T3 levels due to decreased peripheral T4 to T3 conversion due to uremia, malnutrition, illness
	Impaired binding of T3 to thyroid hormone nuclear receptors
	Impaired T3-induced transcriptional activation
Reverse triiodothyronine (rT3)	Normal rT3 levels
Total thyroxine (TT4)	Decreased TT4 levels due to low protein states
Free thyroxine (FT4)	Spurious FT4 levels due to impaired hormone-protein binding associated with uremia, nonthyroidal illness low protein states, medications (indirect FT4 assay methods)
	Impaired FT4 cellular uptake
Thyrotropin (TSH)	Decreased clearance
	Blunted response to TRH
	Decreased pulsatility
	Increased half-life
	Impaired glycosylation

Adapted from Rhee CM, Brent GA, Kovesdy CP, et al. Thyroid functional disease: an under-recognized cardiovascular risk factor in kidney disease patients. Nephrol Dial Transplant. 2015;30(5):724-737.

cortisol levels and exogenous glucocorticoids; free nonesterified fatty acids, and certain medications (e.g., amiodarone). Indeed, cross-sectional data in hemodialysis and peritoneal dialysis patients have shown an inverse association between T3 and IL-6, IL-10, CRP, and albumin, suggesting that low T3 may be a marker of inflammation and malnutrition in these populations.

Reverse Triiodothyronine

Although the D1 and D2 enzymes produce biologically active T3, in nonthyroidal illness there is (1) increased conversion of T4 to reverse T3, a metabolically inactive form of thyroid hormone, and (2) reduced degradation of rT3 to inactive diiodothyronine via the type 3 5'-deiodinase (D3) enzyme, leading to higher rT3 levels. In the general population, rT3 levels are low in hypothyroidism. In dialysis patients, however, rT3 levels are typically normal; at this time, the clinical significance of rT3 in dialysis patients is not known.

Low Thyroxine

Low levels of total T4 (TT4) and FT4 are also commonly reported in patients on dialysis; however, it has been suggested that a proportion of these cases may be falsely low due to the impact of low protein states, uremia, nonthyroidal illness, and medication effects on thyroid functional test accuracy. TT4 levels, which capture both free and protein-bound thyroid hormone, may be depressed in patients with low protein levels given that the vast majority of T4 is protein bound. Furthermore, FT4 levels, which are intended to measure the biologically active form of thyroxine, may be inaccurate in euthyroid dialysis patients as a result of uremia, nonthyroidal illness, and medication effects. In the clinical setting, indirect FT4 assays (e.g., FT4 analog assay or FT4 index) are widely used, which estimate the minute fraction of FT4 using TT4 levels and a binding protein estimate. Although indirect FT4 assays are generally accurate, they are protein–hormone binding dependent. Thus, in conditions where serum protein levels are low (e.g., malnutrition) or circulating substances impair hormone–protein binding (e.g., uremia, nonthyroidal illness, heparin, furosemide), indirect FT4 assays are likely to result in spurious FT4 levels and disease misclassification. In contrast, direct FT4 assays more accurately discern FT4 by physically separating free from protein-bound hormone using equilibrium dialysis or ultrafiltration, followed by FT4 quantification using radioimmunoassay or tandem mass spectrometry. Compared to indirect FT4, direct FT4 levels have been shown to be more strongly correlated with TSH (suggesting more accurate thyroid functional assessment) and to be weakly correlated with albumin (suggesting less confounding by protein–energy wasting) in populations with normal and altered hormone–protein binding (e.g., pregnancy). At this time, direct FT4 assays are currently not available outside of reference laboratories, and their accuracy in dialysis patients requires further study.

Elevated Thyrotropin

TSH is the most sensitive and specific single measure of thyroid function in the general population, and it is typically used to screen, diagnose, and monitor treatment in primary hypothyroidism. TSH levels are normal in nonthyroidal illness, but can be depressed in severe, critically ill states or transiently elevated in the recovery phase of illness.

It should be noted, however, that some TSH alterations may be observed in dialysis patients, including reduced clearance, blunted response to TRH, decreased pulsatility, impaired glycosylation and bioactivity, and increased half-life. In one study of 38 dialysis patients, TSH and FT4 were found to be more reliable indicators of thyroid function versus T3 using various metabolic tests as a proxy for thyroid functional status.

One caveat of the aforementioned tests is that serum levels of thyroid functional tests may not per se reflect tissue levels. However, a biochemical test or physiologic measure that is sufficiently sensitive and specific in measuring thyroid function at the tissue level has not yet been identified. Further efforts are needed to define the optimal approach to thyroid functional testing in dialysis patients.

Thyroid Functional Disease and Outcomes in Dialysis Patients

The cardiovascular system is a major target of thyroid hormone action. Thyroid hormone has both genomic and nongenomic effects on a number of cardiac structural and regulatory proteins, membrane ion channels, and cell surface receptors. As a result, thyroid hormone deficiency has been associated with a diverse range of cardiovascular complications in the general population, including impaired systolic and diastolic function, endothelial dysfunction, dyslipidemia, accelerated atherosclerosis, vascular calcification, and conduction abnormalities leading to malignant arrhythmias (Table 57.6).

In the general population, although few studies have examined the prognostic implications of overt hypothyroidism, there have been many studies examining the association between subclinical hypothyroidism and mortality. Findings across studies have been mixed, likely due to heterogeneous cohort characteristics, alternative definitions of hypothyroidism, and variable adjustment for confounders. Recent data suggest that the subclinical hypothyroidism–mortality association is dependent on underlying cardiovascular risk. There has been a tendency toward positive studies in high cardiovascular disease populations, and NHANES III data have shown that subclinical hypothyroidism and hypothyroidism overall were each associated with higher mortality in participants with heart failure but not in those without heart failure. These findings may have a bearing on dialysis patients who have a high prevalence of structural heart disease and exceedingly high cardiovascular mortality risk.

Low Triiodothyronine and Outcomes

As cardiac myocytes are unable to locally generate T3 from its T4 prohormone, there has been particular interest in T3 as the biologically relevant thyroid hormone metric for cardiovascular endpoints. It was previously hypothesized that thyroid hormone deficiency is a physiologic adaptation and a means to conserve metabolism in dialysis patients in whom hypercatabolism, malnutrition, and dialytic protein and amino acid losses are frequently observed. However, more recent data have shown that low circulating T3 levels are associated with adverse cardiovascular sequelae including decreased systolic function, structural heart disease, arterial stiffness, atherosclerosis,

Table 57.6

Cardiovascular Sequelae of Thyroid Hormone Deficiency

Cardiovascular Sequelae	Mechanism
• Impaired systolic and diastolic function • ↓ cardiac output	• Altered transcription of myocyte contractility and relaxation genes • Alteration of cardiac ion channels • ↓ in peripheral oxygen consumption and requirements • ↓ in blood volume from reduced erythropoietin and RBC synthesis
• Arterial stiffness • Impaired vasoreactivity • ↑ SVR • Diastolic hypertension • Dyslipidemia • ↑ Total cholesterol, LDL, and TG	• ↓ Endothelial vasodilator (nitric oxide, adrenomedullin) synthesis and activity • ↓ Tissue thermogenesis and metabolic activity • ↓ Hepatic LDL receptor density and activity → ↓ fractional clearance of LDL • ↓ Catabolism of cholesterol into bile by cholesterol 7-alpha-hydroxylase enzyme
• Accelerated atherosclerosis	• Dyslipidemia • Hyperhomocysteinemia • Hypertension
• Vascular calcification • Ventricular arrhythmia	• ↓ of matrix Gla and klotho • Changes in cardiac ion channel expression → prolongation of QT interval

and vascular calcification in the dialysis population (Table 57.7). Furthermore, some but not all studies have found that low T3 measured at a single point in time is associated with higher mortality in dialysis patients (Table 57.8). In a study of 210 hemodialysis patients who underwent T3 measurement at baseline and 3-month follow-up, patients with persistently low T3 had a 2.7- and 4-fold higher all-cause and cardiovascular death risk, respectively, compared with those with persistently high levels.

Thyrotropin Elevation and Outcomes

Given concerns about potential confounding by nonthyroidal illness in the aforementioned studies, an enlarging body of literature has examined the association between hypothyroidism defined by an elevated TSH with mortality (Table 57.8). In the first of these studies, among 2715 hemodialysis and peritoneal dialysis patients who underwent TSH measurement at a single-point-in-time, those who were hypothyroid had a 27% higher all-cause mortality risk compared with those who were euthyroid. Yet in a subsequent study of 1000 diabetic hemodialysis patients from the Die Deutsche Diabetes Dialyse Studie (4D Study), subclinical hypothyroidism examined separately or in conjunction with overt hypothyroidism was not associated with sudden cardiac death, cardiovascular events, or all-cause mortality; however, the low prevalence of hypothyroidism (1.8%) in this cohort may have resulted in limited power to detect an association. In the largest study to date, among 8840

Table 57.7

Studies of Thyroid Functional Disease and Cardiovascular Endpoints in Dialysis Patients

Study (Year)	Cohort (n)	Thyroid Metric	Outcome
Cardiovascular Surrogates			
Jaroszynski et al (2005)	HD (52)	↓ FT3	↓ Ventricular depolarization
Zoccali et al (2006)	HD + PD (234)	↓ FT3	↓ LV systolic function ↑ LV mass[a]
Kang et al (2008)	PD (51)	TSH >5 mIU/L + Normal FT4	↓ LV ejection fraction
Tatar et al (2011)	HD (137)	↓ FT3	↑ Atherosclerosis ↑ Arterial stiffness
Tatar et al (2012)	PD (57)	↓ FT3	↑ Arterial stiffness
Saito et al (2012)	HD (52)	↓ FT3	↑ Interstitial edema
Meuwese et al (2013)	PD (84)	↓ FT3	↑ Vascular calcification

Adapted from Rhee CM. Low T3 syndrome in peritoneal dialysis: metabolic adaptation, marker of illness, or mortality mediator? Clin J Am Soc Nephrol. 2015;10(6):917–919.

FT4, free thyroxine; FT3, free triiodothyronine; HD, hemodialysis; LV, left ventricular; PD, peritoneal dialysis; TSH, thyrotropin.

[a]Attenuated to the null after adjustment for IL-6 or serum albumin.

incident hemodialysis patients from a large national dialysis organization, baseline and time-varying hypothyroidism were associated with a 47% and 62% higher all-cause mortality risk, respectively. When examined in finer gradations, higher TSH levels even in the normal range (TSH >3 mIU/L) were associated with a 30% and 42% higher mortality risk in baseline and time-varying analyses, respectively, compared with levels in the low–normal range (TSH 0.5–3 mIU/L). Notably, baseline analyses across BMI subgroups showed that these associations were attenuated to the null in those with BMI ≤20, whereas there was an incrementally stronger hypothyroidism–mortality association across higher BMI categories in time-varying analyses. On the basis of these data, it was hypothesized that hypothyroidism's adverse effects may be nullified in malnourished dialysis patients in whom thyroid hormone deficiency is a physiologic response to reduce catabolism. Given that the observational design of these studies does not establish causality, further study is needed to determine hypothyroidism's role as a mediator of adverse outcomes versus marker of underlying illness versus physiologic adaptation in select dialysis populations (Fig. 57.2).

Treatment Considerations

The 2012 United States Renal Data System Annual Data Report indicates that exogenous thyroid replacement therapy in the form of levothyroxine is the 4th and 12th most commonly prescribed medication among predialysis and dialysis-dependent Medicare Part D recipients, respectively. In the general population, treatment has been shown to reverse diastolic dysfunction, dyslipidemia, endothelial dysfunction, and atherosclerosis. In one study of 4735 patients with subclinical hypothyroidism, levothyroxine treatment was associated with a 39% lower risk of fatal and nonfatal ischemic heart disease events in younger individuals (age 40–70

Table 57.8

Studies of Thyroid Functional Disease and Mortality in Dialysis Patients

Study (Year)	Cohort (n)	Thyroid Metric	Outcome
Mortality			
Zoccali et al (2006)	HD (200)	↓ FT3	↑ All-cause mortality
Enia et al (2007)	PD (41)	↓ FT3	↑ All-cause mortality
Carrero et al (2007)	Dialysis (187)	↓ TT3	↑ All-cause and CV mortality
Fernandez-Reyes et al (2010)	HD (89)	↓ FT3	No association
Ozen et al (2011)	HD (669)	↓ FT3	↑ All-cause mortality[a]
Horacek et al (2012)	HD (167)	↓ FT3	↑ All-cause mortality
Lin et al (2012)	PD (46)	Abnormal thyroid function: 1. TSH >4 mIU/L + Normal FT4, or 2. TSH >4 mIU/L + ↓ FT4, or 3. ↓ TT4, or 4. ↓ TT3	↑ All-cause mortality
Meuwese et al (2012)	HD (210)	1. ↓ TT3 2. ↓ T4	↑ All-cause and CV mortality
Rhee et al (2013)	HD + PD (2715)	↑ TSH	↑ All-cause mortality
Meuwese et al (2013)	PD (84)	↓ FT3	↑ All-cause mortality
Dreschler et al (2014)	HD (1000)	↓ FT3[b]	↑ All-cause mortality during 1st year of observation
Rhee et al (2015)	HD (8840)	↑ TSH	↑ All-cause mortality

Adapted from Rhee CM. Low T3 syndrome in peritoneal dialysis: metabolic adaptation, marker of illness, or mortality mediator? Clin J Am Soc Nephrol. 2015;10(6):917–919.
CV, cardiovascular; FT4, free thyroxine; FT3, free triiodothyronine; HD, hemodialysis; LV, left ventricular; PD, peritoneal dialysis; TSH, thyrotropin; TT3, total triiodothyronine; TT4, total thyroxine.
[b]Study found no association between hypothyroidism (↑ TSH + ↓ or normal FT4) and mortality.

years; n = 3093), but no difference in outcomes among older patients (age >70 years; n = 1642). To date, few studies have examined exogenous thyroid hormone replacement in hypothyroid dialysis patients.

Exogenous T3 Replacement

Previous data have shown that among hemodialysis patients with low T3 levels, exogenous T3 administered at higher than physiologic doses resulted in increased markers of protein degradation, raising concern that thyroid hormone replacement may exacerbate protein–energy wasting, a potent predictor of death in this

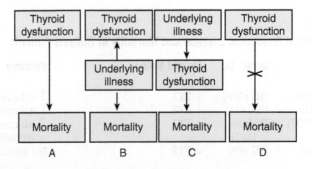

Figure 57.2

Potential Pathways Linking Thyroid Functional Disease and Mortality in Dialysis Patients. (A) Thyroid dysfunction is causally associated with mortality. (B) Thyroid dysfunction is a marker of underlying illness, which in and of itself is associated with mortality. (C) Thyroid dysfunction mediates the association between underlying illness and mortality. (D) Thyroid dysfunction is not associated with mortality in certain populations (i.e., dialysis patients with protein–energy wasting).

population. In the general population, exogenous thyroid hormone treatment of hypothyroidism with T3 alone or in combination with T4 is typically not advised given wide fluctuations in serum T3 levels that may occur because of its rapid gastrointestinal absorption and short half-life (1 day).

Exogenous T4 Replacement

In a single-blind placebo-controlled study of 30 euthyroid hemodialysis patients, exogenous T4 was associated with a reduction in total cholesterol, LDL cholesterol, and lipoprotein levels after 32 weeks of treatment. Although the investigators indicated that treated patients did not develop clinical symptoms of hyperthyroidism, mean thyroid functional test levels rose to thyrotoxicosis ranges. One study examining T4 treatment status and thyroid function at a single point in time found that, compared to patients with normal TSH and no treatment (presumed to be spontaneously euthyroid), those with normal TSH on treatment (presumed to be hypothyroid treated to target) had similar mortality risk, whereas those with high TSH not on treatment (uncontrolled or controlled hypothyroidism) had higher mortality risk.

In light of limited evidence, using a conservative therapeutic approach in dialysis patients akin to that of non-CKD populations who are older or who have underlying cardiovascular disease may be preferred. Although the typical starting dose in young healthy adults is 1.6 μg/kg/day, a lower dose of 25–50 μg/day may be considered in dialysis patients. Given the long 1-week half-life of levothyroxine, steady state is typically achieved 6 weeks after initiation of therapy or dose adjustment. At that time, clinical symptoms should be reevaluated and a repeat TSH level should be measured.

Given their high prevalence of hypothyroidism, frequent use of levothyroxine, and high underlying cardiovascular risk, rigorous longitudinal studies are needed to determine the safety and effectiveness of exogenous thyroid hormone treatment in this population. Levothyroxine has a narrow toxic-to-therapeutic window, and over-replacement or unwarranted treatment may lead to angina, myocardial infarction, atrial fibrillation, increased protein catabolism, and accelerated bone loss. Understanding the impact of thyroid hormone treatment on cardiovascular outcomes and mortality may shed greater light into the causal implications of hypothyroidism in dialysis patients.

CHAPTER 58

Metabolic Abnormalities: Evaluation of Sexual Dysfunction

Biff F. Palmer, MD

Introduction

Sexual dysfunction is a common finding in both men and women with chronic kidney failure. Common disturbances include erectile dysfunction in men, menstrual abnormalities in women, and decreased libido and fertility in both sexes. These abnormalities are primarily organic in nature and are related to uremia as well as the other comorbid conditions that frequently occur in the chronic kidney failure patient. Fatigue and psychosocial factors related to the presence of a chronic disease are also contributory factors.

Sexual Dysfunction in Uremic Men

Erectile dysfunction is one of the most common manifestations of sexual dysfunction in men with chronic kidney disease. The prevalence of this disorder has been reported to be as high as 70%–80% and is similar between patients on hemodialysis and peritoneal dialysis. In addition to abnormalities in blood flow and neural input to the penis, abnormalities in the pituitary-gonadal axis play a prominent role in the genesis of this disorder.

Chronic kidney disease is associated with impaired spermatogenesis and testicular damage, often leading to infertility. Semen analysis typically shows a decreased volume of ejaculate, either low or complete azoospermia, and a low percentage of motility. Histologic findings include damage to the seminiferous tubules and interstitial fibrosis and calcifications in the epididymis and corpora cavernosa. The factors responsible for testicular damage in uremia are not well understood but chronic exposure to phthalates in dialysis tubing may play a role.

The endocrine function of the testes is also abnormal in chronic kidney disease (Table 58.1). Total and free testosterone levels are typically reduced, although the binding capacity and concentration of sex hormone–binding globulin are normal. Low testosterone levels lead to increased plasma concentration of the pituitary gonadotropin, luteinizing hormone (LH), since testosterone normally inhibits LH release through a negative feedback loop. Low serum testosterone levels are associated with increased mortality in dialysis patients. Follicle-stimulating hormone (FSH) secretion is also increased in men with chronic kidney disease, although to a more variable degree such that the LH/FSH ratio is typically increased. FSH release by the pituitary normally responds to feedback inhibition by a peptide product of the Sertoli cells called inhibin. The plasma FSH concentration tends to be highest in those uremic patients with the most severe damage to seminiferous tubules and

Factors Involved in the Pathogenesis of Impotence in Uremic Men

- Vascular system
    - Occlusive arterial disease
    - Veno-occlusive disease and venous leakage
- Neurologic system
    - Impaired autonomic function due to uremia and comorbid conditions
- Endocrine system
    - Gonadal function
        - Decreased production of testosterone
    - Hypothalamic–pituitary function
        - Blunted increase in serum LH levels
        - Decreased amplitude of LH secretory burst
        - Variable increase in serum FSH levels
        - Increased prolactin levels
- Psychological system
- Other factors
    - Zinc deficiency
    - Medications
    - Anemia
    - Secondary hyperparathyroidism

FSH, follicle-stimulating hormone; LH, luteinizing hormone.

presumably the lowest levels of inhibin. It has been suggested that increased FSH levels may portend a poor prognosis for recovery of spermatogenic function following kidney transplantation. Elevated plasma prolactin levels are commonly found in dialyzed men primarily as a result of increased production and to a lesser extent reduced metabolic clearance. Both increased parathyroid hormone and zinc deficiency have been implicated as playing a contributory role in the increased levels.

Gynecomastia occurs in approximately 30% of men on maintenance hemodialysis. This problem most often develops during the initial months of dialysis and then tends to regress as dialysis continues. The pathogenesis of gynecomastia in this setting is unclear. Although elevated prolactin levels and an increased estrogen-to-androgen ratio seem attractive possibilities, most data fail to support a primary role for abnormal hormonal function. Alternatively, a mechanism similar to that responsible for gynecomastia following refeeding of malnourished patients may be involved.

Evaluation of Sexual Dysfunction in the Uremic Man

In evaluating and ultimately treating the impotent kidney failure patient, one must not only consider disturbances in the hypothalamic–pituitary–gonadal axis discussed above but also abnormalities in the sympathetic nervous system and derangements in the arterial supply or venous drainage of the penis. In addition, the psychological effects of a chronic illness and lifestyle limitations may negatively impact sexual function.

A thorough history and physical examination can provide useful information during the initial evaluation of a patient with impotence. A history of normal erectile function prior to the development of kidney failure is suggestive of a secondary cause of impotence. Symptoms or physical findings of a neuropathy as in a patient with a neurogenic bladder would be particularly suggestive of a neurologic etiology. Similarly, symptoms or signs of peripheral vascular disease may be a clue to the presence of vascular obstruction to penile blood flow. One should look for the presence of secondary sexual characteristics, such as facial, axillary, and pubic hair. The lack of these findings and the presence of small soft testicles suggest primary or secondary hypogonadism as the cause of the impotence. Neurogenic and vascular causes are more likely to be associated with normal-sized testicles. Even when the history and physical examination point to a specific abnormality, one must also consider that an individual patient may have more than one factor responsible for the erectile dysfunction, and other causes may need to be ultimately evaluated.

A review of the patient's medications may reveal a drug that could be potentially playing a role in impairing sexual function. Antihypertensive medications are common offenders, with centrally acting agents and beta-blockers being the most commonly implicated agents in causing impotence. The angiotensin-converting enzyme inhibitors or angiotensin receptor blockers are associated with a lower incidence of impotence and represent a useful alternative in kidney failure patients with hypertension. Other drugs commonly implicated include cimetidine, phenothiazines, tricyclic antidepressants, and metoclopramide.

If the history and physical examination reveal no obvious cause, then a psychological cause of erectile dysfunction may need to be considered. Testing for the presence of nocturnal penile tumescence (NPT) has been used in some centers as a means to discriminate between a psychological and organic cause of impotence. The basis for this test is that during the rapid eye movement stage of sleep, males normally have an erection. The assumption is that a man with a psychological cause of impotence would still experience erections while asleep whereas the absence of an adequate erection would make an organic cause more likely. If a patient is found to have nocturnal erections, then psychological testing and evaluation are indicated. It should be noted that NPT testing is not infallible and that if a patient has a normal test and no psychological cause is found, then evaluation for an organic cause should still be pursued.

There are tests that may aid the discrimination between a neurogenic and vascular cause of impotence. Tests used to exclude a vascular etiology of impotence include Doppler studies to measure penile blood flow, measurement of penile blood pressure, and penile pulse palpation. Neurogenic impotence is suggested by detecting a prolonged latency time of the bulbocavernous reflex or confirming the presence of a neurogenic bladder. With the availability of sildenafil (see below) to use as a therapeutic trial, such tests are generally reserved for nonresponders who may eventually be considered for surgical placement of a penile prosthesis.

As discussed previously, hormonal abnormalities are frequently detected in chronic kidney failure patients. Endocrine tests that are useful in the evaluation of an organic cause of impotence include measurement of serum LH, FSH, testosterone, and prolactin levels. It should be noted that only a small percentage of uremic patients will have prolactin levels greater than 100 ng/mL. Imaging studies of the hypothalamic–pituitary region should be performed in patients with levels of greater magnitude in order to exclude the presence of a microadenoma or macroadenoma.

Treatment of Sexual Dysfunction in the Uremic Man

The treatment of sexual dysfunction in the uremic man is initially of a general nature (Fig. 58.1). One needs to ensure optimal delivery of dialysis and adequate nutritional intake. Administration of recombinant human erythropoietin has been shown to enhance sexual function likely through the associated improvement in well-being that comes with the correction of anemia although improvement in the pituitary gonadal feedback mechanism has also been reported. Controlling the degree of secondary hyperparathyroidism with 1,25-dihydroxyvitamin D may be of benefit in lowering prolactin levels and improving sexual function in some patients.

One area that deserves further investigation is the impact of slow nocturnal hemodialysis on sexual function. In a pilot study of five patients undergoing dialysis 6 nights per week for 8 hours each night, serum testosterone levels increased in three patients over an 8-week period. Levels of LH and FSH remained unchanged. In a separate study, the percentage of patients who felt that sexual function was a problem declined from 80% to 29% after 3 months of nightly nocturnal hemodialysis.

Patients with normal NPT testing should be evaluated to determine if there is a psychological component to the impotence. If a problem is found, then a trial of

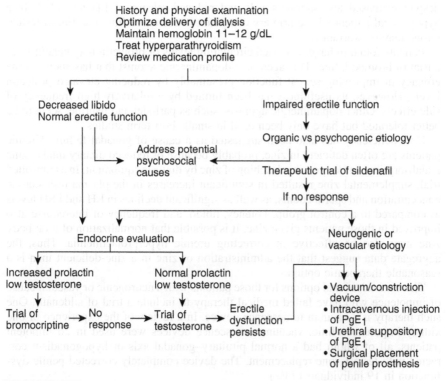

Figure 58.1

Approach to Sexual Dysfunction in Uremic Men.

psychotherapy is warranted. The effectiveness of antidepressant medications and/or psychiatric counseling in chronic kidney failure patients with sexual dysfunction has not been well studied. Use of antidepressant medications can be problematic because many of these agents can cause sexual dysfunction.

It has become common clinical practice to first administer sildenafil to patients who complain of erectile dysfunction and reserve further workup for only those patients who fail to achieve a therapeutic response. A limited number of studies have now been published specifically examining the effectiveness of sildenafil in uremic men with chronic kidney failure. Each of these studies used the International Index of Erectile Function (IIEF) questionnaire as a means to gauge effectiveness of the therapy. The response rate ranged from 60% to 80%. Sildenafil was found to have similar efficacy in patients treated with either hemodialysis or peritoneal dialysis. It should be emphasized that sildenafil is contraindicated in patients who are currently taking organic nitrates. Caution should also be exercised when prescribing this agent to patients with known coronary artery disease. To limit the possibility of hypotension among dialysis patients, some clinicians recommend use of sildenafil on non-dialysis days.

In patients with low circulating levels of testosterone, correcting the deficit generally results in clinical improvement in other forms of gonadal failure. By contrast, administration of testosterone to uremic men usually fails to restore libido or potency, despite increased testosterone levels and reduced release of LH and FSH. In a hypogonadal patient whose primary complaint is decreased libido, a trial of testosterone may be warranted.

Patients found to have increased circulating levels of prolactin may benefit from a trial of bromocriptine. This agent is a dopaminergic agonist that has shown some efficacy in improving sexual function presumably by reducing elevated prolactin levels. However, its usefulness has been limited by a relatively high frequency of side effects. Other dopaminergic agonists, such as parlodel and lisuride, seem to be better tolerated but have only been used in small short-term studies.

Zinc deficiency has also been suggested as a cause of gonadal failure. Uremic patients are often deficient in zinc, probably because of reduced dietary intake, zinc malabsorption, and/or possible leaching of zinc by dialysis equipment. In a controlled trial, supplemental zinc resulted in significant increases in the plasma testosterone concentration and sperm counts, as well as significant declines in LH and FSH levels as compared to a control group. Potency, libido, and frequency of intercourse also improved in those patients given zinc. It is possible that normalization of total body zinc may also be effective in correcting uremic hyperprolactinemia. Thus, the aggregate data suggest that the administration of zinc in a zinc-deficient man is a reasonable therapeutic option.

There are additional options for those patients with a neurogenic or vascular cause of impotence who have failed medical therapy to include a trial of sildenafil. One such therapy is a vacuum tumescence device. In a review of the experience of one kidney impotence clinic, vacuum tumescence devices were used in 26 impotent patients, all of whom had a normal pituitary–gonadal axis or hypogonadism corrected with testosterone replacement. The device completely corrected penile dysfunction in 19 individuals (73%).

Intraurethral administration of alprostadil (synthetic prostaglandin E_1) provides the delivery of prostaglandin to the corpus cavernosum, resulting in an erection sufficient for intercourse. The drug is supplied in an applicator that is inserted in the urethra. Alprostadil can also be injected into the penis shaft, resulting in vasodilation and inhibition of platelet aggregation. The major side effects of intrapenile alprostadil therapy are penile pain, priapism, and bleeding. Given the presence of platelet dysfunction with uremia, intracavernosal injections should be used with caution in patients with end-stage renal disease. Surgical placement of a penile prosthesis is typically considered in patients who fail the less invasive first-line treatments.

A well-functioning renal transplant can restore sexual activity and fertility; however, some features of reproductive function may remain impaired, particularly reduced libido and erectile dysfunction. This improvement occurs in association with normalization of the serum testosterone concentration and, in many patients, an increase in sperm count.

Sexual Dysfunction in Uremic Women

Disturbances in menstruation and fertility are commonly encountered in women with chronic kidney disease, usually leading to amenorrhea by the time the patient reaches end-stage renal disease. The menstrual cycle typically remains irregular with scanty flow after the initiation of maintenance dialysis, although normal menses is restored in some women. In others, hypermenorrhagia develops, potentially leading to significant blood loss and increased transfusion requirements. Women on chronic dialysis also tend to complain of decreased libido and reduced ability to reach orgasm.

Indirect determination of ovulation suggests that anovulatory cycles are the rule in uremic women. For example, endometrial biopsies show an absence of progestational effects and there is a failure to increase basal body temperature at the time when ovulation would be expected. In addition, the preovulatory peak in LH and estradiol concentrations are frequently absent. The failure of LH to rise in part reflects a disturbance in the positive estradiol feedback pathway, because the administration of exogenous estrogen to mimic the preovulatory surge in estradiol fails to stimulate LH release. Pregnancy can rarely occur in advanced kidney failure but some degree of residual kidney function is usually present. As in men with chronic kidney disease circulating levels of prolactin are increased. The secretion appears autonomous and is resistant to maneuvers designed to stimulate or inhibit its release.

Postmenopausal uremic women have gonadotropin levels as high as those seen in nonuremic women of similar age. The age at which menopause begins in chronic kidney failure tends to be decreased when compared to normal women.

Treatment of Sexual Dysfunction in Uremic Women

The high frequency of anovulation leads sequentially to lack of formation of the corpus luteum and failure of progesterone secretion. Because progesterone is responsible for transforming the endometrium into the luteal phase, lack of progesterone is associated with amenorrhea. For patients who desire to resume menses, administration of a progestational agent during the final days of the monthly cycle will usually be successful.

On the other hand, ongoing menses can contribute significantly to the anemia of chronic kidney disease, particularly in those patients with hypermenorrhagia. In this setting, administration of a progestational agent during the entire monthly cycle will terminate menstrual flow. Rarely, a patient may require hysterectomy for refractory uterine bleeding.

It is not known whether the usual absence of menses in women with chronic kidney failure predisposes to the development of endometrial hyperplasia and possible carcinoma. Because these patients are often anovulatory, there is no disruption of the proliferative effect of estrogen by the release of progesterone. It is therefore recommended that women with chronic kidney failure be monitored closely by a gynecologist; it may be desirable in at least some cases to administer a progestational agent several times per year to interrupt the proliferation induced by unopposed estrogen release (Fig. 58.2).

While pregnancy can rarely occur in women on thrice-weekly chronic dialysis, restoration of fertility as a therapeutic goal should be discouraged. More intensive dialysis as achieved by daily nocturnal hemodialysis may allow for improved fertility. In comparison, the abnormalities in ovulation can usually be reversed and successful pregnancy achieved in women with a well-functioning kidney transplant. Uremic women who are menstruating normally should be encouraged to use birth control.

Studies addressing the therapy of decreased libido and sexual function in uremic women are lacking. Amenorrheic hemodialysis patients may have low estradiol levels that can secondarily lead to vaginal atrophy and dryness and result in discomfort during intercourse. Such patients may benefit from local estrogen therapy or vaginal lubricants. Low-dose testosterone may be effective in increasing sexual desire but is rarely used secondary to potential toxicity. Use of a transdermal

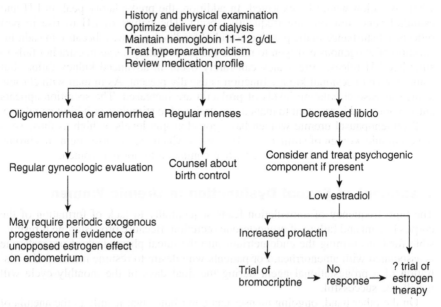

Figure 58.2

Approach to Sexual Dysfunction in Uremic Women.

testosterone patch was recently shown effective in improving libido in nonuremic surgically menopausal women; however, this therapy is not yet approved. Bromocriptine therapy in hyperprolactinemic patients may help in restoring sexual function but has not been well studied. Estrogen supplementation may improve sexual function in those patients with low circulating estradiol levels. Successful transplantation is clearly the most effective means to restore normal sexual desire in women with chronic kidney failure.

SECTION XXII

Uremic Osteodystrophy

CHAPTER 59

Chronic Kidney Disease–Mineral and Bone Disorder

Wei Chen, MD • David Bushinsky, MD

Patients with chronic kidney disease (CKD) often have disturbances in divalent ion metabolism, which include dysregulation of calcium and phosphorus, development of bone disease and extra-osseous calcification, especially in their vasculature. These disturbances were previously referred to as renal osteodystrophy. However, the term *renal osteodystrophy* is primarily a description of altered bone morphology in patients with CKD. In 2006, Kidney Disease: Improving Global Outcomes (KDIGO) proposed a new term called CKD–mineral and bone disorder (CKD-MBD), where CKD-MBD was defined as a systemic disorder of mineral and bone metabolism due to CKD manifested by either one or a combination of the following: (1) abnormalities of calcium, phosphorus, parathyroid hormone (PTH), or vitamin D metabolism; (2) abnormalities in bone turnover, mineralization, volume, linear growth, or strength; and (3) vascular or other soft-tissue calcification.

Pathophysiology of CKD-MBD

CKD-MBD is a complex disorder and involves feedback loops among the kidneys, intestine, bone, and vasculature. It is characterized by phosphate retention and secondary hyperparathyroidism. Before discussing the pathophysiology of secondary hyperparathyroidism, we will briefly review the regulation and action of the hormones that are involved in mineral metabolism: PTH, vitamin D, and fibroblast growth factor-23 (FGF23).

Review of PTH, Vitamin D, and Fibroblast Growth Factor-23

PTH is secreted by the chief cells of the parathyroid glands primarily in response to a fall in arterial blood ionized calcium. PTH also increases in response to a fall in calcitriol (1,25-dihydroxyvitamin D, the activated form of vitamin D) and an increase in serum phosphate. PTH increases the concentration of calcium by increasing bone resorption, enhancing calcium reabsorption from the distal renal tubules and thick ascending limb, and increasing the production of calcitriol, which leads to an increase in intestinal calcium absorption. PTH reduces renal reabsorption of phosphate in the proximal tubule thus lowering serum phosphorus. However, the PTH-induced increase in bone resorption and the calcitriol-mediated increase in intestinal phosphate absorption both can lead to an increase in the level of serum phosphorus.

Cholecalciferol (vitamin D_3) is a fat-soluble steroid that is synthesized in the skin in the presence of ultraviolet light or obtained from the diet. In the liver, it is converted to 25-hydroxyvitamin D by 25-hydroxylase. 25-Hydroxyvitamin D then enters the circulation and is hydroxylated in the proximal tubules of the kidneys to calcitriol (1,25-dihydroxyvitamin D), which is the most biologically active form of vitamin D. Calcitriol production is increased by PTH, a low arterial concentration of calcium and phosphorus. Calcitriol increases intestinal absorption of calcium and phosphate, and at high levels, it induces bone resorption and perhaps renal tubular calcium reabsorption. It also lowers PTH level, leading to less urinary phosphate excretion.

FGF23 is produced in osteocytes and osteoblasts. Its primary stimulus remains unclear but appears to involve phosphorus retention. In kidneys, FGF23 binds to a fibroblast growth factor receptor complex along with klotho, a protein that induces phosphaturia through downregulation of the proximal tubule sodium-phosphate cotransporter and reduces phosphorus absorption by decreasing calcitriol production. FGF23 inhibits PTH secretion by binding to receptors on the parathyroid glands. Elevated levels of FGF23 have been associated with CKD progression, left ventricular hypertrophy, endothelial dysfunction, vascular stiffness, and higher mortality rates in patients with CKD.

Development of Secondary Hyperparathyroidism in CKD

Phosphate excretion decreases as renal function declines. With a constant intake of phosphorus and the majority of phosphorus being absorbed regardless of the level of calcitriol, phosphate is retained. Phosphate retention reduces ionized calcium by directly binding with calcium, as well as by stimulating FGF23 release from osteocytes and decreasing calcitriol synthesis, leading to an increase in PTH. The decreased calcitriol concentration in patients with CKD appears to be secondary to the increase in FGF23 concentration as well as loss of renal function and phosphate retention. The pathophysiology of secondary hyperparathyroidism in patients with CKD is illustrated in Fig. 59.1.

In the 1970s, Bricker and Slatopolsky proposed the "trade-off" hypothesis as a mechanism for the development of secondary hyperparathyroidism. The idea of the "trade-off" hypothesis is that the body pays a biologic "price" (i.e., PTH excess) in order to maintain normal levels of calcium and phosphorus. At some increased level of PTH, this response appears to be maladaptive because although PTH is phosphaturic, it also increases serum phosphorus by increasing bone resorption. As renal function deteriorates, the effect of PTH on urinary phosphate excretion diminishes and the excess PTH exacerbates hyperphosphatemia by increasing bone resorption and leads to significant bone disease.

The temporal sequence of disordered phosphorus metabolism in progressive CKD is demonstrated in Fig. 59.2. The prevalence of hyperphosphatemia, elevated FGF23, and PTH levels increases progressively with worsening kidney function. Our current understanding is that the alterations in FGF23, PTH, and calcitriol are all physiologic responses to prevent the increase in serum phosphorus. An increase in FGF23 is detected first, well before the development of CKD stage 3. Elevated FGF23 levels leads to decreased production of calcitriol and subsequently development of secondary hyperparathyroidism. The serum level of phosphorus begins to increase when estimated glomerular filtrate rate (eGFR) falls below 60 mL/min/1.73 m^2, but remains in a relatively normal range until eGFR is less than 30 mL/min/1.73 m^2. Serum phosphate, FGF23, and PTH levels continue to rise while patients are on dialysis.

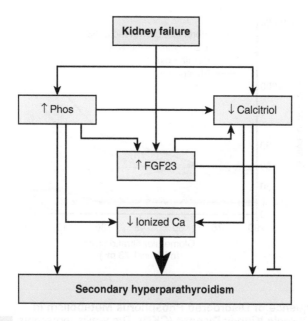

Figure 59.1

Pathophysiology of Secondary Hyperparathyroidism. When renal failure occurs, phosphate retention develops. Phosphate retention ultimately leads to decreased ionized calcium, which promotes PTH release and development of secondary hyperparathyroidism. Phosphate retention reduces ionized calcium by directly binding with calcium, as well as by stimulating FGF23 release from osteocytes and decreasing calcitriol synthesis. The decreased calcitriol concentration in CKD is secondary to the combination of loss of renal function, increase in FGF23 concentration, and phosphate retention. Phosphate retention can also directly stimulate PTH gene expression and increase PTH synthesis independent of the ionized calcium concentration and calcitriol level. Contrarily, elevated FGF23 levels may inhibit the secretion of PTH.

Epidemiology of Disordered Mineral Metabolism

Increased FGF23 levels appear to be independently associated with mortality in both patients with advanced CKD and patients on chronic hemodialysis. In a recent study, among patients with advanced CKD (mean eGFR of 18 mL/min/1.73 m^2), the median FGF23 concentration was 392 RU/mL. Compared to the lowest quartile of FGF23, the two highest quartiles of FGF23 were associated with a significantly elevated risk for all-cause mortality (hazard ratios of 1.76 [95% confidence interval (CI) 1.28–2.44] and 2.17 [95% CI 1.56–3.08]), cardiovascular events, as well as initiation of chronic dialysis. Similarly, among patients on hemodialysis, increasing FGF23 levels was associated with a monotonically increased risk of death. With FGF23 quartile 1 as the reference category, the odds ratio for quartile 3 was 4.5 (95% CI 2.2–9.4) and for quartile 4 was 5.7 (95% CI 2.6–12.6).

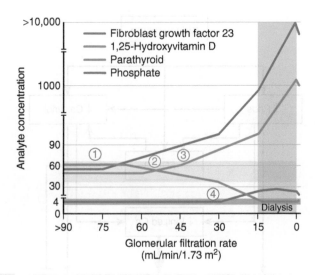

Figure 59.2

Temporal Sequence of Disordered Phosphorus Metabolism in Progressive Chronic Kidney Disease (CKD). The y-axis represents circulating concentrations of the individual analytes with the temporal changes. The individual analytes are color-coded (C-terminal FGF23 [RU/mL] in red; 1,25-dihydroxyvitamin D [pg/mL] in purple, PTH [pg/mL] in green; and phosphate [mg/dL] in blue). Current hypotheses propose increased FGF23 as the earliest alteration in mineral metabolism in CKD (no. 1, red). Gradually increasing FGF23 levels cause the early decline in 1,25(OH)$_2$D levels (no. 2, purple) that free PTH from feedback inhibition, leading to secondary hyperparathyroidism (no. 3, green). All of these changes occur long before increase in serum phosphate levels are evident (no. 4, blue). (Adapted from Wolf M, Forging forward with 10 burning questions on FGF23 in kidney disease. J Am Soc Nephrol 2010;21:1427-1435.)

The relationship between serum calcium, phosphorus, and PTH and mortality is typically a U-shaped curve, with very low and very high levels associated with increased mortality. The data from the Dialysis Outcomes and Practice Patterns Study (DOPPS) from 1996 to 2007 showed that the lowest mortality risk was observed with serum calcium between 8.6 and 10.0 mg/dL (albumin-corrected calcium between 7.6 and 9.5 mg/dL), phosphorus between 3.6 and 5.0 mg/dL, and PTH between 101 and 300 pg/mL. Mortality was the highest when serum calcium was >10.0 mg/dL, phosphorus >7.0 mg/dL, and PTH >600 pg/mL.

In the dialysis population, both hypo- and hypercalcemia are associated with high all-cause mortality, with hypercalcemia more closely associated with cardiovascular mortality. The prevalence of hypocalcemia (calcium <8.5 mg/dL) is ~11% in patients on dialysis. Patients on dialysis develop hypocalcemia due to phosphate retention and reduced calcitriol level. The prevalence of hypercalcemia (calcium >10.2) is slightly lower at ~5%. The causes of hypercalcemia in patients on dialysis include the use of calcium-containing phosphate binders and vitamin D analogs, high dialysate calcium concentration, and development of tertiary hyperparathyroidism. According to the data from DOPPS, serum calcium ≤8.5mg/dL was associated with greater risk of all-cause, but not cardiovascular mortality, while calcium >10 mg/dL was associated with both all-cause and cardiovascular mortality. Adjustment for low serum albumin substantially attenuates the mortality risk associated with low uncorrected calcium and strengthens the risk associated with high uncorrected calcium concentration.

Hyperphosphatemia is associated with high mortality in patients with CKD as well as in the general population. Hyperphosphatemia is a late manifestation of CKD with the prevalence of more than 50% when eGFR is <20 mL/min/1.73 m^2. In an observational cohort using the data of prevalent and incident patients on maintenance hemodialysis or peritoneal dialysis in DaVita dialysis facilities, patients with serum phosphorus ≥6.4 mg/dL had an increased risk of all cause and cause-specific mortality. For all-cause mortality, the adjusted hazard ratios was 1.59 (95% CI 1.47–1.54) for patients on hemodialysis and 1.48 (95% CI 1.34–1.63) for patients on peritoneal dialysis. To study the effect of serum phosphorus levels in individuals without CKD on cardiovascular disease, 3368 participants from the Framingham Offspring study were followed for a mean of 16.1 years. At the end of the follow up period, individuals with the serum phosphorus between 3.5–6.2 had 1.55-fold cardiovascular disease risk (95% CI 1.2–2.07) compared to those with serum phosphorus between 1.6–2.8 while adjusting for age, sex, body mass index, diabetes, hypertension, smoking, cholesterol, eGFR, and inflammatory markers.

Similarly, both hypo- and hyperparathyroidism in patients on dialysis is associated with higher mortality. Analysis using DOPPS data showed that PTH ≤100 pg/mL might be associated with significant greater cardiovascular mortality. More importantly, PTH >600 pg/mL was associated with higher all-cause and cardiovascular mortality. Other subsequent studies have confirmed this finding.

Bone Disease

Bone Disease in CKD

In 2006, KDIGO recommended a new system to describe bone pathology in patients with CKD. This system describes three key histologic features observed in the bone of patients with CKD: turnover, mineralization, and volume. There are four major types of bone diseases that occur in patients with CKD: adynamic bone disease, osteitis fibrosa cystica, osteomalacia, and mixed uremic osteodystrophy (see Table 59.1). Adynamic bone disease is characterized by low bone turnover, which is often the result of excessive PTH suppression. Osteitis fibrosa cystica is characterized by high bone turnover and is due to secondary hyperparathyroidism. In the past two decades, with the development of better phosphorus binders and the use of cinacalcet and vitamin D analogs, the prevalence of osteitis fibrosa cystica has markedly decreased, while the prevalence of adynamic bone disease has increased. Osteomalacia is characterized by low bone turnover and abnormal mineralization. It was once primarily due to aluminum deposition in bone when aluminum-containing phosphate binders were utilized and when aluminum was present in water used for dialysis. Osteomalacia is uncommon now after the discontinuation of high-dose aluminum-containing phosphate binders and incorporation of reverse osmosis system in dialysis water treatment systems. Mixed uremic osteodystrophy is

Table 59.1

Major Types of Bone Diseases in Chronic Kidney Disease

	Turnover	Mineralization	Volume	Etiology
Adynamic bone disease	Low	Abnormal	Low	Excessive suppression of parathyroid glands
Osteitis fibrosa cystica	High	Abnormal	Increased	Secondary hyperparathyroidism
Osteomalacia	Low	Abnormal	Abnormal	Aluminum deposit
Mixed uremic osteodystrophy	High or low	Abnormal	Abnormal	—

characterized by either high or low bone turnover as well as abnormal mineralization. The symptoms of bone disease usually only occur in severe cases and may include bone tenderness, fracture, muscle weakness, and arthritis. Both high- and low-turnover bone diseases are associated with increased fracture risk.

Patients With CKD Have More Hip Fractures

Patients with CKD have more hip fractures compared to patients without kidney disease. This was demonstrated by Nickolas et al using data from the Third National Health and Nutrition Examination Survey, which surveyed the United States non-institutionalized civilian population between 1988 and 1997. Compared to those with eGFR> 100 mL/min/1.73 m^2, participants with eGFR <60 mL/min/1.73 m^2 have a two-fold increase in the likelihood of reporting a previous hip fracture. The risk of hip fractures is even higher in patients on dialysis. According to the United States Renal Data System (USRDS) between 1989 and 1996, the overall incidence of hip fracture was 7.45 per 1000 person years for males and 13.63 per 1000 person years for females. The overall relative risk for hip fracture was ~4.4 for dialysis patients compared with people of the same sex in the general population. Patients on hemodialysis have a higher risk of hip fractures compared to patients on peritoneal dialysis. In the general population, hip fracture is associated with increased mortality. Similarly, in the dialysis population, hip fracture is associated with approximately a two-fold increase in all-cause mortality.

Diagnosing Bone Disease

Bone biopsy with histomorphometric analysis is the gold standard for diagnosing bone disease in patients with CKD and can be very helpful in determining the clinical course and response to treatment. KDIGO recommends that in patients on chronic dialysis, it is reasonable to perform a bone biopsy in various settings including but not limited to: unexplained fractures, persistent bone pain, unexplained hypercalcemia or hypophosphatemia, possible aluminum toxicity, and prior to initiation of bisphosphonate therapy. This recommendation is not graded, and there remains a controversy over the indications for bone biopsy. Overall, bone biopsies are not routinely preformed, and there are several reasons for this. Since aluminum toxicity is now rare and both high- and low-turnover bone disease are associated with increased fracture risk, there are few circumstances (perhaps in the case of determining if bisphosphonate therapy is appropriate) in which the precise knowledge of bone pathology will guide therapy. In addition, few nephrologists are trained to perform bone biopsies.

Besides bone biopsy, there is no other method to adequately predict the underlying bone histology. Although circulating intact PTH levels may indicate the presence and severity of hyperparathyroidism, they are not a strong predictor of the underlying bone disease or useful in defining the type of renal osteodystrophy. Some biochemical markers of bone resorption, such as serum C-telopeptide of type I collagen, have been studied to help diagnose bone disease in CKD, but none has been shown to be useful. Radiographic examination of bone is not adequate. In the general population, dual energy X-ray absorptiometry (DXA) is the clinical standard to screen and stratify fracture risk. In patients with CKD, fracture risk screening by DXA has been controversial. DXA does not have sufficient resolution to either discriminate between cortical and trabecular bone or to determine turnover or mineralization. The data on whether bone mineral density measured by DXA can predict fracture risk are inconsistent. KDIGO does not recommend routine bone mineral density testing in patients on chronic dialysis. Lastly, high-resolution peripheral quantitative computed tomography (HR-pQCT) is a novel imaging tool. It is a noninvasive, low-radiation method to assess three-dimensional bone microarchitecture and volumetric bone mineral density in cortical and trabecular compartments of the distal radius and distal tibia. Since its availability in the mid-2000s, its application in clinical research has increased significantly. However, its utility in clinical practice for fracture prediction remains unclear.

Vascular Calcification

Vascular Calcification and Cardiovascular Mortality

Vascular calcification is common in patients with CKD with a prevalence of ~70%–80%. Multiple studies in patients with CKD have demonstrated that the extent of vascular calcification is an independent predictor of cardiovascular morbidity and mortality. Vascular calcification occurs in both the intima and media of vessel walls. Intimal calcification is an indicator of atherosclerosis. In coronary arteries, it is positively correlated with atherosclerotic plaque burden and contributes to ischemic heart disease. Medial calcification is a characteristic feature of CKD and closely associated with dialysis duration and disordered mineral metabolism. The unique feature of medial calcification in CKD is supported by the presence of vascular calcification in young CKD patients without any traditional risk factors for atherosclerosis and the high prevalence of medial calcification in the epigastric arteries of patients with end stage renal disease (ESRD) at the time of kidney transplantation. Medial calcification causes arterial stiffness and decreases vessel compliance. This loss of cushioning function of arteries may lead to systolic hypertension and increased afterload, resulting in left ventricular hypertrophy and subsequent heart failure. Increased afterload also compromises coronary perfusion and exacerbates ischemic heart disease (see Fig. 59.3). Medial calcification appears to be responsible for calcific uremic arteriopathy or calciphylaxis, which is a systemic calcification of arterioles leading to ischemia and subcutaneous necrosis.

There are several risk factors that predispose patients with CKD to vascular calcification. These include the traditional ones such as older age, diabetes mellitus,

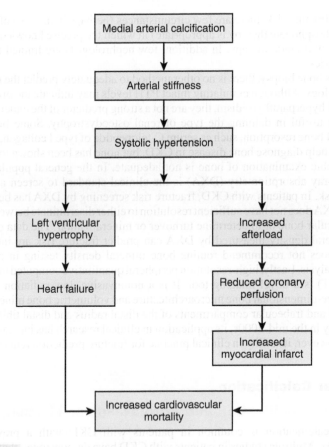

Figure 59.3

Medial Arterial Calcification and Cardiovascular Outcomes. Medial calcification is a characteristic feature of chronic kidney disease (CKD). It causes arterial stiffness and decreases vessel compliance. Loss of cushioning function of arteries may lead to systolic hypertension and increased afterload, resulting in left ventricular hypertrophy and subsequent heart failure. Increased afterload also compromises coronary perfusion and exacerbates ischemic heart disease. All of these contribute to the increased cardiovascular mortality in patients with CKD.

dyslipidemia, and inflammation. There are also risk factors that are more specific to patients with CKD. They are the so-called uremic toxins, dialysis vintage, disordered mineral metabolism, and therapies used to treat hyperparathyroidism in CKD, in particular, calcium-containing phosphate binders and activated vitamin D. Disordered mineral metabolism can lead to vascular calcification, which is an active regulated cell-mediated process. Elevated serum phosphorus can lead to phenotypic transition of vascular smooth muscle cells to osteoblast-like cells and enhanced matrix mineralization, thus promoting vascular calcification.

Diagnosing Vascular Calcification

Current guidelines do not recommend routine screening for vascular calcification. Detection of vascular calcification using any technique has not been shown to have any clinical utility in terms of risk stratification or therapy. Electron-beam computed tomography (CT) is thought to be the gold standard to detect and quantify vascular calcification. The magnitude of coronary artery calcification imaged using electron-beam CT is a strong predictor of cardiovascular mortality. Due to the high dose of radiation exposure, the utility of electron-beam CT is generally limited to research. Plain radiography, although not as sensitive as electron-beam CT, can also be used to detect vascular calcification. The National Kidney Foundation (NKF) Kidney Disease Outcomes Quality Initiative (KDOQI) guidelines suggest using plain radiography as an imaging modality, specifically lateral abdominal radiograph, if a practitioner chooses to assess calcification. There are two scoring systems that have been developed to systemically quantify vascular calcification using plain radiography. They are Kauppila and Adragao Scores. Kauppila scores evaluate lumbar aortic calcification. The segments of abdominal aorta in front of the lumbar spine L1-L4 are assessed. Adragao scores assess calcification in muscular arteries including the iliac, femoral, radial, and digital arteries. Plain radiography of the hands and pelvis are taken. Both high Kauppila and Adragao scores are associated with high cardiovascular mortality in patients with CKD. Since medial calcification can lead to arterial stiffness, ankle-brachial index and pulse wave velocity can also be used to assess vascular calcification.

Bone-Vascular Axis

Current literature suggests that there is a direct biologic interplay between the bone and vascular systems. Numerous epidemiologic studies demonstrate an inverse relationship between vascular calcification and bone density (i.e., patients with lower bone mass are more likely to have more vascular calcification). The relationship is well documented in the general population, postmenopausal women, and dialysis patients, and the association persists after adjusting for age. The mechanism linking bone activity and vascular calcification is complex and not well understood. Vascular calcification is an actively regulated cell mediated process with promoters and inhibitors of calcification. When exposed to a pathogenic environment, vascular smooth muscle cells undergo phenotypic changes to transition to osteoblast-like cells and lay down collagen which may then become mineralized and lead to overt vascular calcification. Several mechanisms have been proposed to explain the link between bone development and vascular calcification: 1) there are several common factors that are involved in bone remodeling and calcification, such as osteoprotegerin and activator of the nuclear factor-kappa B ligand system; 2) atherosclerosis of bone vessels may compromise bone blood supply affecting bone integrity; and 3) circulating complexes released from bone turnover, such as calcium/phosphate may promote vascular calcification.

Treatment

Management of CKD-MBD includes control of phosphorus, calcium, and PTH. It involves optimizing dietary phosphate intake, administration of phosphate binders, use of calcimimetics and vitamin D, and an appropriate dialysis prescription. For patients with severe hyperparathyroidism that is refractory to medical therapies, parathyroidectomy is recommended. In this section, we will discuss treatment targets and dietary phosphate and provide an overview of medical management. Phosphate binders, vitamin D therapy, and parathyroidectomy are discussed in greater detail in subsequent chapters.

Treatment Targets

The NKF/KDOQI guidelines in 2003 suggest the following optimal treatment targets for patients on dialysis: corrected serum calcium between 8.4 and 9.5 mg/dL, serum phosphorus between 3.5 and 5.5 mg/dL, and PTH between 150–300 pg/mL. In 2009, KDIGO (an independent international organization) proposed a different clinical practice guideline for the treatment of CKD-MBD. In 2010, NKF published a commentary summarizing the KDOQI and KDIGO guidelines and put the KDIGO guideline into the context of the supporting evidence and the setting of care delivered in the United States. These guidelines are summarized in Table 59.2. It is important to note that current practice guidelines are largely based on observational studies and expert opinions. There are no interventional randomized controlled trials to demonstrate that correcting the abnormalities in mineral metabolism (serum calcium, phosphorus, and PTH) will improve cardiovascular outcomes and patient survival.

Dietary Phosphate

Phosphorus is ingested from food as a constituent of phosphoprotein, phospholipids, and nucleotide phosphates. The typical Western diet has a high phosphate content, which comes from dairy products and protein sources. The KDOQI guidelines

Table 59.2

Treatment Targets Recommended by the National Kidney Foundation Kidney Disease Outcomes Quality Initiative (KDOQI) 2003 and Kidney Disease: Improving Global Outcomes (KDIGO) 2009 for Patients on Dialysis

	KDOQI	KDIGO	KDOQI Commentary*
Serum calcium	8.4–9.5 mg/dL	Maintain in normal reference range	Mortality risk increases with calcium 9.5–11.4 mg/dL
Serum phosphorus	3.5–5.5 mg/dL	Lower toward normal range	Mortality risk increases with phosphorus 5.0–7.0 mg/dL
Parathyroid hormone (PTH)	150–300 pg/mL	Maintain within ~2–9 times the upper reference limit	Corresponding to PTH of ~130–600 pg/mL; mortality risk increases with PTH 400–600 pg/mL

*KDOQI US Commentary on the 2009 KDIGO Clinical Practice Guideline for the Diagnosis, Evaluation, and Treatment of CKD–Mineral and Bone Disorder (CKD-MBD), published in the *American Journal of Kidney Disease* 2010.

suggest to restrict dietary phosphate to 800 to 1000 mg per day when serum phosphorus levels are >4.6 mg/dL in CKD stages 3 and 4 and >5.5 mg/dL in CKD stage 5. Since protein energy malnutrition is highly prevalent in patients on chronic dialysis, we generally do not recommend dietary protein restriction. Rather, it is important to differentiate the source of protein and phosphate.

In general, animal protein has higher phosphorus bioavailability compared to plant protein. Foods with a high phosphate load include nuts, hard cheeses, egg yolk, meat, poultry, and fish. Plant protein, especially grains, have a lower phosphate-to-protein ratio because most of the phosphate is in the form of phytate, which is not absorbed. Moe et al conducted a crossover trial of 9 patients with a mean eGFR of 32 mL/min/1.73 m^2 to compare the serum phosphorus and other hemostatic response to dietary phosphate intake after ingesting either meat or vegetarian diet of equivalent nutrients and found that 1 week of a vegetarian diet resulted in lower serum phosphorus and FGF23 levels.

In addition to the phosphate load from food, food additives also contribute significantly to phosphate retention in patients with CKD. Phosphorus in the form of phosphate salts (phosphoric acid, pyrophosphate, polyphosphate, and phosphate) is used in industrial food processing as food preservatives and as a color or flavor enhancer. Inorganic phosphate salts from the additives are almost completely absorbed in the gastrointestinal tract. Phosphorus additives are common and the amount of phosphorus load is considerable compared to the phosphorus content in natural food. Leon et al reviewed the food labels of ~2400 best-selling branded grocery products and found that 44% of these grocery items contained phosphorus additive—prepared frozen food (72%), dry food mixes (70%), packaged meat (65%), bread and baked goods (57%), and yogurt (51%). They also sampled meals for 4 days consisting of foods with and without phosphorus additive and found that meals composed mostly of phosphorus additive–containing foods had 736 mg more phosphorus per day compared with meals consisting of phosphorus additive-free foods.

It can be challenging to limit dietary phosphate intake because many foods contain phosphorus. It is crucial to differentiate the source of phosphorus, choose plant protein over animal protein, and to avoid foods with phosphorus-containing additives. Boiling can also reduce the phosphorus content in foods. The degree of mineral loss (calcium, phosphorus, sodium, and potassium) is proportional to the cooking time, amount of boiling water, and the size of the pieces.

Medical Management

Medical management of CKD-MBD includes oral phosphate binders, calcimimetics, and activated vitamin D therapy (Table 59.3). Oral phosphate binders limit the absorption of dietary phosphate and include calcium-containing and non-calcium-containing binders. Calcium-containing binders are less costly compared to non-calcium-containing binders, but they may result in a positive calcium balance and vascular calcification resulting in higher cardiovascular mortality. The impact of calcium load from calcium-containing binders on vascular calcification is greater in the presence of adynamic bone disease. Compared with calcium-containing binders, a recent meta-analysis of available studies suggests that non-calcium-containing binders may decrease mortality in patients with CKD. Jamal et al conducted a systemic review and meta-analysis of articles published between 2008 and 2012 to investigate the effect of calcium-containing binders versus non-calcium-containing

ı

Table 59.3

Medical Treatment of CKD-MBD

Phosphate Binders
Calcium-Containing Binders
Calcium carbonate
Calcium acetate

Non-Calcium-Containing Binders
Sevelamer hydrochloride/carbonate
Lanthanum carbonate
Sucroferric oxyhydroxide
Ferric citrate
Nicotinamide
Aluminum hydroxide/carbonate

Vitamin D Therapy
Vitamin D Derivative
Calcitriol (1,25-dihydroxycholecalciferol)

Vitamin D Analogs
Doxercalciferol
Paricalcitol
Alfacalcidol
Falecalcitriol
22-Oxacalcitriol

Calcimimetics
Cinacalcet

binders on mortality in patients with CKD and found that patients on non-calcium-containing binders had a 22% reduction in all-cause mortality compared with those on calcium-containing binders. Aluminum-containing binders are no longer used because of aluminum toxicity, which can manifest as dementia, osteomalacia, anemia, and arthritis. Iron-based phosphate binders, such as ferric citrate, are newer agents. Ferric citrate appears comparable to sevelamer in terms of phosphorus control and supplies iron, which may help to maintain hemoglobin levels.

Calcimimetics increase the sensitivity of the calcium-sensing receptor on the parathyroid gland to calcium and result in a substantial reduction in PTH and also lower calcium and phosphorus. Because of the hypocalcemic effect of calcimimetics and the risk of symptomatic hypocalcemia, calcimimetics should not be started if serum calcium is <8.4 mg/dL. The EVOLVE (Evaluation of Cinacalcet HCl Therapy to Lower Cardiovascular Events) trial tested the hypothesis that treatment with cinacalcet might reduce the risk of death or nonfatal cardiovascular events in patients undergoing dialysis with moderate to severe hyperparathyroidism. In the unadjusted intention-to-treat analysis, cinacalcet did not significantly reduce the risk of death or major cardiovascular events. Subsequent subgroup analysis showed that cinacalcet decreased the risk of death and major cardiovascular events in older, but not younger, patients on hemodialysis.

Vitamin D derivative (calcitriol) and synthetic vitamin D analogs bind to vitamin D receptors to increase intestinal calcium absorption and bone resorption, thus suppressing PTH. Vitamin D therapy should not be started until serum phosphorus has been controlled (<5.5 mg/dL) and serum calcium is <9.5 mg/dL because vitamin D may increase total calcium and phosphorus and promote vascular calcification. There have been no prospective studies demonstrating that the use of vitamin D or its analogs has any effect on cardiovascular mortality.

Optimal Dialysis Prescription

Phosphate is distributed unevenly in various compartments of the body with only a small amount in the plasma compartment and the majority in muscles, cell walls, and bone. Although hemodialysis can effectively remove phosphate, transferring of phosphate from these spaces to the plasma is relatively slow. Standard hemodialysis (4 hours per treatment) removes approximately as much phosphorus as is absorbed in a single day. However, patients eat 7 days a week and are generally dialyzed 3 days a week. Phosphate clearance can be improved through increasing the frequency of the dialysis treatments. Several studies have shown that patients undergoing short daily or nocturnal dialysis had better phosphorus control and required lower dose of phosphate binders. In peritoneal dialysis (PD), phosphate clearance may be influenced by PD modality (continuous ambulatory PD or continuous cycling PD) and membrane transport type.

Besides use of calcium-containing binders and vitamin D, a high dialysate calcium concentration also contributes to positive calcium balance in patients on hemodialysis. In a crossover study, Basile et al. measured hourly ionized calcium with 3 different dialysate calcium concentrations (2.5, 2.75 and 3.0 mEq/L). They found calcium balance was positive with all dialysate calcium concentrations and increased progressively with a higher dialysate calcium bath. The additional calcium influx to the patient transiently increases arterial blood ionized calcium, which suppresses PTH levels and induces bone mineralization. Once the bone becomes fully mineralized, the additional calcium contributes to calcification in soft tissue such as arterial media. In a randomized controlled trial, patients dialyzed against 1.75 mmol/L calcium bath had a faster progression of coronary artery calcification compared to those dialyzed against 1.25 mmol/L calcium bath. The KDIGO guidelines suggest using 1.25 mmol/L dialysate calcium bath as it results in a relatively neutral calcium balance in the majority of patients during dialysis.

Conclusion

CKD-MBD is a systemic disorder of mineral and bone metabolism manifested by abnormalities of calcium, phosphorus, PTH, FGF23, as well as bone disease and extra-osseous calcification. All of these abnormalities are associated with increased mortality in patients with CKD. Management of this complex disorder includes lowering dietary phosphate intake, administration of phosphate binders, use of calcimimetics, vitamin D, and appropriate dialysis treatments. In the past decade, there have been more data suggesting the potential harmful effect of calcium-containing phosphate binders and use of high dialysate calcium concentrations on vascular calcification, which could contribute to the high cardiovascular mortality in patients with CKD.

C H A P T E R   6 0

Phosphate Management in Patients With End-Stage Renal Disease

Laura Kooienga, MD • Antonio Bellasi, MD • Geoffrey A. Block, MD

Introduction

Achieving adequate control of serum phosphate (P) remains one of the most difficult challenges facing clinicians caring for patients with end-stage renal disease. Despite a global heightened awareness of the causes and consequences of elevated serum phosphate and in spite of advances in therapeutic interventions targeting this mineral disorder, only modest progress has been made toward routinely achieving the international recommendation of a "normal" P level of <4.6 mg/dL. Elevations in P are a key component of what is now referred to as CKD-MBD (chronic kidney disease–mineral and bone disorder), a systemic disorder affecting the skeleton and vasculature and is consistently associated with increased risk of all-cause mortality, cardiovascular mortality, vascular calcification, and valvular calcification. Effective control requires thoughtful attention to all aspects of phosphate homeostasis including diet, dialysis prescription, control of secondary hyperparathyroidism, and individualized prescription of medication to reduce intestinal phosphate absorption.

Phosphate Physiology

Phosphorus is the second most abundant element in the human body after calcium. Approximately 85% of phosphorus is located in bones and teeth, 14% is intracellular, and only 1% is extracellular. In normal adults, the fasting plasma phosphate concentration ranges from 2.5 to 4.5 mg/dL (0.80–1.45 mmol/L); however, the majority of healthy individuals have serum phosphate <4.0 mg/dL. This represents the net balance of daily dietary intake, intestinal absorption, skeletal influx/efflux, cellular redistribution, and urinary phosphate excretion. The recommended dietary allowance of phosphorus is 700 mg/day whereas the average dietary intake according to nutritional database information ranges from 1000 to 1800 mg (18–36 mmol) per day. These estimates however are now suspected to substantially underestimate actual phosphorus intake because of the routine use of phosphate additives in food processing. Recent reports indicate that when compared to phosphorus content measured by ash analysis, nutritional database estimates underestimate content by 35%–100%. Substantial quantities of phosphate in the form of additives have now been reported in commonly prescribed medications and common beverages as well. Foods high in phosphate are typically those also high in protein and include dairy products, meats, eggs, and cereal; however, the bioavailability of meat-based phosphate far exceeds that of plant-based phosphate because of the lack of naturally occurring phytase in the human gastrointestinal tract. Despite equivalent total phosphorus content, Moe et al reported significantly lower P exposure over 24 hours

with plant-based versus meat-based diets in patients with CKD. Given the importance of maintaining adequate total protein intake (1.2 g/kg/day) in patients on
dialysis, we concur with the recent recommendation to go beyond the superficial
assessment of total P content to evaluate both the bioavailability (natural and dependent on cooking method) and P density (mg P/gram protein) as suggested by
Kalantar-Zadeh. Intestinal absorption of phosphate is greatest in the jejunum and
ileum and occurs passively via a paracellular route and actively via a phosphate
sodium-dependent cotransporter (NaPi-2b). Basal phosphate absorption is a linear,
nonsaturable function of oral intake that is normally approximately 70% of ingested;
however, this may go up or down with NaPi-2b regulation by diet or active vitamin
D. Phosphate binder therapy affects only the passive, nonregulated component of P
absorption, a finding likely underlying the similar clinical efficacy of all available
treatments. Renal handling of phosphate occurs primarily by the regulation of
proximal tubule expression of type II-a and type II-c sodium phosphate cotransporter
(NaPi-2a/c). The daily filtered load of phosphate is approximately 4–8 g, and under
normal conditions only 5%–20% of the filtered phosphate is excreted. Parathyroid
hormone (PTH), 1α-25(OH)$_2$D$_3$, and fibroblast growth factor 23 (FGF23) are key
regulators of NaPi-2a/c expression and thus phosphate reabsorption in the renal
proximal tubule. FGF23 levels are extraordinarily elevated in patients receiving
dialysis (10-1000X ULN), and this has emerged as a plausible causative link between
CKD-MBD and cardiovascular disease, with elevated serum FGF23 levels consistently associated with adverse cardiovascular (CV) outcomes, particularly those
related to incident congestive heart failure or sudden death. Human data demonstrate
a linear relationship between FGF23 and left ventricular (LV) mass while animal
and preclinical data demonstrate that FGF23 can cause cardiomyocyte hypertrophy
and left ventricular hypertrophy (LVH) whereas pan-blockade of FGF receptors can
both regress and prevent LVH. These adverse effects are complementary yet distinct
from those seen with elevations in serum phosphate, which is universally recognized
to accelerate the development of vascular calcification and subsequent arterial
stiffening. It may be of clinical relevance that serum calcium, calcium load, and
active vitamin D all stimulate production of FGF23.

Phosphate Binder Therapy

Although elevated phosphate levels are consistently associated with adverse outcomes in multivariable adjusted analyses, there are no randomized controlled trials
demonstrating clinical benefit with their use. Indeed, most clinical trials with phosphate binders are of very short duration (4–12 weeks) although their actual application is long term (years). It remains undetermined if the current practice pattern of
prescribing phosphate binders is associated with net benefit or harm, particularly
when one considers that mean achieved phosphate remains at or above 5.0 mg/dL
in most reports. Several observational studies have reported survival benefits associated with phosphate binder use (independent of serum phosphate) although these are
quite susceptible to bias inherent among dialysis patients who do not require phosphate binders. A variety of agents have been used to create poorly soluble phosphorus
complexes in the intestinal lumen and in doing so limit passive phosphate absorption.
These agents include aluminum salts, calcium salts, magnesium salts, nonabsorbed
polymers, and most recently iron-containing compounds. All of these agents have
demonstrated similar clinical efficacy in reducing serum phosphate in patients

receiving dialysis (though they have not demonstrated efficacy in patients with non-dialysis-dependent CKD); however, each may be associated with side effects and class-specific limitations. As expected, gastrointestinal side effects are particularly common with intestinal phosphate binders.

Heavy Metal Compounds

Aluminum salts are highly effective phosphate binders, independent of pH. Unfortunately, despite limited total systemic absorption, clinical experience from the 1980s demonstrated that long-term use results in dementia, encephalopathy, microcytic anemia, and profound osteomalacia. Thus, in the United States, aluminum salts typically are used only as short-term therapy when other means of controlling phosphate have failed. In some parts of the world, there has been a resurgence of interest in the use of aluminum salts, with careful attention to the aluminum content of water and avoidance of concurrent use of citrate; however, serum aluminum levels are known to be a poor predictor of tissue aluminum levels, and the 2009 KDIGO guidelines do not endorse routine chronic use of aluminum salts.

Like aluminum, lanthanum carbonate (LC) is a heavy metal that potently binds intestinal phosphorus and that has minimal intestinal absorption, the result of which has not been demonstrated to result in clinical adverse effects. Unlike aluminum, it does not appear to cross the blood–brain barrier and therefore the potential for adverse neurologic effect is felt to be extremely low. Treatment with LC at doses of 500–3000 mg/day significantly reduces serum phosphate levels in a dose-related fashion with a significantly lower incidence of hypercalcemia and elevated calcium × phosphorus product when compared with calcium-based binders. LC has an adverse-event profile similar to other phosphate binders though it has clinically been associated with both diarrhea and intestinal obstruction, ileus, and fecal impaction. Use of LC has been reported to reduce FGF23 and in a secondary analysis of a randomized controlled trial was shown to improve all-cause mortality among dialysis patients older than 65 years.

Calcium-Based Compounds

After the discovery of the detrimental effects of aluminum-based binders, calcium-based binders became the most commonly prescribed phosphate binders and, in many parts of the world, remain so today. Calcium carbonate and calcium acetate are widely available, relatively inexpensive, and effective at reducing serum phosphate. However, they have a lower affinity for phosphorus compared with aluminum compounds and hence require larger doses with increased number of pills in order to achieve a satisfactory control of phosphate. In addition, they may provide a large calcium load, particularly if coadministered with concomitant active vitamin D compounds. Calcium acetate is composed of 25% elemental calcium and is effective across a wide range of intestinal pH whereas calcium carbonate is 40% elemental calcium and is less effective at alkaline pH (as in patients receiving H_2 blockers or PPIs). Although current recommendations suggest limiting total daily calcium intake to 1500 mg/day (estimating 500 mg/day from the diet), few data exist to support this target. A recent radio-labeled calcium balance study in patients with CKD stage 3 confirms a substantially positive calcium balance with small doses of elemental calcium while also demonstrating that in patients with this degree of residual renal function, the phosphate binder had no effect on overall phosphate balance. Notably, calcium accumulation has been implicated in the molecular mechanism underlying vascular calcification (VC) with potential synergy with serum phosphate in promoting calcification through enhanced expression of the sodium and phosphate cotransporter Pit-1 on the surface of vascular smooth muscle cells. Despite its near universal application as a "criterion" to approve a non–calcium phosphate binder, there is no rational basis for the common practice of using serum calcium levels to ascertain "safety" of using calcium-based phosphate binders. It is well known that serum calcium levels are effectively maintained within the normal range despite wide variation in calcium intake (low or high) and calcium balance (positive or negative).

Similarly, serum calcium levels poorly predict the risk of progressive VC.

Despite the low cost and widespread availability of calcium-containing binders, they have not significantly improved phosphorus control in patients receiving dialysis over the past two decades. Additionally, they increase the calcium burden, increase the risk of hypercalcemia, and are associated with the development of calcific uremic arteriopathy (formerly known as calciphylaxis). They have been demonstrated to increase the progression of VC and are likely to be associated with increased mortality as reported in a recent meta-analysis by Jamal et al. Although it is unclear whether the effect on mortality is mainly driven by one specific compound, calcium-free phosphate binders reduce the risk of all-cause mortality by 22% when compared to calcium-containing phosphate binders (risk ratio 0.78, 95% CI 0.61–0.98). It is for these reasons that it is our opinion that calcium-based phosphate binders should be considered third-line therapy for the control of serum phosphate. It is unclear based on available data if there is any "safe" dose of exogenous calcium. A recent trend to reduce the dialysate calcium concentration to <2.5 mEq/L in order to provide a theoretical margin of safety with regard to calcium balance has recently been associated with increased adverse events, including heart failure and intradialytic hypotension and cannot be recommended as a routine practice.

Nonabsorbable Polymers

Sevelamer hydrochloride was the first non-aluminum, non-calcium-based phosphate binder developed for the management of hyperphosphatemia in ESRD. This synthetic ion-exchange polymer is as effective as calcium-containing binders and is generally well tolerated, with an adverse event profile similar to placebo. Its major drawbacks are the large pill burden, gastrointestinal side effects, and high cost. However, when compared to other phosphate binders, sevelamer offers several potential advantages, including fewer hypercalcemic episodes, antiinflammatory effect, ability to lower total cholesterol and low-density lipoprotein (LDL) cholesterol, and ability to reduce uric acid levels. Furthermore, in a randomized clinical trial of 200 prevalent HD patients receiving treatment for 12 months with either sevelamer or calcium-based binders, a significant reduction in the progression of coronary artery and aortic calcification was found. In a different study, sevelamer use significantly attenuated coronary artery calcification progression in patients new to hemodialysis when compared to calcium-based binders. Preliminary data in CKD patients not receiving dialysis suggest that sevelamer reduces vascular calcification progression as well as the risk of the composite endpoint of all-cause mortality and dialysis inception (fully adjusted hazard ratio 0.62; 95% confidence interval 0.40–0.97) when compared to calcium carbonate. Notably, these effects seem independent of dietary phosphorus restriction. Finally, a recent study in 466 CKD patients incident to dialysis showed a significant reduction in the risk of cardiac arrhythmias, all-cause cardiovascular mortality, and all-cause mortality but not in the risk of death not related to cardiovascular events in patients treated with sevelamer versus calcium carbonate. These findings are supported by a propensity-matched analysis of U.S. hemodialysis patients that demonstrated a survival benefit associated with sevelamer use as compared to calcium-based phosphate binders. Overall, the available data suggest that the clinical advantages of sevelamer (no systemic absorption, no heavy metal or tissue accumulation, no contribution to calcium load, effective phosphate control, attenuation of vascular calcification and cardiovascular risk, and beneficial impact on lipids, uric acid, and markers of inflammation) solidify its use as a first-line phosphate binder in patients with CKD stage 5. It remains to be seen whether alternative, non-calcium-containing phosphate binders have similar aggregate benefits. Cost and pill burden remain significant obstacles from a global and individual patient perspective.

Magnesium-Based Binders

There is a resurgence of interest in using magnesium salts as potential alternatives to calcium given the inverse association between magnesium and cardiovascular events in the general population and data suggesting that magnesium may have a protective role with regard to vascular calcification. In general, magnesium-based phosphate binders are less potent than most calcium salts and can have significant systemic absorption resulting in increased serum magnesium levels, although a recent observational study has demonstrated that mortality in dialysis patients is highest among those with the lowest serum magnesium. Although the use of magnesium-free dialysate to help avoid hypermagnesemia in the setting of administration of magnesium salts is poorly tolerated, low magnesium dialysate concentrations of 0.6 mg/dL have been used successfully and are tolerated well. Recently, combination magnesium carbonate (60 mg elemental magnesium)/calcium acetate (110 mg elemental calcium) has been approved for hyperphosphatemia management after it was demonstrated to have similar clinical efficacy to other phosphate binders with similar tolerability. Interestingly, this combination magnesium/calcium P binder has been shown to reduce (favorably) the serum propensity to calcify when measured ex vivo. Experimental and clinical data support the notion that magnesium carbonate/calcium acetate effectively lowers serum phosphate and may attenuate vascular calcification progression as well as improve the bone and cardiovascular risk profile.

Iron-Based Therapy

Awareness of the risks associated with calcium-based phosphate binders has hastened the development of alternative treatment options. It has been recognized for many years that iron-based compounds could effectively bind phosphate, and two such compounds have recently been approved for the reduction of phosphate in patients on dialysis.

Sucroferric oxyhydroxide was demonstrated to be as effective in reducing serum P as compared to active control (primarily sevelamer and calcium) but with a substantially reduced pill burden of <4 pills/day. No change in systemic iron parameters were observed (as compared to the effects reported with ferric citrate below), and FGF23 was not assessed. Tolerability was comparable to active control, with the obvious exception of dark stools common to all iron preparations.

Ferric citrate was also compared to active control over a 52-week trial period and demonstrated equivalent P control while simultaneously increasing iron saturation and ferritin. Over the course of the 1-year trial, there was a significant reduction in use of ESA and intravenous iron. Tolerability was again comparable to active control although there were significantly fewer serious adverse events, including a reduced hospitalization for cardiovascular, infectious, and gastrointestinal reasons. FGF23 was not assessed in the phase 3 trials with ferric citrate but was assessed in a phase 2 trial in patients with non-dialysis-dependent CKD and was reduced by approximately 40%. A recent report suggests that total FGF23 is increased in iron deficiency anemia and is reduced with some, though not all, intravenous iron preparations. This suggests that the effect of ferric citrate on FGF23 may in part be related to treatment of iron deficiency.

Future Therapies

Several new or repurposed compounds are being investigated as future phosphate-reducing treatments. Nicotinamide is a nicotinic acid derivative (and component of niacin) that in a rat model has been found to inhibit sodium-dependent phosphorus cotransport via the NaPi-2b transporter located in the intestinal brush border membrane. Several clinical reports have demonstrated the ability of nicotinamide to reduce serum phosphate in patients with CKD though reduced platelet count has been reported as a potential complication. Clinical trials in patients with non-dialysis-dependent CKD are under way to assess the clinical efficacy of nicotinamide. Recently, it has been reported that a non-absorbed inhibitor of the sodium-hydrogen exchanger type 3 (tenapanor) was effective in reducing intestinal sodium and phosphate absorption in healthy volunteers whereas animal data supported a positive effect on attenuating the development of vascular calcification. Phase 1 clinical trials with tenapanor in dialysis patients confirmed the efficacy of this novel compound to reduce serum phosphate when given twice daily unrelated to meals. Finally, a third iron-based compound is being developed as a phosphate binder, adipate-modified iron oxide or PT20, and has reported clinical efficacy in phase 2 trials in patients on dialysis (personal communication).

Dialytic Control of Hyperphosphatemia

Even with optimal dietary phosphorus compliance and appropriate use of phosphate binders in conjunction with conventional thrice-weekly hemodialysis (CHD), neutral phosphate balance is difficult to obtain. Aside from dialysis duration and frequency, the major determinants of dialytic phosphate removal are dialyzer surface area and predialysis serum phosphate level. This is in part due to the complex elimination kinetics of phosphorus. Within the first 60–90 minutes of initiation of hemodialysis, there is a rapid reduction in serum phosphate level, followed by a decreased phosphate gradient between the plasma and dialysate with resulting less efficient transfer. Throughout the duration of the treatment the rate-limiting step in phosphorus removal is the relatively slow movement of phosphorus from the intracellular pools to the extracellular pool. Rebound in serum P begins during the last hour of dialysis, with a large rebound occurring after the termination of dialysis, reaching 70%–80% of predialysis serum phosphate values. Phosphate removal with a standard 4-hour hemodialysis treatment ranges between 600 and 1200 mg (1800–3600 mg/week) and with continuous ambulatory peritoneal dialysis averages 300–360 mg/day (2100–2520 mg/week). This amount is not substantially different by use of different dialyzers, types of renal replacement therapy, or with buffer used in dialysate. Two alternatives to conventional hemodialysis are short daily hemodialysis (defined as 3-hour sessions six times per week) and nocturnal hemodialysis, which is typically performed 3–6 nights per week for 8–10 hours while patients are sleeping. Both alternatives to CHD enhance phosphate removal and in some patients allow for an increased dietary phosphorus intake with a decreased requirement for phosphate binders, if required at all. The small Frequent Hemodialysis Network Trial (total n = 87) demonstrated that more frequent (6×/week) dialysis was associated with no statistical improvement in the primary outcome of death or change in LV mass but did find a benefit on the secondary endpoint of reduction in serum phosphate. A third alternative to conventional hemodialysis, hemodiafiltration, is also associated with modest increases in net phosphate removal and has been associated with improvement in all-cause mortality in a large, randomized controlled trial.

Skeletal Health and Phosphate

Classically attributed to severe tertiary hyperparathyroidism and/or use of vitamin D, phosphate (and calcium) efflux from bone contributes significantly to serum P, and several recent analyses suggest that even "adequately" controlled secondary hyperparathyroidism is contributing substantially to the difficulties in controlling serum phosphate. Li et al describe a nearly linear relationship across the spectrum of PTH between PTH and the risk of hyperphosphatemia and it has been a consistent finding that use of calcimimetic therapy reduces serum phosphate approximately 10% though it has no known effect on intestinal phosphate transport. Similarly, data on biochemical outcomes postparathyroidectomy demonstrate a nearly 50% reduction in serum phosphate (from >6 mg/dL to ≈3.5 mg/dL) 1 month postprocedure. More convincingly, data from a recent phase 1 trial of denosumab, a monoclonal antibody to RANKL that results in immediate inhibition of osteoclast activity, reduced serum phosphate by 1.5 mg/dL at 2 weeks in dialysis patients with baseline PTH <300 pg/mL. When interpreted in the context of the aforementioned postdialysis rebound in serum phosphate to 70% of predialysis values within 12–16 hours postdialysis, it appears that diet and dietary intervention alone are likely to contribute no more than perhaps 30%–35% to achieved serum phosphate. Caution is therefore urged in not labeling dialysis patients as "noncompliant" with P binders or diet on the basis of inadequate P control, and careful attention should be paid to the use of active vitamin D, achievement of adequate control of PTH, and the use of nonstandard dialysis schedules to achieve better P-related outcomes.

Conclusion

Given the substantial body of evidence associating higher phosphate levels in patients with CKD with increased all-cause and CV mortality, it is reasonable to continue to exert sustained effort directed at reducing serum phosphate when it is above 4.5 mg/dL. Beyond the direct benefits of reduction in serum phosphate, there is emerging data that reductions in FGF23 are independently associated with improved survival, and we must begin to consider the effects of our therapy on this important hormone (e.g., both calcium-containing P binders and active vitamin D increase FGF23). The only definitive way to assess whether there is net clinical benefit or harm of phosphate binders will be through randomized controlled trials testing either high versus "normal" achieved serum phosphate or perhaps with placebo controls. Given the lack of demonstrated benefit of current therapy and the clear potential for harm, clinical equipoise certainly exists. Indeed, despite the ongoing clinical standard of care practice, when rigorously evaluated in patients with non-dialysis-dependent CKD, the only placebo-controlled trial of P binders (LC, calcium acetate, and sevelamer) given for 9 months demonstrated minimal efficacy and, for some, clear evidence of harm. There is much to learn about the physiology of phosphate; the contribution of diet and cooking methods to serum phosphate; the impact of phosphate additives in medicine, beverages, and food; and the appropriateness of the current model of delivering adequate dialysis based on urea kinetics.

CHAPTER 61

Use of Vitamin D Sterols and Calcimimetics in Patients With End-Stage Renal Disease

Thanh-Mai Vo, MD • Kevin J. Martin, MD

Secondary hyperparathyroidism and altered bone and mineral metabolism are well-known complications of chronic kidney disease (CKD), which begin early in the course. Detailed investigations over the last several decades have uncovered the major pathogenetic factors involved in the generation and maintenance of these abnormalities.

As the glomerular filtration rate declines, there is, at least, a transient retention of phosphorus, an increase in the levels of fibroblast growth factor 23 (FGF-23), a progressive decrease in 1,25-dihydroxyvitamin D, and the development of skeletal resistance to parathyroid hormone (PTH). These changes contribute to the development and maintenance of secondary hyperparathyroidism.

There are both skeletal and extraskeletal effects (most notably, vascular calcification) that have been associated with these disturbances in mineral metabolism. Accordingly, these abnormalities need to be controlled in patients with decreased kidney function. As a result of a series of careful investigations that have uncovered the pathogenetic factors, therapies have been designed to target these abnormalities in order to control hyperparathyroidism. In general, these measures involve a multifaceted approach targeting the following:

1. Correction of hypocalcemia, if present
2. Control of hyperphosphatemia by dietary restriction and the use of phosphate binders
3. Administration of vitamin D sterols
4. Use of a calcimimetic

Often, these strategies are used in combination to achieve the control of hyperparathyroidism and, with the exception of calcimimetics, may be considered for use early in the course of CKD. It is important to note that calcimimetics are not approved for use in CKD patients who are not on dialysis. Whereas a vitamin D sterol-based approach would be reasonable in patients whose serum calcium values are low to low normal and whose phosphorus levels can be controlled, a calcimimetic-based approach may be more suitable for patients whose serum calcium values are high normal to high and phosphorus values remain above target. Both strategies may be used in combination.

The therapies are adjusted as required in an effort to meet the biochemical laboratory targets as recommended by Kidney Disease: Improving Global Outcomes (KDIGO). Thus, it is recommended that serum calcium values should remain in the normal range, serum phosphorus values should be reduced toward normal, and intact

PTH values should reside between 2 to 9 times the upper limit of normal for the assay used. Trends in intact PTH values should also be considered because an increasing intact PTH even within the target range may require therapy.

Role of Vitamin D Sterol Therapy

Because the decline in active vitamin D production plays a major role in initiating and maintaining secondary hyperparathyroidism, it is rational to include the use of vitamin D sterols as part of its treatment. Because nutritional vitamin D deficiency (low levels of 25-hydroxyvitamin D) commonly occurs early in the course of CKD, it is desirable to correct this deficiency early in this disease process (CKD stage 2 or 3). Current guidelines recommend measurement of 25-hydroxyvitamin D in patients with CKD, and if less than 30 ng/mL, oral supplementation with ergocalciferol or cholecalciferol should be given to achieve 25-hydroxyvitamin D level greater than 30 ng/mL. However, many patients are first seen when kidney disease is advanced, and supplementation with vitamin D (to achieve normalization of 25-hydroxyvitamin D levels) cannot overcome the reduced ability of the remnant kidney to produce the active sterol calcitriol. Accordingly, in advanced kidney disease, it is necessary to use active vitamin D sterols to achieve the desired result.

Calcitriol and other 1α-hydroxylated vitamin D sterols, such as 1α-hydroxyvitamin D_3 (alfacalcidol), 1α-hydroxyvitamin D_2 (doxercalciferol), and 19-nor-$1\alpha,25$-dihydroxyvitamin D_2 (paricalcitol), have been shown to be effective in the control of secondary hyperparathyroidism and improve bone histology. In patients with very elevated levels of PTH and severe nodular parathyroid hyperplasia, the effectiveness of vitamin D sterols may be limited because the expression of vitamin D receptor is decreased in such tissue. Accordingly, it appears rational to initiate treatment of secondary hyperparathyroidism with vitamin D metabolites early in its course before parathyroid hyperplasia has progressed to a refractory stage.

In patients with end-stage renal disease (ESRD), indications for therapy with vitamin D metabolites are more defined; however, hypercalcemia and hyperphosphatemia are frequent complications of therapy. Although 25-hydroxyvitamin D levels are decreased in patients with ESRD and ergocalciferol or cholecalciferol may be given to achieve an increase in 25-hydroxyvitamin D levels, the dosing consequences and benefits of this remains ill-defined. Active vitamin D sterols are increasingly used as oral or intravenous pulses given intermittently (e.g., three times weekly) rather than as continuous oral therapy. In recent years, analogs of calcitriol have been developed and include 22-oxacalcitriol (OCT), 1α-hydroxyvitamin D_2 (doxercalciferol), and 19-nor-$1\alpha,25$-dihydroxyvitamin D_2 (paricalcitol). These analogs have less calcemic activity than the parent compound and yet retain the ability to suppress PTH release in vivo. Formal direct comparisons between these compounds are not available, but it appears that all can be used effectively. In observational studies, a favorable effect on patient mortality has been associated with therapy with active vitamin D sterols; however, the mechanism of the effect has not been defined. Studies in experimental animal models with the use of vitamin D sterols demonstrated beneficial effects in the heart, kidney, and vascular reactivity, however, similar data in patients are currently lacking. The Paricalcitol Capsules Benefits Renal Failure Induced Cardiac Morbidity in Subjects With Chronic Kidney Disease Stage 3/4 (PRIMO) study by Thadhani et al, which was a multinational, double-blind, randomized, placebo-controlled trial, was conducted to test whether the administration of the vitamin D analog paricalcitol would have a beneficial effect on left ventricular mass (using cardiac magnetic resonance imaging) in patients with CKD. PTH levels were reduced when patients were given paricalcitol. Reduction in PTH levels were seen after 4 weeks, and levels were maintained within the normal range throughout the duration of the study. At 48 weeks, however, the change in left ventricular mass index did not differ between the control and treatment groups.

Role of Calcimimetic Therapy

An additional approach to the treatment of hyperparathyroidism in ESRD is the use of the calcimimetic agent cinacalcet hydrochloride. This calcimimetic agent activates the parathyroid calcium–sensing receptor and increases its sensitivity to calcium. In dialysis patients, cinacalcet hydrochloride results in a significant decrease in PTH levels and, when administered daily, can facilitate the control of hyperparathyroidism and help to achieve Kidney Disease Outcomes Quality Initiative (KDOQI) practice guideline targets for calcium, phosphate, and intact PTH. Serum calcium decreases with calcimimetic therapy; thus, cinacalcet is especially useful in patients with marginal or frank hypercalcemia or with hyperphosphatemia and can be used in conjunction with other therapies. If hypocalcemia occurs, then oral calcium supplements may be given; however, the long-term consequences of calcium loading in this situation are not well defined at the present time. Therapy with cinacalcet is often limited by nausea, which may limit compliance with this therapy. A Randomized Study to Evaluate the Effects of Cinacalcet Plus Low Dose Vitamin D on Vascular Calcification in Subjects With Chronic Kidney Disease Receiving Hemodialysis (ADVANCE) has evaluated the effect of cinacalcet on the progression of vascular calcification and appears to suggest that progression of vascular calcification may be attenuated with this approach. The EValuation Of Cinacalcet Hydrochloride (HCl) Therapy to Lower CardioVascular Events (EVOLVE) study, which was a multicenter, prospective, randomized, placebo-controlled trial, sought to examine the effect of cinacalcet therapy on survival in dialysis patients with hyperparathyroidism. This study included 3883 adult patients undergoing dialysis who either received cinacalcet or placebo for management of secondary hyperparathyroidism. Although there was improvement in the PTH levels in those who received cinacalcet, a significant difference in the risk of death or major cardiovascular events was not definitively demonstrated. It is important to note that almost 20% of patients in the placebo group began receiving commercially available cinacalcet before the occurrence of a primary event, which complicates the interpretation of these results.

The agents available, active vitamin D sterols and calcimimetics coupled with effective phosphate binders, can achieve control of secondary hyperparathyroidism and the abnormal bone and mineral metabolism in many cases. Therapy needs to be individualized because of the heterogeneity of the biochemical findings, the burden of disease, and the severity of comorbid conditions. After therapy is initiated, regular monitoring is needed to avoid overcorrection of the abnormalities that may result in conversion of high turnover bone disease (e.g., hyperparathyroidism) to low turnover adynamic bone disease. Such a development may also have serious consequences of extraskeletal, skeletal, and cardiovascular disease.

CHAPTER 62

Parathyroidectomy

Phuong-Chi T. Pham, MD, FASN • Phuong-Thu T. Pham, MD, FASN

The addition of the calcimimetic cinacalcet to the medical therapy for secondary hyperparathyroidism (sHPT) has conferred both better normalization of biochemical parameters (reduction in hypercalcemia and serum parathyroid hormone [PTH] levels) and a significant reduction in the need for parathyroidectomy in dialysis-dependent patients (relative risk, 0.49; 95% confidence interval 0.40–0.59; Cochrane analysis 2014). Nonetheless, medically refractory sHPT and tertiary HPT remain as serious complications in a minority of patients who eventually require invasive therapies.

Invasive parathyroid intervention involves direct percutaneous ablative injection therapy, subtotal or total parathyroidectomy, and combination subtotal parathyroidectomy and percutaneous injection.

As an adjunct to medical therapies and avoidance of surgery, a "pharmacologic parathyroidectomy" technique involving selective medical destruction of large resistant parathyroid glands and nodular hyperplastic tissues may be performed. In this technique, percutaneous ethanol is injected into a selected hyperactive gland in combination with calcitriol pulse therapy. Doppler ultrasonography is subsequently used to monitor the loss of blood supply to the treated gland, an indication of successful hyperactive tissue destruction. Although the procedure may be effective, it is associated with an increased risk of transient recurrent laryngeal nerve palsies. Subsequent trials substituting ethanol with calcitriol to avoid laryngeal nerve injuries yielded similarly successful results by some but not all investigators. The high local calcitriol concentration is thought to induce apoptosis of hyperplastic parathyroid cells while sensitizing the remaining cells to calcitriol and calcium via upregulation of their respective receptors.

The efficacy of direct parathyroid injection therapy, however, is limited to milder disease, smaller parathyroid glands (i.e., <500 mg) with two or less nodular lesions, easily accessible lesions per ultrasonographic guidance, and absence of ectopic glands. Recurrent disease with subsequent conversion to parathyroidectomy has been reported to occur in up to 20% of nontransplant candidates. Continuing exposure of remnant parathyroid tissues to the uremic milieu is thought to be the source for recurrent parathyroid hyperplasia. In addition, the procedure requires accurate technical expertise that may not be universally available. Nonetheless, percutaneous parathyroid injection therapy remains a viable option for selected medically resistant, nonsurgical candidates.

Indications for Parathyroidectomy (Table 62.1)

In general, medically resistant hyperparathyroidism correlates with diffuse hyperplasia or hyperplastic nodular formation or both. As sHPT progresses, the gland

Table 62.1

Indications for Parathyroidectomy*

Nonrenal Transplant Patients
- Elevated intact PTH levels >800 pg/mL associated with hypercalcemia or hyperphosphatemia that are refractory to medical therapy (KDOQI)
- Clinical signs and symptoms associated with refractory hyperparathyroidism
  - Hypercalcemia
  - Uncontrollable hyperphosphatemia
  - Evidence of osteitis fibrosa by bone biopsy, classic radiologic findings, or bone metabolic markers
  - Enlarged ± nodular parathyroid glands (>500 mg)
  - Calciphylaxis
  - Intractable pruritus
  - Progressive calcification of blood vessels
  - Severe skeletal deformity
  - Severe bone pain
  - Anemia resistance to erythropoietin
  - Peripheral neuropathy

Renal Transplant Recipients
- Severe and persistent hypercalcemia ≥11.5 mg/dL for ≥6–12 months and
- Symptomatic and progressive hypercalcemia
  - Nephrolithiasis
  - Persistent osteitis fibrosa
  - Progressive vascular calcification
  - Calciphylaxis
  - Calcium-related renal graft function deterioration

*Indications for parathyroidectomy are opinion based.
KDOQI, Kidney Disease Outcome Quality Initiative; *PTH,* parathyroid hormone.

evolves from a diffuse polyclonal hyperplastic pattern into monoclonal hyperplasic nodules, or tertiary hyperparathyroidism. Cells in the latter have diminished expression of both vitamin D– and calcium-sensing receptors, the binding sites for drug efficacy of active vitamin D and cinacalcet, respectively.

For patients with medically resistant hyperparathyroidism who may not undergo or lack access to direct parathyroid injection therapy, parathyroidectomy may be necessary. The incidence of parathyroidectomy among patients requiring renal replacement therapy has been estimated to range from 3 to 5 per 1000 patient-years during the first 3 to 5 years of dialysis and increases to 30 to greater than 40 per 1000 patient-years after 10 or more years of dialysis vintage.

Based on the Kidney Dialysis Outcome Quality Initiative (KDOQI) clinical practice guidelines, parathyroidectomy is recommended for patients with severe hyperparathyroidism with persistently elevated levels of intact PTH above 800 pg/mL in association with hypercalcemia or hyperphosphatemia who are refractory to medical therapy. Clinical manifestations consistent with medically refractory cases are summarized in Table 62.1. In the case of elevated PTH levels without radiologic evidence of high turnover bone disease, adynamic or aluminum bone disease must be ruled out because parathyroidectomy may worsen the underlying bone disease.

Additionally, noncompliance with medical therapy must be excluded before surgical consideration. The use of ultrasound with color Doppler to distinguish between medically resistant hyperplasia and medically suppressible disease caused by inadequate therapy or noncompliance has been advocated by some investigators. Although both scenarios present with markedly elevated serum intact PTH levels, their respective serial ultrasound with color Doppler findings may be distinct. Parathyroid glandular volume and vascularity reduction, with or without the formation of cystic-like lesions, and echogenicity normalization are observed with intensified medical therapy in suppressible disease in contrast to glandular enlargement and increased vascularity in medically refractory disease. Diagnosis with the former aborts any unnecessary parathyroidectomy. After resistant hyperparathyroidism is confirmed, parathyroidectomy should be promptly performed as safely tolerated to avoid progressive complications.

With a successful renal transplantation, approximately 50% of hyperparathyroidism cases will resolve by 3 to 6 months and most by 1 year. Persistent hyperparathyroidism to require parathyroidectomy, however, occurs at a typical prevalence of 5% but may vary from 1% to 20% among different transplant centers. Persistent hyperparathyroidism after renal transplantation generally reflects a poor functioning graft or tertiary hyperparathyroidism in a normal functioning graft. Indications for parathyroidectomy after renal transplantation include severe persistent hypercalcemia 11.5 mg/dL or greater persisting for more than 6 to 12 months, symptomatic hypercalcemia, nephrolithiasis, persistent metabolic bone disease, vascular calcification or calciphylaxis, and calcium-related renal allograft deterioration (see Table 62.1). Because spontaneous resolution of hyperparathyroidism may not occur rapidly, it is generally advisable to delay any plan for parathyroidectomy to 1 year posttransplant.

Preoperative Considerations

Preoperatively, decisions must be made with regards to the method and utility of radiologic localization of the parathyroid glands, type of parathyroidectomy to be performed, and routine medical management.

Preoperative Localization of Parathyroid Glands

In contrast to primary hyperparathyroidism in which imaging of the abnormal parathyroid glands and localization of the adenoma(s) before the first parathyroidectomy is recommended, a similar approach for sHPT is generally not necessary. Although good radionuclide localization techniques may provide slightly better sensitivity at detecting solitary adenomas than the observed rate of 90% to 95% with experienced surgeons, they provide significantly less sensitivity for detecting multigland hyperplasia, a common presentation of sHPT. Because of the lack of significant added benefit, the use of preoperative localization studies in patients with sHPT is not firmly established and may even be discouraged in some practices for fear of over reliance on imaging findings and resultant negligence in the search for ectopic glands.

For repeat parathyroidectomy because of persistent or recurrent disease or altered neck anatomy secondary to previous neck surgeries, however, preoperative localization is recommended. Functional imaging studies of parathyroid tissues with [99m]technetium- (Tc-) labeled sestamibi with subtraction or washout imaging to delineate parathyroid from thyroid glands are generally the study of choice. High-resolution ultrasonography may be combined to confirm equivocal scans. High-resolution computed tomography (CT) and magnetic resonance imaging have been disappointing and generally not recommended. Whether the introduction of four-dimensional CT, in which the fourth dimension measures temporal changes in hyperactive areas, provides any benefit in preoperative localization in sHPT remains to be defined. The combined use of single-photon emission CT with functional sestamibi imaging may be considered in cases with ectopic sites. Invasive procedures such as venous sampling of PTH or needle aspiration are associated with higher morbidity and cost and are thus rarely used except in difficult reoperative cases in which imaging techniques have failed to localize the abnormal tissues.

Parathyroidectomy Options

Three parathyroidectomy surgical options, including subtotal parathyroidectomy, total parathyroidectomy with autotransplantation (typically into the forearm), and total parathyroidectomy without autotransplantation, have been reported to result in varying success rates. Selection of the specific surgical option is based on expected procedure outcome and patient's clinical course. In general, subtotal parathyroidectomy is the preferred procedure if a patient has a higher chance to develop hypoparathyroidism than recurrent hyperparathyroidism after parathyroidectomy, but total parathyroidectomy with or without autotransplantation is the procedure of choice when the patient is expected to have high risks for recurrent disease.

In younger renal transplant candidates, subtotal parathyroidectomy sparing a generous remnant gland may be preferred because hypoparathyroidism may develop after a successful renal transplant. For older nonrenal transplant candidates with permanent exposure to uremia and a history of exposure to aluminum, total parathyroidectomy with autotransplantation may be preferred to avoid the potential postsurgical complication of hypoparathyroidism and resultant worsening of aluminum bone disease. When hyperparathyroidism recurs with autotransplantation, resection of the autograft in the arm is more easily performed than reexploration for the remnant parathyroid gland within the altered neck anatomy. Despite this surgical advantage, uncontrolled local tissue and vascular invasion as well as transformation into malignant tissue have been reported with autotransplantation. Delayed autotransplantation of cryopreserved parathyroid tissues versus immediate autotransplantation with fresh tissues may be an alternative option. Delayed autotransplantation may be advantageous because it allows for in vitro testing of the parathyroid tissues' potential for autonomous growth and may avert the reintroduction of irrepressible hyperplastic tissues. In addition, the delay may allow for abortion of the procedure in patients who develop recurrent hyperparathyroidism at subsequent follow-up. It must be emphasized, however, that the eventual use of cryopreserved tissues has been reported to be less than 1% to 2%, and the rate of functional autotransplantation has also been noted to be disappointing, particularly at small, inexperienced centers (<20%). The practicality and associated costs of routine parathyroid tissue cryopreservation have been recently questioned.

For permanent dialysis-dependent, nonrenal transplant candidates with no history of aluminum exposure, total parathyroidectomy without autotransplantation may be preferred because the risk of permanent hypoparathyroidism and subsequent aluminum bone disease in the persistently uremic state is relatively low. Several authors have shown that long-term hypoparathyroidism was relatively uncommon, and clinically significant adynamic bone disease was exceptionally rare. The absence of hypoparathyroidism was attributed to the eventual proliferation of unrecognized small embryonic residual parathyroid tissue. Long-term efficacy and safety for the use recombinant parathyroid hormone in the event of chronic hypoparathyroidism following total parathyroidectomy in patients with chronic kidney disease or kidney transplant remain to be studied.

Preoperative Medical Management

In preparation for parathyroidectomy, both hematologic and electrolyte abnormalities should be maximally corrected. In addition, basal levels of calcium, magnesium, phosphate, and intact PTH are obtained. Dialysis-dependent patients should receive anticoagulant-free dialysis the morning of surgery to optimize platelet function and minimize bleeding risks. Patients with severe anemia should receive blood transfusions to further minimize uremic bleeding diathesis. Preoperative vitamin D sterols and calcium supplements have also been advocated to minimize the risk of postoperative hypocalcemia and hypophosphatemia. Reduction or discontinuation of phosphate binders may also be considered to avoid postoperative hypophosphatemia. In addition, preoperative direct or indirect laryngoscopy is recommended to assess vocal cord function in all patients who have had recent alteration in voice quality or previous thyroid or parathyroid operations.

Operative Procedure

A successful parathyroidectomy mandates a meticulous methodical approach and a comprehensive understanding of the embryologic development of the parathyroids as well as their common locations in adulthood. The variability in location of the parathyroid glands is summarized in Table 62.2.

In general, during the operation, the patient is positioned with the neck extended to bring the thyroid and parathyroid glands anterosuperiorly to facilitate the exploration. The deeper structures within the neck are reached from the midline after lifting of the subplatysmal flaps and strap muscles off the thyroid gland. The thyroid lobe is subsequently retracted out of the neck to expose the space between the thyroid gland and the carotid artery, trachea, and esophagus. Both laryngeal nerves are promptly identified before the search for any parathyroid gland. A systematic approach is used to identify the superior followed by the inferior glands. Visualization of all parathyroid glands, including supernumerary glands, is crucial. Excision of fat tissues surrounding the parathyroid glands, bilateral removal of the thymic tongue, and exploration of the carotid sheaths bilaterally are required to uncover supernumerary glands. In total parathyroidectomy with autotransplantation, tissue suitable for grafting is selected after histologic examination of each gland on frozen section. The chosen tissue typically comes from the smallest gland without macroscopically visible nodules. The glandular tissue (50–90 mg) is sliced into approximately 30 1 × 1- × 3-mm pieces to be used for immediate autotransplantation into 20 to 30 pockets in the brachioradial muscle or cryopreserved for delayed autotransplantation. Although more studies and experience are needed, subcutaneous infusion of normal parathyroid tissue has been reported to be a simple approach for parathyroid tissue implantation that could obviate the need for more invasive autotransplantation.

In subtotal parathyroidectomy, the smallest and non-nodular gland is selected for partial resection, and its viability is assured before resection of the remaining glands.

Table 62.2

Common Locations of Parathyroid Glands

	Location	Percentage
Superior glands	Cricothyroidal or juxtathyroidal (within 1 cm superior to the intersection of the RLN and the ITA)	75–80
	Upper pole of thyroid gland	20
	Intrathyroid	2–5
	Retroesophageal or retropharyngeal	1
Inferior glands	Tissue immediately adjacent to thyroid lower pole	40–60
	Tongue of thymic tissue (between the inferior border of the thyroid gland and clavicle)	40
	Intrathyroid	2–5
	Ectopic (migrational path from base of tongue to lower neck)	2
	Anterior mediastinum	1

ITA, inferior thyroid artery; *RLN,* recurrent laryngeal nerve.

Intraoperatively, two valuable tools may be used to optimize surgical outcomes. The most beneficial technical advance has been attributed to the development of a rapid intraoperative PTH assay. The short half-life of PTH ($\approx$3 minutes) and the rapid turnaround time for PTH detection (8–20 minutes) allow surgeons to intraoperatively assess the adequacy of parathyroid tissue resection and the need to search for ectopic glands. Likewise, the rapid PTH assay can prevent excessive glandular tissue removal and postoperative hypocalcemia. The availability of intraoperative PTH measurements, however, is not universally available.

Another technique that surgeons may use intraoperatively to detect hyperfunctioning glands is nuclear mapping with ^{99m}Tc-sestamibi. In this technique, ^{99m}Tc-sestamibi is administered intravenously 2 to 6 hours before surgery. The characteristic differential and late retention of the isotope within the parathyroid tissue may be used to localize the affected glands intraoperatively with a handheld gamma detector. It must be noted, however, that the sensitivity of gamma-probe localization has better sensitivity in detecting adenomas than hyperplastic glands. The best use of nuclear mapping involves cases in which significant scarring has occurred from previous neck surgeries or when ectopic glands are present.

Postoperative Management

In the postoperative period, close monitoring of different electrolytes is required because significant changes may occur (Table 62.3). Hypocalcemia, specifically, occurs in almost all cases. Serum calcium level may decrease by as much as 60% of the preoperative level. The hypocalcemic nadir typically occurs during the first 2 to 4 postoperative days. Restoration to normal calcium level may occur within 2 weeks, but hypocalcemia may remain severe for several months in a subset of patients. In patients undergoing autotransplantation, hypocalcemia may persist until the implanted tissue is able to provide adequate function in 2 to 3 weeks up to 1 year after surgery. Hypocalcemia-associated tetany and seizures have been observed

Table 62.3

Electrolyte and Metabolic Abnormalities Following Parathyroidectomy

Electrolyte and Metabolic Abnormalities		Mechanisms	Onset and/or Duration	Management
Calcium	Hypocalcemia	Hungry bone syndrome	First 2–4 days; Usually normalizes within 2–3 weeks	Calcium, calcitriol supplements
		Failure of autograft function	May recover within 2–3 weeks, but may be permanent	Calcium, calcitriol supplements; Consider implantation of cryopreserved parathyroid tissue
		Inadequate remnant gland	Usually recovers with persistent uremic state (i.e. if no renal transplant)	Calcium, calcitriol supplements; Consider implantation of cryopreserved parathyroid tissue
	Hypercalcemia	Excessive calcium, calcitriol supplements	Days to weeks following surgery	Decrease calcium, calcitriol use
		Missed ectopic gland; Inadequate gland removal	Persistent hypercalcemia	Radiological ± invasive localization
Phosphorus	Hypophosphatemia	Hungry bone syndrome	First 2–4 days to one year	Phosphorus supplement; Encourage high intake of dairy products
Magnesium	Hypomagnesemia	Hungry bone syndrome	First 2–4 days to perhaps one year	Magnesium supplement
Potassium	Hyperkalemia	Vitamin D deficiency and/or hypocalcemia associated reduction in insulin secretion	Within the first 10–12 hours	Glucose and insulin; Hemodialysis for life-threatening hyperkalemia and poor kidney function
Other	Alkaline phosphatase	Hungry bone syndrome	Increases over the first 4 days; Peaks at 7–14 days; Decreases by third week and normalizes by 6 months	Must rule out liver abnormality

to occur more frequently during or closely after dialysis unrelated to the lowest calcium level. We speculate that the degree of blood alkalinization with dialysis and resultant decrease in ionized calcium may be contributory. Rapid correction of metabolic acidosis with dialysis should be avoided if possible.

The abrupt decrease in calcium level after parathyroidectomy in patients with high bone turnover has been attributed to the marked reduction in osteoclastic activity in association with the decrease in PTH levels and unopposed osteoblastic activity, a phenomenon known as "hungry bone syndrome." Other possible associated biochemical alterations include a decrease in serum phosphate and magnesium levels and an increase in serum alkaline phosphatase levels. Reported risks for hungry bone syndrome include severe preoperative bone disease, osteitis fibrosa cystica, "brown tumors," lower initial serum calcium, and younger patient age. Although not universal, preoperative biochemical findings predictive of hungry bone syndrome have been suggested to include higher serum calcium, PTH, and alkaline phosphatase levels and lower serum magnesium and albumin levels.

Early postoperative calcium levels may be used to predict hypocalcemia. Whereas an initial upsloping postoperative calcium curve based on two calcium measurements within the first 24 hours has been shown to be strongly predictive of a stable postoperative calcium level, a steeply downsloping initial calcium curve may predict eventual hypocalcemia. Greater PTH levels correlate well with bone histology and osteoblastic activity and may be used as a surrogate predictor of postparathyroidectomy hypocalcemia.

Strategies to ameliorate postparathyroidectomy hypocalcemia include preoperative administration of an active vitamin D metabolite (e.g., calcitriol 2–4 µg/day 2 days before surgery), close postoperative calcium level monitoring, and aggressive postoperative calcium and calcitriol supplementation.

As soon as the patient can tolerate oral intake, elemental calcium at 1 to 2 g orally three times a day may be given. At 4 hours postparathyroidectomy, a serum calcium level must be obtained. A decrease in serum calcium of greater than 10% is indicative of the need for intravenous (IV) calcium supplement (100 mL of 10% calcium gluconate mixed in 150 mL 5% dextrose mixture to run at 20–30 mL/hr or ≈90 mg/hr of elemental calcium). Otherwise, continuation of oral calcium supplement may suffice. Monitoring of calcium levels should be continued every 6 hours for the next 2 to 3 days and tapered off in frequency when calcium levels stabilize. In emergent cases of symptomatic hypocalcemia, 20 to 30 mL of the above solution mixture may be infused over 10 to 15 minutes followed by a continuous infusion at 20 to 30 mL per hour as deemed necessary by subsequent calcium levels and symptoms. Postoperative continuation of vitamin D is recommended to minimize the mean postoperative reduction in serum calcium as well as the amount of calcium required for supplementation. Both vitamin D and calcium doses should be adjusted to maintain normal calcium levels.

New-onset hypercalcemia after parathyroidectomy is unusual but may occur as a result of excessive calcium and calcitriol supplements. Alternatively, postoperative persistence of hypercalcemia may signify inadequate parathyroid gland removal, missed ectopic glands, or misdiagnosed cause of hypercalcemia. Radiologic localization of the parathyroid glands is required in persistent hypercalcemic cases for surgical reexploration.

Postparathyroidectomy hypophosphatemia is uncommon among patients with renal failure. Nonetheless, hypophosphatemia may occur because of reduced phosphate mobilization from bone and enhanced uptake for bone formation. Patients with significant existing periarticular calcium phosphate deposits may actually benefit from a higher degree of phosphorus mobilization and amelioration of hypophosphatemia. Supplementation with both oral and IV phosphate salts may be used with close monitoring. If the patient has concurrent hypocalcemia, phosphate supplementation must be given in between meals to avoid binding with calcium in the gastrointestinal tract and resultant reduction in calcium absorption. As with hypophosphatemia, postparathyroidectomy hypomagnesemia is uncommon among renal patients but may occur in association with the hungry bone syndrome. Correction of hypomagnesemia to normal range is warranted to avoid other metabolic complications, including poor response to calcium supplementation among those with hypocalcemia.

Hyperkalemia has been commonly observed both intra- and postoperatively. Intraoperative serum potassium levels greater than 7.0 mEq/L have been reported. The onset and degree of hyperkalemia seem to correlate with the time and degree of hypocalcemia, respectively. Although the responsible mechanisms for postparathyroidectomy hyperkalemia have not been elucidated, we propose that vitamin D deficiency and hypocalcemia may induce insulin deficiency and a resultant reduction in intracellular potassium shift. In mice lacking a functional vitamin D receptor, the expression of insulin mRNA has been shown to be suppressed. In addition, hypocalcemia per se may reduce insulin secretion. In patients with moderate or severe hyperkalemia, a trial of IV glucose and insulin (e.g. 1 ampule of 50% dextrose with 5–10 units or regular insulin) may be administered. A low level of 5% dextrose infusion alone has not proved adequate in preventing postparathyroidectomy hyperkalemia. Life-threatening hyperkalemia requires emergent hemodialysis.

Postoperative elevation of plasma bone-specific alkaline phosphatase has also been described. A significant increase may be observed 4 days after parathyroidectomy with a peak value at 7 to 14 days. A decrease in the alkaline phosphatase level is expected to occur by the third postoperative week with normalization by the sixth postoperative month. The postoperative change in plasma alkaline phosphatase level has been attributed to enhanced osteoblastic activity.

Suggested perioperative management guidelines for parathyroidectomy are summarized in Table 62.4.

Other Postparathyroidectomy Complications

In addition to the electrolyte and metabolic disturbances observed after parathyroidectomy, other complications may occur. Direct surgical complications include pain, poor wound healing, formation of a hematoma or seroma, and damage to the recurrent laryngeal nerve with vocal cord paralysis. As previously noted, both hypo- and hyperparathyroidism may be observed postoperatively. Hypoparathyroidism may result from inadequate remnant parathyroid mass or poor function of the remnant tissue caused by infarction. In the setting of hypoparathyroidism, existing undiagnosed aluminum-related osteomalacia may worsen. Persistent hyperparathyroidism may occur secondary to missed accessory glands or incomplete parathyroidectomy and may require reexploration. Proliferation of the remnant tissue may contribute to recurrent hyperparathyroidism, particularly among patients with continuing exposure to the uremic milieu. Finally, in some patients with pre–end-stage renal disease, significant postoperative deterioration in renal function has been reported. Earlier

Table 62.4

Suggested Perioperative Management for Parathyroidectomy

Preoperative Period
- Routine preoperative evaluation
- Normalization of electrolytes as much as possible
- Transfusion with packed red blood cells to maintain hemoglobin >8.5 g/dL
- Start vitamin D supplement (e.g., calcitriol 2-4 μg/day for 2 days before surgery)
- Reduction or discontinuation of phosphate binders
- Dialysis morning of surgery if dialysis dependent
- Imaging of parathyroid glands for reexploration parathyroid surgery or altered neck anatomy

Postoperative Period
- Calcium supplement 1–2 g orally three times a day as soon as oral intake is possible
- Intravenous calcium supplement (1–2 mg elemental calcium/kg body weight/hr)* if poor oral intake or significant hypocalcemia (ionized calcium <3.6 mg/dL or corrected total calcium <7.2 mg/dL)
- Continue with vitamin D supplement (i.e., calcitriol 2 μg/day)
- Electrolyte monitoring[†]
  - Serum ionized calcium levels at 4–6 hours postoperatively, then every 6 hours for 2–3 days, and then every 12–24 hours until stable
  - Serum potassium at 4 hours postoperative; then q every hours for 2 days or until stable
  - Serum phosphate, magnesium at 4 hours postoperative; unless significantly abnormal, recheck levels the next morning
  - Intact PTH level and alkaline phosphatase the next morning; repeat and follow up as clinically indicated

---

*See text for calcium solution mixture and rates of infusion.
[†]Levels of different electrolytes may need to be checked more frequently if they are severely abnormal.
PTH, parathyroid hormone.

---

case reports suggested that aggressive calcium and vitamin D supplementation may have been contributory presumably because of significant renal cortical calcification. More recently, it has been suggested that PTH per se has vasodilatory effects on afferent arterioles and vasoconstrictive effects on efferent arterioles. The acute decrease in PTH levels after parathyroidectomy causes a reversal in renal hemodynamics and hence a fall in glomerular filtration pressure, an effect that may adversely affect patients with marginal renal function.

Finally, it must be noted that despite a reduction in the need for parathyroidectomy in the calcimimetic age, differences in long-term morbidity and mortality between calcimimetic-manageable sHPT and parathyroidectomy are not known. Although most reports suggest improved long-term survival with parathyroidectomy, current data with calcimimetics have not shown similar benefits.

SECTION XXIII

Acquired Cystic Kidney Disease

C H A P T E R 6 3

Acquired Cystic Kidney Disease

Anthony Chang, MD

There are many types of cystic diseases of the kidney, but a specific form often occurs in end-stage renal disease (ESRD) patients. *Acquired cystic kidney disease* (ACKD) is defined by the presence of four or more renal cysts for both kidneys and an absence of any hereditary renal cystic disease. These cysts are associated with potential complications, including significant bleeding and malignant neoplasms.

Epidemiology

Acquired cystic kidney disease is more commonly observed in men and those of African descent. Acquired renal cysts are found in fewer than 10% of predialysis patients with long-standing azotemia (serum creatinine >2.5 mg/dL). However, the incidence increases to 10% to 20% after 1 to 3 years of dialysis and to 90% or greater in those dialyzed for more than 8 to 10 years. These cysts have been reported in patients on either peritoneal dialysis or hemodialysis. Azotemia is the only consistent factor in the development of ACKD.

Pathophysiology

The pathophysiology of acquired renal cysts is uncertain, but numerous etiologic factors have been proposed, including ischemia, intratubular obstruction from casts or calcium oxalate crystals, and interstitial fibrosis leading to extratubular constriction and obstruction. These cysts form from tubules and often remain in communication with one or more tubular segments. The cysts are usually lined by a single layer of epithelial cells, which reveal an increased proliferative capacity, and some may demonstrate epithelial hyperplasia with tufting of the cells. All of these features are suggestive of increased tubular cell growth. The immunophenotype of most cyst-lining cells is often consistent with proximal tubular epithelial cells but can also consist of distal nephron epithelial cells. Cysts tend to be larger and more numerous and to exhibit increased growth in males compared with females. Kidney transplantation reduces the incidence of ACKD because cysts can regress.

There are increased levels of inflammatory cytokines, including interleukin-6 (IL-6) and IL-8 and c-*jun*, in patients with ACKD. The proto-oncogene c-*jun* has been noted to be increased in early cyst formation associated with hyperplastic epithelium. Although c-*jun* activation was not noted uniformly in cystic kidneys with renal cell carcinoma (RCC), other specific growth factors remain to be identified. It is also known that cyst growth is increased by substances that stimulate cyclic adenosine monophosphate (cAMP) and that high levels of cAMP are found in dialysis patients, possibly as a response to parathyroid hormone (PTH). Other potential "renotropic factors" remain to be identified. Of interest, apolipoprotein L1 (*ApoL1*) is expressed in proximal tubular epithelial cells, and microcystic tubular dilation and thyroidization-type tubular atrophy were recently found to be fairly specific features in the kidneys of patients with two *ApoL1* risk alleles (G1 or G2 variants). The specific role of *ApoL1* has not been studied in ACKD, but given the increased incidence in those of African descent, this potential connection may be worth further consideration.

Clinical Course and Complications

The renal cysts of ACKD alone are not worrisome, but there are two important consequences with clinical implications. First, hemorrhage with hematuria is the most frequent complication, occurring in 14% of ACKD patients, and a smaller subset of patients may develop perirenal or retroperitoneal hematomas or rarely renal rupture. Second, the cysts may represent the earliest precursor lesion of RCC because some cysts that are lined by a single epithelial cell layer demonstrate the identical immunophenotype of concurrent neoplasms, when present. Therefore, the risk of developing RCC in this population can be more than 100 times greater than in the general population with normal renal function, but overall, this remains a rare complication with an annual incidence of less than 1%.

In the earliest reports, one third of patients with cysts were found to have neoplasms. Most neoplasms were small, which were classified as renal adenomas based on their size (<5 mm) and may be multifocal and bilateral. Larger neoplasms may represent RCC. There are two common subtypes of RCC in the setting of ACKD: (1) ACKD-associated RCC and (2) clear cell papillary RCC, which are both recognized by the 2016 World Health Organization classification of renal tumors. Other subtypes of RCC, such as conventional clear cell, papillary, and chromophobe, can also occur. ACKD-associated RCC is the most aggressive subtype and has the capacity for nodal metastasis at the time of diagnosis even when the primary mass is less than 3 cm in size, which contrasts with the other subtypes of RCC. Some of these tumors may develop in the native kidneys of patients after kidney transplantation. Tumors have even occurred in pediatric patients who have been on dialysis for a prolonged period.

Diagnosis and Screening

Two imaging techniques have been the mainstays for detection of renal cysts. Ultrasonography is an easy, noninvasive method. However, end-stage kidneys are often shrunken and exhibit marked increased echogenicity, making cysts difficult to detect with ultrasonography. In addition, the low resolution of this technique may preclude the detection of small cysts and tumors (<0.5 cm in diameter) often seen during the early stages of ACKD.

Although computed tomography (CT) scanning is more expensive and difficult to perform, it affords higher resolution, enabling detection of small cysts and tumors in shrunken kidneys. The intravenous (IV) administration of contrast material may further enhance tumor detection (Fig. 63.1). Helical CT with early enhancement rather than delayed enhancement may be superior in the detection of early tumors in ACKD. Magnetic resonance imaging with gadolinium for further evaluation of complicated cystic renal lesions may be the best technique. However, nephrogenic

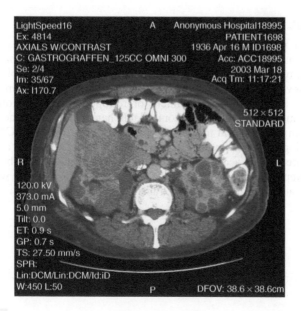

Figure 63.1

Large acquired cystic kidneys with a large tumor in the right kidney. This tumor was found because of gross hematuria and was noted to be metastatic.

systemic fibrosis is a potential devastating complication of gadolinium use, so this particular compound is best avoided in patients with ESRD.

Screening for ACKD and malignant neoplasms is controversial, and guidelines for dialysis patients have not been established. Schwarz and colleagues have recently suggested screening guidelines for kidney transplant patients. They recommend annual ultrasound imaging of native kidneys regardless of ACKD status. The frequency of ultrasound screening would increase with the complexity of renal cysts as detected by imaging. Screening for malignant neoplasms in ACKD patients is projected to achieve only a modest gain in survival over a 25-year period with significant economic costs and possible harm from imaging procedures because of radiation exposure. However, screening may be more beneficial in younger patients and those with fewer comorbidities and longer life expectancies. For this reason, patients are screened yearly in Japan. Other factors to be considered include the duration of azotemia (serum creatinine >2.5 mg/dL for 3–5 years) and the length of time on dialysis. Special consideration should be given to patients awaiting renal transplantation. All such patients should be screened for ACKD and tumors, regardless of the duration of azotemia or dialysis. This screening will identify those patients with tumors before instituting active immunosuppression therapy.

The onset of symptoms such as hematuria or flank pain in a dialysis or chronically azotemic patient should lead to a prompt investigation for ACKD. Males with acquired cysts may need evaluation more frequently.

Treatment

Only a small proportion of ACKD patients develop significant complications. Hemorrhage into cysts or the collecting system is the most common. Usually, this bleeding requires only pain control. Aspirin should be avoided. If bleeding persists or becomes severe, wire-loop embolization remains an option. A similar conservative approach is used for the treatment of retroperitoneal hematomas, although nephrectomy may be needed for uncontrollable hemorrhage or intractable pain.

Nephrectomy is the usual treatment for RCC in the setting of ACKD. However, nephron-sparing surgeries (radiofrequency ablation or cryoablation) and even active surveillance are gaining acceptance, especially in patients who may be poor surgical candidates. Nephrectomy should also be performed in all patients with tumors of any size who are candidates for renal transplantation.

SECTION XXIV

Diabetes

C H A P T E R   6 4

End-Stage Renal Failure in the Diabetic Patient

Mark E. Williams, MD, FACP, FASN

The Diabetic ESRD Population

Diabetes mellitus has emerged as the health epidemic of the 21st century, and with it diabetic kidney disease has become the single most important cause of end-stage renal disease (ESRD) worldwide. Although diabetes-related complications have declined over time, the rates of ESRD have decreased less than the rates of other complications. Furthermore, kidney disease accounts for most of the excessive cardiovascular and all-cause mortality risk associated with diabetes. In 2012, a total of 49,258 Americans with diabetes listed as a primary cause initiated chronic dialysis to treat ESRD and its complications, 43% of the total incident population; of 636,905 prevalent ESRD patients, 38% were attributed to diabetes. (In total, diabetes is present in about 60% of all U.S. dialysis patients.) Of prevalent patients, those with ESRD attributed to diabetes were more likely to be treated with in-center hemodialysis and less likely to have a transplant than other patients (Fig. 64.1). The incidence of ESRD due to diabetes is higher with increasing age, and significantly higher in blacks/African Americans, Hispanics, Asians, and Alaskan natives, compared with whites. This chapter emphasizes features of special importance to the adult ESRD population with diabetes.

Predialysis Care/Dialysis Initiation

Patients with diabetic CKD may develop symptoms such as gastroparesis or neuropathy that mimic those of uremia; may be prone to malnutrition, hyperkalemia, or volume overload; or may develop uremic symptoms earlier than those without diabetes. Conventional wisdom has been that ESRD patients with diabetes require earlier initiation of dialysis than nondiabetics, a "preventive" strategy to slow progression of some complications of diabetes, and to improve outcomes. Although the trend toward early dialysis starts in the general ESRD population reversed, starting in 2009, diabetic patients continue to be among patients in whom dialysis is initiated early. Diabetes strongly predicted early start of dialysis according to the USRDS. As shown in the 2014 USRDS annual data report, patients with diabetes (eGFR 11.6 mL/minute) continue to start dialysis on average with a slightly higher eGFR than those without diabetes (10.9 mL/minute). Recent guidelines continue to support early initiation for patients with diabetes. Relative to other outcomes data, information concerning mortality rates and factors that influence mortality soon after initiation of dialysis in incident dialysis patients is limited. Mortality risk among hemodialysis patients is highest in the first 3–4 months after dialysis initiation. Data

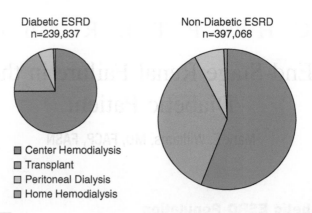

Diabetic ESRD
n=239,837

Non-Diabetic ESRD
n=397,068

☐ Center Hemodialysis
☐ Transplant
☐ Peritoneal Dialysis
☐ Home Hemodialysis

Figure 64.1

Relative populations and treatment modalities for U.S. prevalent ESRD patients, 2012. (Source: USRDS Data Report, 2014.)

on risk/benefit of early initiation in patients with diabetes, however, report mixed results.

Dysglycemia

The maintenance of glucose homeostasis is affected both by diabetes and by kidney failure. The core pathologic defects in diabetes are decreased insulin secretion (type 1) and insulin resistance, impaired insulin secretion, increased hepatic glucose production, decreased glucose uptake by muscle, and increased renal glucose reabsorption (type 2). When kidney impairment progresses, additional alterations occur which may further cause dysglycemia: insulin secretion by the pancreas is reduced, and insulin clearance is diminished. With a molecular weight of 6000, insulin has a high renal clearance through filtration and secretion. Renal insulin clearance is reduced as GFR falls to 15–20 mL/min/1.73 m². Abnormal glucose homeostasis is further affected in uremic individuals by peripheral insulin resistance, involving defective glucose uptake and reduced muscle protein anabolism (but not cellular potassium uptake). Glucose uptake mediated by specific transporter proteins is a major action of insulin. Insulin resistance in CKD is a unique metabolic abnormality induced by factors such as uremic toxins, chronic inflammation, excess visceral fat, oxidative stress, metabolic acidosis, and deficiency of vitamin D and erythropoietin. Improvement with dialysis treatment is due at least in part to removal of uremic toxins. To what extent insulin resistance also contributes to protein–energy wasting through the ubiquitin–proteosome pathway, to atherosclerosis, and to cardiovascular disease remains unclear in ESRD.

The net clinical effect of these defects in diabetic ESRD are variable: insulin resistance in advancing CKD may be offset by insulin retention and poor caloric intake; improvement in insulin resistance by dialysis may be offset by more robust caloric intake as uremia improves. A significant reduction in insulin requirements following a hemodialysis treatment may be anticipated. Although clinical assessment of insulin resistance in diabetic ESRD is not practical, it remains a potential therapeutic target. However, insulin sensitizers, a potential treatment, are either sparingly used or contraindicated in ESRD.

Prediabetes

In recent years, there has been a marked increase in the number of U.S. adults with prediabetes, to at least 35%. In the general population, prediabetes is identified by a hemoglobin A_{1c} (HbA_{1c}) value of 5.7%–6.4%. The risk of diabetes is not linear, but increases with higher HbA_{1c} levels below the diabetic range. Prediabetes is associated with increased risk of all-cause and cardiovascular mortality in the general population. ESRD patients who test in the prediabetic range should have annual monitoring for the development of diabetes, lifestyle interventions, and identification/ treatment of other cardiovascular risk factors such as hypertension, hyperlipidemia, and obesity.

Assessing Glycemic Control in ESRD

Two primary techniques are available for assessing the effectiveness of glycemic management: self-monitoring of blood glucose and hemoglobin A_{1c}. Proposed glycemic control parameters for diabetic ESRD patients are fasting blood glucose of 100–140 mg/dL and 2-hour postprandial blood glucose of <200 mg%. In the general diabetes population, HbA_{1c} is the primary predictor of diabetic complications. HbA_{1c} reflects average blood glucose concentrations over approximately the 3 preceding months, correlates fairly well with blood glucose levels, and has provided evidence in interventional trials of the benefit of tight glycemic control. It does not inform about glycemic variability or hypoglycemia. Current society guidelines continue to recommend an HbA_{1c} target of <7.0% in general, with the caveat that goals must be individualized based on factors such as duration of diabetes, age and life expectancy, and comorbid conditions. Treatment goals for patients with advanced CKD, at least for those with related limited life expectancy and at risk for hypoglycemia, have been extended to above 7% (kdoqi 2012).

However, it should be noted that trials conducted in the past decade have forced a reevaluation of the validity of the HbA_{1c} test in the setting of ESRD, as well as indicating only a weak correlation between it and outcomes in this population. The first source of uncertainty in ESRD is unreliability of the HbA_{1c} test itself. Compared with the general diabetic population, correlation with average glucose levels is weaker. Furthermore, data indicate that HbA_{1c} measurements are misleadingly low in patients with ESRD, resulting in an underestimation of hyperglycemia. The most likely sources of discordance from other glycemic tests in kidney patients are anemia, the use of erythrocyte-stimulating agents, and the administration of intravenous iron. ESAs stimulate the production and release of immature erythrocytes whose hemoglobin appears to have reduced glycosylation. No correction factor to eliminate these effects is currently available.

Achieving Glycemic Control in ESRD

There have been no randomized, clinical trials to evaluate the effects of glycemic control in patients with ESRD. Two large, comparably sized retrospective observational studies with methodological differences have reported on the relationship of glycemic control and outcomes in ESRD patients with diabetes, yielding somewhat conflicting conclusions. Kalantar-Zadeh et al demonstrated, after adjustment for multiple potential confounders, an incremental relationship between higher HbA_{1c} values and higher mortality. A follow-up study indicated that poor glycemic control ($HbA_{1c} \geq 8.0\%$) was associated with high all-cause and cardiovascular deaths. Williams et al was able to establish only a weak and variable relation and only when follow-up was extended to a maximum of 3 years. Findings from the Dialysis Outcomes and Practice Patterns Study (DOPPS) indicated that mortality increased as HbA_{1c} exceeded the 7%–7.9% range. A meta-analysis of nine observational studies and one secondary analysis indicated that higher mortality risk did not occur until the A_{1c} levels were $\geq 8.5\%$. Patients with very low HbA_{1c} levels are also at risk. In a post hoc analysis of the German Diabetes and Dialysis Study (4D Study), each 1% increase in baseline HbA_{1c} was associated with an 18% higher risk of sudden cardiac death, although myocardial infarction events were not affected. Overall, these data suggest that HbA_{1c} ranges of 7%–8% may be optimal. Intensity of glycemic control must be individualized based on potential risks and benefits, with an HbA_{1c} target of closer to 7% for younger, incident ESRD patients, and closer to 8% for longstanding diabetes, older patients, longer dialysis vintage, and with multiple comorbid conditions. Glycated albumin and serum fructosamine have been proposed as alternative measures in ESRD. Their linkage to average glucose levels and their prognostic significance are not well established in ESRD. For real-time assessment, continuous glucose monitoring is increasingly valued, particularly given the potential effects of the dialysis treatment on short-term glycemia.

Diabetic Ketoacidosis/Hyperosmolar Coma

Potentially lethal hyperglycemic crises such as diabetic ketoacidosis (DKA) and hyperosmolar coma occur rarely in ESRD patients with diabetes but may be severe and prolonged when they do occur. DKA is a complex disorder that affects volume status, electrolytes, and acid–base balance. It affects patients with type 1 diabetes and rarely those with new-onset type 2 diabetes. The underlying pathophysiology is that of absolute or relative insulin deficiency, insulin resistance, and increased counterregulatory hormones. Common precipitating causes are omission of insulin doses, myocardial ischemia or infarction, and infection. Making the appropriate diagnosis in the ESRD patient is based on hyperglycemia, positive serum ketones, metabolic acidemia, and an increased anion gap. The diagnosis may be delayed insofar as hyperglycemia may be mild, the plasma reaction for ketones may be negative, and the anion gap may not be affected.

In addition, the clinical presentation of severe hyperglycemia and ketoacidosis are atypical in patients with ESRD. Because osmotic diuresis does not occur, volume contraction is avoided (unless vomiting, diarrhea, or excessive insensible loss occurs). Patients will present with weight gain, thirst, pulmonary congestion, and, in extreme circumstances, coma. However, because the rise in serum osmolality and sodium levels is not marked, there may be few neurologic symptoms. Total body potassium deficit is limited, and hyperkalemia may result. Because excessive urinary phosphate excretion does not occur, hypophosphatemia is not expected. Magnesium deficiency is absent. The bicarbonate deficit may be variable.

It follows that acute management of DKA/hyperosmolar coma should be modified in ESRD patients. Insulin, frequently in low doses, is the only treatment required in many cases. (Current guidelines for treatment of DKA in general recommend against the use of bolus doses of insulin. Aggressive insulin treatment may result in severe and prolonged hypoglycemia.) Administration of large volumes of crystalloid are inappropriate, as patients are already at risk for volume overload. Intravenous crystalloid may be required if gastrointestinal (GI) losses have occurred. Use of bicarbonate is not indicated unless the level is critically low, particularly as it may exacerbate volume overload. No phosphate replacement is needed. Typical indications for urgent dialysis include pulmonary edema and hyperkalemia.

Hypoglycemia

Patients with ESRD are prone to hypoglycemia, sometimes spontaneous, unrelated to hyperglycemia treatment. Declining kidney function leads to reduced renal insulin clearance, and degradation of insulin in peripheral tissues is also decreased. In addition, defenses against hypoglycemia are not intact, because renal gluconeogenesis, a protective source of glucose production from precursor molecules during starvation, is impaired. Patients with ESRD may also have diminished glycogen stores due to suboptimal nutrition. Causes of hypoglycemia found in the absence of diabetes or ESRD, such as adrenal insufficiency, infection/sepsis, alcohol abuse, organ failure, and insulinoma, may need to be considered. (One caveat is that fasting insulin levels may be higher in the presence of ESRD, and serum cortisol levels may be variable.) Although dextrose contained in the dialysate solution may offset falling glucose levels, acute hypoglycemia occurring during or immediately after the dialysis session may still require treatment with oral glucose or intravenous dextrose. If available, 15–20 g of glucose should be administered; in more severe episodes, intravenous dextrose 50%, 10–50 mL. Reduction in insulin or conversion to an oral agent with lower hypoglycemic risk, such as a thiazolidinedione or dipeptidyl peptidase-4 inhibitor, may be necessary, after consultation with the diabetologist. Glucagon kits for emergency use should be prescribed. Long-acting insulin may pose a prolonged risk. Nonselective beta-blockers may mask hypoglycemia symptoms and delay recovery from an episode.

Medications

Oral Hypoglycemic Agents

In recent years, multiple hypoglycemic therapies have become available, with diverse mechanisms of action, primarily for patients with type 2 diabetes. In the general diabetes population, a patient-centered approach (patient preferences, side effects, risk of hypoglycemia, cost) is currently recommended. However, oral therapies for managing diabetes are restricted in the ESRD population. There have been few substantive trials of oral hypoglycemic agents in ESRD. As a result, dosage uncertainties and contraindications make management of the ESRD patient difficult, so that medications are being underprescribed. A selection of recommended oral hypoglycemic agents in ESRD is reviewed in Table 64.1. (Multiple other classes and agents are omitted from the table because their use should be avoided in the ESRD patient. These include other sulfonylureas, biguanides, alpha-glucosidase inhibitors, other incretin-mimetics, and SGLT-2 inhibitors.)

Table 64.1

Selection of Oral Antidiabetic Medications Recommended in ESRD

Class	Compound	Drug Name	Formulations	Mechanism of Action
Sulfonylureas	Glipizide	Glucotrol	5, 10 mg	Close K_{ATP} channels on β-cell membrane
		Glucotrol XL	2.5, 5, 10 mg	
	Glimepiride	Amaryl	1, 2, 4 mg	
Meglitinides	Repaglinide	Prandin	0.5, 1, 2 mg	Close K_{ATP} channels on β-cell membrane
Thiazolidinediones	Pioglitazone	Actos	15, 30, 45 mg	Activate the nuclear transcription factor PPAR-γ
DPP-4 inhibitors	Sitagliptin	Januvia	25, 50, 100 mg	Inhibit the inaction of endogenous incretins by DPP-4
	Saxagliptin	Onglyza	2.5, 5 mg	
	Linagliptin	Tradjenta	5 mg	
	Vildagliptin	Galvus	50 mg	
Incretin mimetics	Liraglutide	Victoza	18 mg/3 mL	Activates GLP-1 receptor

SubQ, subcutaneously.

Primary Physiologic Action	Advantages	Disadvantages	Renal Metabolism/Elimination	ESRD Dose Range
↑Insulin secretion	Common use	Hypoglycemia Weight gain Low durability ?Cardiovascular risk Drug interactions	10% excreted unchanged in urine	2.5–10 mg daily
			Weakly active and inactive metabolites excreted in urine	1–4 mg daily
↑Insulin secretion	↓Postprandial glucose excursions Dosing flexibility Relative safety	Hypoglycemia Weight gain Frequent dosing High cost	Limited excretion of inactive metabolites	0.5–1.0 mg 3× daily with meals
↑Insulin sensitivity	No hypoglycemia Durability of effect Favorable effect on lipid profile	Weight gain Possible fluid retention ?Bladder cancer Fractures High cost	Limited excretion of active metabolites	15–30 mg daily
↑Insulin secretion ↓Glucagon secretion	Well tolerated No weight gain Less hypoglycemia	Effect is modest ?Pancreatitis Urticaria/angioedema	Excreted mostly unchanged in urine	25 mg daily
			Renal excretion of drug and metabolites	2.5 mg daily
			Very limited urinary excretion	5 mg daily
			Some excretion of drug by kidneys	50 mg daily
↑Insulin secretion ↓Glucagon secretion ↓Gastric emptying ↑Satiety	Weight loss No hypoglycemia	GI side effects No experience in renal failure Injection required ?Medullary thyroid cancer ?Pancreatitis High cost Weight loss	Endogenous enzymes throughout the body	0.6–1.8 mg SubQ daily

Insulin

Limitations of the oral hypoglycemic agents make insulin therapy common in the ESRD diabetic patient. In the general population, patients with markedly symptomatic hyperglycemia should already be on an insulin-based regimen. Furthermore, because of the progressive nature of type 2 diabetes, insulin therapy is eventually required in many. As CKD stages progress in type 2 patients, the proportion using oral agents decreases, and insulin use is greater. Insulin therapy in advanced CKD is not fundamentally different from patients without CKD, but insulin requirements may be lower and insulin action more prolonged. Endogenous insulin has a molecular weight of 6000 and is freely filtered by the glomerulus. Additional clearance occurs through tubular secretion. About a quarter of endogenous insulin is degraded by the kidneys, even more so for administered insulin that does not initially pass through the liver. Exogenous agents are primarily cleared by renal elimination. At low GFR levels, insulin clearance decreases to the point that insulin requirements fall significantly, if hypoglycemia is to be avoided.

Glycemic management with insulin in the ESRD patient is certainly made more complex by a number of factors. The general trend toward reduced insulin doses as CKD progresses is further complicated by issues such as improvement in insulin sensitivity with dialysis, increased carbohydrate consumption as appetite improves, and exposure to dextrose in the hemodialysis solution; and, to a far greater extent, peritoneal dialysis fluid for patients on that modality. In a limited euglycemic clamp study, basal insulin requirements fell by 25% on the day after hemodialysis, with no change in bolus requirements. In recent years, dialysate dextrose concentrations for hemodialysis have been reduced by half to 100 mg/dL but still serve the purpose of avoiding glucose loss during the treatment and helping to prevent hypoglycemia. On the day of hemodialysis, insulin needs will depend on food consumption. Insulin requirements in the 24-hour period following hemodialysis are likely to be reduced.

New human insulin–derived analogs have been developed in recent years that reproduce the physiologic basal and prandial insulin secretion in response to glucose (Table 64.2). Whether they can improve glycemic control while reducing hypoglycemia in ESRD remains to be determined. There are few pharmacokinetic data, and an absence of therapeutic guidelines for insulin adjustments in advanced CKD. Rapid-acting analogs such as insulin lispro have a more rapid absorption and onset of action yet shorter duration of action than regular human insulin. Long-acting insulin analogs such as glargine or detemir have delayed absorption. Long-acting insulin for basal coverage, combined with sliding-scale nutritional coverage with short-acting insulin analogs, may be preferable to intermediate NPH insulin. In patients who remain nephrotic, binding of insulin detemir to serum albumin after injection may make the clinical management more difficult. A regimen consisting of noninsulin oral agents and basal insulin is commonly used in type 2 patients. Continuous insulin infusion via an insulin pump may improve glycemic control with less hypoglycemia risk, but experience in ESRD is limited. Management in concert with an expert diabetologist is strongly recommended.

Hemodialysis Access

Current ESRD guidelines call for early fistula placement followed by timely evaluation for maturation, and interventions as needed, as the optimal strategy for most patients, especially those younger than 60 years. It is increasingly recognized that a

Table 64.2					

Profiles of Available Insulins and Insulin Analogs

Insulin Type	Name	Example	Onset of Actions	Peak Effect	Duration
Basal	NPH	Humulin N Novolin N	1–2 h	4–8 h	12–18 h
	Glargine	Lantus	2 h	No peak	20–24 h
	Detemir	Levemir	2 h	3–9 h	16–24 h
Nutritional	Regular	Humulin R Novolin R	30 min	2–4 h	6–8 h
	Lispro	Humalog	5–15 min	1–2 h	4–6 h
	Aspart	Novolog	5–15 min	1–2 h	4–6 h
	Glulisine	Apidra	5–15 min	1–2 h	4–6 h

Summary pharmacokinetic data are from individuals without moderate or severe CKD.

fistula-first strategy is more effective when the likelihood of fistula maturation is high. Patients with vascular disease, including those with diabetes as a comorbidity, are more likely to have maturation failure. USRDS 2011 data indicate that access used for the first outpatient dialysis treatment was a fistula in 17% of those with diabetes as primary cause, and 16% in others. Nonetheless, diabetes is commonly identified as a negative predictor of fistula patency, usability, and access flow rates. In addition to cardiovascular factors, mechanistic pathways may include oxidative stress and altered matrix metabolism. Ischemia distal to the AV access is particularly common in patients with diabetes. Patients with diabetes have a lower mean cumulative access survival in some studies. An extended time for maturation may improve fistula outcomes but data are limited.

Nutrition/Protein–Energy Wasting

Nutritional management in ESRD is addressed in Chapter 61. Current guidelines regarding nutritional management in ESRD focus primarily on protein and energy balance and do not separately address the patient with diabetes. Multiple factors contribute to the nutritional and metabolic status of the diabetic ESRD patient, however, including dietary deficiencies and protein energy wasting, making dietary management of the CKD/ESRD patient more complex in the patient with diabetes. During CKD progression, diabetic patients may manifest generalized malnutrition and protein–energy wasting related to inadequate calorie/protein intake, gastroparesis, intercurrent illness, poor glycemic control, proteinuria, diarrhea, and other factors, compounded by endocrine abnormalities such as insulopenia/insulin resistance. Uremic malnutrition, particularly decreases in serum biomarkers such as albumin and prealbumin, is more prevalent in diabetic ESRD patients and is associated with increased risk of hospitalization and death. Compared with nondiabetics, incident diabetic ESRD patients have higher lean body mass at baseline, followed by accelerated loss during the first dialysis year. Contributors to net protein depletion may include poor glycemic control, deficiency or resistance to the anabolic actions of insulin, and subclinical inflammation. Preservation of muscle mass is the ultimate goal of management of this protein–energy wasting condition in

CKD/ESRD patients. Dietary interventions may include high-protein meals or supplements, or enteral feeding. Concerns about the glycemic burden of nutritional interventions may be a secondary concern. During intercurrent illness, intensive nutritional support may be required. No large randomized clinical trials have evaluated the benefit of nutritional interventions such as protein supplementation, appetite stimulants, and antiinflammatory intervention, on outcomes in diabetic ESRD patients.

Hypertension

There are no well-controlled studies of hypertension management in diabetic ESRD patients. The vast majority of patients will have hypertension, frequently refractory, and per guidelines many will already be on RAAS blockade. The optimal blood pressure target and regimen (including bedtime dosing of medications) in patients with ESRD due to diabetes is not adequately defined. Observational studies of the general ESRD population have suggested a U-shaped relationship between blood pressure and mortality. The association between low blood pressure in particular with mortality appears to be more pronounced in patients with diabetes. In patients with a recent myocardial infarction, beta-blockers are indicated, although the risk of hypoglycemia should be addressed.

Dialysis-Associated Hypotension

In patients with ESRD, intra- and postdialytic hypotension continues to play an important role in morbidity. The basis of development of hypotension in this setting typically involves abnormal reduction in blood volume, defective contraction of resistance vessels, and diminished cardiac output. Drops in systolic and diastolic pressure during and after hemodialysis are both greater in hemodialysis patients who have diabetes, related to poor cardiac performance and small-fiber peripheral neuropathy. The normal compensatory response to erect posture is a modest fall in systolic pressure and increase in diastolic pressure and pulse rate. Orthostatic hypotension, such as occurs following intermittent hemodialysis, may be defined as a fall in systolic blood pressure by 20 mm Hg or more with upright posture. Complications include orthostatic dizziness, stroke, and angina. Evaluation of the diabetic dialysis patient with hypotension should include review of volume status, target weight, hemoglobin/hematocrit, and the cardiac status. Multiple medications may contribute, including alpha-adrenergic blockers, vasodilators, antianginals, antidepressants, narcotics, sedative/hypnotics, antipsychotics, and phosphodiesterase inhibitors. Management of dialysis-associated hypotension in the diabetic patient has evolved, as the use of hypertonic saline and higher dialysate sodium concentrations (>140 mEq/L) have fallen into disfavor. Sitting and standing blood pressures should be closely monitored, and the transition postdialysis from a supine to standing position observed. Potential offending agents must be evaluated. Custom-fitted elastic stockings should be obtained where needed. Fludrocortisone acetate is a synthetic mineralocorticoid that may improve hypotension in ESRD by amplifying catecholamine effects to increase peripheral vascular resistance. Midodrine, a direct alpha-1 adrenoreceptor agonist, is the only peripheral selective agent approved by the FDA for orthostatic hypotension. Midodrine is a prodrug but is rapidly absorbed and its peak action is 1 hour after ingestion. The dose range is 2.5 mg to 10 mg tid.

Potential side effects of midodrine include angina, pilomotor reactions, pruritus, supine hypertension, gastrointestinal complaints, and urinary retention.

Cardiovascular Disease

Because all patients with diabetes have a risk of coronary heart disease equivalent to those who have already had a coronary occlusive event, diabetes is designated as a major risk factor for cardiovascular disease by the American Heart Association (AHA). Cardiovascular disease is listed as a cause of death in roughly two-thirds of individuals with diabetes. Diabetes is considered an independent risk factor for several forms of cardiovascular disease, including atherosclerotic coronary heart disease, cardiomyopathy, and stroke. The heightened cardiovascular risk is exaggerated in those whose diabetes is complicated by chronic kidney disease.

Individuals with both diabetes and ESRD are more likely to have a cardiovascular event (myocardial infarction, heart failure, stroke) than those with either condition alone. Compared with the general population, they are at greater risk of sudden cardiac death. Diabetic ESRD patients are more likely to die after an acute myocardial infarction than are nondiabetics. Assessment of cardiovascular risk through identification of potentially remediable risk factors should be the first step in reducing clinical risk in diabetic ESRD patients. According to the AHA, risk assessment must consider major risk factors (hyperglycemia, hypertension, abnormal serum lipids, smoking) as well as predisposing conditions (family history, physical inactivity, excessive body weight, abnormal obesity pattern).

Practice guidelines increasingly classify ESRD as a coronary risk equivalent. For diabetic ESRD, coronary prevention is therefore secondary prevention. AHA risk assessment for diabetes is meant to include not only low-density lipoprotein (LDL) cholesterol but also triglycerides, low high-density lipoprotein (HDL), and small LDL particles. However, current treatment guidelines pertaining to ESRD do not support initiation of statin therapy in dialysis patients, although they may be continued when dialysis is initiated in those already under treatment. KDIGO and other guidelines indicate that statins for secondary prevention in diabetic ESRD are not effective, although post hoc analyses of AURORA and 4-D trials restricted to the occurrence of cardiac events have suggested benefit with statin therapy. There is no evidence of excessive side effects of statins in diabetic ESRD.

Infection

Clinical evidence points to a higher prevalence of infection in diabetes, related to impaired host defenses such as immune dysfunction caused by the hyperglycemic environment, vascular disease, gastrointestinal dysmotility, and poor antibacterial activity in urine. Examples of infections associated with diabetes include the urinary tract (emphysematous cystitis, pyelonephritis, perinephric abscess, fungal infection), lungs (pneumonia, influenza, tuberculosis), GI system (emphysematous cholecystitis, esophageal candidiasis), and soft tissues (foot infections, necrotizing fasciitis, surgical wound infections). Mortality rates due to sepsis are almost twice as high in diabetes. Diabetes is a proven risk factor for infections in ESRD patients. Hospitalization rates for infection are slightly more common. More common infectious complications include episodes of sepsis and central venous catheter–related infections. In peritoneal dialysis patients, women with diabetes have the highest peritonitis rates. An association with staphylococcal skin colonization is unproven. Mortality caused by sepsis is approximately 50 times greater with diabetic ESRD compared with diabetes in the general population. Diabetic ESRD patients should therefore be considered a high-risk group for the development of infection, including lethal sepsis. Antiinfluenza and antipneumococcal vaccination is strongly recommended, along with routine screening for tuberculosis, regular foot examinations, proper wound care, and aggressive evaluation/management of febrile episodes.

Peripheral Arterial Disease/Foot Ulcers

The patient with diabetes and advanced CKD has three independent risk factors for lower limb complications: peripheral arterial disease, neuropathy, and increased susceptibility to infection. In addition, uremic myopathy may result in wasting of the intrinsic foot muscles and development of high plantar pressures. The prevalence of foot ulcers is five times greater in diabetic ESRD than nondiabetic, and nonhealing foot ulceration usually precedes more serious problems such as severe infection, gangrene, and need for amputation. Unfortunately, dialysis patients are less likely to inspect their feet or attend podiatry clinics and more likely to have potentially foot-damaging behavior such as barefoot walking. Furthermore, neuropathy in patients with diabetes will mask the classic symptom of claudication. Diabetic dialysis patients are more likely to require major amputations (below-knee and above-knee) and to suffer death following amputation surgery.

Lower extremity amputations are preventable through patient education, proper foot hygiene and therapeutic footwear, and regular foot surveillance consisting of full assessment at dialysis initiation followed by monthly foot evaluations for warning signs. The most important factors to be evaluated when confronted with foot ulcers are the presence of peripheral arterial disease, peripheral neuropathy, and foot deformities. Commonly used criteria to identify PAD in the diabetic ESRD patient include assessment of peripheral pulses, Doppler waveforms indicating poor monophasic waveform or the absence of flow, and toe blood pressures. The ankle/brachial index (ABI) is determined by dividing the blood pressure in the ankle by that in the brachial artery. An ABI of ≤0.90 indicates PAD, whereas a falsely elevated value >1.30 suggests a calcified, noncompressible vessel, weakening the sensitivity of ABI in detecting PAD. Thus, when both occlusion and stiffness are present, the diagnostic sensitivity of the ABPI is reduced. In diabetic ESRD, low ABI loses its predictive value because of the high prevalence of arterial stiffness. As a consequence, reliance on the physical examination is even more important.

In the general diabetic population, foot screening combines risk stratification and intervention to prevent complications. Multidisciplinary diabetic foot care should be integrated into the comprehensive dialysis care of the diabetic ESRD patient. Risk factors for major amputations are extensive infection, heel ulcers, poor vascular run-off, and low ejection fraction. Careful patient selection for revascularization or amputation is essential in concert with early referral to the vascular surgeon and foot specialist. Lower extremity revascularization in diabetic ESRD may be complicated by infection, impaired wound healing, increased perioperative mortality rates, and reduced lower extremity salvage and patient survival. Even after successful postamputation rehabilitation, the mortality risk is increased. Endovascular revascularization may be appealing as first-line therapy over open bypass surgery for achieving improved blood flow to the ulcer area. Prevention programs should especially be emphasized for individuals at the highest risk (diabetic ESRD with previous ulceration or amputation).

Neuropathy

Important neurologic complications in diabetic ESRD include cardiovascular autonomic neuropathy (CAN) and diabetic peripheral neuropathy (DPN). Autonomic neuropathy may present with resting tachycardia, fixed heart rate, exercise intolerance, intradialytic hypotension, orthostatic hypotension, or silent myocardial ischemia. Sympathetic overactivity is characteristic of CAN. Mortality in diabetic patients with CAN is significantly increased. The only current method likely to improve CAN is strict glycemic control, particularly in type 1 diabetes. Some studies suggest beneficial effects of hemodialysis on heart rate variability due to CAN. Beta-blockers may provide protection from cardiovascular events. DPN and neuropathic pain may occur in up to half of patients with diabetic ESRD. DPN may also be complicated by neuroarthropathy (Charcot foot) or foot ulceration. Pain may be managed with nonopioids, opioids, and adjuvants. Gabapentin is approved by the FDA and commonly used, but because of renal excretion, the dose must be titrated carefully and limited to a maximum of 1800 mg/day. Signs of toxicity include myoclonus and altered consciousness. The selective serotonin reuptake inhibitor duloxetine is also approved for painful DPN but not recommended in advanced CKD. Opioids are effective but with long-term use cause limiting side effects such as constipation, impaired cognitive function, and tolerance/addiction. Tramadol is relatively well tolerated in doses up to 200 mg/day with no postdialysis supplemental dose required.

Gastroparesis

One of the major causes of protein malnutrition in diabetic ESRD is dysmotility in the gastrointestinal tract. Diabetic gastropathy includes gastroparesis, or delayed emptying of ingested nutrients in the absence of gastric outlet obstruction, and other dyspeptic conditions found in patients with diabetes. Overall, about half of type 1 and a third of type 2 patients have gastroparesis. In the general diabetic population, gastroparesis is associated with protein malnutrition and more frequent hospitalizations. It places patients at risk for weight loss, impaired drug absorption, poor quality of life, and probably increased mortality rates and may be exacerbated by hemodialysis and peritoneal dialysis. Episodes may be triggered by poor glycemic control (which delays gastric emptying), medication intolerance, infections, noncompliance, or other factors. Gastroparesis itself causes nonspecific symptoms of nausea, vomiting, anorexia, early satiety, and postprandial abdominal discomfort. Delayed gastric emptying on scintigraphy is the hallmark diagnostic finding. Complications include electrolyte disturbances, volume depletion, esophagitis, Mallory–Weiss tears, and bezoar formation. Fluctuations in gastric emptying will affect periprandial glucose concentrations and make glycemic control more difficult.

The initial treatment approach includes modification of diet, correction of hyperglycemia, and use of prokinetic agents. Dietary therapy includes low-volume, frequent, soft or liquid meals with low fat and fiber content. Metoclopramide, a dopamine antagonist with central antiemetic and peripheral gastric prokinetic actions, improves the acute effects of gastroparesis in about half of patients, but with a high incidence of dose-dependent tardive dyskinesia. The initial dose is 5 mg preprandial. (A related dopamine antagonist, domperidone, is not approved in the United States but may be available with special IRB approval.) Oral or intravenous erythromycin, used as a promotility agent, accelerates gastric emptying and improves bloating, although the oral formulation may result in its own gastrointestinal side effects. Ondansetron orally may improve intractable symptoms. Options in resistant cases include botulinum toxin injection, gastric stimulation, surgery, or vagotomy. Prompt hospitalization is required in cases of dehydration and diabetic ketoacidosis.

Ophthalmologic Complications

Diabetic retinopathy is a specific microvascular complication of both type 1 and type 2 diabetes. The prevalence of diabetic retinopathy among ESRD patients is high, and the majority of diabetic CKD patients have had laser photocoagulation therapy before reaching ESRD. Background retinopathy may cause visual impairment leading to blindness when the macular area is involved. Even more damaging is proliferative diabetic retinopathy, with neovascularization as well as vitreous hemorrhage. Comprehensive eye examination with high-quality fundus photography by an ophthalmologist is indicated within 5 years of onset of type 1 diabetes and soon after the diagnosis of type 2 diabetes. Frequent eye examinations are recommended but continue to be uncommon among ESRD patients with diabetes, with only one in five receiving two tests per year. In those without retinopathic findings, follow-up should be every 2 years, and in those with retinopathic findings, at least annually. Proliferative diabetic retinopathy may be treated with laser photocoagulation therapy, which is beneficial in preventing further visual loss. Hypertension accelerates progression of diabetic retinopathy, adding to the urgency of treatment of high blood pressure readings in diabetic ESRD patients. Diabetic retinopathy is not a contraindication to aspirin therapy. Heparin in doses required for dialysis anticoagulation does not appear to be associated with acceleration of diabetic retinopathy.

Home Hemodialysis

Available data indicate that patients with diabetes are somewhat underrepresented in the ESRD population on home hemodialysis. The USRDS data report for year 2012 indicates that one-third of patients on home hemodialysis had diabetes as a primary diagnosis. In the Canadian Multicenter Nocturnal Home Hemodialysis Cohort (1994–2006), the entire cohort tended to be younger and less likely to have diabetes than the general ESRD population. Only 12% had diabetes. Diabetes was a powerful predictor of death or treatment failure, however, and was equivalent to the addition of 14.5 years of age.

Peritoneal Dialysis

Peritoneal dialysis is a viable alternative to hemodialysis. USRDS data for year 2012 report that about 6% of prevalent dialysis patients due to diabetes are on this modality, versus about 7% on dialysis with other diagnoses. As in patients without diabetes, selection of a dialysis modality in patients with diabetes is known to depend on factors such as comorbidities, creation of dialysis access, hemodynamic stability, tolerance of the dialysis modality, and functional level. The presence of diabetes modifies both the potential advantages and disadvantages of peritoneal dialysis in ESRD, beyond those for patients without diabetes. Extra advantages include improvement in circulatory stress with its perfusion abnormalities affecting organ systems such as the heart, brain, kidney, and retina and better preservation of residual renal function, which is more likely to be lost in diabetics. Extra disadvantages include the enhanced metabolic effects of obligatory glucose absorption, including hyperglycemia, hyperlipidemia, and obesity; increased accumulation of advanced glycation end products, particularly in the peritoneum itself; and worsening of GI side effects, including esophageal reflux and gastroparesis.

Glucose absorption during peritoneal dialysis commonly exceeds 100 g per exchange. Correlation between the concentration of dialysate dextrose and daily mean glucose concentrations by continuous glucose monitoring has been demonstrated. Higher prescribed peritoneal dialysate glucose may be associated with overall risk of death and with the need to transfer to hemodialysis. Poor glycemic control appears to be associated with incrementally higher mortality in peritoneal dialysis patients with diabetes. Glucose-sparing regimens have been developed in order to reduce the peritoneal and systemic exposure to glucose. Icodextrin, for example, achieves greater ultrafiltration with less glucose exposure. A recent multinational, randomized controlled study supported the use of glucose-sparing (icodextrin, amino acid–based dialysate) compared to dextrose-containing dialysate in diabetic patients. An important caveat is that patients treated with icodextrin are at risk for having overestimation of blood glucose measurements when testing with glucose dehydrogenase/pyrroloquinolinequinone cofactor (GDH/PQQ) glucometers, likely due to assay interference by circulating maltose metabolites of the icodextrin.

Most nephrologists do not currently use intraperitoneal insulin. However, for diabetic patients requiring peritoneal dialysis, the option of adding insulin to peritoneal dialysate solutions prior to infusion provides coverage of dialysate dextrose exposure, allowing some patients to avoid insulin injections and reducing insulin requirements in others. Intraperitoneal insulin is absorbed into the portal system and results in more physiologic delivery than with intermittent subcutaneous injections, better inhibiting hepatic gluconeogenesis and ketogenesis. However, full conversion of subcutaneously treated patients will require up to fourfold more insulin, as absorption to the dialysis tubing is significant. Other possible disadvantages of intraperitoneal insulin include increased risk of bacterial contamination/peritonitis, lowered plasma HDL levels, rare complications of peritoneal fibroblast proliferation, hepatic steatosis, malignant omentum syndrome, and increased cost. The superiority of intraperitoneal insulin has not been uniformly demonstrated. Therefore, these disadvantages have limited the use of intraperitoneal insulin. Use of intraperitoneal insulin appears to have further diminished with the advent of CCPD, out of concern for greater risk of nocturnal hypoglycemia and the lack of information on insulin dosing when placed in substantially larger bag volumes. When intraperitoneal insulin is instituted to cover dextrose exposure during overnight exchanges, regular human insulin is the standard, in incremental doses of 2 to 12 units per liter. For complete conversion of subcutaneous to intraperitoneal insulin, a total dose 3–4 times the subcutaneous dose should be divided among the CCPD bags and any daytime exchange bag. However, the conversion should be gradual and start with one quarter of the ultimate dose. Rapid-acting insulin analogs should be avoided.

Studies comparing patient survival between hemodialysis and peritoneal dialysis for diabetic patients have yielded conflicting results. A frequently cited observational ESRD study (45% with diabetes) indicated higher mortality risk with hemodialysis among younger diabetics with no comorbidities, and lower mortality risk with hemodialysis in older diabetics whether comorbidities were present at baseline or not. A more recent study using more advanced statistical methods also showed a survival disadvantage for diabetics with at least one comorbidity or older than 65 years.

Kidney Transplantation

Although replacement or preemption of dialysis by kidney transplantation presents the best hope for improved survival and quality of life in diabetic ESRD, access to transplantation remains significantly reduced. Living donor kidney transplant counts remain relatively low in diabetic ESRD, although the number of deceased donor recipients with ESRD from diabetes has grown steadily. Compared with about half of patients with ESRD in general, about one-fifth with diabetic ESRD have a functioning transplant. Patient and graft outcomes of patients with diabetes treated with kidney transplantation remain inferior to those without diabetes, primarily related to higher cardiovascular and infection-related deaths. However, a recent retrospective analysis from a large single center suggested that significant reductions in cardiac events and infectious deaths in diabetic recipients was evident in recent years, unrelated to selection of lower-risk candidates, whereas similar improvements were not noted in recipients without diabetic ESRD. Mortality rates after initiation of dialysis increase exponentially after type 1 patients start on dialysis, and preemptive transplantation results in superior outcomes. For patients with type 1 diabetes who may qualify for a kidney transplant, it has therefore been recommended that the patient should be referred for kidney transplantation when their eGFR reaches 25 mL/min/1.73 m^2. It is not yet determined what effect on diabetic dialysis patients the revised national kidney transplant allocation system will have. The system uses the diabetes diagnosis as one factor in a scoring system that calculates expected posttransplant survival to better match potential recipients with available kidneys.

Outcomes

Among hemodialysis patients, the overall hospitalization rate is 1 per approximately 7 months. Patients who have diabetes as their primary cause of ESRD have a higher risk of all-cause hospitalization, about once every 6 months, and a similar degree of risk increase for cardiovascular and infection (but not vascular access infection) causes.

Overall mortality rates for ESRD patients have continued to decline over the past two decades, falling by 25% between 2003 and 2012. However, diabetes continues to carry the highest mortality rates of all primary diagnoses requiring renal replacement therapy. Adjusted survival probabilities after initiation of ESRD treatment begin to be worse for diabetes as primary ESRD cause around 24 months. By 60 months, survival probability is 37%, 6.4 percentage points lower than for hypertension and 16.6% lower than for glomerulonephritis. The mortality rate with type 1 diabetes increases exponentially following transition to dialysis. Patients with diabetic ESRD have the greatest number of comorbid conditions. Cardiovascular disease (acute myocardial infarction, heart failure, stroke, malignant arrhythmias, sudden death), the leading cause of death in the general ESRD population, is twice as common in ESRD patients with diabetes. Increased risk of mortality occurs similarly in patients with diabetes mellitus as primary renal disease and diabetes as a comorbid condition, compared to the prevalent ESRD population.

Quality of Life

Although it is an important issue, few studies have compared health-related quality of life in ESRD patients with and without diabetes. Available data indicate that patients with ESRD secondary to diabetes have worse health-related quality of life and inferior functional status, and lower physical aspects of HRQOL (health-related quality of life). Interventions to improve HRQOL (other than kidney transplantation) require further exploration.

SECTION XXV

Drug Use in Uremia

C H A P T E R 6 5

Principles of Drug Usage in Dialysis Patients

Ali J. Olyaei, PharmD • William M. Bennett, MD

Evolution of the field of dialysis and advances in surgical procedures and access placement have made it possible to treat patients with end-stage renal disease (ESRD) with dialysis therapy for more than 60 years. Improvements in pharmacotherapy and pre- and postdialysis management have contributed to these remarkable advancements. However, uremia may directly or indirectly affect different aspects of drug pharmacokinetics or pharmacodynamics. Most therapeutic agents or their metabolites are completely or partially eliminated by the kidneys.

Patients with chronic kidney disease (CKD) often have a number of comorbidities and require pharmacotherapy to correct or prevent complications of these conditions. In patients with CKD, drug elimination is significantly altered, and elimination of drugs through the kidneys is impaired. In addition, uremia may alter extrarenal drug metabolism. Depending on various factors (e.g., the size of the drug molecule and degree of protein binding), a significant amount of drug removal may occur during dialysis. To prevent toxicity and optimize efficacy, it is critical that these factors be taken into account and appropriate dosage adjustments made when prescribing drugs for dialysis patients. This chapter discusses pharmacologic principles for prescribing drugs in this population and references specific dosage recommendations.

Pharmacologic Principles and Alterations in Uremia

Dosage modification in dialysis patients must take into account the effects of uremia and other factors on a variety of pharmacokinetic parameters, such as drug absorption, volume of distribution, protein binding, and drug metabolism. Drug absorption may be impaired because of delayed gastric emptying or edema of the gastrointestinal (GI) tract, particularly in diabetic patients with gastroparesis. Medications commonly prescribed in dialysis patients may alter drug absorption.

Gastric pH is frequently high because of the use of antacids or H_2 blockers, which may result in decreased absorption of medications requiring an acid milieu. Aluminum- or calcium-containing phosphate-binding antacids may form nonabsorbable chelation products with certain drugs, such as digoxin or tetracycline, with impairment of their absorption.

After absorption and equilibration, individual drugs distribute throughout the body in a characteristic manner. The apparent volume of distribution (V_d) is the quantity of drug in the body (L/kg body weight) divided by the plasma concentration at equilibrium. V_d represents that amount of water in which the drug must have been dissolved to render the observed plasma concentration. Whereas drugs that are highly tissue bound or lipid soluble usually have a large V_d, drugs that are highly bound to circulating proteins are largely confined to the vascular space and therefore usually have a V_d of less than 0.2 L/kg. A variety of disease states, including uremia, may alter the V_d of therapeutic agents. From a practical standpoint, the changes in V_d are usually not clinically significant except for those drugs that have a small V_d (<0.7 L/kg) under normal circumstances.

The degree of drug protein binding may be altered in uremia, with potentially important pharmacologic consequences. It is the unbound or free drug that is pharmacologically active and available for metabolism or excretion. Decreased binding of various drugs has been demonstrated in patients with renal failure. As a result, for any given drug level (bound plus unbound), the proportion of free or active drug is increased. Because both drug elimination and pharmacologic activity are increased for any given dose, the clinical consequences are difficult to predict.

When a medication reaches the systemic circulation, it will be metabolized by the smooth endoplasmic reticulum in the liver, GI tract, and other tissues. Drug metabolism is a complex set of sequences that involves many organs and pathways in the body. The metabolism of a drug by the liver before entering the systemic circulation is called *first-pass metabolism*. With first-pass metabolism, a drug is absorbed into the intestines and enters the portal vein before it reaches the liver for metabolism. After it is metabolized by the liver, the drug then enters the systemic circulation, where it produces an effect on the body. Generally, first-pass metabolism reduces the bioavailability of a given drug, thus decreasing the plasma concentration. In patients with CKD, the addition of phosphate binders, calcium, and iron may interfere with first-pass metabolism and reduce the drug exposure significantly.

In phase 1 metabolism, the oxidase class of enzymes are involved with drug metabolism. This oxidase group is more commonly known as CYP 450 enzymes. When a drug interacts with oxygen, one of the oxygen binds to the drug and the other forms H_2O, causing the drug to become more water soluble. For all of this to occur requires active CYP 450 enzymes. The most common CYP 450 enzyme is CYP 3A4, which metabolizes 50% of all drugs. With CYP 2D6, polymorphisms can affect the rate of drug metabolism. Uremia and kidney disease might affect expression of many of these enzymatic pathways.

With phase II metabolism, the enzymes involved with metabolism are transferases. The enzymes help transfer polar molecules to a drug to make them more soluble. Examples of these enzymes include, glucuronate, glutathione, and sulfate. The product of this reaction is known as a *conjugate*, thus the term *the conjugation reaction*. One of the most well-known medications that uses phase II metabolism is acetaminophen. The most common process for phase II metabolism is glucuronidation conjugation.

The kidneys are the most common route of drug excretion. The drug removal rate is typically expressed as elimination half-life ($t^1/_2$), the time required for the plasma concentration to decrease by 50%. The half-life is dependent on V_d and clearance (renal, hepatic, or other) as expressed by the following formula:

$$t\tfrac{1}{2} = 0.693 \ \mu \ V_d/\text{clearance}$$

As the renal clearance decreases, $t^1/_2$ will increase (assuming that V_d is unchanged). It should be noted that active drug metabolites may also be excreted by the kidney and therefore have a prolonged half-life in renal failure.

Drug Administration

Drugs or their metabolites that are normally excreted by the kidney require dosage modification in advanced renal failure. In general, the loading dose of a drug does not need to be changed unless the V_d is significantly altered. The maintenance regimen may be modified by the interval extension method or dosage reduction. The interval extension method uses the same dose at greater intervals and is useful for drugs with long half-lives. The dosage reduction method reduces the dosage and leaves the interval between doses unchanged. This method generally leads to more constant serum levels.

Monitoring of drug levels can be very useful in guiding drug therapy and in preventing toxicity. Interpretation of drug levels must be made in light of the amount of drug administered, the time elapsed since the last dose, and the route of administration.

After steady-state levels are reached, peak drug levels occur 30 to 60 minutes after parenteral administration or 1 to 2 hours after oral ingestion—and trough levels are drawn immediately before the next dose. In general, peak levels tend to correlate with drug efficacy, but trough levels are used as indicators of toxicity. Drug level monitoring can be expensive and is not always available. Drug level monitoring does not always reduce the incidence of toxicity. Ongoing clinical assessment is important even when drug levels are within the established therapeutic range. Most assays do not distinguish between free and protein-bound drug in the plasma. An increase in unbound drug is common in patients with renal failure. Table 65.1 summarizes the therapeutic drug monitoring in renal insufficiency for drugs for which monitoring of drug levels is routinely recommended.

Renal Function Assessment

The glomerular filtration rate (GFR) is closely correlated with unchanged drug elimination through the kidney and is useful in determining dosage adjustments. The Cockcroft and Gault formula is the most commonly used method of calculating the creatinine clearance (Clcr), which has traditionally been used to approximate the GFR. Both blood urea nitrogen (BUN) and serum creatinine (Scr) are, at best, crude markers of renal function. The Cockcroft and Gault formula (as follows) includes the variables of age (years), ideal body weight (IBW) (kg), and Scr (mg/dL) and calculates the Clcr (mL/min):

$$CrCl = (140 - Age) \times IBW/(Scr \times 72)(\times 0.85 \text{ for females})$$

Patients with acute renal failure should have an assumed Clcr of less than 10 mL/min, and it should be remembered that Clcr overestimates the GFR. A new marker of GFR, iohexol, is currently being used in both the research and clinical settings to more accurately measure renal function without exposing the patient to radiolabeled material. In addition, the Modification of Diet in Renal Disease (MDRD) study recently reported a new formula for estimating renal function. The formula approximates GFR rather than Clcr and therefore may be a more accurate estimate of renal function. The formula uses a creatinine assay (the kinetic alkaline picrate reaction), which is the least subject to artifact interference. GFR was predicted over a wide range of values, including variables for ethnicity and serum albumin

Table 65.1

Therapeutic Drug Monitoring

Drug Name	Therapeutic Range	When to Draw Sample	How Often to Draw Levels
Aminoglycosides (Conventional Dosing) Gentamicin, tobramycin amikacin	Gentamicin and tobramycin: • Trough: 0.5–2 mg/L • Peak: 5–8 mg/L Amikacin: • Peak: 20–30 mg/L • Trough: <10 mg/L 0.5–3 mg/L	• Trough: Immediately before dose • Peak: 30 min after a 30- to 45-min infusion	• Check peak and trough with third dose. • For therapy less than 72 h, levels not necessary. Repeat drug levels weekly or if renal function changes.
Aminoglycosides (24-h Dosing) Gentamicin, tobramycin, amikacin		Obtain random drug level 12 h after dose	After initial dose. Repeat drug level in 1 wk or if renal function changes.
Carbamazepine	4–12 mcg/mL	Trough: Immediately before dosing	Check 2–4 days after the first dose or change in dose.
Cyclosporin	150–400 ng/mL	Trough: Immediately before dosing 12 h after maintenance dose	Daily for first week, then weekly 5–7 d after first dose for patients with normal renal and hepatic function; 15–20 days in anephric patients.
Digoxin	0.8–2.0 ng/mL		
Lidocaine	1–5 mcg/mL	8 hr after IV infusion started or changed	
Lithium	Acute: 0.8–1.2 mmol/L Chronic: 0.6–0.8 mmol/L	Trough: Before AM dose at least 12 hr since last dose	
Phenobarbital	15–40 mcg/mL	Trough: Immediately before dosing	Check 2 wk after first dose or change in dose. Follow-up level in 1–2 months.
Phenytoin	10–20 mcg/mL	Trough: Immediately before dosing	5–7 d after first dose or after change in dose.

Drug	Therapeutic Range	Sampling Time	Monitoring
Free Phenytoin	1–2 mcg/mL		
Procainamide	(A) 4–10 mcg/mL • Trough: 4 mcg/mL • Peak: 8 mcg/mL (B) 10–30 mcg/mL	(A) Trough: Immediately before next dose or 12–18 hr after starting or changing an infusion (B) Draw with procainamide sample	
NAPA (*N*-acetyl procainamide), a procainamide metabolite			
Quinidine	1–5 mcg/mL	Trough: Immediately before next dose	
Sirolimus	10–20 ng/dL	Trough: Immediately before next dose	
Tacrolimus (FK-506)	10–15 ng/mL	Trough: Immediately before next dose	Daily for first week, then weekly
Theophylline PO or Aminophylline IV	15–20 mcg/mL	Trough: Immediately before next dose	
Valproic acid	40–100 mcg/mL	Trough: Immediately before next dose	With third dose (when initially starting therapy or after each dosage adjustment). For therapy <72 hr, levels not necessary. Repeat drug levels if renal function changes.
Vancomycin	• Trough: 5–15 mg/L • Peak: 25–40 mg/L	• Trough: Immediately before dose • Peak: 60 min after 60-min infusion	Check 2–4 after first dose or change in dose

IV, intravenous; *PO*, oral.

concentration, and did not rely on timed urine collections. The MDRD study equation is as follows.

$$GFR = 170 \times (Scr)^{-0.999} \times (Age)^{-0.176} \times (0.762 \text{ if female}) \times (1.180 \text{ if patient is black})$$
$$\times (BUN)^{-0.170} \times (Albumin)^{-0.318}$$

Effects of Dialysis on Drugs

Drug removal during dialysis is an important factor to consider when prescribing drug therapy for a patient with ESRD. A variety of factors affect dialysis drug clearance, including molecular weight, water solubility, degree of protein binding, and membrane clearance. Drugs with molecular weights of more than 500 daltons are poorly cleared by conventional hemodialysis (HD) membranes. In addition, drugs that are highly protein or tissue bound or that are highly lipid soluble are not dialyzed to a significant extent because of their large V_d. The clearance of some molecules of molecular weight of more than 500 daltons may be greater with peritoneal dialysis (PD) than with HD. From a practical standpoint, however, it is unusual for PD to remove drugs that are not also removed by HD.

The use of more permeable membranes, such as polysulfone, is becoming more common. Removal of drugs with relatively low molecular weights and small V_d could conceivably be enhanced with the use of these membranes. Vancomycin removal, for example, is significantly increased when polysulfone membranes are used compared with cuprophane membranes. Thus, supplemental vancomycin administration is required after each dialysis session with a polysulfone membrane to maintain therapeutic vancomycin levels.

Table 65.2

Antimicrobial Agents in Renal Failure

Antimicrobial Agents in Renal Failure

			Dosage Adjustment in Renal Failure		
Drugs	**Normal Dosage**	**% of Renal Excretion**	**GFR >50 mL/min**	**GFR 10–50 mL/min**	**GFR <10 mL/min**
Aminoglycoside Antibiotics					
Streptomycin	7.5 mg/kg q12h (1.0 g q24h for tuberculosis)	60%	q24h	q24–72h	q72–96h

Continuous hemofiltration modalities are gaining popularity in intensive care units for the management of patients with acute kidney injury. In this procedure, convective mass transfer removes solutes and drugs. In general, a drug is significantly removed if it is primarily distributed in the plasma water and is not highly protein bound. Measurement of serum drug levels may be helpful in guiding the need for supplemental dosing with these modalities.

Dosing Tables

Table 65.2 presents key information required for prescribing medications in dialysis patients. Table 65.2 provides information on drugs that require dosing adjustment for patients with ESRD and on the half-lives of the drugs (hours). The adjustment for ESRD applies to patients with renal function poor enough to require maintenance dialysis (GFR generally <10 mL/min). In patients with renal failure, a careful pharmacotherapeutic plan pertinent to each patient's situation should be developed. When the method of adjustment is interval extension (I), the number of hours that should elapse between doses is indicated in Table 65.2. The quantity of the dose should be the same as that given to a patient with normal renal function. On the other hand, when the dose reduction method (D) is recommended, the adjustment refers to the percentage of the dose given to a patient with normal renal function. This dose should be given at the usual dosing interval. Brackets in Table 65.2 indicate the dosage formulation and currently available formulations. However, similar to any clinical guideline, patient-specific factors such as age, disease state, nutrition, and body fluid should be considered during the dosage adjustments.

Comments	Hemodialysis	Continuous Ambulatory Peritoneal Dialysis	Continuous Venovenous Hemofiltration
Nephrotoxic, ototoxic; toxicity worse when hyperbilirubinemic; measure serum levels for efficacy and toxicity			
Peritoneal absorption increases with presence of inflammation			
V_d increases with edema, obesity, and ascites			
For the treatment of TB; may be less nephrotoxic than other members of class	1/2 normal dose after dialysis	20–40 mg/L/d	Dose for GFR 10–50 mL/min and measure levels

Continued

Table 65.2

Antimicrobial Agents in Renal Failure—cont'd

Antimicrobial Agents in Renal Failure

			Dosage Adjustment in Renal Failure		
Drugs	Normal Dosage	% of Renal Excretion	GFR >50 mL/min	GFR 10–50 mL/min	GFR <10 mL/min
Kanamycin	7.5 mg/kg q8h	50%–90%	60%–90% q12h or 100% q12–24h	30%–70% q12–18h or 100% q24–48h	20%–30% q24–48h or 100% q48–72h
Gentamicin	1.7 mg/kg q8h	95%	60%–90% q8–12h or 100% q12–24h	30%–70% q12h or 100% q24–48h	20%–30% q24–48h or 100% q48–72h
Tobramycin	1.7 mg/kg q8h	95%	60%–90% q8–12h or 100% q12–24h	30%–70% q12h or 100% q24–48h	20%–30% q24–48h or 100% q48–72h
Netilmicin	2 mg/kg q8h	95%	50%–90% q8–12h or 100% q12–24h	20%–60% q12h or 100% q24–48h	10% to 20% q24–48h or 100% q48 to 72
Amikacin	7.5 mg/kg q12h	95%	60% to 90% q12h or 100% q12 to 24h	30% to 70% q12 to 18h or 100% q24–48h	20% to 30% q24–48h or 100% q48 to 72h
Cephalosporin					
Oral Cephalosporins					
Cefaclor	250–500 mg q8h	70%	100%	100%	50%
Cefadroxil	500–1 g q12h	80%	100%	100%	50%
Cefixime	200–400 mg q12h	85%	100%	100%	50%
Cefpodoxime	200 mg q12h	30%	100%	100%	100%
Ceftibuten	400 mg q24h	70%	100%	100%	50%

Comments	Hemodialysis	Continuous Ambulatory Peritoneal Dialysis	Continuous Venovenous Hemofiltration
Do not use once-daily dosing in patients with creatinine clearance <30–40 mL/min or in patients with ARF or uncertain level of kidney function	1/2 full dose after dialysis	15–20 mg/L/d	Dose for GFR 10–50 mL/min and measure levels
	1/2 full dose after dialysis	3–4 mg/L/d	Dose for GFR 10–50 mL/min and measure levels
	1/2 full dose after dialysis	3–4 mg/L/d	Dose for GFR 10–50 mL/min and measure levels
May be less ototoxic than other members of class Peak: 6–8 Trough: <2	1/2 full dose after dialysis	3 to 4 mg/L/d	Dose for GFR 10 to 50 mL/min and measure levels
Monitor levels Peak: 20–30 Trough: <5	1/2 full dose after dialysis	15 to 20 mg/L/d	Dose for GFR 10 mg/L to 50 mL/min and measure levels
Coagulation abnormalities, transitory elevation of BUN, rash, and serum sickness–like syndrome			
	250 mg bid after dialysis	250 mg q8–12h	N/A
	0.5 to 1.0 g after dialysis	0.5 g/d	N/A
	300 mg after dialysis	200 mg/d	Not recommended
	200 mg after dialysis	Dose for GFR <10 mL/min	N/A
	300 mg after dialysis	No data: dose for GFR <10 mL/min	Dose for GFR 10–50 mL/min

Continued

Table 65.2

Antimicrobial Agents in Renal Failure—cont'd

Antimicrobial Agents in Renal Failure

Drugs	Normal Dosage	% of Renal Excretion	Dosage Adjustment in Renal Failure		
			GFR >50 mL/min	GFR 10–50 mL/min	GFR <10 mL/min
Cefuroxime axetil	250–500 mg q8 h	90%	100%	100%	100%
Cephalexin	250–500 mg q8 h	95%	100%	100%	100%
Cephradine	250–500 mg q8 h	100%	100%	100%	50%
IV Cephalosporins					
Cefazolin	1–2 g IV q8h	80%	q8h	q12h	q12–24h
Cefepime	1–2 g IV q8h	85%	q8–12h	q12h	q24h
Cefmetazole	1–2 g IV q8h	85%	q8h	q12h	q24h
Cefoperazone	1–2 g IV q12h	20%	No renal adjustment is required		
Cefotaxime	1–2 g IV q6–8h	60%	q8h	q12h	q12–24h
Cefotetan	1–2 g IV q12h	75%	q12h	q12–24h	q24h
Cefoxitin	1–2 g IV q6h	80%	q6h	q8–12h	q12h
Ceftazidime	1–2 g IV q8h	70%	q8h	q12h	q24h
Ceftriaxone	1–2 g IV q24h	50%	No renal adjustment is required		
Cefuroxime sodium	0.75–1.5 g IV q8h	90%	q8h	q8–12h	q12–24h
Penicillin s					
Oral Penicillins					
Amoxicillin	500 mg PO q8h	60%	100%	100%	50%–75%
Ampicillin	500 mg PO q6h	60%	100%	100%	50%–75%

Comments	Hemodialysis	Continuous Ambulatory Peritoneal Dialysis	Continuous Venovenous Hemofiltration
Malabsorbed in presence of H_2 blockers; absorbed better with food	Dose after dialysis	Dose for GFR <10 mL/min	N/A
Rare allergic interstitial nephritis; absorbed well when given intraperitoneally; may cause bleeding from impaired prothrombin biosynthesis	Dose after dialysis	Dose for GFR <10 mL/min	N/A
	Dose after dialysis	Dose for GFR <10 mL/min	N/A
	0.5–1.0 g after dialysis	0.5 g q12h	Dose for GFR 10–50 mL/min
	1 g after dialysis	Dose for GFR <10 mL/min	Not recommended
	Dose after dialysis	Dose for GFR <10 mL/min	Dose for GFR 10–50 mL/min
Displaced from protein by bilirubin; reduce dose by 50% for jaundice; may prolong PT	1 g after dialysis	None	None
	1 g after dialysis	1 g/d	1g q12h
	1 g after dialysis	1 g/d	750 mg q12h
May produce false increase in serum creatinine by interference with assay	1 g after dialysis	1 g/d	Dose for GFR 10–50 mL/min
	1 g after dialysis	0.5 g/d	Dose for GFR 10–50 mL/min
	Dose after dialysis	750 mg q12h	Dose for GFR 10–50 mL/min
	Dose after dialysis	Dose for GFR <10 mL/min	1.0 g q12h
Bleeding abnormalities, hypersensitivity, seizures			
	Dose after dialysis	250 mg q12h	N/A
	Dose after dialysis	250 mg q12h	Dose for GFR 10–50 mL/min

Continued

Table 65.2

Antimicrobial Agents in Renal Failure—cont'd

Antimicrobial Agents in Renal Failure

Drugs	Normal Dosage	% of Renal Excretion	Dosage Adjustment in Renal Failure		
			GFR >50 mL/min	GFR 10–50 mL/min	GFR <10 mL/min
Dicloxacillin	250–500 mg PO q6h	50%	100%	100%	50%–75%
Penicillin V	250–500 mg PO q6h	70%	100%	100%	50%–75%
IV Penicillin					
Ampicillin	1–2 g IV q6h	60%	q6h	q8h	q12h
Nafcillin	1–2 g IV q4h	35%	No renal adjustment is required		
Penicillin G	2–3 million units IV q4h	70%	q4–6h	q6h	q8h
Piperacillin	3–4 g IV q4–6h		No renal adjustment is required		
Ticarcillin–clavulanate	3.1 g IV q4–6h	85%	1–2 g q4h	1–2 g q8h	1–2 g q12h
Piperacillin–tazobactam	3.375 g IV q6–8h	75%–90%	q4–6h	q6–8h	q8h
Quinolones					
Ciprofloxacin	200–400 mg IV q24h	60%	q12h	q12–24h	q24h
Levofloxacin	500 mg PO q24h	70%	q12h	250 q12h	250 q12h
Moxifloxacin	400 mg q24h	20%	No renal adjustment is required		
Nalidixic acid	1.0 g q6h	High	100%	Avoid	Avoid
Norfloxacin	400 mg PO q12h	30%	q12h	q12–24h	q24h
Ofloxacin	200–400 mg PO q12h	70%	q12h	q12–24h	q24h

Comments	Hemodialysis	Continuous Ambulatory Peritoneal Dialysis	Continuous Venovenous Hemofiltration
	None	None	N/A
	Dose after dialysis	Dose for GFR <10 mL/min	N/A
	Dose after dialysis	250 mg q12h	Dose for GFR 10–50 mL/min
	None	None	Dose for GFR 10–50 mL/min
	Dose after dialysis	Dose for GFR <10 mL/min	Dose for GFR 10–50 mL/min
Sodium, 1.9 mEq/g	Dose after dialysis	Dose for GFR <10 mL/min	Dose for GFR 10–50 mL/min
Sodium, 5.2 mEq/g	3.0 g after dialysis	Dose for GFR <10 mL/min	Dose for GFR 10–50 mL/min
Sodium, 1.9 mEq/g	Dose after dialysis	Dose for GFR <10 mL/min	Dose for GFR 10–50 mL/min
Food, dairy products, tube feeding, and Al(OH)$_3$ may decrease the absorption of quinolones			
Poorly absorbed with antacids, sucralfate, and phosphate binders; IV dose 1/3 of oral dose; decreases phenytoin levels	250 mg q12h (200 mg if IV)	250 mg q8h (200 mg if IV)	200 mg IV q12h
L-isomer of ofloxacin: appears to have similar pharmacokinetics and toxicities	Dose for GFR <10 mL/min	Dose for GFR <10 mL/min	Dose for GFR 10–50 mL/min
	No data	No data	No data
Agents in this group are malabsorbed in the presence of magnesium, calcium, aluminum, and iron; theophylline metabolism is impaired; higher oral doses may be needed to treat CAPD peritonitis	Avoid	Avoid	N/A
See above	Dose for GFR <10 mL/min	Dose for GFR <10 mL/min	N/A
See above	100–200 mg after dialysis	Dose for GFR <10 mL/min	300 mg/d

Continued

Table 65.2

Antimicrobial Agents in Renal Failure—cont'd

Antimicrobial Agents in Renal Failure

Drugs	Normal Dosage	% of Renal Excretion	Dosage Adjustment in Renal Failure		
			GFR >50 mL/min	GFR 10–50 mL/min	GFR <10 mL/min
Miscellaneous Agents					
Azithromycin	250–500 mg PO q24h	6%	No renal adjustment is required		
Clarithromycin	500 mg PO q12h		No renal adjustment is required		
Clindamycin	150–450 mg PO q8h	10%	No renal adjustment is required		
Dirithromycin	500 mg PO q24h		No renal adjustment is required		
Erythromycin	250 to 500 mg PO q6h	15%	No renal adjustment is required		
Ertapenem	1 g IV q24h		1 g IV q24h	0.5 g IV q24h	0.5 g IV q24h
Imipenem–cilastatin	250 to 500 mg IV q6h	50%	500 mg q8h	250–500 q8 to 12h	250 mg q12h
Meropenem	1 g IV q8h	65%	1 g q8h	0.5–1g q12h	0.5–1g q24h
Metronidazole	500 mg IV q6h	20%	No renal adjustment is required		
Pentamidine	4 mg/kg/day	5%	q24h	q24h	q48h
Trimethoprim/ sulfamethoxazole	800/160 mg PO q12h	70%	q12h	q18h	q24h
Vancomycin	1 g IV q12h	90%	q12h	q24–36h	q48–72h
Vancomycin	125–250 mg PO q6h	0%	100%	100%	100%
Antituberculosis Antibiotics					
Rifampin	300–600 mg PO q24h	20%	No renal adjustment is required		

Comments	Hemodialysis	Continuous Ambulatory Peritoneal Dialysis	Continuous Venovenous Hemofiltration
No drug–drug interaction with CSA/KF	None	None	None
	None	None	None
Increase CSA/FK level	None	None	None
Nonenzymatically hydrolyzed to active compound erythromycylamine	None	No data: none	Dose for GFR 10–50 mL/min
Increase CSA/FK level; avoid in transplant patients	None	None	None
	Dose after dialysis	Dose for GFR <10 mL/min	Dose for GFR <30
Seizures in ESRD; nonrenal clearance in ARF is less than in chronic renal failure; administered with cilastin to prevent nephrotoxicity of renal metabolite	Dose after dialysis	Dose for GFR <10 mL/min	Dose for GFR 10–50 mL/min
Fewer seizures than with imipenem	Dose after dialysis	Dose for GFR <10 mL/min	Dose for GFR 10–50 mL/min
Peripheral neuropathy, increase LFTs, disulfiram reaction with alcoholic beverages	Dose after dialysis	Dose for GFR <10 mL/min	Dose for GFR 10–50 mL/min
Inhalation may cause bronchospasm; IV administration may cause hypotension, hypoglycemia, and nephrotoxicity	None	None	None
Increase serum creatinine; can cause hyperkalemia	Dose after dialysis	q24h	q18h
Nephrotoxic, ototoxic; may prolong the neuromuscular blockade effect of muscle relaxants	500 mg q12–24h (high FLX)	1.0 g q24–96h	500 mg q12h
Peak: 30–40 Trough: 5–10			
Oral vancomycin is indicated only for the treatment of *Clostridium difficile*	100%	100%	100%
Decrease CSA/FK level; many drug interactions	None	Dose for GFR <10 mL/min	Dose for GFR <10 mL/min

Continued

Table 65.2

Antimicrobial Agents in Renal Failure—cont'd

Antimicrobial Agents in Renal Failure

Drugs	Normal Dosage	% of Renal Excretion	Dosage Adjustment in Renal Failure		
			GFR >50 mL/min	GFR 10–50 mL/min	GFR <10 mL/min
Antifungal Agents					
Amphotericin B	0.5 mg–1.5 mg/kg/day	<1%	No renal adjustment is required		
Amphotec	4–6 mg/kg/day	<1%	No renal adjustment is required		
Abelcet	5 mg/kg/day	<1%	No renal adjustment is required		
AmBisome	3–5 mg/kg/day	<1%	No renal adjustment is required		
Azoles and Other Antifungals					
Fluconazole	200–800 mg IV q24h/q12h	70%	100%	100%	50%
Flucytosine	37.5 mg/kg	90%	q12h	q16h	q24h
Griseofulvin	125–250 mg q6h	1%	100%	100%	100%
Itraconazole	200 mg q12h	35%	100%	100%	50%
Ketoconazole	200–400 mg PO q24h	15%	100%	100%	100%
Miconazole	1200–3600 mg/day	1%	100%	100%	100%
Posaconazole	200 mg q6h	1%	100%	100%	100%
Terbinafine	250 mg PO q24h	>1%	100%	100%	100%
Voriconazole	4–6 mg/kg q12h	1%	100%	100%	100%
Caspofungin	70 mg LD; then 50 mg/day	1%	100%	100%	100%
Micafungin	100–150 mg IV daily	1%	100%	100%	100%
Anidulafungin	200 mg LD; then 100 mg/day	1%	100%	100%	100%
Antiviral Agents					
Acyclovir	200–800 mg PO 5×/day	50%	100%	100%	50%
Adefovir	10 mg q24h	45%	100%	10 mg q48h	10 mg q72h
Amantadine	100–200 mg q12h	90%	100%	50%	q96h–7 days

Comments	Hemodialysis	Continuous Ambulatory Peritoneal Dialysis	Continuous Venovenous Hemofiltration
Nephrotoxic; infusion-related reactions; give 250 cc NS before each dose	q24h	q24h	q24–36h
Increase CSA/FK level			
	200 mg after dialysis	Dose for GFR <10 mL/min	Dose for GFR 10–50 mL/min
Hepatic dysfunction; marrow suppression more common in azotemic patients	Dose after dialysis	0.5–1.0 g/d	Dose for GFR 10–50 mL/min
	None	None	None
Poor oral absorption	100 mg q12–24h	100 mg q12–24h	100 mg q12–24h
Hepatotoxic	None	None	None
	None	None	None
Avoid IV formulation in CKD			
Poor absorption; neurotoxicity in ESRD; IV preparation can cause renal failure if injected rapidly	Dose after dialysis	Dose for GFR <10 mL/min	3.5 mg/kg/d
Renal toxicity	10 mg weekly after HD	No data	No data
	None	None	Dose for GFR 10–50 mL/min

Continued

Table 65.2

Antimicrobial Agents in Renal Failure—cont'd

Antimicrobial Agents in Renal Failure

Drugs	Normal Dosage	% of Renal Excretion	Dosage Adjustment in Renal Failure		
			GFR >50 mL/min	GFR 10–50 mL/min	GFR <10 mL/min
Cidofovir	5 mg/kg weekly ×2 (induction); 5 mg/kg every 2 weeks	90%	Avoid in CKD	No data: avoid	No data: avoid
Delavirdine	400 mg q8h	5%	No data: 100%	No data: 100%	No data: 100%
Didanosine	200 mg q12h (125 mg if <60 kg)	40%–69%	q12h	q24h	50% q24h
Emtricitabine	200 mg q24h	86%	q24h	q48–72h	q96h
Entecavir	0.5 mg q24h	62%	q24h	q48–72h	q96h
Famciclovir	250–500 mg PO q8h–q12h	60%	q8h	q12h	q24h
Foscarnet	40–80 mg IV q8h	85%	40–20 mg q8–24h according to ClCr		
Ganciclovir IV	5 mg/kg q12h	95%	q12h	q24h	2.5 mg/kg q24h
Ganciclovir	1000 mg PO q8h	95%	1000 mg q8h	1000 mg q12h	1000 mg q24h
Indinavir	800 mg q8h	10%	No data: 100%	No data: 100%	No data: 100%
Lamivudine	150 mg PO q12h	80%	q12h	q24h	50 mg q24h
Maraviroc	300 mg q12h	20%	300 mg q12h	No data	No data
Nelfinavir	750 mg q8h	No data	No data	No data	No data
Nevirapine	200 mg q24h × 14d	<3	No data: 100%	No data: 100%	No data: 100%

Comments	Hemodialysis	Continuous Ambulatory Peritoneal Dialysis	Continuous Venovenous Hemofiltration
Dose-limiting nephrotoxicity with proteinuria, glycosuria, renal insufficiency; nephrotoxicity and renal clearance reduced with coadministration of probenecid	No data	No data	Avoid
	No data	No data	No data: dose for GFR 10–50 mL/min
Pancreatitis	Dose after dialysis	Dose for GFR <10 mL/min	Dose for GFR <10 mL/min
		Dose after dialysis	No data
		Dose after dialysis	No data
VZV: 500 mg PO q8h HSV: 250 PO q12h Metabolized to active compound penciclovir	Dose after dialysis	No data	No data: dose for GFR 10–50 mL/min
Nephrotoxic, neurotoxic, hypocalcemia, hypophosphatemia, hypomagnesemia, and hypokalemia	Dose after dialysis	Dose for GFR <10 mL/min	Dose for GFR 10–50 mL/min
Granulocytopenia and thrombocytopenia	Dose after dialysis	Dose for GFR <10 mL/min	2.5 mg/kg q24h
Oral ganciclovir should be used ONLY for prevention of CMV infection; always use IV ganciclovir for the treatment of CMV infection	No data: dose after dialysis	No data: dose for GFR <10 mL/min	N/A
Nephrolithiasis; ARF due to crystalluria, tubulointerstitial nephritis	No data	No data: dose for GFR <10 mL/min	No data
For hepatitis B	Dose after dialysis	No data: dose for GFR <10 mL/min	Dose for GFR 10–50 mL/min
Drug interaction with CYP III-A	No data	No data	No data
	No data	No data	No data
May be partially cleared by HD and PD	Dose after dialysis	No data: dose for GFR <10 mL/min	No data: dose for GFR 10–50 mL/min

Continued

Table 65.2

Antimicrobial Agents in Renal Failure—cont'd

Antimicrobial Agents in Renal Failure

			Dosage Adjustment in Renal Failure		
Drugs	**Normal Dosage**	**% of Renal Excretion**	**GFR >50 mL/min**	**GFR 10–50 mL/ min**	**GFR <10 mL/min**
Oseltamivir	75 mg q12h	99%	75 q12h	75 mg/day	75 mg q48h
Ribavirin	500–600 mg q12h	30%	100%	100%	50%
Rifabutin	300 mg q24h	5%–10%	100%	100%	100%
Rimantadine	100 mg PO q12h	25%	100%	100%	50%
Ritonavir	600 mg q12h	3.50%	No data: 100%	No data: 100%	No data: 100%
Saquinavir	600 mg q8h	<4%	No data: 100%	No data: 100%	No data: 100%
Stavudine	30–40 mg q12h	35%–40%	100%	50% q12–24h	50% q24h
Telbivudine	600 mg PO daily		100%	600 mg q48h	600 mg q96 h
Tenofovir	300 mg q24h		100%	300 mg q48–72h	300 mg q96h
Valacyclovir	500–1000 mg q8h	50%	100%	50%	25%
Valganciclovir	900 mg PO daily or q12h		100%	50%	25%
Vidarabine	15 mg/kg infusion q24h	50%	100%	100%	75%
Zanamivir	2 puffs q12h × 5 days	1%	100%	100%	100%
Zalcitabine	0.75 mg q8h	75%	100%	q12h	q24h
Zidovudine	200 mg q8h, 300 mg q12h	8%–25%	100%	100%	100 mg q8h

Comments	Hemodialysis	Continuous Ambulatory Peritoneal Dialysis	Continuous Venovenous Hemofiltration
	Dose after dialysis		
HUS	Dose after dialysis	Dose for GFR <10 mL/min	Dose for GFR 10–50 mL/min
	None	None	No data: dose for GFR 10–50 mL/min
Many drug interactions	No data: none	No data: dose for GFR <10 mL/min	No data: dose for GFR 10–50 mL/min
	No data: none	No data: dose for GFR <10 mL/min	No data: dose for GFR 10–50 mL/min
	Dose for GFR <10 mL/min after dialysis	No data	No data: dose for GFR 10–50 mL/min
	Dose for GFR <10 mL/min after dialysis	No data	No data: dose for GFR 10–50 mL/min
Nephrotoxic	Dose for GFR <10 mL/min after dialysis	No data	No data: dose for GFR 10–50 mL/min
TTP/HUS	Dose after dialysis	Dose for GFR <10 mL/min	No data: dose for GFR 10–50 mL/min
Granulocytopenia and thrombocytopenia	Dose after dialysis	Dose for GFR <10 mL/min	450 mg/day
	Infuse after dialysis	Dose for GFR <10 mL/min	Dose for GFR 10–50 mL/min
Bioavailability from inhalation and systemic exposure to drug is low	None	None	No data
	No data: dose after dialysis	No data	No data: dose for GFR 10–50 mL/min
Enormous interpatient variation; metabolite renally excreted	Dose for GFR <10 mL/min	Dose for GFR <10 mL/min	100 mg q8h

Continued

Table 65.2

Antimicrobial Agents in Renal Failure—cont'd

Analgesic Drug Dosing in Renal Failure

			Dosage Adjustment in Renal Failure		
Analgesics	**Normal Dosage**	**% of Renal Excretion**	**GFR >50 mL/ min**	**GFR 10–50 mL/ min**	**GFR <10 mL/ min**
Narcotics and Narcotic Antagonists					
Alfentanil	Anesthetic induction 8–40 mcg/kg	Hepatic	100%	100%	100%
Butorphanol	2 mg q3–4h	Hepatic	100%	75%	50%
Codeine	30–60 mg q4–6h	Hepatic	100%	75%	50%
Fentanyl	Anesthetic induction (individualized)	Hepatic	100%	75%	50%
Meperidine	50–100 mg q3–4h	Hepatic	100%	75%	50%
Methadone	2.5–5 mg q6–8h	Hepatic	100%	100%	50%–75%
Morphine	20–25 mg q4h	Hepatic	100%	75%	50%
Naloxone	0.4–2 mg IV	Hepatic	100%	100%	100%
Pentazocine	50 mg q4h	Hepatic	100%	75%	75%
Propoxyphene	65 mg PO q6–8h	Hepatic	100%	100%	Avoid
Sufentanil	Anesthetic induction	Hepatic	100%	100%	100%
Non-Narcotics					
Acetaminophen	650 mg q4h	Hepatic	q4h	q6h	q8h
Acetylsalicylic acid	650 mg q4h	Hepatic (renal)	q4h	q4–6h	Avoid

Comments	Hemodialysis	Continuous Ambulatory Peritoneal Dialysis	Continuous Venovenous Hemofiltration
Titrate the dose regimen	N/A	N/A	N/A
	No data	No data	N/A
	No data	No data	Dose for GFR 10–50 mL/min
CRRT: titrate	N/A	N/A	N/A
Normeperidine, an active metabolite, accumulates in ESRD and may cause seizures; protein binding is reduced in ESRD; 20%–25% excreted unchanged in acidic urine	Avoid	Avoid	Avoid
	None	None	N/A
Increased sensitivity to drug effect in ESRD	None	No data	Dose for GFR 10–50 mL/min
	N/A	N/A	Dose for GFR 10–50 mL/min
	None	No data	Dose for GFR 10–50 mL/min
Active metabolite norpropoxyphene accumulates in ESRD	Avoid	Avoid	N/A
CRRT: titrate	N/A	N/A	N/A
Overdose may be nephrotoxic; drug is major metabolite of phenacetin	None	None	Dose for GFR 10–50 mL/min
Nephrotoxic in high doses; may decrease GFR when RBF is prostaglandin dependent; may add to uremic GI and hematologic symptoms; protein binding reduced in ESRD	Dose after dialysis	None	Dose for GFR 10–50 mL/min

Continued

Table 65.2

Antimicrobial Agents in Renal Failure—cont'd

Antihypertensive and Cardiovascular Agent Dosing in Renal Failure

Antihypertensive and Cardiovascular Agents	Normal Doses			Dosage Adjustment in Renal Failure	
	Starting Dose	Maximum Dose	% of Renal Excretion	GFR >50 mL/min	GFR 10–50 mL/min
ACE Inhibitors					
Benazepril	10 mg q24h	80 mg q24h	20%	100%	75%
Captopril	6.25–25 mg PO q8h	100 mg q8h	35%	100%	75%
Enalapril	5 mg q24h	20 mg q12h	45%	100%	75%
Fosinopril	10 mg PO q24h	40 mg q12h	20%	100%	100%
Lisinopril	2.5 mg q24h	20 mg q12h	80%	100%	50%–75%
Pentopril		125 mg q24h	80%–90%	100%	50%–75%
Perindopril		2 mg q24h	<10%	100%	75%

GFR <10 mL/min	Comments	Hemodialysis	Continuous Ambulatory Peritoneal Dialysis	Continuous Venovenous Hemofiltration
	Hyperkalemia, ARF, angioedema, rash, cough, anemia, and liver toxicity			
25%–50%		None	None	Dose for GFR 10–50 mL/min
50%	Rare proteinuria, nephrotic syndrome, dysgeusia, granulocytopenia; increases serum digoxin levels	25%–30%	None	Dose for GFR 10–50 mL/min
50%	Enalaprilat, the active moiety, formed in liver	20%–25%	None	Dose for GFR 10–50 mL/min
75%	Fosinoprilat, the active moiety, formed in liver; drug less likely than other ACE inhibitors to accumulate in renal failure	None	None	Dose for GFR 10–50 mL/min
25%–50%	Lysine analog of a pharmacologically active enalapril metabolite	20%	None	Dose for GFR 10–50 mL/min
50%		No data	No data	Dose for GFR 10–50 mL/min
50%	Active metabolite is perindoprilat; the clearance of perindoprilat and its metabolites is almost exclusively renal; ≈60% of circulating perindopril is bound to plasma proteins, and only 10%–20% of perindoprilat is bound	25%–50%	No data	Dose for GFR 10–50 mL/min

Continued

Table 65.2

Antimicrobial Agents in Renal Failure—cont'd

Antihypertensive and Cardiovascular Agent Dosing in Renal Failure

Antihypertensive and Cardiovascular Agents	Normal Doses			Dosage Adjustment in Renal Failure	
	Starting Dose	Maximum Dose	% of Renal Excretion	GFR >50 mL/min	GFR 10–50 mL/min
Quinapril	10 mg q24h	20 mg q24h	30%	100%	75%–100%
Ramipril	2.5 mg q24h	10 q12h	15%	100%	50%–75%
Trandolapril	1–2 mg q24h	4 mg q24h	33%	100%	50%–100%
Angiotensin II Receptors Antagonists					
Candesartan	16 mg q24h	32 mg q24h	33%	100%	100%
Eprosartan	600 mg q24h	400–800 mg q24h	25%	100%	100%
Irbesartan	150 mg q24h	300 mg q24h	20%	100%	100%
Losartan	50 mg q24h	100 mg q24h	13%	100%	100%
Telmisartan	20–80 mg q24h		<5%	100%	100%
Valsartan	80 mg q24h	160 mg q12h	7%	100%	100%
Beta-Blockers					

GFR <10 mL/min	Comments	Hemodialysis	Continuous Ambulatory Peritoneal Dialysis	Continuous Venovenous Hemofiltration
75%	Active metabolite is quinaprilat; 96% of quinaprilat is excreted renally	25%	None	Dose for GFR 10–50 mL/min
25%–50%	Active metabolite is ramiprilat; data are for ramiprilat	20%	None	Dose for GFR 10–50 mL/min
50%		None	None	Dose for GFR 10–50 mL/min
	Hyperkalemia, angioedema (less common than ACE inhibitors)			
50%	Candesartan cilexetil is rapidly and completely bioactivated by ester hydrolysis during absorption from the GI tract to candesartan	None	None	None
100%	Eprosartan pharmacokinetics more variable ESRD; decreased protein binding in uremia	None	None	None
100%		None	None	None
100%		No data	No data	Dose for GFR 10–50 mL/min
100%		None	None	None
100%		None	None	None
	Decrease HDL, mask symptoms of hypoglycemia, bronchospasm, fatigue, insomnia, depression, and sexual dysfunction			

Continued

Table 65.2

Antimicrobial Agents in Renal Failure—cont'd

Antihypertensive and Cardiovascular Agent Dosing in Renal Failure

Antihypertensive and Cardiovascular Agents	Normal Doses			Dosage Adjustment in Renal Failure	
	Starting Dose	Maximum Dose	% of Renal Excretion	GFR >50 mL/ min	GFR 10–50 mL/min
Acebutolol	400 mg q24h or q12h	600 mg q24h or q12h	55%	100%	50%
Atenolol	25 mg q24h	100 mg q24h	90%	100%	75%
Betaxolol	20 mg q24h	80%–90%	100%	100%	50%
Bopindolol	1 mg q24h	4 mg q24h	<10%	100%	100%
Carteolol	0.5 mg q24h	10 mg q24h	<50%	100%	50%
Carvedilol	3.125 mg PO q8h	25 mg q8h	2%	100%	100%
Celiprolol		200 mg q24h	10%	100%	100%
Dilevalol	200 mg q12h	400 mg q12h	<5%	100%	100%
Esmolol (IV only)	50 mcg/kg/min	300 mcg/kg/ min	10%	100%	100%
Labetalol	50 mg PO q12h	400 mg q12h	5%	100%	100%

GFR <10 mL/min	Comments	Hemodialysis	Continuous Ambulatory Peritoneal Dialysis	Continuous Venovenous Hemofiltration
30%–50%	Active metabolites with long half-life	None	None	Dose for GFR 10–50 mL/min
50%	Accumulates in ESRD	25–50 mg	None	Dose for GFR 10–50 mL/min
50%		None	Dose for GFR 10–50 mL/min	Dose for GFR 10–50 mL/min
100%		None	None	Dose for GFR 10–50 mL/min
25%		No data	None	Dose for GFR 10–50 mL/min
100%	Kinetics are dose dependent; plasma concentrations of carvedilol have been reported to be increased in patients with renal impairment	None	None	Dose for GFR 10–50 mL/min
75%		No data	None	Dose for GFR 10–50 mL/min
100%		None	None	No data
100%	Active metabolite retained in renal failure	None	None	No data
100%	For IV use: 20 mg slow IV injection over a 2-min period; additional injections of 40 mg or 80 mg can be given at 10-min intervals until a total of 300 mg or continuous infusion of 2 mg/min	None	None	Dose for GFR 10–50 mL/min

Continued

Table 65.2

Antimicrobial Agents in Renal Failure—cont'd

Antihypertensive and Cardiovascular Agent Dosing in Renal Failure

	Normal Doses			Dosage Adjustment in Renal Failure	
Antihypertensive and Cardiovascular Agents	Starting Dose	Maximum Dose	% of Renal Excretion	GFR >50 mL/min	GFR 10–50 mL/min
Metoprolol		50 mg q12h	100 mg q12h	<5%	100%
Nadolol	80 mg q24h	160 mg q12h	90%	100%	50%
Penbutolol	10 mg q24h	40 mg q24h	<10	100%	100%
Pindolol	10 mg q12h	40 mg q12h	40%	100%	100%
Propranolol	40%–160 mg q8h	320 mg/day	<5%	100%	100%
Sotalol	80 q12h	160 mg q12h	70%	100%	50%
Timolol	10 mg q12h	20 mg q12h	15%	100%	100%

GFR <10 mL/min	Comments	Hemodialysis	Continuous Ambulatory Peritoneal Dialysis	Continuous Venovenous Hemofiltration
100%		None	None	None
25%	Start with prolonged interval and titrate	40 mg	None	Dose for GFR 10–50 mL/min
100%		None	None	Dose for GFR 10–50 mL/min
100%		None	None	Dose for GFR 10–50 mL/min
100%	Bioavailability may increase in ESRD; metabolites may cause increased bilirubin by assay interference in ESRD; hypoglycemia reported in ESRD	None	None	Dose for GFR 10–50 mL/min
25%–50%	Extreme caution should be exercised in the use of sotalol in patients with renal failure undergoing hemodialysis; to minimize the risk of induced arrhythmia, patients initiated or reinitiated on sotalol should be placed for a minimum of 3 days (on their maintenance dose) in a facility that can provide cardiac resuscitation and continuous ECG monitoring	80 mg	None	Dose for GFR 10–50 mL/min
100%		None	None	Dose for GFR 10–50 mL/min

Continued

Table 65.2

Antimicrobial Agents in Renal Failure—cont'd

Antihypertensive and Cardiovascular Agent Dosing in Renal Failure

Antihypertensive and Cardiovascular Agents	Normal Doses			Dosage Adjustment in Renal Failure	
	Starting Dose	Maximum Dose	% of Renal Excretion	GFR >50 mL/min	GFR 10–50 mL/min
Calcium Channel Blockers					
Amlodipine	2.5 PO q24h	10 mg q24h	10%	100%	100%
Bepridil	No data	<1%	No data	No data	No data
Diltiazem	30 mg q8h	90 mg q8h	10%	100%	100%
Felodipine	5 mg PO q12h	20 mg q24h	1%	100%	100%
Isradipine	5 mg PO q12h	10 mg q12h	<5%	100%	100%
Nicardipine	20 mg PO q8h	30 mg PO q8h	<1%	100%	100%
Nifedipine XL	30 q24h	90 mg q12h	10%	100%	100%
Nimodipine	30 mg q8h	10%	100%	100%	100%
Nisoldipine	20 mg q24h	30 mg q12h	10%	100%	100%

GFR <10 mL/min	Comments	Hemodialysis	Continuous Ambulatory Peritoneal Dialysis	Continuous Venovenous Hemofiltration
	Dihydropyridine: headache, ankle edema, gingival hyperplasia, and flushing Nondihydropyridine: bradycardia, constipation, gingival hyperplasia, and AV block			
100%	May increase digoxin and cyclosporine levels	None	None	Dose for GFR 10–50 mL/min
Weak vasodilator and antihypertensive		None	No data	No data
100%	Acute renal dysfunction; may exacerbate hyperkalemia; may increase digoxin and cyclosporine levels	None	None	Dose for GFR 10–50 mL/min
100%	May increase digoxin levels	None	None	Dose for GFR 10–50 mL/min
100%	May increase digoxin levels	None	None	Dose for GFR 10–50 mL/min
	Uremia inhibits hepatic metabolism; may increase digoxin levels	None	None	None
100%	Avoid short-acting nifedipine formulation	None	None	None
	May lower BP	None	None	Dose for GFR 10–50 mL/min
100%	May increase digoxin levels	None	None	Dose for GFR 10–50 mL/min

Continued

Table 65.2

Antimicrobial Agents in Renal Failure—cont'd

Antihypertensive and Cardiovascular Agent Dosing in Renal Failure

Antihypertensive and Cardiovascular Agents	Normal Doses			Dosage Adjustment in Renal Failure	
	Starting Dose	Maximum Dose	% of Renal Excretion	GFR >50 mL/min	GFR 10–50 mL/min
Verapamil	40 mg q8h	240 mg/day	10%	100%	100%
Diuretics					
Acetazolamide	125 mg PO q8h	500 mg PO q8h	90%	100%	50%
Amiloride	5 mg PO q24h	10 mg PO q24h	50%	100%	100%
Bumetanide	1–2 mg PO q24h	2–4 mg PO q24h	35%	100%	100%
Chlorthalidone	25 mg q24h	50%	q24h	q24h	Avoid
Ethacrynic acid	50 mg PO q24h	100 mg PO q12h	20%	100%	100%

GFR <10 mL/min	Comments	Hemodialysis	Continuous Ambulatory Peritoneal Dialysis	Continuous Venovenous Hemofiltration
100%	Acute renal dysfunction; active metabolites accumulate, particularly with sustained-release forms	None	None	Dose for GFR 10–50 mL/min
	Hypokalemia or hyperkalemia (potassium-sparing agents), hyperuricemia, hyperglycemia, hypomagnesemia, increase serum cholesterol			
Avoid	May potentiate acidosis; ineffective as diuretic in ESRD may cause neurologic side effects in dialysis patients	No data	No data	Avoid
Avoid	Hyperkalemia with GFR <30 mL/min, especially in diabetics; hyperchloremic metabolic acidosis	N/A	N/A	N/A
100%	Ototoxicity increased in ESRD in combination with aminoglycosides; high doses effective in ESRD; muscle pain, gynecomastia	None	None	N/A
Ineffective with low GFR		N/A	N/A	N/A
100%	Ototoxicity increased in ESRD in combination with aminoglycosides	None	None	N/A

Continued

Table 65.2

Antimicrobial Agents in Renal Failure—cont'd

Antihypertensive and Cardiovascular Agent Dosing in Renal Failure

| Antihypertensive and Cardiovascular Agents | Normal Doses | | | Dosage Adjustment in Renal Failure | |
	Starting Dose	Maximum Dose	% of Renal Excretion	GFR >50 mL/min	GFR 10–50 mL/min
Furosemide	40–80 mg PO q24h	120 mg PO q8h	70%	100%	100%
Indapamide	2.5 mg q24h	<5%	100%	100%	Avoid
Metolazone	2.5 mg PO q24h	10 mg PO q12h	70%	100%	100%
Eplerenone	25 mg/day	200 mg/day	100%	100%	100%
Spironolactone	100 mg PO q24h	300 mg PO q24h	25%	100%	100%
Thiazides	25 mg q12h	50 mg q12h	>95%	100%	100%
Torsemide	5 mg PO q12h	20 mg q24h	25%	100%	100%
Triamterene	25 mg q12h	50 mg q12h	5%–10%	q12h	q12h

GFR <10 mL/min	Comments	Hemodialysis	Continuous Ambulatory Peritoneal Dialysis	Continuous Venovenous Hemofiltration
100%	Ototoxicity increased in ESRD, especially in combination with aminoglycosides; high doses effective in ESRD	None	None	N/A
Ineffective in ESRD		None	N/A	None
	High doses effective in ESRD; gynecomastia, impotence	None	None	None
Avoid	Active metabolites with long half-life; hyperkalemia common when GFR <30, especially in diabetics; gynecomastia, hyperchloremic acidosis; increases serum by immunoassay interference	N/A	N/A	Avoid
Avoid	Usually ineffective with GFR <30 mL/min; effective at low GFR in combination with loop diuretic; hyperuricemia		N/A	N/A
100%	High doses effective in ESRD; ototoxicity	None	None	N/A
Avoid	Hyperkalemia common when GFR <30, especially in diabetics; active metabolite with long half-life in ESRD; folic acid antagonist; urolithiasis; crystalluria in acid urine; may cause ARF	Avoid	Avoid	Avoid

Continued

Table 65.2

Antimicrobial Agents in Renal Failure—cont'd

Antihypertensive and Cardiovascular Agent Dosing in Renal Failure

Antihypertensive and Cardiovascular Agents	Normal Doses			Dosage Adjustment in Renal Failure	
	Starting Dose	Maximum Dose	% of Renal Excretion	GFR >50 mL/min	GFR 10–50 mL/min
Miscellaneous Agents					
Amrinone	5 mg/kg/min daily dose <10 mg/kg	10 mg/kg/min daily dose <10 mg/kg	10%–40%	100%	100%
Clonidine	0.1 PO q12h/ q8h	1.2 mg/day	45%	100%	100%
Digoxin	0.125 mg qod/ q24h	0.25 mg PO q24h	25%	100%	100%
Hydralazine	10 mg PO q6h	100 mg PO q6h	25%	100%	100%
Midodrine	No data	No data	75%–80%	5–10 mg q8h	5–10 mg q8h
Minoxidil	2.5 mg PO q12h	10 mg PO q12h	20%	100%	100%

GFR <10 mL/min	Comments	Hemodialysis	Continuous Ambulatory Peritoneal Dialysis	Continuous Venovenous Hemofiltration
100%	Thrombocytopenia; nausea, vomiting in ESRD	No data	No data	Dose for GFR 10–50 mL/min
100%	Sexual dysfunction, dizziness, portal hypotension	None	None	Dose for GFR 10–50 mL/min
100%	Decrease loading dose by 50% in ESRD; radioimmunoassay may overestimate serum levels in uremia; clearance decreased by amiodarone, spironolactone, quinidine, verapamil; hypokalemia, hypomagnesemia enhance toxicity; V_d and total body clearance decreased in ESRD; serum level 12 h after dose is best guide in ESRD; digoxin immune antibodies can treat severe toxicity in ESRD	None	None	Dose for GFR 10–50 mL/min
100%	Lupus-like reaction	None	None	Dose for GFR 10–50 mL/min
No data	Increased BP	5 mg q8h	No data	Dose for GFR 10–50 mL/min
100%	Pericardial effusion, fluid retention, hypertrichosis, and tachycardia	None	None	Dose for GFR 10–50 mL/min

Continued

Table 65.2

Antimicrobial Agents in Renal Failure—cont'd

Antihypertensive and Cardiovascular Agent Dosing in Renal Failure

| Antihypertensive and Cardiovascular Agents | Normal Doses | | | Dosage Adjustment in Renal Failure | |
	Starting Dose	Maximum Dose	% of Renal Excretion	GFR >50 mL/min	GFR 10–50 mL/min
Nitroprusside	1 mcg/kg/min	10 mcg/kg/min	<10%	100%	100%
Amrinone	5 mcg/kg/min	10 mcg/kg/min	25%	100%	100%
Dobutamine	2.5 mcg/kg/min	15 mcg/kg/min	10%	100%	100%
Milrinone	0.375 mcg/kg/min	0.75 mcg/kg/min	100%	100%	100%

Hypoglycemic Agent Dosing in Renal Failure

| Hypoglycemic Agents | Normal Doses | | | Dosage Adjustment in Renal Failure | |
	Starting Dose	Maximum Dose	% of Renal Excretion	GFR >50 mL/min	GFR 10–50 mL/min
Acarbose	25 mg q8h	100 mg q8h	35%	100%	50%
Acetohexamide	250 mg q24h	1500 mg q24h	None	Avoid	Avoid
Chlorpropamide	100 mg q24h	500 mg q24h	47%	50%	Avoid
Exenatide	5 mcg q12h	10 mcg q12h	No data	100%	Use with caution
Glibornuride	12.5 mg q24h	100 mg q14h	No data	No data	No data
Gliclazide	80 mg q24h	320 mg q24h	<20%	50%–100%	Avoid
Glipizide	5 mg q24h	20 mg q12h	5%	100%	50%

GFR <10 mL/min	Comments	Hemodialysis	Continuous Ambulatory Peritoneal Dialysis	Continuous Venovenous Hemofiltration
100%	Cyanide toxicity	None	None	Dose for GFR 10–50 mL/min
100%	Thrombocytopenia; N/V in ESRD	No data	No data	Dose for GFR 10–50 mL/min
100%		No data	No data	Dose for GFR 10–50 mL/min
		No data	No data	Dose for GFR 10–50 mL/min

GFR <10 mL/min	Comments	Hemodialysis	CAPD	Continuous Venovenous Hemofiltration
	Avoid all oral hypoglycemic agents on CRRT			
Avoid	Abdominal pain, N/V, and flatulence	No data	No data	Avoid
Avoid	Diuretic effect; may falsely elevate serum creatinine; active metabolite has $t_{1/2}$ of 5–8 h in healthy subjects and is eliminated by the kidney; prolonged hypoglycemia in azotemic patients	No data	None	Avoid
Avoid	Impairs water excretion; prolonged hypoglycemia in azotemic patients	No data	None	Avoid
Avoid				
No data		No data	No data	Avoid
Avoid		No data	No data	Avoid
50%		No data	No data	Avoid

Continued

Table 65.2

Antimicrobial Agents in Renal Failure—cont'd

Hypoglycemic Agent Dosing in Renal Failure

	Normal Doses			Dosage Adjustment in Renal Failure	
Hypoglycemic Agents	Starting Dose	Maximum Dose	% of Renal Excretion	GFR >50 mL/min	GFR 10–50 mL/min
Glyburide	2.5 mg q24h	10 mg q12h	50%	100%	50%
Liraglutide	0.6 mg/day	1.8 mg/day	6%	100%	100%
Metformin	500 mg q12h	2550 mg/day (q12h or q8h)	95%	100%	Avoid
Pioglitazone	15 mg q24h	45 mg q24h	3%	100%	100%
Pramlintide	15 mcg	60 mcg daily	No data	100%	No data
Repaglinide	0.5–1 mg	4 mg q8h			
Rosiglitazone	2 mg q24h	8 mg q24h	3%	100%	100%
Sitagliptin	25 mg	100 mg	79%	100%	50%
Tolazamide	100 mg q24h	250 mg q24h	7%	100%	100%
Tolbutamide	1 g q24h	2 g q24h	None	100%	100%
Parenteral Agents					
Insulin		Variable	None	100%	75%
Lispro insulin		Variable	No data	100%	75%

Hyperlipidemic Agent Dosing in Renal Failure

	Normal Doses			Dosage Adjustment in Renal Failure	
Hypoglycemic Agents	Starting Dose	Maximum Dose	% of Renal Excretion	GFR >50 mL/min	GFR 10–50 mL/min
Atorvastatin	10 mg/day	400 mg SR q24h 80 mg/day	<2%	100%	100%
Bezafibrate		200 mg q6h–q12h	50%	50%–100%	25%–50%
Cholestyramine	4 g q12h	24 g/day	None	100%	100%
Clofibrate	500 mg q12h	1000 mg q12h	40%–70%	q6–12h	q12–18h
Colestipol	5 g q12h	30 g/day	None	100%	100%
Fenofibrate	48 g/day	145 g/day	30%	100%	100%
Fluvastatin	20 g/day	80 g/day	<1%	100%	100%

GFR <10 mL/min	Comments	Hemodialysis	CAPD	Continuous Venovenous Hemofiltration
Avoid		None	None	Avoid
Avoid	No data on dialysis			
Avoid	Lactic acidosis	No data	No data	Avoid
100%	Drug interactions	None	None	NA
No data				
100%	Increases LDL	None	None	NA
25%				
100%	Diuretic effects	Avoid	Avoid	Avoid
100%	May impair water excretion	None	None	Avoid
	Dosage guided by blood glucose levels			
50%	Renal metabolism of insulin decreases with azotemia	None	None	Dose for GFR 10–50 mL/min
50%	Avoid all oral hypoglycemic agents on CRRT	None	None	None

GFR <10 mL/min	Comments	Hemodialysis	Continuous Ambulatory Peritoneal Dialysis	Continuous Venovenous Hemofiltration
100%	Liver dysfunction, myalgia, and rhabdomyolysis with CSA/FK	No data	No data	No data
Avoid	No data	No data	No data	
100%		No data	No data	No data
Avoid		No data	No data	No data
100%		No data	No data	No data
50%				
100%		No data	No data	No data

Continued

| Table 65.2 |

Antimicrobial Agents in Renal Failure—cont'd

Hyperlipidemic Agent Dosing in Renal Failure

	Normal Doses			Dosage Adjustment in Renal Failure	
Hypoglycemic Agents	**Starting Dose**	**Maximum Dose**	**% of Renal Excretion**	**GFR >50 mL/ min**	**GFR 10–50 mL/ min**
Gemfibrozil	600 q12h	600 q12h	None	100%	100%
Lovastatin	5 mg/day	20 mg/day	None	100%	100%
Nicotinic acid	1 g q8h	2 g q8h	None	100%	50%
Pravastatin	10–40 mg/day	80 mg/day	<10%	100%	100%
Probucol		500 mg q12h	<2%	100%	100%
Rosuvastatin	5 mg/day	20 mg/day	<5%	100%	100%
Simvastatin	5–20 mg/day	20 mg/day	13%	100%	100%

Antithyroid Dosing in Renal Failure

			Dosage Adjustment in Renal Failure		
Antithyroid Drugs	**Normal Dosage**	**% of Renal Excretion**	**GFR >50**	**GFR 10–50 mL/min**	**GFR <10 mL/min**
Methimazole	5–20 mg q8h	7	100%	100%	100%
Propylthiouracil	100 mg q8h	<10	100%	100%	100%

Gastrointestinal Agent Dosing in Renal Failure

	Normal Doses		
Gastrointestinal Agents	**Starting Dose**	**Maximum Dose**	**% of Renal Excretion**
Antiulcer agents			
Cimetidine	300 mg PO q8h	800 mg PO q12h	60%
Famotidine	20 mg PO q12h	40 mg PO q12h	70%
Lansoprazole	15 mg PO q24h	30 mg q12h	None
Nizatidine	150 mg PO q12h	300 mg PO q12h	20%
Omeprazole	20 mg PO q24h	40 mg PO q12h	None
Rabeprazole	20 mg PO q24h	40 mg PO q12h	None
Pantoprazole	40 mg PO q24h	80 mg PO q12h	None
Ranitidine	150 mg PO q12h	300 mg PO q12h	80%

GFR <10 mL/min	Comments	Hemodialysis	Continuous Ambulatory Peritoneal Dialysis	Continuous Venovenous Hemofiltration
100%		No data	No data	No data
100%		No data	No data	No data
25%		No data	No data	No data
100%		No data	No data	No data
100%		No data	No data	No data
50%				
100%		No data	No data	No data

Hemodialysis	Continuous Ambulatory Peritoneal Dialysis	Continuous Venovenous Hemofiltration
No data	No data	Dose for GFR 10–50 mL/min
No data	No data	Dose for GFR 10–50 mL/min

Dosage Adjustment in Renal Failure

GFR >50 mL/min	GFR 10–50 mL/min	GFR <10 mL/min	Comments
100%	75%	25%	Multiple drug–drug interactions; beta-blockers, sulfonylurea, theophylline, warfarin, and so on
100%	75%	25%	Headache, fatigue, thrombocytopenia, alopecia
100%	100%	100%	Headache, diarrhea
100%	75%	25%	Headache, fatigue, thrombocytopenia, alopecia
100%	100%	100%	Headache, diarrhea
100%	100%	100%	Headache, diarrhea
100%	100%	100%	Headache, diarrhea
100%	75%	25%	Headache, fatigue, thrombocytopenia, alopecia

Continued

Table 65.2

Antimicrobial Agents in Renal Failure—cont'd

Gastrointestinal Agent Dosing in Renal Failure

Gastrointestinal Agents	Normal Doses		% of Renal Excretion
	Starting Dose	Maximum Dose	
Metoclopramide	10 mg PO q8h	30 mg PO q6h	15%
Misoprostol	100 mcg PO q12h	200 mcg PO q6h	
Sucralfate	1 g PO q6h	1 g PO q6h	None

Neurologic/Anticonvulsant Dosing in Renal Failure

Anticonvulsants (290)	Normal Doses		% of Renal Excretion	Dosage Adjustment in Renal Failure		
	Starting Dose	Maximum Dose		GFR >50 mL/ min	GFR 10–50 mL/ min	GFR <10 mL/ min
Carbamazepine	2–8 mg/kg/day; adjust for side effects and TDM		2%	100%	100%	100%
Clonazepam	0.5 mg q8h	2 mg q8h	1%	100%	100%	100%
Ethosuximide	5 mg/kg/day; adjust for side effects and TDM		20%	100%	100%	100%
Felbamate	400 mg/q8h	1200 mg/q8h	90%	100%	50%	25%
Gabapentin	150 mg q8h	900 mg q8h	77%	100%	50%	25%
Lamotrigine	25–50 mg/ day	150 mg/day	1%	100%	100%	100%
Levetiracetam	500 mg q12h	1500 mg q12h	66%	100%	50%	50%
Oxcarbazepine	300 mg q12h	600 mg q12h	1%	100%	100%	100%
Phenobarbital	20 mg/kg/day; adjust for side effects and TDM		1%	100%	100%	100%
Phenytoin	20 mg/kg/day; adjust for side effects and TDM		1%	Adjust for renal failure and low albumin		

Dosage Adjustment in Renal Failure

GFR >50 mL/min	GFR 10–50 mL/min	GFR <10 mL/min	Comments
100%	100%	50%–75%	Increase cyclosporine/ tacrolimus level; neurotoxic
100%	100%	100%	Diarrhea, N/V, abortifacient agent
100%	100%	100%	Constipation; decrease absorption of MMF

Comments	Hemodialysis	Continuous Ambulatory Peritoneal Dialysis	Continuous Venovenous Hemofiltration
Plasma concentration: 4–12, double vision, fluid retention, myelosuppression	None	None	None
Although no dose reduction is recommended, the drug has not been studied in patients with renal impairment; recommendations are based on known drug characteristics not clinical trials data	None	No data	N/A
Plasma concentration: 40–100, headache	None	No data	No data
Anorexia, vomiting, insomnia, nausea	Dose after dialysis	Dose for GFR <10 mL/min	Dose for GFR 10–50 mL/min
Fewer CNS side effects than to other agents	300 mg load; then 200–300 mg after hemodialysis	300 mg qod	Dose for GFR 10–50 mL/min
Autoinduction, major drug–drug interaction with valproate	No data	No data	Dose for GFR 10–50 mL/min
	250–500 mg after dialysis	Dose for GFR <10 mL/min	Dose for GFR 10–50 mL/min
Less effect on P450 compared with carbamazepine	No data	No data	No data
Plasma concentration: 15–40 mg/L, insomnia			
Plasma concentration: 10–20 mg/L, nystagmus, check free phenytoin level	None	None	None

Continued

Table 65.2

Antimicrobial Agents in Renal Failure—cont'd

Neurologic/Anticonvulsant Dosing in Renal Failure

Anticonvulsants (290)	Normal Doses			Dosage Adjustment in Renal Failure		
	Starting Dose	Maximum Dose	% of Renal Excretion	GFR >50 mL/min	GFR 10–50 mL/min	GFR <10 mL/min
Primidone	50 mg	100 mg	1%	100%	100%	100%
Sodium valproate	7.5–15 mg/kg/day; adjust for side effect and TDM		1%	100%	100%	100%
Tiagabine	4 mg q24h, increase 4 mg/day, titrate weekly		2%	100%	100%	100%
Topiramate	50 mg/day	200 mg q12h	70%	100%	50%	Avoid
Trimethadione	300 mg q6h–q8h	600 mg q6h–q8h	None	q8h	q8h–q12h	q12h–q24h
Vigabatrin	1 g q12h	2 g q12h	70%	100%	50%	25%
Zonisamide	100 mg q24h	100–300 mg q12h–q24h	30%	100%	75%	50%

Comments	Hemodialysis	Continuous Ambulatory Peritoneal Dialysis	Continuous Venovenous Hemofiltration
Plasma concentration: 5–20	1/3 dose	No data	No data
Plasma concentration: 50–150; weight gain; hepatitis; check free valproate level	None	None	None
Total daily dose may be increased by 4–8 mg at weekly intervals until clinical response is achieved or up to 32 mg/day; total daily dose should be given in divided doses two to four times daily	None	None	Dose for GFR 10–50 mL/min
	No data	No data	Dose for GFR 10–50 mL/min
Active metabolites with long half-life in ESRD; nephrotic syndrome	No data	No data	Dose for GFR 10–50 mL/min
Encephalopathy with drug accumulation	No data	No data	Dose for GFR 10–50 mL/min
Manufacturer recommends that zonisamide should not be used in patients with renal failure (estimated GFR <50 mL/min) because there has been insufficient experience concerning drug dosing and toxicity; zonisamide doses of 100–600 mg/day are effective for normal renal function; dose recommendations for renal impairment based on clearance ratios	Dose for GFR <10 mL/min	Dose for GFR <10 mL/min	Dose for GFR <10 mL/min–50

Continued

Table 65.2

Antimicrobial Agents in Renal Failure—cont'd

Rheumatologic Dosing in Renal Failure

			Dosage Adjustment in Renal Failure		
Arthritis and Gout Agents	**Normal Dosage**	**% of Renal Excretion**	**GFR >50**	**GFR 10–50 mL/ min**	**GFR <10 mL/ min**
Allopurinol	300 mg q24h	30	75%	50%	25%
Auranofin	6 mg q24h	50	50%	Avoid	Avoid
Colchicine	Acute: 2 mg; then 0.5 mg q6h Chronic: 0.5–1.0 mg q24h	5–17	100%	50%– 100%	25%
Gold sodium	25–50 mg	60–90	50%	Avoid	Avoid
Penicillamine	250–1000 mg q24h	40	100%	Avoid	Avoid
Probenecid	500 mg q12h	<2	100%	Avoid	Avoid
Pegloticase	8 mg IV q2wk	No data	100%	100%	100%
Febuxostat	40–80 mg PO daily	3%	100%	100%	50%
Nonsteroidal Anti-Inflammatory Drugs					
Diclofenac	25–75 mg q12h	<1	50%–100%	25%–50%	25%
Diflunisal	250–500 mg q12h	<3	100%	50%	50%
Etodolac	200 mg q12h	Negligible	100%	100%	100%
Fenoprofen	300–600 mg q6h	30	100%	100%	100%
Flurbiprofen	100 mg q8h–q12h	20	100%	100%	100%
Ibuprofen	800 mg q8h	1	100%	100%	100%
Indomethacin	25–50 mg q8h	30	100%	100%	100%
Ketoprofen	25–75 mg q8h	<1	100%	100%	100%
Ketorolac	30–60 mg load; then 15–30 mg q6h	30–60	100%	50%	25%–50%

Comments	Hemodialysis	Continuous Ambulatory Peritoneal Dialysis	Continuous Venovenous Hemofiltration
Interstitial nephritis; rare xanthine stones			
Renal excretion of active metabolite with $t_{1/2}$ of 25 h in normal renal function; $t_{1/2}$ 1 wk in patients with ESRD; exfoliative dermatitis	1/2 dose	No data	Dose for GFR 10–50 mL/min
Proteinuria and nephritic syndrome	None	None	None
Avoid prolonged use if GFR <50 mL/min	None	No data	Dose for GFR 10–50 mL/min
Thiomalate proteinuria; nephritic syndrome; membranous nephritis	None	None	Avoid
Nephrotic syndrome	1/3 dose	No data	Dose for GFR 10–50 mL/min
Ineffective at decreased GFR	Avoid	No data	Avoid
	No data	No data	No data
May decrease renal function; decrease platelet aggregation; nephrotic syndrome; interstitial nephritis; hyperkalemia			
Sodium retention			
	None	None	Dose for GFR 10–50 mL/min
	None	None	Dose for GFR 10–50 mL/min
	None	None	Dose for GFR 10–50 mL/min
	None	None	Dose for GFR 10–50 mL/min
	None	None	Dose for GFR 10–50 mL/min
	None	None	Dose for GFR 10–50 mL/min
	None	None	Dose for GFR 10–50 mL/min
	None	None	Dose for GFR 10–50 mL/min
Acute hearing loss in ESRD	None	None	Dose for GFR 10–50 mL/min

Continued

Table 65.2

Antimicrobial Agents in Renal Failure—cont'd

Rheumatologic Dosing in Renal Failure

			Dosage Adjustment in Renal Failure		
Arthritis and Gout Agents	**Normal Dosage**	**% of Renal Excretion**	**GFR >50**	**GFR 10–50 mL/ min**	**GFR <10 mL/ min**
Meclofenamic acid	50–100 q6h–q8h	2–4	100%	100%	100%
Mefenamic acid	250 mg q6h	<6	100%	100%	100%
Nabumetone	1.0–2.0 g q24h	<1	100%	50%–100%	50%–100%
Naproxen	500 mg q12h	<1	100%	100%	100%
Oxaprozin	1200 mg q24h	<1	100%	100%	100%
Phenylbutazone	100 mg q6h–q8h	1	100%	100%	100%
Piroxicam	20 mg q24h	10	100%	100%	100%
Sulindac	200 mg q12h	7	100%	100%	100%
Tolmetin	400 mg q8h	15	100%	100%	100%

Sedatives	**Normal Dosage**	**% of Renal Excretion**
Barbiturates		
Pentobarbital	30 mg q6–8h	Hepatic
Phenobarbital	50–100 mg q8–12h	Hepatic (renal)
Secobarbital	30–50 mg q6–8h	Hepatic
Thiopental	Anesthesia induction (individualized)	Hepatic
Benzodiazepines		
Alprazolam	0.25–5.0 mg q8h	Hepatic
Clorazepate	15–60 mg q24h	Hepatic (renal)
Chlordiazepoxide	15–100 mg q24h	Hepatic
Clonazepam	1.5 mg q24h	Hepatic
Diazepam	5–40 mg q24h	Hepatic

Comments	Hemodialysis	Continuous Ambulatory Peritoneal Dialysis	Continuous Venovenous Hemofiltration
	None	None	Dose for GFR 10–50 mL/min
	None	None	Dose for GFR 10–50 mL/min
	None	None	Dose for GFR 10–50 mL/min
	None	None	Dose for GFR 10–50 mL/min
	None	None	Dose for GFR 10–50 mL/min
	None	None	Dose for GFR 10–50 mL/min
	None	None	Dose for GFR 10–50 mL/min
Active sulfide metabolite in ESRD	None	None	Dose for GFR 10–50 mL/min
	None	None	Dose for GFR 10–50 mL/min

Dosage Adjustment in Renal Failure

GFR >50 mL/min	GFR 10–50 mL/min	GFR <10 mL/min	Comments
			May cause excessive sedation, increase osteomalacia in ESRD; charcoal hemoperfusion and HD more effective than PD for poisoning
100% q8–12h	100% q8–12h	100% q12–16h	Up to 50% unchanged drug excreted with urine with alkaline diuresis.
100%	100%	100%	
100%	100%	100%	
			May cause excessive sedation and encephalopathy in ESRD
100%	100%	100%	
100%	100%	100%	
100%	100%	50%	
100%	100%	100%	Although no dose reduction is recommended, the drug has not been studied in patients with renal impairment; recommendations are based on known drug characteristics not clinical trial data
100%	100%	100%	Active metabolites, desmethyldiazepam, and oxazepam may accumulate in renal failure; dose should be reduced if given longer than a few days; protein binding decreases in uremia

Continued

| Table 65.2 |

Antimicrobial Agents in Renal Failure—cont'd

Sedatives	Normal Dosage	% of Renal Excretion
Estazolam	1 mg qhs	Hepatic
Flurazepam	15–30 mg qhs	Hepatic
Lorazepam	1–2 mg q8–12h	Hepatic
Midazolam	Individualized	Hepatic
Oxazepam	30–120 mg q24h	Hepatic
Quazepam	15 mg qhs	Hepatic
Temazepam	30 mg qhs	Hepatic
Triazolam	0.25–0.50 mg qhs	Hepatic
Benzodiazepines		
Benzodiazepine Antagonist		
Flumazenil	0.2 mg IV over 15 sec	Hepatic
Miscellaneous Sedative Agents		
Buspirone	5 mg q8h	Hepatic
Ethchlorvynol	500 mg qhs	Hepatic
Haloperidol	1–2 mg q8 to 12h	Hepatic
Lithium carbonate	0.9–1.2 g q24h	Renal
Meprobamate	1.2–1.6 g q24h	Hepatic (renal)

Antiparkinson Agents	Normal Dosage	% of Renal Excretion
Carbidopa	1 tab q8h–6 tabs daily	30
Levodopa	25–500 mg q12h–8 g q24h	None

Dosage Adjustment in Renal Failure

GFR >50 mL/min	GFR 10–50 mL/min	GFR <10 mL/min	Comments
100%	100%	100%	
100%	100%	100%	
100%	100%	100%	
100%	100%	50%	
100%	100%	100%	
No data	No data	No data	
100%	100%	100%	
100%	100%	100%	Protein binding correlates with α_1 acid glycoprotein concentration
			May cause excessive sedation and encephalopathy in ESRD
100%	100%	100%	
100%	100%	100%	
100%	Avoid	Avoid	Removed by hemoperfusion; excessive sedation
100%	100%	100%	Hypertension, excessive sedation
100%	50%–75%	25%–50%	Nephrotoxic; nephrogenic diabetes insipidus; nephrotic syndrome; renal tubular acidosis; interstitial fibrosis; acute toxicity when serum levels >1.2 mEq/L; serum levels should be measured periodically 12 h after dose; $t_{1/2}$ does not reflect extensive tissue accumulation; plasma levels rebound after dialysis; toxicity enhanced by volume depletion, NSAIDs, and diuretics
q6h	q9–12h	q12–18h	Excessive sedation; excretion enhanced by forced diuresis

Dosage Adjustment in Renal Failure

GFR >50 mL/min	GFR 10–50 mL/min	GFR <10 mL/min	Comments
100%	100%	100%	Requires careful titration of dose according to clinical response
100%	50%–100%	50%–100%	Active and inactive metabolites excreted in urine; active metabolites with long $t_{1/2}$ in ESRD

Continued

Table 65.2

Antimicrobial Agents in Renal Failure—cont'd

Antipsychotics (334,335) Phenothiazines	Normal Dosage	% of Renal Excretion
Chlorpromazine	300–800 mg q24h	Hepatic
Promethazine	20–100 mg q24h	Hepatic
Thioridazine	50–100 mg PO q8h; increase gradually; maximum of 800 mg/day	
Trifluoperazine	1–2 mg q12h. Increase–no more than 6 mg	
Perphenazine	8–16 mg PO q12h, q8h, or q6h; increase–64 mg/day	
Thiothixene	2 mg PO q8h; increase gradually–15 mg/day	
Haloperidol	1–2 mg q8–12h	Hepatic
Loxapine	12.5–50 mg IM q4–6h	
Clozapine	12.5 mg PO. 25–50 daily–300–450 by end of 2 wk	
Maximum: 900 mg/day	Metabolism nearly complete	
Risperidone	1 mg PO q12h; increase to 3 mg q12h	
Olanzapine	5–10 mg	Hepatic
Quetiapine	25 mg PO q12h; increase in increments of 25–50 q12h or q8h; 300–400 mg/day by day 4	Hepatic
Ziprasidone	20–100 mg q12h	Hepatic

Corticosteroids (340)	Normal Dosage	% of Renal Excretion
Betamethasone	0.5–9.0 mg q24h	5
Budesonide	No data	None
Cortisone	25–500 mg q24h	None
Dexamethasone	0.75–9.0 mg q24h	8
Hydrocortisone	20–500 mg q24h	None
Methylprednisolone	4–48 mg q24h	<10
Prednisolone	5–60 mg q24h	34
Prednisone	5–60 mg q24h	34
Triamcinolone	4–48 mg q24h	No data

Dosage Adjustment in Renal Failure

GFR >50 mL/min	GFR 10–50 mL/min	GFR <10 mL/min	Comments
			Orthostatic hypotension, EPS, and confusion can occur
100%	100%	100%	
100%	100%	100%	Excessive sedation may occur in ESRD
100%	100%	100%	Hypotension, excessive sedation
			Do not administer drug IV
			Potential hypotensive effects

Dosage Adjustment in Renal Failure

GFR >50 mL/min	GFR 10–50 mL/min	GFR <10 mL/min	Comments
100%	100%	100%	May aggravate azotemia, Na$^+$ retention, glucose intolerance, and hypertension
100%	100%	100%	Same as above
100%	100%	100%	Same as above
100%	100%	100%	Same as above
100%	100%	100%	Same as above
100%	100%	100%	Same as above
100%	100%	100%	Same as above
100%	100%	100%	Same as above
100%	100%	100%	Same as above

Continued

Table 65.2

Antimicrobial Agents in Renal Failure—cont'd

	Normal Doses		
Anticoagulants	**Starting Dose**	**Maximum Dose**	**% of Renal Excretion**
Alteplase	60 mg over 1 hour then 20 mg/hr for 2 hours		No data
Anistreplase	30 U over 2–5 min		No data
Aspirin	81 mg/day	325 mg/day	10%
Clopidogrel	75 mg/day	75 mg/day	50%
Dabigatran	150 mg PO q12h	150 mg PO q12h	7%
Dalteparin	2500 units SQ/day	5000 units SQ/day	Unknown
Dipyridamole	50 mg q8h		No data
Enoxaparin	20 mg/day	30 mg q12h	8%
Fondaparinux	2.5 mg–10 mg/day		77%
Heparin	75 U/kg load then 15 U/kg/h		None
Iloprost	0.5–2.0 ng/kg/min for 5–12 h		No data
Indobufen	100 mg q12h	200 mg q12h	<15%
Rivaroxaban	20 mg q24h	20 mg q24h	
Streptokinase	25,0000 U load; then 10,0000 U/h		None
Sulfinpyrazone	200 mg q12h		25%–50%
Sulotroban	No data		52%–62%
Ticlopidine	250 mg q12h	250 mg q12h	2%
Tranexamic acid	25 mg/kg q6h–q8h		90%
Urokinase	4400 U/kg load; then 4400 U/kg qh		No data
Warfarin	5 mg/day	Adjust per INR	<1%

ACE, angiotensin-converting enzyme; *ARF,* acute renal failure; *AV,* atrioventricular; *bid,* twice a day; *BP,* blood pressure; *BUN,* blood urea nitrogen; *CAPD,* continuous ambulatory peritoneal dialysis; *CKD,* chronic kidney disease; *ClCr,* creatinine clearance; *CMV,* cytomegalovirus; *CNS,* central nervous system; *ESRD,* end-stage renal disease; *CRRT,* continuous renal replacement therapy; *CSA/FK,* Cyclosporine/tacrolimus; *DVT,* deep vein thrombosis; *ECG,* electrocardiography; *EPS,* extrapyramidal symptoms; *FLX,* high flex; *GFR,* glomerular filtration rate; *GI,* gastrointestinal; *HD,* hemodialysis; *HDL,* high-density lipoprotein; *HSV,* herpes simplex virus; *HUS,* hemolytic uremic syndrome; *INR,* international normalized ratio; *IV,* intravenous; *LD,* loading dose; *LFT,* liver function test; *MMF,* mycophenolate; *N/A,* not applicable; *N/V, nausea or vomiting; NS,* normal saline; *NSAID,* nonsteroidal anti-inflammatory drug; *PD,* peritoneal dialysis; *PO,* oral; *PT,* prothrombin time; *q,* every; *qhs,* at bedtime; *RBF,* renal blood flow; *SQ,* subcutaneous; *SR,* slow release; $t_{1/2}$, half-life; *TB,* tuberculosis; *TDM,* therapeutic drug monitoring; *tPa,* tissue-type plasminogen activator; *TTP,* thrombotic thrombocytopenic purpura; V_d, volume of distribution; *VZV,* varicella zoster virus.

Dosage Adjustment in Renal Failure

GFR >50	GFR 10–50 mL/min	GFR <10 mL/min	Comments
100%	100%	100%	tPa
100%	100%	100%	
100%	100%	100%	GI irritation and bleeding tendency
100%	100%	100%	
100%	50%	No data	
100%	100%	100%	
100%	100%	100%	
100%	75%–50%	50%	1 mg/kg q12h for treatment of DVT; check anti-factor Xa activity 4 h after second dose in patients with renal dysfunction; some evidence of drug accumulation in renal failure
100%	Avoid	Avoid	
100%	100%	100%	Half-life increases with dose
100%	100%	50%	
100%	50%	25%	
100%	75%	Avoid	
100%	100%	100%	
100%	100%	Avoid	Acute renal failure; uricosuric effect at low GFR
50%	30%	10%	
100%	100%	100%	Decrease CSA level and may cause severe neutropenia and thrombocytopenia
50%	25%	10%	
No data	No data	No data	
100%	100%	100%	Monitor INR very closely; start at 5 mg/day. 1 mg vitamin K IV over 30 min or 2.5–5 mg PO can be used to normalize INR

CHAPTER 66

Medication Management

Harold J. Manley, PharmD, FASN, FCCP

Medication management is a patient-centered care process that optimizes safe, effective, and appropriate drug therapy. Medication management is a repeating process that involves patient assessment, creating and implementing a care plan, and follow-up and evaluation (Fig. 66.1). Care is provided through collaboration with patients and their health care teams, including physicians, nurses, pharmacists, dietitians, social workers, and patient care technicians.

An average dialysis-dependent patient has five or six comorbid conditions, requiring 10 to 12 medications resulting in an average 19 pills (range, 17–25 doses) daily. This polypharmacy does not necessarily reflect poor medical management or overuse of medications. However, the sheer number of medications; the presence of renally altered drug disposition; and the challenges involved with tracking, monitoring, managing, and actually taking all these medications place dialysis patients at high risk for medication-related problems (MRPs). In addition to complex polypharmacy, the average dialysis patient also experiences "polyprovider" issues. The typical dialysis patient has nearly five different prescribers (e.g., nephrologist, primary care provider, endocrinologist, cardiologist, gastroenterologist, psychiatrist) and uses several pharmacies (e.g., mail order, specialty, chain drug store, large retailer, food market, or independently owned pharmacy) to obtain access or afford their medications.

In a recent Medicare-managed care study, 405 patients (mean [standard deviation or SD] age, 74 [5.1] years) had a mean (SD) of 2.9 (1.3) prescribing physicians, and 98 (24%) patients reported having experienced an adverse drug event (ADE) in the previous 6 months. In a multivariable logistic regression model, each additional provider prescribing medications increased the odds of reporting an adverse drug event by 29% (odds ratio [OR], 1.3; 95% confidence interval [CI], 1.0–1.6). The number of chronic health conditions was also associated with adverse drug events. Having four or five self-reported chronic conditions doubled a person's odds of experiencing an ADE (OR, 2.1; 95% CI, 1.0–4.1) and having six or more conditions tripled the likelihood of experiencing an ADE (OR, 3.4; 95% CI, 1.6–6.9). The number of prescribing physicians was an independent risk factor for patients self-reporting an ADE. The authors suggest that one possibility for higher ADEs is poor communication among multiple providers.

The complex medical management of various comorbid conditions and the fragmented health care system with inadequate communication among multiple prescribers and pharmacies, as well as the frequent care transitions between ambulatory care sites (e.g., dialysis center, ambulatory primary care practice, ambulatory specialty practice) and the hospital, skilled nursing facility, or long-term care facility places dialysis patients at high risk for MRPs. Previous reports illustrate that risk factors for experiencing MRPs include three or more concurrent disease states,

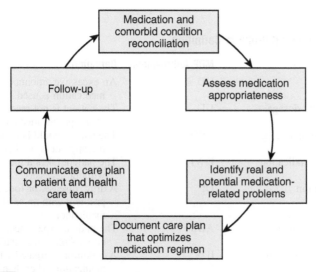

Figure 66.1

Medication management process.

medication regimen changed four or more times during the past 12 months, taking five or more medications or 12 or more doses per day, noncompliance history, drugs that require therapeutic monitoring, and presence of kidney disease or diabetes as a chronic condition. Dialysis patients have all of these risk factors. Providing medication management services is critically important to avoid adverse clinical events and the high costs associated with MRPs, often resulting in avoidable hospitalizations.

Medication-related problems can be classified into nine categories: (1) indication without drug therapy (IWD); (2) drug without indication (DWI); (3) improper drug selection (IDS); (4) subtherapeutic dosage, that is, (5) underdose (UD), (6) overdosage (OD), (7) or adverse drug reaction (ADR); (8) drug interaction (DI; failure to receive drug [FRD]; and (9) inappropriate laboratory monitoring (LAB). Table 66.1 provides examples for each MRP type.

Medication-Related Problems in Dialysis Patients

Most data regarding MRPs in patients with end-stage renal disease (ESRD) pertain to adults undergoing in-center hemodialysis (HD). Over the past 20 years, 11 studies have evaluated MRPs in in-center adult HD patients. Collectively, pharmacists participating in these studies evaluated more than 900 patients and found the average number of MRPs per patient to be 4.5 (range, 2.8–7.2). Pharmacist drug therapy recommendations that address MRPs were implemented up to 96% of time by the medical team.

For peritoneal dialysis (PD) patients, in a prospective, observational study of 42 patients, the mean number of prescription medications was 9.2 and 2.2 for nonprescription medications. Of the patients using antihypertensive agents, 62% used more than one agent, indicating the medication burden and likelihood of MRPs in PD patients is similar to that of patients undergoing in-center HD.

Table 66.1

Medication-Related Problem Definition

MRP	MRP Abbreviation	Definition
Overdose	OD	An excessive amount of the proper medication is used.
Subtherapeutic dosage	UD	The patient is not receiving enough of the proper medication.
Indication without drug	IWD	The patient could benefit from drug therapy but is not being treated.
Drug without indication	DWI	The patient takes a medication without necessity.
Drug interaction	DI	A drug, disease, or food causes a problem with an existing medication.
Adverse drug reaction	ADR	The patient experiences an untoward effect from a medication.
Improper drug selection	IDS	A condition is treated with a medication other than the drug of choice.
Failure to receive drug therapy	FRD	The patient does not receive the medication that is prescribed (nonadherence, cost, or other issues).
Improper laboratory monitoring	LAB	Laboratory monitoring associated with medication therapy is not done or is inadequate.

MRP, medication-related problem.

Pediatric dialysis patients are a subgroup with unique and complex needs regarding medication therapy. These include but are not limited to special dosing (e.g., weight based), need for compounded pharmaceutical formulations, off-label use of medications, sociodemographic issues extending beyond the patients themselves, and adherence issues. In two observational cohort studies conducted at an inpatient setting and outpatient clinic in the United Kingdom, MRPs in pediatric renal patients were characterized via chart review. Two pharmacists each having more than 10 years' experience in tertiary pediatric renal pharmacy practice were involved in collecting the data. A total of 267 MRPs were identified from 266 prescription chart reviews. The incidence of MRPs was 51.2% (203 MRPs, 166 charts; 95% CI 43.2%–60.6%) in hospitalized patients and 32% (64 MRPs, 100 charts; 95% CI 22.9%–41.1%) in outpatients. The number of prescribed medications was the only independent predictor during inpatient treatment (OR, 1.06, 95% CI 1.02–1.10; $p = .002$) with no significant predictors identified at outpatient clinics. The severity level of the MRPs was minor, 53.9% (144 of 267), or moderate, 46.1% (123 of 267). Suboptimal drug effect was the predominant MRP (inpatient, 68%; outpatient, 39%). Prescribing error and patients' medicine-taking behavior were the main contributory factors. The majority of the MRPs in the inpatient setting were resolved.

Another study evaluated the potential scope of MRPs in 283 pediatric patients who made a total of 374 nephrology and hypertension clinic visits. Each visit included a pediatric clinical pharmacist team member. The mean number of interventions by the clinical pharmacist was 2.3 on the first visit. These data suggest that focused MRP evaluation by a pharmacist could potentially be valuable in improving total costs and outcomes in pediatric patients with ESRD.

Identifying and Resolving Medication-Related Problems in Dialysis Patients

Medication management, also called medication therapy management (MTM), is a patient-centered process to create treatment plans centered on each patient's medication-related goals. There are two distinct components to medication management: medication reconciliation and medication review. These two distinct processes are focused on preventing and resolving various MRPs.

1. **Medication and medical problem reconciliation** is the process of creating and maintaining an accurate medical problem and medication list that reflects all current active medical problems and medications the patient is taking and how they are being taken.
2. **Medication review** is the service whereby a clinician evaluates the medication list for appropriateness, effectiveness, safety, and convenience in conjunction with the patient's health status.

Medication Reconciliation

Clinicians need to be aware of what medication regimen(s) a patient is currently taking or previously exposed to before initiating new or modifying existing medication therapy (i.e., medication reconciliation). Therefore, medication reconciliation could be considered the foundation or primary function to be performed before any clinical intervention is implemented.

Regulatory requirements to perform periodic medication reconciliation in dialysis patients do exist. The Centers for Medicare & Medicaid Services (CMS) Conditions for Coverage require that a dialysis patient's comprehensive plan of care include a medication history and should be developed within 30 days of patient admittance to a dialysis facility, *at least annually* for stable patients and *monthly* for unstable patients defined as extended hospitalization (>15 days), frequent hospitalizations (>3 episodes within 30 days), marked deterioration in health status, significant change in psychosocial needs, concurrent poor nutritional status, unmanaged anemia, or inadequate dialysis. Furthermore, medication history is a component of the Measures Assessment Tool. Codified via V506, it states that "medication history" should include a review of the patient's allergies and of all medications, including over-the-counter (OTC) medications and supplements that the patient is taking. The assessment should demonstrate that all current medications were reviewed for possible adverse effects, interactions, and continued need.

Medication reconciliation is an important patient safety initiative to prevent various MRPs. Medication reconciliation is preparatory to any medication assessment or review, care planning, and evaluation. Given the complex pharmacotherapy regimens, multiple prescribers, and utilized pharmacies and frequent care transitions, at each dialysis treatment patients should be asked if they had any additions, deletions, or changes to their medication lists. The medication list should include all prescribed medications, OTC products, vitamins, and herbal products. Medication reconciliation should occur each time a dialysis patient presents for dialysis by a member of the dialysis center's interdisciplinary team. Complete medication reconciliation should occur at periodic intervals (e.g., monthly or bimonthly) but at a minimum with each short-term care plan and after transitions in care. Accurate medication reconciliation does require training, and, ideally, a pharmacist would provide this function or specifically train other members of the dialysis team to do so.

Management of an accurate medication list in dialysis patients is complex because of the high medication and pill burden and the involvement of multiple prescribers. In addition, this population experiences an average of 1.7 hospitalizations per year. The Institute for Healthcare Improvement, Institute of Safe Medication Practices, and The Joint Commission all recognize that gaps in medication knowledge occurring during transitions of care are responsible for up to 50% of medication errors in the hospital and up to 20% of ADEs. In a small single-center study, 65% of MRPs identified in hospitalized dialysis patients were associated with gaps in transfer of medication information among the patients, caregivers, and various health care settings and caregivers. Similarly, in the general population, discrepancies in medication lists generated from comprehensive patient interview and physician-acquired medical history were reported in up to 67% of cases at the time of admission to the hospital.

Medication list discrepancies place dialysis patients at risk for five of the nine MRPs: patient receiving incorrect medication dose (e.g., OD or UD), patient not getting necessary medications (e.g., FRD), patient not getting correct dosage form (e.g., IDS), and patient experiencing an ADE because of unnecessary drug exposure. In a prospective observational study of patients enrolled in a pharmacist clinic at an outpatient HD center, medication record discrepancies were classified and assigned a potential MRP. Over the 5-month period, 215 drug interviews were conducted in 63 patients. A total of 113 drug record discrepancies were identified in 38 patients (60%). Discrepancies (mean ± SD 1.7 ± 1.3; range, 1–7) were identified during 65 drug interviews (30.2%). Electronic drug records were discrepant by one drug record, two drug records, and more than two drug records 60.0%, 26.2%, and 13.8% of the time, respectively. Medication record discrepancies placed patients at risk for ADEs and dosing errors in 49.6% and 34.5%, respectively, of 113 discrepancies.

In a larger, more recent publication, patients at an academic HD unit were interviewed to obtain a best possible medication history in which medication discrepancies were identified, classified, and resolved with the multidisciplinary team. The team also determined discrepancy clinical impact assessment for potential ADEs. A total of 228 patients on HD were interviewed, and 512 discrepancies were identified for 151 patients (3.4 discrepancies per patient). Of these, 174 (34%) were undocumented intentional discrepancies and 338 (66%) were unintentional discrepancies. The unintentional discrepancies were classified as 21% omissions, 36% commissions, and 43% incorrect dose/frequency. Most medication discrepancies were related to a patient taking a medication that was not indicated (25% and risk for ADE), medication required but patient not taking (25% and risk for FRD), patient not willing to take the medication as prescribed (28% and risk for FRD), or incorrect dosing of a drug (20% and risk for OD or UD). Overall, 6% of discrepancies were classified as clinically significant potential ADEs.

Current barriers to providing comprehensive medication reconciliation in most dialysis facilities in the United States includes lack of staff training on the importance and process of medication reconciliation, nonexistent or poor interfaces in electronic health information among care facilities (outpatient dialysis center, hospital, skilled nursing facilities, rehabilitation centers), and the absence of clinical pharmacists in most dialysis facilities.

A consistently applied medication reconciliation process that occurs regularly in the dialysis facility as well as during care transitions could address many of these issues. The medication reconciliation is a person-to-person interaction between a patient (or caregiver) and a health care professional that includes:
1. Collection of an accurate list of all medications the patient is taking
2. Comparison between new medication list and previous list in medical record
3. Reconciliation of medications and resolution of any noted discrepancies

Medication Review

It is important to understand the difference between medication reconciliation and medication review. *Medication reconciliation* is the process whereby an accurate medication list can be constructed and maintained. *Medication review* is the process whereby the patient's medication regimen is evaluated for appropriateness and safety, and it requires advanced clinical pharmacotherapy skills to assess drug therapy in the context of the individual patient's comorbidity, health literacy, and sociodemographic issues (Table 66.2).

Medication review is a multistep process whereby a clinician:
1. Identifies all real and potential MRPs in a patient through clinical assessment of the patient's medical conditions, medications taken, and other available clinical data (e.g., laboratory results, physical exam)
2. Creates and documents a plan of care to resolve or prevent MRPs identified to optimize therapeutic outcomes associated with patient's medication use
3. Communicates any change(s) to the patient's medication regimen to the patient and their care providers
4. Educates patients regarding any change(s) to therapy

In a 2-year randomized, controlled trial of 104 HD patients assigned to receive pharmaceutical care (in-depth bimonthly medication therapy reviews conducted by a clinical pharmacist) or usual care (brief medication therapy reviews conducted by nurse), the former was associated with fewer hospitalizations (1.8 ± 2.4 vs 3.1 ± 3; $p = 0.02$); the trend for reduced length of stay did not achieve statistical significance (9.7 ± 14.7 vs 15.5 ± 16.3 days; $p = 0.06$). A recent study showed that integrated pharmacy services in HD patients receiving Medicare and Medicaid were associated with lower rates of death and hospitalization. Program services were deployed over time and included medication reconciliation and review at the time of program enrollment as well as medication delivery and refill management. In addition, patients had round-the-clock access to pharmacists who provided telephone medication management services. Future studies are needed to measure patient utilization of various pharmacy services and outcomes associated with that utilization.

The Medicare Modernization Act of 2003 created the provision for prescription drug coverage for Medicare beneficiaries through Medicare Part D. Within that provision Medicare prescription drug plans are mandated to provide MTM services to "high-risk enrollees" who meet various eligibility requirements. Eligible beneficiaries for MTM services are enrollees in a specific Part D plan who meet *all* of the following: (1) have multiple chronic diseases, (2) are taking multiple Part D drugs,

Table 66.2

Comparison Between Medication Reconciliation and Medication Review

Medication Reconciliation Process	Medication Review Service
1. Collection of an accurate list of all medications the patient is taking	1. Identifies all real and potential MRPs in a patient through clinical judgment of patient's medical conditions, medications taken, and other available clinical data (e.g., laboratory results, physical exam)
2. Comparison between new medication list and previous list in medical record	2. Creates and documents a plan of care to resolve or prevent MRPs identified in order to optimize therapeutic outcomes associated with patient's medication use
3. Reconciliation of medications and resolution of any noted discrepancies	3. Communicates any change(s) to the patient's medication regimen to the patient and his or her care providers
	4. Educates patient regarding any change(s) to therapy

MRP, medication-related problem.

and (3) are likely to incur $3507 or more annual Part D drug costs in 2017 and subsequent years (drug cost threshold specified by CMS §423.153(d)(1).

About 10% of Medicare Part D plans already target ESRD patients, and it is expected that this percentage will increase in subsequent years since Medicare added ESRD to the current list of targeted conditions. In addition to adding ESRD to the list of targeted medical conditions, Medicare also increased Part D MTM program standardization and requirements and increased beneficiary MTM eligibility through reduction in the threshold of the number of comorbidities and annual expenditure on prescription drugs.

Medicare requires pharmacist involvement in MTM program creation and allows Part D MTM program services be provided by pharmacists or other qualified providers. In 2012, almost all (99.5%) Part D MTM programs used pharmacists to provide the services. Physicians, registered nurses, and support staff (e.g., pharmacy technicians, patient care coordinators or case workers, pharmacy students, and MTM assistants) were used 9.3%, 28.9%, and 64.5% of time, respectively, in the provision of MTM services.

In providing MTM services, the MTM pharmacist will work with the member and physician or other caregiver to establish and achieve drug therapy treatment goals, avoid or minimize undesirable medication effects, and improve clinical outcomes. MTM is a patient-centric and comprehensive approach to improve medication use, reduce the risk of adverse events, and improve medication adherence.

Medicare also mandates that every targeted patient who meets Part D plan criteria for MTM be offered a complete medication review that is documented in a standard format. The Medicare MTM Program Standardized Format (Format) is a written summary of a comprehensive medication review (CMR). A CMR is an interactive person-to-person or telehealth medication review and consultation conducted in real time between the patient or other authorized individual, such as prescriber or caregiver, and the pharmacist or other qualified provider. The CMR is designed to improve patients' knowledge of their prescriptions, OTC medications, herbal therapies, and dietary supplements; identify and address problems or concerns that patients may have; and empower members to self-manage their medications and their health conditions. The pharmacist or qualified provider must assess a patient's medication therapy and create a plan to optimize patient outcomes. Section 10328 of the Affordable Care Act amended section 1860D-4(c)(2)(ii) of the Act to require prescription drug plan sponsors to offer, at a minimum, an annual CMR and required the development of a standardized format for the action plan and summary. Standardization of the format of these documents is expected to improve the quality of the MTM program services and provide consistency in beneficiary communications across differing Medicare Part D programs.

After each interactive CMR, the patient is provided an individualized written "take-away" that includes a personal medication record, reconciled medication list, and medication action plan that includes recommendations for monitoring, education, or self-management. The medication action plan contains specific patient and provider recommendations to address any MRPs identified. The patient provider also receives a copy of the medication action plan for their consideration.

In addition to CMRs, Medicare requires targeted medication reviews (TMRs) to occur at least quarterly in all eligible patients. A TMR may be an interactive person-to-person medication review and consultation but may be delivered via the mail or other means. TMRs should occur at least quarterly and after a sentinel event (e.g., transitions of care, fall event) and are used to assess current medication use, identify unresolved MRPs from the annual CMR, identify new MRPs, and identify patients who have had a transition in care or hospitalization. After each follow-up TMR, a new medication action plan may be created and provided to the patient or provider(s) (or both).

Despite the various efforts to increase patient MTM eligibility and minimum provider requirements for MTM services, there remains significant heterogeneity among the various Part D prescription drug plans regarding patient selection criteria, provider type (e.g., nurse versus pharmacist), and the level of care (e.g., telephone vs person to person). Additionally, fewer than 12% of eligible Medicare Part D beneficiaries actually obtain MTM services.

Nearly all dialysis patients would be eligible for MTM services because their per-beneficiary per-year medication costs (Parts B and D combined) far exceed the $3507 threshold to qualify for MTM services. Despite the high total medication costs experienced by nearly all patients on dialysis, many may still not qualify for MTM services in the current system because Part B costs (e.g., erythropoiesis-stimulating agents [ESAs], calcitriol, intravenous iron) are not included in the qualifying criteria. Congress recently passed legislation delaying the inclusion of oral ESRD-related drugs under the ESRD Prospective Payment System (PPS) or "bundle" from 2014 to January 1, 2024. When this is implemented, the costs of phosphate binders and cinacalcet will financially impact dialysis units and will affect ESRD patient eligibility for MTM services. Because phosphate binders and cinacalcet comprise almost 50% of total Part D costs for dialysis patients, the implications for dialysis patients qualifying for MTM are clear. It is estimated with exclusion of phosphate binders and cinacalcet from Part D costs, fewer than 30% of patients without the low-income subsidy and fewer than 45% of patients with the low-income subsidy will meet the threshold for MTM in 2016. So, although the need for MTM for dialysis patients will not diminish, clearly fewer patients will meet the thresholds for number of medications and cost criteria to qualify for such services when oral ESRD drugs are included in the PPS in 2024.

In addition to the potential loss of eligibility of dialysis patients to participate in MTM offered by Medicare Part D programs, with the inclusion of dialysis-specific oral medications in the bundle, many of these patients will begin receiving prescription medications from multiple pharmacies, further fragmenting medication management services. For many community pharmacists, the only indication that a patient has kidney disease or is dialysis dependent has often been the presence of a phosphate binder or cinacalcet in the medication profile. When these medications will no longer be filled by a patient's community pharmacist, MRPs such as necessary dosage adjustments of other medications may not be identified at the time the prescription is dispensed. Providing medication management services in conjunction and alignment with dialysis services is essential to overcome these challenges.

The dialysis facility can serve as the central medication coordination center and the dialysis health care team as the medication coordination team for each patient. The dialysis facility is the most logical and convenient location for integrated pharmacy services, including medication pick-up, medication reconciliation, and person-to-person medication management services, to occur. This is also a model that could be used by home dialysis patients who make trips to the dialysis center for routine care. Including a clinical pharmacist as an integral part of the dialysis facility team to help provide these medication-related services within the construct of the existing team would substantially facilitate medication management services. In Canada, clinical pharmacy services fund one pharmacist per 100 HD patients, 200 peritoneal or home HD patients, and 300 chronic kidney disease (stages 3–5) patients and has been shown to reduce costs and improve care. Although the structure and costs of the Canadian health care system differ from those in the United States, these data suggest pharmacist-to-patient ratios that are successful in impacting patient outcomes.

Economic Impact

Identification and resolution of MRPs will result in improved patient outcomes and reduced health care expenditures. Reducing MRPs has the potential to generate considerable cost savings to the health care system. It has been estimated that for every $1 spent on detecting and addressing MRPs in the dialysis population, $4 may be saved by the health care system. These cost savings are expected to accrue by lower prescription drug costs from avoidance of unnecessary or inappropriate medications and fewer hospitalizations. Using available data regarding reduced hospital admissions and lengths of stay, a sustainability model could be developed that uses a portion of net savings from Medicare Part A, which could support medication management services under Medicare Part B. Indeed, MRPs in the general population are implicated in approximately 16% of hospital admissions, and 50% of these hospitalizations are potentially avoidable. In one report involving patients with chronic kidney disease, stage 5 medications were implicated in nearly 50% of hospitalizations, considered the sole reason for admission 18% of time, and considered a contributor but not the sole cause for the admission 29% of time. Another report found that nearly 50% of MRPs identified in dialysis patients admitted to the hospital were preexisting, and another 50% occurred during hospitalization (26.7%) or at discharge (25.5%).

Providing medication management services can also increase revenue on the clinic level. Clinics with medication management services may have lower hospitalization rates and thereby fewer missed dialysis treatments. Additionally, approved Current Procedural Terminology (CPT) codes for MTM exist (99605, 99606, 99607), and medication management services could be covered by billing under these codes at standard reimbursement rates. Presently, there is no standard reimbursement rate for each CPT code. Different payers, such as Part D prescription drug plans (PDPs) or commercial health care plans, establish their own payment guidelines and rates for services on a plan-to-plan basis. Reimbursement rates vary based on complexity of medication review and time spent conducting the medication review. A financial analysis of billing for MTM services in a community pharmacy setting found that over a 16-month period, performing 103 CMRs and 88 follow-up TMRs was cost neutral when the pharmacist performed all aspects of the visits. This included pharmacist salary, program support (e.g., computers), and overhead. Additional sensitivity analyses were performed that demonstrated use of ancillary personnel would significantly improve financial gain to the pharmacy.

As previously mentioned, CMS requires Part D PDPs to provide MTM services for high-risk, high-cost patients. Data also suggest that dialysis staff believe medication management services are needed and valuable. Establishing comprehensive medication management services, including face-to-face review by a pharmacist and regularly scheduled medication reconciliation to all dialysis patients, would necessitate compensation for these services. CMS should encourage programs to develop strategic programmatic growth through cost-sharing mechanisms that would allow dialysis organizations to offset additional costs of comprehensive medication management services by sharing in any potential cost reductions (e.g., reduced hospitalizations and clinic visits). The Affordable Care Act created the CMS Innovation Center to test payment and service delivery models, reduce costs, and improve quality. CMS proposes to partner with groups of health care providers and suppliers to form ESRD Seamless Care Organizations (ESCOs) to test and evaluate a new model of payment and care delivery specific to Medicare beneficiaries with ESRD. Participating ESCOs will be clinically and financially responsible for all care offered to a group of matched beneficiaries, not only dialysis care or care specifically related to a beneficiary's ESRD. Medication management is a required component of the proposed ESCOs, and participants in this initiative will be able to provide more data to inform the growth of medication management services for ESRD patients.

Using existing data and data from participating ESCOs, CMS could also consider whether incentivizing dialysis facilities to use medication management services, in the form of MTM or otherwise, by incorporating a metric regarding medication management into the Quality Incentive Program, would be feasible and effective. Indeed, savings from reduction in total costs of care (resulting from, for instance, reduced hospitalizations) could provide a powerful incentive in shared savings.

The current Medicare ESRD prospective payment system does not include the resources to establish and maintain a model of patient care that includes comprehensive medication management services. As health care models are evolving in the general population, there is an opportunity to design and assess innovative models of care in dialysis patients in collaboration with practitioners, dialysis providers, and CMS.

Conclusion

Dialysis patients have complex medication regimens with large pill burdens, use multiple prescribers and pharmacies, and experience many care transitions. MRPs frequently occur in dialysis-dependent patients and are associated with poor outcomes and high cost. Systematic provision of medication management will identify and resolve MRPs and will likely improve patient outcomes and reduce total cost of care.

SECTION XXVI

Rehabilitation and Psychosocial Issues

C H A P T E R 6 7

Physical Activity, Function, and Exercise-Based Rehabilitation for Dialysis Patients

Sharlene Greenwood, PhD • Pelagia Koufaki, PhD

The focus on increasing physical activity for people at risk of developing cardiovascular disease (CVD) is at an all-time high. Rehabilitation, meaning recovering or restoring what is necessary to get on with living, has been a low priority in most dialysis facilities, and the inclusion of integrated rehabilitation programs for dialysis patients is not routinely offered as part of patient care. However, a recently published British Association of Sport and Exercise Science (BASES) expert statement on exercise for people with chronic kidney disease (CKD) suggests that every stable patient with CKD, irrespective of age, gender, comorbidities, or prior exercise experience, should be provided with specific written advice on how to safely and effectively increase physical activity to: (1) enhance confidence and self-efficacy in performing physical activities, (2) attenuate deterioration of physical function and associated limitations in activities of daily living, (3) increase physiologic reserve, (4) reduce comorbid events, and (5) enhance quality of life. The focus of this chapter is on the core principle of exercise for reversing the effects of physical deconditioning and for optimizing physical functioning and quality of life for patients on dialysis.

Definitions

Physical functioning is often used as a term to encompass many concepts. Physical functioning is best defined as an individual's ability to perform activities required in his or her daily life. Physical functioning is determined by many factors, including physical fitness (cardiorespiratory fitness, strength, and flexibility), sensory function, clinical condition, environmental factors, and behavioral factors. *Physical fitness* is a set of attributes people have or achieve that relates to the ability to perform physical activity. One of these attributes is *cardiorespiratory fitness* (often referred to as *exercise capacity*), which relates to the ability of the cardiac, circulatory, and respiratory systems to supply and use oxygen during sustained physical activity.

Physical functioning can be improved with regular physical activity or exercise training. *Exercise* (physical activity) is defined as bodily movement produced by the contraction of skeletal muscle that substantially increases energy expenditure. *Exercise training* is planned, structured, and repetitive bodily movement done to improve or maintain one or more components of physical fitness or to obtain other health benefits. Increased *physical activity* can be considered exercise training, although increased physical activity can also result from unstructured increases in

Table 67.1

Definition of Terms Related to Physical Functioning

- *Physical functioning:* an individual's ability to perform activities required in daily life
- *Physical fitness:* a set of attributes that relates to the ability to perform physical activity (e.g., cardiorespiratory fitness, muscle strength, flexibility)
- *Exercise capacity (cardiorespiratory fitness):* attribute that relates to the ability of the cardiac, circulatory, and respiratory systems to supply and use oxygen during sustained physical activity
- *Exercise (physical activity):* bodily movement produced by muscle movement that substantially increases energy expenditure
- *Exercise training:* planned, structured, and repetitive bodily movement done to improve physical fitness or to obtain other health benefits

movements throughout the day. The use of the term *physical activity* may be less intimidating to dialysis patients who are typically elderly and often frail or chronically fatigued. However, exercise training is appropriate and recommended for dialysis patients because of their extremely low levels of physical functioning and exercise capacity. Table 67.1 outlines these definitions.

Physical Activity and Function

Physical inactivity significantly increases the risk of premature morbidity and mortality in patients requiring hemodialysis (HD). There is an increased age profile of incident HD patients, with a median age of 65 years, and an associated presence of the clinical syndrome of frailty. This syndrome is characterized by persistent fatigue, weight loss, muscle weakness, severe functional limitations, and low physical activity levels, many of which often deteriorate further with the initiation of HD. This translates into impaired capacity to undertake activities of daily living (ADLs), to live independently, and to impaired quality of life. Physical function, regardless of how it is measured, is low in patients at all stages of CKD. Higher levels of physical function and habitual physical activity have been shown to be related to enhanced longevity, less morbidity and lower hospitalization rates, and enhanced quality of life in patients receiving dialysis-based renal replacement therapy.

Exercise Rehabilitation

Exercise rehabilitation has started gaining some attention as an appropriate and safe option to improve physical function and quality of life by aiming to alleviate muscle weakness or dysfunction and unfavorable cardiovascular outcomes. Physical inactivity is a modifiable risk factor, and exercise interventions designed to increase physical activity and reduce sedentary behaviors in patients at risk of CVD may improve health-related outcomes and be cost effective in the longer term. HD therapy enforces regular sedentary behavior three times a week for up to 4 hours at a time. A main facilitator to intradialytic exercise therefore is the reduced time and transport cost burden to patients because exercise time can be incorporated during dialysis therapy. There is also the potential for an improvement in dialysis efficiency and enhanced solute removal.

Current understanding of United Kingdom–based practices indicates that provision of physical activity or exercise programs for patients with CKD appears to be extremely varied across the United Kingdom and is often only an option for patients in an area where research studies are being conducted. Currently, there are four published systematic reviews and meta-analyses that have evaluated the overall effectiveness of exercise interventions on various health-related outcomes in patients from all stages of CKD and after transplantation and in patients on HD only. Koufaki et al recently published a systematic review and synthesis of the research evidence in an attempt to translate the findings from these systematic and meta-analytic reviews, together with any recently published research evidence, to provide some well-informed recommendations on exercise rehabilitation in CKD. Readers are directed to these published reviews for an in-depth analysis of the research literature. Some of the reported benefits of exercise training in dialysis patients are outlined in Table 67.2.

Physical Function Assessment for People With Chronic Kidney Disease

In light of the strong associations among physical function limitations, muscle weakness, physical activity levels, and adverse health outcomes, physical function outcomes should be measured routinely as part of initial and ongoing dialysis patient assessment. The choice of assessment tools will largely be determined by the individual patient's overall health status and willingness to collaborate and staff expertise and equipment availability (because most physiologic function tests require expensive and technically sophisticated devices). It is also important to note that for some patients, physical function or functional capacity assessment and especially determination of peak physiologic capacity may be contraindicated such as in cases of uncontrolled coexisting medical conditions or infections or instability during the dialysis treatment with large fluctuations in body mass, blood pressure, and so on. Furthermore, the choice of type and specific protocol for physical function assessment should be based on the primary purpose of the assessment (e.g., diagnostic, exercise training prescription, risk stratification) and should also take into consideration the specific characteristics of the tests available (e.g., validity, reproducibility, and availability of normative data). Summary information, extracted from the research literature, about the different types of physical function tests used with patients in CKD stage 5 is provided in Table 67.3. For more detailed description of protocols and validity information, interested readers are referred to the review by Koufaki and Kouidi, published in 2010.

In addition to physical function tests, validated patient-reported outcome measures should be obtained to establish the improvement in health-related quality of life (HRQOL), in particular self-reported physical activity status. The Dukes Activity Status Index (DASI) is a self-administered questionnaire that contains 12 components relating to physical activity, which the patient scores his or her perceived level of ability against (Hlatky et al, 1989). In summary, physical function measurement outcomes can be used to:

- Establish degree of functional impairment and identify the optimum timing for interventions.
- Evaluate the presence and severity of symptoms and adverse clinical outcomes such as muscle wasting, angina thresholds, and so on.

Table 67.2		

Studies Relating Physical Functioning and Physical Activity to Outcomes

Measure	Findings	Citation
VO_{2peak}	Patients with VO_{2peak} <17.5 mL/kg/min had more deaths than those with VO_{2peak} >17.5 mL/kg/min. Exercise capacity was the strongest predictor of survival over the 3.5-year follow-up.	Sietsema et al (2004)
Self-reported functioning	Patients with PCS score (SF-36) below the median (<34) were twice as likely to die and 1.5 times more likely to be hospitalized. For every 5-point increase in the PCS, there was a corresponding 10% increase in the probability of survival.	DeOreo (1997)
	Compared with patients with a PCS score (SF-36) >50, those with PCS score <20 had a hazard ratio of 1.97, those with PCS of 20–29 had a hazard ratio of 1.62, and those with a PCS score of 30–39 had a hazard ratio of 1.32. A decline in PCS over 1 year resulted in additional mortality and increased risk of mortality: hazard ratio of 1.25 per 10-point decline in PCS score.	Knight et al (2003)
	PF scale on Duke Health Profile was predictive of survival: difference of 10 points results in 63% greater chance of survival over 1 year.	Parkerson and Gutman (2001)
Physical activity (from USRDS wave 2 form)	Patients who were sedentary at study initiation of dialysis had a 62% greater risk of mortality over 1 year compared with nonsedentary patients.	O'Hare et al (2003)
	Mortality risk was lower for patients who exercised two to three times a week (RR 0.74) or four or five times a week (RR 0.70).	Stack et al (2005)

PCS, physical composite score; *PF*, physical function; *RR*, relative risk; *USRDS, SF-36*, Short Form 36; United States Renal Data System; VO_{2peak}, maximal oxygen consumption.

- Determine safe and effective exercise rehabilitation training zones.
- Evaluate response to therapeutic interventions.

Intradialytic Cycling: A Pragmatic Approach to Encourage Exercise Training

A pragmatic approach to prescription and delivery of intradialytic exercise training may be used as an integrated renal rehabilitation plan in the dialysis unit. The following pragmatic approach to exercise training for dialysis patients was generated by members of the British Renal Society Rehabilitation Network (BRS RN). An

Table 67.3

Summary of Reported Functional Capacity Tools That Can Be Used With Patients on Dialysis for Routine Physical Function Assessment

Method	Measurement Outcomes	Endpoints	Comments
Integrated Exercise Capacity Incremental shuttle walk	• Distance and speed *Usual monitoring tools* • BP and HR • Angina scales • RPE scales	• No increases in BP with increasing workload • BP >220/ 110 mm Hg • Symptoms such as dizziness, angina, lack of responsiveness to oral or visual signs • Patient's request • Equipment failure	• Most patients terminate test because of muscle fatigue, breathlessness, or lack of confidence. • A familiarization session should be provided. • See absolute contraindications to exercise testing. • Reproducibility information is available.
Neuromuscular Capacity Absolute dynamic muscle strength Relative dynamic muscle strength Hand-grip strength	1, 3, 5 maximum repetitions (RM) Max number of repetitions performed at % of RM $Kg.m.s^{-1}$ or max kg achieved	• Patient's request • Inability to continue because of adverse symptom development	• Familiarization sessions may be required. • Whole-body and muscle group–specific warm-up sessions are required. • Muscle function–related measures are strong independent predictors of disease progress and survival. • Reproducibility information available on some indices. • Ease of comparability with a wide range of other chronic conditions.

Continued

Summary of Reported Functional Capacity Tools That Can Be Used With Patients on Dialysis for Routine Physical Function Assessment—Cont'd

Method	Measurement Outcomes	Endpoints	Comments
Functional Capacity Walking tests Sit-to-stand tests Stair climb-descent Squat test Balance Flexibility tests	Walking distance (in meters) incremental shuttle walk, 6-min walk) Walking speed (in m.s^{-1}) Shuttle walk test, 10-m walk, timed up and go STS-5, STS-10 (in seconds), or STS-60 (total number in 60 s) Climbing and descent speed, 2-min stair climbing test Time (s) to perform 10 squats Sit and reach	• Patient's request • Inability to continue because of adverse symptom development	• They objectively measure the patient's capability to perform tasks that relate to ADLs. • Reproducibility information is available for some tests (STS, walking test, stair climb). • A familiarization session may be required. • Assessor and patient friendly • Quick and inexpensive • Minimum interference and inconvenience for patient • Ease of comparability with a wide range of other chronic conditions

ADL, activity of daily living; *BP,* blood pressure; *HR,* heart rate; *RM,* repetition maximum; *RPE,* rating of perceived exertion; *STS,* sit to stand.

From Greenwood SA, Naish P, Clark R, et al. Intra-dialytic exercise training: a pragmatic approach. J Renal Care 2014;40(3):219-226.

understanding of the key components of exercise programing and prescription are integral to the delivery of a safe and effective program.

Patient Suitability for Starting an Exercise Program

The following exclusion criteria should be considered before any patient is accepted for an intradialytic exercise programme:
• Myocardial infarction within 3 months
• Unstable angina

- Acute infection
- Acute orthopedic condition
- Uncontrolled hypertension (blood pressure >180/100 mm Hg)
- Uncontrolled arrhythmia
- Other conditions raising concern over fitness for exercise should be discussed with the patient's physician.
  On-the-day exclusion might also include:
- Symptomatic hypotension
- Low blood glucose
- Cannulation or fistula problems
- Excessive interdialytic fluid gain (>4 kg)

Staffing

Ideally, the responsible nephrologist would prescribe cycling on dialysis when a patient first starts on dialysis with the intention of introducing exercise as a necessary aspect of patient treatment rather than an optional adjunct. The nephrologist is accountable for providing the medical assessment of suitability for the exercise program and ongoing medical support. This then means that a qualified member of staff, whether he or she is a physiotherapist, nurse, or dietitian, would be able to lead patient management in the program. The aim is that the intradialytic cycling becomes a standard component of a HD session for suitable patients. All exercise sessions must be performed in a clinical setting where supervision of appropriately qualified staff and resuscitation facilities are available. Ideally, there should be a "link nurse" for each unit to promote the service and liaise with either the nephrologist or physiotherapists if any concerns arise. In the United States, a significant barrier to provision of intradialysis cycling is the lack of reimbursement for the equipment and necessary staff to oversee the safe provision of this service in the current fee-for-service payment system. As integrated care systems become more common and payment for dialysis treatments are capitated, facilities will have the resources needed to consider the value of such programs for patients in the facility.

Equipment

There are several designs of exercise cycles used in dialysis units, including free-standing models, exercise cycles that attach to the dialysis chair or couch, and models that can be positioned for use on a hospital bed. Examples of this equipment can be found on the BRS's Physical Activity network website (www.britishrenal.org/Physical-Activity). The option chosen may depend on the type of dialysis couch in operation in the dialysis unit or whether patients are dialyzed on hospital beds.

Pragmatic Exercise Prescription

Patients should wear appropriate footwear and adopt a well-supported upper body and lower back body stature that does not overstress the shoulder and lower back muscles (depending on the mode and cycle ergometer) during leg cycling. The first 5 minutes of cycling should be a progressive warm-up (starting slow and increasing intensity), and the final 5 minutes should be a cool-down phase. The intensity should initially be 30% to 50% of the conditioning workload for 3 minutes and then decreased to 20% to 0% for another 3 minutes. The duration and intensity of the exercise prescription should be increased according to patient tolerance using the following steps as a guideline.

1. The initial prescription should be based on the exercise assessment. If using an intradialytic cycle, then this can be used for the assessment. The exercise intensity should aim to be 50% to 60% of what a patient could achieve at baseline assessments. If possible, the patient should achieve 20 minutes during the first dialysis session with a rest in between. Otherwise aim to do 10 minutes cycling, either as five 2-minute or two 5-minute sessions (with short rests in between).

2. Begin to gradually increase the duration of exercise. Aim for 30 to 40 minutes. The aim should be to increase the intensity of the exercise to 70% to 80% over the longer term.

The rating of perceived exertion (RPE) scale or a similar outcome can be used to monitor the patient's perceived intensity level and ensure that the patient is working optimally. If using the RPE scale, the patient should be asked to rate him- or herself during the training time of the program, optimally aiming for an RPE between 13 and 15, "somewhat hard" to "hard." For each exercise session, the resistance, distance, time, and RPE from that session should be recorded, as well as any reasons for stopping or not partaking in the exercise training. This information can be used for progression, to share achievements with patients, and to assess compliance with the program.

Goal Setting

It is important to ascertain a patient's motivation to increasing his or her exercise levels and likeliness to adhere to the program. To do this, behavioral change techniques such as motivational interviewing can help to resolve ambivalence for starting the program and encourage a patient to continue. Goal setting is another important aspect of any exercise program and can be an effective way of improving motivation and the likelihood of achievement. The goals must be specific, measureable, achievable, realistic, and timed (SMART), for example, to be able to walk up one flight of 12 stairs with no rests within 3 months. Ideally, goals should be set at baseline and reassessed at consistent time points, whether it is every 3 or 6 months, by an exercise professional. Practical resources for goal setting can be found at www.cardiosmart.org.

Competence

Training, provided by a physiotherapist or exercise physiologist, to all staff involved in the intradialytic cycling program is important. Staff should be deemed competent to:

- Assess the patient's ability to exercise, including using validated outcome measures.
- Be able to identify when a patient is not suitable to exercise.
- Design an appropriate exercise program based on the exercise assessment.

- Progress the patient's exercise intensity to an individual level using the RPE or an alternative scale.
- Use the equipment safely, adhering to manual handling policies.

Potential Barriers and Solutions to the Provision of Intradialytic Exercise Programs

To successfully implement an intradialytic cycling program and develop a sustainable longer term exercise and physical activity plan, it is crucial to also appreciate the global barriers to implementation and then consider localized barriers that may need to be problem solved within individual HD units. Preexisting exercise beliefs of patients and HD unit staff members can be a strong demotivating factor for exercise. Staff members caring for patients receiving HD therapy may consider patients as "too old" and "too unwell" or "uninterested" to undertake exercise during dialysis. When surveying 100 patients receiving HD therapy, Delgado and Johansen found the main patient barriers to exercise as fatigue on HD days (67%) and non-HD days (40%), shortness of breath (48%), and lack of motivation (42%). Often these identified patient barriers can be solved through considering a holistic patient-centered approach using motivational interviewing techniques to set patient-specific, meaningful, and achievable goals to assist with compliance with the initiation of exercise and the maintenance of longer term exercise behavior. Some other possible non–patient-related reasons for the lack of provision of intradialytic exercise may include lack of physiotherapy expertise, lack of knowledge or incentive among nephrologists, lack of facilities, lack of financial incentives, funding for staff time and equipment, a poor understanding of the benefits of exercise therapy, and a fear of complications.

A number of potential strategies could be used at a local level to tackle some of the potential barriers to implementation of an intradialytic exercise program. Involving members of the renal multidisciplinary team, such as renal-specific physiotherapists or exercise physiologists, who are well equipped to provide specific and individualized exercise prescription while appreciating confounding comorbidities can facilitate a change in the "exercise culture" of a renal unit. Visiting a renal unit with an active intradialytic exercise program may alleviate initial fears about implementing a program. There are also resources available such as the BRS's Physical Activity network website (www.britishrenal.org/Physical-Activity).

Exercising on Nondialysis Days

Although other long-term conditions, such as chronic obstructive pulmonary disease and cardiac disease, routinely offer outpatient exercise-based rehabilitation programs for their patient groups, this approach has not been used extensively for patients with CKD. Renal rehabilitation, either as a supervised exercise program or prescribed exercise programs offered in a gym setting on a nondialysis day, can improve the physical fitness and well-being of participating patients. Kouidi et al compared a supervised training program for HD patients on nondialysis days with exercise during dialysis and demonstrated better improvements in peak oxygen consumption (47% vs 31%) in the supervised program but also a higher dropout rate (33% vs 21%). There is a possible tension with exercising HD patients on nondialysis days because it is perhaps slightly unrealistic to expect patients receiving hospital-delivered HD therapy to attend additional hospital-based exercise classes on nondialysis days.

The Way Forward: Translational Rehabilitation

The evidence for the benefits of physical activity for patients with CKD is accumulating, and encouragement to exercise and lead a physically active lifestyle is included in national CKD management guidelines. The challenge is, quite clearly, how to translate the research findings into routine clinical practice. Strong evidence for the beneficial effects of exercise in nonresearch settings comes from the Dialysis Outcomes and Practice Patterns Study (DOPPS), published in 2010. A cross-section of 20,920 DOPPS participants in 12 countries from 1996 to 2004 was reviewed. Regular exercise was associated with higher HRQOL, better physical functioning, fewer limitations in physical functioning, better sleep quality, less intrusiveness of body pain or anorexia, a more positive affect, and fewer depressive symptoms. The offering of exercise in a unit was associated with 38% higher odds of patients' exercising. Finally, the overall mortality risk was lower in units with more exercisers.

The following are suggestions for ways that might be adopted to facilitate the incorporation of exercise therapy into routine care.

- Education, support, and advocacy should be offered to nephrologists in practice and in training and to nurses.
- Exercise promotion and provision, when feasible based on reimbursement and staffing, should be offered as part of routine care in all renal units.
- Standards of care relating to exercise rehabilitation, endorsed by national and professional bodies should be developed, with an agreed timescale for their implementation. The participation of representative patients' groups (National Kidney Federation in the United Kingdom) should be part of these activities.
- The documentation of functional capacity initially and serially after the start of dialysis should exist in all national registries. In addition, every unit undertaking exercise promotion and delivery should document its effects and associations as part of routine care.
- Funding of well-designed, multicenter research continues to be crucial to provide a better evidence base. Future larger research trials should aim to specifically address the relationship between changes in physiologic function and whether they translate into changes in functional outcome benefits and increased survival.

Areas in which no clear conclusions can be drawn from the current research literature that need to be addressed are the effects of exercise on vascular function and incidence of cardiovascular events, dialysis efficiency, nutritional supplementation, blood pressure, and systemic inflammation.

Thus, although the research evidence base needs enriching, the association between exercise and better outcomes in the dialysis population is sufficiently strong to state the following. It is now time, as has been stated by a number of authors of previous reviews, for nephrologists and their MDT colleagues, for their professional bodies, and for government health departments to recognize the importance of this area of renal care. Exercise rehabilitation for CKD patients should be implemented in renal units in as timely and comprehensive a way as possible.

C H A P T E R 6 8

Physical, Psychosocial, and Vocational Rehabilitation of Adult Dialysis Patients

John H. Sadler, MD

Whatever the cause of chronic renal failure, for most patients, the effects are the same. The insidious progression of symptoms parallels the slow worsening of blood chemistries as glomerular filtration declines. Many patients fail to recognize the change in their vigor and well-being and simply adjust to serial changes. This allows marked losses in exercise capacity and endurance to occur as deconditioning proceeds. Similar slowing of mental processes impairs relationships and communication. Dialysis removes most of the accumulated metabolites but does not restore lost abilities. Those require, at least, exercise and stimulation to recover. This chapter addresses the additional efforts needed to rehabilitate dialysis patients and the reasonable expectations for improvement.

Background

Concern for rehabilitation has a long history in chronic renal failure. Advocates for Medicare benefits for dialysis and transplantation before the 1972 legislation made public assurances of the restored productivity of successfully treated patients, predicting that benefits provided would be returned in part by taxes paid by reemployed patients. Such enthusiasm was appropriate to the patients of that era of severely limited resources: Each was carefully reviewed and accepted because of his or her ability to resume an active life with correction of uremia. Nephrologists reporting these results to encourage funding for dialysis and transplantation did not project what would ensue with open enrollment of all comers into end-stage renal disease (ESRD) therapy.

After implementation of the Medicare ESRD Program in 1973, the dialysis population rapidly expanded—and just as rapidly ceased to be a uniform, motivated, youthful population with little comorbidity. As well, return to productive employment ceased to be the norm. Because the only definition of rehabilitation used was vocational rehabilitation (VR), there was a widely perceived failure of the ESRD Program to fulfill its promise. Many in Congress and elsewhere felt betrayed. Nephrologists were embarrassed, and rehabilitation dropped from the ESRD vocabulary.

In place of rehabilitation, the focus turned to mortality and hospitalization (which also got worse with older, sicker patients)—and to the development of improved technology. By the time the United States Renal Data System (USRDS) was developed, using the Medicare database to shine a unique spotlight on ESRD care, the emphasis had changed from the large numbers of people who survived chronic renal failure with treatment to the number of dialysis patients who had short survival, poor health, or both.

Redefining Rehabilitation

The initial definition of rehabilitation addressed only the restoration of gainful employment, partly because of its potential economic consequences and partly because it was hard data easily used for assessment of outcome. It was widely remarked that in the absence of employment as the standard, no one knew how to define rehabilitation.

Despite those remarks, other medical communities recognized that there are also psychosocial rehabilitation and physical rehabilitation in addition to VR. Efforts to improve and monitor outcomes in those areas were often used by general internists, physiatrists, social workers, exercise therapists, and others. Cardiac rehabilitation has become nearly universal after cardiac injury or surgery.

The ESRD community has many clinicians who always sought to understand the lifestyle and problems of their patients and to help them cope with and improve their lives, but this was individual effort—with no systematic structure, no standards or guidelines, and no national or regional recognition. The results were reported as anecdotes of fulfilling experiences for professionals, as well as successes for patients—but not as clinical trials in medical journals. The impact of these experiences was quite limited.

In 1993, with support from Amgen, the Life Options program was started, and the Life Options Rehabilitation Advisory Council (LORAC), composed of experts in dialysis care and psychosocial research, was established to lead it. The Council's members set out to define an orderly structure for rehabilitation efforts that would include physical, psychosocial, and VR arenas and that would provide guidance to clinicians and facilities undertaking it. This program is not the only such effort, but the organization of ideas and the subsequently reported successful programs make it an easy model for application to most ESRD treatment sites, as well as to other chronic disease settings.

Life Options begins with the "five Es" of renal rehabilitation (Table 68.1). The approach starts with *encouragement*, believing that the person can do better and that

---

Table 68.1

Life Options' Definition of Renal Rehabilitation

- *Encouragement:* Surround the patient with a positive attitude.
- *Education:* Learn about kidney disease and dialysis, and about opportunities and interests.
- *Exercise:* Essential to recover and maintain physical capacity; improves cardiovascular health.
- *Employment:* Maintain or return quickly when possible; understand barriers and benefits.
- *Evaluation:* Repeated assessment of status and changes; important for factual reinforcement (along with regular assessment of functional status and health-related quality of life).

everyone involved will be gratified by the accomplishment, gently (or forcefully, if necessary) stimulating the patient to make the effort to be healthier. The *evaluation* that individualizes the approach can be included in the clinical planning for each patient, required by regulations and routinely documented. This includes education, work history, former and recent activity levels, physical capacity, social support, interests and hobbies, and hopes for the future. Patients need to know that this is happening, need to be informed, and need to make some choices in their plan. Interval reevaluation is important both to adjust the program and to provide everyone involved with a means of measuring what has been accomplished. Recognition of even small steps forward can mean a great deal. Setting a goal individualized to each patient's needs and capacities in clear and measurable terms and noting milestones as each is reached will ensure that all participants are rewarded.

Education begins with each patient learning about renal failure and the dialysis regimen; follows with health improvement goals, functional expectations, and exercise methods; and continues through specific learning to enable progress toward specific goals. Self-management of this regimen and direction is encouraged. Subsequently, this may include outside agencies or individuals. Some patients may not progress past the simplest grasp of their situation, but every patient needs enough knowledge to minimize fear of their disease and its treatment and to lessen dependence on staff and family. The opportunity to learn about subjects of interest may activate patients who have been self-absorbed and passive.

Almost every patient needs *exercise*, because most undergo significant physical deconditioning with loss of capacity and endurance as disease progresses. The "spiral of deconditioning" described by exercise physiologist Patricia Painter is quickly recognized by most patients and clinicians as accurate. Loss of vigor is so gradual the patient often does not recognize it. Exercises to reverse this decline need to be light but regular, composed of repetitions capable of being counted so that there will be a tangible reward through achieving higher counts, which reveal improved physical capacity. Most patients can train themselves to physical capacity near premorbid levels. Painter's work in active dialysis facilities demonstrates improved peak oxygen uptake after successful physical training, an objective measure of improved functioning. A booklet on ESRD-specific exercises is available through Life Options Renal Resource Center, Medical Education Institute, 414 D'Onofrio Dr., Madison WI 53719 (800-468-7777) or www.lifeoptions.org.

Stationary bicycles, treadmills, and other exercise devices are effective and have been installed in a number of dialysis facilities. Some are used before dialysis; others have been adapted for use during the usually boring time spent on dialysis. Exercises during dialysis are usually well tolerated, without disrupting the procedure.

Everyday objects may also be used for exercise. A chair can be used for bracing during movement or for seated leg exercises. Canned goods can be used as dumbbells. Large rubber bands (Therabands) are used as a resistance to pull against. A sandbag can serve as a flexible weight that can be held on a foot to exercise a leg or in a hand to exercise a shoulder. Walking is always a good exercise for those who can. Walking indoors works when weather or neighborhoods discourage going outside. A few steps up and down the stairs are easy to repeat and count, with numbers increasing as exercise builds endurance.

Most of these simple actions build strength for activities of daily living. Periodic reassessment provides the patient with a satisfying reinforcement of accomplishment. It is important to promote expectations of well-being sufficient for continued productive living and independence and then to demonstrate that ability. Counting repetitions is simple. When more quantitative results are sought, the standard 6-minute walk, stand-sit-stand test, or measured grip strength may be used. Loss of confidence may be as limiting as the loss of physical strength. Repeated reinforcement of progress through objective measurements can rebuild confidence.

The goal of *employment* is not realistic for most dialysis patients. Published reports confirm that those already employed can often retain employment or return to it promptly with less difficulty than trying to place an individual in a new job. Success is also related to education level. VR agencies and private employment companies can provide evaluations, arrange some types of training, and make potential employment contacts. The enthusiasm for such services must often come from the patient or the dialysis staff assisting the patient. VR offices are more accustomed to amputees, persons impaired in vision or hearing, or others with more obvious physical deficiencies, and some workers there may be ill at ease with a dialysis patient's problems. The pool of those who want to work or who can realistically become employable may be small, but for those few, even a part-time job can be a great advantage. Working produces income and provides tangible evidence of recognition and personal worth, sets a framework for living through a regular schedule, and helps maintain physical capacity.

A survey of dialysis patients 18 to 55 years old found that more than 30% believed themselves able to work, but fewer than 20% were able to be employed. A favorable economy may improve that situation. The clinical team must realize the potential for employment and support the effort if patients are to succeed. In addition, a number of patients are known to work part time or "off the books" to avoid loss of disability benefits, which compete well with what many can earn. Those unreported jobs are usually out of the ESRD professionals' awareness as well.

Other life-enhancing activities are more widely available than returning to employment. The mean age of dialysis patients is over 60 years, and many are beyond employability. However, some of them can discover useful and rewarding roles as volunteers or as members of other community activities that engage them in life outside their home, distracting them from focusing on health problems. These activities meet a broad definition of rehabilitation. Not just the elderly but the majority of dialysis patients can improve their physical, social, and intellectual functioning through education (in living with dialysis, in crafts, in history, arts, or specific interests) and through exercise during, before, or after dialysis in an entertaining way.

With encouragement, most patients can find ways to incorporate simple physical conditioning into daily activities. Encouragement from many sources (family, staff, volunteers, other patients, and so on) underlies the patient's acceptance and promotion of his or her own health. The clinical team's evaluation of results and feedback to the patient and family of the findings can reinforce the rewards of self-improvement efforts on a number of levels. All of these can aid in establishing groups for shared activity, increasing social interaction, and avoiding isolation.

Every renal clinician can relate stories of individual patients who are not responsive to any effort at motivation, whose noncompliant behavior and self-destructive lifestyle frustrate everyone who comes in contact with them. Such individuals should not be accepted as the norm. Positive support for good habits and visible recognition of self-improvement achieved by other patients help to prevent bad habits from becoming contagious. These failures do not merit emphasis but sometimes can be seen as an object lesson for other patients who would avoid their fate. Expecting effective rehabilitation will not always succeed, but expecting failure fulfills itself easily. For clinicians, the success of some patients can make tolerable the frustration caused by those who are unresponsive, undisciplined, determinedly pessimistic individuals.

Prerequisites to Effective Rehabilitation

Adequate Dialysis and Anemia Control

Fundamental to the promotion of health for dialysis patients is an adequate dose of dialysis. Monitoring to ensure this is routine. The mean measured dose of dialysis as Kt/V or urea reduction ratio is increasing every year. Higher blood and dialysate flows and more powerful dialyzers produce much of the increase, but many patients have to dialyze longer—never a welcome change. Motivation to accept longer treatment must come from learning the importance of good laboratory values and seeing the results in improving health. Learning is a central part of any successful dialysis regimen, and renal clinicians must teach. Nephrologists must lead this effort. Informed patients can accept the choices needed for health and rehabilitation.

Correction of anemia is equally essential to health promotion. Achieving adequate red blood cell (RBC) mass requires sound nutrition, conserving blood in procedures, adequate iron replacement, vitamin supplements, and (for most patients) regular administration of recombinant erythropoietin (EPO) to promote erythropoiesis. Increased RBC mass is important to strength and endurance, general well-being, and relief of some symptoms once thought to be the result of uremia. Exercise capacity improves. Average hematocrits rose sharply when EPO became available and have continued to rise slowly since. That continued rise may be partly due to better monitoring and maintenance of iron stores, to promotion of better nutrition, or to higher doses of EPO. Much of this effort is made pursuing the raised expectations of the clinical renal community. Patients have become more aware of their hematocrit levels and their goals. That awareness provides patients with another milestone of achievement.

Comorbid Conditions and High-Risk Lifestyles

Control of comorbid conditions such as hypertension and heart failure is a routine consideration for the dialysis population because these conditions are frequent in renal failure. Rehabilitation requires each individual to reach his or her optimal health and to realize adequate stability for the confidence to try to expand capabilities. Medications are usually effective for these conditions, but effective sodium and volume restriction and regular physical activity, such as some of the exercises previously mentioned, promote cardiovascular health.

Systematic monitoring of cardiac function through periodic echocardiograms and other testing can guide clinical management and recognize new problems in established cardiac disease. For patients with diabetes, better control of glucose and blood pressure help preserve vision and cardiovascular function even after the onset of renal failure. For those with demonstrated vascular disease, control of serum lipids is important to preserve circulatory function. This often requires cholesterol-lowering medication as well as lifestyle modification. All of these factors merit attention as part of the health plan that underlies rehabilitative efforts. In these days of National

Kidney Foundation Kidney Disease Outcomes Quality Initiative (KDOQI) guidelines, there is always external monitoring of most of these factors.

Beyond specific diseases, many patients are obese, use tobacco, abuse alcohol or drugs, and are passive and inactive. All such behaviors are difficult to change, but a supportive and consistent group of dialysis clinicians, assisted by successful patients, can often motivate change. Repetitive contact makes this encouragement more effective through reinforcement. Specific instruction, counseling, or focused group therapy may be needed outside dialysis. The final responsibility is the patient's, who must make the change effective. These high-risk behaviors are common across the entire population, but when added to the risks of renal failure and its treatment, they pose even greater potential harm to ESRD patients. Clinicians must seek effective messages that help change patient behavior to promote health.

Diet and activity are cultural practices. Changing them requires patients to learn the reason for changes. Repetitive monitoring and reinforcement aid motivation. Damaging habits seen as pleasures are given up more easily with some compensating enrichment of relationships, surroundings, or other pleasures that reward compliance. This is often beyond the reach of dialysis clinicians, but there are some conditions we can change (e.g., schedule and companions during treatment). Other conditions only need to be pointed out emphatically (e.g., weight loss, improved exercise capacity, and better laboratory values).

Depression is common in ESRD patients. It is probably a normal response to having to start dialysis, and it often dissipates as symptoms clear. If exercise can restore vigor, spirits often rise as well. Clinicians need to be sensitive to clues to mood change and depression because these can affect compliance, nutrition, activity, and survival. Patients with physical disease and depression often respond well to antidepressant medication as well as to improved circumstances.

Family Participation

Families may be protective of patients to the point of promoting dependence or preventing activities that can improve their functioning. The family needs to be included in learning and reinforcement of desirable behavior. Families need reassurance that denying a wish that adds to disease is the right thing to do, even if it causes friction. Patients regress behaviorally as they become limited by disease, acting more childlike in many ways. Families have to deal with that behavior more than clinicians, and their easiest coping mechanism may be to yield to requests that break the regimen and promote comorbidity. Older patients in particular may retreat and withdraw, making it difficult to engage them in the social and physical activity necessary to promote health. Family members need to make efforts to break this pattern, but many find it difficult to exercise authority over parents. Support and education from the clinical team can help them understand and act appropriately.

Implementing Renal Rehabilitation

Effective rehabilitation efforts require that everyone endorse the concept and commit to the program. Administration must commit resources of staff time and space to enable these activities. They have to value the goal, or they will not invest to reach it. The medical director and other nephrologists must accept the idea and promote it because attitudes and values often come from the doctors.

Nurses and clinical technicians must consistently reinforce the goal of rehabilitation and encourage the activities leading toward it in their repeated contacts with patients. Consistent positive attitudes move the program forward and improve the atmosphere in the facility at the same time. Social workers can coordinate outside agencies and contacts to assist patients, and their contacts with patients can be most effective in building a positive attitude in them. Because nutrition is fundamental to gaining strength and feeling better, dietitians have opportunities to show patients how learning and following a regimen makes them healthier.

Some individual on the staff, often a social worker or dietitian but also frequently a nurse, must be named responsible for coordinating the rehabilitation program and for monitoring outcomes accomplished. The coordinator must be supported by all staff, not abandoned in the position, because patients often need help from multiple sources to succeed.

The coordinator may lead groups of patients in exercise activities or designate another person to do so if exercise in the facility is undertaken. Any staff member can teach simple exercises for patients to do independently, at home or in dialysis. All staff can help with education, and all staff must consistently encourage patients to make the effort—and then cheer the results. Rehabilitation is a team effort. These steps can be a byproduct of existing practices and contacts. The theory is simple: A group of people consistently believing that trying will accomplish something good for patients can convince patients to make the effort. Then everyone can enjoy the results, and the facility is a more pleasant place.

Evaluation of Outcomes

Employment, as noted in the historical review, is readily documented. Physical improvement is less so. Self-reports from patients are valuable, but it may be useful to observe and count repetitions of simple exercises or to use a standard measurement such as stand-sit-stand (as many times as possible in 30 seconds), the 6-minute walk (probably too time consuming to do for a group), or measured grip strength. Attitudes and increased knowledge are subjective but definite, and they merit notation.

An overall assessment through self-report of a standard health or functional status questionnaire or health-related quality of life form is now a regular practice in dialysis, and the results correlate well with survival and hospitalization and predict behaviors that may affect the course of dialysis. These self-reported data demonstrate good correlations with more conventional clinical outcomes and offer interval assessment of health status that can guide clinicians' efforts to improve functioning and well-being.

Applying these instruments and using the scores obtained to assess progress toward rehabilitation has been recommended as the single most useful indicator of an effective approach to renal rehabilitation in a facility. There are accepted, recognized instruments of considerable experience that may be valuable to a facility in assessing the patient's perception of progress. Used semiannually, such reports give a numerical score that can be followed as an integrated evaluation by the patient of the outcome of care. These results can point out aspects of care that need attention, just as laboratory test results and physical findings can guide the dialysis prescription.

As ESRD patients become "older and sicker," it is easy to give up hope of improvement or accomplishment for many. However, when the five Es are applied as part of dialysis care, every patient has an opportunity to improve him- or herself and become rehabilitated in terms specific to him or her. The results reported in a number of facilities confirm that as attitudes and communication improve demonstrably improved functioning occurs and the staff share in the rewards they have helped patients achieve. When rehabilitation is defined as helping each patient reach his or her highest level of functioning and satisfaction, the goal is reasonable, individually achievable, and beneficial.

Conclusions

The amount of time dialysis patients and staff spend together invariably exerts influence. It can be an opportunity to enrich one another's lives in ways that encourage and reward healthy behavior, leading to rehabilitation as defined here. All such endeavors take time, and current constrained finances in ESRD care make this difficult because time is in short supply. Using milestones and giving guidance toward rehabilitation have to be incorporated into the obligatory contacts of treatment or there will not be time to do these things. Health promotion and rehabilitation have to be a central part of therapy, not an additional or peripheral aspect of care that receives attention only after other steps are complete. When physical, social, and sometimes VR are the goals of treatment, dialysis can become holistic therapy.

Expecting people on dialysis to return to active lifestyles, whether employed or not, is not always successful. However, expecting passivity, depression, and progressive physical deterioration will usually lead to just those outcomes. The social environment in a dialysis facility is conditioned by the expectations of clinicians and their response to good results. Rehabilitation will not occur passively. The matrix of adequate use of effective technology, good nutrition, appropriate medication, and medical monitoring is fundamental to dialysis care and essential for effective rehabilitation. A conscious, organized plan to help each patient improve according to individual capability is the next step toward improved health. Working partnerships between patients and clinicians can succeed in promoting greater health, confidence, and positive attitudes. These attributes are themselves one level of rehabilitation for many patients.

Rehabilitation, and the promotion of optimal health accompanying it, is best seen as the central goal of treatment—not as an addition to treatment. Incorporated into the framework of care in this fashion, it is effectively addressed as part of routine care as much as dialysis, medication, and diet. Once clinicians are comfortable with their knowledge of renal rehabilitation, the contact with patients includes observations, recommendations, instructions, and assessments of their health status without a great increase in contact time.

Programmed exercise before, during, or after dialysis requires some oversight, which will consume time for a staff member able to supervise exercise. Surveys for health and functional status and quality of life measurement are largely self-administered, but scoring and handling require some staff effort. Analyzing and using these results in focusing attention and improving care take thought and practice. Helping patients to make themselves well is achievable. The rewards of improved productive living for patients, improved satisfaction for staff, and stabilizing the patient population (which preserve facility income) make renal rehabilitation a positive experience for all concerned.

CHAPTER 69

Ethical Considerations in the Care of Dialysis Patients

Alvin H. Moss, MD, FACP, FAAHPM

Ethics in the care of patients is about doing the right and good thing. Nephrologists want to do the right thing and treat their patients ethically, but unfortunately, studies show that most nephrologists have not received formal training in the ethics of the care of dialysis patients. The first step in the process of ethical decision making is to identify the ethical questions (Table 69.1). Ethical questions ask what should or ought to be done. In the care of dialysis patients, the following questions are particularly relevant: Who should and **should not** receive dialysis? On what basis should decisions about renal replacement therapy and modality be made? When should a time-limited trial of dialysis be used? When should stopping dialysis be considered? How should a nephrologist respond to a patient's request to stop dialysis? How should a patient who stops dialysis be treated?

Who Should and *Should Not* Receive Dialysis?

The question in the 1960s, "Who should be dialyzed?" morphed in the 1990s into "Who should *not* be dialyzed?" In the 1960s, it was unthinkable that patients with diabetes or older than the age of 75 years would be candidates for dialysis. In 2015, patients with diabetes constitute 45% of incident dialysis patients, and patients older than the age of 75 years are the fastest growing age group in the dialysis population. The growth of the dialysis population has far exceeded the estimates when the Medicare End-Stage Renal Disease (ESRD) Program was established by Congress in 1972.

In the 1960s, the Admissions and Policy Committee of the Seattle Artificial Kidney Center decided who received access to dialysis and lived and who was denied access to dialysis and died. The straightforward answer to the question, "Who should receive dialysis?" from an ethical perspective is that patients with medical indications for dialysis for whom the burdens are likely to outweigh the benefits and who consent to dialysis should receive it. The answer becomes more complicated for a number of reasons. First, not all patients with stage 5 chronic kidney disease (CKD) and an estimated glomerular filtration rate less than 10 mL/min are certain to benefit from dialysis. There is accumulating evidence that stage 5 CKD patients older than the age of 75 years with significant comorbidities may not survive any longer with dialysis than without it. The level of this evidence has risen to the point where the second edition of the clinical practice guideline, *Shared Decision-Making in the Appropriate Initiation of and Withdrawal from Dialysis,* recommends an informed consent conversation in which patients receive information about their diagnosis, prognosis, and all treatment options before a decision about dialysis is

Table 69.1

The Seven-Step Process of Ethical Decision Making in Patient Care

1. What are the ethical questions?
2. What are the clinically relevant facts?
3. What are the values at stake?
4. List options. What could you do?
5. What should you do? Choose the best option from the ethical point of view.
6. Justify your choice. Refer back to the values and give reasons why some values are more important in this case than others.
7. How could this ethical issue have been prevented? Would any policies, guidelines, or practices be useful in changing any problems with the system?

Reproduced with permission from the Renal Physicians Association. *Shared Decision-Making in the Appropriate Initiation of and Withdrawal from Dialysis*, 2nd ed. Rockville, MD: Renal Physicians Association; 2010.

made. Similarly, the American Society of Nephrology (ASN) in its Choosing Wisely Campaign identified one of the five things physicians and patients should question is the possible limited benefit of dialysis to certain older patients. In its Choosing Wisely announcement on April 4, 2012, the ASN stated, "Don't initiate chronic dialysis without ensuring a shared decision-making process between patients, their families, and their physicians. ... Limited observational data suggest that survival may not differ substantially for older adults with a high burden of comorbidity who initiate chronic dialysis versus those managed conservatively."

The clinical practice guideline also identified other groups of patients who should *not* receive dialysis: patients with decision-making capacity who, being fully informed and making voluntary choices, refuse dialysis or request that dialysis be discontinued; patients who no longer possess decision-making capacity who previously indicated refusal of dialysis in an oral or written advance directive; patients who no longer possess decision-making capacity with properly appointed legal agents who refuse dialysis for them or request that it be discontinued; and patients with irreversible, profound neurologic impairments such that they lack signs of thought, sensation, purposeful behavior, and awareness of themselves and the environment.

The guideline also recommended other patients for whom strong consideration should be given to not providing dialysis, that is, those who have a terminal illness from a non–kidney-related cause. For example, a patient who is dying from a metastatic cancer for which no further chemotherapy or radiation therapy is being offered because of a low likelihood of benefit should, in most circumstances, not be started on dialysis. The potentially longer survival time that dialysis might afford is likely to be at the expense of a greatly diminished quality of life with significant pain and suffering as the cancer spreads. This same conclusion also could be reached for patients with end-stage heart or lung disease who, despite the provision of dialysis, might have severe progressive shortness of breath, pain, and a greatly diminished quality of life.

There are also patients whose medical condition precludes the technical process of dialysis because the patients are unable to cooperate with it, for example, a patient with advanced dementia who can only be restrained with great difficulty from pulling out his dialysis needles or catheter or a patient who because of severe cardiovascular instability experiences refractory hypotension during dialysis with loss of consciousness and seizures. Fortunately, the clinical practice guideline identifies these categories of patients and provides practical strategies for deciding with these patients and their legal agents about dialysis.

The publication of the first edition of the *Shared-Decision Making* clinical practice guideline in 2000 was in response to the report of the Institute of Medicine Committee to Study the Medicare ESRD Program, which in its 1991 report recommended the development of a clinical practice guideline "for evaluating patients for whom the burdens of renal replacement therapy may substantially outweigh the benefits." The objectives for the first and second edition of the guideline were strongly motivated by ethical considerations: synthesize available research evidence as a basis for making recommendations about starting, withholding, continuing, and withdrawing dialysis; enhance understanding of the principles and processes useful for and involved in making decisions to withdraw or withhold dialysis; promote ethically as well as medically sound decision making in individual cases; recommend tools that can be used to promote shared decision making in the care of dialysis patients; and offer a publically understandable and acceptable ethical framework for shared decision making among health care providers, patients, and their families. Table 69.2 presents the recommendations in this guideline.

Since the publication of the second edition of the clinical practice guideline in 2010 and the ASN Choosing Wisely recommendations in 2012, there have been additional major studies confirming the previous recommendations and documenting that older patients starting dialysis in the hospital undergo significantly increased intensity of treatment and shortened survival times with a high percentage of remaining life spent hospitalized.

On What Basis Should Decisions About Renal Replacement Therapy and Modality Be Made?

The clinical practice guideline and the ASN Choosing Wisely Campaign recommend a shared decision-making approach for making decisions about dialysis. Shared decision making is the recognized preferred model because it addresses the ethical need to fully inform patients about the risks and benefits of treatment, as well as the need to ensure patient's values and preferences play a prominent role. In shared decision making, the nephrologist is the expert in the patient's diagnosis, prognosis, and treatment alternatives, and the patient is the expert in his or her own history, values, and goals. In the process of shared decision making, physicians and patients reach agreement on a specific course of treatment and share responsibility in the decision based on an understanding of the patient's overall condition and values. Shared decision making is appropriate for making decisions about starting, continuing, and stopping dialysis. Shared decision making achieves the goal of the Institute of Medicine's (IOM's) 2001 report *Crossing the Quality Chasm: A New Health System for the 21st Century* by facilitating individualized, patient-centered care. The IOM defined "patient centered" as "providing care that is respectful of and responsive to individual patient preferences, needs, and values and ensuring that patient values guide all clinical decisions." In fact, shared decision making has been described as the "pinnacle" of patient-centered care. Unfortunately, data from

Table 69.2

Recommendations in the *Shared Decision-Making in the Appropriate Initiation of and Withdrawal From Dialysis*, 2nd Edition, Clinical Practice Guideline

Establishing a Shared Decision-Making Relationship
- Recommendation no. 1: Develop a physician–patient relationship for shared decision making.

Informing Patients
- Recommendation no. 2: Fully inform AKI, stage 4 and 5 CKD, and ESRD patients about their diagnosis, prognosis, and all treatment options.
- Recommendation no. 3: Give all patients with AKI, stage 5 CKD, or ESRD an estimate of prognosis specific to their overall condition.

Facilitating Advance Care Planning
- Recommendation no. 4: Institute advance care planning.

Making a Decision to Not Initiate or to Discontinue Dialysis
- Recommendation no. 5: If appropriate, forgo (withhold initiating or withdraw ongoing) dialysis for patients with AKI, CKD, or ESRD in certain, well-defined situations.
- Recommendation no. 6: Consider forgoing dialysis for AKI, CKD, or ESRD patients who have a very poor prognosis or for whom dialysis cannot be provided safely.

Resolving Conflicts About What Dialysis Decisions to Make
- Recommendation no. 7: Consider a time-limited trial of dialysis for patients requiring dialysis but who have an uncertain prognosis or for whom a consensus cannot be reached about providing dialysis.
- Recommendation no. 8: Establish a systematic due process approach for conflict resolution if there is disagreement about what decision should be made with regard to dialysis.

Providing Effective Palliative Care
- Recommendation no. 9: To improve patient-centered outcomes, offer palliative care services and interventions to all AKI, CKD, and ESRD patients who suffer from burdens of their disease.
- Recommendation no. 10: Use a systematic approach to communicate about diagnosis, prognosis, treatment options, and goals of care.

AKI, acute kidney injury; *CKD,* chronic kidney disease; *ESRD,* end-stage renal disease.
Reproduced with permission from the Renal Physicians Association. *Shared Decision-Making in the Appropriate Initiation of and Withdrawal from Dialysis,* 2nd ed. Rockville, MD: Renal Physicians Association; 2010.

numerous studies of dialysis patients performed between 2006 and 2013 show that shared decision making has been poorly integrated into the process of dialysis initiation for many patients. There is the expectation that dialysis decision making will improve as the recommendations of the ASN and Renal Physicians Association (RPA) are implemented through the use of decision aids incorporating decision science.

When Should a Time-Limited Trial of Dialysis Be Used?

Time-limited trials of dialysis are specifically recommended when the benefit to a particular patient of dialysis is uncertain. The nephrologist may recommend dialysis, and the patient may be hesitant to begin it, or the opposite situation may be the case in which the nephrologist doubts the benefit of dialysis to the patient but the patient or the patient's family requests that dialysis be initiated. In both of these situations, a time-limited trial of dialysis may promote more informed shared decision making and help to resolve conflict about the dialysis decision. Both the nephrologist and the patient (or the patient's legal agent if the patient lacks decision-making capacity) will see how the patient tolerates dialysis and if the patient's overall condition improves with it. Before a time-limited trial of dialysis is begun, the length of the trial and the parameters to be assessed during and at the completion of the trial should be agreed upon so that at the conclusion of the trial the decision about whether dialysis should be continued can be reached according to the predefined parameters. Interestingly, in a 2005 survey of the RPA nephrologist membership, nephrologists who had been in practice longer and who were knowledgeable of the RPA and the ASN *Shared-Decision Making* guideline published in 2000 reported greater preparedness to make end-of-life decisions and use time-limited trials of dialysis. At the initiation of a time-limited trial, it is important for the nephrologist to specify that if the predetermined outcomes are not achieved that dialysis will be stopped and that the focus of the patient's care will be changed to intensive palliative care in which the goal will be the patient's comfort. Depending on the patient's condition, a transition to hospice may be appropriate.

When Should Stopping Dialysis Be Considered?

Strong consideration should be given to stopping dialysis when the goals for which the patient started dialysis are no longer being accomplished. The United States Renal Data System reports that withdrawal form dialysis is the second most common reason for dialysis patient death and the most common reason for withdrawal of dialysis is failure to thrive. An acute medical complication such as a stroke has been found to be the second most common reason for dialysis withdrawal. Common clinical scenarios in which patients or their family members make a decision to stop dialysis include accelerating comorbid illnesses, often with increased frequency of hospitalizations and loss of cognitive function with progression to severe cognitive impairment. A 2014 article by Schmidt, "Dying on Dialysis: The Case for a Dignified Withdrawal" provides a comprehensive checklist for implementation of dialysis withdrawal in patients who are failing to thrive on dialysis.

How Should a Nephrologist Respond to a Patient's Request to Stop Dialysis?

Although most dialysis centers have one or more patients who withdraw from dialysis each year, the majority of nephrology fellows report they have not been taught how to respond to a patient's request to stop dialysis. The *Shared Decision-Making* guideline recommends a systematic approach to responding to such a request (Table 69.3), which determines the reasons or conditions underlying the request; assesses the medical, psychological, social, and spiritual motivations for such a request; and identifies what interventions could be undertaken to address the factors motivating the request. Determination of the patient's decision-making capacity and ruling out depression or encephalopathy are important first steps in the evaluation.

Table 69.3

Responding to a Patient's Request to Stop Dialysis

- Assess the patient's decision-making capacity and whether it is compromised by major depression, encephalopathy, or another disorder. Determine whether the patient's perceptions about dialysis and potential quality and quantity of life are accurate. Does the patient understand what will happen if dialysis is stopped?
- Does the patient really mean what he or she says, or is the decision being made to get attention, control, or help?
- Are there changes that might improve the patient's quality of life, and is the patient willing to continue dialysis while he or she is being made to see if his or her quality of life improves?
- Determine the reasons or conditions underlying the patient or surrogate request for withdrawal of dialysis. Such assessment should include specific medical, physical, spiritual, and psychological issues, as well as interventions that could be appropriate.
- Identify potentially treatable factors such as the following:
  - Underlying medical disorders, including the prognosis for short- or long-term survival on dialysis
  - Difficulties with dialysis treatments
  - The patient's assessment of his or her quality of life and ability to function
  - The patient's short- and long-term goals
  - The burden that costs of continued treatment, medications, diet, and transportation may have on the patient, family, and others
  - The patient's psychological condition, including depression or conditions or symptoms that may be caused by uremia
  - Undue influence or pressure from outside sources, including the patient's family
  - Conflict between the patient and others
  - Dissatisfaction with the dialysis modality, the time, or the setting of treatment
- Depending on the assessment of potentially treatable factors, recommend psychiatric treatment or refer for counseling.
- Encourage the patient (if he or she has decision-making capacity) to discuss reasons for dialysis withdrawal with his or her family or support system.
- If a fully informed patient with capacity who has been offered or undergone treatment for potentially reversible factors still persists in the request for dialysis withdrawal, the patient's request should be honored to respect patient autonomy.
- If the patient lacks decision-making capacity, determine if the surrogate is making decisions according to the patient's prior expressed wishes for his or her current condition or according to what the surrogate determines to be the patient's best interest. If either is the case and there are not potentially treatable factors that could improve the patient's quality of life, agree to the request to respect the patient's autonomous decision when he or she had capacity or to prevent harm from a life in which there is suffering prolonged by dialysis.

How Should a Patient Who Stops Dialysis Be Treated?

Patients who stop dialysis should be informed of their options for care, including palliative care and hospice, and be treated according to their values and preferences for type of treatment and site of treatment (Table 69.4). The average dialysis patient dies about 8 days after dialysis withdrawal, and 94% are dead within 1 month. For this reason, referral to hospice, if desired by the patient, should be made immediately at the time of dialysis withdrawal. Many hospices are willing to meet with the patient

Table 69.4

Comprehensive Treatment of a Patient Who Stops Dialysis

- Meticulous pain and symptom assessment and management
- Psychological, social, and spiritual support to the patient and family
- Shared decision making for informed consent on patient's preferred treatment in the dying process and site of death
- Inclusion of family and legal agent in discussions
- Completion of advance directive specifying patient's preferred decision maker when incapacity occurs and preference for goals of care focused on comfort
- Completion of Physician Orders for Life-Sustaining Treatment (POLST) Paradigm medical orders (in states where available) specifying do not resuscitate (DNR) and comfort measures without readmission to the hospital except if patient cannot be kept comfortable at home
- DNR order and do not hospitalize order except for comfort in states without POLST Paradigm form
- Referral to hospice with patient's permission
- Bereavement support for family after the patient's death
- Dialysis center annual memorial service for families of patients who stop dialysis

and family before formal admission to hospice to provide information. Advance care planning including completion of advance directives, a do-not-resuscitate order, and Physician Orders for Life-Sustaining Treatment (POLST) Paradigm orders (if available in the state where the patient is being treated) are key to ensure that everyone knows the plan of care and that the patient receives his or her desired treatment at the end of life.

The answers, tables, and recommended readings prepare nephrologists to provide dialysis patient care with high ethical standards. For particularly complex cases in which there is conflict, nephrologists may want to request the assistance of an ethics consultation service. Ethics consultation has been found to be helpful in identifying, analyzing, and resolving ethical dilemmas in patient care

C H A P T E R 7 0

Psychosocial Issues in Dialysis Patients

Daniel Cukor, PhD • Melissa Pencille, PhD •
Deborah Rosenthal, PhD • Paul L. Kimmel, MD

Patients' responses to the onset of end-stage renal disease (ESRD) and its continued treatment can alter their course, prognosis, and quality of life (QOL). The psychological landscape shapes the patient's perception of his or her ability to cope with the diagnosis and the treatment's ongoing demands. Patients' state of mind, level of support, understanding of the disease, and adherence behaviors are all factors determining how patients adjust. Although the extent of one's physical illness affects one's psychosocial functioning, conversely, the strength of one's ability to cope can impact the course of medical illness. For example, increased depression and social strain can lead an ESRD patient to a cycle of decreased compliance, increased illness severity, and greater symptom burden. The goal of this chapter is to review the burgeoning scientific literature on psychosocial challenges in ESRD patients treated with hemodialysis (HD), concentrating on psychopathology, sleep disturbance, and barriers to adherence to the medical prescription.

Psychopathology

Depression

Depression is defined by the newest version of the *Diagnostic and Statistical Manual for Psychiatric Disorders* (DSM 5) as being present when an individual displays either a subjective depressed mood most of the day, nearly every day, or a diminished interest or pleasure in activities, both over a 2-week period, plus four of the following additional symptoms: significant weight loss, insomnia, psychomotor agitation or retardation, fatigue, feelings of worthlessness or guilt, diminished ability to think or concentrate, or recurrent thoughts of death. Additionally, these symptoms need to cause impairment to the individual and need to be judged to not be directly related to a medication or medical condition. These last caveats significantly complicate the diagnosis of depression in ESRD patients because patients are typically treated with a variety of medications for kidney disease or other comorbid conditions that may have side effects that mimic depression. Furthermore, uremia, as well as dialysis treatment, often is the cause of symptoms related to the somatic components of the diagnosis of depression, such as fatigue, insomnia, or inability to concentrate.

Despite challenges to the accurate assessment of depression, a rather consistent rate of increased depressive affect of approximately 20% to 30% in HD patients has been reported. The rate is typically somewhat higher if depression is measured using a self-report measure and somewhat lower with more rigorous clinician-administered diagnostic interviews.

Treatment

Despite these relatively high prevalence rates, depression may be undertreated in patients treated with dialysis. There is also a paucity of studies evaluating depression treatment in HD patients. There are generally two types of approaches used for the treatment of depression in HD patients: pharmacologic and nonpharmacologic.

Pharmacologic Treatment

An early study of a selective serotonin reuptake inhibitor (SSRI) randomly assigned 14 chronic HD patients with major depression to either treatment with fluoxetine or placebo. The antidepressant outperformed placebo at 4 weeks but not at 8 weeks. Two observational studies of the effects of antidepressants in 136 peritoneal dialysis (PD) patients reported improvement in depressive symptoms. These studies, however, had no control arm, relatively low percentages of eligible subjects participating, and high medication discontinuation rates. Atalay et al reported that treatment with sertraline (50 mg a day) for 12 weeks led to a decrease in depressive symptoms in 25 chronic PD patients. Similarly, this study did not have a control arm.

In a Korean study, paroxetine and individual supportive counseling were assessed in 34 depressed dialysis patients. There was a statistically significant but clinically mild response to the treatment. This study also suffered from small sample size, lack of a placebo-control group, and absence of follow-up information.

Nonpharmacologic Treatment

Nonpharmacologic treatment interventions for depression in dialysis patients have been evaluated as well. Two primary interventions include cognitive behavioral therapy (CBT) and exercise therapy.

Cognitive Behavioral Therapy

Cognitive behavioral therapy is a type of psychotherapy that helps patients to dissect the relationships among their emotions, cognitions, and behaviors in order to identify and reframe irrational and self-defeating thoughts, which in turn improves their mood and alters their behaviors. CBT can be performed in groups or individually and attempts to empower individuals to control their negative cognitive and behavioral patterns.

Two randomized controlled trials (RCTs) have examined CBT in ESRD patients. Cukor et al compared patients who received 10 CBT sessions administered chair side during regular HD treatments with a wait list control group using a crossover design. CBT resulted in a significant reduction in depressive affect, increased perception of QOL, and better treatment adherence compared with control participants.

Group CBT was also used in an RCT of depressed HD patients compared with standard care. Eighty-five HD patients with a major depressive disorder were randomized. The CBT group demonstrated a more significant reduction in depressive affect at the end of treatment and at follow-up than the standard care group. CBT appears to be a promising intervention for reducing depression in HD patients.

Exercise Therapy

The ability of exercise programs to improve mood in dialysis patients was tested in three recent small studies. Across the studies, depression was significantly but modestly reduced in patients who engaged in physical activity. However, low retention rates across the exercise programs may limit the efficacy of this intervention as a broad-based strategy.

Anxiety

Anxiety disorders are defined by the DSM 5 by overwhelming feelings of fearfulness, dread, and uncertainty. Unlike relatively mild brief anxiety reactions, a true anxiety disorder must last at least 6 months. There was a significant change in the categorization of anxiety disorders with the recent switch to DSM 5. Obsessive compulsive disorders and posttraumatic stress disorders are no longer classified as anxiety disorders. Similar to depression, the assessment of anxiety is complicated by symptoms overlapping with uremia, multiple measurement tools, and imprecise definitions and cut-offs for clinical diagnosis. Anxiety, measured both as symptoms as well as diagnostically, is a relatively common experience for HD patients. Generally, dialysis patients exhibit significantly greater symptoms of anxiety compared with transplant patients and control participants. A systematic review of 55 studies of anxiety symptoms in ESRD patients indicated an overall prevalence rate of 38%, with levels for individual studies ranging from 12% to 52%. Still, numerous studies have demonstrated that the role of anxiety in ESRD patients treated with HD remains underappreciated and understudied. There are no clinical trials testing the efficacy of anxiety treatments in ESRD populations. RCTs are certainly needed because anxiety is associated with a negative impact on general health, QOL, and a variety of psychosocial parameters in both ESRD patients and in the general population.

Psychosocial Issues

Quality of Life

The demanding requirements of dialysis can have a significant and adverse impact on the overall QOL of dialysis patients. Thus, preserving patients' QOL, or their sense of positive well-being, has become an essential component of medical treatment for ESRD. QOL has become more widely accepted as a salient health outcome and measure of treatment efficacy.

Dialysis patients generally face poor health-related quality of life (HRQOL). HRQOL involves the way patients manage their health in several domains (e.g., physical functioning, physical and emotional roles, social functioning, general health perception). Several studies have shown that patients undergoing dialysis are more likely to have compromised physical and emotional functioning. Decreased physical functioning of ESRD HD patients has been associated with an increased risk of death. Increasing physical activity in HD patients has helped improve physical functioning and overall HRQOL and has been associated with other clinical benefits, including more positive affect, better sleep, and less pain.

Psychosocial variables are associated with variability within HRQOL. Depression, anxiety, social support, coping strategies, and health locus of control have all been linked to decreases in HRQOL in dialysis populations.

Social Support

Social support plays an integral role in health outcomes for ESRD patients in general through its influence on access to health care, treatment compliance, and psychological health. Social support refers to the degree to which an individual belongs to a social network in which he or she gives and receives affection, aid, and obligation to and from family members, friends, colleagues, community members, and medical personnel. Stronger social support is related to improved health outcomes and lower mortality for ESRD patients. There is an interrelationship between social support and level of depressive symptoms, perception of illness effects, and overall satisfaction with life.

Sleep Disorders

Sleep disorders are prevalent in ESRD patients, with a higher rate compared with the general population. Walker et al found approximately 80% of ESRD patients receiving HD reported sleep complaints. Hui et al found daytime sleepiness to be the most common sleep problem reported by Chinese PD patients. Sleep problems are found in both HD and PD patients. The reason for increased rates of sleep-related issues and disorders in this population is likely multifactorial. Sleep disorders in ESRD patients may be in part due to restless legs syndrome (RLS), depression, pruritus, uremia, anemia, medications, sleep apnea, and metabolic changes. There is an association between sleep quality and decreased QOL, health-related risks, and mortality in ESRD patients. Insomnia, RLS, periodic limb movement disorder, and sleep apnea syndrome are prevalent in the HD population.

Insomnia

Insomnia is often debilitating and can occur as a primary disorder or be comorbid with medical illness and psychiatric disorders. Symptoms of insomnia include difficulty with sleep initiation, sleep maintenance, or early morning awakening that results in daytime impairment. In the ESRD population, the prevalence of insomnia varies and may be as high as 69% compared with 10% in the general population.

In the general population, insomnia is associated with decreased HRQOL and impairment in cognitive functioning. Severe insomnia has been associated with increased health care utilization, including medical provider visits, number of hospitalizations, and medication use.

Studies using polysomnographic data have demonstrated alterations in the sleep architecture of dialysis patients. Increased amounts of stage 1 and 2 sleep and decreased slow-wave and REM (rapid eye movement) sleep have been reported in HD patients. One study compared ESRD patients receiving HD with non-ESRD matched control participants. The ESRD sample had significantly decreased sleep time and increased frequency of arousals compared with the control group. Parker et al found HD patients to have decreased total sleep time, increased wake after sleep onset, lower sleep efficiency, higher periodic limb movement index, and longer latencies to sleep onset compared with a chronic kidney disease (CKD) group not undergoing dialysis. Decreased quality of sleep is prevalent even in the early stages of CKD.

Insomnia is generally thought of as having predominantly psychological as opposed to biologic etiologies. Therefore, the preferred treatments for insomnia are often behavioral and psychological. Treatment of insomnia in ESRD patients includes sleep hygiene education (establishing a regular sleep schedule, decreasing caffeine intake, implementing regular physical activity, adjusting environmental factors), CBT, and pharmacologic interventions. Cognitive Behavioral

Therapy—Insomnia (CBT-I) is an empirically validated psychotherapy tailored to the treatment of insomnia symptoms. In the general population, RCTs have found CBT to be an effective intervention. In an RCT of 24 PD patients, Chen et al assessed a 4-week trial of CBT and sleep hygiene education versus sleep hygiene education only. Improvement in sleep latency, quality of sleep, daytime dysfunction, and fatigue was noted in the CBT group, measured by the Pittsburgh Sleep Quality Index and Fatigue Severity Scale.

Benzodiazepines have been used to treat insomnia, although concerns over chronic use of these medications include dependency, withdrawal symptoms, sedation, and rebound symptoms. Benzodiazepine–receptor agonists are also frequently prescribed for patients with insomnia. In a study of 195 HD patients, Yeh et al found that benzodiazepines (42.6%) and hypnotics (20%) were the most frequently prescribed psychotropic drugs. Winkelmayer et al found that benzodiazepines and zolpidem were associated with 15% increased mortality in 4024 dialysis patients. Dialysis patients with a diagnosis of chronic obstructive pulmonary disease were 50% more likely to use benzodiazepines or zolpidem and may be at a higher risk of mortality.

Restless Legs Syndrome and Periodic Limb Movement Disorder

Restless legs syndrome, a neurologic disorder, is characterized by unpleasant sensations, usually in the lower extremities, that involve a strong urge to move the legs. RLS symptoms often worsen during periods of inactivity and are temporarily relieved by movement. Symptoms frequently occur in the evening or night and interfere with sleep. The prevalence of RLS in ESRD patients is 30% to 50%.

Treatment for RLS and periodic limb movement disorder (PLMD) in ESRD patients variably includes dopamine agonists and L-dopa gabapentin, as well as behavioral modifications, such as addressing caffeine, alcohol, and nicotine intake and engagement in physical activity. Giannaki et al randomized 24 HD patients with RLS into a progressive exercise training group (45 minutes of cycling during HD sessions, 3 days per week for 6 months with applied resistance) or a no-resistance exercise control group (45 minutes of cycling, 3 days per week for 6 months without resistance). RLS symptom severity significantly decreased in the resistance group compared with the control group. Improving iron deficiency has also been found to reduce RLS symptoms in ESRD patients.

Sleep Apnea

Sleep apnea syndrome (SAS) is a common disorder in ESRD patients, with a reported prevalence of 50% to 70% in this population. Sleep apnea is characterized by disordered breathing during sleep and can be classified as obstructive sleep apnea (OSA) (intermittent closure of the upper respiratory airway); central sleep apnea (CSA) (intermittent loss of respiratory drive); or mixed, which is a combination of the two. Sleep apnea interferes with sleep initiation and sleep maintenance and can lead to daytime somnolence. The prevalence and severity of the disorder may worsen with the progression of decline of renal function in CKD patients. The symptoms of sleep apnea may be difficult to detect in ESRD patients because common symptoms of uremia are fatigue, daytime somnolence, and cognitive dysfunction, which overlap with those of the sleep disorder.

Unruh et al found that HD patients were four times more likely to have disordered breathing compared with control participants matched for age, gender, body mass index (BMI), and race, after adjusting for cardiovascular disease and a history of diabetes. Risk factors for sleep apnea in the general population include age, gender, obesity, genetics, smoking status, craniofacial and upper airway abnormalities, neck girth, and central body fat distribution. In a study of 76 ESRD patients with OSA and 380 OSA patients with normal kidney function, gender and age were comparable. The ESRD sample, however, was generally not obese, and the mean BMI was lower compared with the control group. ESRD patients were less likely to report symptoms, including snoring, apnea during sleep, nonrefreshing sleep, or morning headaches. The ESRD group had decreased snoring intensity compared with the control group, confirmed using polysomnography.

Treatment of sleep apnea includes addressing underlying medical conditions and use of continuous positive airway pressure (CPAP). Nocturnal HD improves sleep apnea in ESRD patients. Hanly et al assessed 14 HD patients who were switched from conventional HD (4-hour sessions 3 days per week) to nocturnal HD (8 hours, 6 or 7 nights per week) and demonstrated a reduction in the frequency of apneas and hypopneas. The apnea-hypopnea index on nights participants were not receiving nocturnal HD was higher than nights when they were undergoing treatment, although it was still lower than when they were receiving conventional HD. Tang et al demonstrated improvement in sleep apnea in patients treated with nocturnal PD compared with continuous ambulatory peritoneal dialysis (CAPD). They attributed this to improved fluid control during sleep.

Hemodialysis Treatment Adherence

The HD prescription is complex, demanding intensive and extensive life changes. Therapy usually includes attending three weekly scheduled HD treatments during which the patient is connected to a machine for 4 hours a session, has a modified diet restricting intake of phosphate and sodium, and is required to take many medications a day. Adherence to this multifaceted regimen may minimize the likelihood of adverse medical outcomes. Durose et al showed that adherence to the dialysis prescription can extend an individual's life in addition to improving the overall QOL.

Unfortunately, however, nonadherence to the dialysis prescription and other medical requirements is a highly prevalent behavior. Approximately 50% of individuals with ESRD undergoing HD do not adhere to their prescribed treatment regimen. Estimates for nonadherence to the HD prescription range from 22% to 86%, depending on the definition and measurement of adherence.

The most common definition of adherence is "the extent to which a person's behaviors in taking medications, following a diet, and/or executing lifestyle changes corresponds with agreed upon recommendations from a healthcare provider." Adherence marks the extent to which patients' behaviors match physicians' recommendations. Nonadherence can be inadvertent (i.e., when patients do not adhere because of lack of understanding, forgetfulness, or miscommunication with health care professionals) or advertent (i.e., when patients actively choose not to follow their regimen). Adherence to dietary and fluid restrictions, medication prescriptions, and the dialysis regimen are important determinants of outcome. Measurement of adherence to each of these aspects is challenging. The assessment tools and indices are not true measures of adherence but rather are often health indicators that can serve as proxy markers for adherence.

Types of Nonadherence

Fluid and Dietary Nonadherence

Fluid and dietary nonadherence may be indicated by biochemical indices, including serum potassium concentration, phosphate levels, blood urea nitrogen (BUN), and interdialytic weight gain (IDWG). There are no standard cut-off levels for potassium and phosphate that define nonadherence. Studies have used a range from 5.5 to 8 mEq/L as markers of potassium nonadherence and a range from 5.5 mg/dL to 7.5 mg/dL as markers of phosphate nonadherence. IDWG has been measured with both absolute and relative values and is increased by high sodium and fluid intake.

The prevalence of HD patient nonadherence to diet and fluid restrictions ranges from 10% to 85%, depending on the various measurement tools used. In the United States, some studies suggest that 10% to 20% of HD patients routinely exhibit high IDWG. Increased IDWG has been associated with lowered effectiveness of dialysis, hypertension, congestive heart failure, pulmonary edema, and death.

Dialysis patients may often have difficulty understanding, assimilating, and following dietary recommendations. Although a typical diet provides approximately 1500 mg of phosphorus per day coming from milk, meat, poultry, fish, cereal, and eggs, the recommended dietary allowance of phosphorus intake for dialysis patients is 700 mg/day. Smith et al explored potential barriers and facilitators to fluid adherence in dialysis patients. They found that knowledge and accurate self-assessment of health were associated with increased adherence. The most common barrier was an overall lack of motivation to restrict fluid. Social support was sometimes a facilitator and sometimes a barrier, depending on the extent to which family members and friends engaged in the patient's treatment and guided and encouraged them to make the necessary lifestyle changes.

Medication Nonadherence

Medication nonadherence in dialysis patients is measured by both objective and subjective means. Objective measures include electronic monitoring, IDWG, and pill counts. Subjective measures include questionnaires completed by the health care provider or completed by the patient.

The prevalence of nonadherence to medication ranges from 21% to 74% in ESRD patients, depending on the type of assessment. Several investigators have explored the barriers to medication adherence in dialysis patients. Feelings of discomfort, forgetfulness, the use of multiple medications (i.e., patients are generally prescribed an average of 10–12 pills per day), fear of drug interactions, medical expenses, lack of knowledge, and poor communication with physicians are barriers to adherence.

Dialysis Prescription Nonadherence

Dialysis prescription nonadherence is also measured by objective (i.e., the number of skipped sessions or numbers of shortened dialysis sessions) and subjective measures (i.e., staff assessments). There are not established standard cut-offs for the level of skipping or shortening behaviors that define nonadherence. For example, skipping one or more dialysis sessions per month has been used to define nonadherence, but others have used higher cut-offs.

Among 182,536 dialysis patients, Chan et al found that patients who missed their scheduled appointments were more likely to be hospitalized. Also, use of public transportation (vs private), holidays, and inclement weather may modify relationships between missed treatments and hospitalizations.

Factors Affecting Hemodialysis Nonadherence

Many factors have been evaluated for their contribution to nonadherence behaviors in patients treated with HD. These include patient characteristics; psychosocial influences, particularly social support, health beliefs, depression, and illness perceptions; and elements of the dialysis environment, including patient–staff relationships, health literacy, and HD knowledge.

Patient Characteristics and Nonadherence

The influence of age, gender, and ethnicity on adherence behaviors in HD patients has been evaluated. Across studies, and regardless of type of recommended treatment, younger patients are more likely to be nonadherent than older patients. Findings regarding gender have been less consistent. Although the majority of the studies examining the role of gender on nonadherence in HD patients have identified men as being less adherent, one study including HD patients from the United States, Japan, and Europe, including France, Germany, Italy, Spain, and the United Kingdom, found that women were more likely to be nonadherent to dietary recommendations. Similarly, ethnic differences in adherent behaviors are inconclusive. One study found blacks to be more nonadherent to the dialysis regimen (i.e., more likely to skip treatments), but other studies found no race differences. In addition to demographic factors, the role of other individual differences, including smoking and education, on HD adherence has been evaluated. Smokers and patients with lower education have been identified as being less adherent to treatment.

Psychosocial Factors and Nonadherence

The relationships between psychosocial factors, particularly social support, or psychological factors, defined by health beliefs, depression, and illness and treatment perceptions, and adherence have also been assessed.

Social Support and Nonadherence

Social support may be a source of positive impact on adherence in HD patients. The influence of perceived social and family support is generally associated with improved adherence behaviors in patients being treated with HD, but some results have been mixed. Several studies found a significant association between social support and adherence to recommended fluid intake, such that those with lower levels of social support were less likely to adhere to dietary recommendations. In contrast, two other studies did not find such a relationship. Three studies found a strong association between lower levels of social support and a greater likelihood of medication nonadherence. Christensen et al found a positive relationship between social support and adherence to the dialysis treatment, such that higher levels of perceived support were associated with adherence to the dialysis treatment. One study found that having less family support was associated with nonadherence, but another found no relationship between the variables.

Health Beliefs and Nonadherence

Health beliefs, particularly feelings of self-efficacy, relate to an individual's perceived ability to perform a certain behavior. These perceptions of self-efficacy may influence whether individuals will attempt certain behaviors and how the behaviors will be carried out.

Patients treated with dialysis who have lower self-efficacy beliefs have been found to be less adherent to treatment than HD patients with higher self-efficacy beliefs. Two studies found patients with lower dietary self-efficacy had higher potassium levels and IDWG. There is also evidence that increasing self-efficacy can lead to improved adherence. An RCT showed that patients who received self-efficacy enhancement training had a greater reduction in IDWG compared with those who did not receive the intervention at all follow-up periods.

Depression and Nonadherence
Several studies have shown that depression predicts lower adherence in dialysis patients. Khalil et al suggested that depressed patients feel hopeless and have a negative self-image and outlook, which in turn manifests as an inability to adhere to treatment.

Illness and Treatment Perceptions and Nonadherence
Illness perceptions refer to the patients' appraisals of how their disease affects their everyday physical and emotional functioning and overall QOL. Treatment perceptions refer to patients' beliefs about medication. Various studies have found that patients with more optimistic illness perceptions have a greater likelihood of adhering to treatment. Similarly, HD patients with positive perceptions about the benefits of medication use are also more likely to be adherent.

Dialysis Environment and Nonadherence
Patient–Physician Dyad and Nonadherence
Trust is an essential quality between the physician and patient because it can either foster or damage patients' treatment adherence behaviors. Allowing open communication between patients and their health care providers and allowing patients to participate in decision making may enhance adherence. One preliminary study found that patients' increased satisfaction with physicians was associated with improved attendance and greater adherence to the treatment. Additionally, frequent patient–physician contact may lead to better adherence in dialysis patients. Findings from Plantinga et al support this hypothesis. They found HD patients who attended clinics with limited patient–physician contact were less satisfied with their care and more likely to be nonadherent to all aspects of their treatment.

Health Literacy and Nonadherence
Health literacy refers to the "ability to obtain, process, and understand basic health information in order to make appropriate health decisions about one's health and medical care." Lower health literacy has been linked to many health complications such as diabetes, poor adherence, and health disparities in various populations, as well as to death in ESRD patients. Lower health literacy is also correlated with poorer QOL. Health literacy may be an important factor in the care of patients with kidney disease.

There are several possible mechanisms through which dialysis patients' literacy level may exert effects on patient adherence. Patients with low health literacy may have low reading comprehension skills or knowledge of their disease that prevents them from fully understanding self-care demands and the medical and dialytic prescription. Although pamphlets are educational and informative, they may be difficult for people with low reading skills to understand. Limited patient knowledge may also affect patients' self-efficacy and their confidence that they can be adherent.

Health literacy may also influence nonadherence behaviors, particularly taking prescribed medications, following dietary recommendations, and attending dialysis appointments. Green et al found patients with low health literacy were more likely to be nonadherent to the dialysis treatment, having more missed dialysis appointments.

Hemodialysis-Specific Knowledge and Nonadherence

The impact of HD-related knowledge on adherence behaviors in HD patients has been examined in a number of studies. The findings, however, are inconsistent. Some studies demonstrate that patients with more knowledge about their disease are more likely to adhere to their treatment regimens. One intervention study that investigated the change in patients' adherence behavior to taking phosphate binders after they were provided with increased knowledge about the binders (compared with those who did not receive phosphate education) found that patients who received the educational intervention had increased adherence rates, from 82.5% in week 1 to 94% at week 13, compared with the adherence rate change from 85.5% at week 1 to 75.9% at week 13 in the control patients. Another intervention study in which patients were given structured educational sessions showed a decrease in IDWG from 2.64 kg to 2.21 kg. Casey et al found that patient education regarding fluid management improved adherence in 48% of the sample group. In another study, patients who received HD-related knowledge had better fluid adherence than those who did not receive the education. In contrast, Tanner et al and Cummings et al found no association between increased HD-related knowledge and adherence behaviors.

Addressing Hemodialysis Nonadherence

Given the high rates of nonadherence in HD patients, effective treatment options to improve adherence have been evaluated. Interventions include an array of educational, biopsychosocial, and behavioral designs to help HD patients, as they experience multiple and necessary lifestyle changes. Effects of the interventions have been mixed. Disparate results are likely due to differences in sample size, patient characteristics, and adherence outcomes assessed in the studies.

Some educational interventions have proved effective for fluid adherence, but others have not. Cupisti et al showed that a dietary intervention and counseling effectively helped HD patients decrease phosphate and calcium intakes. Similarly, Ford et al showed significant improvement in patients' phosphate levels after 6 months when patients were given a 20- to 30-minute diet education program each month. Sullivan et al showed a decline in serum phosphate levels in the intervention group (i.e., those who received a dietary education intervention vs the control group) after 3 months. Another study found an educational program for compliance with dietary restrictions was more effective in lowering phosphate levels in the long term compared with monthly nutrition counseling and information regarding the use of phosphate binders.

However, Schlatter and Ferrans found that a teaching intervention in a group of 29 HD patients with high phosphate levels had no effect on serum phosphate levels despite an increase in phosphate knowledge. Likewise, Long et al and Wells et al found that an educational program increased knowledge but did not improve dialysis patients' adherence. One study that targeted depression symptoms had an effect on

IDWG. Although participants were in the active phase of treatment, their IDWG rates fell to within the target range. However, the adherence behaviors did not continue through the 3-month follow-up, with mean levels of adherence returning to baseline levels.

Thus, knowledge and education alone do not increase adherence. It is possible that tailoring the intervention to the needs and characteristics of individual patients may be more beneficial.

One strategy for improving medication adherence in dialysis patients is to simplify drug regimens. This can be done by either using fixed-dose combinations to allow for once-daily dosing, using drugs that are administered less often, or administering the drugs intravenously at the end of the dialysis session or orally under direct supervision, if possible. Such strategies may often be incompatible with clinical requirements for drug administration, insurance issues, or clinic policies. Another strategy is to include a multidisciplinary approach in which all members of the treatment team (i.e., the patient, nursing and technical staff, administrators, and physician) are engaged and in open communication in order to reduce barriers and enhance adherence. However, caution is warranted because the success of such approaches has not been demonstrated to improve adherence in the HD population; the evidence from the RCTs has shown no difference from usual care practices.

Conclusion

Hemodialysis, although lifesaving, is a taxing, demanding, and often lifelong treatment for patients. Patients' psychological resilience and available resources may be associated with their QOL, psychological health, compliance with treatment demands, and perhaps even symptom burden and survival because untreated depression is a risk factor for poor outcomes. Beyond the direct impact of depression on ESRD, psychosocial factors interact in a complex fashion and may serve to support or inhibit compliance with the dialysis prescription. As physicians' treatment goals increasingly embrace a biopsychosocial perspective, more clinical and scientific attention is required to understand factors that predict mental health, QOL, and treatment compliance in dialysis patients.

The study of the impact of the psychosocial functioning of ESRD patients is still in the early stages of development. However, it is clear that the psychosocial status of the ESRD patient can have a meaningful impact on disease course. There needs to be rigorous inquiry about the strategies that can optimize psychosocial functioning and medical outcomes in patients with ESRD treated with dialysis.

C H A P T E R 7 1

The Care of Elderly Dialysis and End-Stage Renal Disease Patients

Danica Lam, MD • Sarbjit Vanita Jassal, MD

As the proportion of the general population older than the age of 65 years increases, this is mirrored in the dialysis population. In addition to the management of the multitude of targets and complications of end-stage renal disease (ESRD) and dialysis, care of elderly dialysis patients also requires assessment and management of common geriatric syndromes of impairment (often referred to as "geriatric giants") to maximize independence and function and minimize disease and symptom burden. These geriatric syndromes often interact to affect both morbidity and mortality and require some unique considerations in dialysis patients. Many brief screening strategies can be integrated into clinicians' routine dialysis rounds to quickly identify patients who would benefit from further interventions or referrals to other specialists. This chapter also addresses the importance of advance care planning (ACP) in this population.

Cognitive Impairment and Dementia

Cognitive impairment is very common in dialysis patients: in fact, it appears earlier than it does in the general population, and it is more prevalent in dialysis patients when they are compared with age- and gender-matched control participants. This is true of both hemodialysis (HD) and peritoneal dialysis (PD) patients, as well as those undergoing frequent short daily or nocturnal HD. Studies have documented prevalence rates as high as 75% of moderate to severe impairment when patients are systematically screened with standard tests. In addition, studies suggest that the progression of cognitive impairment is accelerated in the presence of renal disease. This has implications for self-care (e.g., adherence to medications and renal diet restrictions) and dialysis modality (e.g., the different challenges in delivering in-center HD vs home dialysis), as well as prognosis and ACP because dementia is a progressive, terminal diagnosis.

Executive Dysfunction

Executive functioning, or problem-solving functions, are part of day-to-day dialysis life. Patients are expected to manage diet and fluid plans, monitor their dialysis access, and detect early signs of infection. Executive dysfunction, as opposed to, for example, memory impairment is one of the cognitive domains more commonly affected in dialysis patients. This might reflect the significant burden of vascular disease in this population. The challenge is that executive dysfunction can present more subtly than frank memory loss, which patients and families may be more likely to bring to the attention of their dialysis team. Studies show that dialysis care providers identify only a tiny fraction of dialysis patients with objective evidence of cognitive impairment on standard testing (as low as 4%), which suggests that systematic application of standard testing might be more effective at identifying these patients.

Screening

The Mini-Mental State Examination (MMSE) is frequently used to screen for cognitive impairment, but it is not very sensitive in certain scenarios, such as in highly educated patients or those with predominantly executive dysfunction (as might be the case in many dialysis patients). It can also be challenging and therefore inaccurate for patients with language or cultural barriers.

The Mini-COG™ is a simple bedside test that may be more practical and useful as a screening test. It consists of only two components: clock drawing (2 points) and a three-item recall (3 points). Scores of 2 of 5 or lower should prompt further cognitive testing.

Other cognitive tests include the Montreal Cognitive Assessment (MOCA) and the Rowland Universal Dementia Assessment Scale (RUDAS), the latter of which is useful for patients with educational, language, or cultural barriers to accurate assessment with other tools. However, these other tests may be less practical in the dialysis unit setting, where time at the bedside can be limited, there is a lack of privacy, and the environment is full of visual and aural distractions.

Management

Management principles in the general population include pharmacologic and non-pharmacologic treatments. In the general population, pharmacologic therapies such as cholinesterase inhibitors in patients with mild to moderate dementia, and the N-methyl-D-aspartate (NMDA) inhibitor memantine in those with moderate to severe dementia show, at best, modest effects at slowing the rate of deterioration (especially in the setting of probable Alzheimer disease). Side effects are dose dependent and include gastrointestinal, neurologic, and cardiovascular side effects related to cholinergic stimulation, the most common being dizziness and drowsiness, but the most concerning in the dialysis population are weight loss, debility, and syncope. Unfortunately, no studies have looked specifically at the risks and benefits of pharmacologic management in dialysis patients, and these treatments add significantly to the drug burden already seen in this population. If trialed in the individual, patients should be monitored not only for clinical effect but also for side effects. These medications should also be discontinued when functional impairment becomes severe.

Cognitive rehabilitation and exercise programs may be useful but can be challenging to organize around dialysis schedules for patients who receive in-center HD. Referral to a geriatric specialist or occupational therapist might be helpful to explore all management options, especially if there are neuropsychiatric symptoms of dementia or as functional impairment emerges. They may also be able to educate and support caregivers, assist with managing pharmacologic options as discussed earlier, and help access community programs to maximize function and safety.

Behavioral and Psychological Symptoms of Dementia

Dementia is a progressive disease that may progress to seeing complex behavioral abnormalities. Sometimes referred to as behavioral and psychological symptoms of dementia (BPSD), patients present aggressively with screaming, hitting, or other unexpected actions. These can be dangerous behaviors for staff, the patient, and other patients, particularly within an HD center, and clear unit policies around the provision of dialysis and around safety plans are advisable when patients begin to manifest these symptoms.

It is advantageous to have previously had discussions with the family about the risk of BPSD. In fact, a diagnosis of cognitive impairment or dementia presents an opportunity for the dialysis team to engage in ACP with patients and their families (see the Advance Care Planning section). Families should be provided with ongoing education and counseling around the natural history of dementia and encouraged to identify opportunities and barriers that impact patient safety and quality of life and to discuss future circumstances under which withdrawal of dialysis would be appropriate.

Depression

Prevalence rates of depression in older adults are probably underestimated. In both the elderly and dialysis populations, depression is associated with functional decline, increased morbidity, increased risk of developing dementia, and decreased survival. Depression can also be a complication of dementia in itself. Although elderly patients with depression are less likely to attempt suicide than younger patients, rates of suicide completion in this population are higher.

Presentation

Depression in older patients may go unrecognized because it often presents "atypically" in this age group. In dialysis populations, up to 30% of cases of depression appear to go unrecognized or untreated. Elderly patients with depression may present predominantly with fatigue, somatic symptoms, or even cognitive impairment. An additional challenge in dialysis patients is the overlap between dialysis- or ESRD-associated symptoms and those considered characteristic of depressive episodes (e.g., low appetite or fatigue). Nevertheless, depression should be considered in the differential diagnosis when patients present with functional decline, cognitive impairment, or nonadherence to therapy.

Screening

A variety of screening tools have been validated in the geriatric population. The Beck Depression Inventory (BDI) has been studied in dialysis patients but is lengthy. The Geriatric Depression Scale (GDS), which takes less time to administer, has also been used in dialysis patients. Both require adjusted cut-off values for determination of depression.

More practical than both of these to administer is the Personal Health Questionnaire-2 (PHQ-2), a sensitive, validated tool to screen for depression in older adults. It is composed of two questions that ask patients about depressed mood or anhedonia. Patients' responses to each question are scored from 0 to 3 (in order of increasing severity). A total score of 3 or higher should prompt the health care provider to go on to the PHQ-9, which can reliably be used to diagnose depression. Both of these tools have also been studied in the dialysis population.

Referral to a psychiatrist, ideally one with expertise in the geriatric or renal populations (or both), should be initiated when there is clinical evidence for depression because the gold standard for the diagnosis of depression remains psychiatric assessment.

Management

There is limited evidence on the effectiveness of traditional therapies for depression when used specifically in dialysis patients. Nevertheless, many commonly used antidepressants can in fact be used in dialysis patients, albeit at reduced doses. Some also have multifactorial benefits in terms of improved appetite (mirtazapine) or chronic pain management (duloxetine). The same caution should be observed as when they are started for any other patients, namely, close follow-up to identify side effects (including QT prolongation), risk factors for falls (see the Instability and Falls section), and changes in suicidal ideation. Unless nephrologists have comfort and experience overseeing this management on their own, usually co-management with a psychiatrist is warranted.

Nonpharmacologic management of depression can also provide benefits. Group cognitive behavioral therapy (CBT) as well as a modified bedside version of CBT have both been studied but require access to health care professionals trained to deliver such therapies. Group CBT can be challenging for in-center HD patients, who may be reluctant or find it challenging to travel routinely to the hospital on a nondialysis day. Bedside CBT has its own challenges, such as protection of privacy, and more intensive resource use. Close collaboration with mental health professionals with an interest in co-managing renal patients may be helpful.

Instability and Falls

In a report published by the National ESRD Patient Safety Initiative in 2011, falls were identified as one of the top five safety issues for dialysis patients. In the general population, increasing age, medical comorbidities (e.g., malnutrition, diabetes, and cardiac disease), cognitive impairment or depression, and polypharmacy are all associated with an increased risk of falls. All of these risk factors exist in abundance in elderly dialysis patients. In addition, elderly dialysis patients are exposed to distinctive risks related to their kidney disease and uremia, as well as the dialysis process itself. Some studies have found decreased physical function immediately after dialysis when measured by such parameters as performance in sit-to-stand and gait initiation. Treatment with PD is similarly associated with an increased fall risk as that seen with HD.

Decreasing the risk of falls can have important consequences for survival. Injury subsequent to a fall can significantly impact mortality (e.g., there is a 20%–25% increase in 1-year mortality after a hip fracture in elderly patients). In dialysis patients, the risk of mortality associated with a hip fracture after a fall may be as high as double that of matched dialysis control participants. Even if a fall does not cause serious injuries, recurrent falls are also associated with a higher risk of mortality. They can also have important implications for functional status because they are associated with an increased fear of falling, decreased independence, and an increased risk of admission to hospital or long-term care.

Screening

A number of screening tools have been used to identify patients at high risk for falls. The Performance-Oriented Mobility Assessment (POMA), for example, is a comprehensive tool that does not require a specialist to administer and could easily be used with a minimum amount of training. Other published studies describe easy-to-use screening checklists that can be applied by any member of the care team such as nurses.

The 2010 Clinical Practice Guideline of the American and British Geriatrics Societies on falls prevention suggests a quick, three-question screen for community-dwelling older patients, which can be used to identify those at increased risk of falls and who therefore might benefit from intervention.
1. Has the patient had two or more falls in the past 12 months?
2. Is the patient presenting with an acute fall?
3. Does the patient report any difficulty with walking or balance?

Individuals who answer yes to at least one of these questions should then undergo a more comprehensive, multidisciplinary assessment (e.g., with referral to a falls prevention clinic), including a home safety assessment (if applicable and available).

Dialysis-Related Risk Factors

Attention to optimizing other geriatric syndromes should be applied to minimize falls risk. In addition, there are dialysis-related factors to address.

Postural Hypotension
In the general population, reducing postural hypotension is associated with a decreased risk of falls when it is part of a multifactorial approach to falls prevention. Patients appear to have increased sway after HD, suggesting a relationship with subclinical postural hypotension. Unfortunately, no controlled trials have been conducted in the dialysis population, who are exposed to the additional complication of dialysis-related hypotension, and in fact, it is not clear if interventions to mitigate orthostatic hypotension postdialysis can reduce the risk of falls. It would be reasonable, however, to pay particular attention to reducing this complication in high-risk dialysis patients, with careful and frequent dry weight assessments and screening for precipitating medications.

Vitamin D Supplementation
The 2010 Clinical Practice Guideline of the American Geriatric Society (AGS) and British Geriatric Society (BGS) recommends vitamin D supplementation in all older patients. Unfortunately, given the complicated nature of the calcium–phosphate axis and renal bone disease in dialysis patients and the absence of evidence specific to this population, it is not clear that this recommendation should be applied broadly to all dialysis patients, especially because many of them are already prescribed calcitriol for hyperparathyroidism.

Biochemical Abnormalities
Electrolyte abnormalities, however brief (e.g., postdialysis), can also be contributing factors. Hyponatremia has been shown to affect cognition and gait and may be associated with an increased risk of fracture after a fall. The same is true of hypokalemia. Dialysis patients also face unique challenges in terms of the muscular dysfunction and mineral and bone disorders associated with ESRD. Anemia and metabolic acidosis

also affect strength and muscle mass and thus might contribute to an increased risk of falls and fractures. Careful attention to these parameters during routine dialysis rounds might be helpful in patients for whom falls screening is positive.

Environmental Risks Within the Dialysis Unit

The dialysis unit itself presents opportunities for decreasing fall risk. Design and efficient use of the unit to minimize clutter and obstacles between dialysis machines and stations, doorways, scales, and so on may be helpful. Other environmental hazards include spills or leakages on floors, poor lighting, and the scales used to weigh patients pre- and postdialysis. Published experiences suggest that it may be helpful to have staff assistance in transfers, ambulation, and weighing for patients who are identified as being high risk for falls and that root cause analysis or other quality improvement methodologies may be effective to minimize an individual dialysis unit's environmental risks for falls.

Polypharmacy

Efforts should be made to optimize polypharmacy and withdraw psychotropic medications (or at least reduce their doses) (see the Polypharmacy and Safe Prescribing section).

Visual Impairment

There is some evidence that visual impairment is more prevalent in elderly dialysis patients than in the general population. Although there is no evidence specifically in the ESRD population, expediting first cataract surgery in patients in whom it is indicated is recommended by the AGS/BGS guidelines, as part of a multifactorial intervention in high-risk patients (see next section).

Multifactorial Management

In addition to the strategies described earlier, exercise programs that include strength training, and balance, gait, and coordination training seem to be effective, particularly as part of multifactorial falls prevention programs. Other possible components of an exercise program include tai chi, endurance training, and flexibility exercises. The AGS/BGS guidelines suggest that programs last a minimum of 12 weeks and involve one to three sessions per week.

Home assessments and modifications implemented by trained health care professionals, such as occupational therapists, are also helpful as part of multifactorial management programs, as are programs that assess and correct issues related to the feet (e.g., ulcers, nail or other deformities) and footwear.

Patients With Cognitive Impairment

Unfortunately, in the setting of community-dwelling older patients with cognitive impairment, it is less clear if any of the above-mentioned strategies are effective.

Immobility and Rehabilitation

Elderly dialysis patients are at significant risk of functional decline, likely as a result of the interaction of multiple factors, such as their increased risk of cognitive impairment, visual impairment, and depression), but also dialysis-related factors, such as postdialysis fatigue, the number of hours routinely spent immobile in a dialysis chair, and renal bone disease. Not only is impaired function or mobility at the time of dialysis initiation associated with an increased risk of mortality but so is functional decline afterward.

Geriatric Rehabilitation

Geriatric rehabilitation is a well-defined area with good evidence for its efficacy. The experience in geriatric dialysis patients is, of course, more limited but would suggest that it can have significant benefits as well.

Inpatient geriatric rehabilitation programs may benefit elderly patients who are at risk of functional decline coincident with dialysis initiation, enabling them to return home after discharge (as opposed to being placed in a long-term care facility) and decreasing their risk of readmission to the hospital. Interdisciplinary rehabilitation teams with an expertise in caring for geriatric patients are usually involved. Setting a regular dialysis schedule that does not conflict with therapy is key, and short daily dialysis (i.e., 2 hours, 6 days a week) may be particularly effective. There is some evidence that, in the above scenario, elderly dialysis patients do as well in inpatient geriatric rehabilitation programs as their nondialysis peers.

Exercise Training

Exercise training on dialysis can involve physiotherapists and occupational therapists in the dialysis unit in programs fortunate enough to have such resources. However, it can also be provided on a routine basis with equipment such as stationary bikes that patients can use while sitting in an HD chair. Intradialytic exercise training programs have been shown to improve physical performance measures such as the 6-minute walk and timed up-and-go tests. Home-based exercise training programs, supervised by allied health in the community, can also be helpful. All age groups of dialysis patients appear to benefit from exercise training, including frail elderly patients.

Polypharmacy and Safe Prescribing

Studies have shown that the median number of pills taken every day by dialysis patients is approximately 20. Pill burden in dialysis patients is further complicated by the frequency of medication dosing throughout the day and the need for phosphate binders to be taken with meals, accurate timing of thyroid hormone replacements, bedtime statins, antihypertensive drugs, and the like. This represents a pill burden more onerous than that seen in other chronic diseases, such as congestive heart failure or diabetes (which, of course, many renal patients also have).

In elderly patients, this can be compounded by functional impairments (e.g., difficulty with pill bottles or blister packs because of decreased manual dexterity, grip strength, or vision), cognitive impairment, and altered pharmacokinetics and pharmacodynamics that put them at increased risk of adverse drug events.

The American Geriatrics Society maintains an updated list of medications that should not be prescribed routinely in geriatric patients. Examples that are commonly prescribed to dialysis patients include benzodiazepines and other sedative-hypnotics, anticholinergic agents (e.g., dimenhydrinate and diphenhydr-amine), and alpha-blockers. Emerging evidence also supports more lenient blood pressure ($\leq$150/90 mm Hg) and glycemic control (HbA1C $\leq$7.5%) in frail elderly patients, albeit with less guidance specific to dialysis patients.

Scheduling medication reviews on a regular basis, as well as after changes in health status or acute admissions, can help to identify changes in prescriptions or adherence, as well as medications that are inappropriate based on drug interactions or lack of benefit. Collaboration with allied health team members, such as occupa-tional therapists, can help to identify simple methods of improving adherence (e.g., alarms and other tools to remind patients of multiple medication administration times) or strategies to organize pills to minimize errors.

Advance Care Planning

Advance care planning is a dynamic process whereby patients, their families or loved ones, and their health care teams explore the patients' goals, values, beliefs, and understanding of their illness and how these interact with medical care, both cur-rently and in the future, particularly as health declines. It includes but is not limited to the development of advanced directives, decisions around resuscitation, and identification and education of the substitute decision maker (SDM). It should be revisited not only when the patient wishes to but also whenever a patient's health status changes or he or she experiences an acute event. In a randomized trial of elderly patients, ACP significantly improved care at the end of life because patients' prior wishes were more likely to be known and respected.

Advance care planning is particularly important in elderly dialysis patients, who have a limited life expectancy compared with nondialysis age- and gender-matched control participants or younger fellow dialysis patients and who often have multiple, complex life-limiting illnesses in addition to ESRD. In 2011, for example, prevalent dialysis patients in the United States older than the age of 70 years had an expected remaining lifetime of 3.6 years compared with 12.2 in the general population in that age group; after age 80 years, this drops to 2.5 years versus 6.7. It is also important to note that reported rates of dialysis discontinuation before death in patients after the age of 75 years range from 24% to 34%.

Compared with patients with heart failure or cancer, elderly dialysis patients spend more days in the hospital and intensive care unit, are more likely to undergo invasive procedures, and are less likely to die in a hospice setting in the last month of life. Although the willingness of patients and families to discuss prognosis can depend not only on individual experiences and preferences but also cultural back-ground, studies indicate that nephrologists usually underestimate patients' desire to discuss prognosis and ACP, and, accordingly, discussions about expected survival and illness trajectory in ESRD or dialysis are rare. The result is a systematic gap in care that can negatively affect communication between dialysis teams and the people for whom they provide care, patients' and families' awareness of what they can expect as the illness progresses, and alleviation of their symptoms and emotional suffering.

Published experiences with ACP as a routine part of renal care include formalized training programs for dialysis teams, dedicated clinics for discussions around ACP, and dedicated team members to facilitate these discussions.

Prognostic Tools

Nephrologists often identify uncertainty around an individual patient's prognosis or disease course as a barrier to discussions about goals of care. A number of studies have assessed various risk factors that confer an increased mortality risk in dialysis patients, and prognostic tools have been developed to help estimate 6-month mortality in this population. Examples of important clinical factors identified by these studies include increased age, low serum albumin, answering "no" to the surprise question, medical comorbidities (especially ischemic heart disease, dementia, or peripheral vascular disease), functional dependence before starting dialysis, a low body mass index, and sentinel events (e.g., amputation or myocardial infarction).

Caution should be used in the application of these tools, however. They are not intended to be used to withhold dialysis from selected patients based on demographics alone but rather should be used as another resource for clinicians, patients, and family members in decision-making around management options as ESRD approaches.

Substitute Decision Makers

It is particularly important to identify and engage SDMs early on in the process of ACP. A significant proportion of elderly dialysis patients are no longer capable near the end of life, given the illness burden and significant risk of cognitive impairment in this population, and SDMs are then asked to make decisions on their behalf. Research in the general population, however, has consistently shown that SDMs and health care professionals do little better than chance alone (if even that well) in predicting what patients' wishes would be in various critical care or end-of-life scenarios, including those that involve decisions about dialysis continuation.

Advance directives have been shown to improve the likelihood that patients will receive the care that they want. They have also been shown to alleviate the anxiety, depression, and other psychological or emotional suffering that SDMs may feel in making such difficult decisions on behalf of patients. Engaging SDMs early on in the ACP process helps to strengthen their relationships with patients and health care teams and to reassure them when the time comes for them to enact their role that they can do so with prior understanding of what their loved one would want.

Nondialytic Management

There is an emerging body of evidence that suggests that nondialysis or Comprehensive Conservative Renal Care (CCRC) may not be inferior to dialysis, either in terms of survival, effect on functional dependence, or quality of life measures, in elderly ESRD patients with significant medical comorbidities or poor functional status. Even if there is a survival advantage purely in terms of numbers, these patients may not gain much in the way of hospital-free days on dialysis. Most of these data are for in-center HD, with somewhat less available in the area of PD, and none for home HD.

For patients who chose CCRC, it is important to reassure them that they will continue to be cared for. Symptom burden in ESRD patients, whether they are on dialysis or not, is high. The most commonly reported symptoms include low energy, pruritus, dyspnea, constipation or nausea, and pain. In stage 5 chronic kidney disease

(CKD) patients managed without dialysis, there is some evidence that symptom burden increases significantly, along with a precipitous functional decline, in the last 1 to 2 months of life. Early co-management with palliative care teams, particularly those with expertise with patients who have nonmalignant diseases or chronic organ failure, may be useful. Further research is needed to demonstrate whether this may in fact confer a survival benefit specifically in CKD/ESRD patients, as has been shown with other patient populations.

Conclusion

Elderly patients initiating dialysis are at increased risk of geriatric syndromic illnesses, such as falls, functional decline, and cognitive impairment. The high morbidity and mortality associated with these illnesses warrant a unique and personalized approach both to dialysis care but also to overall care. Open discussions of expectations, prognosis, and advance care goals are recommended and may allow the clinician to adapt dialysis care goals to the individual.

Pediatric Dialysis

C H A P T E R   7 2

Vascular Access in Children

Rossana Baracco, MD • Deepa H. Chand, MD, MHSA, FASN •
Rudolph P. Valentini, MD

The number of children with end-stage renal disease (ESRD) in the United States tripled over the course of 30 years, with a prevalence of 27 per million in 1980 and 86 per million in 2010. Although renal transplantation has become the most common renal replacement modality for prevalent children with ESRD, hemodialysis (HD) continues to be the most common initial treatment. Of 1161 incident children with ESRD in 2012, almost half of them began treatment with HD.

Although most children with ESRD will receive a kidney transplant, it is likely that they will require decades of treatment for ESRD and will require HD at some point in their lives. Most children on HD in the United States (78.7%) and Europe (60%) are dialyzed with a central venous catheter (CVC); this despite guidelines emphasizing the creation of permanent vascular access, arteriovenous fistula (AVF) or arteriovenous graft (AVG) for long-term HD in children.

Central venous catheters offer the benefit of immediate and painless access and are best suited for acute HD. However, when used long term, CVCs have a high risk of infection and malfunction and place the child at significant risk for central venous stenosis. Recurrent hospitalizations and procedures to replace CVCs not only increase health care costs but also increase missed school days in the life of a developing child, thereby impairing cognitive and social development.

Arteriovenous Fistulas

Arteriovenous fistulas are the ideal vascular access for chronic HD because they allow for high blood flow rates, resulting in efficient and effective dialysis delivery. They also have the best long-term survival and the lowest rate of complications and hospitalizations. Children dialyzed with an AVF have higher albumin levels and higher mean hemoglobin concentrations and require lower doses of erythropoietin compared with children dialyzed with a CVC. In addition to these benefits, children with an AVF can bathe and swim without restrictions. Disadvantages include needling pain and physical changes in the appearance of the arm.

Although the Fistula First Initiative (FFI), sponsored by the Centers for Medicare & Medicaid, did not include pediatric patients, an international pediatric FFI was introduced in 2008 to increase AVF creation in children. Undoubtedly, AVF creation in small patients can be challenging, particularly in children with early onset of chronic kidney disease (CKD), history of multiple hospitalizations, and central line placements with resulting vein stenosis. The early reports of AVF use in children in the 1970s described about 50% immediate failure rates. Over the years, improved surgical expertise, the use of microsurgery techniques in select centers, and institution of multidisciplinary vascular teams have resulted in improved success rates of AVF creation and use in many centers around the world. Patency rates are now similar to those reported in adults, even for small children.

Preparation

Vein preservation is of particular importance for future AVF creation. The need to protect veins for future access should begin upon diagnosis of CKD in a child. Patients and families should be educated on the importance of protecting veins, especially in the nondominant arm. Venipunctures for blood draws and intravenous (IV) lines should be performed at distal sites of the extremities, preferably the dorsum of the hand, whenever possible. Educating the patient and family will empower them to best defend their "venous capital."

Location

In general, "distal before proximal" and "autogenous before prosthetic" principles should be followed when planning an AVF. The nondominant arm is the preferred limb. If vessels on the nondominant arm are not adequate, the dominant arm is then preferred over the lower limb. A wrist AVF (radiocephalic) remains the first choice for chronic HD in children. The surgery involves the cephalic vein, which is anastomosed to the radial artery in an end-to-side fashion. This AVF allows for preservation of more proximal vessels for future access, and it has high long-term patency. The disadvantages include high primary failure rates when microsurgery is not used and long maturation time in young children. The high primary failure rates in small children are attributed to small vessel size, vessel spasm, and poor venous outflow.

If a radiocephalic AVF is not possible or primary failure occurs, the brachial artery can be used in the creation of a brachiocephalic AVF as the next preferred location. A brachiobasilic AVF is another option on the upper arm. Two-stage basilic vein transposition allows for maturation of small veins, which can offer a superior alternative in small children. The basilic vein, located deep in the upper arm, is usually protected from the repeated trauma of previous venipunctures and may be of particular use in children who have small vessels and are not good candidates for a more distal AVF. The arterialized vein, when it has reached a diameter of 6 mm, is moved up to a more superficial position in a second-stage procedure to allow for easier cannulation. This type of AVF has been reported to have high immediate and long-term patency rates. Another alternative is the use of the proximal radial artery. Construction of this AVF involves disruption of venous valves to achieve bidirectional AVF flow. The vein used depends on the patient's anatomy and can include the median antebrachial, median cephalic, median cubital, or deep communicating vein. This type of AVF has a lower risk of steal phenomena than brachial artery fistulas. This type of AVF has been successfully used in children with high patency rates.

Following the "autogenous before prosthetic" principle, some centers create a thigh AVF in preference over an AVG. Saphenofemoral or transposed femoral vein AVFs have been used in children. The main complication of these fistulas is lower extremity edema. Surgical experience and technical expertise are of paramount importance in determining the optimal site for successful AVF creation.

Preoperative Planning

Children with CKD who are expected to be on HD for at least 6 to 12 months should be referred to a vascular surgeon when the glomerular filtration rate drops below 30 mL/min/1.73 m^2. Early referral is important in children, especially small children, because of long maturation times. The overarching goal should be avoidance of CVC. Patients who present with ESRD will require placement of a CVC; however, they should be educated about the risks of CVC and referred as soon as possible to evaluate for AVF placement if they plan to continue with HD.

Pertinent information in a child with ESRD or advanced CKD being evaluated for vascular access placement includes history of prolonged hospitalizations and the location and complications of previous central lines. Symptoms of central vein stenosis could include swelling and discomfort of the extremity or face and presence of collateral veins. It is important to note the dominant arm (right or left handed). Physical examination should focus on the presence of scars from previous catheters, extremity edema, presence of collateral veins, and the presence and quality of arterial pulses. The veins are typically examined with more detail, evaluating their length and determining their elasticity. Elasticity of the vein may be assessed with the use of a proximal tourniquet. An increase in diameter of 50% or greater may be indicative of an adequate vein for AVF creation.

Imaging tests are routinely done by some centers; others choose to perform them in selected patients. Doppler ultrasonography should be done if there are concerns on physical examination. For patients who have a history of previous CVCs and are suspected to have central venous stenosis, it is necessary to perform a venogram. Appropriately aggressive hydration (dependent on severity of CKD and fluid sensitivity of the patient) should be considered to minimize radiocontrast injury and preserve residual renal function. The minimum acceptable vessel diameters for AVF creation are 2.5 mm for veins and 1.5 mm for arteries, although with the use of microsurgery, successful fistulae have been created with vessels of smaller caliber.

Surgical Considerations

Young patients need to be sedated or brought under general anesthesia for creation of an AVF. Cooperative adolescents could tolerate the procedure with local or regional anesthesia.

Microsurgery is used routinely for the creation of AVF in children in some European centers and in selected cases in other centers. Its use is helpful and increases success rates, particularly of distal AVF in young children (younger than 10 years old) with small arteries. Bourquelot et al, Bagolan et al, Sanabia et al, and Gradman et al, who have reported large European series of children with AVF, achieved functioning radiocephalic AVF with very low failure rates and good long-term patency rates even in small patients (<15 kg). These authors strongly advocate for the use of an intraoperative microscope to create distal AVF in children because it allows for precise dissection and use of small sutures and avoids the need for dilation of the vessels and causing arterial spasm.

The use of an inflatable tourniquet on the upper arm when constructing a distal AVF is described by some authors to offer additional advantages such as "preventive hemostasis," which results in avoidance of extensive arterial dissection, decreased use of clamps, and lower risk of damage to the intima.

Perioperative strategies to optimize early AVF function include starting low-dose daily aspirin at least 1 week before surgery, reducing antihypertensive medications in the immediate preoperative period, and directing intraoperative and postoperative fluid management by nephrology to keep blood pressures at or above the 90th percentile for age, height, and gender.

Postoperative Care and Maturation

Hand exercises have shown to improve maturation in adults and should be encouraged after AVF creation in children old enough to cooperate. Low-dose aspirin has been used in some centers as a means to prevent thrombosis; however, there is no evidence currently that this is effective. Maturation times vary widely in pediatric AVF and have been reported anywhere from 3 to 4 weeks to 6 months. Smaller children tend to have longer maturation times. Communication among the nephrologist, vascular access surgeon, and HD nurse is imperative at this stage to determine the timing of the first AVF cannulation. Educating the patient and family on proper care of their AVF is of equal importance, especially regarding the need to avoid inadvertent compression of the involved extremity.

Cannulation

The first few treatments using a new AVF are usually performed with a 17-gauge needle for cannulation in children. In tenuous situations, single-needle cannulation of the arterial portion of the AVF with venous return through the CVC, if in place, can offer an advantage of less vascular trauma. The pain and anxiety of needling an AVF may also be decreased using this approach in young children. Topical anesthetic cream, applied at home or a few minutes before the scheduled HD session, is useful and may be used routinely. The buttonhole technique has been reported to offer less pain. Buttonhole needles are available for cannulation in children; this option has also been used on occasion in adolescents.

Child life specialists may play an important role in cannulation, helping to educate the child and distract him or her during cannulation with age-appropriate toys and activities. Although it is possible that children may experience significant pain during cannulation, only about 20% of children report great discomfort, and fewer than 10% of children report that they would prefer to return to a CVC. Some AVFs may become quite dilated and appear unattractive, especially radiocephalic AVF, which is easily visible in the forearm. Adolescents may become particularly distressed because of these cosmetic features and should be educated, with the emphasis on the many advantages of their AVF.

Complications

Primary failure is the most common complication and is reported in between 20% to 33% in children, although centers that routinely use microsurgery report much lower failure rates of 5% to 10%. Immediate failure is usually secondary to vessel spasm.

Thrombosis usually occurs secondary to venous stenosis and is the most frequent cause of secondary failure. Postdialytic hypotension can contribute to thrombosis, as well as over compression after needle withdrawal or inadvertent extremity compression between dialysis treatments. Pseudoaneurysms and steal phenomena are less frequent complications, as are AVF infection and high-output cardiac failure. Thigh AVFs may cause significant lower extremity edema in children.

Long-Term Care and Monitoring of Arteriovenous Fistulas

Recommendations for monitoring and surveillance of pediatric AVF are extrapolated from adult evidence because studies are lacking. Monitoring of AVF is necessary because stenosis is a common complication and can lead to thrombosis. Children with AVF may be at higher risk because of the smaller caliber of vessels. It is particularly important to preserve functioning vascular access in children to protect potential future access and minimize CVC placement and usage. Monitoring and surveillance of fistulas may detect significant stenosis (>50% of vessel diameter).

Physical examination should be done at each dialysis session; this includes palpation for a thrill or auscultating for bruit. Venous stenosis can be assessed by elevating the arm; the AVF should collapse if there are no outflow stenoses. The augmentation test evaluates the arterial side and is done by completely occluding the access several centimeters beyond the arterial anastomosis and comparing the pulse between the anastomosis and point of occlusion. Problems, including swelling of the extremity, altered thrill, prolonged bleeding after removing needles, difficult cannulation, and aspiration of blood clots, should raise suspicion of AVF malfunction and should lead to further evaluation by diagnostic angiography.

Surveillance methods include static and dynamic dialysis venous pressure monitoring, Doppler ultrasonography, monitoring intra-access blood flow, and assessing for recirculation. Dynamic venous pressures were not found to predict access thrombosis in a small number of children with AVF. Ultrasound dilution is a noninvasive bedside test to monitor vascular access flow. A sensor is attached to the venous and arterial lines each, and reversing the lines creates recirculation. A saline bolus is then injected via the venous needle into the access flow stream. The sensor on the arterial needle samples the diluted blood and detects changes in ultrasound velocity. Both sensors are connected to a computer, which interprets the changes in Doppler velocity and reports access flow in milliliters per minute. In children, access blood flow of less than 650 mL/min/ 1.73 m^2 has been shown to predict more than 50% of access stenosis. Because pediatric HD units are usually small, the cost of specialized equipment for AVF surveillance might be prohibitive, and staff may have to rely on physical examination and venous pressures. A summary of pediatric AVF studies is shown in Table 72.1.

Arteriovenous Graft

Despite AVF being the preferred access for children receiving HD, it may not be the best choice in all situations. AVGs are neither the most common nor the best and as such are not encouraged or discouraged in adults. In recent years, AVG use has been advocated in adult HD patients in certain situations, including previously failed AVF, poor veins, late referral for vascular access placement with the need for early cannulation, and children in whom AVF is not feasible.

Table 72.1

Arteriovenous Fistula Studies in Children

	Weight (kg)	Use of Operative Microscope	Primary Failure (%)	Primary Patency (%)	Secondary Patency (%)	Complications
Bourquelot et al (1990)	18 (4–48)	Yes	10		85% at 2 years 60% at 4 years 70% at 5 years for radiocephalic	19% of distal AVF had venous stenosis
Samabia et al (1993)		Yes	10			
Bagolan et al (1998)	28 (6.5–54)	Yes	5	90	70% for >15 kg, 56% for <15 kg at 4 years	Thrombosis, 26%; stenosis, 4%
Ramage et al (2005)	41.8	No	25		Median survival, 3.14 years	
Gradman et al (2005)	27 (10–60)	Yes	27	96 at 2 years 50 at 1 year	100% at 2 years 50% at 2 years	Thrombosis, 6.4% 0.84 interventions per 12 access months
Briones et al (2010)		No				
Baracco et al (2014)	52 (14.7–113)	No	32.3	42.9	78.1 at 5 years	Thrombosis, 20%; stenosis, 27%

AVF, arteriovenous fistula.

Comparison With Arteriovenous Fistula

Although the AVG is considered a permanent internal access, much like an AVF, there are fundamental differences. The AVG is more prone to thrombosis and has higher infection rates than an AVF, but it can typically be used much sooner than an AVF (weeks versus months, respectively). Primary failure rates are higher with AVFs than with AVGs; however, secondary failure rates are higher with AVGs than AVFs. Sheth et al reported the creation of 24 AVFs and 28 AVGs in 19 and 23 pediatric HD patients, respectively. The primary failure rates were 33.3% and 3.6% in AVF and AVG, respectively. Access stenoses and infection were reportedly higher in AVGs than in AVFs, but thrombotic episodes were not significantly different. In contrast, the morbidity and mortality risk associated with an AVG is similar to that associated with an AVF. Chand et al evaluated dialysis adequacy (Kt/V, urea reduction rates), anemia management, and albumin status based on vascular access type and found no significant differences between AVFs and AVGs.

Composition

Arteriovenous grafts can be composed of a variety of synthetic materials. Ideally, an AVG should be nonimmunogenic, nonthrombotic, easily placed, quickly accessible, durable, and cost effective. Over several decades, AVGs have been manufactured from a variety of materials, including saphenous vein, Dacron, cryopreserved femoral vein, umbilical, bovine, polytetrafluoroethylene (PTFE), and polyurethane. Although the PTFE AVG is the most commonly used, residual punctures caused by cannulation and seroma formation limit its use. Furthermore, because of perioperative graft edema, the PTFE usually cannot be used initially for several weeks. Nagakawa et al first described the modification PTFE graft by inserting a polyurethane graft segment. This composite graft offers the potential advantage of fewer kinks in the graft conduit, thereby improving efficacy and decreasing stenosis. Additional studies involving this composite AVG in adult HD patients showed no significant difference in operating time, blood loss, or postoperative complications. Less kinking was described with the composite AVG compared with the PTFE AVG. Lau et al further described the successful use of the composite AVG in a pediatric HD patient without complications from the time of placement to last use 5 months later. As such, some practitioners have chosen alternative AVGs or modified the PTFE graft. Grimaldi et al reported the successful use of a polycarbonate urethane AVG within 12 hours in a 3-year-old child weighing 12.7 kg. Seven-month follow-up demonstrated continued successful use of the access with some posterior wall AVG alterations, suggestive of mechanical trauma as a result of repetitive cannulations. Flow and treatment efficacy were not compromised. In recent years, various other modifications are being trialed.

Complications

The primary cause of AVG failure is venous stenosis leading to thrombosis at the graft-vein anastomosis. Ramage et al conducted a retrospective study over a 20-year period evaluating long-term complication rates of AVFs compared with AVG in children receiving HD. Intervention rates were reported as 17.8% for AVFs and 33% for AVGs. Reasons for discontinuation of AVG use was infection (20%), thrombosis (73%), and planned termination of use (6.7%). Although infection is rare, it can be serious, requiring graft removal. Other potential complications are similar to those seen with AVF and include steal syndrome, aneurysms, and development of neointimal hyperplasia over time.

Central Venous Catheters

Advantages of a CVC include immediate access for HD and needle-free dialysis. Disadvantages of a CVC include high infection rate, inadequate flows during dialysis caused by malposition and fibrin sheath formation, and restrictions on the child's activities (swimming). Catheters have also been associated with high markers of inflammation in children in the absence of infection. Long-term complications include central venous thrombosis or stenosis, which can prohibit the successful future placement of an AVF.

Characteristics

The ideal CVC is large enough to allow for adequate blood flow of at least 3 to 5 mL/kg/min; however, it should not be so large that it obstructs the vein. The catheter tip should end in the right atrium or at the junction of the superior vena cava and right atrium. When the tip of the catheter does not reach down far enough and stays in the SVC, there may be inadequate blood flow as the entry and exit sites of the catheter press up against the vessel wall.

Acute HD access is usually obtained via an uncuffed, nontunneled CVC. The femoral vein is frequently used in patients who are acutely ill and require emergent HD. This site should only be used for a short period of time (<2 weeks) because it carries an increased risk of infection, particularly in diapered children.

A cuffed, tunneled catheter is placed for chronic HD because uncuffed catheters can easily become dislodged in children and are at higher risk of infection. Dual-lumen catheters are most commonly used; these are typically made of silicone or polyurethane composites. Split catheters, in which the two catheters are of the same length and separated at the distal end, may be useful in small children in whom the distance between the two ends of a dual-lumen catheter are too far apart to position successfully. The Tesio catheter design consists of two separate catheters of different lengths that are placed in a single vein. The catheters are inserted into a central vein independently. This design is available in 7- and 10-Fr sizes and has proven to have superior survival rates and lower infection rates in children.

Location and Placement

The right internal jugular vein is the preferred site for HD CVC. If this site is not an option, alternatives include the right external jugular or left internal jugular veins. Subclavian catheters should be avoided because they have a very high risk of stenosis in children. Even a minor stenosis in the subclavian vein can obstruct flow from the ipsilateral extremity and cause future forearm fistula failure. Therefore, this vein should not be used in children with CKD unless all other options have been ruled out. Whenever possible, a CVC should not be placed on the same side as a constructed and maturing AVF.

Occasionally, a child with longstanding CKD and history of multiple CVCs has no patent central veins available for access. In this circumstance, a translumbar CVC could be a better option than a femoral one. The use of lower limb vessels for CVC placement carries the risk of damaging the iliac veins, which could potentially result in technical challenges for the vascular anastomosis of a future kidney transplant.

Placement of HD catheters in children should be ultrasound guided and performed by either surgeons or interventional radiologists. Ultrasound guidance reduces the risk of immediate complications, especially in patients with anatomic variations of the internal jugular vein. Fluoroscopy typically is used to confirm the position of the catheter tip after the procedure is completed.

Infants and Small Children

Two-catheter HD may sometimes be required in infants, particularly in an emergency situation. The catheters are placed in the femoral veins; the tip of one is positioned in the inferior vena cava and the other in the internal iliac vein to decrease recirculation. This strategy is only useful, however, for a few dialysis sessions. Another option in infants is to use a single lumen catheter and split it into afferent and efferent lines using a Y connector. This allows for higher blood flows compared with a double-lumen catheter of the same size. The blood flow is controlled by two pumps or a single pump and valve to alternate drawing and returning blood. There is some recirculation with this system, which is proportional to the length of the line between the Y connector and the patient.

More recently, successful continuous renal replacement therapy has been performed in ill neonates and infants with cardiac disease using a two–venous sheath technique. The sheaths, most of which were 4 Fr and placed in both femoral veins, provided high blood flows and allowed for uninterrupted dialysis. Catheter options for pediatric patients are listed in Table 72.2.

Long-Term Care

The CVC exit site should not get wet. This limits the ability of the child to be able to swim. Cleaning of the exit site should be performed at least once weekly. A study

Table 72.2

Central Venous Catheter Sizes for Children on Hemodialysis

Patient Weight	CVC
Newborn	7-Fr dual lumen
5–20 kg	8-Fr dual lumen
20–40 kg	7-Fr Tesio (20–25 kg)
	10-Fr dual lumen
	10-Fr split catheter
	10-Fr Tesio catheter
	11.5-Fr dual lumen (>30 kg)
>40 kg	10-Fr Tesio
	11.5-Fr dual lumen
	12.5-Fr dual lumen

Adapted from National Kidney Foundation. KDOQI Clinical Practice Guidelines and Clinical Practice Recommendations for 2006 Updates: Hemodialysis Adequacy, Peritoneal Dialysis Adequacy and Vascular Access. *Am J Kidney Dis* 48:S1-S322, 2006 (suppl 1).
CVC, central venous catheter.

Table 72.3

Care of Hemodialysis Central Venous Catheter

1. Catheters should be accessed only by experienced dialysis personnel.
2. Clean exit site with CHG/alcohol-based solution.
3. When using heparin to lock CVC, 1000 units/mL concentration is preferred.
4. Measure aPTT before any procedure.
5. Avoid flushing catheter in the perioperative period.
6. Avoid using catheter for IV fluids, medications, or blood draws.

aPTT, activated partial thromboplastin time; CHG, chlorhexidine gluconate; CVC, central venous catheter; IV, intravenous.

in children found that cleaning the exit site once weekly versus three times a week was associated with fewer infections; however, this needs to be confirmed with prospective studies. Most centers use a chlorhexidine gluconate (CHG)/alcohol-based solution, which has been shown to be superior to iodine solutions in prevention of infection. Topical antimicrobial ointments such as mupirocin, Polysporin, and povidone-iodine are used on the skin near the exit site to reduce infection.

The CVC lock varies among centers with the majority of pediatric dialysis units using heparin in concentrations from 1000 to 5000 units/mL. Some pediatric units use tissue plasminogen activator, and one has reported use of 4% citrate solution. There have been several cases of children who had hemorrhagic complications from inadvertent anticoagulation with the use of 5000 units/mL heparin lock flush. It has been demonstrated that CVCs can have a substantial amount of leak (~15%) despite strictly adhering to the "lock volume." Because of their small size, children only need a very small amount of high-concentration heparin to become systemically anticoagulated, so they are at particularly increased risk.

Between dialysis treatments, it is preferable to not use the CVC for IV access (fluids, medication administration, or blood draws) unless in the event of an emergency because the risk of infection increases with each time the catheter is accessed. HD catheters should only be accessed by nurses who are trained and experienced in HD. Table 72.3 summarizes recommendations for the care of CVC in children.

Complications

Acute complications when placing a CVC include inadvertent arterial puncture, air embolism, pneumothorax, hemothorax, and bleeding. Most common long-term complications, often leading to removal of CVC, are malfunction and catheter-related bacteremia. Infection rates have been reported from 1.5 to 8.6 bacterial infection episodes per 1000 catheter days. Other long-term complications include vascular thrombosis, central venous stenosis, and fibrin sheath formation. Accidental extraction is another complication that can occur in children.

Antibiotic lock solutions have been reported to decrease exposure to systemic antibiotics when used prophylactically in children at increased risk for CVC related bacteremia. Tobramycin mixed with anticoagulant at a concentration of 5 mg/mL has been used to lock HD catheters one to three times a week.

C H A P T E R 7 3

Infant Hemodialysis

Deborah Stein, MD

Renal replacement therapy for the infant may be provided in the form of hemodialysis or peritoneal dialysis. For infants who require long-term renal replacement therapy as a bridge to renal recovery or transplant, peritoneal dialysis is the preferred modality because of decreased morbidity and mortality. Furthermore, provision of hemodialysis for infants requires additional staff with specialized training.

Hemodialysis is employed in the infant more commonly in the acute setting, or in those infants with comorbidities limiting the use of peritoneal dialysis, such as those with omphalocele, gastroschisis, bladder exstrophy, or pleural–peritoneal connections. Recent abdominal surgery may also preclude the use of peritoneal dialysis. Recurrent peritonitis may limit the utility of peritoneal dialysis if adequate clearance and ultrafiltration cannot be achieved. Infants who require extracorporeal membrane oxygenation (ECMO) can be treated with hemodialysis via the ECMO circuit. Infants undergoing hemodialysis should receive treatments either in an intensive care unit or in a pediatric dialysis unit with high nursing–patient ratio.

The goal of dialysis is to achieve enough clearance and ultrafiltration to allow for ongoing support of the infant as well as to allow for provision of nutrition.

Vascular Access

Hemodialysis requires a central venous catheter, and in infants this poses technical challenges because of their smaller vessel size and the likelihood that they may require vascular access throughout their lifetime if end-stage renal disease is present. Dialysis catheters are stiff and allow for high rates of blood flow. Thus, use of central lines other than those designed for dialysis is not recommended. Historically, umbilical lines were sometimes used for infant hemodialysis access but this has fallen out of favor with the availability of small diameter hemodialysis lines. If umbilical vessels are used, the umbilical artery must have at least a 5-French catheter, and the umbilical vein at least a 7–8-French catheter. In this case, the tip of the umbilical vein catheter should be above the diaphragm, and the tip of the umbilical artery catheter should be below the renal arteries. If umbilical catheters are used for dialysis, the arterial and venous lines cannot be reversed.

The choice of a temporary (uncuffed, nontunneled) versus semipermanent (cuffed, tunneled) hemodialysis catheter depends on whether the infant is expected to require therapy short- or long-term. However, even if the infant is expected to require long-term dialysis, many will be transitioned to PD and, thus in the acute setting, a temporary catheter (uncuffed) is often placed. Placement of a hemodialysis catheter should be performed with fluoroscopy to confirm placement. The line with the largest possible gauge should be placed in order to allow for optimum blood flows. However, placement of a line that is too broad can result in occlusion of the vessel. Available catheters may differ across institutions. Typically, the smallest catheter that can be used for hemodialysis and still maintain adequate blood flow is 7–8 French.

Options for location of placement of HD catheter in infants include internal jugular (IJ), subclavian, and femoral vein. Catheter insertion site should be determined individually as each infant requiring hemodialysis may have specific circumstances precluding one site or another. Use of the subclavian vein should be avoided if a line can be placed in the IJ, as occlusion of the subclavian vein will preclude creation of an arteriovenous fistula when the child is older and may require additional dialysis access. Ideally, the tip of the catheter should be at the right atrial/superior vena cava junction when placed in the IJ or subclavian. Catheters in the femoral vein should have the tip as central as possible. Femoral catheters are associated with an increased risk of infection, and thus should not be used long term. With noncentral placement of catheters, there is an increased risk of recirculation as well as blood flow limitations.

Complications of hemodialysis access include infection, clotting, venous outflow obstruction, and failure of the access, which may be related to placement, kinking, or breaking of the line. Because these complications result in an inability to provide dialysis urgently and may require surgical replacement of the line, dialysis lines should be used only by trained dialysis staff. To maintain patency of the lines, anticoagulation is used during dialysis, and the details of this are reviewed in Chapter 77.

Equipment/Preparation

Equipment for hemodialysis includes the dialysis machines, blood lines, and dialyzer. Each must be carefully considered to provide the safest and most efficient treatment for the infant. Many dialysis machines will now allow low blood flows, although none provides specific indications for infant dialysis, and thus provision of infant dialysis is an off-label use of the machine. Of critical importance in selecting a dialysis machine to use for the infant is the availability of accurate control of ultrafiltration. In the infant, even small volumes of ultrafiltration may result in hemodynamic changes.

One must have information regarding the priming volume of the blood lines and the dialyzer. This should be available on standard packaging. The priming volume of the dialyzer and blood lines should never exceed 10% of patient's blood volume. For small patients, use of blood to prime the circuit is required to avoid hemodynamic compromise and hemodilution. An aliquot of packed red blood cells should be diluted to achieve a priming hematocrit of 35%–45%. Consideration when using blood primes includes the potential for sensitization when exposing an infant to multiple blood donors, which may complicate future transplantation. Donated blood is anticoagulated with citrate, which can lead to hypocalcemia in the infant, and thus serum calcium should be assessed and supplemental calcium provided if indicated. Blood primes also contain a significant amount of potassium and, if possible, one should provide fresh blood or washed red cells to avoid hyperkalemia. At the end of a treatment initiated with a blood prime, blood in the lines is not returned to the patient because this would represent a large-volume transfusion and can lead to hypervolemia, hypertension, and/or pulmonary edema. If the prime volume is less than 10% of the blood volume, 5% albumin may be used. Lines may need to be warmed to prevent hypothermia in the infant undergoing hemodialysis. Frequent temperature monitoring is required.

For infants undergoing hemodialysis, typically the smallest dialysis filter available is appropriate, as smaller filters will still allow for adequate clearance given the low total blood volume. There are currently a wide variety of filters with various blood volumes available, and each institution may have its own preferable filters based on local experience. Given the low number of small children receiving hemodialysis each year, there are no formal studies comparing the safety and efficacy of different dialysis machines and filters in infants.

Dialysis Prescription for the Infant: Special Considerations

Infants undergoing hemodialysis require special considerations when generating the dialysis prescription, with regard to the clearance, blood flow, and other parameters (Table 73.1).

Rapidly lowering the BUN with hemodialysis can result in disequilibrium syndrome. Problems can also arise in infants who are hyperosmolar due to hypernatremia. Thus, a stepwise approach should be used in those with marked uremia or hypernatremia by providing increasing clearance each day to allow for gradual equilibrium. Initial clearance for an infant with significant uremia should be limited to provide 30% urea reduction rate on the first day, followed by sequential increases in urea reduction (30%, 50%, 70%) to avoid disequilibrium. If the desired ultrafiltration cannot be achieved in the same time frame, one can continue with ultrafiltration only to achieve the desired effect. Dialysis initiated for removal of other substances without significant uremia should focus on removal of that particular substance. In this case, maximal clearance should be attempted with each therapy including the initial treatment. If the infant's BUN is very high but clearance for removal of other solutes is required, one can provide mannitol through the dialysis circuit to avoid rapid osmotic changes and thus prevent disequilibrium and cerebral edema.

Blood flow for hemodialysis in the infant should be 6–8 mL/kg/min. However, in the smallest infants, this may still be insufficient to maintain blood flow through the circuit. The lowest blood flow for most machines is 25 mL/min, and thus the blood flow range should be limited to 25–50 mL/min. Higher flow rates in the infant can lead to cardiovascular collapse. Lower blood flows will increase the risk of clotting, and thus if the infant can tolerate blood flows of 50 mL/min this is preferred. At low blood flow rates, the dialyzer clearance of the solute for the blood flow

Table 73.1

Requirements for Infant Hemodialysis Orders

- Dialyzer/Filter size
- Blood flow
- Dialysate flow
- Sodium program
- Prime composition (blood/albumin vs albumin vs saline)
- Anticoagulation
- Length of treatment
- Ultrafiltration parameters
- Blood products and medications to be administered during treatment

through the circuit will be equal to the blood flow rates for calculating the time needed to achieve a particular clearance. After each treatment, using the urea reduction rate achieved, one can back-calculate the actual clearance of urea and use this for calculating the next prescription.

Dialysate flow should be at least 1.5–2 times the blood flow to provide optimal countercurrent gradient for clearance of molecules. In many institutions, the dialysate flow is set at a minimum of 300 or 500 mL/min. Hemodialysis can result in lowering of the infant's core body temperature. Thus, blood lines and dialysate may be warmed to avoid hypothermia. Conversely, in cases of malignant hyperthermia, room temperature or cooled blood lines can be used to lower core temperature.

Anticoagulation for dialysis is discussed in detail in Chapter 77. However, there are specific considerations for the infant undergoing hemodialysis, which will be discussed here. Heparin is used to anticoagulate the system and avoid clotting. Use of heparin poses risks in the neonate, including intracranial hemorrhage and bleeding from surgical sites. Infants with preexisting conditions such as bleeding or recent surgery may require hemodialysis sessions without heparin. In this case, frequent flushes of saline can be provided prefilter to prevent clotting, and the volume of the flushes can be removed by ultrafiltration. Use of citrate for anticoagulation poses the potential risk of hypocalcemia and requires close monitoring.

Although patients receiving chronic hemodialysis typically undergo three sessions each week, the infant undergoing hemodialysis will require more frequent treatments. Infants in the intensive care unit should undergo daily dialysis to allow for more stable metabolic balance and provide ultrafiltration to allow them to receive adequate nutrition without worsening fluid overload.

Ultrafiltration should be limited to no more than 5% of the infant's dry weight in each dialysis session. If more ultrafiltration is required, one can consider use of CRRT to provide slow continuous removal of fluid rather than attempting to remove a large volume of fluid in the time on intermittent dialysis. If ultrafiltration is required despite the need to avoid excessive clearance, such as in the case of significant uremia, dialysate can be stopped once the desired clearance is achieved, and one can continue ultrafiltration alone as noted above. In this case, there will be a small amount of clearance due to solvent drag/convective clearance.

When dialyzing infants, the rate of ultrafiltration volume must be considered relative to the size of the infant and effective circulating volume. In most institutions, ultrafiltration should not exceed 100 mL/hour. Thus, treatment time may be extended beyond that required for clearance, to allow for adequate ultrafiltration. Before and after a treatment, the infant's weight should be measured on an infant scale, as bed scales will not be sensitive enough to detect small changes that are clinically significant in the infant. Furthermore, current dialysis machines may not report precise ultrafiltration volumes, and small margins of error could be significant to the infant undergoing hemodialysis. If the patient becomes hypotensive and volume is required to reestablish effective circulating volume, fluids can be administered in increments of 10–20-mL boluses, in the form of normal saline, 5% albumin, or blood depending on the situation.

High rates of clearance can lead to hypokalemia, hypophosphatemia, and other electrolyte derangements. Close monitoring of electrolytes and repletion as needed, as well as adjustment of dialysate to avoid life-threatening electrolyte abnormalities, is paramount to the care of the infant receiving hemodialysis. Many vasopressors and sedatives will be cleared with hemodialysis. Thus, the primary team should be prepared to increase the doses of these medications while the infant is receiving hemodialysis. Antibiotics and other medications may need to be dose-adjusted when the infant is receiving hemodialysis. Consultation with a pharmacist familiar with such treatments may be useful. Otherwise, drug-dosing resources can be used to determine whether dosing adjustments are required. Medications for which levels are monitored should be assessed after the patient has reached equilibrium, typically 4–6 hours after completion of the HD session.

Blood products and medications often result in large volumes being administered to the infant. Furthermore, these may provide additional potassium and sodium load. Thus, provision of blood products to the infant with renal failure should be done while on dialysis when possible. If other medications require a large volume but are not dialyzed, they can be provided during dialysis and the volume removed by ultrafiltration to result in no net fluid administration to the patient.

When considering dialysis for a toxin ingestion or overdose, it is critical to review the toxin and its metabolites to determine what will be cleared. Substances that are dialyzed most easily are those that are water soluble, low-molecular-weight, and not protein bound. However, some toxins that are protein-bound may have metabolites that are present in a free state, and thus assessment of the utility of dialysis should be undertaken on a case-by-case basis depending on the compound in question. Dialysis performed for indications other than renal failure, such as hyperammonemia, often requires a different approach and may require maximizing clearance beyond that which is recommended for infants with renal failure. In this case, one does not need to consider disequilibrium as the patient is not usually uremic, and removal of the solute or toxin may dictate changes to the dialysis prescription. Dialysis for infants with inborn errors of metabolism is discussed in Chapter 82.

Patients who require hemodialysis in the acute setting may be transitioned to peritoneal dialysis if they will be dependent on renal replacement therapy long term. In such cases, a PD catheter can be placed at the time of HD catheter placement if such information is known, or later. If a PD catheter will be required, it is preferable to place this early to allow for adequate healing prior to use. HD can continue until the PD catheter is healed and ready for daily use.

Intermittent hemodialysis can be provided via the ECMO circuit in the infant requiring ECMO. In this case, higher blood flows can usually be achieved as the flow through the ECMO circuit is on the order of 100 mL/kg/min. When performing dialysis via the ECMO circuit, one must take into account the volume of distribution, which includes the ECMO circuit. Ultrafiltration is usually not performed via the HD circuit in this case as it can be achieved via the ECMO circuit continuously.

Chronic Hemodialysis

The infant requiring chronic hemodialysis is at increased risk of mortality. In this case, meticulous attention to growth and nutrition is required and is best accomplished with the use of a multidisciplinary team to assess all needs of the infant. This team should include a pediatric nephrologist, experienced pediatric dialysis nurses, renal dietitian, social worker, and pharmacist if possible. Infants undergoing hemodialysis who are otherwise not critically ill will still typically require at least four to five sessions per week to allow for adequate nutrition and growth. Urea kinetic modeling is used to determine dialysis adequacy and is described in detail in Chapter 74.

CHAPTER 74

Urea Kinetic Modeling for Hemodialysis Prescription in Children

Avram Z. Traum, MD • Michael J.G. Somers, MD

Chronic Hemodialysis in Children

Although renal transplantation is the optimal treatment for end-stage renal disease (ESRD) in children and adolescents, many pediatric patients nonetheless must spend some time on dialysis. Historically, a much larger proportion of children than adults undergo peritoneal dialysis, but registry data from the United States Renal Data System (USRDS) and the North American Pediatric Renal Trials and Collaborative Studies (NAPRTCS) suggest that the proportion of children with ESRD receiving hemodialysis (HD) is increasing. Currently, about 60% of incident and prevalent dialysis patients younger than 19 years of age receive HD. As a result, clinicians caring for these children are now faced more often with the need to assess HD adequacy and to be cognizant of the value of urea kinetic modeling in formulating HD prescriptions. Moreover, quality measures stipulating HD adequacy standards for children are now endorsed by many health care improvement organizations, and pediatric dialysis adequacy measures have been included in the ESRD Quality Incentive Program administered by the Centers for Medicare & Medicaid Services (CMS) in the United States.

Despite this increased focus on dialysis adequacy in children, limited data on long-term outcomes of dialyzed children continue to exist, especially analyzed in the context of certain standards of adequacy. The original and the updated National Kidney Foundation Kidney Disease Outcomes Quality Initiative (NKF KDOQI) guidelines for HD adequacy acknowledge this issue. They specify that because of limited specific pediatric data, many recommendations are based on extrapolation from the much broader experience in adults. Unfortunately, many outcome measures looking at dialysis adequacy in adults are focused on narrowly assessing mortality rates or specific organ system morbidity over time and do not consider clinical variables of special import to assessing the adequacy and effectiveness of renal replacement therapy in children (e.g., somatic growth and development, cognitive and emotional maturation, and school attendance and performance).

As dialysis adequacy guidelines are applied more broadly to children with ESRD for both clinical care and assessment of quality care, it is incumbent on pediatric clinicians to determine whether adult standards really do define a proper dose of dialysis for children and to then assess further the applicability of these current standards to appropriate long-term outcome measures. Along these same lines, as new methods of assessing dialysis adequacy are proposed and considered, their application and usefulness to children on HD should be analyzed with pediatric-specific data as well.

The Dialysis Prescription in Children

Because clinicians caring for children with ESRD will be prescribing dialysis to patients whose size and weights may vary 20- or 30-fold, there is much more of an individualized focus on the dialysis prescription in children than in adults. For instance, the HD prescription for an 85-kg adolescent will differ dramatically from the treatment given to a 5-kg baby, which will in turn be quite different than the prescription for a 25-kg elementary school student. Because children receiving dialysis are more likely than adults to have broad variations in size and total blood volume (which in turn affect many technical aspects of safe and successful HD provision), the quantity of dialysis a child receives needs to be more precisely calculated and readjusted. Moreover, as the child grows, the prescription must be reformulated cognizant of ongoing changes in total body water and evolving nutritional requirements.

Similar to trends in adults receiving chronic HD, urea kinetic modeling has become more commonly used in pediatric patients both to serve as an objective measure of HD adequacy and to monitor nutritional adequacy by allowing for the determination of protein catabolic rate (PCR). With this approach, urea clearance is used as a surrogate to reflect removal of low-molecular-weight uremic toxins, and the interdialytic rise in urea levels can be used to estimate protein catabolism. The choice of urea as a marker stems from its relatively even distribution over the total body water, its low molecular mass and ensuing ready dialysis clearance, and its status as the principal constituent of nitrogen waste that accumulates in body water. The extent of clearance of urea from body water has been correlated with morbidity and mortality outcomes.

One of the prime advantages of urea kinetic modeling is that it provides quantitative data that are not only reproducible but that can also guide individualization of dialysis prescriptions. Most notably, modeling elucidates disparities between expected or calculated doses of dialysis and actual delivered dialysis. A major disadvantage of kinetic modeling is the need to coordinate obtaining specific data at stipulated time points. Depending on local resources, these maneuvers may be relatively labor and time intensive and may add cost to the chronic therapy. Although the calculations for kinetic modeling are complicated, numerous web-based programs or electronic applications exist that simplify the compilation of necessary data and facilitate computation of overall adequacy rapidly.

There has also been controversy as to whether the adequacy of dialysis is best measured using a single- or double-pool model of estimated volume. In a single-pool model, the clearance of urea from the blood volume may overestimate the dose of dialysis measured by kinetic modeling because blood measurements are performed before effective reequilibration of urea from the intracellular space into the intravascular space (urea rebound). This concern is especially true in children with smaller distributions of urea who are dialyzed with filters with the capability of high rates of solute clearance.

On the other hand, the need for patients to remain for a substantial period after the dialysis treatment is completed to draw a reequilibrated postdialysis blood urea nitrogen (BUN) adds another layer of logistical complexity to utilization of a double-pool model. There are some data suggesting that for the majority of children generally able to achieve relatively high levels of Kt/V, the discordance rate between single-pool and equilibrated values does not impact the ultimate management of adequate dialysis prescriptions.

Clinicians also need to be cognizant that a patient's particular dialysis regimen and each patient's residual renal function need to kept in mind when assessing dialysis adequacy and setting targets for adequacy. For instance, children receiving dialysis four or more times a week or children with substantial native residual function will need to have these extra sessions and their native kidney function included in both the calculation of dialysis adequacy and the setting of dialysis adequacy targets for an individual dialysis session. This necessitates the use of more complex calculations, but again, the ready availability of programs and applications to calculate adequacy and take into account these variables allow for an individualized approach.

Principles of Urea Kinetic Modeling in Children

The theoretical principles of urea kinetic modeling are identical in children and adults. The rate of removal of any solute from the intravascular space using HD can be modeled by considering the intrinsic permeability properties of the dialyzer, circuit specifics such as blood and dialysate flow, and physical and biochemical properties of the solute to be removed. The dialyzer's most important characteristic is its permeability surface area product (generally abbreviated as K_0A), which dependent on the blood flow (K_D) delivered through the dialyzer, defines its potential clearance of the solute in question. This variable defines the dialyzer's ability to remove the solute in question.

The following mass transfer equation can be set up and solved to quantify the physical removal of any solute in question during dialysis.

$$C_T = C_0(e^{-Kt/V}) + G/K(1 - e^{-Kt/V})$$

Here, C_T is the solute concentration at any given time during the dialysis treatment, C_0 is concentration of the same solute at time 0 or dialysis initiation, K is the dialyzer clearance of the solute for the blood flow through the circuit, t is the duration of dialysis in minutes, V is the volume of distribution of the solute, and G is the ongoing generation rate of the solute. Although this equation can be applied to any solute of interest, its application to urea removal is the underpinning of urea kinetic modeling, and the calculated Kt/V has been used as the measure of the dose of dialysis delivered or the fractional clearance of urea for the patient's volume of distribution.

There are a number of applications of this equation toward changes in metabolic balance. If all variables are known, BUN concentration can be calculated for any time point during the dialysis session. Similarly, with the necessary variables known, V and G can be calculated using BUN measurements acquired at varying time points during the dialysis treatment.

When G is known, the PCR can be calculated using the equation

$$PCR = 6.5G + 0.17(Wt)$$

where PCR is expressed as grams of protein per day, G is grams of BUN per day, and Wt is the patient's weight in kilograms. The PCR can be used along with clinical variables such as growth and laboratory parameters such as serum albumin to help assess nutritional adequacy. A PCR near 1 is considered ideal for most children.

Although adequate dialysis helps improve appetite and nutritional intake in patients receiving chronic HD, there is no evidence that higher doses of dialysis improve nutritional status.

Data Collection

Generally, data are collected over a number of HD sessions to calculate V and G. The remaining variables in the equations are known or can be easily determined. For instance, BUN is measured at the start of an HD session (C_0) and at the end (C_T or C_1) and again at the start of the next session (C_2). This pattern helps to define the intradialytic and interdialytic fluxes in BUN, which provide information as to urea reduction rate (URR) during dialysis, residual renal function with accompaning clearance of the solute in question during and between dialysis sessions, and ongoing generation of urea from protein catabolism. The following variables make it possible to predict BUN at any point in time.

* K_D, *dialyzer clearance:* This is a function of the dialyzer (K_0A), blood flow (Q_B), and dialysate flow (Q_D). The measured rather than the prescribed blood flow should be used for calculations.
* K_R, *residual renal function:* This variable is generally measured initially and then at regular intervals unless a change occurs that would suddenly impact residual function, such as nephrectomy. An adequate urine collection is important to ensure a reliable calculation for this measure and can be done over the interdialytic interval. In children who are not yet toilet trained, such collections can be more problematic, but options such as weighing diapers can provide fairly accurate estimates.
* *T (dialysis time) and U (interdialytic interval):* Both of these variables are measured in minutes, and the actual duration of dialysis for the session in question rather than prescribed time should be used in case there was a disparity.

Along with the volume of distribution (V) and the urea generation rate (G), these variables can be used to calculate BUN. Because the times and clearances are either predetermined variables or are easily measured, these can be entered into the appropriate equations to generate V and G. Alternatively, commercial software or Internet-based shareware exists to perform these calculations (Fig. 74.1). These resources greatly facilitate monitoring dialysis adequacy over time in large numbers of patients.

Common Errors in Calculations

As described previously, V is derived using serial measurements of BUN with respect to multiple HD sessions. Although there may be great variability in V between patients, V should remain fairly consistent for calculations on any individual patient. Thus, errors in calculations may be seen when V calculated for any given month or session varies greatly with respect to previous measurements. Common errors impacting the estimate of V include the following.

* *T is misreported:* The duration of the HD session is actually shorter or longer than that prescribed or utilized for the equation.
* *K is erroneous:* The blood flow (Q_B) actually delivered for the treatment being modeled is different than reported, often related to problems with dialysis access such as stenosis, clotting, or recirculation.

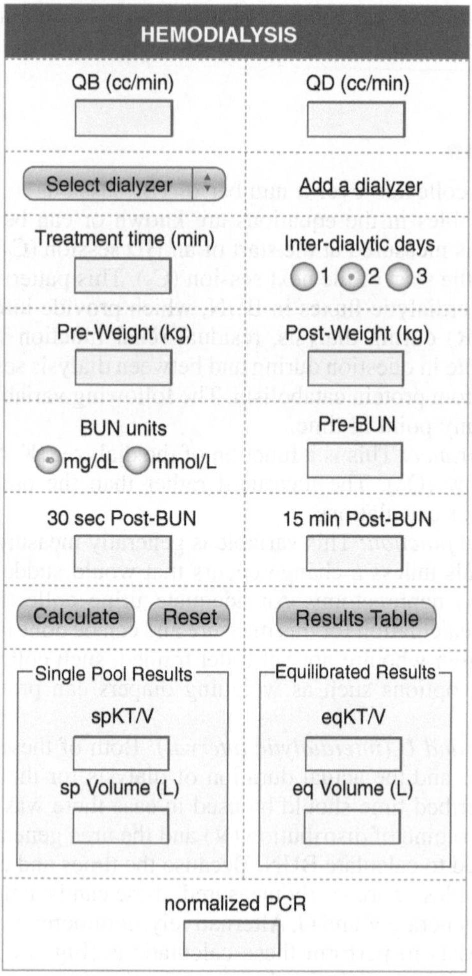

Figure 74.1

Sample dialysis adequacy calculator available as freeware at www.kt-v.net. Similar commercial programs are available for purchase. They facilitate the calculation of Kt/V and greatly reduce the time and effort needed to track doses of dialysis.

- *Measured BUN is wrong:* Either pre- or post-BUN samples are erroneous, generally related to incorrect timing of the samples or incorrect technique obtaining the samples.

Application of Urea Kinetic Modeling

Urea kinetic modeling can provide data about estimated adequacy of HD and nutrition. Although the data can then be used to adjust the dialysis prescription or the child's dietary intake, it must be remembered that the calculated Kt/V is only an estimate of adequacy and that Kt/V within the target range may not necessarily denote optimal dialysis for all children. As with many therapies in children, a better overall measurement of dialysis adequacy would be consideration of the child's composite health, growth, and development while the therapy is ongoing.

Unfortunately, given the need to adjust HD treatments over short spans of time, such long-term global measures of adequacy become supplemental to more immediate assessments such as Kt/V or PCR calculations. The data, nonetheless, can be quite useful in approaching and altering a patient's dialysis care.

For instance, a child found to have a PCR equal to her protein intake would be in neutral nitrogen balance. For an adult, this balance might be acceptable, but for a growing child, it would impact somatic growth and would represent nutritional deficiency. Conversely, a child found with what appears to be high predialysis BUN levels could have high dietary protein intake or may be inadequately dialyzed from previous sessions. In this case, assessing the PCR and Kt/V would differentiate between these situations. Whereas a high PCR could be modified by decreasing the protein intake to a more appropriate level, a low Kt/V could be adjusted by increasing the dialysis time, increasing the blood flow, or assessing the patient's access for technical complications.

National Kidney Foundation Kidney Disease Outcomes Quality Initiative Pediatric Recommendations for Dialysis Adequacy

The NKF KDOQI guidelines suggest that the delivered dose of dialysis should be measured routinely by formal urea kinetic modeling using a single-pool model. The dose of dialysis (Kt/V) should accurately describe the fractional clearance of urea corrected for volume of distribution. These guidelines apply to children with a residual glomerular filtration rate below 5 mL/min on a chronic HD regimen of three treatments weekly. The recommendations do not apply to children receiving dialysis at a different frequency or children with greater residual renal function in whom a standardized Kt/V would need to be used to assess adequacy. In addition, these recommendations do not apply to children with acute kidney injury receiving dialysis or children who are acutely ill and hospitalized receiving dialysis.

The NKF KDOQI guidelines specify that the minimum Kt/V should be 1.2 based on uncontrolled and retrospective reports that point toward improved patient survival with dialysis doses up to Kt/V of 1.2. There have, however, been few studies of the dose of HD as a predictor of outcome in children. One report did suggest that higher Kt/V values in children may facilitate growth, but another looked at mortality and hospitalization rates for dialyzed adolescents and found that teens with Kt/V less than 1.2 had higher hospitalization rates but that rates higher than 1.4 had no added benefit in optimizing outcomes.

To account for variability between prescribed and delivered dialysis doses, the NKF KDOQI adequacy guidelines suggest that the prescribed Kt/V be 1.3 to ensure that a Kt/V of at least 1.2 is delivered. Moreover, the guidelines stipulate that blood sampling be done precisely and in a fashion to minimize recirculation or urea rebound and that the same methodology should be used for all applicable patients in any single dialysis unit to facilitate equivalent levels of care.

These guidelines have been promulgated with the understanding that they may not represent optimal dialysis but are serving as benchmarks for minimal dialysis dose delivery. Especially in children with the added physiologic burden of ongoing growth and development, it has been consensus expert opinion that the delivered dose of dialysis should at least meet these standards. In fact, because achieving higher levels of Kt/V is often easier to reach in small children with lower volumes of distribution than large adults, many pediatric HD patients routinely achieve higher Kt/V levels, but there is still no evidence that targeting these higher levels is of specific benefit.

Although not directly addressed in these guidelines, standardized Kt/V can be measured in children who are receiving intensive chronic HD regimens exceeding three weekly treatments to assess their dialysis adequacy. Standardized Kt/V of at least 2.0 in children receiving intensive HD correlate with a single-pool Kt/V of at least 1.2 measured in children receiving thrice weekly HD.

C H A P T E R 7 5

Hemodiafiltration in Children: An Ultrapure Complete Blood Purification

Michel Fischbach, MD • Ariane Zaloszyc, MD •
Rukshana Shroff, MD, FRCPCH, PhD

Hemodiafiltration (HDF) was initially described in adults and later used in children in the early 1980s in Strasbourg. The initial aim was to improve volume control by adding the stability of hemodynamics with hemofiltration (HF) to the purification capacities of hemodialysis (HD). HDF adds a convective component (HF) to HD, thereby allowing for blood purification combining diffusive mass transport of small uremic toxins and convective mass transfer of larger middle-molecular-weight uremic toxins. The total convective volume achieved over an HDF session is the sum of both the prescribed weight loss and the predetermined ultrafiltration (UF) flow across the filter. This convective volume is replaced milliliter for milliliter with an intravenous (IV) infusion of substitution fluid produced "online" from the dialysate. In online HDF, incoming water is filtered through a reverse osmosis system followed by two disposable membranes in the dialysate circuit to produce "ultrapure" dialysis fluids (both "ultrapure" dialysate and "ultrapure" substitution fluid) with greater than 100-fold lower bacterial and endotoxin levels than the water used for conventional HD. Recent clinical trials in adults on HDF have shown that the total convective volume achieved is an independent predictor of survival. Advances in technology with the availability of dialysis machines that allow controlled UF and smaller dialysis filters and lines have enabled the use of HDF as a safe technique for routine renal replacement therapy in children, largely applied in Europe. In this chapter, we describe the technique, advantages, and clinical studies on HDF in children.

Dialysis: Diffusion, Convection, and Combination Therapy

The removal of uremic toxins by dialysis relies on a combination of the diffusion process and convective mass transport. The diffusive transport of molecules requires the presence of dialysis fluid flowing through the dialyzer, countercurrent to the patient's blood, as is the case in conventional HD. To be optimally efficient, the dialysate flow (in milliliters per minute) with HDF does not need to be higher than 1.5 times blood flow. The convective transport requires UF of fluid (i.e., the convective flow). If the convective flow exceeds the desired weight loss, fluid balance is maintained by an infusion of replacement fluid, as applied in HF. The replacement fluid, also referred to as substitution fluid, can be administered before the filter (predilution), after the filter (postdilution), or both before and after the filter (mixed). HDF combines HD and HF in the same procedure using a highly permeable dialysis membrane. Initially, in the 1980s, only conventional HDF was available (Fig. 75.1), with the replacement fluid industrially prepared using autoclaved plastic bags,

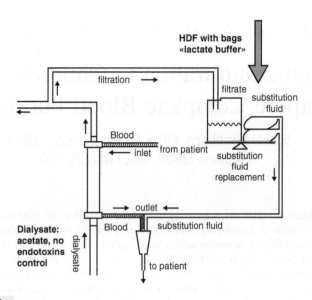

HDF with bags
«lactate buffer»

filtration →

filtrate
substitution fluid

Blood
inlet ← from patient
substitution fluid replacement ↓

→ outlet ←

Blood   substitution fluid
Dialysate:
acetate, no   dialysate
endotoxins
control   to patient

Figure 75.1

Initially in the 1980s, only conventional hemodiafiltration was available, with the substitution fluid industrially prepared using autoclaved sterile plastic bags with lactate buffer. The microbiological purity of the acetate buffered dialysate was only analyzed for bacterial counts. Endotoxin assessment was not available at the time.

entailing both logistical and financial costs. Today, in online HDF, the substitution fluid is prepared through double UF of the dialysate. After the first filtration, ultrapure dialysate is generated, which is then refiltered to create a sterile, nonpyrogenic substitution fluid.

In HD (Table 75.1), the clearance, the diffusive flow of small solutes, mainly depends on the concentration gradient across the dialysis membrane and correlates directly with the rate of the blood flow. The dialysis fluid flow and the mass transfer area coefficient (which includes the dialyzer surface area)—that is, the molecular permeability of the membrane—have an impact on solute diffusive flow, ensuring optimal removal of low-molecular-weight uremic toxins such as urea.

In HF (see Table 75.1), the clearance, the convective flow of a solute, depends on the UF rate, the solute concentration in the plasma, and the solute sieving coefficient (S) (i.e., the molecular permeability of the membrane). The UF flow is mainly dependent on the transmembrane pressure gradient (TMP) applied to the hydraulic permeability of the membranes. For all solutes with S of 1 (i.e., small solutes such as urea), the solute convective flow is equal to the UF rate. Membranes with a sieving curve similar to that of the glomerular basement membrane (i.e., with a steeply falling profile and a cut-off just below the molecular size of albumin) allow the removal of not only small uremic toxins but also of middle-sized and large molecules. Nevertheless, the postdilutional solute convective flow can only be equal to available plasma water flow, which is a fraction of the blood flow. In practice, in postdilution mode, to limit the risks of excessive hemoconcentration, this convective flow is

Table 75.1

Dialytic Solute Removal: Diffusion, Convection, and Combination

Diffusion Process Hemodialysis	Convection Mass Transport Hemofiltration	Combination Hemodiafiltration
Membrane surface area Mass transport coefficient Concentration gradient Blood flow × extraction coefficient	Ultrafiltrate flow (Q_{UF}) Hydraulic permeability Transmembrane pressure (TMP; mm Hg) Membrane surface area Sieving coefficient (S)* Molecular permeability	$K_{HDF} = K_{HD} (1 - Q_{UF} \times S/Q_B) + K_{HF}$ (1) (postdilution; Granger formula) If $Q_{UF} \times S = K_{HF}$ and $Q_B = K_{max}$ Then (1) becomes
$$K_{HD} = Q_B \times \frac{c_i - c_o}{c_i}$$	$$*S = \frac{2\,C_{UF}}{c_i + c_o}$$	$$K_{HDF} = K_{HD} + K_{HF} - \frac{K_{HD} \times K_{HF}}{K_{max}}$$
i, o: in outlet solute concentrations	C_{UF}: ultrafiltrate solute concentration	This shows that if solute removal is maximal with one modality, either HD or HF, there is no/limited gain when using a combination of both modalities.
	$$K_{HF} = \frac{Q_{UF} \times S}{\text{(postdilution)}}$$	For example, if for urea $K_{HDurea} = Q_B = K_{max}$, then $K_{HDFurea} = K_{HDurea}$
	$$K_{HF} = \frac{Q_B \times Q_{UF} \times S}{\text{(predilution)}}$$	
	$Q_B - Q_{UF}$	
K_{HD} hemodialysis clearance	K_{HF} hemofiltration clearance	K_{HDF} hemodiafiltration clearance

HD, hemodialysis; HF, hemofiltration; HDF, hemodiafiltration.

lower than one third of the blood flow. In predilution mode, total plasma water at the filter inlet is the sum of "endogenous" plasma water and reinfusate (i.e., replacement fluid). This enables enhanced UF flow in the dialyzer over the plasma water flow. To improve efficiency in the predilution mode, the convective flow should be high enough to ensure increased solute clearance despite blood dilution. In practice, this is superior to 50% of the blood flow and ideally should be two thirds of or equal to the blood flow. In cases of high hematocrit levels or blood conditions that limit the filtration capacity (e.g., elevated blood protein concentration) or in patients with low blood flow (as is often the case in children), predilution compared with postdilution HDF has been proven to be of significant clinical benefit, with considerably less risk of membrane clotting.

In HDF, the blood purification process is optimized from small to larger molecular weight uremic toxins (Fig. 75.2). Continuously, the diffusive mass transport is completed by the convective mass transport and vice versa in HDF: 1 minute of HDF is equal to 2 minutes of blood purification, 1 minute of HD and 1 minute of HF. However, it must be kept in mind that if the diffusive or convective clearance is maximal for a particular uremic toxin, the addition of HF to HD will not improve its clearance any further. Using highly permeable membranes in HD can achieve a urea clearance nearly equal to the blood flow, so that by adding HF to HD (i.e., performing HDF), urea clearance in HDF is similar to the clearance of urea achieved

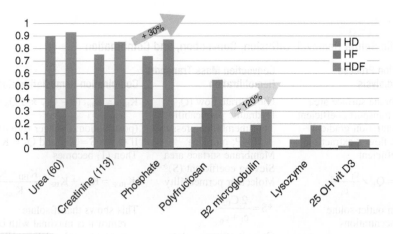

Figure 75.2

Molecular permeability assessed by extraction coefficient of a highly permeable membrane: impact of the dialysis process hemodialysis (HD), hemofiltration (HF), or hemodiafiltration (HDF). In HDF, blood purification process is optimized from small to larger molecular weight uremic toxins.

in HD. The simplified formula clearly shows the limitation of adding HF to HD if clearance is equal to blood flow for a uremic toxin:

$$K_{HDF} = K_{HD} + K_{HF} - (K_{HD} \times K_{HF}/K_{max})$$

K_{maxima} can be considered as nearly equal to blood flow; therefore, if KHD for urea is equal to blood flow, the formula gives:

$$K_{HDF} = K_{HD} + K_{HF} - K_{HF} = K_{HD}$$

Indeed, when HDF was first performed in children, there were concerns about the risk of osmotic dysequilibrium caused by very rapid urea dialytic clearance. In fact, HDF prevented osmotic dysequilibrium and allowed for a higher urea dialytic clearance than tolerated with HD, presumably because of the osmotic stability induced by the continuous iso-osmotic HF substitution fluid inflow.

Optimizing the Determined Convective Volume: Pre-, Post-, or Mixed-Dilution Hemodiafiltration

Depending on the site of replacement substitution fluid relative to the dialyzer, HDF can be pre-, post-, or mixed-dilution HDF, and the achieved convective volume will differ accordingly.

1. **Postdilution HDF,** in which the replacement fluid is infused downstream of the dialyzer, is more widely practiced in adult patients. The convective flow is limited by the hematocrit and plasma protein level: The maximum upper limit of hemoconcentration tolerable is 50% filtration fraction or hematocrit of 50% at the blood outflow (venous flow) of the dialyzer, but in practice at the bedside,

the convective flow is prescribed at lower than one third of the blood flow. Hemoconcentration at high UF rates can result in the deposition of plasma proteins on the membrane surface, clogging the membrane pores and occluding the blood channels of the dialyzer. This can raise the TMP, causing alarms, reducing clearance, and possibly resulting in clotting of the extracorporeal circuit. A filtration fraction up to 30% of the blood flow rate is possible using systems designed to optimize the filtration rate based on automatic adjustment of TMP according to the UF flow rate measurements.

2. **Predilution HDF,** in which the replacement fluid is infused upstream of the dialyzer, allows higher filtration rates than are possible with postdilution HDF. UF rates greater than two thirds of blood flow and up to 100% of the blood flow rate are used to compensate for the decrease in the diffusive gradient of small uremic toxins such as urea caused by blood dilution entering the dialyzer. However, predilution reduces the efficiency of both the diffusive and convective components of solute removal by reducing the solute concentrations in the blood compartment. For equivalent clearance to postdilution HDF, the UF rate in predilution HDF needs to be at least twice that used for postdilution. It is speculated that predilution favors purification of protein-bound uremic toxins, the blood dilution allowing for dissociation of the uremic toxin from the proteins, thereby making it more available for dialytic removal.

   Overall, with new dialysis machines, the convective flow is automatically optimized using either pressure or volume control (Gambro) or using viscosity control (Fresenius Medical Care [FMC]; Autosub+) and thereby is directly dependent on the achieved blood flow. In case of low blood flow or of a risk of clotting (high hematocrit or high protein levels in the blood), predilution is more effective than postdilution because it preserves an effective convective flow throughout the dialysis session.

3. **Mixed-dilution HDF** is a combination of post- and predilution HDF. The replacement fluid is infused both upstream and downstream of the dialyzer. The ratio of the upstream and downstream infusion rates can be varied to achieve the optimal compromise between maximizing clearance and avoiding the consequences of a high TMP and hemoconcentration. Mixed dilution is automatically performed and balanced by the machine with postdilution favored at the start of the session, and thereafter during the dialysis session as hemoconcentration occurs and limits the convective flow, predilution is automatically applied. Mixed HDF is only applicable for children weighing more than 35 kg because of the extracorporeal blood volume of the lines needed for mixed HDF (available with FMC5008 machines).

Internal Hemodiafiltration Versus Online Hemodiafiltration

Every HD performed with a highly permeable membrane is an HDF with a small convective volume equal to the sum of the UF realized to achieve the desired weight loss and the undetermined backfiltration in the dialyzer.

Indeed, in cases in which a highly permeable membrane with a high hydraulic permeability is used, internal filtration occurs with proximal filtration and distal backfiltration in the dialyzer. This results in an apparently neutral fluid balance caused by the UF control system of the machine: The backfiltrated dialysate is then

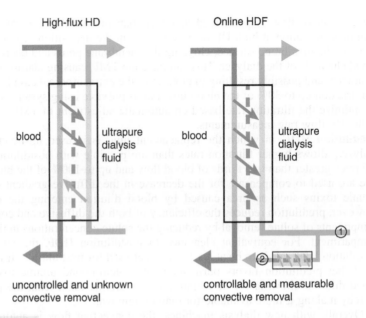

High-flux HD   Online HDF

blood   ultrapure   blood   ultrapure
         dialysis   dialysis
         fluid   fluid

uncontrolled and unknown   controllable and measurable
convective removal   convective removal

Figure 75.3

Schematic representation of high-flux hemodialysis (HD); that is, HD with a highly permeable membrane allowing for an undetermined amount of hemodiafiltration (HDF) and online HDF. Online HDF is represented in postdilution mode (i.e., substitution fluid injected after the filter). In online, HDF, the substitution fluid is prepared through double ultrafiltration of the dialysate. After the first filtration (①), ultrapure dialysate is generated, which is then refiltered (②) to create a sterile, nonpyrogenic substitution fluid. (Courtesy of I. Ledebo with modifications.)

used as a substitution fluid. This gives the benefit of some "internal" convective flow, but at the same time exposes patients to the risks related to using a nonsterile, non–pyrogen-free backfiltered dialysate (Fig. 75.3).

Today, the majority of children throughout the world who receive HD will benefit from high-flux dialysis, that is, conventional HD with high-flux filters (highly permeable membranes). Conversely, HDF is increasingly applied in European pediatric dialysis units. Using online HDF enables the addition of a predetermined convective dialysis dose to the diffusive urea dialysis dose, resulting in a high-efficiency HDF by adding a large convective volume to the HD. The maintenance costs incurred are low. (Dialysate filters need to be changed every 1 to 3 months per machine and are automatically checked by the machine itself.)

Safety and Quality Control in Hemodiafiltration

Because HDF involves large volumes of fluid removed from and added to blood, patients are exposed to risks beyond those associated with routine HD. These additional risks relate to the water purity and control of fluid balance.

Dialysate purity, in terms of microbial contaminants, is measured and defined in colony-forming units (CFUs) and endotoxin units (EUs) in the different fluids used for dialysis. Currently, there are no European norms that address fluid quality for online HDF, and only some countries allow the use of online prepared substitution fluid, but others prohibit the use of online HDF (e.g., the U.S. Food and Drug Administration recommendations). The International Organization for Standardization (ISO) has published a series of standards addressing fluids for HD and HDF (ISO 11663:2009, "Quality of dialysis fluid for HD and related therapies"). In the absence of a clear, detailed EU position, a widely accepted standard for ultrapure dialysis fluid for HDF is defined as having a bacterial count of less than 1 CFU/500 mL and endotoxin contamination of less than 0.05 EU/mL; this is the same quality requirement as for prepackaged IV fluid as defined by the European Pharmacopoeia. With the use of modern technology, a result of less than 0.005 EU/mL is now possible. In practice, many centers across the EU follow the ISO 23500:2011 guidelines and test 500 mL of replacement fluid via the membrane filtration method at least once every 3 months for microbial quality testing.

Importantly, conventional HD with high-flux membranes also achieves some convective clearance, but this is typically low volume, uncontrolled, and not easily measurable. In high-flux HD, loss of plasma water is compensated for by backfiltration of dialysis fluid within the dialyzer, so-called "internal HDF." Depending on the filter size and blood flow rates, the estimated amount of convective transport during high-flux HD in an adult is <10 L/session, but in HDF, 25 to 60 L can be reached, depending on the mode of HDF (pre- or postdilution). Thus, in high-flux HD, as for HDF, sterile, nonpyrogenic substitution fluid is required because it is infused directly into the patient's blood. Standard-quality dialysis fluid (defined as bacterial count <100 CFU/mL; endotoxin <0.50 EU/mL) is not appropriate for use with high-flux HD.

A second important factor related to the dialysate for HDF is its sodium concentration. When high convective volumes are used, particularly in predilution HDF, the dialysate sodium level should be adjusted to the plasma diffusible sodium concentration so that sodium and therefore volume overload is avoided.

The Impact of Hemodiafiltration on Solute Removal

Uremic toxins can be categorized into three groups: free water-soluble low-molecular-weight solutes such as urea, middle-sized solutes such as β_2 microglobulin (β_2-m), and protein-bound solutes such as p-cresol acid. The phosphate ion is small but not "free" because it is surrounded by water molecules; therefore, it has a clearance profile similar to that of the middle-sized molecules.

After reviewing the available literature, which mostly includes studies performed in adult patients, the following can be concluded:
- **Urea:** A change from either low- or high-flux HD to online HDF results, if anything, in a modest increase in small solute clearance, which is of limited clinical significance.
- **Phosphate:** HDF offers improved phosphate control compared with both conventional HD and high-flux HD.
- **β_2-m:** Predialysis β_2-m serum levels are decreased during online HDF; the β_2-m dialytic removal correlates with the convective volume achieved. It should be noted that the enhanced β_2-m dialytic removal with online HDF is associated with

a reduction in factors provoking inflammation and thus generating β_2-m. These factors include the physiologic compatibility of the membrane, the microbial purity of all the dialysis fluids used, and the limitation of back filtration caused by the high convective flow of the HDF process.

Overall, the use of HDF is associated with enhanced clearance of phosphate and β_2-m directly correlated to the convection volume achieved per session.

The convective volume is a surrogate for HDF efficiency. Recent randomized controlled trials (RCTs) in adults have shown that a higher convective volume correlates with improved survival. Nevertheless, the convective volume achieved over an HDF session should be efficient and not risky. "Efficiency" can be tested by the dialytic reduction rate of β_2-m 80% or greater and of $\alpha 1$ myoglobulin 35% or greater. "Risk" can be assessed by the dialytic loss of albumin; this is considered to be less than 5 g albumin per session in adults. These two parameters of membrane permeability are different between the available hyperpermeable membranes, and some membranes have a significantly higher dialysate albumin loss proportional to the prescribed convective volume. All HDF membranes should achieve a β_2-m dialytic reduction rate over 80% and albumin loss less than 5 g per HDF session in adults.

Requirements for Hemodiafiltration in Children

Hemodiafiltration in children requires dialysis machines that allow careful regulation of UF, highly permeable membranes, and ultrapure fluid for replacement of convective flow with equipment allowing for accurate control of fluid balance.

Today almost all new dialysis machines allow for both HD and HDF. In Europe, HDF machines suitable for children are manufactured by Gambro and FMC. All of these machines are suitable for children above 15 kg body weight. Pediatric lines, "baby lines," that are suitable for HDF in children weighing less than 15 kg, would require an extracorporeal volume of less than 80 mL (including both lines and filter) and are available only for the older generation of FMC4008 machines and currently under manufacture for the FMC5008 machine, which became available in 2015.

Only highly permeable membranes are suitable for HDF both in adults and children. Highly permeable membranes are those that allow a defined and enhanced molecular permeability to uremic toxins allowing for more than urea dialytic removal and are defined as membranes characterized by an UF coefficient greater than 20 mL/h/mm Hg/m^2 and a sieving coefficient (S) for β_2-m of greater than 0.6. The UF coefficient (KUF) defines the hydraulic permeability of a membrane and is expressed in mL/min/mm transmembrane pressure: Whereas a low-flux membrane will allow only a small and undetermined convective flow and can be used for HD only, a high-flux membrane allows a larger and predefined convective flow as required for HDF. In practice, the KUF should be high enough to allow 50 mL/m/ m^2 body surface area (equivalent to 2 mL/min/kg body weight) convective flow in postdilution HDF, but membranes with 20 mL/min/mm or greater are frequently used for HDF. Adequate convective transport is achieved by an effective convection volume of at least 20% of the total blood volume processed (in postdilutional HDF).

Writing a Hemodiafiltration Prescription for Children

The dialysis prescription (blood flow, duration of the session, and dialysate flow) should be individually adapted to achieve a urea Kt/V of 1.4 or greater, which is a surrogate for predominantly diffusive blood purification as well as the highest possible convective clearance.

The following points should be considered when writing an HDF prescription for children:

1. HDF requires an optimal arterial blood flow of 5 to 8 mL/min/kg body weight or 150 to 240 mL/m^2 body surface area. This can be achieved through either a fistula or a central venous line.
2. A high-flux membrane with surface area equal to the child's body surface area is used.
3. Dialysate flow of 1.5 times the blood flow is sufficient and adequate to optimize the diffusive blood purification process using highly permeable membranes for HDF.
4. Convective flow is equal to total UF flow, that is, the sum of the weight loss and the replacement fluid (convective dialysis dose per session).
   - Postdilution HDF: The convective flow is one third or less of the blood flow and is limited by the risk of filter clotting. It typically decreases over the dialysis session. (TMP should be limited to <300 mm Hg.)

     Predilution HDF: The convective flow is set at 50% or less of blood flow but optimally can be increased to 75% to 100% of blood flow. This can be done despite the dilution of the blood potentially impacting negatively on urea clearance. β_2-m and phosphate dialytic removal is optimized as is the clearance of uremic protein-bound toxins.
5. Optimal anticoagulation is necessary to prevent filter clotting, particularly in postdilution HDF. A single dose of low-molecular-weight heparin is effective for a 4-hour session. Alternatively, a continuous heparin infusion can be used.
6. The dialysate composition is similar to that used in HD, but careful attention to dialysate sodium concentration is important, particularly when high convective volumes are infused, as with predilution HDF. To avoid the risk of positive sodium balance, the dialysate sodium concentration required is lower than in conventional HD.
7. Replacement fluid that is generated online from the dialysate must be "ultrapure" as discussed earlier. The microbiologic purity (bacterial count and endotoxin level) should be determined regularly at intervals of 1 to 3 months.

Advantages of Hemodiafiltration Over Conventional Hemodialysis: Pediatric Studies

Improved dialysis efficiency and clearance of toxins across a wide molecular weight range: Middle- and large-molecular-weight compounds such as β_2-m that normally accumulate on HD have more than 70% better removal on HDF (see Fig. 75.2). Plasma phosphate has a 30% greater clearance by HDF. Erythropoietin resistance is reduced, possibly as a result of reduced inflammation and removal of erythropoiesis-inhibiting factors (Table 75.2).

1. Improved hemodynamic stability: HDF increases UF and improves intradialytic hemodynamic stability, leading to less intradialytic hypotension and faster recovery time postdialysis.
2. Biocompatibility and reduced inflammation: The use of "ultrapure" dialysate and increased removal of inflammatory cytokines reduces inflammation and oxidative stress, thereby limiting dialysis-related protein wasting.

Table 75.2

Hemodiafiltration With High-Permeable Membranes in Children*

	HD 15 h/wk Cuprophane 12 Months	HDF 9 h/wk PAN 12 Months	HDF 9 h/wk Polysulfone 12 Months
TAc urea (mmol/L)	28 ± 4	18 ± 3	20 ± 2
PCRn (g/kg/j)	0.7 ± 0.2	1 ± 0.1	1.8 ± 0.3
Phosphate (mMol/L)	1.650.28	1.34 ± 0.15	1.15 ± 0.18
Aluminum prescription (g/day)	3	1.5	0.5
Hemoglobin (g/dL)	7.4	8.3	8.9
Need of transfusion per year	5	2	1
Date (yr)	1981	1982	1983

*Hemodiafiltration (HDF) in the era before erythropoietin-stimulating agents were available: children on HDF had a significant reduction in the number of transfusions per year to maintain a hematocrit over 20%.
HD, hemodialysis; PAN, polyacrylonitrile; PCRn, normalized protein catabolic rate;
 TAc, time averaged concentration.

Most important, these benefits of HDF have been associated with improved survival: Three RCTs have shown improved survival on HDF and reduced cardio-vascular mortality when higher convection volumes (>17.4 L and >20 L in the respective studies) are used. In children, HDF leads to impressive catch-up growth with a projected final height approaching target midparental height with daily HDF. Overall, children on intensive daily HDF have symptom-free dialysis sessions, no postdialysis recovery time, no or limited medications, an unrestricted diet, optimized blood purification, and optimized volume control. The dry weight management over a full dialysis week (i.e., daily dialysis) allows the application of the concept of "floating dry weight": Only a safe UF rate (i.e., <1.5 % body weight loss per hour is required); dry weight is attained not obligatory on "Monday" but during the week.

Taken together, all of these benefits of daily intensive HDF lead to an anabolic state, and catch-up growth is seen, with children achieving a normal height, at or above their target midparental height even before kidney transplantation.

Conclusions

Hemodiafiltration is a safe and highly efficient renal replacement therapy that allows diffusive and convective clearance of uremic toxins across a wide molecular weight range. Recent advances in technology have enabled its use as a safe and routine therapy for chronic dialysis even in small children. Careful attention to achieving the highest possible efficient convective volume is important as this is likely to improve patient outcomes.

CHAPTER 76

Home Hemodialysis in Children

Daljit K. Hothi MBBS, MRCPCH, MD • Lynsey Stronach BSc, MSc

The life span of a child on dialysis is 40 to 60 years less than the general population, but that of a pediatric transplant recipient is 20 to 30 years less than the general population. There is no doubt that dialysis is a significant risk factor for mortality and morbidity in children and adults alike. However, over the past decade, there has been a growing consensus of opinion recognizing intensified hemodialysis (HD) regimens, set either in hospital or at home, as a viable, safe, and beneficial therapeutic option in children.

What Is the Optimal Dialysis Dose?

In the Hemodialysis (HEMO) Study comparing high-dose HD versus standard dose HD, the relative risk of death was 0.96. In a secondary analysis, the HD dose showed a significant correlation with body mass index (BMI) and mortality. This raised the possibility of a survival advantage from increasing HD dose in low-BMI patients such as children.

The Dialysis Outcomes and Practical Pattern Study (DOPPS) review of 22,000 adult HD patients from seven countries found that that a higher dialysis dose was an independent predictor of lower mortality on HD with a synergistic survival advantage with treatment time. Therefore, survival was most pronounced by combining a higher Kt/V with longer treatment time, such that for every 30 minutes longer on HD, the relative risk of mortality was reduced by 7%. An Australian and New Zealand Dialysis and Transplantation (ANZDATA) analysis of 4193 patients found that the optimal dialysis dose for survival was a Kt/V greater than or equal to 1.3 and a dialysis session greater than or equal to 4.5 hours.

Such research set the scene for "quotidian home dialysis programs, namely a move away from conventional 4 hours, three-times-per-week dialysis to more frequent or more prolonged dialysis sessions, preferably at home.

Adult Home Hemodialysis Experience

The adult literature on quotidian dialysis practices is consistently positive. Compared with conventional dialysis, increasing frequency, time, or convective clearance is beneficial to the patient. For patients switching to short-daily HD, 33% survived at 6 years and demonstrated reduced hospitalization, fewer vascular access problems, reduced antihypertensive medication burden, lower incidence of left ventricular hypertrophy, improved anemia control, and a reduction in the use of phosphate binders as a consequence of the improved phosphorous clearance.

Nocturnal HD offers superiority over all other quotidian dialysis regimens. It is associated with significant reduction in the risk for mortality or major morbid events compared with conventional HD. During a matched cohort study comparing survival between nocturnal HD and deceased and living donor kidney transplantation, there was no difference in the adjusted survival between nocturnal HD and deceased donor renal transplantation. The proportion of deaths among the three was 14.7% for nocturnal HD, 14.3% for deceased donor transplantation, and 8.5% for live donor transplantation. This is very reassuring for patients who are not eligible for transplantation or those waiting for a transplant. In a comparison with peritoneal dialysis (PD), patients reported a similar perception of control over their kidney disease and did not consider home HD as a more intrusive treatment.

Pediatric Home Hemodialysis Experience

Literature on pediatric home HD is scarce and limited to single-center experiences. Nonetheless, available results are similar to adult data and include pertinent pediatric specific metrics, such as growth.

Tom et al demonstrated improved growth in children without the requirement for growth hormone by dialyzing for 5 hours, three times per week, to yield a single pool Kt/V of 2.0 in combination with a caloric intake at 150% of the recommended daily allowance for age. Goldstein et al delivered six-times-weekly HD at home using the NxStage system in four patients for 16 weeks. All of the children demonstrated progressive reductions in blood pressure (BP) load with concomitant discontinuation of antihypertensive medications in two patients. Serum phosphate levels improved without changes in phosphorus binder medication requirement.

Simonsen et al first described the outcomes for nocturnal HD in four children age 10 to 19 years who were treated with HD for 7 to 8 hours, 6 nights each week for a period of 5 to 55 months. Achieving a weekly Kt/V of 7.2 to 13.6, these children had no fluid or dietary restrictions and required phosphate supplements to avoid hypophosphatemia. Catch-up growth was achieved, and quality of life improved markedly. Subsequently, Geary et al reported on six children age 11 to 17 years on home nocturnal HD. One patient developed a fistula aneurysm from repeated use, in the absence of steal syndrome, and no line disconnections were reported. BP control was variable with two patients with native kidneys still requiring antihypertensives, and three patients became hypotensive requiring prophylactic midodrine to support their BP during ultrafiltration (UF). All patients were completely free from fluid and dietary restrictions, phosphate binders were discontinued, and all patients required supplementation with phosphate in the dialysate in combination with a higher calcium dialysate to prevent a net negative calcium balance. Appetite, well-being, school attendance, and physical and psychological health-related quality of life scores improved in all patients. However, caregivers' feedback did highlight the perceived "burden" of dialyzing at home. Many reflected on the increased intensity of workload that necessitated establishing a new routine within the home. The additional responsibilities evoked anxiety. The mother of one patient was psychologically and emotionally worn out after 1 year and moved to a hybrid program when the patient refused to revert back to in-center dialysis.

Infrastructure

In a cost analysis of daily home nocturnal HD compared with conventional in-center HD, a 27% saving was seen for each patient dialyzed at home despite the increased "disposable" costs of more frequent dialysis sessions. However, this needs to be balanced against the resource commitment of providing a safe and effective home therapy. It requires careful planning, resources, dedicated staff, and an appreciation of risk and governance issues. Programs need to decide on the type of dialysis offered, for example, nocturnal versus short daily treatments, long daily treatments, or hybrid prescriptions. They also need to decide on the type of dialysis machine and water source.

Finances

In pediatrics, diverting care from in-center dialysis beds to the patient's home results in significant savings because of the high staffing costs needed to deliver the 1 : 1 or 1 : 2 nurse-to-patient ratio. This needs to be offset against the initial setup cost to purchase or lease a dedicated dialysis machine for each patient; ideally, to adapt or convert existing rooms or structures into an appropriate training facility; and to employ a dedicated home HD team.

Staffing and Around-the-Clock Support

Home HD remains a relatively new therapy that places a high clinical risk activity in the community directly under the care of parents or other caregivers and patients. To manage this risk, it is crucial to recruit a multidisciplinary team to support the families. The composition of the team will vary depending on resources but at a minimum should include an HD nurse, dialysis technician, nephrologist, dietitian, and social worker. The inclusion of other allied health professionals such as a pharmacist, psychologist, community nurses, local pediatricians, and general practitioner is desirable for optimal support. In addition, it is absolutely essential to have a clear out of office communication pathway and after-hours policy to address families' urgent medical and technical queries while they dialyze their children at home in the evening, on weekends, and at night. To empower and support families further, we recommend providing them with written guidelines for normal ranges for a number of dialysis and physiologic parameters, with clear instructions on how to proceed if parameters fall out of the normal range.

Follow-up is dictated somewhat by geography and medical stability, but when in the community, patients should return to clinic regularly, every 4 to 8 weeks. Between clinics, patients should receive regular phone or email reviews by the nurse specialist.

Training and Education

In principle, home HD should be offered as an equal dialysis option when discussing care pathways with appropriate families. However, before committing to a home therapy, a home assessment needs to be completed. At the time of finalizing suitable training dates, advise the family that a continuous 4- to 6-week time commitment will be necessary. Ideally, we recommend training two people at the outset. We also endorse training or involving the young adult patient immediately, thus promoting independence. Younger children should also be encouraged to learn about the machine setup, access, and dialysis prescription. All families should be offered repeated opportunities to enhance their knowledge and skills after they are home.

Companies supplying the dialysis equipment will often provide considerable teaching materials and expertise. However, in our experience, significant adaptation is often necessary for it to become both safe and relevant to the pediatric population.

Within our center, training is initially started in the HD unit. This is a safety precaution that allows us to rapidly detect and manage acute complications, such as a dialyzer reaction. Ideally, thereafter, training should move quickly to a "family step-down" training facility, co-located within hospital grounds but separate from the dialysis unit, set up to simulate the home environment. If such a facility is not available, training should continue in the regular HD unit, stepping down directly to the patient's home with a higher number of home-assisted or -supported dialysis sessions with the home HD nursing team.

At the end of the training period, the trainee's competency needs to be formally assessed and signed off by the home HD nurse specialist. Within our unit, we also mandate that three or four dialysis treatments are completed unsupervised before discharge, with at least one weekend treatment with no home HD staff on site within the hospital. In an attempt to improve adherence, we also ask the patient and his or her family to sign a treatment contract. After discharge, one of the home HD nursing team travels to the family home for the first dialysis treatment. In addition to providing onsite support, this can also provide an excellent opportunity to engage with the community teams.

Retraining opportunities are offered at minimum every 6 months or are mandated after an adverse event, change in treatment, or dialysis access such as switching from central lines to arteriovenous fistulas.

Remote monitoring is not universally used, but if available, it may alleviate some patient or parental anxieties. Pediatric programs typically use an existing adult facility given the small numbers. Remote monitoring initially required a dedicated phone line and modem, but wireless technology is supplanting this.

Dialysis Equipment

Dialysis Systems Requiring Home Water Conversions

A majority of HD machines that are suitable for home HD require home water conversions in order to produce the large volumes of high-quality dialysate necessary for the dialysis treatment. This cost can sometimes become a barrier to delivering home HD in children when transplantation is the preferred renal replacement therapy and dialysis is viewed as a temporary interim measure. On average, home HD with water conversion is more cost effective than in-center HD if patients stay on dialysis for more than 14 months to offset training and setup costs.

Water conversion requires the installation of a cold water outlet and a drain to allow the carbon filter, reverse osmosis unit, and dialysis machine to be fitted. A system for testing the water quality needs to be put in place. Typically, families test their water for chloride every session and then bring a sample for advanced testing to their monthly hospital clinic visits. The dialysis technician will test for chemicals, endotoxins, and microbiology.

Water conversions, although necessary, can be a source of additional work and anxiety for families because complications such as leaks and blocked drains can occur and need to be addressed as a matter of urgency.

Mobile Hemodialysis System: NxStage

The NxStage System One is a portable home dialysis machine that functions without home water modifications. Dialysate is prepared at home using the NxStage

PureFlow SL integrated water purification and dialysate production system. Purified water is produced in 40- to 60-L batches from ordinary tap and mixed with sterile-filtered concentrate to produce AAMI (Association for the Advancement of Medical Instrumentation) quality, lactate-buffered dialysate. Alternatively, dialysis could be delivered using preprepared 5-L sterile dialysate bags. At Great Ormond Street Hospital, we currently use three NxStage dialysis circuits in the home environment. The first is their standard circuit, CAR-172-C, which is used in children weighing 25 kg or more. This circuit has a preattached polysulfone dialyzer that caused a dialyzer-induced thrombocytopenia in 40% to 60% of our children. These children are now successfully dialyzed at home with the CAR-124-C, a modified continuous venovenous hemofiltration circuit, with a smaller extracorporeal volume that can house an alternative, appropriately sized dialyzer and is suitable for children weighing 20 kg or more. Finally, we have adapted another continuous renal replacement therapy circuit, CAR-125-B, which with an appropriately sized dialyzer can treat children weighing 10 kg or more.

Prescribing dialysis treatment using the NxStage system is very different from standard HD prescriptions because the former relies on the principle of efficient use of dialysate with the spent dialysate being highly saturated. The flow fraction is the ratio of effluent flow (spent dialysate plus UF) divided by blood flow rate and corresponds to the degree of dialysate saturation. When the dialysate saturation approaches 100%, the treatment dose is approximately equivalent to the volume of dialysate used per session. With flow fractions between 30% and 35%, clearance of small molecules such as urea is very efficient achieving dialysate saturations of 90% to 95%. As flow fraction increases clearance falls but to a greater proportion in larger molecules such as creatinine. Therefore, one has to strike a balance between dialysis time, blood flow rates, and flow fraction to preserve dialysate efficiency and both small and middle-molecule clearance. We typically start with a flow fraction of 35% to 40%, dialyzing for 5 hours four times a week with a dialysate volume 70% of the estimated total body water volume per dialysis session.

Patient Selection

As a result of our growing confidence and experiences with home HD, we now have no fixed or absolute patient criteria for home HD except for a commitment to dialyze at home. The referral could be initiated for a number of reasons, including medical, social, or educational or simply patients exercising their rights to choose. Psychosocial involvement may be necessary to ensure families' suitability for home therapies and support them in their decision. Self-care within the HD unit often facilitates the transition to home dialysis by allowing patients and families to gradually build their confidence. We also believe that failed home PD does not preclude the possibility of home HD.

Suggested criteria for accepting patients into a home HD program are listed below. However, specifics may vary among programs.

- Commitment to dialyzing at home. A trained caregiver is not a prerequisite for young adults 16 years of age and older.
- Patient weight 10 kg and above (determined by the combined volume of the extracorporeal circuit and dialyzer)
- Well-functioning vascular access
- No psychosocial concerns that cannot be managed in the community

- Home of a sufficient size to accommodate the dialysis equipment and a month's supply of dialysis consumables
- In consideration of the reverse osmosis dialysis systems at home, the ability to modify the water source
- Family household hygiene that does not compromise the patient's risk of infection
- Child does not live in an area with frequent and prolonged disruptions to electricity supplies. An emergency source of power must be available at all times.

Prescriptions

In our experience, one of the key drivers for families to agree to home HD is the flexibility to perform the HD treatment around their own schedule. The impetus for clinical teams is in improving patient outcomes and quality of life. Attempts to achieve both goals with one dialysis prescription can be difficult, but some useful guides do exist.

Frequent daily dialysis prescriptions typically comprise 2 to 3 hours of dialysis six to seven times per week. Such prescriptions are very useful for working parents who cannot start dialysis until late in the evening or who need to complete treatments early in the evening because of evening work shifts. Such regimens seldom give complete freedom from phosphate binders but can be useful in young children who cannot tolerate long dialysis sessions, in patients on parenteral nutrition or gastrostomy feeds, and for patients who do not tolerate aggressive UF or are not optimally compliant with fluid restrictions. Of all the home dialysis regimes, high-frequency prescriptions are the most expensive in line with the higher dialysis consumables cost.

Alternate-day, prolonged 5- to 6-hour dialysis sessions, typically in the evening, eliminate fluid restrictions and liberalize dietary and phosphate restrictions. Alternate-day therapy frees up more time for the patient and caregiver for social or recreational activities. Such treatments are also associated with an improved sense of well-being. This can come at a cost, especially in young adults, who can become increasingly frustrated about sacrificing their evenings for HD.

Home nocturnal HD prescriptions are typically 8 hours overnight, daily, or on alternate nights. Gentler dialysis prescriptions will virtually eliminate adverse intradialytic symptoms and offers superior clearance of "uremic toxins," particularly phosphate and middle molecules. However, owing to the nonselective nature of HD purification, essential plasma components are also removed, resulting in a theoretical risk of deficiencies. Patients usually have complete freedom from dietary and fluid restrictions, and phosphate binders can be withdrawn, resulting in a reduced medication burden. In patients dialyzing daily, hypophosphatemia is common and can be treated by oral supplements or by adding phosphate to the acid dialysate concentrate as a sodium phosphate (Fleet) enema. To protect against a negative calcium balance, higher dialysate calcium levels of 1.75 mmol/L are recommended from the outset. Some patients may develop persistently low BP, necessitating prophylactic midodrine at the start of dialysis to support the BP, thus allowing UF and reducing the risk of the circuit clotting.

Dialyzing overnight can induce anxiety both in caregivers and children because of fears of disconnection or not hearing machine alarms. Some units have advocated equipping the dialysis machine with a port for downloading treatment data onto a central remote monitoring station via a personal computer or modem. We recommend a baby monitor to amplify the sound of the alarms overnight. Access monitoring is highly recommended using either enuresis alarm pads or more sophisticated monitors such as Hemodialert that are sensitive to fluid and the color red. A cycler base fluid detector that alarms if there are any leaks within the circuit can also be used.

Dialysis Adequacy

Traditionally, dialysis adequacy is assessed by urea clearance quantified as urea reduction ratio or single-pool or equilibrated Kt/V. We believe this is an oversimplification, and the success of a dialysis regimen should be assessed through the combined outcomes of several important endpoints such as cardiovascular health, quality of life, and growth, to name a few. Based on current technology and practices, it is not unrealistic to aim for adequate growth, control of anemia, optimal BP and control of bone and mineral disorders, absence of left ventricular hypertrophy, and excellent psychosocial health.

Conclusion

Hemodialysis is necessary for many children with end-stage renal disease, but outcomes are extremely variable. Quotidian dialysis programs at home are producing results never anticipated in dialysis patients, and even though data are scarce in children, the projected and demonstrable benefits are hard to ignore. We as a pediatric nephrology community have a responsibility to promote, educate, and actively recruit patients into quotidian dialysis programs, based in hospital or at home, to allow a greater proportion of children to receive the therapeutic benefits.

C H A P T E R   7 7

Anticoagulation in Children Undergoing Hemodialysis

Martin Kreuzer, MD • Dieter Haffner, MD

Extracorporeal blood purification techniques are associated with clotting of the extracorporeal circuit; therefore, with the exception of some coagulation disorders, anticoagulation is mandatory. In pediatric practice, the relative surface area of the extracorporeal circuit is increased in relation to its blood volume. The use of smaller lumen diameter lines provides greater surface contact. Passage of blood through the extracorporeal circuit results in activation of leukocytes, macrophages, lymphocytes, platelets, and the complement cascade. Monocyte activation, especially in the presence of activated platelets, results in surface expression and local release of tissue factor, thus activating the coagulation cascade promoting thrombosis in the extracorporeal circuit. In pediatric patients, smaller lumen in catheter, needle, and circuit tubing results in higher resistance, more turbulent flow, and limited blood flow rates compared with adults. The type of blood purification technique has implications for the choice, use, and handling of anticoagulants: In intermittent hemodialysis (HD), anticoagulants are only needed for about 4 hours to prevent the circuit from clotting. In continuous procedures, the need for and potential risks of anticoagulants are present for a considerably longer period of time.

General Considerations

In pediatric practice, most centers use unfractionated heparin (UFH) for treatment in patients without increased risk of hemorrhagic complications because it is inexpensive and easy to handle. Some centers use low-molecular-weight heparins (LMWH) instead because of better predictability.

In patients with heparin-induced thrombocytopenia (HIT) type II (and children with type I), alternatives to heparins are recommended. In noncritically ill children with HIT, we favor argatroban, a reversible direct thrombin inhibitor (DIT) with a considerably short half-life and only few adverse effects.

Data from adults as well as children strongly indicate regional citrate anticoagulation in patients who are actively bleeding or at risk of bleeding (e.g., within 3 days of a bleeding episode; a surgical wound; accidental wound, or tonsillectomy within the past week; or <2 weeks from a cerebral or retinal hemorrhage).

Long-term anticoagulation in continuous renal replacement therapy needs strict anticoagulation management and frequent anticoagulation monitoring, especially in critically ill children.

Very small children (<10 kg body weight) need stringent anticoagulation monitoring. Because of a very slow blood flow and smaller lumen lining, they need higher anticoagulant dosing and thus have an increased risk of hemorrhagic complications.

Unfractionated Heparin

The anticoagulant most commonly used is UFH. It consists of a large series of glycosaminoglycans, which interact with antithrombin. Although heparin effectively reduces coagulation cascade activation and thrombin formation, it can also directly activate platelets, which results in microthrombi deposits on the dialyzer wall.

> (!) For efficient use of heparin, antithrombin is needed. Heparin is an ineffective antico-agulant in patients with low plasma antithrombin levels (e.g., children with severe liver impairment or with an inborn antithrombin deficiency). If necessary, administer antithrombin to keep levels within a normal range.

Heparin is a systemic anticoagulant, with an action time of 3 to 5 minutes. It is not removed by dialysis and only partially by plasma separation. About 35% is excreted via the kidney; therefore, half-life is increased to 50 to 70 minutes in patients with acute kidney injury or end-stage renal disease. The disparity in half-life is greatest in the extremes of age and weight, especially in children weighing less than 10 kg. Heparin is a very negatively charged molecule that adheres well to plastics.

> (!) It is important to use a properly diluted heparin solution to prevent adherence of heparin only to the inner lining of the tube. Use a minimum heparin infusion velocity of 2.0 mL/h!

Heparin can be used in children without risk of bleeding. A loading dose of 25 to 50 IU/kg or 300 to 1000 IU/m^2 (maximum, 2000 IU) should be administered followed by a maintenance dose of 10 to 30 IU/kg/h. Loading dose (or no loading dose) had no effect on occurrence of hemorrhagic complications in children with increased bleeding risk (see the Regional Citrate Anticoagulation section). In inter-mittent HD, the infusion is stopped some 30 minutes before the end of the dialysis, especially in children with shunts, to prevent excess bleeding from the puncture site.

Because there is variability between batches of UFH, bedside monitoring of its effects are crucial. Monitoring can be easily performed by using bedside whole-blood activated clotting time (ACT). The activated partial thromboplastin time (aPTT) can be used but needs a laboratory test. The aim is a 1.2- to 2-fold of baseline or upper normal value.

> (!) With every 10-second aPTT prolongation, the risk of bleeding complications is increased by 50%!

Although the introduction of heparin has been one of the major advances in the history of HD, its side effects can be significant. The most severe of these is bleeding. Heparin can cause allergic reactions because it is derived from pork or bovine intestine. However, with long-term use, heparin can cause osteoporosis and exacer-bate hyperkalemia (by antagonizing aldosterone) and can result in alopecia and abnormal liver function test results.

(!) In case of severe bleeding complications, heparin activity can be quickly reversed: Use 1 mg protamine for every 100 IU of heparin.

Occasionally, patients can develop HIT. The more severe (antibody-mediated) type II reaction usually develops when the patient has been exposed to large doses of heparin. Type II can be observed in 2% to 3% of patients about 5 to 10 days after exposure by a significantly decreased thrombocyte count (<50,000/μL). Instant withdrawal of heparin in type II of HIT is mandatory. Generally, in children with HIT, alternatives to UFH should be used for anticoagulation.

(!) On dialysis, the need for a significantly increasing heparin dosage to achieve sufficient anticoagulation can be a clue to subclinical HIT (type I). Thrombocyte count can be normal or only slightly decreased. In these cases, HIT should be checked.

Low-Molecular-Weight Heparins

Low-molecular-weight heparins were developed to improve the predictability of anticoagulant effects by cleavage of UFH. They are not a single entity, so they vary in their relative effects on inhibiting factors IIa and Xa.

Compared with UFH, LMWH have been reported to be more effective in reducing extracorporeal clotting and fewer hemorrhagic complications.

Low-molecular-weight heparins are mostly cleared by the kidneys. So their half-life is considerably prolonged in renal failure (with enoxaparin having the longest with about 28 hours), and they are not an option for short-term dialysis sessions (<2 hours). In addition, they tend to accumulate in patients undergoing daily dialysis (e.g., small children). They are, in general, administered as one dose at the start of dialysis (for dosage, see Table 77.1). The dosage depends on the LMWH used as well as on frequency and duration of HD sessions. A single bolus may not always provide sufficient anticoagulation for a very long dialysis session (e.g., overnight

Table 77.1

Pediatric Dosing Recommendations for Low-Molecular-Weight Heparins During a Standard 4-Hour Dialysis Session*

Anticoagulant	Half-Life* (h)	Pediatric Dose	Anticoagulation Target
Tinzaparin	4.5	50 IU/kg	Anti–factor Xa activity 0.2–0.4
Dalteparin	5	40 IU/kg	(–0.6) IU/mL
		<15 kg: 1500 IU	
		15–30 kg: 2500 IU	
		30–50 kg: 5000 IU	
Reviparin	5	85 IU/kg	
Nadroparin	5	114 IU/kg	
Enoxaparin	27.7	24–36 mg/m^2	
		0.5–1.0 mg/kg	

*Note that half-lives vary with residual renal function.

dialysis or continuous procedures). Some proportion of the LMWH bolus may be lost via the filter because of its lower molecular weight compared with UFH. Coating the dialyzer surface with vitamin E reduces the loss and may lead to dose reduction.

Monitoring effectiveness (and risk) of LMWH is one of the major drawbacks to its use. Because of an only modest effect on thrombin, only anti-Xa activity can be monitored. Peak levels of 0.4 to 0.6 IU/mL should be achieved, as well as levels below 0.2 IU/mL at the end or immediately after dialysis.

Heparin-induced thrombocytopenia may rarely develop with LMWH. Because of cross-reactions, LMWH should not be used in patients with a history of HIT type II. If bleeding does occur, it is mostly more severe compared with UFH. Because protamine has only a moderate effect on LMWH, fresh-frozen plasma (FFP) may be required in severe hemorrhagic complications.

(!) Protamine does not effectively antagonize the action of LMWHs! In an emergency (e.g., severe bleeding complications), use FFP.

Systemic Anticoagulants as Alternatives to Heparins

Proteoglycans, or DITs, should be used for anticoagulation in patients with HIT. Proteoglycans are naturally occurring anticoagulants produced by many species. In current clinical practice, danaparoid (a mixture of heparan sulfate, dermatan sulfate, and chondroitin) is the most commonly used proteoglycan for systemic anticoagulation. Predominantly, it performs an anticoagulant activity against factor Xa. Compared with other anticoagulants for treating patients with HIT, danaparoid has been reported to be more effective in preventing thrombosis by preventing activation of platelets by HIT type II antibodies. The main disadvantage of danaparoid is the long half-life of about 30 hours in kidney injury. Thus, monitoring and adjusting the loading dose should not only depend on anti–factor Xa activity at the end of the dialysis session but also on anti-Xa activity before the start of the subsequent dialysis session. Pediatric dosing recommendations are given in Table 77.2.

Lepirudin is a recombinant form of the natural anticoagulant hirudin (from the medical leech). It is mainly excreted by the kidneys; thus, it has a significantly increased half-life in dialysis patients of longer than 35 hours, with reports of longer than 100 hours. Lepirudin is a small molecule and therefore dialyzable, with greater clearance using high-flux filters or hemodiafiltration. Pediatric dosing recommendations are given in Table 77.2. Lepirudin can be monitored by aPTT aiming for a ratio to baseline of less than 1.5 before the dialysis session and 1.5 to 2.0 during the session. Unfortunately, the relationship of plasma lepirudin levels and aPTT is not linear, and a small increase in aPTT may reflect a major increase in lepirudin concentration, with a significantly increased risk of bleeding. Thus, most centers recommend further investigations if aPTT exceeds the 1.5-fold of normal values using either the ecarin clotting test or plasma lepirudin concentration. Because lepirudin is an irreversible thrombin inhibitor, there is no simple antidote, and in the case of serious hemorrhagic complications FFP and activated factor VII concentrates are needed.

Argatroban is a reversible DIT. It is a synthetic peptide derived from arginine. Argatroban is licensed by the Food and Drug Administration for the treatment of

Table 77.2

Alternative Options to Heparin in Cases of Heparin-Induced Thrombocytopenia

Anticoagulant	Loading Dose	Maintenance Dose	Monitoring	Dose Adjustment
Danaparoid	1000 + 30 IU/kg for age younger than 10 years or 1500 + 30 IU/kg for age older than 10 years	None	Predialysis anti-Xa <0.30 IU/L	Reduce dose by 250 IU if predialysis anti-Xa >0.3 and <0.5 and stop if >0.5 IU/L.
Argatroban	—	0.7 µg/kg/min (liver disease, 0.2 µg/kg/min)	aPTTr target 2.0–2.5 check after 2 h	Adjust if required by 0.25 µg/kg/min and recheck aPTTr.
Lepirudin	0.2–0.5 mg/kg 5–30 mg	—	Hirudin 0.5–0.8 µg/mL aPTTr 1.5–2.0	Adjust dose for subsequent dialysis.

aPTTr, ratio of therapeutically prolonged activated partial thromboplastin time (aPTT) and baseline aPTT or normal value.

HIT in children in the United States. Patients are treated with a continuous infusion. Pediatric dosing recommendations are given in Table 77.2. Argatroban is mainly metabolized in the liver. The half-time is about 50 minutes. Because of protein binding (54%), argatroban is only partly removed by dialysis, and consideration should be given to reducing the dose toward the end of the dialysis session to prevent prolonged bleeding from the puncture site. Argatroban is highly selective for thrombin (circulating and fibrin bound). In contrast to the anticoagulants mentioned previously, there are no reports on antibody formation against argatroban. Again, there is no antidote, and in case of serious bleeding, FFP and activated factor VII concentrates are needed.

(!) In critically ill children, the clearance of argatroban is significantly reduced by about 50% compared with healthy adults! Do not use argatroban in children with cholestasis because it is mainly secreted by bile and excreted with the feces.

Regional Anticoagulation With Citrate

Citrate is a potent regional anticoagulant. It decreases free (ionized) serum calcium by forming chelate complexes. Thus, calcium is no longer available for the activation of tenase and prothrombinase complexes within the coagulation cascade. This effect is easily reversed by calcium substitution. This mechanism provides the means for regional anticoagulation exclusively in the extracorporeal blood circuit.

Anticoagulation with citrate introduces a degree of complexity to the treatment. In any form of HD, a calcium-free dialysate is needed. If trisodium citrate is used, dialysate sodium concentration has to be decreased. Citrate has a half-life of only a few minutes and is mainly metabolized to bicarbonate in the liver (and skeletal muscles). Thus, during prolonged dialysis sessions, alkalosis may occur, and bicarbonate levels of the dialysis fluid have to be decreased. With modern dialysis machines used during intermittent HD, both sodium and bicarbonate levels of the dialysate can be easily adapted to accommodate these needs. This remains more complicated when using continuous techniques.

(!) Modern dialysis machines are fitted with a pump for citrate infusion controlled automatically by blood flow. If using *additional* pumps to the dialysis machine for infusion of citrate or calcium, be sure to have a stable blood flow and to immediately pause the external pumps in case the blood pump stops. A significant citrate bolus injection into a central venous catheter immediately depletes ionized calcium within the ventricles and may result in sudden cardiac arrest.

The citrate infusion must be adjusted to the blood flow to achieve a postfilter ionized calcium concentration of 0.20–0.30 mmol/L (0.80–1.20 mg/dL) to prevent clotting within the circuit, which equates to a predialyzer citrate concentration of about 4–6 mmol/L (77–115 mg/dL). A 4% trisodium citrate (TSC 4%) and a 3% acid citrate dextrose (ACD) solution are available. We recommend using ACD solution, which is widely available for stabilizing blood products. With ACD solution, dosing in children is quite simple: Choose a prefilter infusion rate of the ACD solution (in milliliters per hour) that is two times the blood flow (in milliliters per minute) or a relationship of 1:30.

The effect of citrate is reversed by calcium infusion. Depending on the patient's situation (e.g., hypocalcemia in critically ill children) and the dialysis technique, recommendations on calcium substitution are not easy to provide. Using 10% calcium gluconate solution (with 0.23 mmol/L calcium or ~1.0 mg/dL) one should start the calcium solution (in milliliters per hour) with a quarter of blood flow (in milliliters per minute) or a relationship of 1:15. In continuous hemofiltration, the substitute usually contains calcium. Hence, an additional calcium substitution is needed only in one third of the patients. Regional citrate anticoagulation in hemofiltration is only possible with a postfilter dilution technique (Fig. 77.1). Check the patient's ionized calcium level before dialysis. If it exceeds 1.30 mmol/L (5.20 mg/dL), start without calcium infusion and begin substitution only if the patient's ionized calcium levels decrease below 1.10 mmol/L. If hypocalcemia is present (ionized calcium <1.00 mmol/L or 4.00 mg/dL), start with a much higher calcium infusion rate (e.g., double the amount mentioned earlier using a relationship to blood flow of 1:7.5). The aim is to keep the patient's ionized calcium levels within the physiologic range (1.00–1.30 mmol/L or 4.00–5.20 mg/dL).

(!) Calcium substitution should never be connected to the venous air trap. Turbulence in blood flow and contact with air result in immediate formation of clots.
   Be aware that a perivascular leakage of calcium-containing solution will lead to severe tissue necrosis and damage!

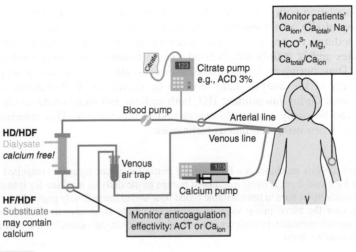

Figure 77.1

Regional citrate anticoagulation. ACD, acid citrate dextrose; HD, hemodialysis; HDF, hemodiafiltration; HF, hemofiltration.

Regional citrate anticoagulation is more complex compared with other anticoagulation techniques because not only does adequacy of anticoagulation need to be monitored (which can be by postdialyzer ionized calcium or ACT) but also for patients' safety, several serum parameters have to be monitored, including ionized calcium level; the ratio of total calcium and ionized calcium (as a marker for citrate intoxication); and sodium, bicarbonate, and magnesium levels. We recommend monitoring of postfilter ionized calcium and patients' ionized calcium levels every 15 minutes within the first hour of initiation of treatment and hourly thereafter. The estimated volume load of the citrate and calcium solution has to be added to ultrafiltration anticipated to prevent hyperhydration.

(!) A total calcium to ionized calcium ratio greater than 2.4 has been associated with a more than 30-fold higher mortality rate in patients with regional citrate anticoagulation 4 weeks later. A ratio greater than 2.4 equals citrate intoxication! Discontinue citrate infusion.

Under normal circumstances, regional citrate anticoagulation is effective in intermittent HD for up to 5 hours. In the case of pediatric apheresis therapy, it is important to realize that the citrate and calcium solution fluid load can be substantial, and apheresis therapy does not provide the possibility of fluid removal. Citrate anticoagulation becomes more difficult with continuous procedures. Over the period of continuous hemofiltration with regional citrate anticoagulation, there will be an accumulation of sodium, bicarbonate, and sometimes citrate and total calcium levels. Sodium and bicarbonate accumulation can be handled with the use of a predilution 5% glucose solution. In more severe cases, the standard substitute solution in continuous hemofiltration can be replaced (partially or totally) by an infusion solution containing less sodium, alkali, or both.

(!) Children have lower muscle mass than adults; therefore, citrate is predominantly metabolized in the liver. Regional citrate anticoagulation is not safe in children with impaired liver function! In anhepatic children (e.g., the first days after liver transplantation), it is difficult to use citrate anticoagulation!

Other Regional Anticoagulants

Prostacyclin is the most potent of the prostanoids, which are naturally occurring anticoagulants and have very short half-lives of only a couple of minutes. Prostanoids (especially prostacyclin) are also potent pulmonary and systemic vasodilators, which produce side effects. Flushing and hypotension are commonly observed side effects, and prostanoids should not be used in children with hemodynamic instability. The systemic side effects of prostacyclin can be significant! Hypotension can be avoided by ensuring that patients are not hypovolemic and by infusing prostacyclin starting at a rate of 0.5 ng/kg/min before the start of dialysis and increasing the dose over a few minutes (aim for 5.0–10.0 ng/kg/min). Because the half-life is in minutes, any hypotensive episode can readily be reversed by stopping the infusion. Prostanoids mainly block platelet activation, so they do not have any measurable effect on standard laboratory coagulation assays. Therefore, measuring a coagulative effect and monitoring efficacy are not possible.

Central Venous Line Locks and Treatment of Clotted Catheters

In most centers, central venous lines are locked with UFH, either neat or diluted to 1000 to 2500 IU/mL. The lock places the patient at an increased risk of bleeding because of systemic infusion of part of the anticoagulant. Thus, undiluted heparin cannot be recommended in children. An accidental flushing of the locked catheter may cause a serious hemorrhagic complication.

Citrate has become a potent alternative as a catheter locking agent. A 5% sodium citrate lock is equally efficient in preventing catheter dysfunction as a 10% citrate lock. In a higher concentration (30%), it may also prevent bacterial growth and biofilm deposition. In contrast to heparin, it is not a problem to slowly flush the lock if the line cannot be aspirated.

In patients with hypercoagulability, a heparin or citrate lock alone may not be sufficient to maintain catheter patency. A regular instillation of urokinase or tissue plasminogen activator (tPa) once a week or every fortnight is helpful in preventing catheter clotting. Clotted catheters can regain patency with urokinase (5000 IU/mL) or tPa (1 mg/mL). Some patients undergoing intermittent HD may need LMWH (enoxaparin 0.1–0.5 mg/kg) administered subcutaneously on days without dialysis to prevent clot formation at or within the catheter. Because of a prolonged half-life of LMWHs in kidney injury, monitoring of anti-Xa activity (aim <0.2 IU/L) before dialysis is necessary.

C H A P T E R 7 8

Peritoneal Dialysis Catheter Placement in Children

Walter S. Andrews, MD • Bradley A. Warady, MD

Peritoneal dialysis (PD) is the predominant initial dialytic modality for children with end-stage renal disease (ESRD). This is especially true for children who have acquired ESRD during their first decade of life. Reasons for the preferential selection of PD in children have included its ability to greatly reduce the need for dietary restrictions, its simplicity of operation, the lack of a need for routine blood access, and the ability of the child to attend school on a regular basis.

For there to be successful PD, there must be successful function of the peritoneal catheter. The catheter should provide reliable and rapid dialysate flow rates without leakage of dialysate. Although significant improvements have occurred in catheter insertion and care over time, the PD catheter is still described as the Achilles' heel of PD because of the potential for catheter-related complications. This chapter explores the key characteristics of the peritoneal catheter, the primary surgical techniques for placement, and the most common catheter-related complications in children.

Types of Peritoneal Catheters

The catheters commonly used for chronic PD are constructed of soft material, such as silicone rubber or polyurethane. The key elements of the catheters are the unique intraperitoneal configurations (curled or straight), number of Dacron cuffs (one or two), and the subcutaneous tunnel configuration (straight or "swan neck"). If one includes the orientation of the catheter exit site on the abdomen as yet another variable, more than 20 different combinations of catheter characteristics are actually possible as documented in the 2011 annual report of the North American Pediatric Renal Trials and Collaborative Studies (NAPRTCS). The first description of placement of a chronic indwelling catheter for PD was in 1968 by Tenckhoff, and the Tenckhoff catheter still remains the one most often used today.

A review of the NAPRTCS registry of PD catheter insertions between 1992 and 2010 revealed that most were either Tenckhoff curled (62.1%) or Tenckhoff straight (25.9%) catheters. The increased utilization of a curled catheter may be related to its potential advantages over a straight catheter, which include (1) better separation between the abdominal wall and the bowel, (2) more catheter side holes available for inflow and outflow, (3) less inflow pain, (4) less of a tendency for migration out of the pelvis, (5) less prone to omental wrapping, and (6) potentially less trauma to bowel. Despite these theoretical advantages, no definitive data in the pediatric literature support the use of a curled catheter over a straight catheter. On the other hand, neither a review of the NAPRTCS data nor a review of available prospective studies provides any evidence of an association between intraperitoneal PD catheter configuration and the development of peritonitis or exit-site infections (ESIs) or tunnel infections (TIs).

The next catheter characteristic to consider is the number of Dacron cuffs on the catheter. If a single-cuff catheter is used, it is recommended that the cuff be positioned between the rectus sheaths and not in a superficial position. In one series, this approach decreased the incidence of subsequent peritonitis by nearly 37% compared with subcutaneous placement of the cuff. When a second cuff was added to secure the catheter's position and to hopefully help prevent bacterial migration, there were initial reports of extrusion of the second cuff. These extrusions were believed to occur because of either excessive torque on the catheter as a result of a steep angle between the exit site and the abdominal wall portion of the catheter or because the outer cuff was less than 2.0 cm from the exit site. Cuff extrusion often resulted in the development of an ESI and the occasional need for shaving of the cuff from the catheter. Although there are very few reports describing the incidence of distal cuff extrusion with double-cuff catheters in children, outer cuff extrusion rates between 4.8% and 8% have been reported. This may be the reason that nearly 51% of the catheters in the NAPRTCS database are single cuff. Several studies, however, have documented a higher incidence of ESIs and peritonitis with single-cuff catheters. Based on these data, the use of a double-cuff Tenckhoff catheter has been recommended in the "Consensus Guidelines for the Prevention and Treatment of Catheter-Related Infections and Peritonitis in Pediatric Patients Receiving Peritoneal Update: 2012."

The shape of the extraperitoneal portion of the catheter can also vary: It can be straight or can have a preformed angle (e.g., swan-neck configuration), in which there is an inverted U-shaped arc (170–180 degrees) between the deep and the superficial cuffs. The latter configuration was originally described by Twardowski et al and has been recommended by many pediatric programs as a significant improvement in catheter design. Although the cumulative NAPRTCS data report a swan-neck or curved tunnel in only 26% of catheters, data recently collected by the International Pediatric Peritoneal Dialysis Network (IPPN) revealed that more than 64% of incident catheters were of the swan-neck variety.

The purposes of the catheter arc are to allow the catheter to exit the skin in a downward-pointing direction and to allow the distal end of the catheter to enter the peritoneal cavity in an unstressed condition (i.e., without too much torque because of the synthetic material's memory), thereby decreasing the chance for its migration out of the pelvis and the development of early drainage failure. A modification of this catheter type is the swan-neck presternal catheter. The major difference between the swan-neck presternal catheter and the standard swan-neck catheter is that the presternal catheter has a very long subcutaneous portion, and the catheter typically exits over the anterior chest wall. This catheter has been successfully used when it is necessary to make the exit site remote from the abdomen, such as in patients with stomas.

One additional advantage of the swan-neck catheter is that it allows a downward-pointing exit site, which may be associated with a decreased likelihood for the accumulation of dirt and debris within the catheter tunnel, prompting the development of a TI or peritonitis. An upward-facing exit site emerged as an independent risk factor for peritonitis in an analysis by Furth et al of the 1992 through 1997 NAPRTCS data. More recently, the 2011 NAPRTCS data revealed that a straight catheter tunnel was associated with a peritonitis rate of 1 in 16.2 patient-months, but the rate associated with a swan-neck/curved downward facing tunnel was only 1 in 23.9 patient-months.

In summary, in children, because of the lack of prospective, randomized studies designed to evaluate PD catheter characteristics, it is impossible to conclude that one catheter characteristic is superior to another based on definitive evidence. However, NAPRTCS data suggest that the time to the first peritonitis episode is longer when a PD catheter is used that has:

- Two cuffs compared with one
- Swan-neck compared with straight configuration
- Downward-pointing exit site compared with lateral or upward exit site

However, these data have not yet been replicated worldwide. As such, the continued collection of this type of information in registries such as the NAPRTCS and the IPPN and by collaboratives such as the Standardized Care to Improve Outcomes in Pediatric ESRD (SCOPE) is mandatory if the optimal catheter characteristics for children are to be determined.

Preoperative Surgical Considerations

All patients who are going to undergo PD catheter placement require careful preoperative evaluation. One factor that has been repeatedly cited in the literature as being associated with an increased risk for postplacement PD catheter migration is constipation. Constipation is common in patients with chronic kidney disease (CKD) and must be addressed preoperatively with the use of either laxatives or an enema. If an enema is used, attention to its phosphorus content is imperative to prevent the development of hyperphosphatemia.

A careful physical examination is required to determine if the patient has any evidence of inguinal or umbilical hernias. In children who receive PD, the incidence of hernias is inversely proportional to age with an overall frequency of 8.0% to 57.0%. The highest frequency of inguinal hernias occurs within the first year of life because of the high incidence of a patent processus vaginalis and a higher intraabdominal pressure related to the presence of dialysis fluid. They are often bilateral and require surgical correction. If a hernia is found, it can be fixed either before or at the time of insertion of the PD catheter.

A critical portion of planning the catheter placement procedure is deciding the most appropriate location of the exit site. In babies, the exit site is typically placed outside the diaper area to help prevent contamination; in older children, it should be either above or below the belt line (an issue ideally discussed with the patient and parent in the preoperative setting). The presence of a vesicostomy, ureterostomy, colostomy, or gastrostomy will also influence the exit-site location. The exit site must be planned so that it is on the opposite side of the abdomen from the stoma sites. If this is not possible, the catheter may need to exit on the chest to get as much distance as possible between the stoma and the exit site. Placement of the exit site on the chest wall with a downward orientation has successfully limited the number of infections in such high-risk situations in children and adults.

Preoperative showering or bathing with an antiseptic soap or chlorhexidine wipes may help to reduce the risk of postoperative infection. Administration of an antibiotic within 60 minutes before skin incision for PD catheter placement has been shown in several studies to decrease the incidence of peritonitis after placement of a PD catheter in children and adults. Interestingly, these studies have shown that any class of antibiotic is associated with a reduction in peritonitis. Currently, we use a first- or second-generation cephalosporin unless the patient is known to be colonized with methicillin-resistant *Staphylococcus aureus* (then clindamycin is used) as has been recommended in the pediatric and adult guidelines.

Routine prophylaxis with vancomycin is not recommended in order to try to avoid the development of vancomycin-resistant organisms. An adult study did, however, report superior results with prophylactic vancomycin versus a cephalosporin. If the child has a lower gastrointestinal stoma, we often add a single dose of an aminoglycoside antibiotic. Some programs, including our own, also screen the patient for *Staphylococcus aureus* nasal carriage before catheter placement. If results are positive, a course of intranasal mupirocin (twice daily for 5 days) is recommended.

Omentectomy and Fibrin Sealants

The data on the use of an omentectomy to prevent PD catheter occlusion are fairly convincing. If an omentectomy is performed, the incidence of catheter occlusion is about 5% compared with an occlusion rate of 10% to 22.7% in patients without an omentectomy. In a recent single-center study of 101 pediatric PD patients who underwent reoperation for infection or malfunction of their PD catheter, lack of omentectomy was the only independent risk factor on multivariate analysis to be associated with catheter revision. Others have published similar pediatric experiences, on occasion also noting a significantly lower peritonitis rate in patients who underwent an omentectomy. These positive outcomes are presumably related to a lower frequency of omental plugging of the catheter, leading to less catheter manipulation and therefore a decreased risk of infection. Omentectomy is currently performed by at least 59% of North American surgeons placing chronic PD catheters and is performed at insertion of 82.4% of PD catheters included in the Italian pediatric PD registry. We and others believe that an omentectomy is a fairly simple procedure that can be carried out at the initial operation with little morbidity and should be strongly considered in all cases.

Fibrin sealant has been used in a variety of surgical specialties for its ability to be an effective sealant. The use of fibrin sealant in PD has been reported to be both effective in treating established leaks and, when used at the time of catheter implantation, may help prevent the development of initial peritoneal leaks. Our experience with fibrin sealant supports both of these assertions. We apply fibrin sealant around the internal cuff and down the tunnel between the inner and outer cuffs.

Surgical Techniques

Since Moncrief and Popovich first reported the use of continuous ambulatory peritoneal dialysis (CAPD), there have been a number of modifications of the technique for implantation of the PD catheter. The complications of dialysate leakage, dislocation of the catheter, erosion or extrusion of the cuffs, ESI, TI, and peritonitis have in one way or another influenced the surgical technique. To decrease the incidence of these complications, emphasis needs to be placed on careful surgical technique and on the surgical skill of the operator.

Multiple studies have now shown that the best results will be obtained if the catheters are inserted by surgeons who have developed an interest and an expertise in the procedure. The two most common PD catheter insertion techniques are open and laparoscopic, both of which permit direct vision of the peritoneal cavity, which is necessary in complicated patients with a history of abdominal surgery and the potential for adhesions. Other approaches include blind placement using the Tenckhoff trocar, blind placement using a guidewire (Seldinger technique), and the minitrocar peritoneoscopy placement technique. A review of recent literature on the topic reveals multiple papers addressing the pros and cons of the laparoscopic versus open techniques for PD catheter insertion. Currently, there are no data that show the superiority of one technique over the other.

Open Technique

Proponents of the open technique suggest that compared with the laparoscopic technique, the former approach does not require any specialized equipment; is less expensive; and in some situations in adults, can be conducted under local anesthesia.

As previously mentioned, the insertion site of the PD catheter in our hands is generally determined such that the exit site is downward facing and is above the diaper area in infants. In older children, the exit site should be either above or below the beltline, with it preferably placed below the beltline in very large children so that the catheter will reach into the pelvis. If the patient has the potential for having a gastrostomy in the future, the catheter exit site is positioned on the right-hand side of the abdomen. Otherwise, the catheter is placed on the left-hand side of the abdomen to avoid any interference with the future transplant incision. The most frequently performed open technique uses an incision over the rectus muscle. A lateral insertion through the rectus is generally deemed preferable to the midline because of the thinness of the midline in children and a decreased propensity for postoperative leakage in children when the rectus incision is used.

A 2-cm transverse skin incision is made just lateral to the umbilicus. The anterior rectus sheath is exposed, and a 2-cm longitudinal incision is created in the middle of the sheath. The rectus muscle is split in the direction of its fibers, and the posterior sheath is opened longitudinally. A partial omentectomy is then carried out under direct vision. The catheter is threaded over a stiffening wire to allow its placement deep in the pelvis, a few degrees to the right of midline to help prevent obstruction to flow in the setting of a full rectum. The posterior sheath is closed, and the inner cuff is fixed to the posterior sheath as part of this closure. The inner cuff is positioned within the rectus muscle, and the anterior sheath is then closed tightly around the catheter with a second purse-string suture.

The lateral opening through which the catheter is tunneled should be kept small to decrease the risk of dialysate leakage. The catheter is then tunneled out to the skin, and the outer cuff is situated 2.0 cm from the catheter exit site. As mentioned previously, shorter distances between the exit site and outer cuff predispose to cuff extrusion, but greater distances lead to formation of a deep sinus tract, granulation tissue formation, and an increased risk for the development of a TI.

before closing the skin, three or four dialysate exchanges (10–15 cc/kg) should be conducted in the operating room (OR) to make sure that there is free flow of fluid both into and out of the abdomen through the catheter. If there are any issues with flow in the OR, the catheter location needs to be reevaluated and corrected. A poorly functioning intraoperative catheter will continue to be a poorly functioning catheter postoperatively.

Laparoscopic Technique

With the introduction of laparoscopy, techniques have been developed that facilitate the percutaneous placement of a PD catheter under direct vision. The true advantage of laparoscopy is not just the ability to watch the placement of the catheter but also the ability to perform additional procedures that will enhance the catheter's longevity such as omentectomy, adhesiolysis, rectus sheath tunneling, and an evaluation for indirect inguinal hernias. Several studies have reported decreased catheter migration, decreased accidental injury to bowel, longer catheter survival, and a decreased incidence of peritonitis associated with the laparoscopic technique. An additional advantage of the laparoscopic technique is that it allows the use of much smaller peritoneal incisions, which decreases the chance for dialysate leakage.

In 2014, the Society of American Gastrointestinal and Endoscopic Surgeons (SAGES) published guidelines for the insertion of PD catheters. These guidelines along with a commentary by Crabtree yielded several technical recommendations: laparoscopic ports should not be placed in the midline (increased risk for hernias), rectus sheath tunneling should be performed without pelvic anchoring sutures (decrease catheter migration), perform omentectomy or omentopexy and perform adhesiolysis if necessary, use an intraoperative irrigation test of the catheter, and suture close all port sites. The laparoscopic technique does require more expertise and more equipment and is more expensive than the open method.

As with the open technique, the catheter insertion and exit sites are marked before incision with consideration of the patient's size, exit-site orientation, and possible future need for a gastrostomy. Under general anesthesia, a vertical incision is made in the umbilicus, and the umbilical fascia is sharply incised. Using blunt dissection, the peritoneum is entered, and (depending on the size of the child) a 3- or 5-mm port is placed. A corresponding 3- or 5-mm laparoscope is then inserted, and the abdomen is insufflated. A 3- or 5-mm instrument is then inserted through a stab wound at the marked catheter exit site. The abdomen is then inspected, and any adhesions can be lysed in preparation for catheter insertion. The omentum can then be extracted from the abdomen through the stab wound or the umbilicus and then removed by the use of electrocautery. We believe that a complete omentectomy is not absolutely necessary as long as a substantial amount of the omentum is removed.

After the omentectomy has been performed, a 1- to 2-cm transverse incision is made in the skin over the midportion of the rectus sheath at the premarked peritoneal catheter insertion site. This is carried down to the anterior rectus sheath. A small hole is made in the anterior sheath, and an expandable laparoscopic sheath loaded in a Veress needle is inserted down to the posterior rectus sheath. Under direct vision, the Veress needle is then slid along the posterior rectus sheath toward the pelvis for about 3 to 5 cm depending on the size of the patient. The Veress needle is then introduced into the abdomen at the distal end of the tunnel. The addition of the tunnel to the insertion technique has decreased our incidence of catheter migration and has been reported to decrease the incidence of catheter leakage. The Veress needle is then removed, leaving the sheath behind. A guidewire is then inserted through the sheath, and its tip is positioned into the pelvis under direct vision. The port is then removed and, using a peel-away sheath technique, a 20-Fr sheath is then inserted into the abdomen over the guidewire. The PD catheter is then placed on a stiffener and inserted into the pelvis under direct vision. The pneumoperitoneum is maintained by pushing the proximal cuff of the PD catheter into the sheath, thereby preventing gas loss. After the catheter has been positioned in the pelvis, the sheath is removed.

As the sheath is being removed, the inner cuff is positioned to lie between the anterior and posterior portions of the rectus sheath. The anterior rectus sheath is then closed around the catheter with two purse-string sutures of 3-0 polydioxanone (PDS). The abdomen is also carefully inspected for evidence of indirect hernias. If these are identified, they are fixed after completion of the PD catheter insertion. The camera and all ports are then removed, and the umbilical fascia is repaired.

At the previously marked catheter exit site, a deep subcutaneous tunnel is created between the catheter exit site and the catheter entrance site using a 20-Fr sheath dilator or a tendon passer. The catheter is then pulled through the tunnel, positioning the outer cuff so that it is at least 2.0 cm from the exit site. The skin exit site should be tight around the catheter. At this point, fibrin sealant is injected around the catheter at the level of the anterior rectus sheath and then down the tunnel between the outer and inner cuffs. We believe that this helps ensure a leak-free closure. As with the open technique, three or four dialysate exchanges (10–15 cc/kg) should be conducted in the OR to make sure that there is free flow of fluid both into and out of the abdomen. If there are any issues with flow in the OR, the catheter location needs to be reevaluated and corrected. The entrance site of the catheter is then closed in two layers. The exit site of the catheter is dressed, and the catheter is secured to prevent local trauma, but no fixation suture is used at the exit site.

Postimplantation Care

The exit site of the catheter is a potential site of infection after PD catheter placement. In an attempt to address this issue, Moncrief has suggested that the external portion of the catheter should initially remain buried beneath the skin in a subcutaneous pocket for 4 to 6 weeks. Twardowski et al, on the other hand, have merely recommended that initially the exit site should be covered with several layers of sterile gauze and kept dry. Some oozing from the exit site is common, and the gauze can wick this away from the skin.

An occlusive dressing should *not* be used. Occlusive dressings tend to trap fluid at the exit site, predisposing to bacterial growth and subsequent infection. Trauma to the exit site, usually from repeated catheter motion, needs to be minimized. The catheter should be covered with a dressing, and dressing changes should not occur more often than once per week until the exit site is healed. Ideally, specially trained staff should conduct the dressing changes, which allows a consistent aseptic technique to be followed. Submersion of the exit site should be avoided to prevent colonization with waterborne organisms. We use this technique at our program, and it has prevented the development of early ESIs in virtually all cases.

Timing of Catheter Use

Some controversy exists as to whether the catheter should be used immediately after placement or whether a timed period (e.g., break-in period) should elapse before its use to facilitate healing and help prevent the development of complications such as leakage and infection. The 1998 International Society for Peritoneal Dialysis (ISPD) catheter guidelines recommended a dialysis-free period of 10 to 15 days after catheter insertion, the Clinical Practice Guidelines for Peritoneal Access recommend 5 to 10 days, and the European guidelines recommend at least 2 weeks whenever possible. All groups discourage the routine practice of peritoneal flushing to check for catheter patency and function.

Although the available data might suggest a preference for delayed catheter usage without regular flushing of the catheter, there is no definitive evidence for any particular break-in period, although the SCOPE collaborative will soon publish prospective data on this issue. A delay in dialysis initiation may be most important for the youngest infants who appear to have the greatest risk for leakage and subsequent catheter revision based on data from the IPPN. Of course, when early usage is necessary, efforts should be made to minimize any increase in the intraperitoneal pressure by using small exchange volumes with the child in the supine position and using a cycling device.

Mechanical Complications

Mechanical complications are generally thought to be the second most common reason (after infection) for catheter failure overall but the most common reason during the initial year on PD. The mechanical complications include obstruction of the catheter by omentum, migration of the catheter out of the pelvis, and blockage of the catheter by fibrin or clots. When omental blockage does occur, laparoscopic removal of the involved omentum can typically be easily accomplished.

Migration of the catheter out of the pelvis can lead to either poor dialysate inflow or outflow or pain with dialysis. One approach to repositioning the catheter is through the use of interventional radiology techniques, in which a guidewire is used to move the catheter back to a workable position in the abdomen. Using this technique, Savader et al reported a durable patency rate of 50% was achieved in patients who experienced an early (<30 days) catheter malposition, but the durable patency rate was 82% in patients with late (>30 days) malposition. The complication rate was low (3%), with only a single episode of peritonitis. More recently, preliminary data from the IPPN revealed a recurrence of catheter malfunction within 3 months of repositioning in 15% of subjects. Comparison of success rates from multiple reports is somewhat difficult because of differences in the techniques used and the period of follow-up.

Our center has used a laparoscopic approach to reposition catheters. In patients who have had no previous abdominal procedures besides the peritoneal catheter placement, we create a pneumoperitoneum by insufflating through the malpositioned PD catheter. After a pneumoperitoneum is achieved, a 3-mm port is placed in the left upper quadrant, and a 3-mm laparoscope is inserted. A stab wound is then made in the right upper quadrant, and a 3-mm grasper is inserted. The catheter is then manipulated under direct vision and is repositioned back into the pelvis. Any adhesions that are encountered during the repositioning of the catheter are lysed at the same time. In addition, we have used this technique to free catheters that have become encased in adhesions. This technique avoids a large incision in the peritoneum, thus allowing a rapid return to dialysis.

Catheters that are functioning poorly but have not migrated out of the pelvis can be occluded by either fibrin or a blood clot. Tissue plasminogen activator (tPa) has been shown to be very effective in unblocking these catheters. Two mg of tPa is reconstituted in 40 cc of normal saline and is instilled in the catheter for 1 hour. This has resulted in the restoration of patency in 57% of the catheters.

Exit-Site Infection, Tunnel Infection, and Peritonitis

Catheter ESIs and TIs and peritonitis are a significant cause of catheter failure. In a review of the NAPRTCS data from 1992 to 1997, the incidence of ESIs and TIs increased from 11% at 30 days post catheter insertion to 30% by 1 year after catheter insertion. The Italian PD registry documented catheter infections as the most common catheter-related complication, with a prevalence of 73.2% and an incidence of one episode per 27.4 patient-months.

Whereas the goal in all cases should be prevention of catheter related infection by following published recommendations and by regular monitoring of the catheter with the use of an exit-site scoring system, when an infection occurs, medical management is typically successful. In general, oral antibiotic therapy is recommended. When antibiotic therapy of an ESI is unsuccessful or the infection has been accompanied by a TI, intravenous or intraperitoneal routes for antibiotic therapy should be considered.

Surgical approaches to therapy have included unroofing and cuff shaving. In an additional report, Wu et al have described a technique in which the authors were able to preserve the intraperitoneal portion of the dialysis catheter and simply excise the external infected portion of the catheter. They reported 26 catheter revisions in 23 patients with 100% resolution of the infection without interruption of PD. To date, we have not had to use this technique, but it is intriguing to consider it for patients in whom interruption of PD would be extraordinarily difficult.

The more standard surgical intervention for infection would be complete removal of the catheter when there is refractory peritonitis, fungal peritonitis, or a refractory catheter ESI or TI. Preservation of the peritoneum should always take precedence over preservation of the catheter. In patients in whom the infection is caused by a gram-positive organism and the dialysate white blood cell count is less than 100/mm^3, catheter removal and replacement can occur as a single procedure under antibiotic coverage. In contrast, refractory peritonitis, fungal peritonitis, and gram-negative infections mandate that there be at least a 2- to 3-week interval between catheter removal and reinsertion.

Complications With Peritoneal Dialysis Catheter Removal

An interesting short report by Korzets et al makes the case that the removal of a PD catheter can be associated with significant complications. In their series of 40 catheter removals, 10 (25%) of the procedures were associated with complications (and 8 of these required further surgical intervention). Half of their complications were related to bleeding. Their usual technique was to remove the PD catheters under local anesthesia, which they thought contributed significantly to their complication rate. In children, any permanently placed PD catheter needs to be removed in the OR. The surgeon removing the catheter must be aware of the device type and implant procedure and recognize that the more complex the catheter design, the more difficult the removal. In essence, the removal of a PD catheter is a real operation that requires strict attention to detail to prevent annoying but potentially significant complications that could require a return to the OR.

The peritoneal catheter is the lifeline for the patient receiving PD. Successful peritoneal access requires a comprehensive approach starting with catheter selection through insertion and finally long-term care of the catheter. The establishment of a PD catheter "team" (nephrologist, surgeon, and nurse) that is focused on the management of these patients leads to better long-term experiences for patients and their families.

C H A P T E R 7 9

Prescribing Peritoneal Dialysis in Children

René G. VanDeVoorde III, MD

Peritoneal dialysis (PD) became a more available therapy for children in the 1960s such that it was no longer considered "experimental" by the early 1970s. Further advances have been made in the size of catheters and tubing and the technology of automated cyclers, which has made PD more adaptable to a variety of patient needs. This would seem to make PD a potentially optimal modality for children with end-stage renal disease (ESRD) requiring dialysis because they have different primary etiologies of renal disease, come in different sizes, and have different daily demands. However, despite this relative indication of its use in children, the percentage of pediatric dialysis patients on PD seems to be decreasing in the United States. This chapter hopes to set a framework of considerations when discussing PD as a potential modality for children.

Initiation of Dialysis in Children

Indications for initiating renal replacement therapy (RRT) in children are based on clinical, biochemical, and psychosocial parameters, which should be individualized for each patient. These parameters may vary based on the child's age, as both biochemical norms and the developmental needs of the child can change, as well as the primary etiology of chronic kidney disease (CKD). An infant with renal dysplasia and a serum phosphorus level of 6 mg/dL is desirable, but if the infant is not gaining weight, it is very worrisome. Whereas an adolescent with lupus nephritis would benefit from lower phosphorus levels, weight gain may put them at certain cardiovascular risk. Inappropriate nutrition in children may allow for "normal" laboratory results (e.g., potassium, urea) and manifest not with weight loss but with growth failure. Therefore, a regular global assessment of the child with advanced CKD with particular attention to growth and development is warranted.

Objective criteria for initiation of dialysis in children have been iterated in the most recent Kidney Diseases Outcomes Quality Initiative (KDOQI) guidelines on PD adequacy. KDOQI's recommendation is that dialysis initiation should be considered in pediatric patients when their estimated glomerular filtration rate (GFR) is 15 mL/min/1.73 m^2 or less and recommended in pediatric patients with a GFR of 8 mL/min/1.73 m^2 or less. European guidelines have shared this objective threshold (GFR <15 mL/min/1.73 m^2) for consideration of dialysis.

However, both guidelines recommend that the pediatric patient's clinical course takes precedence over any estimates of kidney function. Initiation of dialysis should be considered at higher GFR levels if the patient has findings or symptoms that are refractory to medication or dietary management. Similarly, dialysis does not have to be started at lower GFR levels if the patient has normal laboratory values and is otherwise asymptomatic. Metabolic disturbances seen in pediatric patients include hyperkalemia, hyperphosphatemia, metabolic acidosis, and azotemia, though normal serum values for potassium are slightly higher for infants and normal values for phosphorus are higher into preadolescence. The clinical findings may include fluid overload, hypertension, malnutrition, and growth failure. Because there is a preponderance of nonglomerular disorders causing ESRD in children, urine output may be preserved, and fluid overload and hypertension, which is almost universally seen in adults with ESRD, may not even occur in some pediatric patients. Growth failure in children can be particularly difficult to detect if not cognizant to its findings. It may manifest with a static weight during a period when a child would normally be gaining, or a decrease in height velocity, a measure unique to children that varies greatly by growth stage. Other symptoms of ESRD in children may include nausea, vomiting, and decreased energy levels. Frank neurologic symptoms of uremia are rare in children but may present with more subtlety such as decreased levels of concentration and attentiveness. Diminished school performance and decreased daily activity levels should be screened as well.

Similar to KDOQI recommendations in adults with CKD, patient and caregiver education about RRT options should occur as the patient advances into stage 4 CKD. The timing of the education should ideally allow the patient and caregivers to decide on a dialysis modality, if needed, and for any advanced access planning. This should include anticipatory planning for other surgeries that may be needed in the pediatric patient, such as feeding tube placement, native nephrectomy, or major urologic procedures. The education should be conducted by a multidisciplinary team, including dialysis nurses, social workers, and dietitians, who may also assess the patient and caregiver's comprehension of the risks, benefits, and demands of the available treatment options. The education should present nonbiased information on hemodialysis (HD), PD, and transplant to the patient and family but unavoidably may be influenced by the experiences of the multidisciplinary team.

Factors to Consider in Modality Choice in Children

When evaluating the dialysis modality options for pediatric patients, it is important to weigh both the medical and social needs of the individual patient. The most recent KDOQI recommendations on dialysis adequacy conspicuously did not list any indications or contraindications for PD in adults, unlike previous versions. However, in the pediatric recommendations, there were still some patients for whom PD is clearly indicated (Table 79.1). Infants and small children can be especially prone to vascular access complications secondary to their small size. Additionally, this same population may require more frequent dialysis than older patients because of their dependence on fluids for nutrition and therefore benefit from a more frequent dialysis modality such as PD. PD is also medically indicated in patients who cannot establish vascular access, receive anticoagulation, or safely tolerate rapid fluid removal. For a pediatric patient who lives far from a pediatric HD center and may not be large enough to dialyze at a local adult center, PD would be indicated to avoid the potential family disruption created by constant travel for regular HD treatments.

The only absolute contraindications to PD in children are conditions that compromise the abdominal cavity (congenital anomalies) or peritoneum (see Table 79.1). The relative contraindications to PD in children include scenarios that

Table 79.1

Indications and Contraindications of Peritoneal Dialysis in Children

Indications
Infants and young children
Hemodynamic instability
Lack of vascular access sites
Contraindications to anticoagulation
Residing long distance from pediatric hemodialysis center

Contraindications (Absolute)
Gastroschisis, omphalocele, or bladder exstrophy
Diaphragmatic hernia
Unsuitable peritoneum because of extensive adhesions or malignancy
Peritoneal membrane failure

Contraindications (Relative)
Lack of adequate caregiver support
Pending abdominal surgery(-ies)
Imminent (<3 months) kidney transplant
Caregiver or older patient preference

may compromise the peritoneum (abdominal surgery), the success of a home therapy (lack of caregiver capability or desire), or the need for long-term treatment (imminent transplant). Other medical conditions that affect the anterior abdominal wall, such as prune belly syndrome or presence of an ostomy (gastrostomy, colostomy, vesicostomy, or ureterostomy), do not preclude consideration of PD. The increased risk of infection in patients with ostomies may be mitigated by appropriate PD catheter placement and vigilant exit-site care. Observational data suggest that PD may also be an acceptable modality in patients who have a ventriculoperitoneal shunt.

After evaluating the patient and caregivers for possible indications or contraindications to PD, any discussion about dialysis modalities should highlight the advantages and disadvantages of PD (Table 79.2). There are no direct comparative studies of PD to HD in children to suggest superiority of one modality over the other, so the critical issue for families often becomes one of quality of life. However, there are some distinct differences in medical outcomes between the two modalities. Similar to the case in adults, residual renal function is better preserved in children receiving PD, which conveys certain benefits in terms of fluid and middle-molecule clearance. Likewise, pediatric PD recipients have lower all-cause mortality than HD patients, which is likely a product of renal function preservation. Cardiovascular morbidity, as measured by hospitalization rates for related complications, is also reduced in children on PD compared with those on HD.

The other distinct, and often cited, advantage of PD is the flexibility it affords as a home therapy option available to children. Because there are options for automated treatments at night, it facilitates regular school attendance in children while also allowing caregivers to work during the day. The greater frequency of treatment, nearly every day (or night), may permit less dietary restriction of fluid or phosphorus. However, these same advantages come at a potential price. The shift of the burden of responsibility to perform treatments from the in-center medical professional to

Table 79.2

Advantages and Disadvantages of Peritoneal Dialysis in Children

Advantages
Preservation of residual renal function
Decreased all-cause mortality and cardiovascular risk
Lower rates of bacteremia and septicemia
Greater daytime patient and family independence (school attendance, parental work schedules)
Tailored prescription to individual patient and family lifestyle preferences
Fewer dietary and fluid restrictions
No need for vascular access and needlesticks

Disadvantages
Higher risk of infections and hospitalizations
Risk of hernia development (≤40%)
Risk of caregiver burnout
Body image disturbances
Greater nighttime restrictions

---

the at-home provider can increase the potential stress on the caregivers and the home environment. Nighttime treatments can be complicated by patient discomfort or machine alarms, keeping both the patient and caregiver awake, and lead to physical fatigue. Additionally, the regimented nature of the modality lends itself to quickly lead to burnout. This, in turn, can lead to poor adherence to infection prevention measures or to even performing treatments themselves. Thus, provider burnout may increase one of the physical risks of PD while also negating one of the modality's advantages.

One of the distinct disadvantages of PD is a higher overall rate of hospitalization and infections. This higher rate of infection has not been directly associated to provider burnout because the rates of access-related infections are reportedly the same between PD and HD in the United States, but most pediatric nephrologists can likely recount anecdotes of when a caregiver recalls a deviation from the PD regimen, subsequently leading to an infectious complication. Because of this potential risk of home provider burnout, a thoughtful evaluation of the patient and family's medical condition, social motivations, existing support system, and physical and economic capabilities by the multidisciplinary team of physician, nurses, social workers, and other health professionals (psychologists, child life specialists) is warranted. An assessment of the home environment should also be considered, if PD is being considered, to confirm the availability of electricity, water, telephone, and physical space to perform treatments safely. Discussions with the caregivers should also acknowledge that chronic PD is merely one form of treatment in the continuum of RRTs, not the "end all, be all," because up to 20% of pediatric PD patients will need to change to HD at some point.

Prescription Components

The prescribing of PD historically has been performed empirically, with family lifestyle and dialysis center preferences often being the predominant determinants.

However, with advances in the size and safety of equipment as well as improved automated technology, there are increased options available with PD so that it may be tailored to the individual patient's needs, such as age, size, and residual renal function, in addition to lifestyle. Thus, the PD prescription should take into account its clinical impact, including overall patient safety, in addition to its psychosocial impact.

The PD alternatives available in children are similar to those in adults, with both manual and automated options. Continuous ambulatory peritoneal dialysis (CAPD) entails manual exchanges during the day with a long dwell occurring overnight to provide continuous solute removal. It has been prescribed to children throughout the world because it is less costly to perform, so it may be preferred for some patients for this reason. CAPD is generally more effective in children with residual renal function. With the advances in connection technology, there is now a reduced risk of infectious complications associated with accessing the PD catheter frequently during the day in CAPD. However, there are limited options to the volumes of PD solution bags, making CAPD difficult in smaller patients who will have more variable fill volumes. Also, the inconvenience of manual exchanges during the day make it less desirable for some patients, which likely contributes to its low usage rate. One North American dialysis registry showed that CAPD was used in only 25% to 30% of all new pediatric PD patients.

Automated PD, in which a cycler performs the exchanges, has been the preferred modality in children because it allows for a variety of treatment options while also minimizing the work of and risk of error by its operator. Modern cyclers have programming options that allow for very small (60-mL) volumes of exchange, low flow rates, concomitant use of different dialysates, and variation in drain volumes. There are three automated options used with most cyclers. Nightly intermittent peritoneal dialysis (NIPD) entails automated exchanges at night without a last fill, so no effective dialysis is done during the day. This lack of a daytime exchange provides less clearance of middle-sized molecules but allows for normal intraperitoneal pressure during the day with less risk of hernias and feelings of fullness, which may be desirable in younger patients who have feeding difficulties. The addition of a last fill converts NIPD to continuous cycling peritoneal dialysis (CCPD), which has greater clearance but also has more protracted exposure of the peritoneum to glucose and increased dialytic losses of amino acids and protein. Tidal PD is a variation of automated PD with incomplete emptying of the peritoneal cavity with each exchange. This can provide more continuous exposure to dialysate but is often used more to alleviate drain pain or abate any mechanical drainage issues.

There are some physiologic advantages of using automated PD in addition to its conveniences. Because exchanges take place at night, while the patient is recumbent, there is recruitment of a greater amount of functional peritoneal surface area, allowing for greater clearance for the volume of dialysate. Additionally, intraperitoneal pressure is lower when lying down than when upright, so there may be better tolerance of fill volumes and possibly less hernia risk.

The determining factors for choice of dialysate solution, fill volumes, and dwell times in pediatric patients are similar to those in adults, with few exceptions. More biocompatible solutions are preferred, if available. Bicarbonate-based dialysate has been associated with less inflow pain and better correction of acidosis compared with lactate-based solutions in children on PD. Solutions with lower glucose concentration are preferred as long as adequate fluid removal is provided. Other osmotic agents, including amino acids and glucose polymers such as icodextrin, have been used in children, although icodextrin is not as effective with fluid removal in younger children compared with older children and adults.

Goal fill volumes in children should be based off the patient's body surface area. In children older than 2 years of age, the recommended fill volume is 1000 to 1200 mL/m^2 per exchange, similar to adults. However, in children younger than 2 years of age, the recommended fill volume is only 600 to 800 mL/m^2 per exchange because the peritoneal membrane surface area is much greater per unit of weight in infants than in adults. Because there is a much higher rate of hernias seen in children, up to 40%, a graduated increase in fill volumes up to the recommended range, while being mindful of this risk, may be conducive in children. The optimal dwell times for children are best determined by evaluating the peritoneal membrane's transport characteristics, such as by the peritoneal equilibration test (PET). Because this evaluation should not be performed until a few months after the initiation of PD, its results will be unknown at the advent of PD but should be sought during the course of therapy.

One aspect of the PD prescription that often gets overlooked and is essential to sustained use of the modality is the training of the home providers. Because PD is a quotidian regimen, it is recommended that a minimum of two caregivers should be trained how to properly perform PD, with expectations that the nonprimary provider(s) regularly place the patient on and off PD to minimize the risk of burnout to the primary caregiver. Children who are the age of assent (11 years of age and older) and developmentally appropriate should participate in their own care and may also be instructed, but the ultimate responsibility of care rests with the adult caregivers. The goals of home PD training are to instruct the caregivers on how to safely perform the procedure and to recognize and treat the complications of PD. There should be overall objectives of the training, but the instruction itself should be tailored to the caregivers' learning needs. The duration of training will vary, based on the learners, but it should allow for ample opportunities to practice and demonstrate the procedures being taught. Prolonged training, as done in some countries, is associated with improved outcomes such as lower infectious complications, so it may be advantageous if the patient's clinical condition would allow for it. The timing of the training can also be critical, but it is preferably done when the patient is not admitted to the hospital to minimize any potential distractions to the caregivers.

Prevalence of Peritoneal Dialysis Use in Children

Worldwide, PD continues to be the most popular dialysis modality in children. Estimates range from 50% to 70% of children receiving dialysis in North America and Europe, with even higher percentages presumed in developing countries, although accurate global demographic data are lacking. Some of this presumption is based off the rapidly expanding number of dialysis patients in developing nations, most of whom are adults, with the growing proportion of these patients receiving PD. However, it is also based off the presumptive costs of dialysis therapy because PD is considerably less expensive than HD, especially in younger children. Chronic PD therapy has been shown to be practiced successfully, although with some regional variation, throughout the world.

Despite several features that would make PD more ideally suited for the pediatric population, recent trends suggest that it is being prescribed less in children and may no longer be the dialysis modality of first choice in the United States. The North American Pediatric Renal Trials and Collaborative Studies (NAPRTCS) registry has collected data on children receiving dialysis at children's hospitals across North America since 1992. Data from its most recent report have shown that the percentage of children receiving PD, compared with HD, in North America has been steadily declining, from 65.3% in 1992 to 55.7% in the years 2008 to 2010. Additionally, United States Renal Data System (USRDS) data have revealed HD to be the most common initial therapy for ESRD in children age 0 to 19 years, and since 1994, it has also been more prevalent than PD in this population. Similarly, Canadian Organ Replacement Registry (CORR) data have shown a steady decrease in the prevalent use of PD in their pediatric ESRD population since the 1990s, but HD prevalence has remained about the same.

The discrepancy between NAPRTCS and USRDS prevalence data potentially reflects some of the differences between pediatric academic institutions and adult dialysis units because it is estimated that 25% of all pediatric dialysis patients receive their care at nonpediatric centers. Therefore, referral to a pediatric-based dialysis unit may increase the use of this modality in a population for which it may be more suited. However, trend data showing less prevalent PD among pediatric institutions are also worrisome that there is less comfort with this modality or a changing demographic of pediatric patients. If it is the former, then perhaps greater education of patients, caregivers, and prescribers may ensure the most appropriate prescribing of this modality in this more ideally suited population.

CHAPTER 80

Nutritional Management of Children Undergoing Peritoneal Dialysis

Rebecca Thomas, MD • Bethany Foster, MD, MSCE

Nutritional management is a key component of the care of children treated with peritoneal dialysis (PD). This includes regular assessment of nutritional status, as well as development and implementation of a dietary prescription. Optimal nutritional management requires collaboration among the child, the caregivers, a renal dietitian, and other members of the multidisciplinary pediatric nephrology team. The goals are to achieve normal growth, development, and body composition and to avoid the complications associated with malnutrition. Although growth failure is recognized as one of the distinctive features of children with chronic kidney disease (CKD), it is not inevitable. Adequate growth is achievable and is a good indication of adequate nutrition over the long term. Because height has an important impact on self-esteem and perceived quality of life, normal final adult height should be the goal for all children.

It is useful to consider both the patterns and drivers of growth in healthy children when approaching children treated with PD. The infancy phase of growth is dominated by nutrition, the childhood phase by growth hormone, and the pubertal phase by sex hormones. Children with CKD may have disturbances in all of these factors, including a delay in the transition from the infancy phase to the childhood phase (which results in a slower than normal growth velocity). In infancy, poor caloric intake caused by anorexia is the main contributor to growth impairment, but energy intakes for older children with CKD are usually normal relative to size. A much larger proportion of the daily energy requirement is devoted to growth in infants than in older children. Poor appetite may result from a combination of factors, including thirst for water rather than food, administration of unpleasant medications, disordered gastric motility, and dysregulation of appetite-regulating cytokines and hormones.

It is important to note that not all abnormalities in growth and body composition in children treated with PD are related to inadequate nutrition. Other factors may also play a role in the wasting—or "cachexia"—that may occur in CKD, including systemic inflammation, endocrine perturbations, and abnormal neuropeptide signaling.

Assessment of Growth and Nutritional Status

Growth Parameters

The recommended frequency of assessment of growth and nutritional status depends on the age of the child (Table 80.1) and should be individualized according to clinical status. On average, growth assessment should be done twice as often in children

Recommended Parameters and Frequency of Nutritional Assessment for Children With Stages 2 to 5 and 5D Chronic Kidney Disease

Measure	Minimum Interval (Months)		
	Age 0 to <1 Year	Age 1–3 Years	Age >3 Years
Dietary intake	0.5–2	1–3	3–4
Height or length for age percentile/SDS	0.5–1	1	1–3
Height or length velocity for age percentile/SDS	0.5–1	1–2	6
Estimated dry weight and weight for age percentile/DS	0.25–1	0.5–1	1–3
BMI for height age percentile/SDS	0.5–1	1	1–3
Head circumference for age percentile/SDS	0.5–1	1–2	1–3

BMI, body mass index; SDS, standard deviation score.

Adapted, with permission, from National Kidney Foundation. KDOQI Clinical Practice Guideline for Nutrition in Children with CKD: 2008 Update. *Am J Kidney Dis.* 2009;53(suppl 2, recommendation 1, table 1):S16

with CKD compared with healthy children. Basic measurements include weight for age, stature for age (recumbent length in children younger than 24 months, standing height for those older), and head circumference (in children 3 years and younger). It is recommended that the World Health Organization (WHO) growth charts be used as a reference from birth to 2 years because these standards represent ideal growth (which should be the goal for children with CKD). After age 2 years, there is minimal difference between the U.S. Centers for Disease Control and Prevention (CDC) reference curves and WHO growth standards. Calculation of body mass index (BMI) is useful to see if the child's weight for height places him or her in an at-risk category (underweight, overweight, or obese). When plotting BMI relative to age in a child with growth or maturational delay, this may result in inappropriate underestimation of his or her BMI compared with peers of similar height and developmental age. This problem can be avoided by expressing BMI relative to height age rather than chronologic age in children with CKD. Height age is the age at which the child's height would be at the 50th percentile. Although the primary focus of nutritional assessment in children on PD has been typically been to identify undernutrition, it is important to note that more recently evidence has shown that obesity is an emerging problem.

Weight assessment can be challenging in children on PD because of changing volume status. "Dry weight" (i.e., euvolemic weight) should be estimated based on blood pressure, presence of edema, response to ultrafiltration, and serum albumin. The volume of the daytime dialysate dwell must be subtracted from the measured weight.

Dietary Intake

Information about dietary intake provides useful indices of nutrient quantity and quality. It is important to estimate total daily intake of calories, macronutrients (carbohydrate, protein, and fat), vitamins, and minerals. The most clinically feasible methods of determining usual dietary intake are the prospective 3-day dietary diary and the retrospective 24-hour recall (done three times, one weekend day + two weekdays). The retrospective 24-hour recall, although limited by its inability to capture the day-to-day variability in intake, may be more suitable for adolescents, in whom underreporting is common with 3-day dietary histories. A skilled dietitian will consider the following in a comprehensive dietary history.

Feeding history includes information on who is involved with preparation and offering of food (supervised or unsupervised child vs primarily from caregivers); how the food is prepared; how the feed is delivered (e.g., enteral feeding devices, oral); how frequent feeds are (daytime or nighttime); and any oral aversions, swallowing difficulties, or reflux or vomiting.

Elements of the *diet history* include any dietary or fluid restrictions, compliance with these restrictions, and appetite changes affecting intake.

Other important clinical information includes urinary output, usual body weight (and trends), food stability (capacity of family to afford feeds consistently), level of activity, and current dialysis prescription (may impact nutritional requirements based on glucose concentration of dialysis fluids and intake; e.g., early satiety because of daytime dwell volumes).

Physical Examination

A thorough physical examination is an important part of the nutritional assessment. The hydration status, presence or absence of edema, and blood pressure can provide useful guides as to the true dry weight. Signs of nutritional deficiency should be noted. The skin may be dry with excess flaking and uneven pigmentation, and the hair may be brittle, dry, and easily shed. Angular cheilosis and stomatitis, hepatomegaly, and certain neurologic abnormalities may each point to vitamin deficiencies. Genu deformities of the limbs, thickened wrists, costochondral beading (the rachitic rosary), and thickening of the wrists may point to vitamin D–deficient rickets.

Adequacy of Dialysis

It is important to remember that inadequate dialysis may result in poor appetite, nausea, deranged biochemical indices, hypertension, and edema. Dialysate clearances of urea normalized to total body water (Kt/V_{urea}) and the creatinine (CCr) normalized to body surface are measures of dialysis adequacy. Target Kt/V is at least 2.1 to 2.2 per week. Studies in children treated with hemodialysis (HD) showed that catch-up growth was achievable when higher than standard doses of HD were used ($Kt/V > 2.0$ per treatment). It is not known whether enhanced PD clearance would also result in better growth; achieving clearances much higher than recommended would be very difficult with PD because of limitations in feasible hours of treatment and fill volumes.

Dietary Prescription

Energy

Energy requirements for children treated with PD should be considered to be 100% of the estimated energy requirements for chronologic age. Children younger than 3 years old with length- or height-for-age standard deviation score below −1.88 and failing to achieve expected weight gain and growth when receiving estimated energy requirements for chronologic age should be prescribed an energy intake relative to height age. Estimated energy requirement calculations should be individualized (Table 80.2) and take into consideration the child's level of physical activity (Table 80.3) and the calorie contribution from PD fluid.

A balance of calories from carbohydrate and unsaturated fats within the physiologic recommended ranges is suggested (Table 80.4).

Table 80.2

Equations to Estimate Energy Requirements for Children at Healthy Weights

Age	EER (kcal/d) = Total Energy Expenditure + Energy Deposition
0–3 mo	EER = (89 × Weight [kg] − 100) + 175
4–6 mo	EER = (89 × Weight [kg] − 100) + 56
7–12 mo	EER = (89 × Weight [kg] − 100) + 22
13–35 mo	EER = (89 × Weight [kg] − 100) + 20
3–8 y	Boys: EER = 88.5 − 61.9 × Age (y) + PA × (26.7 × Weight [kg] + 903 × Height [m]) + 20
	Girls: EER = 135.3 − 30.8 × Age (y) + PA × (10 × Weight [kg] + 934 × Height [m]) + 20
9–18 y	Boys: EER = 88.5 − 61.9 × Age (y) + PA × (26.7 × weight [kg] + 903 × Height [m]) + 25
	Girls: EER = 135.3 − 30.8 × Age (y) + PA × (10 × weight [kg] + 934 × Height [m]) + 25

EER, estimated energy requirement; PA, physical activity coefficient

Reprinted with permission from Equations to Estimate Energy Requirements for Children at Healthy Weights, Dietary Reference Intakes for Energy, Carbohydrate, Fiber, Fat, Fatty Acids, Cholesterol, Protein, and Amino Acids (macronutrients), 2005. By the National Academy of Sciences, Courtesy of the National Academies Press, Washington, D.C.

Table 80.3

Physical Activity Coefficients for Determination of Energy Requirements in Children Ages 3 to 18 Years

	Level of Physical Activity			
Gender	Sedentary	Low Active	Active	Very Active
	Typical ADLs only	ADLs + 30–60 min of daily moderate activity (e.g., walking at 5–7 km/h)	ADLs + ≥60 min of daily moderate activity	ADLs + ≥60 min of daily moderate activity + an additional 60 min of vigorous activity *or* 120 min of moderate activity
Boys	1.0	1.13	1.26	1.42
Girls	1.0	1.16	1.31	1.56

ADLs, activities of daily living.

Accepted Macronutrient Distribution Ranges

Macronutrient	Children 1–3 Years	Children 4–18 Years
Carbohydrate	45%–65%	45%–65%
Fat	30%–40%	25%–35%
Protein	5%–20%	10%–30%

Lipids
In children and adolescents on PD therapy, reported rates of dyslipidemia vary from 29% to 87%. Given the high risk of CVD in children with CKD, nutritional counseling should suggest use of sources of unsaturated fat rather than saturated or trans fats, and when possible, to choose complex carbohydrates over simple sugars. Both primary and secondary prevention studies provide strong evidence that the consumption of fish and fish oils rich in EPA (eicosapentaenoic acid) and DHA (docosahexaenoic acid) reduces cardiovascular disease morbidity in adults. There are, however, safety concerns, including prolonged bleeding times, difficult glycemic control in patients with diabetes, and environmental contaminants in fish oil products. At this time, there is inadequate evidence to recommend routine use of omega-3 fatty acids to treat hypertriglyceridemia in children with CKD.

Fiber
Dietary fiber is found in most vegetables, fruits, and whole grains, which may be restricted in low potassium and phosphorus diets. Meeting dietary fiber recommendations may thus be more difficult in patients with CKD when intake of these foods is limited. Constipation may lead to technical problems with PD; therefore, when dietary intake does not suffice, fiber should be added via the various mineral and electrolyte-free powdered forms of fiber available (e.g., Benefiber).

Protein
Protein requirements vary with age (Table 80.5) and may be higher during recovery from an acute illness (e.g., peritonitis) and in children with proteinuria. Peritoneal permeability for protein shows large interpatient variability but can be assessed in each patient by calculating daily PD protein losses. Peritoneal protein losses decrease with age from an average of 0.28 g/kg in the first year of life to less than 0.1 mg/kg in adolescents. The recommendation from the 2008 Kidney Disease Outcomes Quality Initiative (KDOQI) guidelines refers to stable children on PD.

Many meat-based protein sources contain significant amounts of phosphate; this should be calculated in the daily phosphate intake. The use of protein supplements to augment inadequate oral intake should be considered in children on PD who are unable to meet requirements through their regular diet alone.

In adults treated with PD, dietary protein intake can be estimated by determination of the protein equivalent of nitrogen appearance (PNA), calculated by measuring the urea nitrogen content of urine and dialysate and multiplying by a constant (6.25 – The number of grams of protein per 1 g of nitrogen). In children, body size–adjusted

Table 80.5

Recommended Dietary Protein Intake in Children With Stage 5D* Chronic Kidney Disease

Age	Recommended Intake (g/kg/day)
0–6 mo	1.8
7–12 mo	1.5
1–3 y	1.3
4–13 y	1.1
14-18 y	1.0

*In children younger than 3 years or children with stunted growth (length/height for age <−1.88 standard deviation score [SDS]), protein requirements should be estimated initially using chronologic age but may be reestimated using height age if there is suggestion of inadequate protein intake.

Adapted, with permission, from National Kidney Foundation. KDOQI Clinical Practice Guideline for Nutrition in Children with CKD: 2008 Update. *Am J Kidney Dis.* 2009;53(suppl 2, recommendation 5, table 12):S49

formulas to estimate PNA have also been developed but are not in common use. There are concerns about their validity in highly anabolic or catabolic states. However, similar concerns exist with the use of PNA in adults. Theoretically, PNA should provide an objective estimate of protein intake in children similar to in adults.

Calcium and Vitamin D

Normal skeletal development depends on adequate calcium intake and normal metabolism. In CKD, multiple factors contribute to impaired calcium homeostasis. These include decreased intestinal absorption of calcium as endogenous production of calcitriol (1.25-dihydroxyvitamin D) declines, decreased spontaneous calcium intake, and decreased vitamin D receptor expression. Intestinal calcium absorption may be boosted by increasing calcium intake (diet or tube feeds and calcium-containing phosphate binders) and by supplementation with α-calcidiol or calcitriol. Calcium salts should be taken between meals and separately from iron supplementation to achieve maximum effects. The calcium content of dialysis fluids may also affect calcium load.

Although negative calcium balance is initially the main concern in children on PD, excess supplementation may result in vascular and other soft tissue calcification. It is therefore recommended to limit total oral and/or enteral calcium intake (Table 80.6). This may include use of non–calcium-containing phosphate binders in children with elevated calcium–phosphate product.

It is suggested that serum 25-hydroxyvitamin D levels be measured at least yearly. If the serum level is below 30 ng/mL (75 nmol/L), the child should be supplemented with ergocalciferol (vitamin D_2) or cholecalciferol (vitamin D_3). After commencement of or alteration in vitamin D doses, serum levels should be repeated in 1 month.

Phosphate

The recommended intake of phosphate for patients on PD with elevated parathyroid hormone (PTH) but serum phosphate concentration in normal reference range is

Table 80.6

Recommended Calcium Intake for Children With Chronic Kidney Disease

In milligrams of elemental calcium per day (mg/day)

Age	DRI	Upper Limit (Healthy Children)	Upper Limit Stage 5D CKD (Dietary + Phosphate Binders)
0–6 mo	210	Not determined	≤420
7–12 mo	270	Not determined	≤540
1–3 y	500	2500	≤1000
4–8 y	800	2500	≤1600
9–18 y	1300	2500	≤2500

CKD, chronic kidney disease; DRI, Dietary Reference Intake.

Adapted, with permission, from National Kidney Foundation. KDOQI Clinical Practice Guideline for Nutrition in Children with CKD: 2008 Update. *Am J Kidney Dis.* 2009;53(suppl 2, recommendation 7, table 20):S61

Table 80.7

Recommended Maximum Oral and Enteral Phosphorus Intake for Children With Chronic Kidney Disease

Age	DRI (mg/d)	Recommended Phosphorus Intake (mg/day)	
		High PTH and Normal Phosphorus	High PTH and High Phosphorus
0–6 mo	100	≤100	≤80
7–12 mo	275	≤275	≤220
1–3 y	460	≤460	≤370
4–8 y	500	≤500	≤400
9–18 y	1250	≤1250	≤1000

PTH, parathyroid hormone.

© All rights reserved. Dietary Reference Intakes. Health Canada, 2005. Adapted and Reproduced with permission from the Minister of Health, 2016.

100% of the Dietary Reference Intakes (DRI) for age for healthy children. Serum phosphate levels should be evaluated in conjunction with serum calcium and PTH levels (Table 80.7). In children on PD, the target range for PTH is two to three times that of healthy children (or ≈200–300 pg/mL). If both the serum PTH and serum phosphate are above the recommended reference ranges, then reducing dietary phosphorus intake to 80% of the DRI is suggested. Elevated phosphate levels can stimulate hyperparathyroidism and defects in bone mineralization and bone resorption. Subnormal serum phosphate levels should also be avoided because rickets may occur as a result in infants and children.

Micronutrients: Vitamins and Trace Elements

Micronutrients are essential components of a balanced diet and contribute to adequate growth and development in children. Children with CKD are at risk of micronutrient deficiencies because of inadequate intake, poor gastrointestinal absorption, and abnormal renal metabolism. Those on PD are at increased risk of deficiency from dialysis-related losses. Target intake for micronutrients is in general 100% of the DRI. The KDOQI guidelines (2008) recommend the administration of a water-soluble vitamin supplement.

Fluids and Electrolytes

Fluid and electrolyte requirements vary based on primary kidney disease, residual kidney function, and renal replacement therapy modality.

Fluid

On average, 80% of an individual's total water intake is derived from drinking water and the other 20% from food. Children with oliguria or anuria should limit their daily fluid intake to avoid complications of volume overload (most notably hypertension). Attempts at fluid restriction may be futile if salt (± sugar) intake is not simultaneously restricted. High sodium intake will lead to increased extracellular fluid (ECF) osmolality, which will then stimulate thirst.

Daily fluid restriction = Insensible fluid losses + Urine output − Amount to be deficited.

(This calculation should also take into account a reasonable expected amount of daily weight gain.)

Sodium

Children with polyuria (usually secondary to obstructive uropathy and renal dysplasia) will have polydipsia and a salt-wasting state. Sodium wasting results in volume depletion and impaired growth (as sodium supports normal expansion of the ECF volume needed for muscle development and mineralization of bone). Infants on PD may also experience substantial sodium losses via dialysate, even when anuric, because of the large peritoneal membrane surface area for body weight. Infants on PD should have sodium balance calculated and sodium supplementation considered.

Children on PD with hypertension (systolic or diastolic pressure ≥95th percentile or prehypertension (systolic or diastolic blood pressure ≥90th percentile and <95th percentile) may require sodium restriction as part of a comprehensive strategy for volume and blood pressure control. Restriction of sodium is usually within the range of 1 to 2 mmol/kg/day but should be individualized. Measures to decrease salt intake include:

1. Consuming fresh instead of canned or processed foods
2. Reducing or eliminating salt added to foods at the table
3. Substituting fresh herbs and spices for salt when cooking
4. Decreasing fast food intake
5. Avoiding, when possible, medications with high sodium content (e.g., antacids, laxatives, nonsteroidal antiinflammatory drugs, sodium polystyrene sulfonate).

Potassium

The vast majority of potassium excretion occurs via urinary losses; only about 10% occurs through intestinal losses. When the kidney loses its ability to filter potassium, limiting dietary potassium becomes an integral part of management of

CKD. The risk of hyperkalemia can also be increased by acidosis, urinary obstruction, medications (angiotensin receptor blockers, angiotensin-converting enzyme inhibitors, potassium-sparing diuretics), hemolysis (blood transfusions and tumor lysis), and urinary obstruction. Both hyper- and hypokalemia cause alterations in skeletal, myocardial, and smooth muscle contractility, and cardiac arrhythmias may result.

Some children on continuous PD may actually develop hypokalemia. For this subgroup, potassium may need to be supplemented orally or via addition to dialysis fluids.

Carnitine

L-carnitine has an important role in the regulation of fatty acid metabolism and adenosine triphosphate (ATP) formation in various organs. It is a biologically active amino acid derivative that may be deficient in children on HD, and some data support L-carnitine supplementation in this population. Far less information exists on the relationship between PD and carnitine deficiency. There is insufficient evidence to conclude that carnitine supplementation is required in the PD population; further studies are needed.

Delivery of Nutrition

Supplemental nutritional support, preferably by the oral route, should be given to children on PD whose usual energy intake fails to meet requirements resulting in suboptimal growth or weight gain for age. If oral supplementation fails, nasogastric or gastrostomy tube feeding should be considered. The schedule of tube feeding (top-up boluses versus overnight continuous gavage) and the formula will depend on age, significant gastroesophageal reflux, and nutrient requirements. The majority of infants on PD will require tube feeding. In the relatively rare situation in which an older child requires tube feeding, it may be beneficial to have the majority of tube feeds overnight to encourage daytime hunger and oral intake and allow for normalization of daytime activities. Gastrostomy tube feeding has some advantages over nasogastric tube feeding such as decreased risk of gastroesophageal reflux and of maxillary and nasal inflammation, less social stigma (because the gastrostomy is not visible), and avoidance of negative oral stimulation. There is no evidence of increased bacterial or fungal peritonitis in children with established gastrostomy tubes (ideally placed before PD catheter placement).

Use of Recombinant Human Growth Hormone Therapy

The growth hormone–insulin-like growth factor 1 (IGF-1) axis is an important regulator of growth and metabolism. Abnormalities in this axis resulting in growth hormone resistance have been noted in children with CKD. These abnormalities include decreased expression of the growth hormone receptor, impaired signal transduction of the growth hormone receptor, decreased production of IGF-1, and decreased activity of IGF by inhibitory IGF-binding proteins. Clinical studies support the efficacy of recombinant human growth hormone therapy in patients on PD. Earlier treatment results in better response. Recombinant human growth hormone therapy should be considered if growth failure (height velocity for age standard deviation score (SDS) <−1.88 or height velocity for age <third percentile)

persists beyond 3 months despite treatment of nutritional deficiencies and metabolic abnormalities. Linear growth targets should take into account the genetic predisposition via midparental height calculations.

Summary

The nutritional assessment of children on PD is a complex process that must be individualized. Frequent monitoring and dietary modifications may be necessary. With a team approach including a dietitian, nephrologist, renal nurses, parents or other caregivers, and patients, normal growth patterns can be achieved.

CHAPTER 81

Peritoneal Dialysis in Neonates and Infants

Joshua J. Zaritsky, MD, PhD • Bradley A. Warady, MD

Introduction

Peritoneal dialysis (PD) has long been considered an effective treatment modality for neonates and infants with severe acute kidney injury (AKI) and is the dialysis modality of choice for patients in this age group with end-stage renal disease (ESRD). Its popularity and success largely derive from its simplicity and effectiveness as a means of removing solute and fluid in even the smallest patients, and because it is a well-tolerated procedure by most patients.

Peritoneal Dialysis as a Renal Replacement Modality for AKI

There is limited literature documenting the etiology of AKI that results in the need for acute PD in this population. However, some generalizations can be made. In most cases, congenital malformations such as renal dysplasia or posterior urethral valves do not compromise kidney function so severely that dialysis is required in the newborn period. Instead, acquired renal disorders, usually related to perinatal asphyxia, hypoxia, sepsis, or hypovolemia make up the majority of insults that mandate acute replacement therapy. Very rarely, acute vascular events such as renal artery or renal vein thrombosis are to blame, but these insults usually have to affect both kidneys to result in AKI requiring dialysis.

Despite the growing popularity of continuous renal replacement therapy (CRRT), survey results of pediatric nephrologists provide evidence that PD remains the predominant acute dialysis modality for children <2 years of age. Access can be placed emergently at the bedside in patients who are too unstable to undergo a surgical procedure. Additionally, PD can typically be performed safely and effectively in patients with cardiovascular instability as a result of the inherent gradual and continuous provision of both ultrafiltration and solute clearance characteristic of the procedure. Finally, PD offers the additional advantage of not requiring systemic anticoagulation, in contrast to hemodialysis (HD) and CRRT.

There are rare absolute contradictions to PD in neonates such as omphalocele, diaphragmatic hernia, or gastroschisis, all scenarios in which there is essentially the lack of a functional peritoneal cavity. Relative contraindications to PD include the presence of severe pulmonary disease since the increased intraabdominal pressure associated with PD could further compromise pulmonary function, or a history of extensive abdominal surgery because of the possible presence of adhesions and a compromised peritoneal cavity. The presence of a vesicostomy or colostomy, or the diagnosis of polycystic kidney disease is not a contraindication to PD, although the risk of peritonitis may be greater in this setting. With these issues in mind and given the lack of prospective trials comparing the outcomes of neonates and infants with AKI stratified by dialysis modality, the decision regarding dialysis modality selection always needs to factor in local resources and expertise along with the patient's clinical status.

Peritoneal Dialysis Access in AKI

The two most commonly placed accesses for acute PD are the percutaneously placed Cook catheter and the surgically placed Tenckhoff catheter. The Cook catheter offers the advantage of bedside placement by a nephrologist or intensivist via the Seldinger technique. Because only local anesthesia is required, it can be placed promptly, even in an unstable patient. However, its use has been associated with a high rate of complications, such as leakage of dialysis fluid from the catheter entry site on the abdominal wall and catheter obstruction. Chadha et al in a single-center retrospective study of infants and young children with AKI found that by day 6 of dialysis, only 46% of Cook catheters were functioning without complications. In comparison, they found that more than 90% of surgically placed Tenckhoff catheters were free of complications at the same time point. Thus, the authors suggested that if acute dialysis is expected to be required for more than 5 days, a Tenckhoff catheter should either be placed initially or elective replacement of the Cook catheter with a Tenckhoff catheter can be performed in a timely manner. Subsequently, the same center reported promising results with the use of a multipurpose percutaneous catheter (Cook Mac-Loc Multipurpose Drainage catheter) in a small cohort of infants with AKI who experienced a mean complication-free catheter survival of approximately 11 days. This catheter continues to be used with good success at one of the author's centers; additional data on this experience are forthcoming.

The most important consideration for the successful placement and function of a Tenckhoff catheter in this population is the experience of the surgeon. This can be particularly problematic at centers caring for a small number of patients overall, where the need to provide dialysis to a very young infant may be a rare event. Because of the importance of the access and the desire for the outcome of placement to be complication free, the surgical placement should be limited to only a few surgeons per center; on rare occasion, it may be preferable to refer the patient to another, more experienced center for access placement, in a manner similar to what has been recommended for vascular access.

Prescription Considerations for AKI

In the acute setting, the prescription of PD is guided by the need for low dialysate fill volumes to prevent dialysate leakage and to keep the intraperitoneal pressures as low as possible to avoid any respiratory embarrassment. Typically, initial dialysis fill volumes for neonates/infants should be approximately 10 mL/kg body weight (300 mL/m^2) and are increased as clinically warranted and tolerated. Because these low volumes result in a rapidly diminished dialysate osmotic gradient and resultant limited ultrafiltration, dwell times of 1 hour or less are frequently used. Dwell times as short at 20 minutes have also been used in neonates when rapid removal of small solutes is desired. Despite the inefficiency introduced by using low dialysate volumes, adequate solute clearance and ultrafiltration rates can be achieved if exchanges are performed around the clock. Golej et al reported a case series of 116 neonatal and pediatric patients who underwent low-volume PD in whom the mean ultrafiltration rate was 2.8 mL/kg/hour. A negative fluid balance was accomplished in 53% of patients, despite the presence of hemodynamic instability in a majority of the subjects. Several patients who presented with hyperkalemia and metabolic acidosis did require the use of higher dwell volumes to adequately control the biochemical abnormalities.

In extreme cases of hyperphosphatemia or hyperammonemia, continuous-flow PD (CFPD) has been employed. CFPD requires placement of two intraperitoneal catheters, with one catheter used for influx and another for efflux of dialysate. In this manner, the transport potential of the peritoneal membrane is maximized by maintaining the highest possible solute concentration gradient. Dialysate flow rates of up to 300 mL/hour in patients as small as 3 kg have been described using this technique.

The lower dialysate fill volume employed in the neonate generally necessitates the use of manual exchanges early in the course of PD, in contrast to an automated cycling device. Advantages of manual exchanges include the low expense and technical simplicity. Neonatal or PICU nurses can be trained to perform manual exchanges, which avoids the need for a dialysis nurse to continuously supervise therapy. Indeed, the combination of simplicity, low cost, and efficacy makes PD with the use of manual exchanges in the neonatal setting an attractive option for centers with limited resources. There are several commercially available manual exchange sets (Baxter, Deerfield, IL; Fresenius, Waltham, MA; Gesco International, San Antonio, TX; Medionics International, CA; Utah Medical Products, Midvale, UT), which minimize the risk of contamination and allow for the warming of dialysate before it is instilled into the patient.

In contrast to manual exchanges, there are automated cyclers that permit the accurate delivery of a fill volume as low as 60 mL, with low-flow drainage modes to avoid unnecessary alarms (Home Choice Pro, Baxter). Practically, automated peritoneal dialysis (APD) can be performed using the cycling device without a substantial recirculation volume in the dialysis tubing when the fill volume is more than 100 mL. The volume of fluid within the dialysis tubing of a "low volume" set is approximately 19 mL.

Standard commercially available dialysis solutions are employed in the acute setting with the choice of dextrose concentration (1.5%, 2.5%, or 4.25%) driven by the need for ultrafiltration. The choice of PD solutions is also largely dependent on their availability in different regions of the world. In the United States, only lactate-buffered solutions are available, whereas bicarbonate-buffered solutions, which are presumably more biocompatible, are available in Europe and other geographic regions. Lactate-based solutions should be avoided in neonates/infants with severe acidemia as lactate needs to be converted by the liver to the effective base.

The Chronic Setting: ESRD

Peritoneal Dialysis as a Renal Replacement Modality for ESRD

Many of the same considerations that favor PD as a renal replacement modality for AKI apply in the setting where long-term dialysis is needed. The high rates of both infectious and mechanical complications of HD when provided to the youngest infants makes its use over long periods of time impractical in most situations. For patients receiving HD for extended periods of time, access revision rates for young infants are estimated at 40%. Couple these issues with recognition that long-term HD access in a neonate or infant consists of a central venous catheter, a practice that is accompanied by a significant potential for stenosis of central veins and the resultant inability to create a fistula in the future for patients who face a lifetime of ESRD care, and one can fully understand the preferential selection of PD as the chronic dialysis modality of choice for neonates and infants.

Chronic PD is particularly advantageous compared with HD for the neonatal/infant patient for reasons other than access. Meeting the nutritional needs of neonates can be challenging, especially with the severely oliguric/anuric patient who must receive formula volumes as high as 150 mL per kg of body weight per day. The relative ease with which the fluid status can be managed with PD on a daily basis precludes the fluctuations of body volume and, potentially, blood pressure inherent to intermittent HD. Multiple studies have also suggested that better growth rates can be achieved in patients on PD compared to HD. Recent data from the North American Pediatric Renal Trials and Collaborative Studies (NAPRTCS) do show improvements in height SDS scores at 24-month follow-up of patients who initiated PD at less than 1 year of age, whereas SDS scores remain unchanged for those on HD. Finally, PD promotes gradual expansion of the abdominal cavity in preparation for successful renal transplantation. This takes on added importance when one considers that parents of these young children often serve as living donors and mandate the need to insert an adult-sized kidney into a recipient who may have a body weight of only 10 kg.

Peritoneal Dialysis Access for ESRD

Long-term PD mandates the surgical placement of a Tenckhoff catheter. As in the setting of AKI, the most important consideration for its successful placement and function in the neonate and infant with ESRD is the experience of the surgeon. If complications such as dialysate leakage are to be avoided, placement of the catheter 2–3 weeks before its eventual use is ideal so that there is an opportunity for ingrowth of the Dacron cuffs of the catheter into surrounding tissues. The provision of fibrin sealant at the peritoneum as a means of achieving a tight closure when a delay in PD initiation is not possible has been practiced. Additional considerations in the chronic setting are the orientation of the subcutaneous tunnel of the catheter, the exit-site orientation and location, the potential need for an omentectomy and timing of placement with respect to concurrent or future placement of a gastrostomy tube (G-tube).

Observational data from the NAPRTCS suggest that Tenckhoff catheters with a downward-pointed exit site are associated with the best peritonitis rates, a characteristic (along with the possible preference for two cuffs) that should be considered for all chronic PD catheters placed in neonates and infants because of the increased rates of peritonitis they experience compared with older children. The catheter exit site should also be placed outside of the diaper area and away from any potential ostomy site (eg, on the right side of the abdomen for any patient in whom G-tube insertion is possible) with the superficial cuff located approximately 2 cm from the skin surface. Occasionally, this necessitates placement of the exit site on the chest wall. Given the small size of the neonatal/infant patient, these requirements can be difficult to accommodate and, as noted above, require a very skilled and experienced surgeon.

As suggested above, one additional unique consideration in this age group is the timing and location of catheter placement relative to G-tube placement in order to accommodate nutritional requirements (see below). The catheter exit site should ideally be placed at a distance (often the contralateral side) from the site of a current or potential gastrostomy to decrease the risk of contamination and possible peritonitis. Likewise, it is recommended that when possible, the PD catheter be placed either simultaneously with or after placement of a G-tube to avoid contamination of the peritoneum from gastric contents and the possible development of peritonitis. When the catheter placement precedes G-tube placement, the latter procedure should take place under prophylactic antibiotic and antifungal therapy.

Prescription Considerations in ESRD

Historically, the prescription of PD in infants was based on the perception that the pediatric peritoneal membrane, especially in infants, had different solute transport properties than that of an adult. This was in large part based on the results of early studies in which dialysis fill volumes were based on body weight. When scaled to body weight, the surface area of the infant peritoneal membrane is almost twice that of a 70-kg adult. Thus, the use of weight-based volumes results in a relatively low fill volume, which in turn, results in more rapid solute equilibrium and the inaccurate perception of an inherent increased solute transport capacity. In contrast, the provision of a fill volume in young children scaled to body surface area (BSA) takes into consideration the age-independent relationship of BSA to peritoneal surface area and makes possible the accurate assessment of membrane transport capacity during the performance of a peritoneal equilibration test (PET). Indeed, when Warady et al based fill volumes on BSA, the peritoneal membrane transport capacity in children was similar across the pediatric age range and to adults.

Whereas it is important to prescribe the fill volume scaled to BSA to optimize solute equilibration and ultrafiltration, it is equally important not to provide too large a fill volume that may lead to an excessive increase in intraperitoneal pressure (IPP) (>18 cm H_2O). The latter development can result in reduced dialysis efficiency because of enhanced lymphatic uptake, in addition to poor tolerance by the patient. Accordingly, the recommended maintenance fill volume for patients below age 2 years is limited by patient tolerance and is generally 600–800 mL/m^2. This is in contrast to a volume of approximately 1100–1200 mL/m^2 that is recommended for older children and adolescents. As mentioned earlier, a smaller, manually delivered volume is typically used when the neonate is started on dialysis and is progressively increased to the limits noted above.

In the chronic setting, an initial empiric dwell time of 1 hour is often used in infants, although consideration has to be made for clearance of larger molecules that would be favored by longer dwell times. Phosphate removal is less of a consideration in these patients compared with older children, as neonates and infants characteristically receive formula with a low phosphorus content or breast milk and may actually require supplemental phosphorus. As in older children and adults, the final determination of dwell time should take into account the characteristics of the individual's peritoneal membrane via standardized testing of solute transport capacity (peritoneal equilibration testing), as well as clinical and laboratory measures of dialysis adequacy.

As in the acute setting, the choice of PD solutions is largely dependent on their availability. Despite the lack of firm data, there is a concern that the standard lactate-buffered solutions with glucose may have negative consequences on long-term membrane performance because of their low pH and the presence of glucose degradation products (GDPs). Given that these patients have many years of ESRD therapy in their future, the use of the new, more biocompatible dialysis solutions may prove to be particularly beneficial to the pediatric patient population. Data in neonates and young children on the subject are very limited. (See Canepa et al for a recent review.)

Icodextrin (Extraneal), a colloidal osmotic agent that is employed in place of dextrose, is available in the United States in contrast to other new solutions, but is rarely used in infants. Whereas Boer et al showed that in 11 children (median age 10.3 years) a 12-hour exchange with 7.5% icodextrin produced ultrafiltration comparable to a 3.86% dextrose solution, Dart et al reported poor ultrafiltration in very young children (median age 2.8 years) with its use. This poor efficacy was due to enhanced absorption of icodextrin across the peritoneal membrane with half of the patients showing substantial absorption, even when dwell times were reduced from 10 to 6 hours. van Hoeck also noted that the use of a long exchange with icodextrin could place a child into a negative amino acid balance.

It can be difficult to precisely determine the efficiency or "adequacy" of dialysis with chronic PD in children. Although small molecule clearance measurements in the form of urea kinetic modeling (Kt/V_{urea}) are widely used, it must be emphasized that the current National Kidney Foundation K/DOQI guidelines on PD adequacy, which recommend a total Kt/V_{urea} of ≥1.8 for children, are largely opinion based. Because a large, prospective study correlating solute removal and clinical outcome in pediatric patients treated with PD has not been conducted, care must always be taken to individualize therapy, even in cases of "adequate" or even high urea clearance. This is particularly true for the neonatal/infant patient population. Parameters that should be taken into consideration include linear growth and weight gain, increase in head circumference, and neurocognitive/psychomotor development.

An additional qualitative target of dialysis adequacy in the neonate and infant are the avoidance of hypovolemia and sodium depletion. Infants receiving PD experience excessive sodium losses across the peritoneal membrane because of the need for high ultrafiltration rates in relation to body weight. Both breast milk and standard formulas contain 7–8 mmol of sodium per liter, which is inadequate for replacement of ongoing losses. Without adequate supplementation (≈3–5 mEq/kg/day), the consequences of the resultant hyponatremia and low intravascular volume can be catastrophic and include both blindness due to anterior ischemic optic neuropathy and cerebral edema. Finally, both sodium and protein losses can have a negative impact on growth. Specifically, neonates and infants can experience excessive losses of protein via PD with studies demonstrating average losses of 250 mg of protein per kg of body weight or almost twice the peritoneal protein losses seen in older children. In order to avoid the negative consequences of protein depletion, current guidelines recommend a dietary protein intake of at least 1.8 g/kg/day for the first 6 months of life, taking into account the dietary reference intakes (DRIs) and peritoneal losses. Of note, protein losses can be higher with the use of alternative PD regimens such as tidal PD.

Outcome in ESRD

Even with surgically placed Tenkhoff catheters, chronic catheter survival remains suboptimal. Data from the Italian PD registry reported a 50% 1-year catheter survival rate in patients less than 6 months of age and an 83.7% 1-year catheter survival rate for those 6–24 months of age. Infectious complications including exit-site infections and peritonitis also occur at a higher rate in neonates and infants. Although peritonitis rates for patients 0–2 years of age have improved from a rate of 1 to 0.79 episodes per patient-year over the last decade, they remain higher than the annualized rate of 0.6 seen in older children.

Most importantly, whereas mortality data have improved in children on dialysis over the past few decades, the highest mortality rates are seen in those patients who receive PD during the first year of life. The most recent NAPRTCS results, based on data collected from 2000 to 2012, shows a 3-year overall patient survival of 82.5% for patients who initiate dialysis during the first year of life. In comparison, children aged 2–5 years at dialysis initiation have a higher overall survival of 92% at 3-year follow-up, and those older than 12 years have a survival rate of nearly 95%. Data from four separate international registries show a slightly lower survival rate for those patients who initiate dialysis within the first month of life, with 2- and 5-year survival rates of 81% and 76%, respectively. What persists, however, is the finding that the most important predictor of mortality in this PD patient age group remains the presence of nonrenal disease. Wood et al clearly showed that comorbidities such as anuria and pulmonary hypoplasia were associated with the greatest risk of mortality in infants undergoing dialysis. A recent publication of the IPPN examining 1830 patients aged 0–19 years found that the presence of at least one comorbidity was associated with a 4-year survival of 73% versus 90% in those without a comorbidity ($p < .001$). Data on the influence of comorbidities on survival are likely impacted by regional differences, because countries with a lower gross national income appear to be more restrictive in terms of making PD available to very young patients and those with significant extrarenal complications.

Conclusion

The last two decades have witnessed tremendous advances in the care of the neonate/infant requiring renal replacement therapy. Peritoneal dialysis, because of its simplicity and effectiveness, remains a popular modality for neonates with severe AKI and is the dialytic modality of choice when treating neonates/infants with ESRD. There have been notable improvements in patient survival, although complications remain high, especially in those infants with comorbidities. All of these issues highlight the need for a multifaceted approach to care to minimize or prevent complications and in turn promote growth, development, and readiness for transplant.

C H A P T E R 8 2

Dialysis in Inborn Errors of Metabolism

Euan Soo, MBBS, MRCPCH, FHKAM (Paed), FHKCPaed, PDipMDPath • Franz Schaefer, MD, PhD

Inherited dysfunction of amino and organic acid metabolism usually manifest in the early neonatal period by neurologic abnormalities such as irritability, somnolence, and, eventually, coma. In urea cycle defects or in organic acidemias, these symptoms are mainly due to excessive hyperammonemia, which may cause irreversible neuronal damage. In disorders of branched-chain amino acid metabolism such as maple syrup urine disease (MSUD), prolonged accumulation of leucine and/or its metabolites (2-ketoisocaproic acid) may lead to severe permanent neurotoxicity.

During the past three decades, the prognosis of these previously lethal disorders has been considerably improved by the introduction of several therapeutic principles.
1. The de novo synthesis of toxic metabolites can be suppressed by a high caloric supply inducing a state of anabolism and reduced proteolysis.
2. In hyperammonemic disorders, new medications that utilize alternative metabolic pathways to reduce neurologic effects. These include sodium benzoate, sodium phenylbutyrate, carbaglutamate, and various vitamins and cofactors.
3. Specific dietary modifications such as a diet low in branched-chain amino acids in MSUD.
4. Finally and most importantly, the accumulation of the small, water-soluble neurotoxic metabolites can be rapidly reversed by dialytic removal.

Because the brain damage induced by neurotoxic metabolites is directly correlated with the duration of exposure to the neurotoxic metabolites, neonatal metabolic crises are considered emergency dialysis indications requiring use of the most readily available and effective dialysis modality.

Currently available dialytic regimens include
- Peritoneal dialysis (PD)
- Intermittent hemodialysis or hemodiafiltration (IHD/IHDF)
- CRRT (including CAVH, CVVH, CAVHD, CVVHD)

A large body of experimental and clinical evidence suggests that the clearance achievable by PD is much less than that obtained by HD. Historically, HD machines were not created for patients weighing less than 15 kg, which meant that for this unique population group, machines were often difficult to use, required large-bore central venous access, and were operated solely off-label. Because technological advances have improved the suitability of extracorporeal blood purification techniques for neonates, they are now the therapy of choice in appropriately equipped and experienced centers. In 2012, the Cardio-Renal Pediatric Dialysis Emergency

Machine (CARPEDIEM) was designed and has successfully performed CRRT for infants less than 3 kg. It offers the advantage of extracorporeal dialysis, as well as additional advantages of smaller venous access down to 4 Fr, without sacrificing clearance or causing hemolysis. In addition, the accurate flow monitoring provides benefits to patient safety, though large-scale randomized controlled trials are not available to demonstrate advantages in survival neurological sequelae.

Although extracorporeal dialysis remains the treatment of choice, PD remains an alternative in cases where extracorporeal dialysis is contraindicated. To improve clearance rates in PD, continuous-flow PD has been introduced as a method to more effectively dialyze neonates, though it is still not a mainstream technique used.

Techniques of Metabolite Removal

In patients with *MSUD*, the low endogenous clearance of leucine and other branched-chain keto and amino acids (BCAA) is insufficient to reverse the accumulation of BCAA that occurs during catabolic states. BCAA clearances several times above the endogenous disposal rate are achieved with PD, and continuous extracorporeal blood purification techniques yield two- to threefold greater metabolite removal rates than PD. Although CVVH, CVVHD, and CVVHDF have all been shown to be feasible, only HD has demonstrated a significant reduction of dialysis time requirements in comparison to PD.

In *hyperammonemic* metabolic crises, experimental evidence suggests that ammonium is more efficiently removed by extracorporeal techniques than by PD. Clinical studies have shown that normalization of blood ammonium levels usually cannot be achieved in less than 24 hours by PD, and dialysis is typically required for 2–5 days. CVVH usually reduces blood ammonium concentrations by 90% within 10–12 hours. The most efficient toxin removal method is clearly achieved by CVVHD. The superiority of CVVHD over CVVH is evident from the fact that ammonium clearance with CVVH cannot be greater and is usually considerably less than the *plasma* flow rate through the dialyzer. In contrast, an ammonium clearance close to dialyzer *blood* flow can be achieved by CVVHD, as shown in Fig. 82.1.

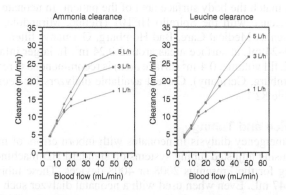

Figure 82.1

Effect of Blood and Dialysate Flow Rate on Ammonium and Leucine Removal by Hemodialysis in a Neonatal Setting.

IHD reliably decreases blood ammonium concentrations by 75% within 3–4 hours. However, repeated sessions are frequently required because of residual or rebound hyperammonemia. Moreover, the use of IHD in neonates and young infants is usually limited by the size of the extracorporeal volume and the rapid depletion of other small solutes such as phosphate. Hence, CVVHD until complete normalization of blood ammonium levels should be considered the treatment of choice when very high dialysate flow rates can be ensured. When not possible, a combination of first IHD followed by CVVHD as maintenance therapy is recommended.

Extracorporeal Blood Purification

Dialysis Equipment

Catheter
The choice of catheter has to draw a balance between the aim of achieving an adequate blood flow and the risks of catheter insertion in a newborn. Ideally, a blood flow of 150 mL/min/m^2 should be attained, that is, 30–35 mL/min in the mature neonate. This goal can be reached by inserting a 6.5-Fr double-lumen catheter (eg, Gambro 6.5 Fr, 3.5 inch) into the internal jugular or a femoral vein. This catheter size provides excellent blood flow rates (ie, 30–40 mL/min), but insertion may be difficult in small neonates. Alternatively, two 5-Fr single-lumen catheters (eg, Medcomp 5 Fr, 3.0 inch) can be inserted in different femoral or jugular veins. Although umbilical catheters are unsuitable for dialysis because of their high flow resistance, 6.5-Fr hemodialysis catheters have occasionally been inserted into an umbilical vessel in neonates within the first few postnatal days.

4-Fr double-lumen catheters have been used successfully with the CARPEDIEM machine (see later) to dialyze infants of less than 3 kg body weight. However, the efficacy of the system for ammonia clearance has not yet been reported.

Dialyzer
Polysulfone dialyzers are preferred because of their superior biocompatibility and lower anticoagulation requirements. The surface of the dialyzer membrane should approximately match the body surface area of the patient. In neonates, we have had excellent experience with the Spiraflo HFT02 (Bellco, Mirandola, Italy) and the FX-Paed (Fresenius Medical Care, Bad Homburg, Germany) filter, which have fill volumes of 19–24 mL at surface areas around 0.24 m^2. In larger infants, the Fresenius F3 (28 mL fill volume, 0.4 m^2 surface area) is recommended (Fresenius Medical Care, Bad Homburg, Germany). Current available dialyzers for neonates are summarized in Table 82.1.

Dialysis Device and Tubing
In principle, emergency dialysis in neonates with inborn errors of metabolism can be performed using adjusted tubing systems on standard HD machines, such as the neonatal tubing for the Fresenius 2008 or 4008 devices. These tubing sets have a fill volume of 47 mL. Even when used with a neonatal dialyzer such as the Spiraflo HFT02, the total volume of the extracorporeal system is 72 mL, which exceeds 10% of the estimated blood volume of an average neonate. Another disadvantage is that an incorrect blood flow rate is displayed when small-volume neonatal tubes are used. Moreover, as a result of the fixed high dialysate flow rate of 300–500 mL/min,

Table 82.1

Commercially Available Filters for Neonatal CRRT: Main Characteristics

Filter	Manufacturer	Surface (m²)	Membrane	Priming (mL)
Miniflow 10	Gambro-Lundia	0.045	AN69	3.5
Minifilter	Minntech	0.07	Polysulfone	6
CARPEDIEM 1	Bellco	0.075	Polysulfone	27.2 (circuit)
CARPEDIEM 3	Bellco	0.245	Polysulfone	41.5 (circuit)
HF20	Gambro-Lundia	0.20	AN69	60 (circuit)
FX-paed	Fresenius	0.2	Polysulfone	18

critical depletions of phosphate, amino acids, and other solutes not present in the dialysis fluid may occur with prolonged use of this technique.

Devices designed for continuous renal replacement treatment are better suited for acute dialysis in children. When considering the choice of a device in a neonate, the extracorporeal volume and accurate flow controls are important. Given the small blood volume of small neonates, volumes larger than 10% estimated blood volume (80 mL/kg) require circuit priming with blood. With very low flow rates, the percentage of error of a few milliliters per minute can be disastrous and cause unforeseen fluid overloading or shock. Current available devices are compared in Table 82.2.

Anticoagulation

Heparin has traditionally been the anticoagulant of choice, and the doses required are at 1000–2000 E/m² with a continuous infusion of 400 E/m²/h during dialysis. Activated coagulation times (ACT) of 140–200 s are targeted, monitoring it hourly. With the further increased risk of intraventricular hemorrhage in small neonates, regional citrate anticoagulation (RCA) has become a popular choice to anticoagulate the circuit. In order to set it up, a separate central venous line is required for calcium substitution. Our center is currently using a 3% ACD-A solution and a 10% calcium gluconate solution as the calcium substitute. Care must be taken not to replace the calcium via the postfilter circuit as this can lead to circuit clotting. Initial formulae to calculate rates of citrate and calcium replacement are as follows:

$$\text{Citrate flow rate (mL/h)} = \text{blood flow rate (mL/min)} \times 2$$

$$\text{Calcium flow rate (mL/h)} = \text{blood flow rate (mL/min)}/4$$

The target ionized calcium levels are 0.20–0.30 mmol/L (0.8–1.2 mg/dL) in the postfilter circuit and within the normal range for a patient 1.1–1.3 mmol/L (4.4–5.2 mg/dL). Adjustments of 25% are made when the calcium levels are not within target levels with rechecking after 5–10 minutes of adjustment. Care must be noted that adjustments will more likely be needed in the neonatal circuits because of the increased circuit citrate required consequent to blood priming and also immaturity of the liver function due to the age and the metabolic disease.

Table 82.2

Main Commercially Available Monitors for Pediatric and Neonatal CRRT: Main Characteristics

Monitor	Manufacturer	Pediatric Lines	Neonatal Lines	Total Extracorporeal Volume (mL)[a]	Blood Pump Range (mL/min)	Blood Flow Step-by-Step Increase (mL/min)	Fluid Turnover Range (mL/h)
Prismaflex	Gambro-Lundia	Y	–	60	20–100	2	50–2500
Multifiltrate	Fresenius	Y	–	72	10–100	2	10–7000
Aquarius	Baxter	Y	–	82	10–200	2	50–11,000
Plasauto Sigma	Asahi	Y	Y	70–87	1–400	1	10–12,000
CARPEDIEM	Bellco	Y	Y	27–42	2–50	1	10–300

[a]Prismaflex equipped with HF20 circuit. Others with FX-Paed.

Management Guidelines

To achieve maximal treatment efficacy, blood flow should be set to the maximal value operated by the machine without stimulating alarms, which should be set as wide as possible. The dialysate flow rate required to achieve maximal clearance is determined by the blood flow rate achieved. In a neonatal dialysis simulation study using a Spiraflo HFT02 filter, we found a linear relationship between blood flow and ammonium and leucine clearance up to the maximal blood flow rate usually achievable in neonates (ie, 30 mL/min) with a dialysate flow rate of 5 L/hour (see Fig. 82.1). As a rule of thumb, extraction of these metabolites is maximal when dialysate flow exceeds blood flow by at least a factor of two. This target can easily be achieved by passing bag dialysis fluid along the filter utilizing the filtration/substitution pump system of a pediatric CRRT device equipped for high dialysate flow rates, such as the Asahi Sigma Plasauto. If only CRRT devices with lower maximal dialysate flow rate are available, an initial period of intermittent HD with 300-mL/min dialysate flow rate should be provided, optionally switching to CVVHD or CVVH once ammonium levels have decreased to a less toxic range. The dialysis fluid should contain glucose and potassium at plasma concentrations and serum phosphorus levels should be monitored closely.

During treatment, dialysis efficacy can be monitored by measuring metabolite clearance using the formula:

$$\text{Clearance (mL/min)} = \text{blood flow (mL/min)} \times (C_{pre} - C_{post})/C_{pre},$$

where C_{pre} and C_{post} are the pre- and postdialyzer metabolite blood concentrations.

The major complications to consider when dialyzing neonates or small infants with metabolic crises are clotting of the extracorporeal system and hemodynamic instability, each of which can cause treatment interruptions and hence hazardous delays in the removal of toxic metabolites. To prevent this, heparin or RCA are recommended as described previously.

To prevent clotting, heparin should be administered at a dose sufficient to increase the ACT to 120–150 seconds. We use an initial bolus of 1500 IU/m² followed by continuous infusion of 300–600 IU/m²/hour. Anticoagulation should be monitored by hourly ACT measurements. Coagulation requirements are inversely related to the blood flow rate.

Hypotensive episodes and osmotic dysequilibrium occur less frequently than in neonates and infants dialyzed for renal failure, because dialysis is usually isovolemic and the accumulated metabolites are osmotically less active than the urea accumulated in uremia. However, hemodynamic instability is common in patients with prolonged duration of hyperammonemia because of urea cycle disorders but can be minimized by prefilling the system with blood and using appropriate extracorporeal tubing and dialyzer membranes with a total fill volume as small as 35 mL.

Whereas heating of dialysis fluids and bloodlines is generally required in neonatal dialysis to prevent hypothermia, therapeutic cooling to 34°C core temperature has been applied successfully to attenuate ammonia generation in neonates with metabolic crises. Whether this novel therapeutic concept will result in reduced dialysis need and improved outcomes remains to be proven.

HD should be continued until clinical improvement and complete normalization of the accumulated metabolite levels (ammonium, leucine) have been achieved. Because unknown amounts of pharmacologic scavengers are cleared by highly efficient extracorporeal blood purification, supplemental doses of these substances may be required during or after IHD.

Peritoneal Dialysis

Because of the lower toxin clearance, peritoneal dialysis is generally not recommended and should only be considered when extracorporeal techniques are prohibited by vital sign contraindications or technical limitations.

Catheter

Stylet catheters can be placed immediately but bear a high risk for the subsequent development of leakage or outflow obstruction. Catheter leakage requires a reduction of dwell volumes or catheter replacement, and outflow obstruction may result in an increased intraperitoneal residual volume, both causing a further decrease of the peritoneal clearance. Thus, careful catheter insertion is a prerequisite for successful PD, and a slight delay for surgical implantation of a single-cuff Tenckhoff catheter may be justified.

Dialysis Prescription

Prescription of fill volumes must be balanced between maximizing toxin removal and adverse effects of increased intraperitoneal pressure (respiratory problems, catheter leakage). Fifteen to 30 mL/kg body weight appears to be an adequate compromise. Short dwell times (30–60 minutes) increase metabolite clearance but also ultrafiltration rates. The use of bicarbonate-buffered dialysate solutions, commercially available in many countries, may help to stabilize acid–base balance and prevent lactic acidosis in neonates.

CHAPTER 83

Neurocognitive Functioning in Children Undergoing Dialysis

Divya G. Moodalbail, MD, • Stephen R. Hooper, PhD

Chronic kidney disease (CKD) is defined as structural or functional abnormality of the kidneys leading to slow and progressive worsening of kidney function that is typically irreversible. CKD is a major public health problem worldwide. The reported prevalence of CKD in children is anywhere between 15 and 74.7 cases per million. Children with CKD are at significant risk for morbidity, mortality, school failure, and decreased quality of life, along with grave danger for development of kidney failure by the third decade of life. End-stage renal disease (ESRD) is advanced kidney disease requiring some form of renal replacement therapy, either dialysis or renal transplant. In 2008, the incidence of ESRD in children within the United States was as high as 15 per million.

This chapter provides a detailed accounting of the empirical literature devoted to a key area that has been increasingly related to CKD over the past several decades, that is, neurocognitive functioning in pediatric CKD, with a particular focus on dialysis. Major databases (PsychLit, MEDLINE, WorldCat, ArticleFirst, PubMed, Ovid MEDLINE) were searched. Designated search terms included *neurocognition* AND *chronic kidney disease, neurocognition* AND *dialysis, cognitive functioning* AND *kidney disease,* and *neurodevelopment* AND *chronic kidney disease.* The chapter reviews eight studies published since 1990 that address neuropsychological functioning in children with CKD, with special attention being devoted to the impact of dialysis on cognitive functioning. We conclude the chapter by providing suggestions that might help achieve better understanding of this significant complication of kidney disease in children.

Cognitive Function in Pediatric Chronic Kidney Disease

Similar to other chronic conditions, studies of children with CKD suggest increased risk for developmental delays, particularly for toddlers and children with ESRD. About 25% of young infants and toddlers with CKD have reported global developmental delays, with the severity of neurocognitive deficits being greater in those with earlier age of onset of CKD, prolonged duration of CKD, and presence of other comorbid medical conditions. Because much cognitive development and learning occur during childhood and early adolescence, it is critical to investigate conditions that have a negative impact on these functions.

Moodalbail et al provided a recent review highlighting a dozen published neuroradiology studies linking cognitive deficits and affective disorders with CKD. These studies documented presence of brain atrophy, cerebral density changes, white matter hyperintensities, and changes consistent with cerebrovascular disease such as cerebral microbleeds, silent cerebral infarction, and cortical infarction in patients with CKD. Similarities in regional cerebral blood flow between patients with CKD and those with affective disorders were noted as well. This comprehensive review reinforced the notion that children with CKD are at significant risk for incurring neurocognitive difficulties, if not impairment, and that there may be multiple neurologic underpinnings to these difficulties that could be linked to kidney disease.

Dialysis and Its Effects on Neurocognition

When compared to the typically developing population without a chronic disease, children with ESRD, despite optimal management, are known to have cognitive impairments. In patients on dialysis, presence of hypertension, anemia, suboptimal nutrition, microvascular disease, and seizures are known to negatively affect neurocognitive performance. Additionally, for those children with CKD who progress to dialysis, a variety of adverse neurocognitive outcomes have been reported. These include lower intellectual functioning, executive functioning deficits, memory and attention problems, and associated learning difficulties and developmental difficulties. In particular, infancy is a vulnerable period associated with rapid development and growth of the nervous system and, hence, infants on dialysis therapy are the ones with greatest risk for disruption of their development, perhaps resulting in delay or impairment.

Various studies spanning the past three decades have reported significant associations between neurocognitive dysfunction and ESRD, with some studies reporting developmental delays in up to 65% of infants with ESRD. Earlier studies from the 1970s and 1980s reported neurotoxicity and associated neurocognitive effects such as seizures, encephalopathy, and speech delays with use of aluminum-containing phosphate binders in children on dialysis. By 1990, treatment regimen was modified for dialysis patients in order to eliminate aluminum and aluminum-containing medications from the standard practice in dialysis. In that regard, the use of erythropoietin since the early 1990s has improved anemia management in ESRD and reduced anemia-related cognitive deficits in this patient population.

Types of Dialysis and Their Impact on Cognition

For patients with ESRD, the three primary treatment options are hemodialysis (HD), peritoneal dialysis (PD), and kidney transplantation. The HD procedure involves perfusion of blood and dialysate on opposite sides of a semipermeable membrane which results in removal of substances from the blood by diffusion and convection. Ultrafiltration removes excess free water. The peritoneal dialysis (PD) procedure involves instillation of dialysate into the peritoneal cavity via a peritoneal catheter. The peritoneal membrane acts as the semipermeable membrane across which diffusion and ultrafiltration occur, which, in turn, facilitate the removal of substances from the blood. Ultrafiltration and fluid removal are both achieved via an osmotic pressure generated by various concentrations of dextrose or icodextrin. Although dialysis is a necessary medical treatment in patients with ESRD, emergent data also have begun to show the potential negative impact of these dialysis procedures on cognitive functioning. As can be seen in Table 83.1, there have been a number of studies examining the neurocognitive functioning of children and adolescents receiving some form of dialysis.

Table 83.1

Cognitive Functioning in Children and Adolescents With End-Stage Renal Disease (ESRD) on Hemodialysis or Peritoneal Dialysis

Author/Date	Sample Description	Study Design	Test to Assess Cognitive Function and Ability	Main Findings
Davis et al (1990) (CKD with conservative management, dialysis combined)	Total n = 37 children (M 25, F 12) undergoing primary transplant evaluation Mean age at transplant 17.6 ± 7.1 months (range, 6–30 months) 20 on dialysis at pretransplant evaluation 17 managed conservatively at pretransplant evaluation	Longitudinal prospective testing before and after renal transplantation	Bayley Mental Development Index or Stanford–Binet Intelligence Quotient	Mental Developmental Index improved from pretransplant (mean ± SD, range: 77.0 ± 21.3, 50–116) to posttransplant (mean ± SD, range: 91.4 ± 20.6, 50–117) Psychomotor Developmental Index improved from pretransplant (mean ± SD, range: 68.7 ±11.7, 50–86) to posttransplant (mean ± SD, range: 85.6 ± 15.5, 65–109)
Fennell et al (1990) (CKD with conservative management, HD, PD, Tx combined)	56 CKD patients 27 conservative management 7 HD 12 CAPD 10 Tx 56 age-, sex-, and race-matched healthy controls Mean age at testing 13.4 years Mean age of onset of CKD 6.5 years Mean duration of CKD 8.4 years	Longitudinal study with repeat testing at 6-month intervals for up to 4 testing periods	A series of neuropsychological tests designed to measure cognitive function	Visuomotor skills: poor visuomotor performance in CKD patients Immediate recall or short-term memory: decreased in CKD Learning: decreased in CKD Verbal ability: decreased in CKD Attention: no differences between CKD and controls

Continued

| Table 83.1 |

Cognitive Functioning in Children and Adolescents With End-Stage Renal Disease (ESRD) on Hemodialysis or Peritoneal Dialysis—cont'd

Author/Date	Sample Description	Study Design	Test to Assess Cognitive Function and Ability	Main Findings
Lawry et al (1994) (CKD with conservative management, HD, PD, Tx combined)	Total n = 24 children 11 CKD patients 5 HD 3 CCPD 1 CAPD 2 CKD 13 transplant patients	Cross-sectional study to assess cognitive function and ability in CKD patients in comparison with transplant recipients	WJ-R standardized achievement test that measured mathematics, reading, and written language achievement in relation to school performance WISC-R and WAIS-R for measurement of verbal and performance abilities	Transplant patients did better on achievement tests of written language ($p = .04$) and in school performance in English compared with dialysis patients ($p < .05$)
Hulstijn-Dirkmaatt et al (1995) (CKD with conservative management, HD, PD combined)	Total n = 31 children (M 18, F 13) Mean age: 2.5 years (range 0.3–5.0 years) at the first assessment 15 CKD with conservative management (mean age 29.2 ± 19.0 months) 16 dialysis, CAPD/HD (mean age 31.0 ± 17.8 months)	Longitudinal, prospective 3-year study with repeated measurements	Bayley Developmental Scales (mental scale only) and McCarthy Developmental Scales (verbal, perceptual-performance and quantitative scales, respectively)	Overall study population DI (mean 78.5, SD 19.5) delayed compared with normal population (mean 100, SD 16) CAPD/HD group DI (mean 67.6, SD 17.3) delayed when compared to CKD group (mean 90.3, SD 14.3), $p = .001$

Study	Sample	Study type	Tests	Results
Mendley and Zelko (1999) (CKD with conservative management, HD, PD combined)	Total n = 9 children (M 5, F 4) Pre-Tx modality 5 PD, 3 HD, 1 conservative Mean age at pre-Tx testing: 14.2 ± 3.5 years Mean age at post-Tx testing: 15.8 ± 3.8 years Mean age at onset of ESRD: 11.7 ± 2.2 years Mean duration of ESRD prior to Tx: 3.44 ± 2.9 years	Pre- and Post-Tx repeat measures	Repeatable tests before and after Tx: PASAT, Stroop Color-Word Naming Test, Buschke Selective Reminding Test, Meier Visual Discrimination Test, Grooved Pegboard test, WISC-III or WAIS-R	Reaction time: mental processing speed improved 1 year post-Tx ($p = .008$) Memory: working memory improved 1 year post-Tx ($p = .016$) Attention: sustained visual attention improved 1 year post-Tx ($p = .039$)
Brouhard et al (2000) (Dialysis and Tx combined)	62 ESRD patients Mean age: 13.7–60.44 years 26 on dialysis and 36 transplant 62 sibling-controls Mean age: 13.7–60.38 years	Cross-sectional, multicentric study	Standardized achievement and intelligence quotient (IQ) tests WRAT used to measure achievement in domains of spelling, reading, and arithmetic	Patients with significantly lower average IQ percentile than their siblings (31 ± 4 vs 44 ± 5, respectively; with normal = 50). Patients with lower achievement test scores than their siblings (spelling: 88.7 ± 4 vs 94.6 ± 2; arithmetic: 88.5 ± 2 vs 94.0 ± 2; reading: 91.9 ± 2 vs 100 ± 3). Increased time on dialysis predicted lower scores on achievement tests.

Continued

Table 83.1

Cognitive Functioning in Children and Adolescents With End-Stage Renal Disease (ESRD) on Hemodialysis or Peritoneal Dialysis—cont'd

Author/Date	Sample Description	Study Design	Test to Assess Cognitive Function and Ability	Main Findings
Warady et al (1999) (PD only)	Total n = 28 children who started PD ≤3 months of age All patients on calcium carbonate phosphate binder 27 of 28 were on supplemental nasogastric tube feeds	Retrospective single-center study	Formal neurodevelopmental evaluation	24 of 28 (86%) patients received their initial kidney transplant at a mean age of 2.1 ± 0.8 years Mental developmental scores: i) At 1 year of age: 22 of 28 (79%) patients in average range; 1 (4%) child was significantly delayed ii) Retesting at ≥4 years of age, 15 of 19 (79%) in average range; 1 (5%) in impaired range. iii) Retesting at ≥5 years of age, 15 of 16 (94%) attended school full time and in age-appropriate classrooms

| Ledermann et al (2000) and Madden et al (2003) (PD only) | Total n = 16 children on CAPD or CCPD (M 14, F 2) Mean age at PD initiation: 0.34 year (range, 0.02–1 year) Mean duration of PD: 17.3 months (range, 1–59 months) | Retrospective single-center study | Age-appropriate psychometric measures Griffiths Mental Development test if ≤6 years of age) WISC-R if ≥7 years of age Strengths and Difficulties Questionnaire to test psychological adjustment | Development: 25% school-age children with general developmental delay (attributed to perinatal asphyxia) 25% children <5 years of age had general delays Cognition: IQ: 67% in average range, 87% in low average range. Mean IQ 86.5 (range 50–102). Psychological adjustment: 50% of the children in borderline/abnormal category for psychological difficulties Attention: 50% with hyperactivity problems Social-behavioral: 43% displaying conduct problems |

ESRD, end-stage renal disease; F, female; HD, hemodialysis; M, male; PASAT, Paced Auditory Serial Addition Test; PD, peritoneal dialysis; SDQ, Strengths and Difficulties Questionnaire; Tx, transplant; WJ-R, Woodcock-Johnson–Revised; WISC-III, Wechsler Intelligence Scale for Children–Third Edition; WISC-R, Wechsler Intelligence Scale for Children–Revised; WAIS-R, Wechsler Adult Intelligence Scale–Revised.

Findings in Infants and Toddlers

In infants and toddlers, mental and motor developments, as components of overall development, are used to assess neurodevelopmental status. In their prospective study, Hulstijn-Dirkmaatt et al compared the cognitive development of 15 toddlers with CKD on conservative management to 16 children with ESRD on dialysis (patients on PD or HD combined). Although both the groups had a lower Developmental Index (mean = 78.5, SD = 19.5) compared with the normal population (mean = 100, SD = 16), children with CKD had a significantly higher Developmental Index compared with dialysis-dependent children (mean = 90.3, SD = 14.3). In a retrospective single-center study, Lederman et al evaluated development in children who started PD as infants. General developmental delay was noted in two of eight (25%) young children, and hyperactivity was described in 50% of the patients. Warady et al retrospectively reviewed the cases of 28 children who started PD during early infancy and noted that 21% (6 of 28 children) had below average mental development when tested at 1 year of age, with 1 child being severely delayed. Based on these studies, it appears that general developmental delay can be seen in as many as 20%–25% of dialysis-dependent children below 5 years of age, and that ongoing developmental surveillance of infants, toddlers, and preschoolers receiving dialysis should be a part of their standard of care.

Findings in Older Children and Adolescents

In older children receiving dialysis, a similar pattern of findings has emerged. Davis et al conducted neuropsychological testing of 37 children with CKD before and after renal transplantation; 20 (55%) of these children were on dialysis at pretransplant evaluation, and the rest were managed conservatively. No significant difference was noted in mean developmental (mental and psychomotor) scores between patients undergoing dialysis and those not undergoing dialysis at the time of testing (mean = 78.8, SD = 18.9, vs mean = 80.4, SD = 14.6, respectively). However, significant improvements in cognitive and psychomotor functions were noted following successful renal transplantation. Significant individual improvement in occipitao frontal head circumference standard deviation score also was noted in 24 children after renal transplantation (p <.001). The investigators concluded that successful renal transplantation earlier in life in children with CKD can result in improved brain growth, along with significant improvements in cognition and psychomotor function.

A series of neuropsychological tests were administered in 56 patients with CKD (all treatment modalities combined, of whom 12 were on PD and 7 were on HD) and 56 age-, race-, and gender-matched healthy controls. Compared with healthy controls, the CKD group had poor visuomotor performance with decreased recall, short-term memory, learning, and verbal abilities. The investigators reported no differences in measures of sustained attention between children with CKD and matched healthy controls. However, mean cognitive test scores were reported for the CKD group as a whole (all treatment modalities combined) with no information available on scores for the dialysis group. Conversely, Mendley and Zelko documented longitudinal improvements in sustained visual attention (pretransplant mean = 2.19, SD =1.29 vs posttransplant mean = 2.95, SD = 1.33, p = .04), decision speed (pretransplant mean = 2.28, SD = 0.72 seconds vs posttransplant mean = 1.64, SD = 0.31 seconds, p = .008), and working memory, 1 year posttransplant in a group of nine children with CKD. All treatment modalities were combined in this study, with about 90% of the CKD patients being managed on dialysis (five of nine patients on PD, three on HD), whereas one was managed conservatively and received pre-emptive renal transplant.

Lawry and colleagues reported lower IQ and achievement test scores in children and adolescents with CKD when compared to age- and gender-matched patients with renal transplant. The investigators reiterated the importance of regular cognitive and achievement testing for children with CKD so that the areas of deficit can be addressed early on by the schools. Brouhard et al compared standardized achievement and IQ test scores in 62 ESRD patients (dialysis and transplant combined) and their sibling controls. Approximately 42% (26 patients) of the sample were on some form of dialysis therapy. The ESRD patients had significantly lower average IQ percentiles and lower achievement test scores than their siblings. Additionally, increased time on dialysis was a predictor of lower scores on achievement tests. The investigators concluded that patients' lower academic achievement could be due to underlying kidney disease, lower intelligence, and school absences.

Summary and Conclusions

For those children with kidney disease who progress to dialysis, a variety of adverse neurocognitive outcomes have been reported. Based on the literature review as noted in Table 83.1, lower intellectual functioning, executive functioning deficits, memory and attention problems, and associated learning difficulties have been reported in children on dialysis. These findings are important in that they indicate the presence of significant risk for cognitive difficulties or impairments for children receiving dialysis. What is not known, however, is the genesis of these difficulties or whether one form of dialysis may create more risk than another. The studies reviewed for this chapter point to key needs in the literature, particularly with respect to teasing out the differential impact of dialysis modalities on cognitive functioning in children. The studies also point to the strong possibility of increased risk of cognitive difficulties for younger children who may require dialysis; however, this developmental concern also requires further study.

From a clinical perspective, the studies reviewed clearly suggest the presence of general developmental delays, with rates up to 25% of dialysis-dependent children below 5 years of age. Clinically, this observation stresses the importance of tracking developmental milestones regularly in infants, toddlers, and preschoolers receiving dialysis as part of their standard of care. Along with the nephrology team, a multi-disciplinary approach involving developmental specialists, such as a clinical psychologist and a developmental pediatrician, is critical in order to identify and address cognitive issues early on in these patients. For older patients, the need for detailed neuropsychological assessment also may be in order as part of their standard of care. Although the studies reviewed comprised children receiving different types of dialysis and, generally, relatively small sample sizes, there was a consistent trend across all of the studies for the findings to suggest the presence of cognitive delays or impairments. As children with CKD begin to move into the range of ESRD severity, it would be important for regular surveillance of their neurocognitive status to occur, particularly once a dialysis modality is necessary.

Despite the initial findings produced from this literature, there are a number of future needs/directions that could advance our knowledge in this field. First, most of these studies (as noted in Table 83.1), though focusing on dialysis-related neurocognitive difficulties, suffer from small sample size. Second, the literature on older children reveals that most of these studies have mixed populations of children with CKD, with a combination of ages, thus hindering efforts to determine if there are developmental time periods where dialysis can have a more profound negative impact on cognitive functions. Third, nearly all of the available studies included samples receiving different modalities of renal replacement therapy, but the sub-samples were too small to analyze, thus not permitting a direct comparison of the effects of different dialysis modalities on cognitive functioning. Finally, outside of examining patients pre- and posttransplant, there were no longitudinal studies that examined the long-term effects on a child's neurodevelopmental status, thus leaving questions pertaining to whether the effects of dialysis are transient, linked to the presence of worsening CKD via a Gordian knot, or in some fashion contribute to the exacerbation of the disease by exerting a negative impact on the neurologic systems subserving cognitive abilities. Consequently, there are many remaining scientific questions to be addressed and, at present, it is difficult to make any clear conclusion about the specific effects of dialysis on neurocognition in children.

Given the high number of children with kidney disease, expected long-term survival of pediatric CKD patients, and availability of established guidelines to initiate and continue dialysis, a focused, adequately powered scientific approach toward better understanding the impact of dialysis on neurodevelopmental status is warranted. Larger samples of specific subtypes of dialysis should be studied, with sensitivity to age and developmental parameters being carefully considered. Further, future research should focus on potential risk factors, such as anemia, hypertension, age of onset of kidney disease, and duration of ESRD, etc., to advance our knowledge of the effect of modifiable mediators of cognitive deficits in children on dialysis. In the meantime, the general finding across studies that many children on dialysis, regardless of modality, are at risk for disruption in their cognitive functioning should encourage the inclusion of formal developmental surveillance into their medical management and routine standard of care.

C H A P T E R   8 4

Growth in Children With End-Stage Renal Disease

Rose M. Ayoob, MD • John D. Mahan, MD

Introduction

Growth is a complex biologic process dependent on adequate nutrition as well as the integrated homeostasis of metabolic and endocrine pathways. Growth failure has long been recognized as one of the most common and profound complications seen in pediatric patients with chronic kidney disease (CKD). Growth impairment may be seen in up to 50% of children with moderate to severe renal dysfunction (CKD 3–5). Despite available treatments including renal replacement therapy, 30%–60% of children with end-stage renal disease (ESRD) ultimately have reduced adult height. Data from the North American Pediatric Renal Trials and Cooperative Studies (NAPRTCS) 2011 annual report included 7039 patients and provided patient characteristics and height data for children at initiation of maintenance dialysis. Baseline height scores for children at dialysis initiation were 1.60 standard deviation scores (SDS) below appropriate age- and sex-adjusted height levels. During the first 36 months of dialysis, mean changes in height SDS (z scores) for patients stratified by age continued to lag for all but children <2 years of age (Fig. 84.1) and the absolute height deficits were worse for younger patients and males.

Although a trend toward improved final adult height for children with CKD has been noted over the last decade, mean final height in several studies of patients with CKD stage 3–5 still ranges between −0.6 and −3.5 SD. Children who required dialysis during childhood manifest the greatest adult impairment in height. This outcome is a significant burden for these young adult survivors of childhood CKD. Broyer et al studied the social outcomes of 244 adults who had received kidney transplants as children with ESRD (mean age at transplantation 11.9 ± 4.0 years) and found that better adult height correlated with higher educational attainment, better employment rates, more successful marriages, and greater rates of independent living. Rosencrantz reported the quality of life in 29 adults with childhood-onset ESRD and found that their mean adult height SDS was low at −1.56 ± 1.55; 36% were dissatisfied with their adult height (compared with 4% of healthy controls); and that height dissatisfaction correlated with poorer quality of life.

Patients receiving renal transplants and/or treatment with recombinant human growth hormone (rhGH) show better mean final height than those patients who continued on long-term dialysis and/or did not receive concomitant rhGH therapy. Young age at onset of ESRD, long duration of renal failure, male gender, and the presence of congenital nephropathies are the most relevant risk factors for decreased final adult height.

Complicating the approach to understanding and treatment of growth failure in children with CKD is its multifactorial pathogenesis in most affected children.

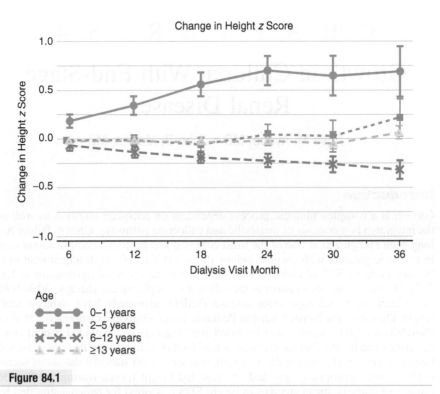

Figure 84.1

Mean Change in Height *Z* Score Reported by Age Group During the First 36 Months After Dialysis Initiation. (Reproduced from North American Pediatric Renal Trials and Collaborative Studies 2011 annual report [online]. http://www.NAPRTCS.org.)

Congenital and acquired renal abnormalities can exert effects early or late on their growth and development. Clinical manifestations due to decreased renal function can be highly variable and may result in diverse complications, including fluid and electrolyte abnormalities, metabolic acidosis, abnormal bone metabolism, and malnutrition that can affect growth. In addition, children undergo various medical interventions and different modes of renal replacement therapy at different times during their growth and development. Growth in children with CKD may therefore be influenced by (1) patient genetic factors and nonrenal comorbidities; (2) specific aspects of the timing, type, and severity of the underlying renal disorder; (3) specific types and severity of CKD complications; and (4) the impact of the different types and timing of renal therapies.

The impact of growth failure in children with CKD can be profound. Chronically malnourished children display behavioral changes such as irritability, apathy, and attention deficits. Growth failure in children with CKD has been associated with an increased incidence of hospitalizations as well as a reported threefold increased risk of mortality associated with growth impairment in children requiring dialysis. Furth evaluated the risk of death in a cohort of 2306 patients with CKD from the NAPRTCS

2002 report. Eligible patients were aged 21 years or younger and had available height data at initiation of dialysis. Fig. 84.2 shows patient survival stratified by standardized height (height z score < or >–2.5) and age (≤ or >1 years), two known risk factors for mortality in this population. Taller children (z score >–2.5) had a lower risk of death than shorter children (z score <–2.5) in both age groups. Significant impairments in both psychosocial and psychological development as well as decreased quality of life (QOL) scores have been documented in children with ESRD and growth failure.

Growth Patterns

Physiologic growth patterns can be divided into the periods of infancy, midchildhood, and puberty. Adequate nutritional intake is the most important requirement for growth during the first 2 years of life where growth and neurologic development are recognized to be more directly dependent on caloric intake than in older age groups. In midchildhood, growth is driven by the somatotropic hormone axis. During puberty, the gonadotropic hormone axis has an additional influence on growth by stimulating growth plate chondrocytes, modulating growth hormone (GH) secretion from the pituitary gland and directly affecting all somatic cells. The growth pattern typically seen with congenital chronic renal failure and the sequence of primary growth factors are depicted in Fig. 84.3.

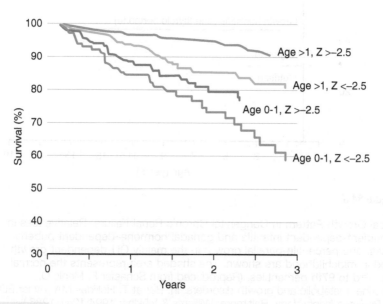

Figure 84.2

Association of Growth Failure and Survival in Children With Chronic Kidney Disease. (Reproduced from Furth, SL, et al., Growth failure, risk of hospitalization and death for children with end-stage renal disease. Pediatr Nephrol, 2002;**17**(6):450-455.)

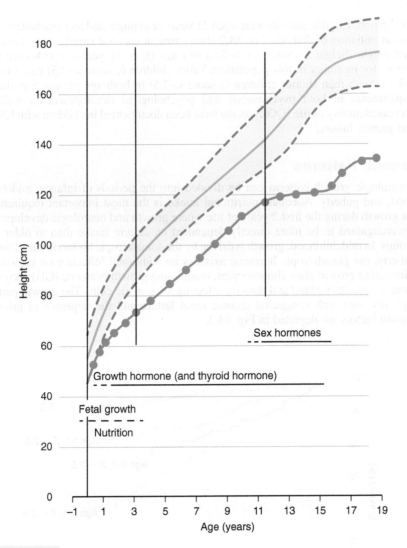

Figure 84.3

Typical Growth Pattern in Congenital Chronic Renal Failure. Relative loss in the nutrient-dependent infantile and gonadal hormone–dependent puberty phases, and percentile-parallel growth in the mainly GH-dependent growth period in midchildhood are shown. The shaded area represents the normal range, 3rd to 97th percentiles. (Reproduced from Schaefer F, Mehls O. Endocrine, metabolic and growth disorders. In: Barrat T, Holliday MA, Avner ED, eds. *Pediatric Nephrology*. Baltimore: Williams & Wilkins; 1994:1241-1286.)

Children with congenital renal disorders, where renal impairment is present in the first two years of life, are particularly affected because 33% of final adult height is normally attained during the first 2 years of life. Despite the initial delay in infancy, growth progresses steadily through childhood but typically at a lower rate. Height velocity again decreases during the last 2–3 years of prepubertal growth resulting in further growth impairment. In such children the pubertal growth spurt is often delayed and decreased in magnitude which results in further loss of growth and reduced final adult height.

Assessment of Growth

Because growth failure is a common concern in children with CKD, anthropometric measurements must be incorporated into the routine care of these children. In fact, these anthropometric values should be considered as a *fifth vital sign* for the child with CKD evaluated in the outpatient setting. Regular assessment of head circumference (until 3 years of age), height, weight, and body mass index (BMI) permits early detection of failing growth and provides opportunities for earlier focused interventions. Height (length for children not standing yet), weight, and BMI must be measured and recorded at each routine health care visit. Plotting these values on age- and gender-appropriate growth charts, and calculating percentiles and SDS, allows detection of concerning measures or trends. Calculating the height velocity SDS score can facilitate determination of suboptimal growth before the height value is out of the normal range.

Growth failure is defined as height and/or weight below the third percentile (<–1.88 SDS) for age and gender. BMI below the third percentile (<–1.88 SDS) for age and gender is also an important marker of growth failure. Although detection of height, weight, or BMI below –1.88 SDS is a clear sign of growth failure, earlier detection of a disturbing growth pattern (eg, height velocity SDS <–1.88) can provide opportunities for early interventions.

Growth Failure in CKD

There is no single cause of growth failure in most children with CKD; multiple factors often are in play (Table 84.1). Although genetic and nonrenal comorbidities exert significant effects on growth, understanding the influence of nonmodifiable and modifiable renal factors helps fully define the mechanisms operant in growth failure in a specific child with CKD.

Underlying Renal Disease

The earlier in life CKD occurs, the more likely the child is to have growth failure. Congenital renal dysplasia or hypoplasia with or without urinary tract obstruction is the most common cause of ESRD during infancy and childhood. Renal dysplasia is often associated with significant water and electrolyte losses, which contribute to poor growth. Children with chronic glomerulopathies may show decline in growth rates even with only mild renal insufficiency. Known risk factors for growth delay also include the nephrotic state and a history of glucocorticoid use. Among the various causes of renal disease, children with nephropathic cystinosis or primary hyperoxaluria show the most markedly compromised final adult heights.

Table 84.1

Factors Affecting Growth in Children With CKD

Genetic Factors/Parental Height

Nonrenal Comorbidities
- Neurologic disorders
- Genetic conditions
- Heart disease
- Gastrointestinal/liver disorders
- Neoplasia/cancer treatments

Renal Nonmodifiable Factors
- Age of CKD onset
- Level of GFR
- Residual renal function
- Type of renal disorder
- Corticosteroid therapy

Renal Modifiable Factors
- Excessive water and/or salt losses
- Poor caloric/protein intake
- Malnutrition-inflammation syndrome
- Metabolic acidosis
- Anemia
- CKD–mineral bone disorder
- GH/IGF-1 resistance
- Gonadotropin abnormalities

CKD, chronic kidney disease; GFR, glomerular filtration rate; GH, growth hormone; IGF-1, insulinlike growth factor 1.

Protein–Energy Malnutrition

The most important cause of poor growth in children with CKD is inadequate energy and/or protein intake. Normal infants and children are particularly vulnerable to malnutrition due to their typical low nutritional stores and high energy demands; the presence of CKD can further complicate meeting these essential needs. Protein–energy malnutrition is common in dialysis patients, with as many as one-third of patients showing mild or moderate malnutrition and 1/10th having severe malnutrition. The term "malnutrition–inflammation complex syndrome" (MICS) has been used to describe the association between chronic inflammation and malnutrition in dialyzed children and adults. Possible causes of MICS include comorbid illnesses, oxidative stress, nutrient loss through dialysis, anorexia, induction of cytokines during exposure to bioincompatible dialysis materials, and uremic toxins.

Metabolic Acidosis

Metabolic acidosis usually occurs as glomerular filtration rate (GFR) falls below 50% of normal but intake of protein/acid load as well as catabolism also contributes to its development. Metabolic acidosis is associated with decreased linear growth and increased protein breakdown in children with CKD. In experimental uremia models, metabolic acidosis suppresses GH secretion and reduces serum IGF-1 levels, triggers resistance to anabolic actions of GH, inhibits albumin synthesis, increases calcium efflux from bone, and augments protein degradation. Alterations of protein metabolism by metabolic acidosis in children with chronic renal failure results in increased glucocorticoid production that can impair growth.

CKD–Mineral Bone Disorder

Skeletal disturbances due to CKD–mineral bone disorder (CKD-MBD, formerly termed renal osteodystrophy) can contribute to uremic growth failure. Abnormalities in bone cells and bone structure can be seen in both high and low bone turnover forms of CKD-MBD. Secondary hyperparathyroidism causes destruction of growth plate architecture, epiphyseal displacement, and metaphyseal fractures, all leading to impaired longitudinal growth. Growth arrest may occur as a result of severe destruction of the metaphyseal bone architecture.

Anemia

Long-standing anemia in CKD patients may lead to profound systemic consequences such as anorexia and catabolism due to altered energy metabolism. Anemia may suppress growth secondary to poor appetite, intercurrent infections, cardiac complications, and reduced oxygen supply to cartilage and has been associated with delayed growth.

Endocrine Dysfunction

The growth hormone–insulinlike growth factor 1 (GH–IGF-1) axis is an important regulator of growth and metabolism in children, and significant abnormalities in this axis occur in children with CKD (Fig. 84.4). In the normal state, GH production and release by the anterior pituitary are regulated by hypothalamic GH-releasing hormone and somatostatin, with circulating GH and IGF-1 levels providing negative feedback to the hypothalamus. Release of GH is also stimulated by the GH-releasing peptide ghrelin, which is expressed by the stomach and hypothalamus. Circulating GH stimulates production and release of IGF-1, primarily from the liver. Most circulating IGF-1 is bound to IGF-binding protein (IGFBP) 3 and acid-labile subunit (ALS); less than 1% of IGF-1 occurs in the free or bioactive form. Circulating free IGF-1 mediates many of the biologic effects of GH, including stimulation of longitudinal bone growth and regulation of renal hemodynamics.

Children with CKD have multiple abnormalities of the GH–IGF-1 axis (Fig. 84.4). These include increased circulating levels of GH, as a result of increased pulsatile release and reduced renal GH clearance, counterbalanced by reduced responsiveness to endogenous GH and IGF-1. Uremic GH and IGF-1 resistance impairs linear bone growth and many cellular processes. An important mechanism for GH resistance in CKD involves a defect in the postreceptor GH-activated Janus kinase 2 (JAK2) signal transducer and activator of the transcription (STAT) pathway (Fig. 84.5). Decreased density of GH receptors in target organs may also play a role in GH resistance in children with CKD as suggested by reduced circulating levels of growth hormone–binding protein (GHBP), a product of proteolytic cleavage of the GH receptor, in proportion to the severity of renal dysfunction.

IGF-1 resistance is also exacerbated by increased levels of circulating IGFBPs 1, 2, 4, and 6, because of decreased GFR, that reduce bioavailable IGF-1. Increased proteolysis of IGFBP 3 also decreases IGF-1 available for the formation of IGF 1–ALS–IGFBP 3 complexes. The sum of these abnormalities results in impaired GH and IGF-1 effects on growth in children with CKD.

The gonadotropic hormone axis is also altered in adolescent patients with CKD. Decreased renal clearance of gonadotropins leads to elevated gonadotropin levels

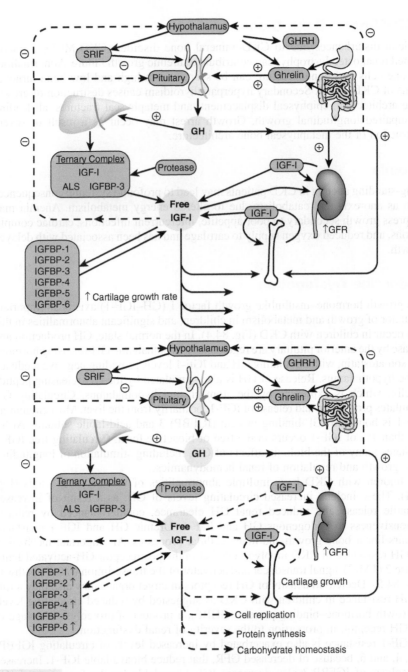

Figure 84.4

The Growth Hormone–Insulinlike Growth Factor 1 (GH–IGF-1) Axis in Normal Children and Children With Chronic Kidney Disease.

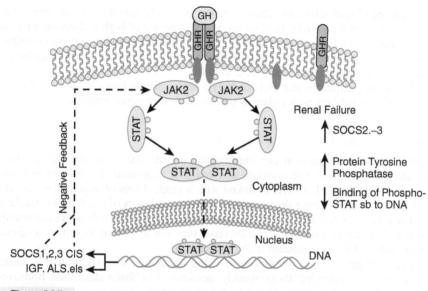

Figure 84.5

Growth Hormone–Mediated Janus Kinase/Signal Transducer and Activator of the Transcription Signal Transduction.

and reduced pituitary secretion of bioactive luteinizing hormone. In uremia, increased levels of sex hormone–binding globulins significantly lower free testosterone. Total testosterone levels are also reduced in these children. Serum testosterone is not positively correlated with the rate of GH secretion, as is the case in healthy children; in fact, GH secretion rates are lower than expected at each level of testosterone in boys with CKD. These physiologic abnormalities also contribute to pubertal growth impairment in adolescents with CKD.

Treatment

General Measures

In infants and young children with CKD, the most important measure to avoid growth failure is to provide adequate energy and protein intake. In general, initial target energy intake for children treated with maintenance dialysis (MD) should be between 80% and 100% of the recommended daily allowance (RDA) of healthy children. Provision of adequate energy for growth may require supplementary feeding through a nasogastric tube or gastrostomy. Children treated with maintenance hemodialysis (HD) should have initial dietary protein intake based on RDA for chronologic age and an additional increment of 0.4 g/kg/day. Children treated with maintenance peritoneal dialysis (PD) should have initial dietary protein intake based on RDA for chronologic age plus an additional increment based on anticipated peritoneal losses.

The beneficial effect of correction of acidosis on growth retardation was initially described in children with renal tubular acidosis and normal renal function. Growth is better in CKD children with serum bicarbonate >22 mmol/L, and therefore it is recommended that serum bicarbonate levels below 22 mmol/L be corrected in all children treated with CKD. In children on MD, the use of high sodium bicarbonate concentrations in dialysate as well as oral administration of sodium citrate or sodium bicarbonate should be individualized to maintain steady-state serum bicarbonate levels to at least the target goal of 22 mmol/L.

Providing adequate water and electrolyte replacements based on observed losses is essential in patients with polyuria and/or salt-losing nephropathies.

Dialysis and Intensified Dialysis

Although dialysis treatment can improve the uremic state, longitudinal growth is usually not improved with standard conventional treatments. In children and adolescents, long-term PD or HD is linked with a gradual loss of standardized height. Several large studies have documented mean annual losses of 0.2–0.8 SD standardized height in such children. As in standard HD, catchup growth is not commonly observed in children on PD. Residual renal function is a more important predictor of growth on PD than standard dialytic clearance.

Catch-up growth may be enhanced using intensified dialysis protocols, either short daily or extended thrice-weekly sessions. Fischbach described improved growth when intensified HD (3 hours, 6 days per week) treatments were combined with recombinant human growth hormone (rhGH) with an average increase in growth velocity from 3.8 cm/year at baseline to 8.9 cm/year during the intervention. The benefit of intensified HD may result from improved clearance of uremic toxins. This additional clearance may also better address malnutrition–inflammation and metabolic acidosis leading to improved appetite, tissue anabolism, and better growth.

Transplant

Only successful kidney transplantation is able to restore the conditions for normal growth compromised by the uremic state. However, growth rates after transplantation vary widely, from further deterioration of standardized height in some children to complete catch-up growth in others. In a NAPRTCS analysis, the mean effect of transplantation before puberty on final adult height was no improvement, 0 SDS, confirming that the relative height achieved *at time of transplantation* is the most important predictor of final adult height. Whereas pubertal patients tend to lose relative height following transplantation, good potential for posttransplant catch-up growth exists in patients younger than 6 years. Infant allograft recipients typically exhibit excellent spontaneous growth rates, with a relative height gain of +1.5 SD within first 2–7 years following transplant. Despite development of minimal steroid and steroid withdrawal protocols, catch-up growth in pubertal patients continues to lag behind that seen in prepubertal children. A recent German study demonstrated that despite improved growth in many children after transplant in the era of less steroid therapy and less rejection episodes, mean final adult height was still low at −1.65 SDS and more than 33% of the adults had height <−1.88 SDS.

Growth Hormone Therapy

Treatment of growth failure in children with CKD must be based on a thorough evaluation and therapy directed toward modifiable factors associated with growth

Table 84.2

Rationale for the Use of rhGH in Children With CKD and Growth Failure

Improvement in linear growth and final adult height
Increased muscle mass and bone density
Better physical and social functioning
Improvement in psychosocial development
Decrease in overall morbidity and mortality
Decrease in hospitalizations
Reduced number of school days missed
Improved perception in overall health related quality of life

rhGH, recombinant human growth hormone; CKD, chronic kidney disease.

impairment. Recombinant GH (rhGH) therapy should be considered for any child with CKD 2–5 experiencing poor linear growth despite correction of modifiable factors that may adversely affect growth. Provision of exogenous rhGH is able to overcome the effects of GH and IGF-1 resistance. In addition to promoting growth, rhGH therapy provides other benefits to children with CKD. GH treatment–related anabolic effects include improvements in body weight, mid-arm circumference, improved bone mineral density, and better lipid profiles. Table 84.2 lists additional benefits of rhGH in children with growth failure and CKD.

The algorithm in Fig. 84.6 for the evaluation and treatment of growth failure in children with CKD summarizes a logical approach to rhGH therapy in children with CKD. Once metabolic and nutritional factors affecting growth have been properly addressed over a 3- to 6-month period, children who have not established normal growth velocity or achieved normal height for age should be evaluated for rhGH therapy. Height SDS, height velocity SDS, absolute height velocity, pubertal stage, and bone age should be assessed before treatment to confirm patient eligibility and provide baseline determinations for monitoring growth while receiving rhGH treatment. Baseline hip and knee x-rays, funduscopic examination, blood chemistries, parathyroid hormone (PTH) levels, and thyroid studies should be performed prior to treatment initiation. Ongoing monitoring for adverse events should be performed.

Following comprehensive pretreatment evaluation, children with no other cause for poor growth may be initiated on rhGH at 0.05 mg/kg/day (0.35 mg/kg/week or 28 IU/m^2/week) administered by subcutaneous injection. GH stimulation tests are not needed for children with CKD who experience poor growth after proper treatment of all modifiable factors that can affect growth. Throughout rhGH therapy, children must be monitored regularly (typically every 3–4 months) for dose modification based on weight gain, response to therapy, adverse events, and complicating factors that may further affect growth. Higher doses of rhGH may be required during puberty for some patients, and adolescents with CKD who receive "pubertal doses" of rhGH (up to 0.7 mg/kg/week) may demonstrate better height velocity and improvement in final adult height. Because rhGH administration increases plasma IGF-1 levels, and many of the growth-promoting effects of GH are mediated by IGF-1, it has been suggested that a relationship might exist between plasma IGF-1 concentrations and catch-up growth in children with rhGH therapy. In children with

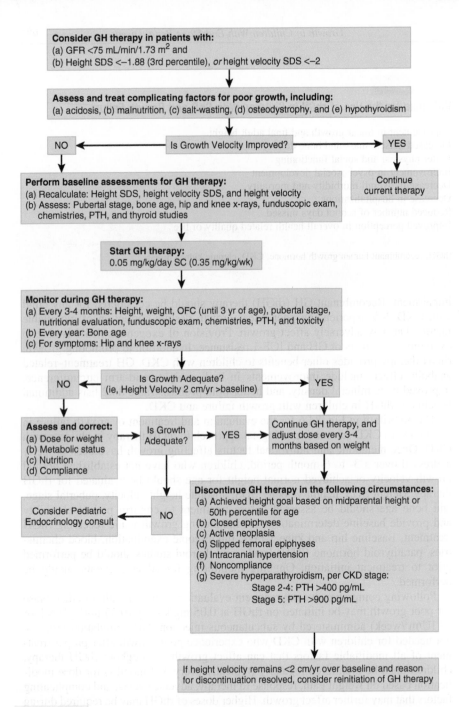

Figure 84.6

2006 Consensus Conference Algorithm for Evaluation and Treatment of Growth Failure in Children With Chronic Kidney Disease. (Reproduced from Mahan JD, Warady BA. Assessment and treatment of short stature in pediatric patients with chronic kidney disease: a consensus statement. Pediatr Nephrol. 2006;21(7):917-930.)

CKD receiving rhGH, serum IGF-1 may be a useful measure of therapeutic efficacy and adherence to therapy. Recombinant GH therapy should be discontinued when the epiphyses close or if the child's height goal has been achieved (based on mid-parental height or 50th percentile for age). It should be temporarily discontinued in the presence of active neoplasia, slipped capital femoral epiphyses, benign intracranial hypertension, severe hyperparathyroidism (PTH >900 pg/mL for stage V CKD and >400 pg/mL for CKD 2–4), nonadherence with treatment, or at the time of renal transplantation. Close monitoring of growth should continue after discontinuing rhGH therapy, because reinitiation of rhGH may be appropriate if the height velocity decreases and the reasons for the discontinuation of rhGH are resolved.

Patients with CKD experience complications with both the timing of and the duration of the normal pubertal growth spurt compared with healthy children. Multiple clinical studies in growth-retarded prepubertal children with CKD before dialysis have shown that treatment with rhGH increases height velocity during the first treatment year almost twofold compared with baseline or placebo-treated

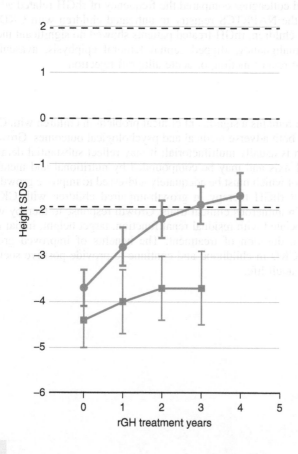

Figure 84.7

Superior Efficacy of Growth Hormone Treatment in Children With CKD Stages 2–4 (n = 19, Circles) vs Dialysis (n = 6).

children. No acceleration in bone maturation was observed in these studies; therefore, predicted adult height steadily increased during treatment with rhGH. Additional studies have shown that the response to GH is significantly less in dialyzed children compared to children with earlier CKD as shown in Fig. 84.7. In addition, the cumulative height gained during treatment with rhGH was positively affected by the duration of therapy as well as the initial target height deficit and negatively affected by the duration of dialysis. The relative height gain attained during therapy with rhGH appears to be maintained until the final height is achieved in patients undergoing renal transplant. In Hokken–Koelega's retrospective study of 52 children who underwent renal transplantation before the age of 15 years and did not receive rhGH therapy, the median height SDS was below the third percentile for age at the time of first dialysis, decreased significantly during dialysis, and did not improve following renal transplantation. The final adult height of these patients remained below the third percentile for age for 77% of the males and 71% of the females.

In the largest study to address side effects with rhGH therapy in children with CKD, Fine and colleagues compared the frequency of rhGH-related adverse events in patients in the NAPRTCS registry to untreated children with CKD. Compared with untreated children, rhGH-treated patients showed no significant increase in the incidence of malignancy, slipped capital femoral epiphysis, avascular necrosis, deterioration of renal function, or acute allograft rejection.

Summary

Growth failure remains a significant clinical problem in children with CKD and has been linked to both adverse medical and psychological outcomes. Growth failure in this population is usually multifactorial; it may reflect substantial derangements of the GH–IGF-1 axis and may be compounded by nutritional and metabolic abnormalities, each of which must be adequately addressed to improve growth. The safety and efficacy of rhGH therapy in growth-impaired children with CKD has been demonstrated in numerous clinical trials. Growth response to therapy with rhGH is positively associated with residual renal function, target height, initial target height deficit, and the duration of treatment. The benefits of improved growth impact children with CKD in childhood and continue to provide positive social and other outcomes into adult life.

C H A P T E R 8 5

Adequacy of Peritoneal Dialysis/ Assessing Peritoneal Function in Pediatric Patients

Vimal Chadha, MD • Bradley A. Warady, MD

The provision of dialysis to a child with stage 5 chronic kidney disease (CKD) (GFR <15 mL/min/1.73 m^2) constitutes only one element of the comprehensive management of this debilitating disease. It is apparent that to achieve the best possible outcome, optimal management of anemia, secondary hyperparathyroidism, renal osteodystrophy, acidosis, fluid balance, hypertension, dyslipidemia, nutrition, and growth are equally important and are considered by many as pertinent parameters of dialysis adequacy, in addition to solute removal by dialysis. It is also important to recognize that successful management of all these issues is interdependent. Interestingly, although the therapeutic endpoints of many of these clinical issues are relatively well defined, there is no consensus on what constitutes adequate dialysis.

In adults, dialysis adequacy is currently characterized by urea removal (small solute clearance) with specific quantitative targets based on the evidence of an association between solute clearance and patient morbidity/mortality. The same cannot currently hold true for children because of the low mortality rate experienced by patients in this age group and the absence of any well-substantiated correlations between their clinical status and the efficiency of dialysis. Furthermore, the provision of evidence-based pediatric PD adequacy guidelines is hampered by a crucial epidemiologic issue; because stage 5 CKD remains a relatively uncommon disease in children and a significant proportion of patients receive a kidney transplant soon after developing end-stage renal disease (ESRD), no long-term pediatric outcome study is adequately powered to detect an effect of the delivered PD dose on pediatric patient outcome. Accordingly, the revised pediatric component of the National Kidney Foundation's–Kidney Disease Outcomes Quality Initiative (NKF-K/DOQI) Peritoneal Dialysis Adequacy guidelines suggest that the clinical "wellness" of the individual patient should remain an important treatment goal and an important means by which the adequacy of care should be assessed. An understanding of the basic concepts of dialysis adequacy and key issues from the K/DOQI publication are reviewed in this chapter.

Adequate versus Optimal Dose of Dialysis

The concept of adequate dialysis was born more than 30 years ago when a systematic analysis of the National Cooperative Dialysis Study (NCDS) involving adult hemodialysis patients revealed that the relationship between dialysis dose and patient outcome was not linear, and increasing the dialysis dose beyond a certain threshold does not result in any additional beneficial outcome. Likewise, although an adequate dose of PD might best be defined as the minimum dose, in terms of the quantity of solute removed, below which a clinically unacceptable rate of negative outcomes occur, the optimal dose of dialysis is that dose above which no significant reduction in negative outcomes or improvement in positive outcomes occur to justify the additional patient burden or cost. Therefore, the optimal dose lies somewhere between the minimal effective (adequate) dose and the maximal dose, or the dose above which there are clearly no additional benefits. However, and as noted above, it is difficult to define the optimal PD dose in children with confidence because of the absence of definitive data correlating dialysis dose to patient outcome. Thus, the recommended clinical practice is, in essence, to provide the most dialysis that can be delivered to the pediatric patient within the constraints of social and clinical circumstances, quality of life (QOL), and cost.

The provision of adequate dialysis must take into account the choice of PD modality and an individualized prescription based on the desired solute clearance and the volume removal (ultrafiltration) required to maintain optimal fluid balance and achieve nutritional/metabolic goals.

Prescription of Peritoneal Dialysis

Choice of Peritoneal Dialysis Modality

Both continuous ambulatory peritoneal dialysis (CAPD) and automated peritoneal dialysis (APD) are used by children, although the latter is the preferred PD modality, in large part because its use is characterized by freedom from dialysis procedures during the daytime hours. The provision of an APD cycling device is associated with an increased cost and a slight increase in complexity relative to CAPD. APD has classically been divided into APD with a day-dwell, also known as continuous-cycling peritoneal dialysis (CCPD), and dry-day APD, also known as nocturnal intermittent peritoneal dialysis (NIPD).

An alternative form of APD is tidal peritoneal dialysis (TPD) which uses an initial fill volume followed by partial drainage at periodic intervals. Initially, the principal purpose of TPD was to enhance clearance of small solutes; however, it is primarily used now to minimize pain during drainage of dialysate from the peritoneal cavity. Largely as a result of its complexity and high cost, TPD is not widely used.

As both CAPD and APD modalities can provide adequate clearances, the former is often used effectively in developing countries because of substantial cost savings. In wealthier countries, the use of APD predominates in infants, children, and adolescents.

Initial Dialysis Prescription

The initial prescription should take into account the patient's body surface area (BSA), exchange dwell time, the residual renal function (RRF), and the desired fluid removal. In view of the age-independent relationship between peritoneal surface area and BSA, the use of BSA as a scaling factor for the prescribed fill volume is recommended. Whereas the target range for the fill volume of patients greater than 2 years of age is 1000–1200 mL/m^2 BSA, the initial prescribed volume should be somewhat lower for smaller infants (600–800 mL/m^2 BSA) and the fill volume should be increased in a stepwise manner, as tolerated by the patient. To optimize small-solute clearance, minimize cost, and possibly decrease the frequency of exchanges, one should first increase the instilled volume per exchange (maximum 1400 mL/m^2 BSA) as tolerated by the patient, before increasing the number of exchanges per day. The volume of the supine exchange(s) should be increased first as this is the position with the lowest intraabdominal pressure. Objective evidence of patient tolerance may require assessment of the intraperitoneal pressure.

The PD prescription process should also take into account the peritoneal membrane transport characteristics as defined by the peritoneal equilibration test (PET) (vide infra), which helps define the frequency of exchanges and dextrose concentration of dialysate (1.5%, 2.5%, or 4.25%) required (along with RRF, if it exists) to achieve the targeted solute and fluid removal. It should be recognized that it is often impractical to consider the provision of a dialysis prescription solely based on kinetic data and achieved solute clearance without reference to social constraints such as school attendance and the working schedule of parents.

Patients receiving APD, usually remain on the cycler for 8–10 hours during the nighttime, and maintain a daytime fill volume that is typically one-half the nocturnal fill volume. The use of NIPD, characterized by the absence of any daytime dwell, can be considered in pediatric patients who are clinically well, whose combined dialysis prescription and RRF achieves or exceeds the target solute clearance, and who are without evidence of hyperphosphatemia, hyperkalemia, hypervolemia, or acidosis. Patients who do not meet these criteria and receive cycler dialysis are generally prescribed CCPD.

Patients receiving CAPD perform 3–5 daily exchanges using a double-bag PD solution with a Y-set disconnectable system. Drainage of spent dialysate and inflow of fresh dialysis solution are performed manually, relying on gravity to move fluid into and out of the abdomen. The initial fill volume can be 600–800 mL/m^2 during the day, and 800–1000 mL/m^2 overnight. When there is inadequate ultrafiltration overnight because of rapid glucose absorption, higher dextrose concentration or an icodextrin-based PD solution can be employed for the prolonged nighttime exchange.

Peritoneal Equilibration Test

The peritoneal equilibration test (PET) was developed as a clinically applicable means of characterizing solute transport across the peritoneum and is the most common technique used in children to assess the peritoneal membrane transport capacity and guide the prescription process. The procedure yields data necessary to determine the fractional equilibration of creatinine and glucose between dialysate and blood expressed as the dialysate to plasma (D/P) ratio for creatinine and the ratio of dialysate glucose to initial dialysate glucose (D/D$_O$). The test exchange volume should be 1000–1100 mL/m^2 when the procedure is conducted in children. The provision of a smaller volume, which may be necessary in young infants, may result in more rapid equilibration and the artifactual appearance of an inherently more rapid membrane transport capacity. Although the specific details of the PET are discussed in Chapter 31, it is important to highlight the fact that glucose in high concentration (as occurs in dialysis fluid) interferes with the measurement of creatinine by the photometric method. The resulting creatinine value is falsely elevated. Accordingly, the creatinine concentration in dialysis fluid should either be measured by the enzymatic assay method in which there is no glucose interference, or the creatinine values must be corrected for glucose interference by determining a correction factor for the individual laboratory.

It has been suggested that a patient's initial PET evaluation should be performed approximately 1 month after dialysis initiation to facilitate categorization of a patient's transport capacity in the most accurate manner. Patients are categorized as high, high average, low average, or low solute transporters based on a comparison of their data to reference norms. A child who is classified as a rapid transporter is likely to dialyze most efficiently in terms of solute and water removal by using short, frequent dialysis cycles as in APD. On the other hand, a low or low average transporter may benefit most from a schedule that includes longer dwell times as in classical CAPD. Attention to these prescription issues may be particularly important to children because of the high incidence of cardiac disease and the goal of achieving euvolemia and normotension (vide infra). Whereas routine repetition of the PET evaluation is not indicated, repeat testing should be considered when there is clinical/biochemical evidence of suboptimal dialysis or when clinical events have occurred (e.g., repeated peritonitis) which may have altered the membrane transport capacity.

Personal Dialysis Capacity Test

The personal dialysis capacity (PDC) test is based on the three-pore model of solute and fluid transport across the peritoneum. The PDC test describes the peritoneal membrane transport characteristics by functional parameters, which are calculated based on data obtained from several exchanges of different duration and performed with PD solutions of different glucose concentration over a day. The test calculates the following three parameters:

1. The effective peritoneal surface area, or unrestricted pore area over diffusion distance $(A_0/\Delta X)$, corresponding to the diffusion capacity for solutes and comparable to the D/P value of the PET.
2. Absorption, that is, the final rate of fluid reabsorption from the abdominal cavity, primarily representing the lymphatic flow.
3. The large-pore flow, which represents the rate of protein-rich fluid passing through the large pores from blood to dialysate. A large-pore flow that is higher than expected according to the total vascular surface area is a sign of an inflamed peritoneal membrane.

Mass Transfer Area Coefficient (MTAC)

The MTAC is an additional measure of solute transport capacity and is the most precise means of estimating intrinsic peritoneal membrane permeability to a specific solute. Unlike the D/P ratio determined with the PET, the MTAC is essentially independent of dialysis mechanics such as the fill volume and the dialysate dextrose concentration. Whereas most clinicians have been reluctant to use the MTAC to characterize peritoneal membrane solute transport capacity largely because of the complexity of the calculations involved, computer technology has made determination of the MTAC much easier.

Measurement of Peritoneal Dialysis Dose

A valid and reproducible measure of the dose of PD is essential to determine the quantity of dialysis delivered to an individual patient. The total (RRF + dialysis) weekly Kt/V_{urea} and the total weekly creatinine clearance (C_{Cr}) are the best available measures of PD dose and both have been used in clinical practice. Nevertheless, determination of dialysis and urine Kt/V_{urea} alone is currently recommended for follow-up based on the simplicity of the calculation and the fact that studies in adult patients on PD have not provided any evidence of a benefit in terms of patient outcome when expressing clearance in any manner other than Kt/V_{urea}.

Kt/V_{urea} is a measure of the amount of plasma cleared of urea during the sampling period ($K*t$) normalized to total body water (TBW) or V, the volume of urea distribution. The total weekly Kt/V_{urea} is calculated as follows:

$$Weekly\ Kt/V = \frac{D_{ur} \times V_D + (U_{ur} \times V_u)}{P_{ur} \times V} \times 7$$

where D_{ur}, U_{ur}, and P_{ur} are the dialysate, urinary, and plasma concentrations of urea; V_D and V_U the 24-hour dialysate and urine volumes; and V the urea distribution volume.

In the calculation of Kt/V_{urea}, it is most important to use an accurate estimate of V. Traditionally, anthropometric prediction equations based on height and weight such as those of Mellits and Cheek have been used to estimate V. However, such equations were established in healthy populations, and subsequent studies have revealed that the use of these equations routinely overestimates V (or TBW) in pediatric patients receiving PD. In contrast, the determination of TBW by heavy water ($H_2{}^{18}O$ or D_2O) dilution in 64 pediatric patients receiving PD has allowed for the development of accurate TBW prediction equations. The gender-specific equations are as follows:

$$Males:TBW = 0.010 \times (height \times weight)^{0.68} - (0.37 \times weight)$$

$$Females:TBW = 0.14 \times (height \times weight)^{0.64} - (0.35 \times weight)$$

Gender-specific nomograms to estimate TBW that are based on these equations are shown in Tables 85.1 and 85.2.

Because the height × weight parameter also predicts BSA, it has been possible to simplify the prediction equations by utilizing BSA as determined by the Gehan and George equation (vide infra). Although slightly less precise than the best-fitting equations, these equations might be considered more "user friendly":

$$Males:TBW = 20.88 \times BSA - 4.29$$

$$Females:TBW = 16.92 \times BSA - 1.81$$

In obese and malnourished patients, the TBW calculation should be based on the patient's ideal body weight so as to avoid overdialysis in the former, and underdialysis in the latter group of patients.

Table 85.1

Male Total Body Water (L) Nomograms

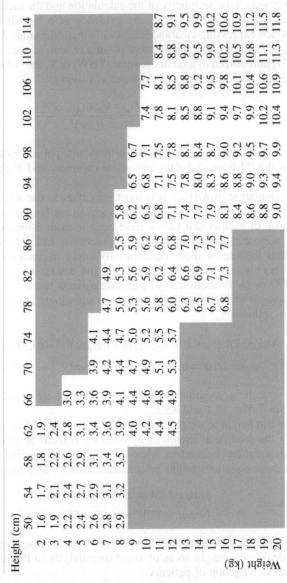

Weight (kg)	\ Height (cm) 50	54	58	62	66	70	74	78	82	86	90	94	98	102	106	110	114
2	1.6	1.7	1.8	1.9													
3	1.9	2.1	2.2	2.4													
4	2.2	2.4	2.6	2.8	3.0												
5	2.4	2.7	2.9	3.1	3.3												
6	2.6	2.9	3.1	3.4	3.6	3.9	4.1										
7	2.8	3.1	3.4	3.6	3.9	4.2	4.4	4.7	4.9								
8	2.9	3.1	3.4	3.9	4.1	4.4	4.7	5.0	5.3	5.5	5.8						
9		3.2	3.5	4.0	4.4	4.7	5.0	5.3	5.6	5.9	6.2	6.5	6.7				
10				4.2	4.6	4.9	5.2	5.6	5.9	6.2	6.5	6.8	7.1	7.4	7.7		
11				4.4	4.8	5.1	5.5	5.8	6.2	6.5	6.8	7.1	7.5	7.8	8.1	8.4	8.7
12				4.5	4.9	5.3	5.7	6.0	6.4	6.8	7.1	7.5	7.8	8.1	8.5	8.8	9.1
13								6.3	6.6	7.0	7.4	7.8	8.1	8.5	8.8	9.2	9.5
14								6.5	6.9	7.3	7.7	8.0	8.4	8.8	9.2	9.5	9.9
15								6.7	7.1	7.5	7.9	8.3	8.7	9.1	9.5	9.9	10.2
16								6.8	7.3	7.7	8.1	8.6	9.0	9.4	9.8	10.2	10.6
17											8.4	8.8	9.2	9.7	10.1	10.5	10.9
18											8.6	9.0	9.5	9.9	10.4	10.8	11.2
19											8.8	9.3	9.7	10.2	10.6	11.1	11.5
20											9.0	9.4	9.9	10.4	10.9	11.3	11.8

Table 85.1

Male Total Body Water (L) Nomograms—cont'd

Weight (kg) \ Height (cm)	106	110	114	118	122	126	130	134	138	142	146	150	154	158	162	166	170	174	178	182	186	190
20	10.9	11.3	11.8	12.3	12.7	13.2	13.6	14.0	14.5	14.9	15.3	15.7										
22	11.4	11.9	12.4	12.8	13.3	13.8	14.3	14.7	15.2	15.7	16.1	16.6										
24	11.8	12.3	12.9	13.4	13.9	14.4	14.9	15.4	15.9	16.4	16.8	17.3	17.8	18.3	18.7							
26	12.2	12.8	13.3	13.9	14.4	15.0	15.5	16.0	16.5	17.0	17.5	18.0	18.5	19.0	19.5							
28	12.6	13.2	13.8	14.4	14.9	15.5	16.0	16.6	17.1	17.7	18.2	18.7	19.3	19.8	20.3	20.8	21.3					
30	13.0	13.6	14.2	14.8	15.4	16.0	16.6	17.1	17.7	18.3	18.8	19.4	19.9	20.5	21.0	21.6	22.1					
32	13.3	14.0	14.6	15.2	15.8	16.5	17.1	17.7	18.3	18.8	19.4	20.0	20.6	21.2	21.7	22.3	22.9	23.4	24.0			
34	13.6	14.3	15.0	15.6	16.3	16.9	17.5	18.2	18.8	19.4	20.0	20.6	21.2	21.8	22.4	23.0	23.6	24.2	24.7			
36	13.9	14.6	15.3	16.0	16.7	17.3	18.0	18.7	19.3	19.9	20.6	21.2	21.8	22.4	23.1	23.7	24.3	24.9	25.5	26.1	26.6	
38	14.2	14.9	15.7	16.4	17.1	17.8	18.4	19.1	19.8	20.4	21.1	21.8	22.4	23.0	23.7	24.3	24.9	25.6	26.2	26.8	27.4	
40			16.0	16.7	17.4	18.1	18.8	19.5	20.2	20.9	21.6	22.3	23.0	23.6	24.3	24.9	25.6	26.2	26.9	27.5	28.1	28.8
42			16.3	17.0	17.8	18.5	19.2	20.0	20.7	21.4	22.1	22.8	23.5	24.2	24.9	25.5	26.2	26.9	27.5	28.2	28.8	29.5
44			16.6	17.3	18.1	18.9	19.6	20.4	21.1	21.8	22.6	23.3	24.0	24.7	25.4	26.1	26.8	27.5	28.2	28.8	29.5	30.2
46			16.8	17.6	18.4	19.2	20.0	20.8	21.5	22.3	23.0	23.8	24.5	25.2	26.0	26.7	27.4	28.1	28.8	29.5	30.2	30.9
48			17.1	17.9	18.7	19.5	20.3	21.1	21.9	22.7	23.5	24.2	25.0	25.7	26.5	27.2	27.9	28.7	29.4	30.1	30.8	31.5
50			17.3	18.2	19.0	19.8	20.7	21.5	22.3	23.1	23.9	24.7	25.4	26.2	27.0	27.7	28.5	29.2	30.0	30.7	31.5	32.2
52						20.1	21.0	21.8	22.6	23.5	24.3	25.1	25.9	26.7	27.5	28.2	29.0	29.8	30.6	31.3	32.1	32.8
54						20.4	21.3	22.1	23.0	23.8	24.7	25.5	26.3	27.1	27.9	28.7	29.5	30.3	31.1	31.9	32.7	33.4
56						20.7	21.6	22.5	23.3	24.2	25.0	25.9	26.7	27.6	28.4	29.2	30.0	30.8	31.7	32.4	33.2	34.0
58						20.9	21.8	22.8	23.7	24.5	25.4	26.3	27.1	28.0	28.8	29.7	30.5	31.4	32.2	33.0	33.8	34.6
60						21.2	22.1	23.1	24.0	24.9	25.8	26.7	27.5	28.4	29.3	30.1	31.0	31.8	32.7	33.5	34.4	35.2
62						21.4	22.4	23.3	24.3	25.2	26.1	27.0	27.9	28.8	29.7	30.6	31.5	32.3	33.2	34.0	34.9	35.7
64						21.7	22.6	23.6	24.6	25.5	26.4	27.4	28.3	29.2	30.1	31.0	31.9	32.8	33.7	34.5	35.4	36.3
66									24.8	25.8	26.8	27.7	28.6	29.6	30.5	31.4	32.3	33.2	34.1	35.0	35.9	36.8
68									25.1	26.1	27.1	28.0	29.0	30.0	30.9	31.8	32.8	33.7	34.6	35.5	36.4	37.3
70									25.4	26.4	27.4	28.4	29.3	30.3	31.3	32.2	33.2	34.1	35.1	36.0	36.9	37.8
72									25.6	26.6	27.7	28.7	29.7	30.7	31.6	32.6	33.6	34.5	35.5	36.4	37.4	38.3
74									25.9	26.9	27.9	29.0	30.0	31.0	32.0	33.0	34.0	34.9	35.9	36.9	37.8	38.8
76									26.1	27.2	28.2	29.3	30.3	31.3	32.3	33.3	34.4	35.3	36.3	37.3	38.3	39.3
78									26.3	27.4	28.5	29.5	30.6	31.6	32.7	33.7	34.7	35.7	36.7	37.7	38.7	39.7
80									26.5	27.6	28.7	29.8	30.9	31.9	33.0	34.1	35.1	36.1	37.1	38.2	39.2	40.2

Table 85.2

Female Total Body Water (L) Nomograms

Weight (kg) \ Height (cm)	50	54	58	62	66	70	74	78	82	86	90	94	98	102	106	110	114
2	2.0	2.1	2.2	2.4													
3	2.4	2.6	2.8	2.9													
4	2.8	3.0	3.2	3.4	3.6												
5	3.1	3.3	3.5	3.8	4.0												
6	3.3	3.6	3.8	4.1	4.3	4.6	4.8										
7	3.5	3.8	4.1	4.4	4.8	4.9	5.2										
8	3.7	4.0	4.3	4.6	4.9	5.2	5.5	5.5	5.7		6.6						
9				4.9	5.2	5.5	5.8	5.8	6.1	6.4	7.0	7.3	7.6				
10				5.1	5.4	5.8	6.1	6.1	6.4	6.7	7.4	7.7	8.0	8.3	8.6		
11				5.3	5.6	6.0	6.4	6.4	6.8	7.1	7.7	8.1	8.4	8.7	9.0	9.3	9.6
12				5.4	5.8	6.2	6.6	6.7	7.1	7.4	8.0	8.4	8.7	9.1	9.4	9.7	10.0
13								7.0	7.3	7.7	8.3	8.7	9.1	9.4	9.8	10.1	10.4
14								7.2	7.6	8.0	8.6	9.0	9.4	9.7	10.1	10.5	10.8
15								7.4	7.8	8.2	8.9	9.3	9.7	10.0	10.4	10.8	11.2
16								7.6	8.0	8.5	9.1	9.5	9.9	10.3	10.7	11.1	11.5
17								7.8	8.3	8.7	9.3	9.8	10.2	10.6	11.0	11.4	11.8
18											9.6	10.0	10.5	10.9	11.3	11.7	12.2
19											9.8	10.2	10.7	11.1	11.6	12.0	12.5
20											10.0	10.4	10.9	11.4	11.8	12.3	12.7

Table 85.2

Female Total Body Water (L) Nomograms—cont'd

Weight (kg)	\ Height (cm) 106	110	114	118	122	126	130	134	138	142	146	150	154	158	162	166	170	174	178	182	186	190
20	11.8	12.3	12.7	13.2	13.6	14.0	14.5	14.9	15.3	15.7	16.1	16.5										
22	12.3	12.8	13.3	13.7	14.2	14.7	15.1	15.6	16.0	16.4	16.9	17.3										
24	12.8	13.3	13.8	14.3	14.8	15.2	15.7	16.2	16.7	17.1	17.6	18.0	18.5	18.9	19.4							
26	13.2	13.7	14.2	14.8	15.3	15.8	16.3	16.8	17.3	17.8	18.3	18.7	19.2	19.7	20.1							
28	13.6	14.1	14.7	15.2	15.8	16.3	16.8	17.3	17.9	18.4	18.9	19.4	19.9	20.4	20.9	21.3	21.8					
30	13.9	14.5	15.1	15.7	16.2	16.8	17.3	17.9	18.4	18.9	19.5	20.0	20.5	21.0	21.5	22.0	22.5					
32	14.3	14.9	15.5	16.1	16.6	17.2	17.8	18.4	18.9	19.5	20.0	20.6	21.1	21.7	22.2	22.7	23.2	23.7	24.3			
34	14.6	15.2	15.8	16.4	17.0	17.7	18.2	18.8	19.4	20.0	20.6	21.1	21.7	22.3	22.8	23.4	23.9	24.4	25.0			
36	14.8	15.5	16.2	16.8	17.4	18.1	18.7	19.3	19.9	20.5	21.1	21.7	22.3	22.8	23.4	24.0	24.5	25.1	25.6	26.2	26.7	
38	15.1	15.8	16.5	17.1	17.8	18.4	19.1	19.7	20.3	21.0	21.6	22.2	22.8	23.4	24.0	24.6	25.1	25.7	26.3	26.9	27.4	
40			16.8	17.4	18.1	18.8	19.5	20.1	20.7	21.4	22.0	22.7	23.3	23.9	24.5	25.1	25.7	26.3	26.9	27.5	28.1	28.6
42			17.0	17.7	18.4	19.1	19.8	20.5	21.1	21.8	22.5	23.1	23.8	24.4	25.0	25.7	26.3	26.9	27.5	28.1	28.7	29.3
44			17.3	18.0	18.7	19.5	20.2	20.9	21.5	22.2	22.9	23.6	24.2	24.9	25.5	26.2	26.8	27.4	28.1	28.7	29.3	29.9
46			17.5	18.3	19.0	19.8	20.5	21.2	21.9	22.6	23.3	24.0	24.7	25.3	26.0	26.7	27.3	28.0	28.6	29.3	29.9	30.5
48			17.8	18.5	19.3	20.0	20.8	21.5	22.3	23.0	23.7	24.4	25.1	25.8	26.5	27.2	27.8	28.5	29.2	29.8	30.5	31.1
50			18.0	18.8	19.6	20.3	21.1	21.8	22.6	23.3	24.1	24.8	25.5	26.2	26.9	27.6	28.3	29.0	29.7	30.4	31.0	31.7
52						20.6	21.4	22.1	22.9	23.7	24.4	25.2	25.9	26.6	27.4	28.1	28.8	29.5	30.2	30.9	31.6	32.2
54						20.8	21.6	22.4	23.2	24.0	24.8	25.5	26.3	27.0	27.8	28.5	29.2	29.9	30.7	31.4	32.1	32.8
56						21.1	21.9	22.7	23.5	24.3	25.1	25.9	26.6	27.4	28.2	28.9	29.7	30.4	31.1	31.9	32.6	33.3
58						21.3	22.1	23.0	23.8	24.6	25.4	26.2	27.0	27.8	28.5	29.3	30.1	30.8	31.6	32.3	33.1	33.8
60						21.5	22.4	23.2	24.1	24.9	25.7	26.5	27.3	28.1	28.9	29.7	30.5	31.3	32.0	32.8	33.5	34.3
62						21.7	22.6	23.4	24.3	25.2	26.0	26.8	27.7	28.5	29.3	30.1	30.9	31.7	32.4	33.2	34.0	34.8
64						21.9	22.8	23.7	24.6	25.4	26.3	27.1	28.0	28.8	29.6	30.4	31.3	32.1	32.9	33.6	34.4	35.2
66									24.8	25.7	26.5	27.4	28.3	29.1	30.0	30.8	31.6	32.4	33.2	34.1	34.9	35.7
68									25.0	25.9	26.8	27.7	28.6	29.4	30.3	31.1	32.0	32.8	33.6	34.5	35.3	36.1
70									25.2	26.1	27.0	27.9	28.8	29.7	30.6	31.5	32.3	33.2	34.0	34.9	35.7	36.5
72									25.4	26.4	27.3	28.2	29.1	30.0	30.9	31.8	32.7	33.5	34.4	35.2	36.1	36.9
74									25.6	26.6	27.5	28.4	29.4	30.3	31.2	32.1	33.0	33.9	34.7	35.6	36.5	37.3
76									25.8	26.8	27.7	28.7	29.6	30.6	31.5	32.4	33.3	34.2	35.1	36.0	36.8	37.7
78									26.0	27.0	27.9	28.9	29.9	30.8	31.7	32.7	33.6	34.5	35.4	36.3	37.2	38.1
80									26.2	27.2	28.1	29.1	30.1	31.1	32.0	33.0	33.9	34.8	35.7	36.7	37.6	38.5

As noted previously, the measurement of dialysis delivery also requires the determination of RRF and BSA. It is important to recognize that greater RRF has repeatedly been shown to be associated with superior patient survival in adults. In children, the presence of RRF has also been shown to be associated with improved height SDS. The RRF is calculated as the glomerular filtration rate (GFR) by determining the average of the clearance of urea and creatinine as follows:

$$RRF = \left[\frac{U_{cr} \times V_u}{P_{cr}} + \frac{U_{ur} \times V_u}{P_{ur}} \right] \Big/ 2$$

where U_{cr} and P_{cr} are urinary and plasma concentrations of creatinine, U_{ur} and P_{ur} are urinary and plasma concentrations of urea, and V_u is the 24-hour urine volume. This method mathematically balances the tubular secretion of creatinine and the tubular reabsorption of urea that is characteristic of CKD. During the first few years of dialysis therapy, RRF often contributes appreciably to total solute and water removal. The loss of RRF is the major cause of a decreasing total (dialysate and RRF) clearance in PD subjects followed longitudinally and must be compensated by changes in the dialysis prescription to maintain the desired level of total clearance.

The determination of BSA has been commonly derived using the method of DuBois and DuBois, and most of the currently available data are based on this method. However, in an independent comparison, the Gehan and George method was preferred because more than 400 subjects, including many children, were used to define this formula; in contrast, only 9 subjects were used to define the formula of DuBois and DuBois. The respective formulae are as follows:

DuBois and DuBois method: $BSA(m^2) = (71.84 \times Wt(kg)^{0.425} \times Ht(cm)^{0.725})/10,000$

Gehan and George method: $BSA(m^2) = 0.0235 \times Wt(kg)^{0.51456} \times Ht(cm)^{0.42246}$

Adequacy Recommendations

Clinical "wellness" of the pediatric patient is an important parameter of PD adequacy, and adequate dialysis is likely provided if a patient's status is characterized by adequate growth, maintenance of normal serum chemistries, good blood pressure control and nutritional status, and adequate psychomotor development. Despite this fact, solute clearance and ultrafiltration (fluid removal), only two of the complex functions carried out by the healthy kidney, are the parameters most commonly utilized to assess dialysis adequacy.

Solute Clearance

As mentioned above, the latest K/DOQI guidelines recommend the use of Kt/V_{urea} alone as the solute clearance measurement to characterize dialysis adequacy. Few studies have been conducted with results that have contributed to the establishment of a recommended target clearance. The ADEMEX study, the largest longitudinal study of adult CAPD patients to date, did not demonstrate any clinical benefit associated with a Kt/V_{urea} of >1.7/wk, whereas studies by Lo et al have provided evidence for a recommended minimal Kt/V_{urea} of >1.7/wk and an optimal Kt/V_{urea} of 1.8/wk based on survival data in anuric adult CAPD patients. Because no similar large-scale studies have been performed in children and clinical experience supports the recommendation that solute clearance targets in children should meet/exceed those of adults, the latest recommendations for children are as follows:

- For patients with RRF (defined as urine Kt/V_{urea} of >0.1/wk): The minimal dose of total (peritoneal and kidney) small-solute clearance should be a Kt/V_{urea} of at least 1.8/wk.
- For patients without RRF (defined as urine Kt/V_{urea} of <0.1/wk) or in those in whom RRF is unable to be measured accurately, the minimal dose of small-solute clearance should be a peritoneal Kt/V_{urea} of at least 1.8/wk.

Current guidelines do not set different targets for continuous and noncontinuous forms of PD such as NIPD, nor do they set different targets based on peritoneal transport status.

However, regardless of the delivered dose of dialysis, if a patient is not doing well and has no other identifiable cause other than kidney failure, a trial of increased dialysis is indicated.

Maintenance of Euvolemia

Achievement of euvolemia is an exceptionally important adequacy target because of the high prevalence of hypertension and cardiovascular disease in children receiving PD. Optimization of the fluid status requires knowledge and understanding of a patient's ultrafiltration capacity and RRF. In patients who are hypertensive or in whom there is evidence of volume overload, ultrafiltration should generally be positive for all daytime and nighttime exchanges. An effort should be made to determine the lowest possible dialysate dextrose concentration required to achieve the desired ultrafiltration volume so as to hopefully help preserve peritoneal membrane function. This is best conducted with knowledge of the patient's peritoneal membrane transport capacity as derived from the PET. Patients who are characterized as high/rapid transporters and who are unable to achieve the ultrafiltration necessary for blood pressure control with standard dialysis solutions should be considered candidates for use of an icodextrin-based dialysis solution. Additional factors that may help maintain euvolemia include dietary sodium and fluid restriction, and even diuretics in patients with RRF, as was recently demonstrated by the International Pediatric Peritoneal Dialysis Network (IPPN). On the other hand, in patients who are polyuric, negative net daily ultrafiltration from PD may be desirable because of its potential to replenish decreased intravascular volume and improve RRF. When negative net daily ultrafiltration is not possible, provision of additional fluids is recommended. It is thus reasonable to suggest that fluid status, rather than fluid removal, should be the primary goal for adequate dialysis therapy.

Timing and Frequency of Solute Clearance and Ultrafiltration Measurement

For patients initiating dialysis for the first time and/or patients with substantial RRF, the initial measurement of total clearance should be performed within 4 weeks of the initiation of PD. For patients transferring from another renal replacement therapy to PD and/or for patients who do not have substantial RRF, the initial measurement of the delivered dose of PD should be made within 2 weeks of PD initiation to help prevent a prolonged period of underdialysis. The measurement of total Kt/V_{urea} should be performed when the patient is clinically stable (e.g., stable weight, stable BUN and creatinine concentrations) and at least 4 weeks after the resolution of peritonitis.

The total solute clearance should be measured once during the first 6 months of therapy and at least once every 6 months thereafter. As mentioned earlier, modification of the measurement schedule may be necessary if the dialysis prescription has been changed or there have been clinical events (e.g., protracted/repeated peritonitis) that may have altered the function of the peritoneal membrane. The measurement of RRF should be performed a minimum of every 3 months until the residual Kt/V_{urea} is <0.1, when its contribution to total clearance becomes negligible, a change in the dialysis prescription to compensate for the loss of RRF should be followed by a repeat assessment of the solute clearance. Finally, the patients' record of PD effluent volume should be reviewed monthly with particular attention to the drain volume from the overnight dwell of CAPD and the daytime dwell of CCPD.

Adjusting the Dialysis Prescription by Computer Modeling

Computer-based dialysis modeling may help tailor the PD prescription to the desired solute removal, transport type, body size, and lifestyle, etc. Kinetic modeling programs use peritoneal membrane transport capacity test data from the standard PET (PD Adequest, Baxter Healthcare) and the Personal Dialysis Capacity test (PACK PD, Fresenius; CDC Gambro) to help in prescription management. These have been validated for clinical use in pediatrics. The major advantage of the computer assistance is the flexibility and speed with which prescription options can be determined. Kinetic modeling may be especially important for APD therapies because of the variety of prescription modifications that are inherent to this modality. Whereas an increase in the fill volume is generally the most effective approach to increase the delivered dose of dialysis, computer-assisted kinetic modeling can also be used to determine the likely impact of changes in the exchange frequency or the addition of a daytime exchange, characteristics that influence dialysis adequacy and QOL. It needs to be emphasized that even with the use of computer assistance, actual solute clearance measurements are mandatory to confirm the delivered dialysis dose.

Summary

The adequacy of PD is only one aspect of the global management of the stage 5 CKD patient. Clinicians formulating the PD prescription designed to achieve dialysis adequacy in children should be well versed in the properties of CAPD and APD, the value and limitations of Kt/V_{urea} as a measurement of adequacy, the assessment of peritoneal transport characteristics in children, and the use of computer technology to adjust the dialysis prescription. While the clinical correlates of adequate or optimal dialysis in children are currently not yet defined as they are in adults, it must be emphasized that the achievement of numeric targets should never be considered the sole determinant of adequate care. Kt/V_{urea} is only a measure of delivered dialysis dose and cannot and should not be equated to dialysis adequacy. It should be seen as the minimum dose of dialysis required to keep the patient healthy. Dialysis adequacy should rightly be assessed by the patient's well-being. The recent introduction of tools specifically designed to evaluate QOL in children with kidney disease provide the means to assess another important outcome parameter. In the patient who is otherwise thriving, failure to achieve specific numeric targets may not be an indication to alter the dialysis prescription or modality. Alternatively, it is important to recognize that grossly inadequate solute clearance may occur in patients who show only subtle clinical signs of inadequate dialysis, such as a deteriorating nutritional state. Clinical features that may be suggestive of inadequate dialysis and factors that may contribute to this outcome are listed in Tables 85.3 and 85.4, respectively. In the end, individualizing the prescription is the key to improving patient outcome with long-term PD therapy (Fig. 85.1).

Table 85.3

Outcome Measures That May Be Associated With Inadequate Dialysis

- Lack of subjective feeling of well-being
- Clinical or biochemical signs of malnutrition (e.g., low body mass index [BMI], low serum albumin)
- Poor growth/poor response to recombinant growth hormone
- Developmental delay
- Poor school performance
- Poor response to anemia management
- Poor control of renal osteodystrophy
- Excessive calcium × phosphorus product
- Uncontrolled hypertension
- Congestive heart failure

Table 85.4

Factors Contributing to Inadequate Dialysis

- Loss of residual renal function
- Prescription inadequate for peritoneal membrane transport characteristics
- Reduced peritoneal surface area due to extensive intraabdominal adhesions
- Loss of membrane solute transport/ultrafiltration capacity due to peritonitis
- Noncompliance with PD prescription
- Poorly functioning PD catheter

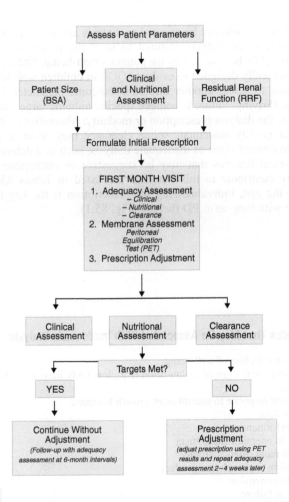

Figure 85.1

Algorithm for PD Prescription Management.

C H A P T E R   8 6

Continuous Renal Replacement Therapy in Pediatric Patients

David T. Selewski, MD, MS • Patrick D. Brophy, MD, MHCDS

Introduction

There have been a myriad of changes in the practice and application of continuous renal replacement therapy (CRRT) to pediatric patients over the past two decades. The evolution of CRRT in pediatric patients has occurred in parallel to changes in the recognition and epidemiology of acute kidney injury (AKI) in pediatric patients. The etiology of AKI had been largely related to hemolytic uremic syndrome, primary renal diseases, or sepsis. Over the last two decades, the etiology of AKI in industrialized countries has transitioned to being secondary to other conditions or critical illnesses including congenital heart disease, sepsis/multiorgan dysfunction, bone marrow transplant, neonatal critical illness, and nephrotoxic medications. Utilizing modern definitions of AKI, recent studies have shown that AKI is most common in critically ill children with an incidence of 10%–24.5%. In the most critically ill patients, such as those requiring mechanical ventilation, the incidence of AKI is as high as 82%. AKI has been shown to be associated with adverse outcomes including prolonged hospitalization, mechanical ventilation, and increased mortality. With the recognition of the impact of AKI on outcomes, the importance of the provision of renal replacement therapy in children has become clear.

In determining modality choice for the provision of RRT in pediatric patients, the provider may use hemodialysis, peritoneal dialysis, or CRRT. When considering the choice of modality, one must take into account a number of factors including the goal of therapy, patient characteristics, and institutional expertise. Over the last 30 years CRRT has become the modality of choice for providing RRT in critically ill children. There are a number of advantages of CRRT, including slower and more controlled fluid removal, which in turn avoids larger fluid shifts that may occur with other modalities (hemodialysis). CRRT also allows for improved metabolic control and the provision of adequate nutrition relative to other modalities. Furthermore, CRRT is capable of providing cumulative solute clearance similar to if not superior to intermittent hemodialysis with the benefit of improved hemodynamic tolerance. As a result, a detailed understanding of pediatric CRRT is critical to the care of critically ill children.

At its core, the application of CRRT to children involves the same basic principles applied to adults with a number of considerations unique to children to ensure safe and adequate therapy. Pediatric patients require special consideration in all aspects of CRRT, including but not limited to indication, nutrition, vascular access, dose, anticoagulation, membrane choice, adaptation of adult equipment, and extracorporeal blood volume. There are also unique pediatric indications and populations that are more commonly seen in pediatrics, including those with inborn errors of metabolism, those on extracorporeal membrane oxygenation, and neonates.

Indication and Timing of Initiation

The indications for the initiation of CRRT are similar in children as those in adults including severe acidosis, severe electrolyte abnormalities, severe uremia, intoxications, and fluid overload. An additional indication worth discussing is the inability to provide adequate nutrition. Children with AKI are frequently volume and, therefore, nutritionally restricted in an attempt to avoid the need for RRT. This conservative approach to AKI care reduces the ability to provide adequate nutrition to the pediatric patient. Given that the provision of proper nutrition to advance the anabolic process is key to clinical improvement, it is now recognized that the institution of CRRT to effectively "make room" for adequate nutritional supplementation is a cornerstone of pediatric critical care. Thus nutritional provision is a true indication for CRRT initiation. Additional indications seen in pediatric patients include intoxications and inborn errors of metabolism. Other considerations for the institution of CRRT include the expected trajectory of the underlying disease, the degree of organ dysfunction including the presence of systemic inflammation, and the potential solute burden (tumor lysis syndrome).

The prospective pediatric CRRT Registry (ppCRRT) has provided the most comprehensive evaluation of the indications for CRRT initiation. Briefly, the ppCRRT registry was a prospective multicenter observational study formed to describe current practices in pediatric CRRT. The registry was closed in 2005 enrolling 370 patients and provides the most comprehensive data on pediatric CRRT. This registry shows that fluid overload was the indication in 78% of critically ill children receiving CRRT, including 46% for combined fluid/electrolyte, 29% fluid overload in isolation, and 3% for the prevention of fluid overload. Other indications within the registry included electrolyte abnormalities (13%) and intoxications/inborn errors of metabolism (9%). These indications mirror those of a diverse group of single-center studies that consistently demonstrate fluid overload/ fluid management as a primary indication for CRRT in 70%–80% of the cases of CRRT. The impact of the degree of fluid overload at CRRT initiation warrant further discussion.

The pioneers of pediatric CRRT have been at the forefront of the study of the prognostic significance of fluid overload at CRRT initiation as a predictor of outcomes. In 2001, Goldstein et al evaluated the outcomes of children requiring CRRT and demonstrated that the degree of fluid overload at CRRT initiation was significantly higher in nonsurvivors (16% vs 34%, $p = .03$). This study used the cumulative fluid balance from intensive care unit admission to calculate fluid overload based on the following equation:

$$\%FO = \{Sum\ of\ Daily(Fluid\ in - Fluid\ out)/ICU\ Admission\ Weight\} * 100$$

These findings have been confirmed in a number of single-center and multicenter studies (Table 86.1). The largest of these studies included 297 patients from the ppCRRT registry, which showed increased mortality with increasing degrees of fluid

Table 86.1

Fluid Overload and Outcomes in Pediatric Continuous Renal Replacement Therapy

Author, Year	Population Size	Study Design	Method of FO Measurement	Main Findings
Goldstein, 2001	21	Retrospective, single-center	FO% from ICU admission to CRRT initiation	FO% at CRRT initiation was associated with increased mortality (16% survivors vs 34% nonsurvivors)
Gillespie, 2004	88	Retrospective, single-center	FO% from ICU admission to CRRT initiation	FO >10% at CRRT initiation associated with increased mortality (OR 3.0)
Foland, 2004	113	Retrospective, single-center	FO% from up to 7 days before CRRT initiation	Higher FO% at CRRT initiation associated with increased mortality (7.8% survivors vs 15.1% nonsurvivors)
Hayes, 2009	76	Retrospective, single-center	FO% from ICU admission to CRRT initiation	FO% at CRRT initiation was associated with increased mortality (7.3% survivors vs 22.3% nonsurvivors), FO%>20% at CRRT initiation associated with increased mortality (OR 6.1) and prolonged hospitalization
Sutherland, 2010	297	Prospective multicenter registry data	FO% from ICU admission to CRRT initiation	At CRRT initiation, FO characteristics: 51.5% with <10% FO, 17.2% with 10%–20% FO, and 31.3% with ≥20% FO. Higher FO% (continuous) and FO% >20% at CRRT initiation associated with increased mortality (OR 8.5)
Selewski, 2011	113 (50 on ECMO and CRRT)	Retrospective, single-center	FO% from ICU admission to CRRT initiation	Higher FO% at CRRT initiation associated with increased mortality in patients on ECMO and general pediatric critical care (5% survivors vs 23% nonsurvivors)

CRRT, continuous renal replacement therapy; ECMO, extracorporeal membrane oxygenation; FO, fluid overload; ICU, intensive care unit.

The following references support Table 86.1:

Goldstein SL, Currier H, Graf C, et al. Outcome in children receiving continuous venovenous hemofiltration. *Pediatrics.* 2001;107:1309-1312.

Gillespie RS, Seidel K, Symons JM. Effect of fluid overload and dose of replacement fluid on survival in hemofiltration. *Pediatr Nephrol.* 2004;19:1394-1399.

Foland JA, Fortenberry JD, Warshaw BL, et al. Fluid overload before continuous hemofiltration and survival in critically ill children: a retrospective analysis. *Crit Care Med.* 2004;32:1771-1776.

Hayes LW, Oster RA, Tofil NM, Tolwani AJ. Outcomes of critically ill children requiring continuous renal replacement therapy. *J Crit Care.* 2009;24:394-400.

Sutherland SM, Zappitelli M, Alexander SR, et al. Fluid overload and mortality in children receiving continuous renal replacement therapy: the prospective pediatric continuous renal replacement therapy registry. *Am J Kidney Dis.* 2010;55:316-325.

Selewski DT, Cornell TT, Lombel RM, et al. Weight-based determination of fluid overload status and mortality in pediatric intensive care unit patients requiring continuous renal replacement therapy. *Intens Care Med.* 2011;37:1166-1173.

overload at CRRT initiation controlling for severity of illness (29.6% mortality for fluid overload <10%, 43.1% for 10%–20% fluid overload, and 65.6% with >20% fluid overload). In each of the studies, mortality is significantly increased at CRRT initiation when the patient is 10%–20% fluid overloaded. Although firm recommendations cannot be made about an absolute FO cutoff for the consideration of the initiation of CRRT, experts agree that fluid overload of 10%–20% consideration should be made for intervention.

Although the contribution of cumulative fluid overload at CRRT initiation has become clear, the optimal timing of CRRT initiation remains a highly studied topic. To fully grasp the decision making and risk stratification in children, it becomes important to further describe the disease characteristics of critical illness unique to children. Pediatric patients have been shown to develop multiorgan dysfunction early in the course of their critical illness. This was demonstrated in a study by Proulx et al that showed that 87% of children with multiorgan dysfunction had their peak organ dysfunction score within 72 hours of admission. Furthermore, epidemiologic data have shown that AKI most commonly occurs early in the ICU course in children. The epidemiologic data on the timing of initiation of CRRT in the adult literature has shown an association between late CRRT initiation and poor outcomes. Recently, a single-center retrospective analysis in pediatric patients has shown that the median timing of initiation of CRRT was later in nonsurvivors (3.4 days vs 2 days, $p = .001$). As a result, there is an effort under way to develop a "renal angina" scoring system to risk-stratify children on admission to the ICU with the hope of early identification of the patients who will go on to require CRRT during their critical illness. The optimal timing of initiation of CRRT remains a top research priority.

Mechanism of Clearance and Options for Therapy

The current CRRT devices allow for multiple therapeutic choices. To fully appreciate the strengths and weaknesses of these options, an understanding of the basic concepts of diffusion and convection is necessary. The human kidney relies on both convective and diffusive clearance to maintain homeostasis, with convection occurring in the glomerulus and diffusion in the tubules.

Diffusion refers to the movement of solutes down a concentration gradient across a semipermeable membrane. Diffusion favors the movement of smaller particles (<500 Daltons) down a large concentration gradient. The rate of diffusion of a solute is governed by concentration, membrane permeability, membrane surface area, and solute characteristics (size and charge). Convection describes the movement of solute across a semipermeable membrane with solvent in response to a transmembrane pressure gradient. This concept is frequently referred to as "solvent drag," where solvent and solute move together across the membrane. As a result, convection results in the production of an isotonic ultrafiltrate. Convection favors the movement of larger molecules and provides the theoretical benefit of middle molecule clearance.

Ultrafiltration utilizes a transmembrane pressure gradient to drive solvent through a semipermeable membrane to achieve fluid removal. The determinants of ultrafiltration rate include membrane permeability, membrane surface area, and pressure gradient. Ultrafiltration is classically associated with convective therapies, but also occurs during dialytic therapies with fluid removal.

The following equations describe solute clearance in diffusion and convection.

Diffusion:

Solute transport is governed by $Jd = DTA \, (dc/dx)$, where

Jd = solute flux, D = diffusion coefficient, T = solution temperature, A = membrane surface area, dc = concentration gradient between compartments, and dx = membrane thickness

Convection:

Filtration is governed by $Q_f = K_m \, TMP$, where

Q_f = filtration rate (mL/h), K_m = membrane permeability coefficient, and TMP = transmembrane pressure (mm Hg) {TMP = $P_b - P_{uf} - p$, where P_b = hydrostatic pressure of blood, P_{uf} = hydraulic pressure of the dialysate/ultrafiltrate compartments, and p = protein oncotic pressure}

Solute transport is governed by $Jc = UF(x)_{uf}$, where

UF = ultrafiltrate volume and $(x)_{uf}$ = solute x concentration in the ultrafiltrate

Convective treatment clearance is represented by $K_c = Q_f \, (x)_{uf}/(x)_{Pw}$, where

Q_f = Uf rate and $(x)_{uf}/(x)_{Pw}$ = ratio of ultrafiltrate and plasma water solute concentrations (or the Sieving coefficient)

During ultrafiltration, the passage of solute is based on the membrane sieving coefficient. For molecules that pass freely, the sieving coefficient is 1 and for those that do not pass the coefficient approaches 0. The diffusion coefficient describes the extent to which solute passes across a semipermeable membrane during dialysis (see above). For some smaller molecules, the diffusion coefficient and sieving coefficient are the same, whereas for larger molecules such as vancomycin the sieving coefficient is greater than the diffusion coefficient. For molecules where the sieving coefficient is greater than the diffusion coefficient, there may be a theoretical advantage to convective therapies. This provides the theoretical basis for convective clearance removing larger molecules (middle molecules including cytokines such as tumor necrosis) as a treatment for systemic inflammatory processes.

The description of the variety of CRRT modalities depends on the type of vascular access and the modality or modalities delivered. Historically, CRRT was developed using arterial and venous access (CAVH); this is generally not currently practiced with regularity. This has been replaced with pump-driven venovenous access. The current modalities are determined by the type of clearance desired (convection, diffusion, or both) and include continuous venovenous hemofiltration (CVVH), continuous venovenous hemodialysis (CVVHD), and continuous venovenous hemodiafiltration (CVVHDF).

CVVH (Fig. 86.1A) utilizes convective clearance with high ultrafiltration rates. The ultrafiltrate produced is replaced by a physiologically appropriate sterile replacement fluid, which may be delivered either pre- or postfilter. Solute clearance is driven by membrane surface area and blood flow rate. The rate of ultrafiltration is the major determinant of clearance. A theoretical advantage to giving prefilter replacement fluid is that it may decrease the incidence of clotting in the filter as it dilutes the blood entering the filter, but comes at the expense of reduced solute clearance. If the replacement fluid is given postfilter, there may be an increased risk of clotting secondary to hemoconcentration across the filter. This becomes problematic when the filtration fraction across the filter approaches 25%–30%.

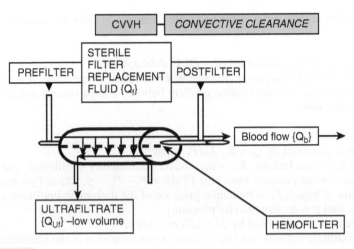

Figure 86.1 A

(A) Continuous Venovenous Hemofiltration.

CVVHD (Fig. 86.1B) offers primarily diffusive solute clearance through the use of dialysis fluid that runs countercurrent to the blood flow within the filter. The clearance is determined primarily by blood flow rate, dialysate rate, and membrane surface area, with a contribution of convective clearance from ultrafiltration. The diffusive clearance in CVVHD differs from intermittent hemodialysis in that the dialysate flow rate is slower than the blood flow rate, which allows for equilibration of solutes. Therefore, the dialysis rate in CRRT approaches the creatinine clearance, which is an important difference from intermittent hemodialysis. In this modality, there is some convective clearance provided by patient fluid removal via ultrafiltration. The ultrafiltration is directly related to fluid removal titrated to the desired

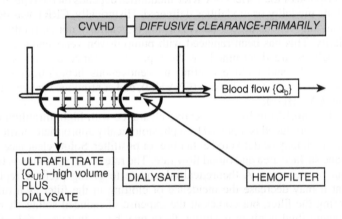

Figure 86.1 B

(B) Continuous Venovenous Hemodialysis.

patient weight loss plus removal of obligate fluids (medication drips, TPN, etc.). As a result of ultrafiltration, this modality may have convective clearances of up to 17%.

CVVHDF (Fig. 86.1C) offers both convective and diffusive solute clearance through the combination of dialysis fluid and filter replacement fluid. This combination technique may offer an improved clearance rate of some intoxicants and middle molecules. Replacement fluid can be administered either pre- or postfilter with the caveats mentioned above.

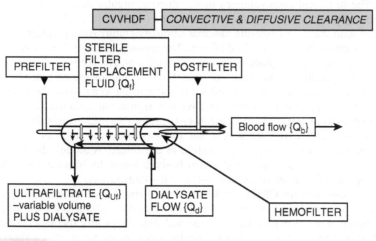

Figure 86.1 C

(C) Continuous Venovenous Hemodiafiltration.

There are currently no firm recommendations in terms of the modality of choice to deliver CRRT. The ppCRRT registry noted significant practice variation with regards to modality choice across centers with 48% CVVHDF, 21% CVVH, and 30% CVVHD. In certain clinical situations such as sepsis, modalities that employ convective clearance may provide a benefit. This is based on the clearance of middle molecules and a potentially beneficial effect on disordered inflammation. At this time, there is only a single study in pediatric stem cell patients that suggests convective clearance may provide benefit over primarily diffusive therapies.

Access

The provision of vascular access that is of the appropriate location and size is the most important aspect to performing adequate Pediatric CRRT. In general, one wants to maintain a venous pressure of less than 200 mm Hg. Although recirculation is commonly discussed with hemodialysis, this is less of an issue because of the continuous nature of CRRT. Classically, dual-lumen catheters were sufficient for CRRT but with the trend toward citrate anticoagulation, double-lumen access with an additional separate central line has become necessary. This occurs because of the need for an additional central line for calcium infusion back to the child when citrate anticoagulation is used in CVVHD (see section on anticoagulation). The two key components to consider with vascular access for CRRT in children are location and size.

Vascular access can be placed in internal jugular, femoral, or subclavian veins to successfully provide CRRT. In the evaluation performed by the ppCRRT group, internal jugular catheters had significantly longer circuit survival when compared to subclavian or femoral catheters. The advantage of the internal jugular catheter is that it is independent of the patient's motion, delivers adequate blood flow with insignificant resistance, and appears to be associated with lower infection rates. The historical disadvantages of the internal jugular catheter were related to concerns of pneumo- or hemothorax at the time of placement. These concerns have lessened with the use of bedside vascular ultrasonography during placement, which is now the recommended standard of care. The femoral line may have less complication risks at the time of placement, but the disadvantages are risk of thrombosis of the vein complicating future renal transplant options and increased risk of infection. Furthermore, unless the catheter resides in the inferior vena cava, the catheter can be sensitive to patient movement and require significant sedation or paralysis in order to perform CRRT. Many nephrologists prefer to avoid using subclavian catheters because of the risk of subclavian stenosis, as some patients may develop end-stage renal disease requiring a fistula in the future. Although the location for vascular access is made on an individual basis, a hierarchy of access as follows is generally accepted: internal jugular →femoral →subclavian.

Blood flow rates for CRRT are determined by the size of the child, the machine used, and the vascular access pressures. The size of the catheter is the limiting factor in the blood flows that may be achieved and thus frequently dictates the limits of CRRT dose. Flow characteristics of vascular access demonstrate that a short, large-bore access has less flow resistance than a longer, smaller internal lumen access, which is consistent with the Poiseuille law. The ppCRRT group evaluated catheter size and demonstrated that 5-Fr catheters had significantly lower circuit survival (20 hours) than catheters of other sizes. The average circuit life of 20 hours using a single double-lumen 5-Fr catheter makes the delivery of adequate CRRT impossible and as such should be avoided. In practice, most small neonates can have access achieved with a double-lumen 7-Fr catheter. Table 86.2 provides suggested sizes of vascular access by patient weight.

Finally, before acute catheter placement, the team should consider the potential duration of therapy. If prolonged renal replacement therapy is a possibility, consideration should be made for tunneled catheter placement. These catheters have been

Table 86.2	
Suggested Size and Selection of CRRT Vascular Access for Pediatric Patients	
Patient Size	**Catheter Size and Source**
Neonate	Dual-lumen 7.0 French
3–6 kg	Dual-lumen 7.0 French or triple-lumen 7.0 French
6–30 kg	Dual-lumen 8.0 French
>15 kg	Dual-lumen 9.0 French
>30 kg	Dual-lumen 10.0 French or triple-lumen 12 French

shown to have less dysfunction, lower rates of infections, fewer thrombotic complications, and better catheter survival.

Prescription

With the recent advances in CRRT equipment, there has been an expansion in the capability and flexibility to prescribe CRRT in children. Classically, compared with intermittent hemodialysis, CRRT is thought to provide lower-efficiency clearance. Over the course of a full day, CRRT is capable of providing clearances similar to intermittent hemodialysis. Newer CRRT machines are capable of running at blood flow rates as high as those of intermittent hemodialysis machinery. In prescribing CRRT, it is important to understand the rate-limiting principles in comparison to intermittent hemodialysis. At its core, the basic principles that limit clearance and prescription in CRRT and intermittent hemodialysis still persist. The clearance in intermittent hemodialysis is limited by blood flow, as the dialytic rates are greater than blood flow rates by 1.5–2 times. In CRRT, the clearance is limited by the rate of dialysis (CVVHD) or replacement fluid delivery (CVVH).

The blood flow prescribed is dependent on the vascular access (discussed above), CRRT machine, and the size of the patient. The recommended blood flow rates in children are prescribed based on weight and range from 3 to 10 mL/kg/min. Our practice is to prescribe 5 mL/kg/min of blood flow in patients greater than 10 kg. The prescription in infants and neonates less than 10 kg may require higher blood flow rates to generate the appropriate access and return pressures to successfully perform CRRT utilizing adult machines. Typically, the minimum blood flow is 35–50 mL/min irrespective of patient size.

The dose of CRRT has remained a hotly studied topic throughout nephrology in children and adults. An early study by Ronco et al comparing a high dose of ultrafiltration (35 mL/kg/h) to lower dose (20 mL/kg/h) demonstrated benefit in critically ill patients. Subsequent to this, there were several studies evaluating higher dose CRRT with mixed results. There have been two randomized trials evaluating high-dose CRRT in adults that have failed to show benefit of higher doses of CRRT. There have not been any such studies in children to date. Based on these studies, the recommended delivered dialysis dose is 20–25 mL/kg/h. This group recognized that patients with sepsis and AKI may represent a special population that may benefit from higher-dose CRRT. Furthermore, this population may benefit from convective therapies to allow for improved middle molecule clearance.

In prescribing CRRT in children, one should consider the total delivered CRRT dose, which is composed of replacement fluid (pre- or postfilter) and countercurrent dialysate rate. Although adult studies prescribe CRRT dose based on weight, it is common to prescribe based on body surface area in children. A starting delivered dialysis dose of 2 L/h/1.73 m^2 is common, which roughly gives a urea clearance of 30 mL/min/1.73 m^2. In prescribing CRRT, it is important to realize that the dose prescribed differs from the dose delivered. This can result from technical issues surrounding CRRT, including filter clotting, circuit malfunction, and bag changes and trips to imaging units (i.e., computed tomography studies). Furthermore, studies in critically ill patients have shown that the delivered dose may be up to 30% lower than was prescribed. In patients where predilution (CVVH or CVHDF) is prescribed, this can lower the clearance by as much as 35%. As a result, it may be necessary to prescribe higher doses to achieve the desired delivered CRRT dose.

Table 86.3

Filter Characteristics

Hemofilter	Membrane	Surface Area (m²)	Filter Priming Volume (mL)
M 60	AN-69	0.6	93
HF 20*	PAES	0.2	60
M 100	AN-69	0.9	152
HF 1000	PAES	1.1	165
HF 1400	PAES	1.4	186

*Not FDA approved in the United States.

When managing the pediatric patient on CRRT, it is important to consider substances that are beneficial to the patient that are also cleared during CRRT. When a pediatric patient is placed on CRRT one must consider the clearances of medications including antibiotics. Higher clearances can result in lower drug levels, and as a result many medications need increased dosing. In the care of patients on CRRT, drug levels should be followed when possible and the involvement of a clinical pharmacist is paramount. Similarly, higher levels of clearance result in increased clearance of amino acids and can negatively impact the nutritional status. As a result, children, particularly the smallest ones, require supplementation with amino acids with doses of 3–4 g/kg/day. Similarly, higher doses of CRRT can lead to electrolyte abnormalities, such as hypophosphatemia, depending on the composition of replacement and/or dialysis fluids. To prevent this and adequately manage patient nutritional supplementation, the support of a dietitian is ideal to manage children on CRRT.

In prescribing and managing CRRT in the smallest pediatric patients, there are a number of special considerations. One must appreciate the implications of the extracorporeal volume of the CRRT circuits (Table 86.3) relative to the patient's blood volume. The typical blood volume in infants <10 kg is 80 mL/kg, and 70 mL/kg in larger children. As a result, a large proportion of the blood volume can be extracorporeal at any given time, and children on CRRT can develop significant hypothermia (which may mask fevers). To prevent hypothermia, the use of patient warmers, heating pads applied to circuit tubing or manufacturer-specific blood warmers, and control of the room temperature should be employed. Ideally, the extracorporeal volume of the CRRT circuit should be <10% of the patient's blood volume. Under circumstances where the patient's circuit volume is in excess of 10% of the patient's total blood volume, blood priming is necessary. The packed red cells obtained from most blood banks possesses a high hematocrit (around 50%–60%) and needs to be reconstituted to around 30% with 0.9% saline in order to avoid clotting the circuit. Further considerations about CRRT dose should be made in the smallest children who receive citrate anticoagulation (see below).

Solutions

Consideration of both convective (CVVH) as well as diffusive (CVVHD) therapies (see section on prescriptions and anticoagulation) needs to be made when determining what type of solution to employ. Furthermore, the standards and approvals by the FDA differ for dialysis solution and replacement solution. The FDA in the United States considers anything that is placed into the vascular space a drug, and dialysis

Table 86.4				

Comparison of Common Solutions

Electrolyte (mmol/L)	PrismaSate (Gambro)	ACCUSOL (Baxter)	Duosol (Braun)	Prismasol (Gambro)
Na (mEq/L)	140	140	140	140
Ca (mEq/L)	0/2.5/3.5	3.5	3	0/2.5/3.5
K (mEq/L)	0/2/4	0–4	0–4	0/2/4
Mg (mEq/L)	1/1.5	1.0–1.5		0/1/1.2/1.5
Cl (mEq/L)	102–120	109.5–116.3	109–113	106–121
Phos (mmol/L)	0	0	0	0
L-Lactate (mEq/L)	3	0	0	3
Bicarb (mEq/L)	22/32	30–35	35	22/32
Glu (mg/dL)	0/110	0–100		0/100
FDA OK	Y (D)	Y (D)	Y (D)	Y (FRF)

Each company now has an FDA-approved assortment of available solutions for CRRT. This list is simply representative and not exhaustive.
For further information, please seek information from the company.

solutions are not considered drugs but, rather, devices as these are not infused intravascularly.

There are a number of commercially available solutions that can serve as dialysis or replacement solutions (Table 86.4). Previously, when choosing solutions one could choose from those buffered primarily with lactate or with bicarbonate. Several studies have since demonstrated that bicarbonate-based solutions are superior. Bicarbonate-based buffered solutions are now the standard of care for dialysate and replacement solutions and are recommended in the KDIGO guidelines. It is worth noting that a number of these solutions continue to contain small amounts of lactate. Commercially available solutions contain varying amounts of sodium, potassium, glucose, magnesium, calcium, and phosphorous. These may be phosphorus or calcium based. It makes no difference whether phosphorus or calcium is used. However, with the phosphorus-based solutions, calcium must be infused and with the calcium-based solution phosphorus must be infused to the patient. Calcium-free dialysate is used when citrate anticoagulation is employed. It is important to appreciate that the patient's electrolytes will approximate the composition of the CRRT solutions over time. As a result, diligent monitoring of electrolytes is necessary. It is common in CVVHDF to use the same fluid for replacement and dialysis as a safety measure.

In the appropriate clinical scenario, specific adjustments to solutions or types of solutions may be used to achieve the goals of care. In hyperosmolar states, a sodium concentration of 150 mEq/L or 160 mEq/L may be utilized to prevent rapid osmotic shifts. Similarly high sodium concentrations may be utilized as part of a neuroprotective strategy in the right clinical scenario. When performing CVVHDF, one may consider the utilization of normal saline or sodium bicarbonate as postfilter replacement to correct the pH.

Anticoagulation

Activation of the clotting cascade occurs in CRRT circuits because of contact of the circulating blood with artificial surfaces. This can be exacerbated by low blood flow rates, turbulent blood flow, and high hematocrits. Anticoagulation is employed to prevent clotting and provide the prescribed CRRT dose. The most common anticoagulants used are unfractionated heparin and citrate. In adult studies, citrate anticoagulation has been shown to be superior at prolonged filter life with less bleeding complications. In 2005, the ppCRRT group presented the largest study to date evaluating the anticoagulation practices in 138 patients, which showed centers used heparin (37%), citrate (56%), and no anticoagulation (7%) for CRRT. This study showed that there was no difference in circuit life in those receiving heparin (44.7±27.1 hours) versus citrate (44.7±35.9 hours) anticoagulation, but did show that both were superior to no anticoagulation (27.2±21.5 hours). This study also suggested that there were fewer bleeding complications in children receiving citrate anticoagulation.

The decision to perform anticoagulation in the most critically ill children with underlying sepsis and disseminated intravascular coagulopathy or liver failure warrants further discussion. Historically, the approach of no anticoagulation has been utilized in these patient populations. Many of these patients have a paradoxical coagulopathy, are on continuous fresh-frozen plasma replacement, and have platelet infusions to correct the underlying coagulopathy, which will in turn promote clotting of the CRRT system. As a result, we discourage the approach of using no anticoagulation in these patients and suggest modifying protocols in these patients. Based on the published data, it is clear that anticoagulation is necessary to deliver CRRT, and either heparin or citrate can be used in children.

Heparin anticoagulation has been used in dialytic therapies for children for decades. Heparin is infused in the CRRT system prefilter and is used to anticoagulate the system. Heparin's anticlotting potential is then measured by measuring a post-filter PTT or an activated clotting time (ACT). The advantage of measuring an ACT is that it can be monitored at bedside. The target PTT is 1.5 times normal, and the target ACT is 180–220 seconds. This is usually accomplished by initially giving 20–30 units/kg bolus followed by a continuous drip of 10–20 units/kg/h of heparin. The advantage of heparin is the historical use and familiarity by many nephrologists. The disadvantage of heparin is that it is infused into the patient and can be associated with anticoagulation of the patient. Further, heparin can be associated with heparin-induced thrombocytopenia (HIT), which can facilitate an increased risk of bleeding. In many patients with multiorgan system failure requiring renal replacement therapy, systemic heparinization may be a detriment and should be avoided secondary to increased risk of bleeding.

Citrate-based regional anticoagulation regimens rely on the ability of citrate to chelate ionized calcium, thus removing a critical component for activation of both coagulation cascades and platelets. Citrate is infused into the arterial limb of the CRRT circuit and creates a hypocalcemic environment at the filter. The majority of calcium-citrate complexes are dialyzed through the filter during dialysis and lost in the effluent. Patient hypocalcemia is avoided by infusing calcium back into the patient via a separate central access independent of the CRRT system. In larger triple-lumen catheters, calcium can be infused in the most distal lumen but should be done cautiously. Any calcium–citrate complexes that return to the patient are then metabolized in the mitochondria of the liver, kidney, or skeletal muscle. Each citrate molecule is metabolized to 3 molecules of bicarbonate.

Regional citrate anticoagulation involves two processes. The first process is to deliver citrate into the arterial limb of the circuit to achieve target CRRT filter ionized calcium between 0.20 and 0.40 mmol/L, immediately postfilter. The second process is to deliver calcium back into the patient to target a physiologic level between 1.10 and 1.30 mmol/L. Although many protocols exist, either a 4% trisodium citrate (TSC) solution or an anticoagulant dextrose solution A (ACD-A, Baxter Healthcare, Deerfield, IL) solution are available. An equimolar amount of ACD-A has a lower amount of citrate (67% TSC and 33% citric acid). The most frequently cited pediatric protocol utilizes ACD-A. This protocol starts with an infusion rate based on patient blood flow:

$$\text{ACD-A infusion rate (mL/h)} = \text{blood pump rate (mL/min} \times \text{min/h)} \times 1.5$$

Calcium is then returned to the patients by using an 8% calcium infusion (8 g calcium chloride/1 L normal saline) using a separate central access. The infusion rate is as follows:

$$\text{Calcium chloride infusion rate (mL/h)} = \text{blood pump rate (mL/min} \times \text{min/h)} \times 0.6$$

Following the initiation of CRRT circuit, systemic ionized calcium and central calcium/electrolytes are drawn every 6 hours to monitor anticoagulation and for systemic side effects. Protocols are then used to adjust citrate and calcium infusion rates based on a sliding scale.

Regional citrate anticoagulation does have the potential for metabolic complications, including metabolic alkalosis, hypernatremia, hypocalcemia, hyperglycemia, and citrate toxicity. Citrate anticoagulation may result in metabolic alkalosis as a result of the metabolism of citrate to bicarbonate. This is of particular concern when dialysate and replacement solutions with higher bicarbonate solutions are utilized. This can be managed by either increasing the clearance by increasing the CRRT dose, the utilization of a replacement normal saline solution (pH 5.4–5.8, starting at 25% citrate rate), or adjustment of total parenteral nutrition. Hyperglycemia is more frequent in the smaller infants because of the glucose in the ACD-A solution (2.45 g/dL), and these patients require close monitoring.

Citrate toxicity can develop in patients and is termed citrate lock. This occurs when the delivery of citrate exceeds the clearance (dialysis and metabolism) of excess citrate and is typified by low ionized calcium, elevated total serum calcium, and an anion gap acidosis or alkalosis. Citrate toxicity can be monitored by monitoring the total serum calcium to ionized calcium ratio and occurs at a ratio of 2.5 (mmol/L) or 10 (if total calcium measured in milligrams per deciliter). Patients at the highest risk for the development of these complications include those with impairment of the organ systems that metabolize citrate (liver and muscle). If there is evidence of citrate accumulation, it is reasonable to increase the clearance by increasing the CRRT dose early in the course. If more severe toxicity is present, the citrate infusion can be held, typically for 15–30 minutes, and restarted at 70% of the previous dose. Regional citrate anticoagulation can be safely performed in children with liver failure by using modified protocols that typically start at a lower citrate infusion rate.

When citrate anticoagulation is used in children, particular care must be paid to infants less than 10 kg. These infants require a blood flow that is higher than the typical 5 mL/kg/min in order to make the CRRT machines function properly. As a result, in protocols where the citrate is dosed based on blood flow, these children receive higher citrate infusion rates by weight than older children. To prevent citrate accumulation and toxicity, it is common to start these children at higher CRRT doses to provide adequate clearance. Our practice is a minimum CRRT dose of 600 mL/h.

Membrane and Filter

When selecting the appropriate filter for pediatric patients, one needs to take into account the filter size and biocompatibility. The surface areas in CRRT filters are smaller than the surface area of HD dialyzers. CRRT filters are chosen based on the equivalent body surface area related to the patient's weight (Table 86.3). As a rule, the filters are permeable to nonprotein-bound solutes with a relative molecular mass less than 40,000 (although this is dependent on the filter fibers of the specific hemofilter). CRRT membranes have improved in terms of biocompatibility over the past decades.

The current standard of care is to utilize biocompatible membranes to perform CRRT. The filter options that are available include those composed of acrylonitrile (AN-69, Baxter, Lakewood, CO) versus polysulfone. When considering the filter to utilize one must take into account the risks and benefits of each filter. The AN-69 membrane has a potential benefit in septic patients by providing better cytokine clearance. The drawback to the AN-69 membrane is its association with the "bradykinin release syndrome" (described below). The polysulfone-based filters are not associated with the bradykinin release, but are not available in the appropriate infant sizes in the United States.

The bradykinin release syndrome occurs when blood is exposed to the AN-69 membrane resulting in activation of pre-kallikrein and Hageman factor, resulting in production of the potent vasodilator bradykinin. This membrane reaction is pH dependent and potentiated by angiotensin-converting enzyme inhibitors. In smaller patients who require blood priming, this presents as a potential cause of hypotension because most blood-bank blood has a pH of about 6.3 and has the bioactive components required to trigger the bradykinin release phenomenon. One approach to this reaction is to bypass the hemofilter by giving the blood postfilter, synchronizing a saline prime of the filter, and a bicarbonate infusion to the filter (30 mEq over 15 minutes). This, along with judicious use of bicarbonate boluses to the filter during startup, has allowed for the safe use of this membrane. Although the membrane reaction can be avoided and treated with appropriate interventions, some institutions have chosen to avoid the AN-69 membranes altogether and utilize larger filters in infant patients.

Nutrition

Although CRRT readily allows for optimization of nutritional support in patients with high catabolic states, it also contributes to the development of a negative nitrogen balance through the loss of free amino acids and peptides across hemofilters. Patient nutrition should be tailored to meet their overall needs with the aim of promoting an anabolic state. It is clear that improved nutrition is associated with decreased morbidity in such patients. Currently, we suggest 2.5–3.5 g/kg/day of protein (target BUN 40–60 mg/dL) and a daily caloric intake 20%–30% above normal resting energy expenditure.

Inborn Errors of Metabolism

Hyperammonemia represents a true emergency and warrants prompt treatment. The utilization of CRRT for treatment of inborn errors of metabolism (such as urea cycle defects) is standard practice. In children with hyperammonemia, treatment protocols classically began with a run of intermittent hemodialysis followed by a transition to CRRT in order to prevent the usual rebound associated with intermittent HD. More recently, using modern CRRT devices, treatment protocols have been developed utilizing CRRT at doses of 8 L/h/1.73 m^2 without an initial hemodialysis run. This regimen may provide benefit by avoiding hypotension that may be associated with hemodialysis runs in critically ill neonates. If a metabolic cocktail such as sodium benzoate is required, the dose may need to be increased in order to accommodate the increased clearance these cocktails have with CRRT. In general, we have found doubling the infusion rate to be adequate and should involve consultation with pharmacists and geneticists.

Extracorporeal Membrane Oxygenation

Extracorporeal membrane oxygenation (ECMO) is a lifesaving therapy for neonates and children with severe, reversible, cardiopulmonary failure. A multitude of studies in adults and children have shown that AKI is common in patients on ECMO with an incidence frequently in excess of 60%–70%. As a result, the children frequently require renal replacement therapy. The indications for renal replacement therapy for children on ECMO are similar to other critically ill children. Similar to other pediatric patient populations, fluid overload is a common indication for the initiation of CRRT in children on ECMO. In a single-center study, the degree of fluid overload at CRRT initiation while on ECMO was shown to be significantly different between survivors (FO 24.5% at initiation) and nonsurvivors (FO 38% at initiation). A recent single-center study by Paden et al demonstrated that nearly 100% of survivors have renal recovery following CRRT on ECMO and are discharged without requirement for renal support therapy in a pediatric population.

Although a full description of the CRRT on ECMO is outside of the scope of this text, there are a number of important points that make CRRT on ECMO unique. The ECMO circuit provides anticoagulation by systemic heparinization and access capable of blood flow rates generally in excess of 100 mL/kg/min. The two options for performing CRRT on ECMO include an in-line hemofilter or an in-line CRRT machine (please see recommended reading for a comprehensive article). A systemic comparison of the two options has not been performed and the choice is frequently institutional in nature and may depend on the construct of the ECMO circuit. One concern with utilizing the in-line filter is that fluid removal is frequently measured by using an infusion device. These devices have been shown to be less accurate than CRRT machines and this can be particularly problematic in the smallest children.

Intoxications

Use of CRRT in combination with HD for treatment of intoxication (lithium, carbamazepine, and vancomycin) is quite successful, decreasing (and in most cases eliminating) the need for older more complex techniques such as charcoal hemoperfusion.

Conclusion

CRRT has become the modality of choice for the provision of renal replacement therapy in the most critically ill children and has been shown to be both safe and effective in pediatric patients. Although many advances have been made over the last several decades, there remain many important questions about the exact timing, dose, and modality of CRRT to perform. Although exact recommendations on these topics cannot be made, it is agreed on that the institution of center-specific protocols and procedures is necessary to provide safe CRRT. The successful provision of CRRT in pediatric patients requires the cooperative effort among pediatric critical care physicians, nephrologists, nurses, and pharmacists to care for our sickest patients.

C H A P T E R   8 7

Prevention and Treatment of Bone Disease in Pediatric Dialysis Patients

Katherine Wesseling-Perry, MD

Childhood and adolescence are crucial times for developing a healthy skeletal and vascular system; alterations in bone modeling/remodeling or vascular biology in youth carry consequences that severely impact quality of life as well as life span. In childhood, chronic kidney disease (CKD) causes disordered regulation of mineral metabolism with subsequent alterations in bone modeling, remodeling, and growth. Similar to the adult population, cardiovascular disease is the leading cause of mortality in children with kidney disease, and abnormal mineral metabolism, bone disease, and its therapies are closely linked to cardiovascular pathology. Together, these alterations are termed "CKD–mineral and bone disorder" (CKD-MBD).

Pathogenesis of Abnormal Mineral Metabolism in CKD

Role of Fibroblast Growth Factor 23

As early as stage 2 CKD (glomerular filtration rate [GFR] between 60 and 90 mL/min/1.73 m^2), circulating levels of fibroblast growth factor 23 (FGF23) begin to rise in adults and children. Increased levels of FGF23 are due to a combination of decreased renal excretion, changes in degradation, and increased osteocytic production. Oral phosphate loading stimulates FGF23 production; however, phosphate-independent mechanisms, including a decrease in the expression of membrane-bound Klotho (a coreceptor for FGF23 signaling), iron deficiency–mediated stimulation of FGF23 transcription, increased levels of cleaved αKlotho, and inflammation likely also contribute.

The effects of increasing FGF23 on mineral metabolism are multiple and include the induction of renal phosphate excretion by reducing expression levels of the renal phosphate cotransporters, NaPi2a and NaPi2c, the suppression of renal 1α-hydroxylase activity, and the stimulation of the 24-hydroxylase, enhancing the metabolism of the biologically active 1,25(OH)$_2$D. With progressive CKD, rising FGF23 values result in a decline in 1,25(OH)$_2$D levels. Recent evidence suggests that FGF23 may also regulate parathyroid hormone (PTH) secretion; in vitro and in vivo experiments indicate that FGF23, by activating mitogen-activated protein kinase (MAPK) pathways in the parathyroid gland, also directly suppresses PTH release.

Role of 1,25(OH)$_2$D

In CKD, reduced circulating 1,25(OH)$_2$D contributes to secondary hyperparathyroidism and parathyroid gland hyperplasia in a number of ways: through decreased intestinal calcium absorption, decreased binding to the vitamin D receptor (VDR), decreased VDR expression, and reduced calcium sensing receptor (CaSR) expression. 1,25(OH)$_2$D itself increases *VDR* gene expression in the parathyroid glands, further suppressing *PTH* gene transcription. 1,25(OH)$_2$D$_3$ also increases the expression of the CaSR, the expression of which is reduced in hyperplastic parathyroid tissues obtained from patients with secondary hyperparathyroidism. Thus, low levels of calcitriol may allow parathyroid cells to proliferate whereas the administration of calcitriol may suppress proliferation of parathyroid cells.

Role of 25(OH)D

25(OH)vitamin D (25(OH)D) deficiency is prevalent in patients with CKD, as a result of multiple factors: many are chronically ill with little outdoor (sunlight) exposure; CKD dietary restrictions, particularly of dairy products, curtail the intake of vitamin D–rich food and lead to decreased dietary calcium intake; and patients with CKD (particularly those with darker skin pigment) display decreased skin synthesis of vitamin D$_3$ in response to sunlight compared with individuals with normal kidney function. Proteinuric diseases further exacerbate vitamin D deficiency in the CKD population, as 25(OH)D, in combination with vitamin D–binding protein, is lost in the urine. Increased catabolism of 25(OH)vitamin D through the 24-hydroxylase may also play an important role in the development and maintenance of 25(OH)vitamin D deficiency. Low levels of 25(OH) D also contribute to the development of secondary hyperparathyroidism, both directly and through limiting substrate for the formation of 1,25(OH)$_2$D. Apart from its conversion to 1,25(OH)$_2$ D$_3$, 25(OH)D may have its own effect on tissues. 25(OH)D is converted inside the gland to 1,25(OH)$_2$ D$_3$, directly suppressing PTH through parathyroid gland–specific 1α-hydroxylase. Supplementation with ergocalciferol has been shown to decrease serum PTH levels and to delay the development of secondary hyperparathyroidism in pediatric patients with CKD.

Role of Phosphorus

Phosphorus retention and hyperphosphatemia are also important factors in the pathogenesis of secondary hyperparathyroidism, but only in late stages of CKD. Hyperphosphatemia lowers blood ionized calcium levels as free calcium ions complex with excess inorganic phosphate; the ensuing hypocalcemia stimulates PTH release. Phosphorus also enhances the secretion of FGF23, thereby impairing renal 1α-hydroxylase activity, which diminishes the conversion of 25(OH)D to 1,25(OH)$_2$D$_3$. Finally, phosphorus can directly enhance PTH synthesis by decreasing cytosolic phospholipase A2 (normally increased by CaSR activation), leading to a decrease in arachidonic acid production with a subsequent increase in PTH secretion and, in vitro, phosphorus increases the stability of the PTH mRNA transcript (Fig. 87.1).

Alterations in the Parathyroid Gland Calcium Sensing Receptor Expression

Alterations in parathyroid gland CaSR expression also occur in secondary hyperparathyroidism, thereby contributing to parathyroid gland hyperplasia. The CaSR is a seven-transmembrane G protein–coupled receptor with a large extracellular

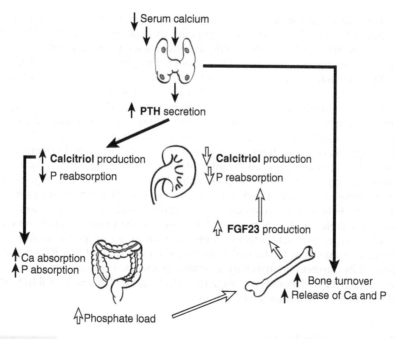

Figure 87.1

Pathogenesis of Secondary Hyperparathyroidism in CKD.

N-terminus, which binds acidic amino acids and divalent cations. Low extracellular calcium levels result in decreased calcium binding to the receptor, a conformational relaxation of the receptor and a resultant increase in PTH secretion, whereas activation of the receptor by high levels of serum calcium decrease PTH secretion. The expression of the CaSR is reduced by 30% to 70% as judged by immunohistochemical methods in hyperplastic parathyroid tissue obtained from human subjects with renal failure. Decreased expression and activity of CaSR have been linked to decreased responsiveness in PTH secretion because of altered calcium levels, resulting in an insensitivity to serum calcium levels with subsequent uncontrolled secretion of PTH.

Role of Skeletal Resistance to Parathyroid Hormone

Resistance of the skeleton to the hypercalcemic action of PTH is another potential cause of hyperparathyroidism in patients with renal insufficiency. In vitro and in vivo experimental data indicate that amino-terminally truncated PTH fragments antagonize the calcemic actions of the full-length PTH molecule (PTH(1-84)). Synthetic PTH(7-84) with or without a mixture of other carboxyl-terminal PTH fragments inhibits the calcemic effect of PTH(1-34) in vivo in rats and dialysis patients with hyperparathyroid bone disease because of increased levels of PTH(1-84), have increased circulating levels of PTH(7-84), and are resistant to the calcemic actions of PTH(1-34).

Current data suggest that first-generation immunometric assays (IMAs) for measuring PTH (1st PTH-IMA) overestimate the concentration of PTH(1-84) in circulation by 40%–50% in both healthy individuals with normal renal function and those with varying degrees of CKD. Although Faugiere et al suggested that 2nd PTH-IMA and, mainly, the ratio between PTH(1-84)/amino-truncated PTH fragment (calculated from the differences in PTH levels determined between 1st and 2nd PTH-IMAs) could be a better predictor of bone turnover than 1st PTH-IMA, these findings were not confirmed by subsequent investigations, and current data do not yet support the claim that 2nd PTH-IMAs provide an advantage over 1st PTH-IMAs for the diagnosis of the different subtypes of renal bone diseases. Furthermore, the variation in PTH assays between manufacturers makes interpretation of their values, and their relationships to bone turnover, difficult to assess. More recently, discrimination between nonoxidized and oxidized forms of PTH have shown promise in improved prediction of adverse outcomes in dialysis patients. These assays are not currently available for clinical practice, however, and their value as predictors of the different subtypes of renal osteodystrophy as well as the response to therapeutic interventions remains to be defined. Current guidelines suggest that PTH values, as determined by current commercially available assays, be maintained within a broad range—between 2 and 9 times the range for individuals with normal renal function—in patients treated with maintenance dialysis.

Renal Osteodystrophy

Abnormalities in Bone Turnover, Mineralization, and Volume

Renal bone disease is a common complication of CKD and is nearly universal at the start of dialysis therapy. Although the term "CKD–mineral and bone disorder" (CKD-MBD) refers to the alterations in mineral metabolism and their effects on both the cardiovascular and skeletal systems in the CKD population, the term "renal osteodystrophy" is used specifically to describe the bone pathology defined by bone histomorphometry that occurs as a complication of CKD. Traditionally, such lesions have been characterized according to alterations in bone turnover, ranging from high bone turnover (secondary hyperparathyroidism, osteitis fibrosa) to lesions of low bone turnover (adynamic bone disease and osteomalacia). However, alterations in skeletal mineralization and volume are also common in pediatric patients in CKD and may contribute to outcomes such as fractures, skeletal deformities, and poor growth, which persist despite normalization of bone turnover. Bone histomorphometry is the gold standard for the diagnosis of different types of bone diseases associated with CKD, providing measures of bone turnover, mineralization, and volume, and all may be altered in patients with CKD, occurring concomitantly with alterations in circulating levels of PTH, calcium, phosphorus, 1,25D, 25OHD, and FGF23.

Turnover

Abnormalities in bone turnover, driven by circulating PTH concentrations, are prevalent in both adults and pediatric patients with advanced stages of CKD. PTH activates the PTH/PTHrP receptor on osteocytes and osteoblasts, thereby directly increasing the cellular activity of osteoblasts and, indirectly, the activity of osteoclast. Skeletal resistance to PTH develops as CKD progresses, because of multiple factors including, although likely not limited to, the accumulation of circulating PTH fragments and downregulation of the PTH receptor; however, excessive levels of PTH result in increased resorption of bone matrix and release of mineral into the circulation. Prolonged exposure to elevated PTH levels and increases in bone turnover may lead to peri-trabecular fibrous changes in bones; thus, the renal osteodystrophy associated with prolonged secondary hyperparathyroidism is often termed "osteitis fibrosa cystica." A state of low-turnover bone disease (adynamic renal osteodystrophy), defined as decreased bone formation rate in conjunction with decreased cellular activity and an absence of excessive osteoid accumulation, is most common in adult dialysis patients. This condition may occur, especially in children treated with maintenance dialysis, because of overaggressive therapy with active vitamin D sterols and calcium salts. In addition to the increased risk for fractures and vascular calcifications that is observed in adults with adyamic bone, this form of bone disease in children treated with dialysis is associated with a further decline in growth.

Although bone turnover is undoubtedly affected by changes in circulating PTH in advanced CKD, recent data from animals and humans have suggested that changes in bone turnover occur before alterations in circulating mineral, PTH, or vitamin D concentrations are apparent and that these changes are mediated in large part by alterations in osteocyte biology. Data from mice suggest that low bone turnover occurs in early CKD, independent of measurable changes in mineral ion homeostasis and increased osteocytic sclerostin expression appears related to these early changes in bone turnover. Sclerostin is an inhibitor of Wnt signaling–mediated bone turnover; thus, increases in its expression result in suppression of bone formation and the development of adynamic bone in early stages of CKD. PTH, however, suppresses sclerostin expression and, as moderate to severe CKD develops, rising PTH levels inhibit skeletal sclerostin expression, allowing bone formation rates to rise.

Mineralization

Although renal osteodystrophy has traditionally been defined by lesions in bone turnover, alterations in skeletal mineralization are also prevalent in children with CKD. Increases in unmineralized bone (osteoid) in conjunction with delayed rates of mineral deposition are common. Defective mineralization that is associated with low to normal bone turnover is termed "osteomalacia." The histomorphometric characteristics of osteomalacia include the presence of wide osteoid seams, an increased number of osteoid lamellae, an increase in the trabecular surface covered with osteoid, and a diminished rate of mineralization or bone formation, as assessed by double tetracycline labeling. Fibrosis is often absent. Defective mineralization in combination with increased bone formation rates is termed "mixed uremic osteodystrophy" and is characterized by wide osteoid seams, prolonged mineralization times, bone marrow fibrosis, and increased bone formation rates. Patients with mixed lesion often display high serum PTH and alkaline phosphatase levels along with lower serum calcium levels.

Although the mechanisms of skeletal mineralization are incompletely understood, factors such as 25(OH)D deficiency and altered FGF23 metabolism have been implicated in their pathogenesis. In the general population, nutritional 25(OH)D deficiency results in osteomalacia, and a similar phenotype may occur in patients with CKD. Phosphate depletion, as may occur with frequent dialysis, may also result in osteomalacia. FGF23 may also play a role; both overexpression and ablation of

FGF23 in mice with normal renal function are associated with abnormal mineralization of osteoid, although by different mechanisms. The phosphaturic effect of increased FGF23 may cause rickets and osteomalacia through an insufficiency of mineral substrate. The mechanisms leading to impaired mineralization in FGF23-null animals, which have severe hyperphosphatemia and normal or elevated serum calcium levels, remain uncertain; however, osteomalacia in these animals suggests that FGF23 may play a direct role in skeletal mineral deposition. Although the ramifications of defective mineralization remain to be established, increased fracture rates and bone deformities are prevalent in pediatric CKD patients despite adequate control of bone turnover. These complications may be due, in part, to alterations in bone mineralization.

Volume

Because PTH is anabolic at the level of trabecular bone, high levels of serum PTH are typically associated with increases in bone volume, trabecular volume, and trabecular width. However, bone volume may also be low (termed "osteoporosis"), particularly in individuals with underlying age-related bone loss or in those treated with corticosteroids. Low bone volume is rare in the pediatric CKD population.

Cardiovascular Disease

Cardiovascular disease is the most common cause of mortality in patients with all stages of CKD, with young (i.e., 20- to 30-year-old) dialysis patients displaying the same rates of mortality from cardiovascular disease as 80-year-old individuals in the general population. Cardiovascular disease is not limited to the adults, but is also common in children with CKD. In addition to traditional risk factors for cardiovascular disease (i.e., hypertension and smoking) found in the general population, risk factors for vascular disease in predialysis CKD and dialysis patients include hypercalcemia, hyperphosphatemia, elevated levels of the calcium × phosphorus product, and treatment with high doses of calcium salts and vitamin D sterols. In contrast to the calcified atherosclerotic plaques that develop in the vascular intima of aging individuals with normal kidney function, uremia facilitates calcification of the tunica media. This form of calcification is associated with decreased distensibility of blood vessels, causing a rigid "lead pipe" pathology that is associated with increased risk for congestive heart failure. Carotid ultrasound measurement of intima medial thickness (IMT) has been validated for the assessment of cardiovascular pathology in children, with increased thickness associated with worsening disease. The prevalence of vascular changes in children with early CKD—patients who not only lack the mineral metabolism-associated risk factors common in the dialysis population but who also lack traditional adult risk factors such as obesity, diabetes, hypertension, and smoking—suggest that factors unique to CKD and independent of circulating mineral content contribute to vascular disease.

The mechanisms by which vascular calcification develop in CKD remain to be fully elucidated. In patients with compromised renal function, the entire smooth muscle layer surrounding arteries may be replaced not only by calcium deposits but by tissue that resembles bone. In patients with CKD, core binding factor-1 (Cbfa1) is thought to trigger mesenchymal cell to osteoblast transformation. Expression of the sodium-dependent phosphate transporters PIT-1 and PIT-2 likely contributes to the increased calcification and upregulation of pro-mineralization factors such as osteopontin, bone sialoprotein, osteonectin, alkaline phosphatase, type I collagen, and bone morphogenic protein-2 (BMP-2), which is potentiated by the uremic milieu, whereas expression of calcification inhibitors, such as fetuin A and matrix Gla protein, is suppressed. Elevated circulating values of FGF23 have also been linked to cardiovascular disease in patients with all stages of CKD, and recent experimental data have defined a direct role for FGF23, independent of changes in mineral metabolism, on pathologic changes in cardiac myocytes. FGF23 levels are often hundreds- to thousands-fold higher in patients with renal failure compared with those detected in individuals with normal kidney function, and these values have been associated with an increased prevalence of left ventricular hypertrophy and with premature mortality in adults with all stages of CKD. Recent experimental data have demonstrated that these associations may reflect a direct effect of FGF23 on the myocardium that induces myocyte hypertrophy.

Clinical Signs and Symptoms

Growth Retardation

Growth retardation is the hallmark of CKD in children. Growth failure worsens as renal function declines; the average height of children with even mild CKD (GFR 50–70 mL/min/1.73 m^2) is 1 standard deviation (SD) below the average for healthy children. Moderate CKD (GFR 25 to 49 mL/min/1.73 m^2) is associated with a height SD of −1.5, and, at the time of initiation of dialysis, the mean height SD is −1.8. Boys, younger patients, and those with prior renal transplants are at greatest risk for growth failure. Acidosis has been linked to delayed linear growth in patients with renal tubular acidosis and normal renal function, and its correction often leads to acceleration in growth velocity. Calcitriol deficiency, secondary hyperparathyroidism, and bone deformities also contribute to growth retardation; however, the optimal target values for PTH that maximize growth remain controversial. Treatment for secondary hyperparathyroidism with large, intermittent doses of calcitriol and calcium-based phosphate binders has been shown to reduce bone formation and suppress osteoblastic activity in both adults and children. However, adynamic bone disease may develop and linear bone growth decrease, despite serum PTH levels in the K/DOQI recommended range during intermittent vitamin D sterol therapy. GH resistance contributes to impaired linear growth in renal failure. Children who are treated with maintenance dialysis respond less well to rhGH therapy than do children with less severe CKD; the mechanisms for differences in response to GH therapy remain to be determined. Notably, bone formation rate increases out of proportion to changes in PTH values during treatment with rhGH, complicating the noninvasive assessment of renal osteodystrophy during therapy.

Skeletal Deformities and Pain

Genu valgum is the most common skeletal deformity in pediatric patients. Young children may exhibit exaggeration of the physiologic varus alignment. Radiographic features associated with vitamin D deficiency include metaphyseal widening of the wrist and ankle, craniotabes, and rachitic rosary. Pathologic or stress fractures may arise if the bones remain bowed and weak. The prevalence of slipped capital femoral epiphysis has declined over the past two decades because of better control of secondary hyperparathyroidism. Skeletal pain can accompany limping or problems with weight bearing.

Myopathy

Muscle involvement can range from muscle wasting, diffuse pain, weakness, and numbness to contracture of the extremities. The exact etiology for the myopathy described in renal failure is still unclear, but rapid fluid removal, electrolyte imbalance, low calcitriol, and the presence of calcific uremic arteriolopathy or calciphylaxis may contribute. There are no diagnostic tests available, and muscle biopsy may show severe atrophy without inflammation or the presence of calcification of small and medium-sized vessels.

Prevention and Treatment of CKD-MBD

To minimize complications in the skeleton and to prevent extraskeletal calcifications, particular attention must be made to alterations of bone and mineral metabolism in CKD. The specific aims of management of CKD-MBD are (1) to maintain blood levels of serum calcium and phosphorus near normal limits, (2) to prevent hyperplasia of the parathyroid glands and to maintain serum PTH at levels appropriate for stage of CKD (Table 87.1), (3) to avoid the development of extraskeletal calcifications, and (4) to prevent or reverse the accumulation of toxic substances such as FGF23, aluminum, and β_2-microglobulin.

Dietary Manipulation of Calcium and Phosphorus

As active vitamin D levels fall during the progression of renal disease, calcium absorption in the gut and kidney diminishes and hypocalcemia develops with advanced CKD stage. Patients with untreated CKD commonly ingest as little as 400–700 mg of elemental calcium per day in their diet. Calcium-rich foods such as dairy products, unfortunately, also are high in phosphorus. Thus, increasing dietary

Table 87.1

PTH Values

Stage	Treatment Target Range
3	KDIGO: Upper Limit of Normal
	KDOQI: 35–70 pg/mL
4	KDIGO: Upper Limit of Normal
	KDOQI: 70–110 pg/mL
5	KDIGO: Upper Limit of Normal
	KDOQI: 200–300 pg/mL
5D	KDIGO: 2–9 times Upper Limit of Normal
	KDOQI: 200–300 pg/mL
	European Children: 2–3 times Upper Limit of Normal

Sources: KDIGO: Kidney Int (2009) 76(suppl 113):S1-S130; KDOQI: Am J Kidney Dis (2003) 42(4 suppl 3):S1-S201; European Guidelines: Pediatr Nephrol (2006) 21:151–159.

consumption of calcium to meet daily needs is accompanied by excessive intake of phosphorus, which cannot be excreted in the face of renal failure.

The development of hyperphosphatemia occurs in the vast majority of patients with advanced renal insufficiency. Hyperphosphatemia and an elevated calcium–phosphorus ion product have been reported as independent risk factors for vascular calcification and mortality in adult dialysis patients. Thus, treatment goals include maintaining serum phosphorus levels within normal limits for age and avoiding a calcium–phosphorus ion product above 55 mg^2/dL^2. The average phosphorus intake of both adults and children in the U.S. population is approximately 1500–2000 mg/day, and 60%–70% of the dietary intake is absorbed. In the early stages of renal failure, mild dietary phosphate restriction is sufficient in preventing hyperphosphatemia and may also modulate the progressive rise in circulating FGF23. However, strict adherence to dietary phosphate restriction is often difficult because low-phosphate diets are unpalatable, especially to older children and adults, and because phosphorus intake is directly linked to protein intake, with 10–12 mg of phosphorus accompanying each gram of protein. Adequate protein intake is necessary for growth in children and for maintenance of lean body mass in adults. Current dietary recommendations suggest that children, depending on age, ingest anywhere from 1 to 2.5 g/kg/day.

Patients treated with dialysis require dietary phosphorus restriction, in addition to phosphate-binder therapy, because standard prescription peritoneal dialysis and hemodialysis remove insufficient amounts of phosphate (300–400 mg/day for peritoneal dialysis and 800 mg/treatment for hemodialysis) to maintain normal serum phosphorus levels (Table 87.2). The use of daily, slow, continuous hemodialysis in some centers has been associated with excellent control of serum phosphorus levels, often allowing phosphate-binding agents to be discontinued. Indeed, some patients have developed hypophosphatemia and have required the addition of phosphorus to the dialysate solution to prevent the long-term consequences of hypophosphatemia.

Phosphate-Binding Agents

Phosphate-binding agents reduce intestinal phosphate absorption by forming poorly soluble complexes with phosphorus in the intestinal tract. Aluminum-containing

Table 87.2

Normal Values for Serum Phosphorus, Total Calcium, Blood Ionized Calcium, and Alkaline Phosphatase Concentrations

Age (Years)	Serum Phosphorus (mg/dL)	Serum Total Calcium (mg/dL)	Blood Ionized Calcium (m/M)	Alkaline Phosphates (IU)
0–0.25	4.8–7.4	8.8–11.3	1.22–1.40	
1–5	4.5–6.5	9.4–10.8	1.22–1.32	100–350
6–12	3.6–5.8	9.4–10.3	1.15–1.32	60–450
13–20	2.3–4.5	8.8–10.2	1.12–1.30	40–180

Source: KDOQI.

phosphate binders were used frequently in the past, but long-term treatment led to bone disease, encephalopathy, and anemia. The use of aluminum-containing phosphate binders, therefore, should be restricted to the treatment of patients with severe hyperphosphatemia (>7 mg/dL) associated with hypercalcemia or an elevated calcium–phosphorus ion product, because both conditions will be aggravated by calcium-containing compounds. In such cases, the dose of aluminum hydroxide should not exceed 30 mg/kg/day, and the lowest possible dose should be given only for a limited period of approximately 4–6 weeks. Plasma aluminum levels should be monitored regularly. Concomitant intake of citrate-containing compounds should be avoided, because citrate enhances intestinal aluminum absorption and increases the risk for acute aluminum intoxication.

To avoid aluminum-related bone disease and encephalopathy, the use of aluminum-free phosphate binders has been advocated. Among these, calcium-containing salts are used worldwide for control of hyperphosphatemia and serve as an additional source of supplemental calcium. Several calcium salts, including calcium carbonate, calcium acetate, and calcium citrate, are commercially available. Calcium carbonate is the most commonly used compound, and studies in adults and children have shown its efficacy in controlling serum phosphorus levels. The recommended dose is proportional to the phosphorus content of the meal and is adjusted to achieve acceptable serum levels of calcium and phosphorus. Large doses of calcium carbonate may lead to hypercalcemia, particularly in patients treated concomitantly with active vitamin D sterols or those with adynamic bone. Hypercalcemia usually is reversible with reductions in the dose of oral calcium salts, dose of vitamin D sterol, and dialysate calcium concentrations. To avoid the development and progression of cardiovascular calcifications, it is currently recommended that elemental calcium intake in adults should not exceed 2 g/day, with less than 1500 mg of calcium given as calcium-containing phosphorus binders. Although calcium requirements in children are not well defined, intake should be considered in light of age-based guidelines (Table 87.3).

Table 87.3

Recommended Daily Dietary Intake for Calcium

Age Range (Years)	Adequate Intake (mg/day)	Tolerable Upper Level (g/day)
0–0.5	200	1
0.5–1.0	260	1.5
1–3	700	2.5
4–8	1000	2.5
9–13	1300	3
14–18	1300	3
19–30	1000	2.5
31–50	1000	2.5
51–70 males	1200	2
51–70 females	1200	2

Source: Institute of Medicine, National Academy of Sciences. *Dietary Reference Intakes for Calcium, Phosphorus, Magnesium, Vitamin D, and Fluoride.* Washington DC: National Academy Press 2011.

To limit the vascular calcification risks associated with the use of calcium salts and the bone and neurologic toxicity associated with aluminum hydroxide, alternative phosphate binders have been developed. Sevelamer, a calcium- and aluminum-free hydrogel of cross-linked poly-allylamine, has been shown to lower serum phosphorus, the calcium–phosphorus ion product, and PTH without inducing hypercalcemia in adult patients treated with hemodialysis. Sevelamer also halts the progression of vascular calcification, although these lesions increase during calcium-containing binder therapy in adult hemodialysis patients. In addition to its effects on serum phosphorus levels, sevelamer has been shown to decrease concentrations of total serum cholesterol and low-density lipoprotein cholesterol, but to increase high-density lipoprotein levels. These effects may offer additional benefits in reducing cardiovascular complications in patients with end-stage renal disease.

Other alternative phosphate-binding agents include magnesium, iron, and lanthanum compounds. Magnesium carbonate lowers serum phosphorus levels, but magnesium-free dialysate solutions should be used in those treated with dialysis. Large doses, however, result in diarrhea, limiting the use of this compound as a single agent. Iron compounds, such as stabilized polynuclear iron hydroxide and ferric polymaltose complex, have proved to be effective phosphate binders in short-term studies in adults with CKD. Clinical trials have demonstrated that lanthanum carbonate also effectively controls serum phosphorus and PTH levels without increasing serum calcium values. Lanthanum carbonate lowers serum phosphorus and PTH levels without causing hypercalcemia, adynamic bone disease, or osteomalacia. However, lanthanum is a heavy metal that accumulates in different organs in animals with normal renal function, and additional long-term studies are therefore needed to confirm the absence of toxicity before this agent is recommended for widespread use in pediatric CKD patients.

Vitamin D Therapy

Despite dietary phosphate restriction, the intake of phosphate-binding agents, the use of an appropriate level of calcium in dialysate solution, and an adequate intake of calcium, progressive osteitis fibrosa cystica due to hyperparathyroidism develops in a significant number of uremic patients. Treatment with active vitamin D sterols is aimed at controlling serum PTH levels and the resultant high-turnover bone disease. Current evidence indicates that two main issues should be considered with respect to vitamin D therapy: first, treatment for 25(OH)D deficiency, a common finding in patients with renal disease, in itself may reverse hyperparathyroidism. Second, treatment with active vitamin D sterols, by inhibiting the formation of prepro-PTH and by activating the CaSR, is useful in pharmacologically reducing PTH levels.

Assessment and Treatment of 25(OH)D Deficiency

Although current guidelines are controversial, with the Institute of Medicine suggesting that 25(OH)vitamin D values be maintained above 20 ng/mL, current recommendations from the National Kidney foundation stratifies vitamin D deficiency into three categories: (1) severe deficiency, defined as a serum level less than 5 ng/mL; (2) mild deficiency, equivalent to serum concentrations of 5–15 ng/mL; and (3) vitamin D insufficiency, with levels between 16 and 30 ng/mL. Thus, ergocalciferol treatment should be initiated in patients with CKD when 25(OH)D levels fall below 30 ng/mL.

Severe deficiency (<5 ng/mL) should be treated with 50,000 IU orally, once a week for 12 weeks, then 50,000 IU orally once a month for a total of 6 months. Alternatively, 500,000 IU may be given as a single intramuscular dose. Serum 25(OH)D levels in the range of 5–15 ng/mL (so-called mild deficiency) should be treated with 50,000 IU of ergocalciferol orally once a week for 4 weeks, followed by 50,000 IU orally once a month for a total of 6 months. Vitamin D insufficiency (serum levels between 16 and 30 ng/mL) should be treated with 50,000 IU of ergocalciferol orally once a month for 6 months. In D-deficient patients, serum 25(OH)D levels should be rechecked after completion of the 6-month course of therapy.

Treatment With Active Vitamin D Sterols

Active vitamin D sterols act through a variety of pathways to decrease PTH production—by increasing calcium absorption in the gut and kidney, by binding to the CaSR, by increasing skeletal sensitivity to PTH, and by altering prepro-PTH transcription. Calcitriol (Rocaltrol) has been used widely for many years to control secondary hyperparathyroidism in both adults and children. The efficacy of daily oral doses of calcitriol for the treatment of patients with symptomatic renal osteo-dystrophy has been documented in several clinical trials. Bone pain diminishes, muscle strength and gait–posture improve, and osteitis fibrosa frequently resolves partially or completely. Active vitamin D therapy has been associated with protective effects on both the heart and the kidney. Active vitamin D sterols ameliorate cardiac hypertrophy, improve cardiac systolic function, and decrease proteinuria. Doses of oral calcitriol in most clinical trials have ranged from 0.25 to 1.5 μg/day. In patients with CKD, initial doses are determined by target PTH levels and specific stage of kidney disease. In dialysis patients, $1,25(OH)_2D_3$ given thrice weekly by IV injection or by oral pulse therapy is effective in reducing serum PTH levels. Dosage regimens range from 0.5–1.0 μg to 3.5–4.0 μg three times weekly or 2.0–5.0 μg twice weekly. Low doses should be used initially, and dosage adjustments should be based on frequent measurements of serum calcium, phosphorus, and PTH levels.

Oral 1α-$(OH)D_3$ (alfacalcidol) undergoes 25-hydroxylation in the liver to form calcitriol, and this agent is used widely in Europe, Japan, and Canada. Calcitriol and 1α-$(OH)D_3$ are similarly effective for the treatment of secondary hyperparathyroid-ism in patients with CKD. 19-Nor-1 a,$25(OH)_2D_2$ (paricalcitol) is effective in con-trolling serum PTH levels in adult patients with CKD stages 3 and 4, as well as in dialysis patients. 1α-$(OH)D_2$ (1α-D_2, doxercalciferol) is as effective as calcitriol in the control of secondary hyperparathyroidism in pediatric patients.

Calcimimetics

Cinacalcet, an allosteric activator of the calcium-sensing receptor, reduces serum PTH levels and the calcium–phosphorus ion product in adult patients; thus, calci-mimetic therapy may provide an additional option for the reduction of both PTH levels and cardiovascular disease. Although early case reports suggested that calci-mimetic therapy could also reduce vascular calcification burden in dialysis patients, a recent prospective trial in 3883 adults with advance secondary hyperparathyroid-ism (the EVOLVE trial) failed to demonstrate a beneficial effect of calcimimetics on either CV events or on mortality. Owing to the presence of the calcium-sensing receptor on the growth plate, these agents are not approved and should be used with caution in growing children.

Parathyroidectomy

Patients with severe hyperparathyroidism often are unresponsive to vitamin D therapy, developing hypercalcemia and hyperphosphatemia without reduction in PTH values or parathyroid gland size. Clinical features that indicate the need for parathyroidectomy are as follows: the presence of hyperplasia and/or hypertrophy of the parathyroid glands (as documented by the presence of biochemical and radiographic features and, if necessary, the findings of osteitis fibrosa cystica on bone biopsy), elevated serum PTH levels unresponsive to vitamin D sterol therapy, persistent hypercalcemia, pruritus unresponsive to dialysis or other medical treatment, progressive extraskeletal calcification, severe skeletal pain or fractures, and calciphylaxis. Aluminum-related bone disease must be ruled out first in patients receiving low-dose calcitriol with persistent hypercalcemia. Other causes of hypercalcemia, such as sarcoidosis, malignancy-related hypercalcemia, intake of calcium supplements, and the presence of adynamic/aplastic bone lesions not related to aluminum, should also be considered.

When the decision has been made to perform parathyroid surgery, it is essential to avoid a marked postoperative fall in serum calcium levels caused by the "hungry bone" syndrome. Because of the severity of the bone disease, this fall can be much more marked and prolonged than after parathyroidectomy for primary hyperparathyroidism. Patients should receive daily oral calcitriol (0.5–1.0 μg) or some sort of intravenous active vitamin D sterol for 2–6 days before parathyroid surgery and during the postoperative period to stimulate intestinal calcium absorption and to maximize the effectiveness of oral calcium salts. Within 24–36 hours after surgery, marked hypocalcemia with serum calcium levels below 7–8 mg/dL may develop; thus, calcium gluconate should be initiated at a rate of 100 mg of calcium ion per hour in the operating room. Serum calcium should be measured every 4–6 hours and the calcium gluconate infusion rate increased if the serum calcium level continues to fall. The infusion rate may exceed 200 mg/h. Enteral calcium carbonate is initiated once the patient is able to tolerate oral intake, and doses as high as 1.0 g (elemental calcium) given four to six times daily, along with vitamin D sterol in excess of 1.0–2.0 μg/day (for calcitriol, doses of other agents vary according to their potency), are often needed for patients with marked hypocalcemia. Serum phosphorus levels may fall to subnormal levels postoperatively; phosphate treatment will markedly aggravate the hypocalcemia, and patients should not be treated with phosphate unless serum phosphorus falls to below 2.0 mg/dL.

Growth Hormone Therapy

Recombinant human growth hormone (rhGH) should be considered in children with growth failure that does not respond to optimization of nutrition, correction of acidosis, and control of renal osteodystrophy. Serum phosphorus and PTH levels should be well controlled prior to the initiation of rhGH in children with CKD. Serum phosphorus levels should be less than 1.5 times the upper limit for age and PTH levels less than 1.5 times the upper target values for the CKD stage before rhGH therapy is begun. GH therapy will increase serum PTH levels during the first months of therapy; therefore, serum PTH levels should be monitored monthly. Current recommendations suggest that GH therapy should be discontinued temporarily if PTH levels exceed three times the upper target value for the CKD stage; however, it is important to note that growth hormone also directly increases bone formation rate, independent of PTH values, thus distorting the relationship between PTH and bone formation rate.

Summary

Understanding of bone disease in kidney disease has increased over the years, but the clinical strategies currently employed to prevent the development of bone disease in children are still evolving. The management of bone disease in children should start early and should include correction of hypocalcemia, maintenance of age-appropriate serum phosphorus (Table 87.2), treatment of metabolic acidosis, and maintenance of serum intact PTH levels within the current recommended target ranges (Table 87.1). The primary aim in the early treatment of secondary hyperparathyroidism in children with CKD is to protect the young skeleton against the effects of progressive kidney disease and to prevent the development of parathyroid gland hyperplasia.

CHAPTER 88

Management of Anemia in Children Undergoing Dialysis

Carlos E. Araya, MD • Joshua Zaritsky, MD, PhD

Introduction

Anemia management appears to be on the cusp of dramatic changes because of development of novel erythropoiesis-stimulating agents (ESAs) and new understandings of iron metabolism. As the adverse effects of erythropoietin have become more apparent and concerning, there has been a push to optimize ESAs and iron therapy. This chapter will review the basic management of anemia in children undergoing dialysis and should provide a practical approach to the day-to-day management of anemia in children who require renal replacement therapy.

The anemia of chronic kidney disease (CKD) is most often normocytic and normochromic. It is primarily due to the decreased production of endogenous erythropoietin (EPO) and, to a lesser degree, decreased responsiveness to the hormone, shortened red blood cell survival, blood loss from frequent blood draws, and the hemodialysis procedure. Patients with CKD have a gradual decline in hemoglobin (Hb) over time as the level of glomerular filtration rate (GFR) declines. If left untreated, anemia of CKD has not only been associated with a multitude of adverse symptoms but also to higher morbidity, increased hospitalization days, and mortality in both adult and children.

Definition of Anemia

Anemia is defined as a decrease in red blood cell mass. In practice, anemia is determined by a low Hb and hematocrit (Hct) level relative to normative values based on gender and age. The World Health Organization has published Hb thresholds to classify individuals as anemic. Reference Hb concentration values have also been published using data from the U.S. National Health and Nutrition Examination Survey III (NHANES III) which included patients from age 1 year and older. The National Kidney Foundation–Kidney Disease Outcomes Quality Initiative (NKF-KDOQI) definition of anemia has been taken from the NHANES III report. The Kidney Disease: Improving Global Outcomes (KDIGO) guidelines define anemia if the Hb concentration is <11 g/dL in children 0.5–5 years, <11.5 g/dL in children 5–12 years, and <12 g/dL in children 12–15 years. Hemoglobin rather than Hct is considered a more accurate indicator of anemia because it is not affected by storage of the blood sample at room temperature, is more accurate in patients with hyperglycemia, is not affected by changes in plasma water, and is more reproducible when different automated counters are used.

Prevalence of Anemia in Chronic Kidney Disease

Anemia is associated with CKD of any cause and the severity of the anemia is related to the degree of loss of GFR. This association has been reported in both adults and children. In a single-center, cross-sectional study of 366 children and adolescents with CKD, approximately 31% of patients with stage 1 and 29% of patients with stage 2 CKD reported prevalent anemia, defined as Hb <12 mg/dL, whereas 66% of patients with stage 3 and 93% of patients with stages 4 and 5 CKD were anemic. Among children in the 2006 End Stage Renal Disease Clinical Performance Measures Project, 98% of 801 prevalent pediatric peritoneal dialysis patients were prescribed ESA.

In the Chronic Kidney Disease in Children Prospective Cohort Study (CkiD), the investigators found a linear decline in Hb below a threshold iohexol-determined GFR of 43 mL/min per 1.73 m^2, independent of age, race, gender, and underlying diagnosis. The Hb declined by 0.3 g/dL for every 5 mL/min per 1.73 m^2 decrease in GFR. Because serum creatinine-based estimated GFR may overestimate measured GFR in children, anemia may be seen even at early stages of CKD.

The Effects of Anemia

The symptoms of anemia of CKD typically manifest gradually as the decline in Hb occurs slowly. Patients may report fatigue, weakness, decreased exercise tolerance, loss of appetite, dizziness, pallor, tachycardia, tachypnea, or chest pain.

Severe anemia in children with CKD has been associated with increases in cardiac workload and left ventricular hypertrophy (LVH). In a retrospective study that included pediatric dialysis patients, 75% of the children were noted to have LVH, but those with severe LVH had a significantly lower Hb level. Diastolic dysfunction has also been reported in children with CKD and has been associated with anemia. Treatment of anemia with ESA has been reported to have beneficial effects on cardiac parameters. In a blinded, crossover study of children undergoing peritoneal and hemodialysis, patients were assigned to ESA or placebo. ESA produced a rise in mean Hb from 6.9 to 11.5 g/dL, which was associated with a significant fall in the cardiac index. Some patients had a reduction in the thickness of the interventricular septum and left ventricular posterior wall, but this did not reach statistical significance after 24 weeks. Cardiac performance also improves with correction of anemia. In this study, children with end stage renal disease (ESRD) performed treadmill tests before and 1 and 6 months after ESA administration. There was a decrease in heart rate, decrease in resting oxygen consumption, and increase in exercise time.

Anemia of CKD is associated with higher morbidity, higher risk for hospitalization, and increased mortality. In an analysis of the North American Pediatric Renal Transplant Cooperative Studies (NAPRTCS) database, which included 1942 patients, a multivariate analysis demonstrated anemia (Hct <33%) to be associated with a 52% higher risk of death (adjusted RR 1.52, 95% CI 1.03–2.26, $p = .037$). The presence of anemia was also associated with an increased risk for prolonged hospitalization, irrespective of dialysis modality.

Anemia also affects growth in children. An evaluation of the CKD registry of the NAPRTCS was used to evaluate factors associated with short stature in children with CKD. A total of 5615 patients were entered into the registry during the studied period, and investigators found that anemia (Hct below 33%) was an independent risk factor for short stature. In a retrospective study, catch-up growth was independently associated to Hb and ESA therapy. However, others have not found that correction of anemia with ESA improves the growth of children with CKD.

Anemia has been shown to cause changes in cognitive function such as increases in reaction times and impairment in immediate and delayed memory. In another study, investigators evaluated the Wechsler intelligence score in 22 children with anemia of CKD treated with ESA. The investigators found that the Wechsler intelligence score increased in 11 children from 92 ± 16 to 97 ± 17 over the 12-month period ($p = .007$).

Anemia of CKD has a negative impact on several aspects of health-related quality of life. In a study of adolescent patients with CKD stages 1–5 including transplantation patients, anemic patients reported greater limitations in the quality of life questionnaire domains relating to (1) physical functioning, (2) limitations in schoolwork or activities with friends as a result of physical health, and (3) parental impact in time and family activities when compared to children without anemia.

Testing for Anemia

The main cause of anemia in CKD is decreased production of endogenous erythropoietin levels. Therefore, the initial laboratory evaluation is aimed at identifying other factors that may be contributing to the anemia. In particular, if the severity of anemia is disproportionate to the degree in renal dysfunction, there is evidence of iron deficiency or there is evidence of leukopenia or thrombocytopenia. The NFK-KDOQI Guidelines recommend the following tests in the initial assessment of anemia: a complete blood count (CBC), absolute reticulocyte count, serum ferritin and serum transferrin saturation (TSAT), or content of Hb in reticulocytes. The KDIGO Guidelines suggest the same tests plus the addition of serum vitamin B_{12} and folate levels.

The CBC provides information about the severity of the anemia and adequacy of bone marrow function. Hemoglobin rather than Hct should be the standard measure for assessing anemia. For hemodialysis patients, the midweek predialysis sample is optimal. For peritoneal dialysis patients, the timing of the sample is not critical as plasma volume does not fluctuate significantly. In addition to the Hb, the red blood cell indices provide valuable information. The anemia of CKD is in general normocytic and normochromic. Macrocytosis may indicate folate or vitamin B_{12} deficiency, whereas microcytosis may indicate iron deficiency or inherited disorders of Hb formation. Leukopenia and thrombocytopenia indicate a generalized disorder of the bone marrow such as myelodysplasia. Abnormalities of the white blood cell count and differential or platelet count is not usual in anemia of CKD and may indicate other conditions.

The reticulocyte count is used to determine effective erythropoietic activity. Erythropoietin levels are not routinely measured.

Testing for Iron Deficiency

Although there are multiple laboratory tests aimed at determining iron status of a patient, the KDIGO and the NKF-KDOQI anemia workgroups have recommended that ferritin and the TSAT be the primary indices used. When compared to a functional gold standard of iron deficiency or an anatomic one (bone marrow stained for iron), most adult studies using a cutoff of 100 ng/mL have shown a sensitivity between 35% and 48%. In contrast, serum ferritin's specificity using the same cutoff is quite high (75%–100%), indicating that most CKD patients with levels below 100 ng/mL are truly iron deficient.

The diurnal and interlaboratory measurement variation of serum iron severely limits its value in determining iron deficiency. Instead, the circulating iron available for erythropoiesis is measured by the TSAT. It is calculated by dividing the total serum iron (the vast majority of which is bound to transferrin) by the total iron-binding capacity (TIBC), which reflects the total amount of transferrin in serum. Using a cutoff of 20%, TSAT's sensitivity ranges from 59% to 88% whereas its specificity is slightly lower, 63%–78%.

Currently the KDIGO 2012 practice guidelines for pediatric CKD 5D recommend intravenous (IV) iron administration during ESA therapy to maintain a serum ferritin greater than 100 ng/mL and a TSAT greater than 20%. These guidelines remain unchanged from the previous 2006 NKF-KDOQI guidelines for children. Given the lack of pediatric data, these recommendations are largely based on adult guidelines. One exception is the continued use of the lower 100 ng/mL ferritin cutoff for pediatric hemodialysis patients whereas for adult hemodialysis patients that cutoff had risen to 200 ng/mL in the 2006 NKF-KDOQI guidelines. In fact, in the KDIGO 2012 guidelines, the focus on adults has moved away from a lower limit with the recommendation that iron be given if the TSAT is ≤30% and the ferritin ≤500 ng/mL. Given the poor sensitivity of serum ferritin (especially at levels >200 ng/mL) and the safety concerns of superphysiologic ferritin levels, the upper limit of ferritin remains undefined. Although the KDIGO workgroup stated that "iron should not routinely be administered" above these levels, there is flexibility for a "therapeutic trial" of up to 1000 mg in patients with low Hb on high ESA doses.

In an attempt to address the limitations of serum ferritin and TSAT, several other markers of iron status have been proposed and examined. To date, reticulocyte Hb (Chr Hb) content appears to be the most promising, showing improved sensitivity and specificity over ferritin and TSAT in adult studies. CHr Hb is a measure of the amount of Hb in reticulocytes, and thus given the very short life span of reticulocytes (1–2 days) it should reflect how much iron is available for incorporation into new red blood cells. Additionally, CHr Hb is available on many of the current multi-channel hematology analyzers that do complete blood counts. The current NKF-KDOQI guidelines include CHR Hb measures (cutoff 29 pg/cell) but have not been extended to pediatric CKD because the cutoff values remain unclear.

Two other measures of iron status that bear mentioning include percentage of hypochromic red cell and soluble transferrin receptor. Percentage of hypochromic red cells is a measure of the Hb concentration in RBCs by taking into account the absolute amount of Hgb as well as the size of the RBC. Although its utility is likely compatible to CHr Hb, its use in the United States has been hampered because of the need for rapid analysis as red cells tend to expand while they are stored. Soluble transferrin receptor (sTFR) levels reflect the expression of membrane transferrin receptors on premature erythroblasts and thus reflect the need for iron. In a situation where erythropoiesis has been stimulated by an ESA and the patient does not have sufficient iron sTFR levels rise, however, sTFR also provides an estimate of the erythroblast mass in the bone marrow. Thus, an ESA-treated patient may have a high sTFR due to iron deficiency or increased erythroblastic activity or a combination of both. Studies of sTFR in adult CKD have been mixed, and no clear cutoff has been established.

Vitamin and Mineral Deficiency

Vitamins and minerals play critical roles in erythropoiesis. The B vitamins are water-soluble and thus are removed during dialysis. Deficiency of vitamin B_{12} causes megaloblastic anemia because vitamin B_{12} is required for DNA synthesis. Individuals who are deficient have large erythrocytes because of the abnormal maturation process. Vitamin B_{12} is found only in products derived from animal sources; thus, vegetarians are at greater risk of becoming vitamin B_{12} deficient. Patients with gastrectomy, surgical removal of ileum, or chronic malabsorption disorder are more likely to have vitamin B_{12} deficiency. Vitamin B_{12} deficiency occurs rarely in patients receiving hemodialysis.

Folic acid deficiency also causes a macrocytic anemia indistinguishable from vitamin B_{12} deficiency. Pyridoxine (vitamin B_6) deficiency causes a microcytic anemia that can be easily confused with iron deficiency.

Vitamins developed for dialysis-dependent patients are excellent sources of the water-soluble B vitamins. The addition of 0.25 mg/month of vitamin B_{12} may be necessary in selected patients. A weekly dose of 2–3 mg of folic acid and 100–150 mg of vitamin B_6 is recommended for adult hemodialysis patients receiving ESA therapy.

Vitamin C (1–1.5 g/week) was shown to overcome functional iron deficiency in patients with high ferritin levels. The potential increase of oxidative stress induced by IV iron therapy may be blunted by concomitant administration of vitamin E (1200 IU).

Copper is an essential component of several enzymes that are required for blood formation. Factors that are associated with copper deficiency include prolonged diarrhea, premature birth, excessive zinc intake and Menkes kinky hair syndrome that is due to a genetic defect in copper absorption. Copper deficiency causes an anemia that is very similar to iron deficiency. Cobalt, a critical component in the vitamin B_{12} molecule, is required in trace amounts for erythropoiesis. Cobalt deficiency is very rare.

Erythrocyte-Stimulating Agents

The ESAs includes all agents that augment erythropoiesis through direct or indirect action on the EPO receptor and they have become the hallmark of therapy for anemia of CKD. Overall, ESA therapy has been regarded as beneficial in attenuating the effects of anemia, as described earlier in this chapter. Furthermore, ESA treatment also reduces the need for blood transfusions and minimizes transfusion-associated risks (transmission of blood-borne viral infections, allosensitization, reactions, and transfusional hemosiderosis).

Presently, ESAs available include epoetin alfa and epoetin beta, which are considered short acting, and darbepoetin and methoxy polyethylene glycol-epoetin beta, which are long acting. The choice of short-acting or long-acting ESA will depend on patient-specific issues as there is no evidence to suggest that one formulation is superior to another in terms of patient outcomes.

The initiation of ESA therapy in adults is considered when the Hb concentration falls below 10 g/dL. In children, there are limited data in order to recommend an

Hb threshold. The KDIGO guidelines recommend basing the initiation of ESA after considering all potential benefits and potential harms. The goal of ESA therapy is to increase the Hb at a rate of 1–2 g/dL per month with a target Hb of 11–12 g/dL. The Hb should not exceed 13 g/dL in ESA-treated patients. The NKF-KDOQI Guidelines recommend that children on dialysis who initiate ESA therapy have their Hb monitored every 2 weeks. Once the target Hb level has been reached and the patient is on a stable ESA dose, monitoring every 4 weeks is recommended. Hemoglobin levels should be followed more closely after making a significant change to the ESA dose. Dose adjustments are indicated if the Hb is rapidly approaching or is above the target level, if the Hb increases by more than 1.3 g/dL in a 2-week period, or if the Hb fails to increase 1.6–2 g/dL over a period of 8 weeks.

ESA can be given intravenously or subcutaneously. The route of administration of ESA will be determined by patient-oriented issues, treatment setting, efficacy considerations and the class of ESA being prescribed. For patients undergoing peritoneal dialysis, subcutaneous administration is the only route feasible. For those patients undergoing hemodialysis, intravenous or subcutaneous administration is possible. In children, subcutaneous injections are uncomfortable and the IV route is generally recommended for those patients on hemodialysis.

The dose of ESA in children will vary depending on the age of the child, the route of administration, and the mode of dialysis. Epoetin alfa and epoetin beta dosing usually start at 50 IU/kg body weight three times per week. However, young children will require higher EPO doses. Data from NAPRTCS reported that children younger than 1 year of age received an average of 350 IU/kg/week, those 2–5 years of age received 275 IU/kg/week, those 6–12 years of age needed 250 IU/kg/week, whereas those older than 12 years needed 200 IU/kg/week. A reduction in dosing is possible when EPO is given subcutaneously rather than intravenously. Children on hemodialysis require higher EPO doses per week compared with children on peritoneal dialysis. It has been proposed that this is due to greater blood loss during hemodialysis treatment.

Darbepoetin alfa is a hyperglycosylated form of EPO. It differs as it contains 5 N-linked oligosaccharide chains instead of 3 chains. Pharmacokinetic studies in children show that the half-life of darbepoetin in children is similar to adults. Following IV administration to patients receiving dialysis, the terminal half-life was reported to be 22 hours and approximately threefold longer than that of epoetin alfa. Following subcutaneous administration, the average terminal half-life was 42 hours. Dosing usually starts at 0.45 µg/kg body weight (dosing range 0.25–0.75 µg/kg body weight) once every 1–2 weeks. Investigators have proposed a conversion dose of erythropoietin alfa to darbepoetin to be 0.5 µg for every 200 IU of erythropoietin alfa rather than the 1 µg/200 IU conversion recommended by the manufacturer. In an open-label study involving patients aged 1–18 years of age, darbepoetin was reported to be noninferior to EPO in the treatment of anemia of CKD.

Methoxy polyethylene glycol-epoetin beta is an erythropoietin continuous receptor activator with increased half-life when compared to erythropoietin. Following an IV administration of 0.4 µg/kg body weight to CKD patients receiving peritoneal dialysis, the terminal half-life was 134 ± 65 hours (mean $\pm$ SD). After a subcutaneous administration of 0.8 µg/kg to CKD patients receiving peritoneal dialysis, the terminal half-life was 139 ± 67 hours. The initial dose is 0.6 µg/kg of body weight every 2 weeks administered subcutaneously or intravenously. Its safety and efficacy have not been rigorously evaluated in children. In one study, 16 children on peritoneal dialysis were converted to subcutaneous methoxy polyethylene glycol-epoetin beta scheduled every 2 weeks. The follow-up period was 6 months. The medication dose was increased from 0.86 ± 0.33 to 1.67 ± 0.4 µg/kg at month 3 and was 1.6 ± 0.67 µg/kg at the end of the study. The Hb levels were maintained and no adverse events were observed during the protocol.

Lack of Response to ESA

Erythropoietin resistance or failure to respond to ESA is recognized with the inability to maintain a constant Hb level with increasing doses of ESA (typically in excess of 500 IU/kg/week), or if there is a decrease in Hb levels with the use of a constant ESA dose. The etiology of ESA resistance includes infection/inflammation (probably mediated in part by high hepcidin levels), absolute iron deficiency, secondary hyperparathyroidism, chronic blood loss, vitamin B_{12}/folate deficiency, use of angiotensin-converting enzyme inhibitors or angiotensin-receptor blockers, malnutrition, underdialysis, hemoglobinopathies, and rarely antibody-mediated pure red cell aplasia. Some of the conditions that cause hyporesponsiveness are reversible and addressing the implicating factors will result in improved response to ESA. Furthermore, not all causes of failure to respond to ESA are readily apparent, and some patients require evaluation for the more unusual causes listed above.

Risk of Adverse Outcomes

Hypertension is the most common adverse effect attributed to ESA therapy. Patients can experience de novo hypertension or worsening of chronic hypertension. In children, an increase in antihypertensive therapy occurred in 30% of those treated with ESA. Several mechanisms have been considered in the pathogenesis of ESA-induced hypertension. These include the possible role of the rise of Hct and erythrocyte mass, changes in production or sensitivity to endogenous vasopressors, alterations in vascular smooth-muscle ionic milieu, dysregulation of production or responsiveness to endogenous vasodilatory factors, a direct vasopressor action of EPO, and finally arterial remodeling through stimulation of vascular cell growth. If the hypertension is significant, temporary discontinuation or reduction in the dose of ESA as well as administration of antihypertensive treatment may be indicated.

There are no controlled clinical trials in children that have evaluated other outcomes such as risk of death, stroke, congestive heart failure, thrombosis of hemodialysis vascular access, and other thromboembolic events with regards to ESA use or higher Hb targets as in the adult population.

Iron Therapy

Oral Iron Supplementation

Iron supplements are necessary to meet the demand for increased erythropoiesis during ESA therapy in children with CKD. The current KDIGO guidelines again closely follow adult recommendations and state that oral therapy is likely adequate for non-dialysis and peritoneal dialysis patients while hemodialysis patients likely require IV iron therapy (see below). However, some investigators have advocated for oral iron therapy in pediatric hemodialysis patients. One small randomized trial of 35 pediatric hemodialysis patients demonstrated that although IV iron did result in increased ferritin levels, it did not show a significant advantage over oral iron in terms of maintaining adequate iron stores for erythropoiesis. It is important to note that at the beginning of this trial all patients were iron replete by current KDIGO standards. Additionally, most adult studies of hemodialysis patients have shown that IV iron is superior to oral iron.

Oral iron is usually dosed at 3–6 mg/kg/day of elemental iron given twice daily with a maximum dose of 300 mg/day. Generally the dose should be taken at least 2 hours before or 1 hour after phosphate binders and food to maximize absorption. Coadministration of iron with other medications such as phosphate binders and antacids limits its absorption due to changes in gastric pH. As an aside, oral iron preparations can be used as phosphorus binders but have not been widely marketed as such. High-dose vitamin C has been found to enhance the iron absorption in the gut but has the potential side effect of oxalate deposition in the presence of decreased kidney function. Compliance with oral iron therapy in children can be limited by gastrointestinal intolerance, which is dose related and occurs in up to 20% of patients. Additionally, the use of the oral suspension can cause teeth discoloration and staining.

There are a multitude of oral iron preparations available, with varying amounts of elemental iron including ferrous sulfate, ferrous fumarate, ferrous gluconate, ferrous succinate, iron polymaltose, and polysaccharide-iron complex. Ferrous sulfate is the most commonly prescribed iron compound containing 65 mg of elemental iron per 325-mg tablet. There are very limited data comparing the efficacy of one preparation versus another in CKD patients. One small study of 46 adults on hemodialysis randomized patients to receive 200 mg of elemental iron daily in one of four preparations (1) Chromagen (ferrous fumarate), (2) Feosol (ferrous sulfate), (3) Niferex (polysaccharide iron complex), or (4) Tabron (ferrous fumarate). Although the Tabron group tended to have the highest percentage of patients with a TSAT >20% followed by Feosol, Chromagen, and Niferex groups, these differences were not statistically significant. Importantly, despite intensive compliance monitoring during the study the mean Hct remained less than 30% and the mean TSAT remained less than 20% in three of the four groups, reinforcing the poor efficacy of oral iron supplementation in hemodialysis patients.

Recently there has been growing interest in the use of oral ferric citrate as both a phosphate binder and an iron supplement. Studies indicate that in adults, ferric citrate is safe and effective as a phosphorus binder with common adverse effects of diarrhea, nausea, vomiting, and constipation. Its use also appears to increase iron stores and reduced need for IV iron and ESA use while maintaining Hb levels in adult hemodialysis patients. There are few data describing its use in child.

Intravenous Iron Supplementation

As stated above, the current KDIGO guidelines recommend IV iron as the preferred route of administration in hemodialysis patients. These recommendations are based on both adult and pediatric data. Specifically, evidence in adult patients comes from several randomized controlled trials comparing IV to oral iron that demonstrated that IV iron administration is superior to oral iron in hemodialysis patients. In pediatric patients, there are several prospective randomized trials showing that IV iron is effective at repleting and maintaining iron store in children on hemodialysis. In the case of pediatric peritoneal dialysis patients, IV iron is often only administered after the patient has not shown response to a course of oral iron. This is likely a function of the overall decreased need for iron in peritoneal dialysis patients because of their much smaller obligate blood loss, the lack of easy IV access, and inconvenience of the small but frequent dosing strategies used in hemodialysis patients.

In general, treatment with IV iron is broken down in a loading phase where consecutive doses are given in order to replete the patient's iron stores and then a maintenance phase where a smaller dose is given once a week. Currently four iron preparations are available for parenteral use in dialysis patients within the United States (Table 88.1) with a fifth (ferric carboxymaltose) approved for use in nondialysis patients. Additionally, iron isomaltoside is available in Europe. These different preparations avoid the toxicity of an iron salt by complexing it with a carbohydrate (i.e., dextran, sucrose, or gluconate). Before the iron within these parenteral compounds can be used directly for erythropoiesis, it must first be processed by the reticuloendothelial system.

Iron dextran, a complex of ferric oxyhydroxide with polymerized dextran, was the first parenteral formulation to become available for the treatment of iron deficiency. Until recently, it was the only parenteral compound that had the advantage of a single infusion up to 1 g, which is both convenient and cost-effective. However, its popularity has decreased due to the FDA black box warning of potential fatal anaphylaxis, which has been estimated at 0.6%–0.7%. Hence, a test dose of 10–25 mg is required before the full infusion to check for the possibility of an allergic response. Other reported adverse reactions that are not thought to be immune mediated include delayed reactions of hypotension, arthralgias, myalgias, malaise, abdominal pain, nausea, and vomiting. Of the two forms currently marketed within the United States, INFeD and DexFerrum, InFed appears to have a lower incidence of adverse effects.

Sodium ferric gluconate, a complex of sodium ferric gluconate in sucrose that was FDA approved in 1999, has a lower rate of adverse reactions, with no fatal hypersensitivity reactions reported to date. Ferric gluconate has had an allergy event

Table 88.1

IV Iron Table

Intravenous Iron Preparation	Dose	Frequency	
		Loading	Maintenance
Iron dextran INFeD: 50 mg/mL (2-mL vials) DexFerrum: 50 mg/mL (2-mL vials)	4 mg/kg/dose not to exceed 100 mg Test dose: Child <10 kg: 10 mg Child 10–25 kg: 15 mg Child >25 kg: 25 mg	3 times weekly for a total of 8–10 dialysis sessions	Once a week
Sodium ferric gluconate Ferrlecit: 12.5 mg/mL (5-mL vials)	1.5–3 mg/kg/dose not to exceed 125 mg	3 times weekly for a total of 8 dialysis sessions	Once a week
Iron sucrose Venofer: 20 mg/mL (5-mL vials)	1–4 mg/kg/dose not to exceed 100 mg	3 times weekly for a total of 10 dialysis sessions	Once a week

reporting rate of 3.3 episodes per million doses compared to 8.7 with iron dextran, and although when it was first marketed a test dose was recommended, that recommendation has been dropped. An international prospective multicenter trial of 66 pediatric patients investigated the safety and efficacy of ferric gluconate at both a 1.5- and 3-mg/kg dose over eight consecutive doses in pediatric hemodialysis patients on ESA therapy. Both dosing regimens resulted in significant increases in mean Hb, Hct, transferrin saturation, serum ferritin, and reticulocyte Hb content with no unexpected adverse reactions reported. Another multicenter study of 23 pediatric hemodialysis patients showed that a weekly ferric gluconate dose of 1 mg/kg was effective as a maintenance regimen.

Iron sucrose, a complex of iron hydroxide and sucrose, was FDA approved in 2000. Several studies have demonstrated its effectiveness and like ferric gluconate is well tolerated with minimal adverse effects. Dosing in children is 1–4 mg/kg weekly for 12 weeks. In a study by Morgan et al, iron sucrose was successfully used in pediatric hemodialysis patients at a dose of 2 mg/kg/week. No adverse events were reported even when patients with suspected iron deficiency received a single loading dose of 7 mg/kg (maximum of 200 mg), followed by 2 mg/kg/week. Another study of 14 pediatric hemodialysis patients concluded that a dosage of 1 and 0.3 mg/kg/dialysis were sufficient for loading and maintenance therapy, respectively.

Ferumoxytol was approved by the FDA in 2009. It is a novel iron oxide nanoparticle with a polyglucose sorbitol carboxymethylether coating. Although it was initially approved as safe and effective in adult CKD patients when administered as a single rapid dose of up to 510 mg, there have been 79 reports of anaphylactic reactions resulting in 18 deaths. Thus, the FDA in 2015 issued a black box warning that ferumoxytol must be given as a diluted IV infusion over a minimum of 15 minutes. Data describing its dosing and use in pediatric patients are lacking.

Finally, ferric carboxymaltose, a polynuclear iron(III)-hydroxide carbohydrate complex, was approved by the FDA in 2013 for use in nondialysis adult CKD patients. Although there are no data describing its use in children, there have been studies indicating its efficacy in adult dialysis patients.

Intradialytic Iron Supplementation

Ferric pyrophosphate citrate (FPC) is a low-molecular-weight iron salt that can be administered via the dialysate where it crosses the hemodialyzer membrane and enters the blood. Because it donates iron directly to transferrin, unlike the iron compounds above, it does not require processing by macrophages and in theory could bypass reticuloendothelial blockade. Adult studies have indicated that it could effectively deliver sufficient iron to replace ongoing losses and maintain the Hb level, leading to its approval by the FDA in 2015. Treatment with FPC did not increase ferritin, possibly reflecting that it does not increase iron stores and thus carries less risk of iron overload. It is currently being investigated as a new means of meeting the increased maintenance iron requirements of pediatric patients receiving hemodialysis.

Iron Safety

Although the use of ESAs, often at high doses, has been embraced by nephrologists, iron therapy has been approached rather conservatively. Ironically there are now important safety concerns with the use of ESAs while the data linking iron administration to poorer outcomes remains lacking. Much of the discomfort with iron administration can be attributed to problems of iron overload as a result of multiple transfusions during the pre-ESA era. In addition, several observational studies have described an association between high serum ferritin levels and infection or mortality. However, the acute phase reactant behavior of ferritin remains a large confounding factor as increased ferritin levels do not necessarily reflect iron status and instead may simply be due to increased levels of inflammation present in CKD patients. Thus, the link between high ferritin levels and infection and mortality may be an epiphenomenon. Indeed, although no randomized controlled study of whether IV iron therapy leads to an increased risk of infection or death has been performed, a retrospective epidemiologic study of 50,000+ hemodialysis patients found that iron administration was associated with improved survival. Finally, many of the concerns regarding the adverse effects of iron, including oxidative stress, are based on in vitro studies. Regardless, when one considers the benefits of improved response to ESA agents, the overall risk benefit ratio favors the use of IV iron in hemodialysis patients.

As far as the upper limit of ferritin, most investigators agree that extremely high levels (>2000 ng/mL) are reflective of simple iron overload or hemosiderosis. Levels of greater than 1200 ng/mL are still associated with increased mortality risk even after adjustment for markers of malnutrition and inflammation. Thus, most clinicians would feel uncomfortable with the use of IV iron at these high ferritin levels. In contrast, it remains unclear if therapy with IV iron is warranted at ferritin levels between 500 and 1200 ng/mL even when the TSAT is less than 20%. The results of the DRIVE study did demonstrate that IV iron therapy in patients with a serum ferritin between 500 and 1200 ng/mL resulted in a 25% reduction in ESA dose. Additionally, the large retrospective study of 50,000+ dialysis patients mentioned above showed that the greatest ESA responsiveness occurred in patients with a TSAT of 30%–50% and a ferritin level of 800–1200 ng/mL. However, the lack of randomized controlled trials comparing the safety and efficacy of targeting ferritin levels greater than 500 ng/mL versus less than 500 ng/mL has led to the KDIGO guidelines reemphasizing the old NKF-KDOQI guidelines that "when ferritin level is greater than 500 ng/mL, decisions regarding IV iron administration should weigh ESA responsiveness, Hgb and TSAT level, and the patient's clinical status."

C H A P T E R 8 9

Assessing Quality of Life in Pediatric Patients Undergoing Dialysis

Stuart L. Goldstein, MD • Shari K. Neul, PhD

Introduction

Advances in medical care now afford increased survival of and improved treatment outcomes for youth undergoing dialysis. However, pediatric patients on dialysis generally have poor psychosocial outcomes compared to youth with other chronic conditions. As a result, health-related quality of life (HRQOL) functioning is now considered an essential component for optimal patient care provision for youth undergoing dialysis. Although pediatric end-stage renal disease (ESRD) and the dialysis treatment continue to carry a heavy disease burden for youth and their families, HRQOL assessment offers the medical team an important opportunity to collaborate with patients and their families in negotiating important developmental phases that impact chronic disease management and long-term psychosocial outcomes. This chapter reviews factors that impact HRQOL functioning, as well as the evolution of, best practices for, and future directions regarding assessment of HRQOL in pediatric patients undergoing dialysis.

Factors Impacting HRQOL Functioning

Previous studies indicate that HRQOL functioning in pediatric patients with ESRD is on par with youth newly diagnosed with cancer undergoing chemotherapy and radiation. ESRD youth are at risk for suboptimal academic, social, and psychological functioning, as well as face challenges in young adulthood to complete their education, secure employment, experience intimate relationships, and live independently. Pediatric ESRD carries a significant disease burden for patients, not only requiring complex, invasive medical management and intensive self-care regimens but the prospect of undergoing recurrent cycles of life-sustaining treatments and a future inevitably overshadowed by a life-limiting disease. Moreover, these factors translate into a broader burden placed on parents and siblings, impacting family psychosocial and financial well-being. Medical management requires highly proficient and coordinated care, with a specialized and technically capable team to optimize dialysis prescriptions and procedures to achieve and sustain improved functional health status and thereby better HRQOL functioning. Patient characteristics, such as age (i.e., developmental level); executive functioning and planning skills; disease severity, knowledge, beliefs, and experience; degree of self-efficacy, socioemotional support, and adjustment and coping skills; level of autonomy versus shared responsibility between adolescents and parents for medical self-care tasks; and family and environmental stressors versus resources influence a patient's ability to initiate and sustain efforts to be medically adherent, prevent medical complications and hospitalizations, communicate and interact effectively with their health care team, and enhance HRQOL functioning. Assessment of HRQOL functioning aims to identify these patient, disease, and treatment factors; however, until somewhat recently, limited options for assessment tools existed.

Evolution of HRQOL Assessment

In 2008, the United States Centers for Medicare and Medicaid Services (CMS) issued its mandate that assessment of HRQOL in pediatric dialysis patients occur at least once per year. However, little guidance was offered regarding which measure(s) to choose, and how to manage assessment results and develop interventions to improve and track HRQOL outcomes. Although validated assessment measures that assess global and disease-specific aspects of HRQOL functioning have been in use for adults with ESRD (e.g., Short Form 36 Health Survey (SF-36) and Kidney Disease Quality of Life [KDQOL™]), only global measures of HRQOL functioning had been available for use with pediatric patients. Initially, assessment of HRQOL functioning in pediatric dialysis patients focused on global domains (e.g., the Child Health and Illness Profile: Adolescent Edition [CHIP-AE], the Children's Health Questionnaire [CHQ], and the Pediatric Quality of Life Inventory [PedsQL]), as no disease-specific measures were yet developed. To fill this gap, the first ESRD-specific measure of HRQOL functioning in pediatric patients was developed and validated: PedsQL 3.0 ESRD Module. (Refer to Table 89.1 for an overview of HRQOL assessment tools used with pediatric patients undergoing dialysis.) Initial studies utilizing the PedsQL 3.0 ESRD Module and its companion measure, the PedsQL 4.0 Generic Core Scales, revealed that patients with ESRD receiving dialysis

Table 89.1				
Pediatric HRQOL Measurement Tools Studied in Pediatric Patients on Dialysis				
Instrument	**Domains**	**Respondent**	**Ages**	**Items**
Child Health Questionnaire (CHQ™)	14	Child Parent proxy	5–18 parent 10–18 child	87 child 28, 50 parent
Pediatric Quality of Life Inventory (PedsQL™ 4.0)	4	Child Parent proxy	2–17 parent 5–7 interview 8–12 child 13–17 teen	23
Child Health & Illness Profile – Adolescent Edition (CHIP-AE)	5 general 14 subdomains	Adolescent	11–17	108
Generic Children's QOL Measure (GCQ)	Perceived self Preferred self	Child	6–14	25
PedsQL 3.0 ESRD Module	7	Child Parent proxy	2–17 parent 5–7 interview 8–12 child 13–17 teen	34

reported worse HRQOL functioning than healthy controls and transplant recipients, with both patient and parent HRQOL ratings being lower than any pediatric chronic illness cohorts previously assessed. Agreement between patient and parent ratings was fairly low, as is fairly typical in most pediatric research examining perceived functioning. Numerous additional studies of HRQOL in pediatric ESRD have enriched our understanding of how patients on dialysis, as well as pre-ESRD and transplant recipients, fare. However, as the rule rather than the exception, researchers employ a variety of or create their own measures while using diverse methodologies and sample sizes to assess HRQOL. Thus, there is now a plethora of descriptive information available that cannot easily be integrated and summarized. Further, the majority of these studies are cross-sectional in design, thus making it difficult to track changes in HRQOL functioning over time. A recent study examining longitudinal change in global and disease-specific HRQOL functioning in pediatric dialysis patients revealed that patient HRQOL ratings were generally better compared with parent ratings of a child's functioning. Patient age, gender, length of time on dialysis, and ESRD history (medically managed prior to vs emergently diagnosed with ESRD) impacted parent and patient perceptions of HRQOL functioning. Parents of older children and those on dialysis longer reported worse HRQOL functioning on multiple global domains. Female patients reported worse emotional functioning and increased appearance-related concerns. Patients medically managed prior to ESRD reported less disease burden compared with their parents whereas those emergently diagnosed fluctuated relative to their parents in how they perceived the burden of ESRD over time. Finally, parents reported significant worsening of academic functioning over time attesting to the impact of school concerns on HRQOL functioning. In brief, availability of global and ESRD-specific HRQOL measures that contain developmentally appropriate content and which contain patient self-report and parent-proxy versions affords clinicians the opportunity to gather both a more comprehensive and nuanced picture of patient functioning. As the assessment of HRQOL functioning in pediatric dialysis patients becomes more sophisticated, consideration of best practices and caveats are important, as is broadening the scope of HRQOL assessment to include methods for intervention planning and tracking of HRQOL outcomes.

Best Practice Considerations and Caveats

The 2008 CMS mandate indicates that a standardized survey be used to assess patient physical and mental functioning and delineates psychosocial elements in the patient plan of care to include factors such as education about quality of life, psychosocial risks/benefits related to access type, and addressing other issues as needed to help patients achieve and sustain appropriate psychosocial functioning. Although these guidelines offer some direction, implementing these in a pediatric dialysis setting requires that various practical and methodological considerations be considered when devising a "best practices" approach to HRQOL assessment. Patient characteristics such as age, cognitive development level, and maturity impact understanding of item content, the ability to have insight into and then reflect on one's experience to respond to the items, and how proximal (e.g., in-the-moment thoughts, dialysis side effects, time of day) versus more distal factors (e.g., underlying disease and impact on cognitive processing, chronic family stress) may differentially affect ratings at the time of assessment. Program-level factors, such as staff availability and familiarity with measure administration and interpretation, financial resources to purchase HRQOL tools and cover staff efforts, and acceptance by all members of the dialysis team can impact how the overall assessment process is implemented and sustained.

Methodological considerations have important implications for whether and how direct patient care regarding HRQOL functioning can be effectively managed. Such matters can include but are not limited to whether to assess global and/or ESRD-specific aspects of HRQOL functioning and obtain patient and/or parent-proxy reports; how frequently to administer tools and implications for respondent fatigue and practice effects; and how to interpret change in HRQOL scores across time. Much has been written on the methodological and practical implications for determining whether change in HRQOL scores is clinically meaningful. The minimal clinically important difference (MCID) score is generally defined as the smallest change in a score on a domain that patients perceive as beneficial and may compel a change in treatment as long as bothersome side effects and excessive cost will not be incurred. Caveats have been raised, however, whether one is examining a minimally important change (MIC) versus a minimally detectable change (MDC), as the distinction is important and has implications for data interpretation and clinical decision making.

Another concern for interpreting HRQOL scores is the phenomenon of response shift, which refers to the change in an individual's internal standards in terms of how one accommodates to a chronic illness and its impact on one's life, as well as what is considered as most valuable in terms of activities that comprise HRQOL functioning, across time. This has significant relevance for pediatric patients undergoing dialysis in terms of how effects of ESRD and its treatment affect these youth and how this in turn changes how and what they value is important to them and their perception of HRQOL functioning across various domains and over various periods of time. Consequently, teasing apart response shift phenomena from normative, developmental changes in pediatric dialysis patients is likely to be difficult but important to consider from a methodological perspective in longitudinal HRQOL assessment efforts. Research design and statistical approaches, such as growth curve modeling, have been studied and considered as potential tools in addressing this issue; however, additional research is needed in pediatric populations.

Broadening the Scope to Include Intervention Planning

Careful consideration of the above issues in developing a programmatic approach to HRQOL assessment should help to lay the important groundwork for broadening the scope of assessment to include intervention planning and tracking. This can likely be achieved via use of patient-reported outcome (PRO) processes and patient-centered care practices. HRQOL functioning is a PRO, and HRQOL assessment is increasingly being incorporated into routine dialysis care for adults with HRQOL PRO benchmarks proposed for applying this information to patient-centered care practices that promote patient involvement in their own care and medical decision making, such as identifying intervention or treatment needs and determining satisfaction with care. In pediatric patient care, the utility of PROs in HRQOL assessment remains relatively understudied. Little exists in the pediatric literature connecting HRQOL assessment findings to patient-centered care practices and in turn to subsequent HRQOL outcomes. Methods need to be devised that can be easily integrated into various clinical settings for sharing HRQOL assessment results with patients and caregivers in easy-to-understand language and graphical displays, discussing information about available resources and mutually identifying ways to address HRQOL needs, and then seeking feedback on whether addressing needs positively influences HRQOL functioning. Implementing such patient-centered care practices as patients are admitted to chronic dialysis treatment and throughout their tenure in the program can serve to promote optimal health and HRQOL functioning, successfully prepare youth for transition to adult care services, and contribute to improving long-term psychosocial and health outcomes.

Future Directions

HRQOL assessment is now considered a key component in the standard of care for pediatric patients undergoing dialysis. A wealth of descriptive information currently exists regarding the multifaceted nature of HRQOL functioning in the pediatric ESRD population. As the study of HRQOL functioning in these youth evolves, clinicians and researchers alike have ample options for pioneering HRQOL assessment efforts that will benefit youth undergoing dialysis and their families. Areas ripe for study include developing and validating measures that assess parent and sibling HRQOL functioning; advancing methodological and statistical approaches to HRQOL assessment, such as multimethod efforts combining qualitative and quantitative procedures and growth curve modeling to track longitudinal outcomes and maturational influences; and computerized adaptive HRQOL assessment that can tailor administration of items based on a patient's unique responses to each item and at an age-appropriate difficulty level to more closely approximate the respondent's actual HRQOL functioning level. Furthermore, also needed is the development or adaptation of HRQOL measures that can be used on an international level to facilitate large, multicenter/intercontinental studies examining the impact of clinical drug trials and treatment approaches (e.g., intensified hemodialysis programs) on HRQOL functioning. Finally, developing and incorporating measures that assess HRQOL functioning from an adaptive, psychosocial-growth perspective will be important, as many youth with ESRD are resilient and thrive in the face of living with a burdensome, life-limiting condition. Identifying factors that facilitate and sustain such resiliency can translate into identifying medical and psychosocial intervention targets and promoting improved HRQOL functioning. HRQOL assessment of pediatric patients undergoing dialysis has advanced tremendously within recent years and continues to offer much opportunity for further groundbreaking research and clinical application to garner the data to convince third-party payers and legislators to invest in innovative (albeit costly) treatment approaches, fund professionals who can further augment the effectiveness of interdisciplinary care, and deliver optimal patient care to improve long-term health and psychosocial outcomes for youth with ESRD.

C H A P T E R 9 0

Immunization in Children Undergoing Dialysis

Jodi M. Smith, MD, MPH • Thor A. Wagner MD

Infections are a source of significant morbidity and mortality in the pediatric dialysis population. Despite this, vaccination rates in the end-stage renal disease (ESRD) population are significantly lower than for the general population. To limit vaccine-preventable infections in this high-risk population, it is critical that pediatric nephrologists monitor the immunization status of their patients and maintain compliance with vaccines and new recommendations. This chapter reviews immunization recommendations for patients on dialysis, how to prepare dialysis patients for transplant, and how to maintain readiness for patients on the transplant list. In addition, evidence of vaccine responsiveness in the pediatric population is presented.

Vaccine Schedule: Current American Academy of Pediatrics Recommendations

In general, patients on dialysis should receive the standard immunizations according to the time frames suggested by the Advisory Committee on Immunization Practices (ACIP), American Academy of Pediatrics (AAP), and American Academy of Family Physicians (http://www.cdc.gov/vaccines/schedules/hcp/imz/child-adolescent.html). Routine childhood immunizations currently include vaccination against diphtheria, *Haemophilus influenzae* type B (Hib), hepatitis A and B, human papillomavirus, influenza, measles, mumps, *Neisseria meningitidis,* pertussis, polio, rotavirus, rubella, *Streptococcus pneumoniae*, tetanus, and varicella.

Numerous studies document the safety of vaccination of dialysis patients. Killed or component vaccines have not been associated with any deterioration in dialysis efficacy. Live-virus vaccines have also been shown to be safe in the pediatric dialysis population.

There are several vaccines (e.g., hepatitis B, influenza, and pneumococcus) with specific recommendations in the AAP Red Book for individuals with chronic kidney disease (CKD).

Summary of Recommendations From 2015 Red Book for Children With End Stage Kidney Disease, Including Transplant Candidates

Children and adolescents with chronic kidney disease or ESRD, including kidney transplant candidates, should receive all vaccinations as appropriate for age, exposure history, and immune status based on the annual immunization schedule for immunocompetent people. Patients 2 years or older with these conditions also should have received, or should be given as a candidate for kidney transplant, a dose of PPSV23, if not previously given. (Patients with ESRD should receive PPSV23 if they have not received a dose within 5 years and have not received two lifetime doses.) PCV13 is administered if not previously received, even for those 6 years or older. When PCV13 and PPSV23 both are indicated, PPSV23 should be given at least 8 weeks after the last PCV13 dose. Kidney transplant candidates who are hepatitis B surface antibody (anti-HBs) negative should receive the hepatitis B vaccine (HepB) series followed by serologic testing and further doses if serologic test results are negative (as indicated for an immunocompetent vaccinee who remains seronegative). Patients 12 months or older who have not received hepatitis A vaccine (HepA), did not complete the vaccination series, or who are seronegative should receive the HepA vaccine series. The measles, mumps, rubella (MMR) vaccine can be given to infants 6 through 11 months of age who are kidney transplant candidates and who are not immunocompromised, repeating the dose at 12 months or more if still awaiting a transplant that will not occur within 4 weeks of vaccination. Living kidney donors should have up-to-date vaccination status. Household members of these patients should be counseled about risks of infection and should have vaccination status made current.

Hepatitis B

Hepatitis B vaccination is recommended for all chronic hemodialysis (HD) patients. Vaccination is also recommended for patients with CKD before they reach end stage renal disease. Compared with immunocompetent individuals, HD patients are less likely to have protective levels of antibody after vaccination with standard vaccine dosages. Protective levels of antibody developed in 67% to 86% of HD patients who received three or four doses in various dosages and schedules. Higher seroprotection rates have been identified in patients with chronic kidney disease who were vaccinated before reaching end stage and starting dialysis. Based on this, higher vaccine dosages or an increased number of doses are recommended for those on HD. Testing after vaccination is recommended for HD patients to determine their response to the vaccine. Testing should be performed 1 to 2 months after administration of the last dose of the vaccine series by using a method that allows determination of a protective level of anti-HBs (e.g., >10 mIU/mL). If the patient has anti-HBs levels of less than 10 mIU/mL after the primary vaccine series, he or she should be revaccinated with a second hepatitis B vaccination series. Administration of three or four doses on an appropriate schedule followed by anti-HBs testing 1 to 2 months after the third dose is usually more practical than serologic testing after one or more doses of vaccine. For HD patients, the need for booster doses should be assessed annually by testing for antibody to hepatitis B surface antigen. A booster dose should be administered when anti-HBs levels decline to less than 10 mIU/mL.

Influenza Vaccine

Children with kidney failure are identified to be at high risk for severe complications of influenza. Therefore, annual influenza vaccination is recommended with the inactivated vaccine. Live attenuated influenza vaccine is not generally recommended for children on dialysis. To allow time for production of protective antibody levels, vaccination should ideally occur before the onset of influenza activity in the community. Therefore, vaccination should start as soon as vaccine is available.

Pneumococcal Vaccine

For children ages 2 to 5 years on dialysis or posttransplant:
1. Administer one dose of PCV13 if any incomplete schedule of three doses of PCV (PCV7, PCV13, or both) were received previously.
2. Administer two doses of PCV13 at least 8 weeks apart if unvaccinated or any incomplete schedule of fewer than three doses of PCV (PCV7, PCV13, or both) were received previously.
3. Administer one supplemental dose of PCV13 if 4 doses of PCV7 or other age-appropriate complete PCV7 series was received previously.
4. The minimum interval between doses of PCV (PCV7 or PCV13) is 8 weeks.
5. For children with no history of PPSV23 vaccination, administer PPSV23 at least 8 weeks after the most recent dose of PCV13.
   For children ages 6 to 18 years on dialysis or posttransplant:
1. If neither PCV13 nor PPSV23 has been received previously, administer one dose of PCV13 now and one dose of PPSV23 at least 8 weeks later.
2. If PCV13 has been received previously but PPSV23 has not, administer one dose of PPSV23 at least 8 weeks after the most recent dose of PCV13.
3. If PPSV23 has been received but PCV13 has not, administer one dose of PCV13 at least 8 weeks after the most recent dose of PPSV23.

For children ages 6 to 18 years on dialysis or posttransplant who have not received PPSV23, administer one dose of PPSV23. If PCV13 has been received previously, then PPSV23 should be administered at least 8 weeks after any prior PCV13 dose.

A single revaccination with PPSV23 should be administered 5 years after the first dose.

Special Situations

In patients on intravenous immunoglobulin (IVIG), vaccines are not generally recommended (with the exception of seasonal influenza vaccine) because efficacy of the host humoral system is often in question, and the vaccine would have to compete against the antibody in the IVIG, which should have good titers for most vaccine-associated pathogens.

In heavily immunosuppressed patients, live vaccines are usually not recommended. For the purpose of the AAP Redbook, high-level immunosuppression is defined as receiving daily corticosteroid therapy at a dose of 20 mg or more (or >2 mg/kg/day for patients weighing <10 kg) of prednisone or equivalent for 14 days or longer or receiving certain biologic immune modulators, for example, tumor necrosis factor-alpha (TNF-α) antagonists (e.g., adalimumab, certolizumab, infliximab, etanercept, and golimumab) or anti–B-lymphocyte monoclonal antibodies (e.g., rituximab). Low-level immunosuppression is defined as receiving a lower daily dose of systemic corticosteroid than for high-level immunosuppression for 14 days or more or receiving alternate-day corticosteroid therapy and receiving methotrexate at a dosage of 0.4 mg/kg/week or less, azathioprine at a dosage of 3 mg/kg/day or less, or 6-mercaptopurine at a dosage of 1.5 mg/kg/day or less.

Household Vaccination

In an effort to protect the dialysis patients from infection, especially if live vaccines are contraindicated for the patient, every effort should be made to ensure that all household contacts are fully vaccinated per standard vaccine schedules.

Live Organ Donor Vaccination

If time permits, potential live organ donors (who may not be household members) should also be fully vaccinated per standard vaccine schedules.

Preparing for Transplantation in the Dialysis Patient

Achieving immunity to vaccine-preventable childhood infections before renal transplantation is critical. Ideally, all routine immunizations should be up to date before referral for transplant. Particular attention and priority should be given to the live-attenuated vaccines (MMR and varicella) that are generally not recommended after organ transplantation. If no immunization records are available, routine immunizations should be "caught up" according to the recommendations of the AAP and ACIP guidelines. Special considerations are noted in the sections that follow.

Live Vaccines

Of note, live vaccines are less effective if given after IVIG.

Varicella Vaccine

Administer a two-dose series of varicella vaccine at ages 12 through 15 months and 4 through 6 years. The second dose may be administered before age 4 years, provided at least 3 months have elapsed since the first dose. If the second dose was administered at least 4 weeks after the first dose, it can be accepted as valid. Immunity to varicella zoster virus (VZV) should be assessed in dialysis patients, and seronegative patients should be reimmunized before transplantation. VZV vaccine may be given as early as 9 months of age if early transplant is anticipated. It can be given simultaneously with MMR or at least 4 weeks later. It is generally recommended that transplant not occur for a minimum of 4 to 6 weeks after immunization with Varivax because of the live viruses it contains.

Measles, Mumps, Rubella Vaccine

Administer a two-dose series of MMR vaccine at ages 12 through 15 months and 4 through 6 years. The second dose may be administered before age 4 years, provided at least 4 weeks have elapsed since the first dose. Immunity to measles and rubella should be assessed before transplantation in dialysis patients. Immunity to mumps remains more challenging and potentially concerning in view of recent epidemics of mumps both in Europe and the United States but in general can be assumed to be present in the face of adequate responses to measles and rubella. Seronegative patients should be reimmunized before transplant. MMR is approved for use down to 6 months of age and could be given if early transplant is anticipated, but such patients should still receive the two-dose series when they are older than 1 year of age. Two catch-up doses may be given at least 1 month apart. In general, patients should not undergo transplantation for a minimum of 4 to 6 weeks after immunization with MMR due to the live viruses it contains.

Rotavirus

The live rotavirus vaccine series is recommended for all infants. The series must be initiated before 15 weeks of age and completed before 8 months of age. As a live vaccine, it is not recommended for immunocompromised patients. Because infant dialysis is uncommon, the need for rotavirus vaccination in dialysis patients is likely to be low and should be considered on a case by case basis.

Recombinant and Inactivated ("Killed") Vaccines

DTap, Tdap, and dT Vaccines

Children age 2 months to 7 years should be vaccinated according to the routine immunization schedule: Administer a 5-dose series of diphtheria, tetanus, pertussis (DTaP) vaccine at ages 2, 4, 6, 15 through 18 months, and 4 through 6 years. The fourth dose may be administered as early as age 12 months, provided at least 6 months have elapsed since the third dose. However, the fourth dose of DTaP need not be repeated if it was administered at least 4 months after the third dose of DTaP. The fifth dose of DTaP vaccine is not necessary if the fourth dose was administered at age 4 years or older. Patients should receive the tetanus, diphtheria, pertussis (Tdap) booster by age 11 to 12 years and then every 10 years thereafter. For the catch-up vaccination schedule and for information about the appropriate use of Tdap and Td in older patients, please see the Centers for Disease Control and Prevention (CDC) and ACIP recommendations.

Poliovirus Vaccine

A total of four doses of inactivated trivalent polio vaccine are recommended for all children: Administer a four-dose series of IPV at ages 2, 4, 6 through 18 months, and 4 through 6 years. The final dose in the series should be administered on or after the fourth birthday and at least 6 months after the previous dose. The first three doses can be given a month apart in children older than 6 years of age who have not received any vaccines. Oral polio vaccine is no longer recommended in the United States and should not be administered to children awaiting transplantation.

Haemophilus influenzae Type B Vaccine

Administer a two- or three-dose Hib vaccine primary series and a booster dose (dose three or four depending on vaccine used in primary series) at age 12 through 15 months to complete a full Hib vaccine series. One booster dose (dose three or four depending on vaccine used in primary series) of any Hib vaccine should be administered at age 12 through 15 months. The number of vaccinations required and the catch-up immunization schedule with Hib vaccine is influenced by the specific vaccine product used; please see the CDC and ACIP guidelines for more detail.

Pneumococcus Vaccine

Administer a four-dose series of PCV13 vaccine at ages 2, 4, and 6 months and at age 12 through 15 months. Dialysis patients are at higher risk of pneumococcal disease and should receive additional vaccination as summarized in Table 90.1, which outlines the recommendations for immunization against *Streptococcus pneumoniae*, the pneumococcal conjugate vaccines (PCV-7 and/or now PCV-13, Prevnar), and the 23-valent pneumococcal polysaccharide vaccine (23PS, Pneumovax).

Table 90.1

Recommendations for Pneumococcal Vaccination

Age	Previous Doses	Recommendations
<23 mo	None	• PCV7 at 2, 4, 6, 12–15 mo.
24–59 mo	4 doses of PCV7	• 23PS at 24 mo, 6–8 weeks after last dose of PCV7.
		• Booster: 23PS, 5 y after first dose of 23PS.
23–59 mo	1–3 doses of PCV7	• 1 dose of PCV7, followed 6–8 weeks later with one dose of 23PS.
		• Booster: 23PS 5 years after first dose of 23PS.
24–59 mo	1 dose of 23PS	• 2 doses of PCV7 (6–8 weeks apart) beginning 6–8 weeks after last 23PS.
		• Booster: 23PS 5 years after first dose of 23PS.
24–59 mo	None	• 2 doses of PCV7, 6–8 weeks apart.
		• 1 dose of 23PS, 6–8 weeks after last PCV7.
5–10 y	None	• One dose of PCV7 and one dose of 23PS 6–8 weeks apart.
>10 y	None	• 23PS only. Unless overly immunocompromised; then one dose PCV7 and one dose 23PS 6–8 weeks apart.

Hepatitis A Vaccine
Initiate the two-dose HepA vaccine series at 12 through 23 months; separate the two doses by 6 to 18 months. In those older than 2 years old not previous vaccinated, a total of two doses given 6 months apart is recommended.

Hepatitis B Vaccine
A three-dose series should be administered to all children beginning at birth and concluding by 6 months of age. Catch-up immunization should be initiated for all children as soon as possible because of the high risks associated with hepatitis B infection in patients receiving HD or posttransplant. Response to vaccination can be assessed by determining the antibody level at 1 to 2 months after the third dose, and if it is less than 10 mIU/mL, the patient can receive up to three more doses. Please see the earlier section that describes repeating the hepatitis B vaccine series.

Influenza Vaccine
Routine annual influenza vaccination is recommended for all children older than 6 months of age. All close contacts, including siblings, parents, caretakers, or other household members, should also be vaccinated. Trivalent inactivated influenza vaccine without preservatives (Fluzone, Sanofi Aventis) should be administered intramuscularly as early in the fall season as possible to children awaiting transplantation to offer protection against influenza. Two doses are required if the initial vaccination is occurring when the child is younger than 9 years of age.

Meningococcal Vaccine
One dose of meningococcal vaccine is recommended for all adolescents. With high-risk conditions (e.g., functional or anatomic asplenia, complement deficiency, HIV infection, eculizumab exposure), vaccination in infancy followed by boosters

every 5 years is recommended. Many new meningococcal vaccine formulations and subtypes have been approved recently, and the recommended age ranges have been revised. The CDC and ACIP recommendations should be reviewed for the most up-to-date guidelines.

Human Papillomavirus

Administer a three-dose series of HPV vaccine to all adolescents age 11 through 12 years. Either HPV4 or HPV2 may be used for girls, and only HPV4 may be used for boys. The vaccine is approved for use starting at age 9 years old. To maximize the efficacy of vaccination, consider vaccinating dialysis patients at age 9 years to increase the chance of completing the series before they are immunosuppressed for organ transplantation.

Updating Immunizations for Dialysis Patients Awaiting Transplant

The immunization status of patients on the transplant waiting list should be monitored and updated as appropriate. Hepatitis B antibody status should be assessed with annual antibody testing and vaccine readministered using either brand of commercially available vaccine (Recombivax HB or Energix) when antibody levels decline below 10 mIU/mL. Recommendations using Recombivax vaccine include a repeat dose 1 to 2 months after the third dose if the antibody levels decline below 10 mIU/mL.

Patients should receive the Tdap booster by age 11 to 16 years and then every 10 years. The influenza vaccine should be given annually once a year to both the patient and his or her family. For additional details about Tdap boosters, please see the CDC and ACIP recommendations.

Vaccine Response in the Dialysis Population: What Is the Evidence?

Because of multiple disturbances of host defenses, patients with CKD can demonstrate suboptimal vaccine responses. Defective host responses can result from the uremic state and protein losses in nephrotic syndrome, the underlying cause of ESRD and its therapy, or the dialysis itself. These factors have been demonstrated to impact virtually every aspect of the host immune system. Antibody responses to currently recommended immunizations in pediatric dialysis patients have been monitored, and the results are variable. In general, these studies identify two main issues in the dialysis population: suboptimal antibody response and waning immunity. In the setting of suboptimal antibody responses, repeat vaccinations with an increased dose can be considered. The issue of waning immunity demands rigorous follow-up of patients (with revaccination as indicated).

Diphtheria and tetanus antibody responses to vaccine have been studied by the Pediatric Peritoneal Dialysis Study Consortium in eight infants on peritoneal dialysis (PD). Seven of the eight infants had protective levels of IgG to both of the toxoids for up to 24 months postvaccination. A less than optimal response to the MMR vaccine was seen in 10 pediatric dialysis patients, with 8 of 10 responding to measles vaccine, 5 of 10 to mumps, and 8 of 10 to rubella. A study of infants immunized while on PD found that 5 of 8 children demonstrated protective antibody titers to rubella. One center demonstrated that a protocol of early MMR vaccination induced immunity in most infants with chronic renal failure and those on PD. Because of variable responsiveness to the various elements of the vaccine, it is recommended that antibody titers be verified previous to transplant.

The responsiveness to the conjugate Hib vaccine was studied in 10 children on PD, with 9 of 10 children younger than 42 months developing protective antibody levels. Serial measurements did reveal declining antibody levels in 2 subjects. Monitoring of antibody levels in high-risk infants and children should be considered.

An open-label multicenter prospective clinical trial to evaluate the safety and immunogenicity of a two-dose regimen of varicella vaccine was conducted by the Southwest Pediatric Nephrology Study Group in 96 children ages 1 to 19 years with chronic renal insufficiency on dialysis. Nearly all children (98%) seroconverted 1 to 2 months after the second dose of the two-dose regimen. At 1, 2, and 3 years' follow-up, all evaluable patients maintained VZV antibody, including 16 who received a transplant. No significant vaccine-associated adverse events were seen. This and other studies confirm that varicella immunization in children on dialysis results in a high rate of seroconversion and persistence of protective antibody titers. More widespread use of the vaccine before renal transplantation is recommended.

In the adult CKD population, the poor antibody responses to the hepatitis B vaccine led to the recommendation that these patients receive higher doses of the vaccine. The Southwest Pediatric Nephrology Group evaluated the responsiveness to the hepatitis B vaccine in 78 pediatric patients with CKD (22 predialysis, 42 chronic dialysis, and 14 transplant). Ninety-one percent of 66 patients who received three doses of the vaccine had a protective antibody titer of 10 mIU/mL or more. The seroprotective rates were 100% in the predialysis group, 94% in the dialysis group, and 64% in the transplant population. The conclusion of the study was that a regimen of three 20-mcg doses of Recombivax HB was suitably immunogenic for children not on immunosuppressive therapy. It is recommended that this vaccine be administered before the progression to ESRD if feasible.

The response to the trivalent inactivated influenza vaccine was studied in a group of pediatric patients with CKD (15 predialysis, 10 dialysis, and 17 renal transplant). There was no significant difference in the seroconversion rates and percentage of patients with protective hemagglutination-inhibition titers between study groups and control participants, suggesting that CKD patients benefit from influenza immunization.

Pneumococcal infection is an important cause of sepsis during childhood, and responses to the multivalent conjugate pneumococcal vaccine have been studied. The antibody response to pneumococcal serotypes 3 and 14 after administration of the pneumococcal polysaccharide vaccine was evaluated in 10 pediatric patients on PD. Evaluation of antibody responses at 1 month and 1 year postvaccination found that the majority of patients retained protective IgG levels. Seven of these 10 patients maintained protective levels at 5 years postvaccination.

Summary

Morbidity and mortality from vaccine-preventable illness are significant concerns in the pediatric dialysis population. However, children with ESRD are often under the care of numerous physicians at multiple sites where vaccinations are administered, and the vaccine history in these complex patients may be overlooked. Pediatric dialysis patients should receive routine childhood vaccinations on a timely schedule, and every effort should be made to complete the vaccination program before transplantation using an accelerated schedule if necessary.

Increased adherence to vaccine recommendations has been observed when the nephrologist assumes responsibility for the administration and surveillance of immunizations. In addition, ensuring that family members are up to date with their immunizations will help to maximize the preventive benefits of this intervention. Small studies in pediatric dialysis patients demonstrate vaccine responsiveness, but an important issue still not well studied is the duration of the immunity after vaccination in this patient population. Thus, it is important for practitioners to be diligent, measure titers when possible, and revaccinate to maintain the health of this vulnerable population.

CHAPTER 91

Prevention and Treatment of Cardiovascular Complications in Children Undergoing Dialysis

Mark M. Mitsnefes, MD, MS

Cardiovascular Mortality in Children on Maintenance Dialysis

In the general pediatric population, death due to cardiac disease is less than 3%. Yet data from the United States Renal Data System (USRDS) from the early 2000s indicate that in children with end-stage renal disease (ESRD), as in adults, mortality from cardiovascular disease (CVD) accounts for almost half of all causes of death and is approximately 10 to 20 times higher than in the general population. Reports from international registries have confirmed that CVD is the leading cause of death in children with ESRD and in adults with childhood onset of chronic kidney disease (CKD). The Australia and New Zealand Dialysis and Transplant (ANZDATA), the Dutch national cohort study (LERIC), and a large German study report that 40% to 50% of all deaths are from cardiovascular or cerebrovascular causes.

Recent USRDS analysis of more than 20,000 pediatric ESRD patients followed over 2 decades with follow-up to 2010 demonstrated that mortality rates for children and adolescents treated with dialysis improved between 1990 and 2010. Despite significant improvement in patient survival, mostly because of a decrease in cardiovascular and infectious disease mortality, CVD remains the worldwide largest obstacle to long-term survival of children and adolescents with CKD. Not surprisingly, the American Heart Association's guidelines for cardiovascular risk reduction in high-risk pediatric patients stratified pediatric CKD patients in the "highest risk" category for the development of CVD.

Of the specific causes of cardiovascular deaths, cardiac arrest is the most common followed by arrhythmia and cardiomyopathy. These causes are different from those of adults. In adults, coronary artery disease (CAD) and congestive heart failure from cardiomyopathy are two leading causes of mortality from CVD. The mortality from these causes is extremely low in children and adults younger than 30 years of age. The high rate of sudden death in children, especially in infants with ESRD, is poorly understood and warrants further investigation. The risk factors and pathogenic mechanisms leading to CVD in adults who had the onset of CKD in childhood are better understood than are those producing cardiac morbidity and mortality in children. This chapter focuses on prevention of the "classic" form of CVD as seen in adults who developed CKD in childhood.

Development of Cardiovascular Disease in Children With Chronic Kidney Disease

The conventional thinking is that two groups of risk factors are responsible for accelerated CVD in adults with CKD. First, compared with the nonuremic population, there is an overrepresentation in uremic patients of classical risk factors (e.g., diabetes, hypertension, and hyperlipidemia). A majority of the adults who develop ESRD do so as a complication of diabetes or generalized atherosclerosis. Often cardiac disease antedates the onset of CKD in these patients. Second, there are numerous uremia-related risk factors such as dyslipidemia, anemia, inflammation, infection, abnormal calcium phosphorus metabolism, and oxidative stress that may singly or in concert trigger the development of CVD. Many of the same risk factors are present in high frequency in children on dialysis, making them extremely susceptible to CVD.

Two parallel processes are involved in the development of CVD in children with CKD. The first is cardiomyopathy. It is initially manifest by disorders of the left ventricle (LV), which lead to adoptive LV remodeling. Two types of LV remodeling are recognized. Concentric LV hypertrophy (LVH) results primarily from pressure overload as occurs with hypertension. Eccentric LVH has been related primarily to volume overload as frequently seen in patients on dialysis or with anemia. It is likely that the effects of hemodynamic overload on the LV are augmented by other nonhemodynamic LVH-generating causes such as high levels of fibroblast growth factor 23 (FGF23), sympathetic hyperactivity, systemic inflammation, and local production of angiotensin II. With time, a maladaptive phase of LVH develops characterized by decreased capillary density, decreased coronary reserve and subendocardial perfusion, a tendency to arrhythmia, and the development of myocardial fibrosis. All of this leads to myocyte death and, finally, to diastolic and systolic dysfunction. Symptomatic cardiomyopathy is very rare in children, but early abnormalities of cardiac structure and function can be seen frequently. LVH develops when CKD is mild or moderate in children and progresses as renal function deteriorates. LVH is very common (52%–75%) during long-term dialysis. Both concentric and eccentric geometric patterns of LVH are present in these patients, suggesting that, as in adults with ESRD, the mechanism of LVH in advanced CKD in children is volume and pressure overload. LVH is prevalent in both children on hemodialysis (HD) and peritoneal dialysis (PD). Small retrospective studies suggest that with good blood pressure (BP) control, LVH will regress in young patients on dialysis. In contrast to adults, in whom systolic dysfunction is frequently associated with early cardiac failure and decreased survival, systolic LV function is usually preserved in children. On the other hand, these children may develop LV diastolic dysfunction, often the initial manifestation of abnormal of cardiac function.

The second process involves accelerated vascular injury which manifests by arterial hypertrophy and stiffness. This leads to arterio- and atherosclerosis. Children on dialysis have a high prevalence of asymptomatic vascular disease as demonstrated by abnormal carotid intima-medial thickness (IMT), diminished arterial wall compliance, and coronary artery calcification. This eventually leads to symptomatic (ischemic) CAD in young adults with childhood onset of ESRD. In ESRD patients, a variety of factors have been associated with the development of atherosclerosis. Many of these factors are similar to those involved in the development of cardiac hypertrophy and include hypertension, dyslipidemia, abnormal calcium–phosphorus metabolism, chronic inflammation, and others.

Evaluation and Treatment Recommendations

The overall strategy in prevention of cardiovascular complications in children with advanced CKD is avoidance of long-term dialysis. The goal is to prevent development and delay the progression of cardiomyopathy and atherosclerosis. Even though kidney transplantation poses continuous cardiovascular risk (hypertension, hyperlipidemia, allograft dysfunction), it eliminates many uremia-related risks, reduces risk of cardiac death by approximately 80%, and prolongs life span by 20 to 30 years. A recent study showed that graft failure after a first kidney transplant was associated with almost a five times higher mortality rate compared with children with a functioning graft. Having maintenance dialysis even for a few months before transplant was also associated with a worse survival in this study. Thus, preemptive kidney transplantation should be the ultimate goal to minimize cardiovascular morbidity and mortality. For patients who must have long-term dialysis, the strategy is directly linked to achievement of adequate dialysis outcomes, which include aggressive monitoring and management of hypertension, dyslipidemia, calcium–phosphorus metabolism, anemia, nutrition, systemic inflammation, and other dialysis complications.

Echocardiographic Evaluation

Kidney Disease Outcomes Quality Initiative (KDOQI) Clinical Practice Guidelines for Cardiovascular Disease in Dialysis Patients recommend that children have echocardiographic evaluation for the presence of cardiac disease (cardiomyopathy and valvular disease) at the time of initiation of dialysis therapy. As already discussed, the most common cardiac diagnosis in children on chronic dialysis is hypertrophic cardiomyopathy or LVH. There is no uniform definition of LVH in children, which makes it difficult to establish specific targets for left ventricle mass (LVM). The most commonly used definition of LVH is based on the 95th percentile of LVM indexed to height raised to the power of 2.7 ($g/m^{2.7}$). If LVH is diagnosed at time of initiation of dialysis, routine echocardiographic monitoring every 6 months is advisable. If the initial echocardiogram is normal, yearly echocardiographic follow-up is suggested. Echocardiography is also important to monitor cardiac function. Shortening fraction, index of systolic function, is routinely calculated from echocardiographic parameters. Systolic dysfunction is rare in children on dialysis, but if discovered, the patient should be evaluated by a cardiologist.

Hypertension

The target BP in children with CKD should be less than the 90th percentile adjusted for age, gender, and height or less than 120/80 mm Hg, whichever is lower. About three quarters of children entering maintenance dialysis therapy have a BP above the 95th percentile or uncontrolled hypertension, and, in almost all, the BP is above the target level of the 90th percentile. It is especially troubling that hypertension is unlikely to improve during long-term dialysis. Hypertension is frequent with both

HD and PD but is reported to be more frequent in hemodialyzed children. Poor BP control in children on maintenance dialysis is multifactorial, but the major cause is fluid overload. Thus, the first step in the diagnosis and management of hypertension should be evaluation of volume status. Unfortunately, many children on dialysis do not achieve their dry weight. Volume status assessment in young patients is frequently not accurate. This is one of the reasons that the frequency of hypertension is higher in young children. In addition, correct assessment of BP is difficult in small children; consequently, it is frequently underdiagnosed and therefore not adequately treated.

Another group of children that presents with significant fluid overload and therefore with hypertension is adolescents, who are almost always noncompliant with fluid and salt restriction. Chronic fluid overload with secondary hypertension is the major cause of high prevalence of LVH in children on chronic dialysis. Thus, aggressive management of fluid overload and achievement of dry weight is the most effective treatment of hypertension and LVH in children on chronic dialysis. For children on HD, longer and more frequent dialysis sessions and sometimes even intermittent ultrafiltration might be needed to improve volume status.

In most children, the achievement of dry weight results in normalization of BP and a significant decrease in the use of antihypertensive medications. If BP remains elevated despite adequate volume control, antihypertensive medications should be optimized. Angiotensin-converting enzyme inhibitors or angiotensin II receptor blockers should be considered as a first line of therapy in children on dialysis because of their renal and cardioprotective effects. Addition of calcium channel blockers or beta-blockers should be tried next. It is important to remember that if effective dry weight is not achieved, antihypertensive medications, especially vasodilators and beta-blockers, will likely not be effective and may further impair the ability to remove fluid. If BP is still inadequately controlled after achieving dry weight and maximizing the use of BP medications, bilateral nephrectomy should be strongly considered.

Achievement of normal daytime office BP measurement does not necessarily predict the absence of hypertension. Patients with CKD frequently have undetected nighttime hypertension. Children who have normal BP measurements in the dialysis unit might benefit from ambulatory BP monitoring to assess the presence of nighttime hypertension.

Dyslipidemia

Dyslipidemia is very prevalent in children on chronic dialysis and is characterized by low high-density lipoprotein (HDL) and high triglyceride levels. Many children also have increased total cholesterol and low-density lipoprotein (LDL). Kidney Disease: Improving Global Outcomes (KDIGO) recommends evaluation of dyslipidemias in adolescents upon presentation with CKD stage 5 (glomerular filtration rate <15 mL/min/1.73 m^2 or on dialysis), at 2 to 3 months after a change in treatment or other conditions known to cause dyslipidemias, and at least annually thereafter. Reasons to repeat lipid measurements after 2 to 3 months of stage 5 CKD include changes in kidney replacement therapy modality, treatment with diet or lipid-lowering agents, immunosuppressive agents that affect lipids (e.g., prednisone, cyclosporine, or sirolimus), and other changes that may affect plasma lipid levels. The assessment of dyslipidemias should include a complete fasting lipid profile with total cholesterol, LDL, HDL, and triglycerides. The definition of dyslipidemia differs in children and adults. Hyperlipidemia in children is defined as lipid levels greater than the 95th percentile for age and gender. The normative data for lipids in children and adolescents currently used are from Lipid Research Clinics Program from the National Institutes of Health published in 1980 and can be found in most recent KDIGO guidelines for management of dyslipidemias in CKD.

For adolescents with stage 5 CKD and a level of LDL of 130 mg/dL or more, KDOQI recommends treatment to reduce LDL to less than 130 mg/dL. If LDL is less than 130 mg/dL, fasting triglycerides are 200 mg/dL or more, and non-HDL cholesterol (total cholesterol minus HDL) is 160 mg/dL or more, treatment should be considered to reduce non-HDL cholesterol to less than 160 mg/dL. All children with dyslipidemias should follow the recommendations for therapeutic lifestyle changes (TLC), which include diet modification with reduction in saturated fat intake and increase in fiber intake and moderate physical activity. Adolescents should be counseled about avoiding smoking. Unfortunately, noncompliance with TLC is one of the major problems in the management of dyslipidemia in adolescents. Pediatric nephrologists must also recognize that appropriate caloric intake, including calories from fat, should be emphasized to avoid malnutrition and ensure normal growth and development, especially in young children.

If LDL cholesterol is 160 mg/dL or more and non-HDL cholesterol is 190 mg/dL or more, statin therapy is recommended in children older than age 10 years. The age limitation is based on the concern that starting a statin at younger age might interfere with sexual maturation because steroid hormones are all derived from cholesterol. Published reports over the past 5 years, mostly concerning children with familial hypercholesterolemia, indicate that statins are safe and can be used in children as young as 8 years of age with no impact on sexual development. However, these studies do not provide long-term safety data. The concern for delayed puberty is one of the reasons that the criteria for statin therapy initiation is different from recommendations in adults in whom statin therapy is initiated at lower levels of LDL cholesterol and non-HDL cholesterol. Although it is prudent to be cautious, the decision to start drug therapy should be guided by the child's overall cardiovascular risk profile. As discussed earlier, children with CKD, especially those on chronic dialysis, are extremely susceptible to develop accelerated atherosclerosis and premature CAD. Because of this risk, the potential benefit from statin therapy might be more important than the risk of delayed puberty. Thus, initiation of statin therapy at lower than currently recommended cholesterol levels might be warranted.

Abnormal Calcium–Phosphorus Metabolism

The Working Group on Cardiovascular Disease in Dialysis Patients recommends maintaining calcium (Ca) and phosphorus (P) levels within the normal range and the Ca $\times$ P product below 55 mg^2/dL^2 in children on chronic dialysis. These recommendations are based on adult studies, demonstrating that hyperphosphatemia and increased Ca $\times$ P product are strongly correlated with cardiac calcification and increased cardiac morbidity and mortality. The majority of children on chronic dialysis are hyperphosphatemic and, as a result, require phosphate-binding therapy. Studies of children and young adults on chronic dialysis determined that the cumulative dose calcium-based phosphate binders and the administration of active vitamin D preparations are strong determinants of arterial stiffness, coronary artery calcification, and metastatic calcinosis. This may represent risk factors for CVD that are, perhaps, even more important than hypertension and dyslipidemia. Therefore, use of non–calcium-based phosphate binders, careful monitoring of serum calcium level, and appropriate adjustment of the dose of vitamin D to avoid hypercalcemia are essential in the management of children on dialysis to prevent development and progression of cardiovascular abnormalities.

Anemia

Studies in adult dialysis patients have identified anemia as a risk factor for patient morbidity and mortality. The studies from the North American Pediatric Renal Transplant Cooperative Study (NAPRTCS) indicate that anemia is very common and is frequently undertreated in children on chronic dialysis. The NAPRTCS data also showed that anemia is present in more than half of children entering maintenance dialysis and is associated with a 52% higher risk of death in chronically dialyzed children. A few small single-center pediatric studies determined that anemic children more frequently have LVH than those with normal hemoglobin and that treatment of severe anemia with erythropoietin results in a significant reduction of LVM index. Recent analysis from Pediatric Peritoneal Dialysis Network (IPPN) indicated that anemia remains a significant problem despite almost universal use of erythropoiesis-stimulating agents (ESAs). In their analysis, ESA resistance was associated with inflammation, fluid retention, and hyperparathyroidism. Importantly, anemia and high ESA dose requirements independently predicted mortality.

The hemoglobin level of 11.0 g/dL represents the value below the 5th percentile for boys younger than 5 years; 11.5 g/dL for boys 6 to 8 years; 12.0 to 12.5 g/dL for boys 9 to 14 years; and 13.5 for boys 15 to 19 years. For girls of all ages, the lower limits of normal values are 11 to 12 g/dL. Current KDOQI guidelines for treatment of anemia recommend keeping the hemoglobin level above 11 g/dL by using an appropriate iron therapy and recombinant erythropoietin. In the opinion of the Working Group, there is insufficient evidence to recommend routinely maintaining hemoglobin levels above 13 g/dL. These target levels are about 2 g/dL less than the mean hemoglobin values for children in each age category. They are based on adult data showing that higher hemoglobin levels in hemodialyzed patients with heart disease were associated with increased rate of nonfatal myocardial infarction (MI). Because symptomatic CVD including MI is extremely rare in children, the results from these adult studies and therefore current hemoglobin targets might not be applicable to pediatric patients. Unfortunately, for recombinant erythropoietin therapy reimbursement in children with CKD, Medicare and insurance companies follow current KDIGO guidelines to keep the upper limit of hematocrit level at 36%. These guidelines apply even to children who are not yet on dialysis, possibly putting them at risk for CVD before initiation of chronic dialysis therapy.

Malnutrition and Inflammation

Adequate nutrition is an essential part of dialysis care. Malnutrition is frequent in children on chronic dialysis, especially in young patients and those who require long-term dialysis. Failure to thrive and hypoalbuminemia are significant risks of death in pediatric patients with ESRD. Recent studies in adults on chronic HD place the malnutrition–inflammation complex at the center of a debate about the role of traditional and nontraditional risk factors for poor cardiovascular outcome. This issue emerged after publication of a series of articles describing the phenomenon of "reverse epidemiology." The studies have shown that in adults on chronic HD, low BP, low body mass index (BMI), and low serum cholesterol are often correlated with an unfavorable clinical outcome. Thus, whereas traditional risk factors of CVD are correlated with an unfavorable outcome in the general population and patients with CKD not yet on dialysis, in hemodialyzed patients, mild hypertension, hypercholesterolemia, and overweight appear to be protective and associated with an improved survival. It has been speculated that malnutrition–inflammation–atherosclerosis complex underlies, at least partly, the phenomenon of reverse epidemiology because malnutrition causes a low BMI and hypocholesterolemia. Whether these results could be applied to pediatric patients is not clear at this time. However, they suggest that more emphasis should be placed on the assessment and management of nontraditional cardiovascular risks in dialyzed children.

Dialysis Adequacy

One of the important reasons that children on dialysis still have very high rates of traditional and CKD-related risk factors and related cardiovascular abnormalities is how we approach dialysis adequacy numbers. Unfortunately, achieving recommended Kt/V_{urea} does not necessary lead to control of the above problems. Data from the Centers for Medicare & Medicaid Services End-Stage Renal Disease Clinical Performance Measures (CPM) Project indicate that 89% of patients receiving HD and 87% of patients receiving PD achieved the recommended modality-specific Kt/V. Yet one third of children had uncontrolled anemia, and almost half had low serum albumin. Using the same database, another study showed that two thirds of HD patients had uncontrolled hypertension and an elevated $Ca \times P$ product. These studies, as well as epidemiologic data on cardiac death in both PD and HD, clearly indicate that current dialysis adequacy recommendations based on Kt/V_{urea} are not adequate to decrease CVD morbidity in children with ESRD. Unlike in adults, there have been no randomized pediatric studies examining the role of more frequent or nocturnal HD on cardiac outcomes. However, small single-center studies of frequent or nocturnal dialysis indicate clinically important improvement in children' health, including growth, hypertension, cardiac hypertrophy, and function. Taking the potential for a longer and possibly more productive life, the benefits of more frequent and longer dialysis treatment might be much more far reaching in children than in older adults.

C H A P T E R   9 2

Surgery in Children With End-Stage Renal Disease

Michael L. Moritz, MD • Ron Shapiro, MD

Children with end-stage renal disease (ESRD) on dialysis provide unique challenges regarding surgical management. In addition to the standard perioperative issues encountered in an adult dialysis patient or in an otherwise healthy child, children on dialysis have many unique issues related to their underlying disease that resulted in ESRD. Dialysis is relatively uncommon in children, with only about 1000 children in the United States on dialysis compared with more than 400,000 adults. Whereas the major cause of ESRD in adults is diabetes and hypertension, these diagnoses are not major causes of ESRD in children. The causes of ESRD in children are numerous and heterogeneous, with the majority of cases being caused by congenital anomalies of the kidney and urinary tract (CAKUTs), cystic kidney diseases, and primary and secondary glomerulonephritis and nephrosis. These underlying diseases can have a variety of systemic manifestations and multiorgan system involvement, which need to be taken into consideration in preoperative planning. In addition, ESRD is a systemic disease in children, resulting in a number of problems, such as growth retardation, developmental delay, electrolyte disturbances, metabolic bone disease, anemia, cardiovascular disease, and immunologic dysfunction, all of which can complicate surgical management. The types of surgical procedures frequently encountered in children on dialysis can be quite different from those in an otherwise healthy child and include a variety of potential urologic procedures, gastrostomy tube placement, dialysis access procedures, native nephrectomies in preparation for transplantation, renal transplantation, and allograft nephrectomy. Dialysis patients also have special considerations related to anesthesia and pain control. The special surgical considerations as they apply to children on dialysis are discussed in this chapter.

Preoperative Surgical Evaluation

An integral part of the preoperative surgical evaluation is to ascertain the underlying cause of the ESRD and to assess if it is associated with extrarenal complications that may have an impact on the surgery (Table 92.1). Frequent causes of ESRD in children are congenital anomalies of the kidney and urinary tract. These conditions can be syndromic occurring as a part of VATER (vertebral anomalies, anal atresia, cardiac defects, tracheoesophageal fistula or esophageal atresia, renal and radial anomalies, and limb defects) syndrome, CHARGE (coloboma of the eye, heart defects, atresia of the nasal choanae, retardation of growth or development, genital or urinary abnormalities, and ear abnormalities and deafness) syndrome, prune belly syndrome, and trisomies. These conditions are frequently associated with congenital heart disease, gastrointestinal obstructions, and airway problems. Patients with

Table 92.1

Renal Diseases Associated With Serious Extrarenal Complications in Children on Dialysis

Renal Disease	Extrarenal Complication
Obsructive Uropathy	
Posterior urethral valves	Pulmonary hypoplasia
Sina bifida	Paralysis, scoliosis, hydrocephalus, seizures, fecal incontinence
Prune belly syndrome	Abdominal muscle deficiency, bilateral cryptorchidism, hypoplastic or dysplastic prostate, malrotation, anorectal malformations
Cystic Kidney Disease	
Autosomal recessive polcystic kidney disease	Congenital hepatic fibrosis, portal hypertension, pulmonary hypoplasia
Autoimmune Diseases	
Systemic lupus erythematosus	Mucocutaneous, musculoskeletal, hematologic, neurologic, pulmonary, cardiac, gastrointenstinal involvement
Granulomatosis with polyangitis/ microscopic polyangitis	Mucocutaneous, upper and lower airway involvement
Inherited Nehropathies	
Alport's syndrome	Sensorineural hearing loss, ocular manifestations, leiomyomatosis, arterial aneurysms
Nephronophthisis	Retinitis pigmentosa, hepatic fibrosis, situs inversus
Cystinosis	Ocular, hepatic, thyroid, pancreatic, muscular, neurologic, and gonadal involvement
Denys-Drash syndrome	Wilms tumor, male pseudohermaphroditism
Multiple Congenital Anomaly Syndromes	
VATER association	Verterbral defects, imperforate anus, tracheoesophageal fistula, cardiac defects, limb anomalies
CHARGE association	Coloboma, cardiac defects, choanal atresia, genital anomalies, ear anomalies
Brachio-oto-renal syndrome	Branchial sinus, preauricular pit or tags, microtia or anotia, hearing loss
Other	
Mitochondrial disorders	Myopathy, seizures, neuropathy, ataxia, retinitis pigmentosis, ophthalmoplegia, lactic acidosis, strokelike episodes, pancreatic insufficiency, cytopenia, hepatic dysfunction, cardiac conduction abnormalities, cardiomyopathy, diabetes mellitus
Oxalosis	Oxalate deposition in heart, blood vessels, joints, bone, retina

severe obstructive uropathy or renal failure at birth may have had oligohydramnios and have a component of pulmonary hypoplasia. Even if there is no readily apparent lung disease at the time of surgery, it can manifest postoperatively with difficulties during extubation and coming off ventilatory support. Many of these children may have been on extracorporeal membrane oxygenation (ECMO) and now have limited vascular access because of previous ECMO cannulas. An important cause of obstructive uropathy in children is spina bifida. These children frequently have ventriculo-peritoneal shunts, seizure disorders, bladder augmentation surgeries, or bladders that are colonized with bacteria. These are important considerations when considering peritoneal dialysis (PD) and renal transplantation. An important cause of ESRD in children is autosomal recessive polycystic kidney disease, which can be associated with congenital hepatic fibrosis, portal hypertension with esophageal varices, and splenic sequestration. An increasingly common cause of ESRD in children is ischemic events from perinatal complications in neonates. These children frequently have cerebral palsy, a history of chronic lung disease, and previous bowel surgery related to necrotizing enterocolitis.

The most important causes of ESRD in adolescents are primary or secondary glomerulonephritis and nephrosis. These children may have been on long-term immunosuppression with steroids or continue to require steroids for a secondary vasculitis and could be at risk for adrenal insufficiency and require perioperative stress dose steroids. Some children with nephrosis may still be nephrotic, spilling large amounts of protein in the urine. All of these conditions have surgical implications and may influence the modality of dialysis and vascular access placement chosen. The causes of ESRD with systemic manifestations in children are too numerous to discuss individually, and many are quite rare, such as oxalosis, atypical hemolytic uremic syndrome, cystinosis, and mitochondrial disorders, but they can have an impact on the perioperative management and need to be taken into consideration (see Table 92.1).

Perioperative Management

Fluid Therapy

Unlike adults on dialysis, children on dialysis may have significant residual renal function and native kidney urine output (Table 92.2). This needs to be taken into consideration when choosing both the composition and quantity of perioperative maintenance intravenous fluids (IVFs). The quantity of residual urine output should

---

Table 92.2

Renal Diseases Associated With Significant Residual Urine Output in Dialysis Patients

Obstructive uropathy
Renal dysplasia
Reflux nephropathy
Cystic kidney diseases
Nephronophthisis
Cystinosis

be assessed on any child on dialysis undergoing surgery. Obstructive uropathy and renal dysplasia are the most common conditions associated with significant residual urine output. These children frequently have an acquired nephrogenic diabetes insipidus and can make large volumes of urine. The volume status of children should be assessed before starting IVFs. Children with oligo-anuric renal failure with signs of fluid overload before surgery should probably be dialyzed before surgery. Those who are not fluid overloaded are probably better off not receiving any IVFs preoperatively unless there is a prolonged period of NPO. If fluids are given, they should be restricted to a rate of approximately 400 mL/m^2/24 hour or 25% of the rate calculated by the Holiday-Segar formula, which is approximately equal to insensible losses. It is safest to give the fluids as 0.9% sodium chloride with dextrose. Patients with ESRD by definition have impaired free water excretion and are at risk for developing hyponatremia. Hypotonic fluids should be avoided because of the potential for developing hyponatremia. Potassium should not be added to the IVFs because of the potential for developing hyperkalemia. Patients with significant residual urine output need a higher IVF rate. Unless they are hypernatremic, with a sodium above 145 mEq/L, hypotonic fluid should probably be avoided. Electrolytes should be closely monitored. The optimal intraoperative fluid is matter of debate. There is concern that using a large amount of 0.9% NaCl intraoperatively may result in a dilutional acidosis with an accompanying hyperkalemia. Some data suggest that using a balanced electrolyte solution such as lactated Ringer's solution or Plasmalyte-148 may result in less acidosis and hyperkalemia even though these fluids have physiologic concentrations of potassium. Insufficient data exist to make a definitive recommendation, but Plasmalyte-148 may be the preferred intraoperative fluid because it has 50 mEq/L of alkali with 5 mEq/L of potassium and is devoid of calcium, so it will not interfere with blood products. Close attention should be given to the volume of intraoperative fluids to avoid fluid overload and its associated complications of hypertension, pulmonary congestion, and heart failure. It is easier to give additional fluids in the postoperative period if necessary rather than to do emergent postoperative dialysis for fluid overload.

Electrolyte Management

Electrolyte abnormalities are frequently encountered in children on dialysis. The major electrolyte complications are hyperkalemia, acidosis, hyperphosphatemia, and hypocalcemia. The best way to prevent these complications is to ensure that the patient is properly dialyzed in reasonable proximity to the surgical procedure, ideally within 24 hours. Preoperative chemistries should be drawn on the day of surgery to ensure that there are no serious electrolyte abnormalities going into surgery and that there is adequate time to respond to and treat the electrolyte abnormality. The most serious electrolyte abnormality is hyperkalemia. Children on dialysis are notoriously difficult to draw blood on through a peripheral vein, and an elevated potassium in a properly dialyzed child may be an artifact of a hemolyzed specimen. A suspected hemolyzed specimen should be repeated with a whole-blood potassium from a free-flowing vein sent to the blood gas laboratory or as an iStat. These values come back within minutes and are less likely to be hemolyzed. A truly hyperkalemic patient should be placed on a cardiac monitor, set to lead two, looking for electrocardiographic (ECG) changes of hyperkalemia. Electrocardiographic changes of hyperkalemia include "peaked" T waves and a shortened QT interval progressing to lengthening of the PR interval and loss of P waves and then to widening of the QRS complex, culminating in a "sine wave" morphology and death if not treated. Hemodialysis (HD) is the definitive treatment for hyperkalemia with ECG changes. Because there can be a delay in instituting HD or starting PD, temporizing measures may be needed. If severe ECG changes are present, calcium should be administered to stabilize the myocardium and reverse cardiac conduction abnormalities. The acute management of hyperkalemia involves shifting potassium intracellularly. The administration of insulin and glucose or a β_2-adrenergic agent such as albuterol are acceptable first-line therapies because both agents can lower the serum potassium by 0.6 to 1 mEq/L within 30 minutes and have an additive affect when given together. Hypertonic sodium bicarbonate is not recommended in the treatment of acute hyperkalemia in dialysis patients. It has not only been shown to be ineffective, but it may actually result in an increase in serum potassium and could aggravate hypocalcemia, fluid overload, and hypertension. The potassium exchange resin sodium polystyrene (Kayexalate) has a limited role in the management of postoperative hyperkalemia in dialysis patients. The onset of action is 2 to 3 hours as a retention enema and 6 hours via gastric administration. It also runs the risk of serious intestinal complications in postoperative patients with an ileus, although sorbitol-free preparations may reduce the risk substantially. Newer exchange resins are currently in clinic trials and may have a role.

Hypertension

Hypertension, defined as systolic blood pressure (SBP) or diastolic blood pressure (DBP) greater than the 95th percentile for gender, age, and height on repeated measurement, is common in children on dialysis. The etiology of hypertension is multifactorial and is related to fluid and sodium overload, renal disease, and medications, including exogenous erythropoietin. The most serious complication of hypertension is symptomatic hypertension in which there is an acute elevation in the SBP accompanied by neurologic symptoms such headache, blurred vision, coma, seizures, or cardiopulmonary symptoms such as congestive heart failure and pulmonary edema. This complication is best avoided by appropriate perioperative management. Numerous measures should be taken to avoid the development of perioperative hypertension: Blood pressure (BP) should be under control with medication before elective surgery, antihypertensive medications should not be held in the perioperative period, patients should be appropriately dialyzed before and after surgery, excess IVFs should be avoided, hypertonic sodium bicarbonate should be avoided, blood products should be used sparingly, nonsteroidal antiinflammatory drugs (NSAIDs) should be avoided, and attention should be paid to adequate pain control.

Children on dialysis frequently have chronic hypertension, and significantly elevated BPs can be well tolerated without apparent neurologic symptoms. If the hypertension is acute or severely elevated to well above the 99th percentile systolic, symptoms may develop. Before acute pharmacologic management is instituted, the BPs should be repeated using a properly sized BP cuff in the upper extremity and pain control and agitation or anxiety should be addressed. If an elevated BP persists, the patient should be evaluated for signs of extracellular fluid overload. Effective short-acting antihypertensive medications that can be given in the recovery room or in a nonacute care (non–intensive care unit [ICU]) setting without an arterial line are the intravenous agents hydralazine and labetalol and the oral agents isradipine and clonidine. The patient's chronic oral antihypertensive medications should be resumed as soon as possible, and consideration should be given to dialyzing the patient. Consideration should be given to transferring patients with refractory hypertension to the ICU for close monitoring and the use of a continuous intravenous antihypertensive medication such as nicardipine or labetalol.

Infectious Complications

Children on dialysis may be at increased risk for perioperative infections, and consideration should be given to administering appropriate perioperative antibiotics to prevent peritonitis, a tunneled dialysis catheter infection, and surgical site infections. There are no published guidelines for the need for antibiotic prophylaxis in dialysis patients, but consideration should be given on a case-by-case basis depending on the surgical procedure and the patient's risk factors. Antibiotic prophylaxis should be given for all patients undergoing a PD catheter placement. Strong consideration should be given for prophylactic antibiotics in PD patients undergoing endoscopy or colonoscopy and gastrointestinal or urologic surgical procedures. The peritoneum should be drained in PD patients undergoing surgery, and children with obstructive uropathy should have a Foley catheter placed. HD patients with a tunneled dialysis catheter or vascular graft should probably receive antibiotic prophylaxis for dental procedures. Dialysis patients on immunosuppressive medications may also benefit from prophylactic antibiotics.

Bleeding Complications

Children with ESRD on dialysis are at risk for both thrombotic complications, because ESRD is a hypercoagulable state, and bleeding complications related to platelet dysfunction. The major risk of bleeding though comes from the use of unfractionated heparin for systemic anticoagulation during HD and from high concentration heparin solutions to lock HD catheters to maintain catheter patency. Heparin has a half-life of 0.5 to 2 hours in dialysis patients, so they can be expected to be anticoagulated for 4 to 6 hours after dialysis. If a patient requires HD in close proximity to a surgical procedure, systemic anticoagulation should be avoided altogether, or the lowest dose of heparin possible should be used.

Children on HD are also at risk for postoperative bleeding complications from inadvertent anticoagulation from high-concentration heparin flush lock solutions of 5000 to 10,000 units/mL. Heparin can either leach from side holes of the catheter or be inadvertently administered when accessing and flushing the catheter. Flushing catheters with high-concentration heparin solutions should be avoided in the perioperative period. If there is the possibility that an HD catheter may need to be used intraoperatively for vascular access, it should either be flushed with 100 units/L heparin, or small volumes of normal saline can be run to maintain catheter patency after careful removal of the heparin from the catheter. A child on HD with postoperative bleeding should have the activated partial thromboplastin time checked to evaluate for inadvertent anticoagulation.

Anemia

Anemia is a frequent complication of children on dialysis. The etiology of anemia is multifactorial, including: renal disease, iron deficiency, frequent blood draws, hemolysis, blood loss associated with HD, and decreased red blood cell (RBC) survival.

Special attention should be paid to correcting anemia with erythropoietin-stimulating agents and iron before surgery to avoid blood transfusions. Perioperative blood transfusions are best avoided in the child on dialysis because blood transfusion can lead to hyperkalemia; volume overload; citrate toxicity with metabolic alkalosis and hypocalcemia; and most important, human leukocyte antigen (HLA) sensitization. United States Renal Data Systems (USRDS) data suggest that the risk of sensitization is substantial for patients receiving blood transfusions. There are no data to suggest that the use of leukocyte-reduced blood products decreases the likelihood of sensitization in potential future kidney transplant candidates (although it would seem to be beneficial because filtered packed RBCs have had 99% of the white blood cells removed, better than washed RBCs, which have 90% of the white cells removed). For these reasons, KDIGO guidelines reserve the use of blood transfusion for urgent treatment of anemia when rapid correction is required to a stabilize the patient's condition because of acute hemorrhage or when rapid preoperative hemoglobin correction is required. Blood transfusions should be based on a case-by-case basis, weighing the risks and benefits and not an arbitrary hemoglobin value.

Pain Control

Postoperative pain management is challenging in children on dialysis because renal insufficiency affects the pharmacokinetic properties of most pain medications, altering the clearance, excretion, and volume of distribution. The magnitude of the effect of renal insufficiency on drug metabolism and whether it is cleared by peritoneal or HD varies depending on the agent. A modified World Health Organization (WHO) ladder has been suggested to treat pain in patients with ESRD and has been demonstrated to achieve adequate pain control in 96% of patients (Fig. 92.1). The nonopioid acetaminophen is the safest agent to treat pain in children on dialysis. The terminal half-life of the metabolites is prolonged in patients with renal failure, so the dosing interval should be increased to 6 to 8 hours. In addition, acetaminophen is dialyzable with HD, so supplemental dosing may be needed. NSAIDs should be used with caution in patients on dialysis with residual renal function or renin-mediated hypertension in order to preserve residual renal function and not aggravate hypertension. If preservation of renal function is not a concern, ibuprofen is the preferred NSAID because it is metabolized in the liver, and its active metabolites do not accumulate in renal failure. Ketorolac should be avoided in patients with renal insufficiency because its active metabolites accumulate and do not appear to be dialyzable. Lidocaine and fentanyl patches along with Voltaren cream may be useful adjuvants for localized pain. Opioid use requires great care when administered to children on dialysis because not all are safe in renal failure. Renal failure affects both the dose and interval of administration of opioids, so lower than recommended doses should be used and titrated up slowly with an extended dosing interval. Table 92.3 outlines the preferred medications to be used in dialysis patients. The preferred opioids are hydromorphone, fentanyl, and methadone. Opioids to be avoided are morphine, codeine, meperidine, and propoxyphene because their metabolites are neurotoxic, renally excreted, and accumulate in renal failure.

Surgical Considerations

There are a variety of surgical procedures that are relatively common in children on dialysis that are unrelated to placement of access for dialysis and renal

Step 3, Severe Pain (7-10)

Hydromorphone
Methadone
Fentanyl
Oxycodone
± *Nonopioid analgesics*
± *Adjuvants*

Step 2, Moderate Pain (5-6)

Hydrocodone
Oxycodone
Tramadol
± *Nonopioid analgesics*
± *Adjuvants*

Step 1, Mild Pain (1-4)

Acetaminophen (Acet)
± *Adjuvants*

"Adjuvants" refers either to medication that are coadministered to manage an adverse effect of an opioid, or to so-called adjuvant analgesics that are added to enhance analgesia such as steroids for pain from bone metastases. Adjuvants also includes medicationn such as anticonvulsants for neuropathic pain.

Figure 92.1

The World Health Organization's three-step analgesic ladder modified to exclude drugs unsafe in renal failure. (From Baraksoy AS, Moss AH. *J Am Soc Nephrol* 2006;17:3198-3203.)

transplantation (Table 92.4). When performing these surgeries, consideration must be given to how they will interfere with ongoing dialysis or with future dialysis and transplantation. This is particularly so as it relates to PD. Any intraperitoneal surgery has the potential for causing adhesions and may interfere with future PD. Intraabdominal surgeries will also interfere with ongoing PD and pose a risk for peritonitis. For minor surgical procedures, such as a (nonlaparoscopic) herniorrhaphy, PD may only need to be interrupted for 1 to 2 days, but with major intraabdominal surgery, PD may be need to be interrupted for as long as 2 weeks. PD cannot be resumed if intraperitoneal drains are in place. A gastrostomy tube should not be placed in close proximity to the PD catheter to avoid the risk of peritonitis. Urologic surgeries in infants with CAKUTs should take into consideration the future placement of a PD catheter and eventual renal transplantation. Blood vessels should be preserved for future HD access and renal transplantation.

Table 92.3

Pain Medications in End-Stage Renal Disease

Preferred

Actaminophen
Hydromorphone
Fentanyl
Methadone
Gabapentin
Pregabalin

Use With Caution

Tramadol
Hydrocodone and oxycodone
Desipramine and nortriptyline

Avoid Using

Meperidine
Codeine
Morphine
Propoxyphene

Table 92.4

Common Surgical Procedures in Children on Dialysis (Not Dialysis Access)

Procedure	Setting
Gastrostomy tube	Infants
Vesicostomy	CAKUTs
Bladder augmentation	CAKUTs
Ureteral reimplantation	
Ureterostomy	
Native nephrectomy	CAKUTs
	ARPKD
Bowel obstruction or lysis of adhesions	History of peritoneal dialysis or intraabdominal renal transplant
ECMO	Neonate with pulmonary hypoplasia
Transplant nephrectomy	Failed renal transplant

ARPKD, Autosomal recessive polycystic kidney disease; CAKUT, congenital anomalies of kidney and urinary tract; ECMO, extracorporeal membrane oxygenation.

Summary

Children on dialysis present with additional challenges when undergoing surgery because of the systemic manifestations of renal disease and the frequent extrarenal complications of childhood renal disease. Particular care is required with perioperative fluid management and with appropriate analgesia. Surgical procedures in children should take into consideration current and future needs for dialysis and renal transplantation.

CHAPTER 93

Infectious Complications in Children Undergoing Dialysis

Pamela Singer, MD, MS • Christine B. Sethna, MD, EdM

Infectious complications are a major cause of morbidity and mortality in children on peritoneal dialysis (PD) and hemodialysis (HD). This chapter reviews the major infectious risks of each modality, proposed preventive strategies and treatment guidelines, and areas for further development.

Peritoneal Dialysis

Epidemiology

Peritonitis is the most significant cause of morbidity in children on PD. Peritonitis is the leading cause of hospitalization, termination of PD, and death among chronic PD patients. The International Pediatric Peritonitis Registry (IPPR), formed by a consortium of 44 dialysis centers across the globe, showed an incidence of 1.4 ± 0.8 peritonitis episodes per patient over a 38-month analysis period. The North American Pediatric Renal Trials and Collaborative Studies (NAPRTCS) registry reported an annualized peritonitis rate of 0.64, or 1 episode per 18.8 patient months over the 1992 to 2010 period. Recent data from the SCOPE (Standardizing Care to Improve Outcomes in Pediatric ESRD) collaborative showed an annualized peritonitis rate of 0.47 or 1 episode every 27.95 months.

Higher rates of peritonitis are seen with younger age, black race, incontinence, and presence of a gastrostomy tube (G-tube). Use of a plastic rather than titanium catheter adapter was associated with significantly higher rates of peritonitis. Preliminary analysis of SCOPE outcome data has identified touch contamination, defined as accidental disconnection or contamination during treatment or via defective PD equipment, as an independent risk factor. for peritonitis. Although some of these risk factors are nonmodifiable, strategies are now being developed to standardize catheter care practices in order to obtain the best outcomes in PD with the lowest incidence of peritonitis.

Microbiology

Causative pathogens of peritonitis vary extensively by locale. Analysis from the IPPR showed that whereas gram-positive peritonitis is more common in Europe, *Pseudomonas* spp. were eight times more common in the United States. Furthermore, in North America, culture-negative peritonitis accounted for 11% of episodes, but in Mexico, it accounted for a full 67%. Table 93.1, taken from an IPPR analysis, shows the differences in causative agents grouped by region. Geographic differences

Table 93.1

Causative Agents of Peritonitis Grouped by Region, Based on Data From the International Pediatric Peritonitis Registry

	All	USA	Mexico	Argentina	Western Europe	Eastern Europe	Turkey	Asia	P Value*
Patients (n)	378	74	9	23	125	42	96	9	
Fungal	10 (3%)	3 (4%)	0 (0%)	0 (0%)	4 (3%)	1 (2%)	2 (2%)	0 (0%)	NS
Coagulase-negative staphylococci	85 (22%)	11 (15%)	1 (11%)	1 (4%)	32 (26%)	**16 (38%)**	23 (24%)	1 (11%)	<.01
Staphylococcus. aureus	78 (21%)	10 (14%)	**4 (44%)**	5 (22%)	34 (27%)	6 (14%)	19 (20%)	0 (0%)	<.05
Streptococci	31 (8%)	7 (9%)	1 (11%)	0 (0%)	13 (10%)	3 (7%)	5 (5%)	2 (22%)	NS
Enterococci	20 (5%)	1 (1%)	0 (0%)	1 (4%)	8 (6%)	2 (5%)	9 (9%)	0 (0%)	.05
Other gram-positive organisms	21 (6%)	8 (11%)	0 (0%)	1 (4%)	4 (3%)	2 (5%)	5 (5%)	1 (11%)	NS
Pseudomonas spp.	28 (7%)	**12 (16%)**	0 (0%)	**3 (13%)**	2 (2%)	1 (2%)	7 (7%)	3 (33%)	<.0005
Other gram-negative organisms	105 (28%)	22 (30%)	3 (33%)	**13 (57%)**	28 (22%)	11 (26%)	26 (27%)	2 (22%)	NS

*P <.05 in the last column indicates significant heterogeneity among regions; individual regions differing significantly from average percentage are marked in bold.
NS, Not significant.
From Schaefer F, Feneberg R, Aksu N, et al. Worldwide variation of dialysis-associated peritonitis in children. *Kidney Int* 2007;72:1374-1379.

are thought to be due to both environmental factors, as well as differences in regional practices regarding chronic catheter care.

Currently, there seems to be a general trend toward more gram-negative and fewer gram-positive infections overall. This may be due to improvement in technique, as well as implementation of *Staphylococcus aureus* colonization eradication regimens. For example, whereas the IPPR analysis showed more than 60% gram-positive peritonitis, in the SCOPE data, approximately 40% of peritonitis cases were caused by gram-positive organisms, with about 20% each of gram-negative and culture-negative peritonitis. The most commonly isolated bacteria isolated from IPPR data were coagulase-negative staphylococci (central nervous system [CNS]) followed by *Enterobacter, Enterococcus,* and *Streptococcus.* Common gram-negative isolates included *Escherichia coli* and *Klebsiella, Proteus,* and *Pseudomonas* spp. Fungal infections represent another important source of peritonitis, 2% to 5% of all cases, and typically have a more severe course.

Preventive Strategies

Based on data from the approximately 500 episodes of pediatric peritonitis in the IPPR, the International Society of Peritoneal Dialysis (ISPD) published updated pediatric guidelines for management of peritonitis in 2012. Similarly, the SCOPE collaborative has devised three "bundles" related to evidence-based practices for PD care in the areas of catheter insertion, PD training, and follow-up catheter care. In preliminary data analysis, adherence with these bundles has been shown to significantly reduce the rate of peritonitis.

With regards to the surgical placement of PD catheters, recommendations have been made regarding the type of catheter, surgical technique, and perioperative care. Based on observational studies, ISPD guidelines recommend the use of a coiled double-cuff rather than single-cuff Tenckhoff catheter inserted in the lateral or downward facing position. No sutures should be used to anchor the catheter at the exit site because these represent a nidus for infection. A titanium adapter should be placed because plastic adapters were shown to have higher rates of peritonitis.

Perioperative antibiotic administration at the time of insertion is associated with a decreased rate of early infection. A first-generation cephalosporin to cover skin flora is recommended because of the increased risk of antibiotic resistance with vancomycin.

In the immediate postoperative period, care is taken to avoid risk factors for infection. This includes immobilization of the exit site with a nonocclusive gauze and tape dressing. Dressings should be changed only once a week under sterile conditions until the exit site is well healed unless the dressing becomes saturated with fluid or visibly dirty. Furthermore, only trained PD nurses should change a PD catheter dressing during this period. Finally, sponge baths should be used until the catheter site is fully healed, avoiding the exit site area. Ideally, the catheter should not be used for at least 14 days after insertion to allow adequate healing time.

Training recommendations focus on the need for a 1 : 1 ratio of PD nurse trainer to patient or family trained. Goals of training include the ability to safely perform all required PD procedures, the ability to recognize contamination and infection, and knowledge of the appropriate responses to these complications. Furthermore, the guidelines emphasize the need for written materials to supplement the training process, as well as a posttraining assessment to ensure competency.

Beyond the perioperative period, sterile technique remains critical in the avoidance of infection. As with all infection prevention strategies, handwashing is a crucial component of preventive care. An initial washing with soap and water is recommended followed by use of an alcohol-based gel. Daily or alternate-day dressing changes, the use of an antiseptic cleansing agent such as chlorhexidine, and administration of a topical antibiotic ointment such as mupirocin or gentamicin have been associated with fewer infections. Gentamicin may be preferable to mupirocin because of its efficacy against *Pseudomonas* spp. When breaks in sterile technique are identified during the PD process, prophylactic antibiotics are indicated to minimize the risk of peritonitis. Prophylaxis is indicated for 1 to 3 days via the intraperitoneal (IP) route.

Future procedures represent another point of risk for infection. Therefore, ISPD guidelines recommend prophylactic antibiotics during dental procedures and genitourinary and gastrointestinal surgeries. In addition, the abdomen should be drained of PD fluid before the procedure to reduce the risk of development of peritonitis. Finally, in some procedures with high risk of bacterial translocation, withholding PD for 1 to 2 days if possible may be beneficial.

G-tube placement represents a significant source of concern because it is associated with higher rates of peritonitis and is frequently needed in PD patients to assist in appropriate nutrition. If at all possible, GT placement should be done before or at the time of PD catheter placement. If a GT is placed after PD has been instituted, the open surgical technique is preferable over the laparoscopic approach because it enables immediate suturing of the stomach to abdominal wall, minimizing the amount of gastric leakage. Appropriate antibiotic prophylaxis should be given, and PD should be withheld for at least 1 day. Antifungal prophylaxis is also indicated in the situation of GT placement because of an observed increased risk of fungal peritonitis.

Diagnosis of Peritonitis

Peritonitis should be suspected whenever a cloudy effluent is present. Fever, abdominal pain, abdominal distention, and vomiting are other commonly seen symptoms that should raise suspicion. In these settings, culture and cell count of PD fluid should be tested. The diagnosis of peritonitis is empirically made in the setting of a PD fluid cell count of 100 white blood cells (WBCs)/mm^3 or more with at least 50% polymorphonuclear cells (PMNs). Because a cell count may show a false-negative result in the absence of an adequate dwell time, ideally, the fluid should be collected after at least 2 hours of dwelling.

The ideal method for culturing PD fluid is to centrifuge a large volume of PD fluid (50 mL) in order to obtain a sediment, which is incubated on culture media. This method results in the lowest rate of culture-negative peritonitis. Alternatively, PD fluid can be injected into blood culture bottles for incubation.

Management of Peritonitis

Intraperitoneal antibiotic administration represents the mainstay of management for peritonitis. IP administration achieves a rapid, high concentration of drug levels at the site of infection, and absorption from the peritoneal cavity generally results in therapeutic blood levels as well. Most antibiotics are administered continuously, given as a constant dose per liter injected into the dialysate, with the subsequent total amount received dependent on the patient's dialysis prescription. Based on the pharmacokinetic profiles of various antibiotic agents, as well as the patient's residual renal function, dosing can sometimes be done intermittently rather than continuously. In these cases, drug levels should be checked to determine a redosing schedule. Table 93.2 shows commonly used antibiotics and their recommended dosing.

Empiric treatment should begin with both gram-positive and gram-negative coverage and should be adjusted accordingly based on culture results. Cefepime has adequate coverage of both gram-positive and gram-negative organisms and is recommended as first-line treatment. Alternatively, a first-generation cephalosporin plus ceftazidime (a third-generation cephalosporin) or an aminoglycoside can be used in combination. In patients with a history of methicillin-resistant *S. aureus* (MRSA) or in centers with high rates of MRSA (>10% of all *S. aureus* infections) vancomycin should be started empirically with any regimen pending culture results. Figs. 93.1 and 93.2 show recommended treatment strategies based on culture results.

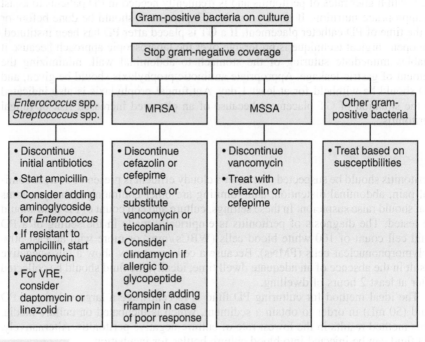

Figure 93.1

Treatment strategy for gram-positive peritonitis. MRSA, Methicillin-resistant *Staphylococcus aureus*; MSSA, methicillin-sensitive *Staphylococcus aureus*; VRE, vancomycin-resistant enterococcus. (From Warady BA, Bakkaloglu S, Newland J, et al. Consensus guidelines for the prevention and treatment of catheter-related infections and peritonitis in pediatric patients receiving peritoneal dialysis: 2012 update. *Perit Dial Int* 2012;32(suppl):S29-S86.)

Table 93.2

Pharmacologic Agents and Dosing Regimens for Treatment of Peritonitis

Antibiotic Dosing Recommendations for the Treatment of Peritonitis

Antibiotic Type	Therapy Type		Intermittent*
	Continuous*		
	Loading Dose	Maintenance Dose	
Aminoglycosides (IP)[†]			
Gentamicin	8 mg/L	4 mg/L	
Netilmicin	8 mg/L	4 mg/L	Anuric: 0.6 mg/kg
Tobramycin	8 mg/L	4 mg/L	Nonanuric: 0.75 mg/kg
Amikacin	25 mg/L	12 mg/L	
Cephalosporins (IP)			
Cefazolin	500 mg/L	125 mg/L	20 mg/kg
Cefepime	500 mg/L	125 mg/L	15 mg/kg
Cefotaxime	500 mg/L	250 mg/L	30 mg/kg
Ceftazidime	500 mg/L	125 mg/L	20 mg/kg
Glycopeptides (IP) [‡]			
Vancomycin	1000 mg/L	25 mg/L	30 mg/kg: Repeat dosing: 15 mg/kg every 3–5 days
Teicoplanin[§]	400 mg/L	20 mg/L	15 mg/kg every 5–7 days
Penicillins (IP)[†]			
Ampicillin	—	125 mg/L	—
Quinolones (IP)			
Ciprofloxacin	50 mg/L	25 mg/L	—
Others			
Aztreonam (IP)	1000 mg/L	250 mg/L	—
Clindamycin (IP	300 mg/L	150 mg/L	—
Imipenem-cilastin (IP)	250 mg/L	50 mg/L	—
Linezolid (PO)	Age <5 years: 30 mg/kg/ day divided into three doses Age 5–11 years: 20 mg/ kg/day divided into two doses Age ≥12 years: 600 mg/ dose twice daily	—	—

Table 93.2

Pharmacologic Agents and Dosing Regimens for Treatment of Peritonitis—cont'd

Others			
Metronidazole (PO)	30 mg/kg/day divided into 3 doses (maximum, 1.2 g/day)	—	—
Rifampin (PO)	10–20 mg/kg/day divided into two doses (maximum, 600 mg/day)	—	—

Antifungals			
Fluconazole (IP, IV, or PO)	6–12 mg/kg every 24–48 h (maximum, 400 mg/day)	—	—
Caspofungin (IV only)	70 mg/m^2 on day 1 (maximum, 70 mg/day)	50 mg/m^2/day (maximum, 50 mg daily)	—

*For continuous therapy, the exchange with the loading dose should dwell for 3 to 6 hours; all subsequent exchanges during the treatment course should contain the maintenance dose. For intermittent therapy, the dose should be applied once daily in the long dwell unless otherwise specified.

†Aminoglycosides and penicillins should not be mixed in dialysis fluid because of the potential for inactivation.

‡In patients with residual renal function, glycopeptide elimination may be accelerated. If intermittent therapy is used in such a setting, the second dose should be time-based on a blood level obtained 2 to 4 days after the initial dose. Redosing should occur when the blood level is below 15 mg/L for vancomycin, or below 8 mg/L for teicoplanin. Intermittent therapy is not recommended for patients with residual renal function unless serum levels of the drug can be monitored in a timely manner.

§Teicoplanin is not currently available in the United States.

IP, Intraperitoneal; IV, intravenous; PO, oral.

From Warady BA, Bakkaloglu S, Newland J, et al. Consensus guidelines for the prevention and treatment of catheter-related infections and peritonitis in pediatric patients receiving peritoneal dialysis: 2012 update. *Perit Dial Int* 2012;32(suppl):S29-S86.

The duration of antibiotic treatment for peritonitis depends on the organism isolated and severity of the infection. For CNS and *Streptococcus* spp., a 2-week course of treatment is considered sufficient. Because *S. aureus* peritonitis is frequently more severe, a 3-week course is recommended. *Enterococcus* spp., although it usually causes a mild infection, is typically treated for 2 to 3 weeks because the initial empiric treatment often does not cover the bacteria. In settings of gram-negative peritonitis other than *Pseudomonas* spp., the treatment regimen is generally 2 weeks. However, in cases of *Pseudomonas* spp. or other extended spectrum β-lactamase (ESBL)–producing species, a 3-week course is recommended. *Pseudomonas* spp. has the ability to create a biofilm within the catheter lumen, increasing the risk of treatment failure. For that reason, the addition of an aminoglycoside to the treatment regimen is recommended for synergy.

Fungal peritonitis is almost always preceded by bacterial infection and antibiotic use, whether for peritonitis or other infection. It is frequently more severe than that caused by bacterial infection, with higher rates of associated catheter loss, membrane

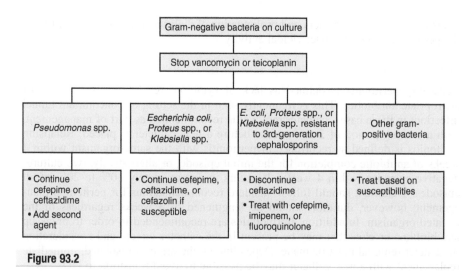

Figure 93.2

Treatment strategy for gram-negative peritonitis. (From Warady BA, Bakkaloglu S, Newland J, et al. Consensus guidelines for the prevention and treatment of catheter-related infections and peritonitis in pediatric patients receiving peritoneal dialysis: 2012 update. *Perit Dial Int* 2012;32(suppl):S29-S86.)

failure, and mortality. Multiple studies in the adult population examining the use of prophylactic antifungal administration at the time of antibiotic use demonstrated lower rates of fungal peritonitis in those who received prophylaxis. Therefore, prophylaxis with either nystatin or fluconazole is recommended at times of antibiotic therapy. In the event that a fungal peritonitis occurs, the ISPD recommends early catheter removal, with treatment for 2 weeks or longer after complete clinical resolution has been achieved. Early catheter removal has been shown to decrease the risk of peritoneal membrane failure. A minimum of 2 to 3 weeks is suggested before placement of a new catheter, necessitating a temporary switch in modality to HD. Antifungal treatment is generally with systemic fluconazole.

Culture-negative peritonitis represents another management challenge. The IPPR reported rates of 31% culture-negative peritonitis. The ISPD 2012 guidelines recommend continuing empiric coverage for 2 weeks in these settings. Although the IPPR reported very high rates of clinical improvement after 72 hours of treatment in culture-negative peritonitis, when improvement does not occur, patients should be recultured, and consideration of catheter removal should be made. Centers that have higher than 20% culture-negative rates should be encouraged to review their culture techniques with staff.

Adjunctive Therapies

In addition to appropriate antimicrobial therapy, adjunctive treatments may be useful in the management of peritonitis. There is evidence to suggest that heparin added to the dialysate during peritonitis may have a beneficial effect on treatment outcomes and catheter patency. This is due to the anticoagulant and antiinflammatory properties of heparin. Other strategies to improve outcomes include reduction of dwell volumes for pain management and prolongation of dialysate dwell times to optimize the peritoneal milieu for bactericidal activity.

Refractory and Relapsing Peritonitis

Refractory peritonitis is defined as lack of symptom resolution after 5 days of appropriate antibiotics. This is frequently seen in the setting of concomitant tunnel infection; in these cases, catheter removal is recommended as part of management, with a waiting period of 2 to 3 weeks before a new catheter is placed. Relapsing peritonitis is defined as recurrence of peritonitis with the same organism within 4 weeks of antibiotic completion for the initial episode, or alternatively, two culture-negative episodes within 4 weeks. It occurs in approximately 10% to 20% of all episodes. Treatment should follow standard recommendations for peritonitis management; however, duration should be lengthened to 3 weeks regardless of the isolated organism. In addition, fibrinolytics are recommended in order to break up any biofilms or clots that may be present in the catheter lumen, and consideration of catheter removal must be made. Depending on the organism isolated, immediate replacement with a new catheter may be possible to avoid transition to HD.

Catheter-Related Infections

In addition to peritonitis, catheter-related infections can occur in children on PD. Catheter tunnel infections (TIs) or exit-site infections (ESIs) may occur alone or in conjunction with peritonitis. TIs usually present with redness, tenderness, and edema along the subcutaneous part of the catheter with or without drainage. The diagnosis of ESI is made on the basis of a scoring system proposed by Schaefer et al (Table 93.3), taking into account the presence of swelling, redness, crusting, pain, and secretions, with or without the isolation of a pathogenic organism. A score of 2 or more along with a positive exit site culture, or of 4 or more without a culture, is considered diagnostic. *S. aureus* and *Pseudomonas* spp. represent the most common causes of catheter-related infections. Oral antibiotic treatment of ESIs is generally acceptable, and for TIs, it can be oral, intravenous (IV), or IP. Treatment duration is generally 2 to 4 weeks and for at least 7 days after resolution of external symptoms. First-generation cephalosporins or ciprofloxacin (which has anti-*Pseudomonal* activity) is recommended as empiric oral treatment pending culture results. A TI or ESI

Table 93.3

Exit-Site Scoring System for Infection

	0	1	2
Swelling	None	Exit site only (<0.5 cm)	Including part or all of the tunnel
Crust	None	<0.5 cm	>0.5 cm
Redness	None	<0.5 cm	>0.5 cm
Pain on pressure	None	Slight	Severe
Secretion	None	Serous	Purulent

From Schaefer F, Kaus G, Muller-Wiefel DE, et al. Intermittent versus continuous intraperitoneal glycopeptide/ceftazidime treatment in children with peritoneal dialysis-associated peritonitis. The Mid-European Pediatric Peritoneal Dialysis Study Group (MEPPS). *J Am Soc Nephrol* 1999;10: 36-145.

in the presence of peritonitis is considered a definitive indication for catheter removal.

Postperitonitis

After an episode of peritonitis, ISPD guidelines recommend retraining of PD providers and a home visit to identify the root cause of the infection.

Hemodialysis

The majority of children receiving HD do so via a central venous catheter (CVC). Although arteriovenous (AV) fistulas and grafts are feasible and preferred in children, in part because of a significantly lower infection rate, they are underused because of a variety of factors, including patient size, lack of personnel skilled in microsurgical technique, and expectation of an expedited kidney transplant.

Fewer data are available regarding catheter-related infections in children on HD than in PD. Although one of the objectives of the SCOPE collaborative is to collect this information, results have not yet been made available. Furthermore, no consensus guidelines exist regarding practices for catheter care. Nevertheless, some pediatric data from single-center studies are available, and information has also been applied from adult data and from general guidelines on pediatric venous catheter care.

Epidemiology and Risk Factors

In multiple studies, the average rate of infection leading to catheter failure is about 1.1 to 1.6 episodes per 1000 catheter days. Risk factors for catheter-related infections include young age, colonization with *S. aureus*, elevated ferritin levels, hypoalbuminemia, and immunosuppression. Tunneled cuffed catheters are associated with lower infection risk than temporary catheters. Interestingly, femoral catheters have been shown in more than one study to have infection rates similar to nonfemoral catheters. Although subclavian catheters have shown lower rates of infection, they are often not used because of the risk of stenosis.

The most commonly isolated bacteria in catheter-related bloodstream infections (CRBSIs) are *S. aureus* and coagulase-negative Staph such as *S. epidermidis*.

Preventive Measures

As with PD catheters, HD-related catheter infections can include ESIs, TIs, and bloodstream infections. ESIs are defined as inflammation confined to the area surrounding the exit site within 2 cm along with a positive exudate culture. TIs are defined as inflammation along the tunnel superior to the cuff, beyond 2 cm from the exit site. The Infectious Disease Society of America (IDSA) defines CRBSIs infections as the same organism growing from a peripheral vein culture and culture from the catheter hub, or alternatively, as two positive blood cultures from different catheter lumens if a peripheral blood culture was not obtained. The patient should also have clinical manifestations of infection such as fever or chills and no other apparent source of infection. Small studies have demonstrated a lower incidence of ESIs, TIs, and bloodstream infection in patients using chlorhexidine for exit-site care as opposed to povidone-iodine; therefore, this should be used for exit-site care.

Some recommend catheter dressing changes with every dialysis session, but other centers use once-weekly regimens. Furthermore, catheters should be managed only by trained dialysis nurses, and sterile technique, including wearing a mask, should be used whenever the catheter is accessed. Catheter exit sites must be covered with sterile gauze and are not allowed to get wet between catheter dressing changes. Semipermeable polyurethane dressings enable bathing and showering without soaking the dressing and are gaining in popularity; however, a recent Cochrane database review of six studies found a higher rate of infection with these dressings compared with gauze and tape. The Biopatch, a chlorhexidine-impregnated catheter dressing, has been shown to reduce ESIs in some studies.

Prophylactic topical antibiotics and use of antibiotic catheter lock solutions are not routinely recommended because of the risk of inducing resistant strains of bacteria. However, heparin locks, which have both anticoagulant and antimicrobial activity, are recommended and reduce the risk of clot formation and infection.

Treatment of Infection

Exit-site infections can generally be treated with topical antibiotics, but tunnel infections and CRBSIs require IV antibiotics. Initial empiric treatment with either vancomycin or nafcillin as well as a third-generation cephalosporin is recommended pending culture results. Broader empiric coverage for *Pseudomonas* spp. and fungi may be considered in high-risk patients. Antibiotics should be administered through the catheter, or alternatively, through a peripheral vein along with antibiotic locks to the catheter. The duration of treatment is generally considered sufficient with 10 to 14 days of appropriate antibiotics, although the Kidney Disease Outcomes Quality Initiative (KDOQI) guidelines recommend at least 3 weeks of therapy for CRBSI. The date of first negative culture is considered the first day of antibiotic treatment. Tables 93.4 and 93.5 show antibiotic guidelines for patients on HD.

Table 93.4

Antibiotic Dosing Guidelines for Patients on Hemodialysis

Empirical dosing pending culture results
Vancomycin plus empirical gram-negative rod coverage based on local antibiogram data
or
Vancomycin plus gentamicin
(Cefazolin may be used in place of vancomycin in units with a low prevalence of
   methicillin-resistant staphylococci)
Vancomycin: 20-mg/kg loading dose infused during the last hour of the dialysis session and
   then 500 mg during the last 30 min of each subsequent dialysis session
Gentamicin (or tobramycin): 1 mg/kg, not to exceed 100 mg after each dialysis session
Ceftazidime: 1 g IV after each dialysis session
Cefazolin: 20 mg/kg IV after each dialysis session
For *Candida* infection: An echinocandin (caspofungin 70-mg IV loading dose followed by
   50 mg IV daily; IV micafungin 100 mg IV daily; or anidulafungin 200-mg IV loading dose
   followed by 100 mg IV daily); fluconazole (200 mg orally daily); or amphotericin B

IV, Intravenous.
From Mermel LA, Allon, M, Bouza E, et al. Clinical practice guidelines for the diagnosis and
   management of intravascular catheter-related infection: 2009 update by the Infectious Disease
   Society of America. *Clin Infect Dis* 2009;49(1):1-45.

Table 93.5

Antibiotic Lock Dosing for Hemodialysis Catheter Infections*

Antibiotic and Dosage	Heparin or Saline, 1 U/mL
Vancomycin, 2.5 mg/mL	2500 or 5000
Vancomycin, 2.0 mg/mL	10
Vancomycin 5.0 mg/mL[†]	0 or 5000
Ceftazidime, 0.5 mg/mL	100
Cefazolin, 5.0 mg/mL	2500 or 5000
Ciprofloxacin, 0.2 mg/mL[‡]	5000
Gentamicin, 1.0 mg/mL	2500
Ampicillin, 10.0 mg/mL	10 or 5000
Ethanol, 70%[§]	0

*These antibiotic lock solutions will not precipitate at the given concentrations. Cefazolin is the preferred agent for treatment of methicillin-susceptible staphylococci, and vancomycin is the preferred agent for treatment of methicillin-resistant staphylococci. Ceftazidime, gentamicin, or ciprofloxacin can be used for treatment of gram-negative microorganisms. Ampicillin is the preferred agent for infections caused by ampicillin-sensitive enterococci, and vancomycin is the preferred agent for treatment of ampicillin-resistant enterococci other than vancomycin-resistant enterococci. The use of an ethanol lock can be considered for the treatment of a mixed gram-positive and gram-negative infection.

[†]Vancomycin at 5 mg/mL is more efficacious than at 1 mg/mL in eradicating staphylococci embedded within biofilm. A precipitate appears when mixing 10 mg/mL of vancomycin with 10,000 IU/mL of heparin; however, by agitating the solution for -10 s, the precipitation resolves and the solution remains precipitate free for 72 hours at 37°C. The lock solution in 2500 IU/mL heparin can be made as follows: Using vials containing 50 mg/mL of vancomycin in water, remove 2 mL and dilute in 8 mL 0.9% NaCL, resulting in 10 mg/mL of vancomycin. Place 1 mL of 5000 IU/mL heparin in a glass test tube and mix with 1 mL of the 10-mg/mL vancomycin solution.

[‡]The maximum concentration of ciprofloxacin is limited because of precipitation at higher concentrations.

[§]An in vitro study demonstrated the compatibility of ethanol 70% and silicone or polyether urethane catheters.

From Mermel LA, Allon, M, Bouza E, et al. Clinical practice guidelines for the diagnosis and management of intravascular catheter-related infection: 2009 update by the Infectious Disease Society of America. *Clin Infect Dis* 2009;49(1):1-45.

NA, Not applicable.

Up to 75% of infections can be treated without catheter removal; however, removal is indicated when symptoms do not improve or when bacteremia and ESI occur together. Furthermore, the IDSA guidelines recommend catheter exchange for *S. aureus*, *Pseudomonas*, and fungal infections.

Future Steps

The continued use of databases and registries to collect information on HD- and PD-related infections is needed. The results of these must be continuously analyzed in order to devise appropriate guidelines regarding catheter care for prevention of infection. On a local level, hospitals should be encouraged to create antibiograms of catheter-related infections in order to implement the most appropriate treatment regimens while minimizing the risk of further antimicrobial resistance. Finally, a stronger push for fistula placement in children on chronic HD is recommended in order to reduce rates of catheter-related infections.

CHAPTER 94

Adherence and Transition in the Pediatric Dialysis Patient

Sarah E. Duncan, MA • Rachel A. Annunziato, PhD

Overview of Adherence

To manage their disease, children undergoing dialysis must follow a treatment regimen that includes diet, fluid intake, medication, and dialysis prescriptions. The complex nature of this treatment regimen provides multiple ways in which patients may be nonadherent, and research suggests that nonadherence rates range from 17% to 43% in this population. Although the consequences of severe nonadherence (i.e., failure to undergo dialysis) are obvious, the implications of more subtle nonadherence are less understood. Limited research suggests that hyperphosphatemia and hypotension may result from nonadherence, but because these are generally asymptomatic, dialysis patients are unlikely to be immediately aware of these consequences. The following presents an overview of methods for assessing adherence, risk factors for nonadherence, and strategies for addressing nonadherence in children receiving dialysis.

Evaluating Nonadherence

Identifying patients who are nonadherent to the dialysis treatment regimen may be challenging because there is currently no gold standard for assessing adherence in this population. The multifaceted nature of the treatment requirements also complicates how adherence is evaluated. The most frequently used measures include objective (physiologic and behavioral) as well as subjective methods (patient, parent, and clinician ratings) as described below.

1. **Physiologic measures:** Laboratory tests measure dietary adherence, and interdialytic weight gain (IDWG) assesses adherence to both sodium and fluid restrictions. The primary benefit of these physiologic measures is that they are considered objective measures of adherence; however, these measures also suffer from several limitations. First, there is no consensus on the specific cut-off points that should be used to distinguish adherence from nonadherence. Additionally, variables other than adherence to the treatment regimen may influence these physiologic indicators. Medication, residual kidney functioning, and dialysis adequacy impact laboratory tests. Similarly, nutritional state, dry weight, and residual kidney functioning can also affect IDWG. Furthermore, the objectivity of IDWG may be compromised for children who are receiving dialysis at home because weight information primarily comes from the family rather than health care staff.

2. **Behavioral measures:** Behavioral components of the dialysis treatment regimen include attendance of appointments and dialysis sessions and time spent

undergoing dialysis. These can be measured through analysis of attendance logs or home dialysis use. Although inventory checks have historically been used to measure home dialysis adherence, these tend to be time consuming and labor intensive, and electronic monitoring has become a viable alternative. The Baxter HomeChoice PRO Card is a computer chip that records the frequency and length of dialysis sessions, the amount of dialysis fluid used, and the number of cycles completed for each dialysis session. The advantage of these behavioral measures is that, unlike physiologic measures, they are not confounded by other factors. However, as with the physiologic measures, a clear consensus has not been reached on the appropriate cut-off point for determining nonadherence.

3. **Subjective reports:** Subjective reports include clinician, patient, and parent reports about adherence behaviors. Clinician reports ask a member of the child's treatment team to determine an adherence rating based on his or her knowledge of the child and clinical expertise. This method allows for a more comprehensive view of adherence than the physiologic measures, but caution must be exercised because the relationship among the clinician, the child, and the family may influence perceptions of adherence. Parent and child reporting are advantageous because of their practicality; these reports are inexpensive and simple to administer. However, they are prone to the same problems with subjectivity and response bias as clinician reports, and adherence levels tend to be higher using self-report than physiologic measures. One way to address some of the response bias inherent in self-reporting is to use parent and child reports simultaneously and compare the two measures for discrepancies.

In conclusion, although monitoring adherence is an important goal for clinicians working with pediatric dialysis patients, there is no single measure that is capable of completely assessing nonadherence. Our recommendation is to use a combination of the above measures to achieve the most comprehensive picture of adherence but to keep in mind the limitations of each.

Variables Associated With Nonadherence

A number of patient, family, and illness characteristics have been associated with adherence in pediatric dialysis patients. Brownbridge and Fielding's (1994) seminal study of 60 children and adolescents with end-stage renal disease (ESRD) found that older age was associated with poorer adherence across indicators of fluid intake restriction, following dietary guidelines, and medication regimen adherence. Poorer adherence in older children and adolescents may be related to an increased desire for autonomy characteristic of this developmental period. Additionally, older age signals the transition of health care responsibilities to the patient (including the transfer to adult care settings), which may negatively impact adherence.

Given the major role families have in caring for a child on dialysis, it is not surprising that family characteristics are also related to adherence rates. Brownbridge and Fielding found that nonadherence was associated with low socioeconomic status and single-parent households. Studies examining adherence in pediatric diabetes and transplant patients have found that adherence rates are higher in children whose parents take on and maintain more active roles in assisting with health care management. Parents who care for their child without the support of a second parent living in the home or who have a lower socioeconomic status may have greater difficulty providing adequate parental supervision of the child's dietary, fluid intake, and medication regimens as well as providing the child with food consistent with his or her dietary restrictions.

Treatment and illness history variables are also associated with lower adherence rates. Brownbridge and Fielding's work suggested that children who had a longer duration of dialysis, higher number of hospitalizations, and other comorbid medical problems had poorer adherence. Additionally, Silverstein et al's (2014) study of 22 pediatric dialysis patients pointed to dialysis type as having an impact on adherence rates. On average, children who received peritoneal dialysis (PD) reported experiencing perceived barriers to adherence significantly more often than children who received hemodialysis (HD). Importantly, although there was a trend toward higher rates of adherence in HD patients compared with PD patients, this was not statistically significant. This pattern may occur because some medication can be administered during dialysis for HD patients, although further research on a larger sample is needed to explore this relationship. Other factors, including treatment regimen side effects, are recognized as having important implications for adherence in other chronically ill pediatric populations and thus also need to be further studied in relation to pediatric dialysis adherence.

Finally, Brownbridge and Fielding's work also suggested that the psychological well-being of both the parent and the child is associated with adherence. Higher levels of parent- and child-reported dialysis-related stress as well as reports of extreme parent and child reactions to the diagnosis were all associated with lower levels of adherence to the treatment regimen. Furthermore, assessments of more general psychopathology found that higher parental depression scores and higher child anxiety scores were related to lower adherence rates, and these findings are consistent with Pai and Ingerski's review of adherence in other chronically ill pediatric populations.

Addressing Adherence

The modifiable factors associated with adherence provide meaningful targets for intervention, yet empirical studies of interventions to improve adherence in pediatric dialysis patients are lacking. To begin to address adherence problems, Pai and Ingerski provide a useful resource of educational, organizational, and behavioral strategies that have been studied in other chronically ill populations. Still, further research must be done to examine the effectiveness of these strategies in pediatric dialysis patients specifically.

Educational interventions aim to increase knowledge about the child's illness, how the illness is treated, and the importance of treatment adherence. Education should be provided at the time of diagnosis, the start of treatment, and periodically throughout treatment, particularly when there are changes in the regimen or in the child's health. Importantly, some research indicates that parental education, rather than patient education, is more closely related to adherence, underscoring the importance of including parents in educational interventions. A study of adult dialysis patients suggests the applicability of educational strategies to the dialysis population. Forty-two patients were educated about the importance of adherence and were informed that their dialysis usage would be monitored using the Baxter HomeChoice PRO Card. Adherence rates were higher in this sample than in a previous study conducted by the same researchers in which the sample did not receive the education or monitoring program. Although caution must be exercised in the interpretation of these results because the study was not designed with a control group, it suggests the promise of educational strategies for improving adherence in dialysis patients specifically.

Organizational approaches for improving adherence include strategies such as maintaining a pill box for the child and keeping it in a set place at home. Reminders and tracking strategies may also be beneficial for the family. For example, setting a daily alarm serves as a reminder to take (or administer) the medication, and using a calendar to track appointments and medication schedules may help to reduce the number of missed appointments or doses.

Behavioral interventions include reinforcing the use of organizational strategies and adherence behaviors and encouraging the discussion of adherence problems. Daily logs to record adherence and barriers and facilitators of this behavior may be used to identify and address circumstances that challenge adherence. Chaining, or linking medication administration to another regularly performed activity such as eating a meal, may also facilitate adherence. Finally, encouraging parental involvement in the treatment regimen may also improve adherence rates. Research with pediatric diabetes patients suggests behavioral interventions that involve the entire family are effective at increasing adherence rates. One study of 104 families randomized participants to treatment as usual, to an educational support group, or to Behavioral Family Systems Therapy (BFST). BFST provides patients with communication and problem-solving training, functional-structural family therapy, and cognitive restructuring. Adherence rates were significantly higher for patients assigned to BFST and the educational support group compared with the treatment-as-usual group, with BFST showing significantly higher adherence rates than the educational support group.

Overall, behaviorally focused interventions that include components of educational and organizational strategies appear to be the most effective interventions for addressing adherence in chronically ill pediatric populations. Importantly, psychological interventions should also be considered as potentially viable ways to address adherence problems in pediatric dialysis patients. As indicated in earlier, depressive symptoms and anxiety symptoms in parents and children may negatively impact rates of adherence. Recognizing and addressing these symptoms through psychotherapy may help to increase adherence, although research must be conducted on these types of interventions in pediatric dialysis patients specifically. Finally, the period of transition to adulthood may be a particularly vulnerable one that deserves special attention. This process is described in more detail next.

Overview of Transition

During adolescence, patients begin a transition toward adulthood. This is a long-term process involving the acquisition of self-managed care. It is likely that transitioning to self-managed care is a significant part of adolescent nonadherence. As this transition progresses, at some specific point, patients must transfer to an adult setting. The timing of transfer often varies based on patient and site-specific factors. Below, an overview of transition and transfer for pediatric dialysis patients is provided. Recent empirically supported approaches to addressing transition are presented followed by a discussion of functional outcomes during this time.

Transitional Procedures for Pediatric Dialysis Patients

There is a great deal of variation among dialysis centers in transitional procedures. For example, patients may be transferred anywhere between ages 16 and 26 years. At some sites, strict guidelines dictate when patients transfer; at others, this process is individualized. The importance of preparing patients for transition, that is, assuming a greater role over their health care, early in adolescence has been recommended. Yet adolescence is known to be a high-risk period for nonadherence. At the same time as patients are getting ready to leave pediatrics, they may be extremely vulnerable to disruptions in their health care management. Indeed, a seminal paper by Watson described a sample of 20 transferring renal transplant recipients. Over a 36-month follow-up period, 7 patients (35%) lost their graft. It appeared that patients struggled with shifting to a new team and managing their health care responsibilities such as medication taking and appointment attendance during this time.

The results of a survey conducted by Bell of 58 pediatric dialysis centers in North America and Europe highlighted specific problem points for transferring patients. Only one third of the responding centers reported having a transition program, but most expressed a need for one. Respondents were asked if their adult counterparts had supports in place for patients exhibiting nonadherence; this was only the case for 26% of the centers. However, some elements of preparation appeared stronger. For example, most sites reported that their patients were able to visit and choose their adult dialysis center before transfer and that resources were available to assist with changes in benefits. Self-management was assessed as well. Fewer than 20% of respondents reported that their adolescent patients were self-managing their care as measured by making appointments and filling prescriptions autonomously at least 60% of the time, although patients' mastery of PD administration was better (48% could do so 60% of the time).

As highlighted by these data, several distinct challenges may emerge during the transfer process. These include systematic patient and family barriers to a smooth, successful transfer. At the systematic level, there are issues specific to each service as well as overall considerations. On the pediatric side, scarce resources or inattention to transition or transfer may lead to poor planning and preparation. These concerns are faced on the adult side as well; staff may be less accustomed and equipped to meet the special needs of young adult patients. Overall, there may be a lack of coordination between pediatric and adult units, which certainly disrupts this process. Patients may be resistant to leaving familiar, trusted providers, a sentiment that is often echoed by family members as well. In the face of such challenges, patients may not be able to form connections with their new providers easily, and this could translate into disengagement and nonadherence.

Evidence-Based Strategies for Transfer

Given these modifiable problem points to a successful transition and transfer, many solutions have been proposed. However, until recently, the literature on transition to adulthood and specifically the actual transfer part of this overall process were limited by minimal data to inform interventions. Now according to a recent technical brief by the Agency for Healthcare Research and Quality (AHRQ), a handful of studies describe data-driven approaches to improving transfer in end-stage organ failure patients, although none yet on dialysis patients specifically. Although these studies have been specific to transplant recipients, important lessons can be derived from them. On a larger scale, there are now data to suggest the utility of transition clinics for ESRD patients. Some caution should be exercised in interpreting findings because these studies have all been retrospective without random assignment to control conditions; nonetheless, results are promising.

The AHRQ described three studies that supported the use of transition clinics. In one study, outcomes for renal transplant recipients seen in a transition clinic ($n = 12$) were compared with a historical control group, pretransition clinic ($n = 34$). Patients were treated in the transition clinic every 4 to 6 months until transfer while also being seen in the pediatric transplant clinic. During this time, patients had access to a range of team members (a pediatric nephrologist, renal nurse, youth health specialist, renal pharmacist, renal dietitian, and social worker). The transition clinic emphasized several self-management goals, including identifying a primary care provider, demonstrating medication knowledge, recognizing signs of rejection and infection, appraisal of ability to self-manage, and awareness of reproductive health issues. Outcomes were compared between the groups for a 2-year period after transfer. In the pretransition group, 24% of patients either died or lost their graft and had to begin dialysis versus none in the transition clinic group. Cost estimates suggested similar expenditures between the two groups but substantial additional costs because of induction of dialysis and death in the historical controls.

Two other studies reviewed by the AHRQ described transition clinics with additional services. In the first study, an integrated pediatric and young adult joint transition clinic and care pathway was established for pediatric nephrology patients in two London hospitals. Patients were seen jointly by pediatric and adult teams from 15 to 18 years of age in preparation for transfer at the age of 18 years. Additionally, a young adult clinic was established within the adult unit and later at a student college and sports center to encourage peer interaction among patients. A first group of 9 patients had transferred before the implemented transition program, and a second group of 12 patients received the revamped services. Data on acute organ rejection, morbidity, and hospital admissions were collected between 1 and 60 months after transfer. Results indicated that 6 transplants were lost in the earlier group (67%), but no transplant losses were observed in the second group. The second study of 66 pediatric kidney transplant patients compared three different transition models offered. The first approach, Model 1 ($n = 26$), was a young adult clinic led by a specialized adult nephrologist. Model 2 ($n = 15$) involved a phase of alternate appointments with an adult nephrologist in private practice over 1 to 2 years before transfer in conjunction with three yearly visits to the adult transplant clinic within the university hospital. Model 3 ($n = 25$) was the same as model 2, minus the connection to the adult clinic. Data were collected 1 year before and 1 year after transfer, using serum creatinine levels, episodes of acute rejection, immunosuppressive therapy, use of steroids, and patient satisfaction as the main outcome measures. Results showed no changes in most clinical outcomes before and after transfer among the three models. However, Model 1 was associated with fewer changes in immunosuppressive therapy, and patients in this group reported the greatest satisfaction (100% compared with 64% in Model 2 and 78% in Model 3).

Finally, as reviewed by the AHRQ, it was found that a less costly "transition coordinator" approach may be an effective way to improve outcomes during transfer for pediatric liver transplant recipients. The transition coordinator role includes preparing patients for self-managed care and transfer before shifting service location and continuing to support patients and both teams afterward. In a prospective study of this approach, patients who used the transition coordinator (*n* = 20) displayed stable adherence throughout the 2-year study period. Among the 20 enrolled patients, there were no deaths versus 4 of 14 (29%) deaths in a historical control group.

Functional Outcomes

Finally, in addition to gauging clinical outcomes during transition and transfer for pediatric dialysis patients, it is important to consider functional outcomes as well. A large study based in the Netherlands compared children with chronic illnesses, including those with ESRD, with healthy norms on a comprehensive measure of developmental milestones (the Course of Life Questionnaire). The ESRD cohort consisted of both transplanted patients and those on dialysis. Findings suggested that adolescents with ESRD lagged behind the normative sample and other chronic illness groups. Specifically, ESRD patients achieved fewer milestones in the domains of autonomy (e.g., employment, traveling alone), social development, and psychosexual development. Interestingly, though, "risky" behaviors that are often common among young adults were also less likely in the ESRD sample. Although rarely discussed in transitional programming, findings indicate the need to include functional outcomes in ongoing efforts.

Conclusions

Pediatric dialysis patients face a complex treatment regimen with high rates of nonadherence. Although monitoring nonadherence is also challenging, at present, multimodal assessment can assist in identifying at-risk patients. To date, treatment of nonadherence in pediatric populations generally and specifically in dialysis has yielded few empirically supported approaches, but behaviorally focused interventions that include components of educational and organizational strategies appear to be the most promising. Such techniques can be feasibly implemented within routine clinical care as well. Finally, patients may be especially vulnerable to nonadherence as they progress through a transition to adulthood. This involves both shifting to self-managed care and ultimately leaving pediatrics. Recently, research has begun to emerge demonstrating the utility of services to improve the transfer process, which has been sorely lacking previously.

The Pregnant Patient

C H A P T E R   9 5

Pregnancy in Dialysis Patients

Susan Hou, MD

Frequency of Pregnancy in Dialysis Patients

Fertility is markedly reduced in dialysis patients. The only survey with responses from all dialysis units was done in Belgium and reported pregnancies in 0.3% of women of childbearing age. The Australia and New Zealand Dialysis and Transplant Registry (ANZDATA) includes the participation of almost 100% of dialysis units in these two countries. Reporting pregnancies from 1966 to 2008, the registry found a rate of pregnancy of 2.07 per 1000 patient years. There is a general impression that the frequency of pregnancy is increasing in dialysis patients, but ANZDATA is the only source with data supporting that impression. The ANZDATA registry notes an increase from 0.54 and 0.67 pregnancies per 1000 year in 1976 to 1985 and 1986 to 1995 respectively, to 3.3 per 1000 patient years from 1996 to 2008. Surveys done in Saudi Arabia, the United States, and Japan give rates of conception of 1.4%, 0.55% and 3.4% respectively. The United States Renal Data System (USRDS) Coordinating Center puts the frequency of conception in U.S. dialysis patients slightly higher at 1% per year, noting a constant rate of conception over the 10 years from 1991 to 2001. Of note is that the frequency of conception in hemodialysis (HD) patients is two to three times higher than in peritoneal dialysis (PD) patients (0.55% vs 0.25% per year) in the American Registry. The difference between HD and PD is also noted in ANZDATA. The frequency of conception is dramatically higher (14.5%) in women doing nocturnal HD receiving 36 hours per week of dialysis. There is one report of a pregnancy that occurred after ovarian stimulation and artificial insemination, which resulted in fetal demise. Little has been done to try to reverse infertility in women on dialysis because pregnancy outcomes have been poor.

None of the surveys takes into account whether patients are sexually active or using contraception. They also do not take into account reasons for infertility other than renal failure, such as prior treatment with cyclophosphamide. The likelihood of pregnancy in sexually active women who are not using contraception is higher than indicated by the surveys.

The reasons for the rarity of pregnancy in dialysis patients are not well understood. One report indicates that 42% of premenopausal women on dialysis have menses, although their menses are often irregular. Dialysis patients frequently have anovulatory periods. Loss of pulsatile luteinizing hormone and hyperprolactinemia were common in the past but may be less common with current dialysis regimens. Careful studies of hormonal changes in women dialyzed with current regimens are needed.

It is not clear whether the difference in the frequency of conception between HD patients and continuous ambulatory peritoneal dialysis (CAPD) patients is the result of endocrine differences or in some way related to PD itself. It is possible that hypertonic dextrose damages the ovum or that the volume of fluid in the

Table 95.1

Management of Pregnant Dialysis Patients

Dialysis Regimen
Hemodialysis
- Dialysis time: $\geq$20 h/wk; as close to 40 h/wk as possible
- Dialysis bath: 2.5 mEq/L calcium; 25 mEq/L bicarbonate; 3.0–3.5 mEq/L potassium. May require addition of phosphorus. Adjust based on weekly measurements of electrolytes, calcium, and phosphorus.
- Heparinization: Stop heparin only for vaginal bleeding.

Peritoneal Dialysis
- Increase total dialysis by 50%.
- Combine cycler and daytime exchanges.
- Hospitalize patient for bloody dialysate.
- Treat peritonitis with penicillins and cephalosporins.
- Decrease exchange volume for comfort.
- Increase exchange frequency or add HD if exchange volume is reduced.
- Hold PD 2 days to 2 weeks after C-section. Restart with small exchange volumes.

Hypertension
- Maintain BP <140/90 mm Hg.
- Measure home BP twice daily on nondialysis days.
- Assess volume status, and treat with a trial of fluid removal.
- Avoid ACE inhibitors and angiotensin receptor blockers even in the first trimester.
- First-line drugs: α-methyldopa, labetalol, calcium channel blockers
- Second-line drugs: other beta-blockers, hydralazine, clonidine
- Start aspirin 81 mg/day.

Anemia
- Increase erythropoietin dose to maintain Hgb 10 g/dL.
- Weekly CBC, monthly iron studies
- Ferric gluconate to maintain iron saturation >15% (pregnancy category B)
- Transfuse for hemoglobin <7 g/dL.

Diet
- Increase dose of water-soluble vitamins fourfold.
- Sodium restriction for weight gain >2 L between treatments
- Protein: 1.5 g/kg + 10 g/day
- Adjust potassium and phosphorus based on chemistries.
- Adjust dry weight after weekly examination of volume status.

ACE, Angiotensin-converting enzyme; BP, blood pressure; CBC, complete blood count; HD, hemodialysis; Hgb, hemoglobin; PD, peritoneal dialysis.

intraperitoneal space interferes with transport of the ovum from the ovary to the fallopian tubes or compresses the fallopian tubes, interfering with movement of the ovum through the tubes. (See Table 95.1)

Contraception

Although the frequency of conception in dialysis patients is lower than for women using any type of birth control, sexually active women who have normal periods should use contraception if they do not wish to become pregnant. The use of oral contraceptives is safe in most dialysis patients, but these drugs should be avoided in patients with lupus and patients with problems with vascular access clotting. There is some concern that intrauterine devices may be associated with increased bleeding because of heparin use with HD. Commonly used barrier methods of contraception are safe and effective. Women with regular menses are more likely to conceive, but in at least one instance, a woman conceived after 9 years of amenorrhea. Pregnancy has occurred in women who have been on dialysis as long as 20 years and fully one fourth of the pregnancies reported in the Japanese series occurred after 10 years on dialysis. Repeat pregnancies in women who become pregnant on dialysis are not uncommon. In the 318 women whose pregnancies are recorded by the National Registry for Pregnancy in Dialysis Patients (NPDR), 8 became pregnant twice, 8 became pregnant three times, and 1 conceived four times.

Diagnosis of Pregnancy in Dialysis Patients

A high index of suspicion is required to make the diagnosis of pregnancy because amenorrhea is frequent in dialysis patients, and nausea and fatigue are often attributed to other problems. Soft signs of pregnancy may be an increase in erythropoietin requirements and difficulty with fluid removal. Because β-human chorionic gonadotropin (hCG) is removed by the kidney, β-hCG levels in dialysis patients are higher at each stage of gestation than in women with normal renal function. Borderline positive hCG levels can be seen in nonpregnant dialysis patients. The stage of gestation must be determined by ultrasonography rather than by quantitative β-hCG levels. Because β-hCG levels are higher than expected for gestational age, a high β-hCG level without a fetal heart beat may be erroneously interpreted as a nonviable pregnancy or hydatidiform mole.

Outcome of Pregnancy in Dialysis Patients

In 1980, the European Dialysis and Transplant Association reported 115 pregnancies in dialysis patients. Of those that were not electively terminated, only 23% resulted in surviving infants. Success rates for pregnancy in dialysis patients have improved somewhat since then. In Saudi Arabia, 30% of pregnancies resulted in surviving infants. The NPDR recorded 236 pregnancies not electively terminated in women who were receiving dialysis at the time of conception. Of the total, 41.5% resulted in surviving infants. Of the 165 pregnancies that reached the second trimester, 57% resulted in surviving infants. Sixteen percent of 117 live-born infants died in the neonatal period, 7.2% of pregnancies reaching the second trimester resulted in stillbirth, and 22% resulted in spontaneous abortion. The four induced abortions performed in the second trimester were done for life-threatening maternal problems (three hypertension and one critical aortic stenosis) rather than for social reasons or anticipated problems. Stillbirth appears to be less common in intensively dialyzed patients. Similar outcomes were seen in the Japanese report, with 60% of 60 pregnancies not electively terminated resulting in surviving infants. Prematurity accounted for most of the neonatal deaths. The high frequency of late pregnancy losses is an ongoing source of heartbreak for women who become pregnant and elect to continue their pregnancies. A recent report from the nocturnal HD program in Toronto had a rate of live births of 86.4% in 22 pregnancies.

Infant survival is only one measure of pregnancy success. Many of these infants are premature or small for gestational age. Eighty-five percent of infants born to women who conceived after starting dialysis reported to the NPDR were born prematurely (mean gestational, age 32.4 weeks). Thirty-six percent weighed less than 1500 g at birth, and 28% were small for gestational age. Their neonatal course was complicated by respiratory distress and other complications of prematurity. Eleven of 116 live-born infants and one stillborn infant reported to the NPDR were noted to have congenital anomalies. Eleven of 49 infants for whom follow-up data were available had long-term medical or developmental problems, most of which appear to be the result of prematurity rather than an azotemic intrauterine environment. The Japanese survey found a 4.4% rate of cerebral palsy and a 4.4% rate of cerebral atrophy in infants born to dialysis patients. The known increase in developmental abnormalities in very small infants and infants delivered 3 or more months preterm would lead us to expect a large number of problems in follow-up of these infants.

The outcome of pregnancy for women who conceive before starting dialysis is better than for those who conceive after starting dialysis, with infant survival being 77.7%.

Maternal Complications

There have been three maternal deaths reported to the NPDR. One death resulted from lupus cerebritis in a woman who started dialysis after conception. There were two deaths in women who conceived after starting dialysis, one as a result of hypertension and one from unknown causes. All three infants survived. Death of the mother before the child reaches adulthood is common.

Hypertension

Approximately 80% of dialysis patients who become pregnant have either a blood pressure (BP) greater than 140/90 mm Hg or require antihypertensive medication at some time during pregnancy. In more than half of hypertensive pregnant dialysis patients, the BP exceeds 170/110 mm Hg. In a series of 69 women in whom BP measurements were available, there were 6 intensive care unit (ICU) admissions for accelerated hypertension in addition to the 1 death. On nondialysis days, the patient should check her BP twice daily. The first line of treatment for hypertension is assessment of volume status and a trial of volume removal. If there is concern that volume removal will compromise uterine blood flow, fetal monitoring can be done during dialysis. Dialysis treatments during which fetal monitoring is done generally are carried out in an inpatient obstetric unit.

Drug Therapy

If volume removal does not control the BP, a wide variety of antihypertensive medications have been used safely in pregnancy. The major groups of drugs contraindicated in pregnancy are angiotensin-converting enzyme (ACE) inhibitors and angiotensin receptor blockers. ACE inhibitors are associated with renal dysplasia, oligohydramnios, and pulmonary hypoplasia when used in the second and third trimester. One paper reports an increase in congenital anomalies in infants exposed to ACE inhibitors in utero during the first trimester. α-Methyl dopa and hydralazine have been used in pregnant women for more than 40 years and are considered safe. Labetalol and calcium channel blockers are widely used alternatives. Calcium channel blockers may cause profound hypotension when used in conjunction with magnesium. Dialysis patients are at increased risk for preeclampsia, but the diagnosis is hard to make because many of the signs and symptoms can be either caused by renal failure or distorted by it. Hyperreflexia or only transient response to fluid removal, and antihypertensive drugs may signal the development of preeclampsia. Measurements of antiangiogenic factors to differentiate between preeclampsia and other causes of hypertension during pregnancy in women with renal disease is an area of active investigation. Dialysis patients may benefit from low-dose aspirin for prevention of preeclampsia. The risk of life-threatening hypertension persists for 6 weeks after pregnancy with 2 of the above mentioned ICU admissions occurring several weeks postpartum.

Anemia

Normal pregnancy is accompanied by a 40% to 50% increase in plasma volume and a 30% increase in red blood cell mass, mediated by increased erythropoietin. Normal hemoglobin in a pregnant woman is 11 g/dL. Dialysis patients dependent on exogenous erythropoietin have a more profound drop in hemoglobin as plasma volume increases. We previously recommended increasing the erythropoietin dose as soon as pregnancy is diagnosed. With increased concern about negative effects of erythropoietin, we now suggest increasing the dose by 25% when the hemoglobin reaches 10 g/dL or below. Further dose adjustments can be made on the basis of weekly complete blood counts. Normal pregnancy requires 700 to 1400 mg of additional iron. Ferric gluconate has been designated category B in pregnancy.

Peritonitis

There are few reports of peritonitis in pregnant PD patients. In three case reports of peritonitis during pregnancy, two resulted in premature labor with one stillbirth. Of six episodes reported to the pregnancy registry, five pregnancies resulted in surviving infants, and one resulted in spontaneous abortion remote from the time of infection. The contact of the fallopian tubes with the peritoneal fluid leads to a high risk of either ascending or descending infection. There is one case report of a postpartum uterine infection resulting in peritonitis requiring catheter removal. Penicillins and cephalosporins are the preferred antibiotics for treating peritonitis. Clindamycin can be used in penicillin-allergic women. Amphotericin can be used for fungal peritonitis. Other antibiotics and antifungal agents are used if considered necessary for the mother's safety.

Dialysis Regimen

Dialysis Modality

There is no difference in infant survival between HD and PD patients (43.9% vs 50%), but the outcome for HD patients dialyzed 20 or more hours per week may be better than the outcome for PD patients. For women starting dialysis during pregnancy, HD is usually preferable. A peritoneal catheter can be placed at any time during pregnancy, but the increased intraabdominal pressure may increase the risk of a dialysate leak.

Hemodialysis

It has been common practice to increase the amount of dialysis in pregnant women. Although information on the effect of dialysis regimens on pregnancy outcome is limited, there is increasing evidence that outcome is improved when the amount of dialysis is increased to 20 or more per week. Infant survival in women dialyzed more than 20 hours per week was 79% compared with 44% in women dialyzed less than 20 hours per week ($p <.05$). Infants of mothers dialyzed 20 or more hours per week are less likely to be born prematurely. Seventy-seven percent of infants born to mothers dialyzed more than 20 hours per week were born at more than 32 weeks' gestation compared with 37.5% of infants born to women receiving less dialysis. The 22 pregnancies in 17 nocturnal HD patients reported from Toronto are a small group but the outcomes are much better than other groups. The nocturnal dialysis patients are all cared for by the same team so that first trimester abortions are less likely to be missed. They are cared for by an obstetric group for whom pregnancy in dialysis patients is no longer an unusual event. The infant survival rate is 86.4%. These women received an average of 40 hours per week of dialysis. There is one report of 100% fetal survival with 1.5 to 3.5 hours of dialysis daily, but this group contains a large number of women who started dialysis after conception. There was also an improvement in polyhydramnios with the increased dialysis dose in this cohort.

The advent of short daily dialysis revealed some of the electrolyte abnormalities that will be seen with intensified dialysis. Hypokalemia may occur, and a 3 or 3.5 mEq/L potassium bath may be required. Some patients no longer require phosphate binders, and, in rare cases, phosphorus has to be added to the bath. The target bicarbonate for a pregnant woman is 18 to 20 mEq/L because of the respiratory alkalosis associated with pregnancy. It may be necessary to decrease the dialysate bicarbonate to 25 mEq/L. With severe alkalosis, hemodiafiltration can be done, replacing ultrafiltered fluid with a bicarbonate-free solution. A dialysate calcium of 2.5 mEq/L is usually enough to provide the 30 g of calcium necessary to calcify the fetal skeleton. All adjustments should be made based on weekly measurements of electrolytes, calcium, and phosphorus.

Heparin does not cross the placenta. The lowest dose of heparin possible should be used, but efforts to dialyze the patient without heparin frequently result in blood loss from clotting of the extracorporeal circuit. It is reasonable to use heparin as long as there is no vaginal bleeding.

Peritoneal Dialysis

Because conception is unusual in PD patients, there are no data on the efficacy of different dialysis regimens. It is reasonable to attempt to increase the amount of dialysis delivered by 50%. The increase may require combining a cycler with several daytime exchanges. Maintaining such a dialysis regimen becomes more difficult late in pregnancy because abdominal discomfort may require decreasing the exchange volume. In some instances, PD has been supplemented by HD.

If a pregnant woman has blood in the peritoneal fluid, she should be hospitalized to evaluate the cause. Hemoperitoneum may signal an impending spontaneous abortion or placental separation. In one instance, severe blood loss occurred when the peritoneal catheter lacerated a dilated vessel on the surface of the uterus.

Diet

The increase in dialysis time usually allows the pregnant woman to eat without dietary restrictions, but the diet should be reviewed frequently with the renal nutritionist. Early in pregnancy, it may be difficult to maintain adequate calorie and protein intake. Caloric intake should be 35 g/kg plus an additional 300 calories for the pregnancy. Protein intake should be 1.5 g/kg plus 10 g for the pregnancy. The dose of water-soluble vitamins should be increased because of the increased requirements in pregnancy and the increased removal with intensive dialysis. The folate dose should be increased to 4 mg/day because folate deficiency during pregnancy is associated with neural tube defects. Dietary potassium and the use of phosphate binders can be guided by weekly laboratory measurements. Sodium restriction may be necessary if there are excessive weight gains between treatments.

We do not prescribe a specific overall weight gain because there is a risk that this would be achieved by inadequate fluid removal at dialysis. The best approach is careful assessment of the volume status by a physician on a weekly basis with adjustment of the dialysis regimen to achieve euvolemia.

Obstetric Considerations

Premature Labor

The greatest cause of fetal loss in pregnant dialysis patients is premature delivery. There is a continuum from second trimester spontaneous abortions to premature births. β-Agonists, indomethacin, calcium channel blockers, and magnesium have been used as tocolytics. Indomethacin is effective particularly in women with polyhydramnios, but the time the dialysis patient requires for treatment for premature labor usually exceeds the recommended time for using the drug. The fetus needs to be monitored for right heart strain. There may be a loss of residual renal function with the use of indomethacin. Magnesium is also suited for short-term use. If magnesium is used either for premature labor or for preeclampsia, the patient should not receive a continuous magnesium infusion but rather a loading dose with supplementation after dialysis. In PD patients, intraperitoneal magnesium has been used to treat premature labor. There is no experience with progestational agents in dialysis patients, but any effective treatment for premature labor that is not contraindicated in renal failure should be attempted in these women because they are at higher risk of premature delivery than almost any other group of pregnant women. None of the agents is suitable for long-term use in women whose premature labor occurs remote from term.

Frequently, there is marked cervical dilatation with relatively mild contractions. Incompetent cervix is enough of a problem that measurement of cervical length should be incorporated into obstetric care. In the 22 pregnancies in nocturnal HD patients, 4 had cervical shortening.

Cesarean delivery need only be performed for the usual obstetric indications. When it is performed in a PD patient, it can be done extraperitoneally. Dialysis has been resumed as early as 24 hours after delivery, but most obstetricians and nephrologists treat the patient with HD for 2 weeks postpartum to avoid incisional leaking.

The baby can be expected to have an osmotic diuresis after delivery and should be monitored in a neonatal ICU and given appropriate fluid and electrolyte replacement.

Conclusions

Pregnancy in dialysis patients is associated with serious maternal risks and with a high fetal loss rate. With careful monitoring of BP, hemoglobin, and serum chemistries, maternal risk can be minimized. With intensive dialysis and improved treatment for premature labor, the success rate for pregnancy in dialysis patients can be expected to improve. Care of the patient requires close cooperation of obstetricians, nephrologists, and neonatologists, but meticulous observation and care by the dialysis staff is the most important prerequisite for success.

Miscellaneous Areas of Clinical Importance

C H A P T E R 9 6

Treatment of Poisoning With Extracorporeal Methods

Marc Ghannoum, MD • Darren M. Roberts, MD, PhD

More than 2 million poisonings were reported to the American Association of Poison Control Centers in 2013. Outcomes are generally favorable, and supportive measures alone are sufficient to manage the majority of poisonings. In selected situations, gastrointestinal (GI) decontamination, timely administration of antidotes, and elimination enhancement treatments may be administered to prevent or reverse toxicity. Urine alkalinization was reported in 0.5% of cases, and multiple-dose activated charcoal was used in 0.06% and extracorporeal treatments (ECTRs) such as hemodialysis (HD) in 0.1% of all cases. However, the number of poisoned patients being treated with HD and related ECTRs is increasing each year, and the types of poisonings being treated are also changing with time. This prompts review and consideration of the indications for ECTRs and operational characteristics that maximize the effect of such treatments.

General Overview of the Treatment of the Poisoned Patient

Background

The range of drugs, chemicals, and natural toxins that can induce poisoning is vast, as are their manifestations. Whereas acute poisoning follows intentional self-poisoning or prescribing or dosing error, chronic poisoning most commonly follows a prescribing or dosing error such as a drug interaction or intercurrent conditions such as impaired kidney function.

Initial Treatment

The initial steps to the treatment of a poisoned patient are resuscitation, close observation, and supportive care. Careful attention to these basic critical care skills is central to management of any poisoned patient, in view of the potential for multisystem manifestations, especially when the incriminating poison is unknown. When the poison exposure is confirmed, toxicity should be anticipated so that necessary interventions can be instituted. Patients who are clinically unstable, or may become so, should be managed in a critical care environment. Early intubation is commonly required for airway protection and is often performed preemptively. Hypotension may be cardiogenic, hypovolemic, or distributive in nature, depending on the poison, and resuscitation, inotrope or vasopressor support is guided by the specific etiology. Supportive care may also include correction of poison-induced dysrhythmias, hypothermia or hyperthermia, and seizures according to current recommendations (reviewed elsewhere).

Risk Assessment

After resuscitation, a detailed risk assessment is required to guide further treatment. The risk assessment is a detailed cognitive process that incorporates consideration of the exposure (type and amount), time since the exposure, resources required such as critical care support, antidotes, and access to ECTRs in a clinically reasonable time frame. This may be supported by blood tests, such as the anion gap, an osmolal gap, or a poison concentration. The risk assessment guides the duration of observation, place for admission, and treatments required. For example, it may prompt transfer to another institution for the purpose of treatment with ECTR. Prompt communication with a regional poison center may advise on various elements of the risk assessment and offer valuable expertise on management issues.

Decontamination

Decontamination is defined as prevention of absorption of a poison. This may be dermal if relevant (e.g., chemical spills) or GI, for which various therapeutic options are available. When GI decontamination is required, activated charcoal 1 to 2 g/kg enterally is usually the preferred agent for most poisons. Its effect is limited to use with organic nonpolar poisons. Its main beneficial effect is within 1 hour of ingestion, although delayed administration may have a role with massive exposures, sustained-release preparations, or poisonings associated with delayed gut transit (e.g., opioid agonists or anticholinergic drugs).

Whole-bowel irrigation using polyethylene glycol 1 to 2 L/h enterally is sometimes used in the treatment of poisonings with sustained-release medications; massive exposures; or those that are not adsorbed to charcoal, such as metals including lithium, iron, and lead. Gastric lavage, cathartics, and forced emesis have a minimal role in the majority of poisonings.

Antidotes

Antidotes are available for a range of poisons and can reverse or reduce toxicity, such as naloxone for opioid poisoning, alcohol or fomepizole for toxic alcohols, oxygen for carbon monoxide, chelators for certain metals, sodium bicarbonate for sodium channel blocking agents, methylene blue for methemoglobinemia, and others.

In the event that an ECTR is required for the treatment of such a poisoning, it is necessary to ascertain whether the ECTR will remove the antidote so that the antidote dosage can be adjusted accordingly. Otherwise the antidote dosage may result in therapeutic failure; this has been demonstrated for *N*-acetylcysteine, ethanol, and fomepizole.

Enhanced Elimination

A final but important consideration in the medical treatment of poisoning is the potential benefit of enhanced elimination. Here, treatments increase the total clearance of the poisoning, with the aim of shortening the duration or severity of poisoning.

Multiple doses of activated charcoal (MDAC) are recommended to enhance the elimination of a number of poisons, including carbamazepine, dapsone, quinine, phenobarbital, and theophylline. MDAC may also facilitate elimination of cardiac glycosides, phenytoin, aspirin, colchicine, and amatoxin. The specific mechanism of action may not be completely understood but may relate to interruption of entero-hepatic circulation, enteral dialysis, or interfering with a prolonged absorption phase.

Urinary alkalinization with sodium bicarbonate can enhance the elimination or reduce nephrotoxicity of some poisons. Increasing urine pH either promotes solubility of the poison, or in the case of weak acids (i.e., with a dissociation constant, pKa, slightly lower than the urinary physiologic pH), it increases the proportion of poison that is ionized, which enhances urinary elimination. An important practical application of urine alkalinization is for salicylate, chlorophenoxy herbicides (e.g., 2-methyl-4-chlorophenoxyacetic acid, 2,4-dichlorophenoxyacetic acid), and to a lesser extent for methotrexate, myoglobin, and fluoride. It has also been used in phenobarbital poisoning, but the effect is less than that of MDAC, and the effect of both treatments simultaneously appears to be less than that of MDAC alone, so it is only used if MDAC cannot be given (e.g., because of ileus). Potential complications associated with urine alkalinization are alkalemia, hypokalemia, hypocalcemia, hypernatremia, and volume overload.

Extracorporeal treatments can significantly enhance the elimination of a range of poisons (as well as their metabolites), and these are discussed later in this chapter.

Characteristics of a Potentially Dialyzable Toxin

In the context of treating poisoning, it is necessary to understand key principles that promote solute removal by ECTR. This reflects properties of the poison, and these are defined by its physicochemical and pharmacokinetic parameters. Factors governing poison removal are the same as those for uremic toxins.

Physicochemical

Smaller-sized molecules are more effectively removed by ECTRs. Previous filter technology limited removal of poisons to those that were less than approximately 500 daltons, but current membranes allow removal of poisons with molecular weight up to 10,000 daltons by HD and 50,000 daltons by hemofiltration (HF). Protein-bound poisons cannot cross most filters or dialyzers because the size of the complex exceeds the cutoff of most filters. In contrast, protein binding is less of a barrier to achieving a high clearance if hemoperfusion (HP) cartridges are used. A particular consideration in poisoning is that protein binding can become saturated at very high concentrations (such as is the case for salicylate and valproic acid), resulting in a relatively higher concentration that is unbound to plasma proteins and therefore crosses the HD filters to a more significant extent than that noted at lower concentrations.

Pharmacokinetics

Extracorporeal treatments are useful if they enhance elimination because there is a significant increase in total clearance relative to endogenous clearance. The larger the proportion that extracorporeal clearance increases total clearance, the more useful the procedure. Poison clearance achieved by an ECTR is at best 400 mL/min, but it is usually much lower. Various factors influence endogenous clearance, including organ injury, when it has an impact on the route of metabolism and elimination of the compound. For example, a number of medicines are predominantly eliminated by the kidneys, so clearance is reduced in the context of impaired kidney function. Endogenous clearance may also vary depending on nutrient availability, when the nutrient is a cofactor in the catabolism of the poison (e.g., folate or folinic acid and methanol). Specific guidance regarding what constitutes potentially significant extracorporeal versus endogenous clearance may depend on the type of poison, time since presentation, and mechanism of toxicity. Additionally, because ECTRs remove poison directly from the intravascular space, poisons that exhibit a low volume of distribution (<1–2 L/kg) are best suited for extracorporeal removal. However, ECTR is useful only if the decrease in blood concentration results in a decrease of the poison concentration at the site of toxicity.

Choice of Extracorporeal Treatment

Although the favored extracorporeal modalities for the correction of uremia usually involve the use of intermittent HD, peritoneal dialysis (PD), or continuous renal replacement therapy (CRRT), several other ECTRs have been advocated for enhancing the elimination of poison (Table 96.1). Ultimately, the choice of an ECTR will depend on the poison's physicochemical characteristics, the patient's condition, comorbid conditions, and local availability of ECTRs.

Hemodialysis

During HD, poison diffuses from the blood into a countercurrent dialysate, both of which are separated by a semipermeable membrane (Table 96.2). Characteristics of poison removal by HD include a low molecular size (<10,000 Da), a low volume of distribution, and a low protein binding (<80%).

Hemodialysis has several distinct advantages over other ECTRs in the management of acute poisonings: Common poisons have a low molecular size (<1000 Da) and are ideally suited for HD elimination. HD also corrects conditions associated with certain poisonings such as acute kidney injury (AKI), volume overload, acid–base abnormalities, and electrolyte disturbances. HD is more widely available, less costly, and less often fraught with complications compared with HP or plasma exchange, for example.

Hemoperfusion

During HP, blood passes over a charcoal-coated column (resins are no longer available in the United States) on to which poison is adsorbed. HP is better suited for larger molecules and for protein-bound poisons than HD but cannot adsorb alcohols and most metals. Charcoal cartridges are seldom available in dialysis units and are approximately 10 times more expensive than a high-flux dialyzer. Cartridges can also nonselectively adsorb glucose, platelets, calcium, and white blood cells, which may have clinical repercussions in poisoning situations. This nonselective binding of plasma components may contribute to early saturation of the cartridge, requiring

Table 96.1

Summary of Extracorporeal Treatments*

Technique	Process	Protein Binding Cutoff	Molecular Cutoff (Da)	Maximal Clearance	Relative Cost	Complications	Comments
Hemodialysis	Diffusion	<80%	<10,000	400 mL/min	+	+	Correction of uremia and acid–base/E+ disorders
Hemoperfusion	Adsorption	<95%	<50,000	350 mL/min	++	+++	Saturation of cartridge
Hemofiltration	Convection	<80%	<50,000	400 mL/min	++	+	Correction of uremia and acid–base/E+ disorders
Therapeutic plasma exchange	Centrifugation, separation, filtration	None	<1,000,000	50 mL/min	+++	+++	
Albumin dialysis	Diffusion, adsorption	<95%	<300,000	400 mL/min	+++	++	Liver replacement support
Exchange transfusion	Centrifugation, separation, filtration	None	None	10 mL/min	++	++	Simpler in neonates Correction of hemolysis
Peritoneal dialysis	Diffusion	<80%	<5000	15 mL/min	++	++	

*All extracorporeal treatments above are less likely to be useful for poisons that have a high volume of distribution or a high endogenous clearance.

Table 96.2

Factors That May Enhance Poison Clearance During Hemodialysis

Larger surface area of dialysis membrane
High-flux dialyzer
High blood and dialysate flow
Increased ultrafiltration rate (with replacement solution)
Increased time on dialysis
A vascular site that has less recirculation
Two dialyzers in series
Two distinct extracorporeal circuits

it to be replaced every 2 to 3 hours to maintain high clearances. HP can also cause hemolysis; to prevent this, the circuit requires more systemic anticoagulation than with HD, and the blood flow must be limited to less than 350 mL/min.

The role of HP has recently come into question when comparing poison clearances from HP to those achieved with high-efficiency dialyzers. In addition, HP does not allow for correction of uremia and electrolyte or acid–base disturbances. For these reasons, HD is generally preferred in almost all settings when HP is considered indicated.

Hemofiltration

During HF, solute and solvent are removed by solute drag, a process known as convection, and replaced by a physiologic solution (see Chapter 27). Poisons that are eliminated by HD will also be eliminated by HF. Although dialyzers do not allow passage of poisons that are larger than 10,000 Da, hemofilters have a cutoff of approximately 50,000 Da. This has relatively little clinical relevance in toxicology considering that the overwhelming proportion of drugs and poisons have a molecular size below 1000 Da. However, some data suggest that myoglobin may be cleared by HF, which is notable because rhabdomyolysis is noted to occur from some poisonings.

Continuous Renal Replacement Therapy

Continuous techniques (see Chapter 28) are a popular choice for the management of AKI in the critical care setting. These modalities are attractive because net fluid removal can be extended over 24 hours instead of the usual 4 hours, thereby reducing the risk of hypotension. However, this advantage appears marginal in most poisonings in which fluid overload is rarely present. Another popular argument for continuous techniques is the avoidance of the usual increase in poison blood concentration after ECTR ("rebound"). When rebound is caused by redistribution of poison from intracellular or extravascular compartments to the plasma, this surge in plasma concentration may be balanced by a decrease in poison concentration away from its toxic compartments if this is located extravascularly. It is therefore disputable if rebound from this scenario would be clinically detrimental. If concerning, for example, with dabigatran in which the rebound may increase bleeding risk, the rebound can be minimized by a prolonged dialysis session, by a switch to CRRT, or with a subsequent dialysis session. Although the postulated advantages for CRRT may be disputed, their major downside is lesser poison clearance by virtue of lower blood and effluent flows. This underlies present recommendations supporting a preference for high-efficiency intermittent ECTR unless local factors prevent the use of intermittent high-efficiency dialysis.

Peritoneal Dialysis

The role of PD in acute poisoning remains dubious because more efficient techniques are able to offer poison clearances that are more than 10-fold greater than those obtained with PD. PD should only be considered in severe poisonings involving infants or when other modalities are unavailable.

Therapeutic Plasma Exchange

Therapeutic plasma exchange (TPE) is a process by which plasma is separated from blood cells, discarded, and then replaced by either albumin or fresh-frozen plasma. Plasma clearance during plasma exchange is usually limited to 50 mL/min. The role of TPE in the treatment of acute poisoning is not well defined, but this method should only be considered for poisons that are highly protein bound (>95%) or in poisons with a molecular size over the cutoffs accepted for HF or HP (>50,000 Da), such as monoclonal antibodies. Adverse outcomes from plasma exchange involve complications associated with placement of the vascular access, bleeding, hypocalcemia, and hypersensitivity reactions to the replacement plasma proteins.

Exchange Transfusion

Exchange transfusion (ET) is a treatment in which whole blood is removed and replaced with transfused blood products. Poison clearance is very limited during ET (10–15 mL/min); however, ET does not require a central venous access and sophisticated machinery, so it may be considered in settings where HD is not available, especially in infants, in whom ET is easier to perform in this population.

Liver Support Devices (Albumin Dialysis)

Liver support devices (LSDs) were developed to support liver function in the context of fulminant hepatic failure or cirrhosis. These devices theoretically remove albumin-bound toxins and xenobiotics better than the more commonly used diffusive and convective techniques. However, preliminary clearance data do not show any superiority for LSDs in poisonings to theophylline, valproic acid, or phenytoin. Because of their very limited availability and high cost (>$10,000 per treatment), they are usually reserved temporarily as a bridge to liver transplantation or spontaneous remission rather than for their capacity to eliminate poison. Several reports describe the use of LSDs in toxin-induced hepatotoxicity, especially to *Amanita* mushroom and acetaminophen, although the practical applicability of these techniques remains uncertain.

Technical Considerations

Poisoned patients have clinical characteristics that differ from those with either AKI or end-stage renal disease. The application of any ECTR should therefore reflect these differences.

Vascular Access: A double-lumen central catheter is required for administering most forms of ECTRs. The femoral site is often preferred for its simplicity but has more recirculation than subclavian or jugular sites.

Choice of Hemodialyzer, Filter, and Adsorber: The dialyzer or hemofilter should have a molecular size cutoff above that of the poison. High-efficiency dialyzers with the larger surface areas will improve clearance of low-molecular-size poisons. With respect to HP, the only column available in the United States is the Gambro Adsorba 300c, a coated activated charcoal cartridge.

Anticoagulation: Heparinization of the dialysis circuit (via unfractionated heparin or low-molecular-weight heparin) should be considered to prevent clotting and maintain patency of the circuit. In patients at high risk of bleeding, saline flushes can be used instead of anticoagulation. For HP, heparin is also used to reduce the risk of hemolysis and is usually required in greater quantities than HD.

Blood, Dialysate, and Effluent Flow: These should all be maximized according to the capabilities of the machine to maximize clearance.

Dialysate Composition: As mentioned, poisoned patients may not share the same metabolic characteristics as those with renal failure. Bicarbonate, sodium, calcium, and magnesium need to be adjusted in the dialysate bath (or replacement fluid) to the requirement of the poisoned patient. Phosphate may also be added to the bath to avoid hypophosphatemia.

Duration of Extracorporeal Treatment: A single 6-hour ECTR will usually suffice to substantially lower blood levels of most xenobiotics, although the length of the procedure will ultimately depend on the efficacy of the procedure used and the body burden of poison to remove.

Patient Disposition: Many poisoned patients die before initiation of dialysis. If the risk analysis on a suspected toxic exposure suggests that a patient may require dialysis, prompt communication with a dialysis unit and consideration of preemptive transfer to one may be required even if the patient does not yet meet criteria for blood purification. Because significant delays may occur between the time a decision is taken to perform ECTR and the time when it is initiated, a dialysis nurse should be rapidly contacted and a temporary dialysis catheter installed as early as possible. Logistics and clinical status may require transfer of the patient to the intensive care unit (ICU). After ECTR, serial poison concentration and clinical status should be monitored for a period long enough to account for redistribution or ongoing absorption ($\approx$12–24 hours). The catheter should remain in place until the physician is convinced that additional sessions are unnecessary.

General Principles Regarding the Use of Extracorporeal Treatment in the Treatment of Poisoning

The decision to initiate any form of blood purification must take into account the patient's clinical status, the benefit expected from ECTRs, and poison-related factors.

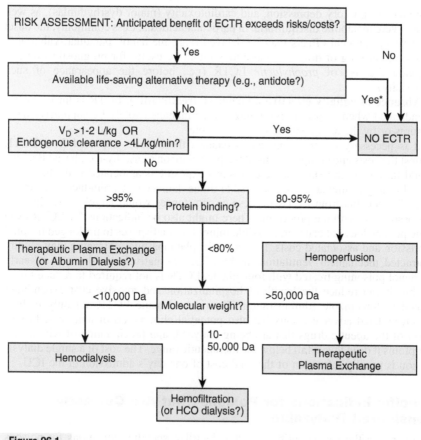

Figure 96.1

Stepwise approach to extracorporeal treatment in poisoning contexts.
(Reproduced with permission from Ghannoum M, Roberts DM, Hoffman RS,
et al. A stepwise approach for the management of poisoning with extracorporeal
treatments. *Semin Dial* 2014;27(4):362-370.)

Absolute indications for ECTR are summarized in Fig. 96.1 and include the following (all must be present):

1. **The ECTR must be able to remove the poison to a significant extent:** This
   has been discussed earlier. Specifically, the poison is dialyzable if (a) it readily
   passes through the extracorporeal membrane, (b) it has a low volume of distribution, and (c) clearance by ECTR represents a significant portion of total body
   clearance. In addition, the extent of removal also reflects ECTR-related factors
   such as membrane type, membrane surface area, and blood and dialysate flow
   rates (see Table 96.1).
2. **The risk of severe poisoning must be present.** ECTR should be considered
   when life-threatening conditions resulting from a poisoning are either present or
   are expected to occur. Clinical signs include neurotoxicity (e.g., repeated seizures,

coma), respiratory depression, and cardiotoxicity (major dysrhythmias), as well as severe metabolic disequilibria, in particular acidosis. Less commonly, the onset of severe clinical effects may be delayed (e.g., methanol, paraquat, valproate), and monitoring of drug concentrations might be useful for prognostication and guide the use of *prophylactic* ECTR (i.e., before the appearance of such toxicity).

3. **Absence of equally effective alternative treatment(s)**. ECTR is uncommonly indicated when a specific poisoning can be managed solely by supportive measures or by the administration of an antidote.

It is necessary for the clinician to balance the benefits expected from ECTR against the costs and complications of the procedure on a case-by-case basis: Benefits would far outweigh risks when the poison's exposure is associated with short-term mortality (e.g., salicylates) or irreversible tissue damage (e.g., blindness for methanol). The benefits from ECTR in these circumstances would largely outweigh any risk associated with the procedure. There might also be indications for ECTR even if the poison does not cause irreversible injury but predisposes to prolonged hospital admission and associated costs. For example, phenobarbital poisoning may require protracted mechanical ventilation in the ICU. Alternatively, in the case of early methanol poisoning treated with fomepizole, ECTR is not required to reduce toxicity, but it can reduce the length of hospitalization and massive cost expenditure related to fomepizole administration. The risks of acute ECTR not only include catheter-related adverse events but also potential elimination of antidotes, loss of effect of therapeutic drugs that are being dialyzed, and precipitation of withdrawal symptoms if drug levels fall below the therapeutic range. The cost of a single dialysis session is usually a fraction of the total cost of one day's admission in the ICU.

Specific Indications for Poisons That Are Currently Considered Dialyzable

Incorporating the various principles stated earlier, specific indications for poisons that are commonly considered potentially amenable to enhanced elimination by ECTR are presented in Table 96.3. This reflects recent consensus statements by the Extracorporeal Treatments in Poisoning Workshop (EXTRP) workgroup (http://www.extrip-workgroup.org), but it is an area of ongoing research and review. Other publications have identified other drugs and poisons that have been treated with ECTR, including poisoning from paraquat, baclofen, pregabalin, and dabigatran for which ECTR may also be considered. In contrast, there are no indications for ECTR for tricyclic antidepressant, digoxin, benzodiazepine, or ethanol poisoning and the indications for phenytoin poisoning remain debated.

Table 96.3

Summary of Recommendations for Extracorporeal Treatment in Poisons Amenable to Extracorporeal Removal

Poison	Indications Poison Concentration	Clinical and Laboratory	Choice of ECTR	Cessation of ECTR When	Other Considerations
Acetaminophen	>1000 mg/L	Metabolic acidosis, coma	HD > CRRT	Clinical improvement	Dose of NAC should be at least doubled. Coadminister MDAC.
Barbiturates (long acting)	Increasing or persisting (barbiturate)	Coma, mechanical ventilation, shock	HD > HP/ CRRT	Clinical improvement	
Carbamazepine		Refractory seizures, life-threatening dysrhythmias, prolonged coma, respiratory depression requiring mechanical ventilation, toxicity despite MDAC	HD > CRRT/ HP	Clinical improvement *or* carbamazepine <10 mg/L	MDAC therapy should be continued.
Dabigatran		Active bleeding and abnormal coagulation parameters	HD > CRRT	Significant improvement of coagulation parameters and bleeding cessation	Closely monitor coagulation parameters and clinical signs of bleeding after ECTR.
Lithium	>5.0 mEq/L	Decreased LOC, seizures, dysrhythmias, impaired kidney function	HD > CRRT	Clinical improvement *or* Li <1.0 mEq/L	
Ethylene glycol	>50 mg/dL (if ethanol used) >30 mg/dL (if no antidote used)	Shock, coma, seizures, anion gap >24 mmol/L, AKI	HD > CRRT	Clinical improvement AND ethylene glycol <10 mg/dL	ECTR may not be required if normal kidney function. The dose of antidotes (ethanol or fomepizole) must be adjusted during ECTR.

Continued

Table 96.3

Summary of Recommendations for Extracorporeal Treatment in Poisons Amenable to Extracorporeal Removal—cont'd

Poison	Poison Concentration	Indications Clinical and Laboratory	Choice of ECTR	Cessation of ECTR When	Other Considerations
Metformin	>90 mg/dL	Shock, failure of standard supportive measures, decreased LOC, (lactate) >20 mmol/L, pH <7.0	HD > CRRT	lactate <3 mmol/L *and* pH >7.35	Repeat sessions using HD or CRRT. Closely monitor lactate and pH for additional ECTR courses.
Methanol	>70 mg/dL (if fomepizole used) >60 mg/dL (if ethanol used) >50 mg/dL (if no antidote used)	Coma, seizures, new vision deficits, pH ≤7.15, anion gap >24 mmol/L	HD > CRRT	Clinical improvement *and* methanol <20 mg/dL	The dose of antidotes (ethanol or fomepizole) must be adjusted during ECTR. Folic acid should be continued during ECTR.
Salicylates	>90 mg/dL	Altered mental status, ARDS, impaired renal function, pH ≤7.20	HD > HP > CRRT	Clinical improvement AND salicylate <20 mg/dL	ET may be used in children/ Coadminister MDAC.
Theophylline	>100 mg/L (acute exposure) >60 mg/L (chronic poisoning)	Seizures, life-threatening dysrhythmias, shock, clinical deterioration despite optimal care, GI decontamination cannot be administered	HD > HP > CRRT	Clinical improvement *or* theophylline <15 mg/L	Coadminister MDAC.
Valproic acid	>900 mg/L	Cerebral edema, coma, shock, acute hyperammonemia, pH ≤7.10, respiratory depression	HD > CRRT/ HP	Clinical improvement or VPA <100 mg/L	

AKI, Acute kidney injury; ARDS, acute respiratory distress syndrome; CRRT, continuous renal replacement therapy; ECTR, extracorporeal treatment; ET, exchange transfusion; GI, gastrointestinal; HD, intermittent hemodialysis; HP, hemoperfusion; LOC, level of consciousness; MDAC, multiple doses of activated charcoal; NAC, N-acetylcysteine; VPA, Valproic Acid.

C H A P T E R 9 7

Preventive Care in End-Stage Renal Disease

Jean L. Holley, MD

Preventive care of dialysis patients encompasses general medical care issues as well as dialysis-specific issues that are detailed in preceding chapters. In this chapter, aspects of general medical preventive care are discussed as they apply to chronic dialysis patients. The transplant status of a patient will affect some of these issues; for example, recommendations for cancer screening and immunizations will in part depend on the patient's transplant status, and when relevant, this will be noted. Individual patient recommendations for preventive care are based on the individual patient's prognosis and risk factors. The suggestions for appropriate preventive care for dialysis patients that follow need to be individualized for specific patients by their nephrologists and dialysis care providers. Preventive care can be categorized into immunizations, infection prevention, screening, health care counseling, advance care planning (ACP) and supportive care, and disease monitoring. Each of these is discussed in this chapter.

Immunizations

Table 97.1 lists the Centers for Disease Control and Prevention (CDC) recommendations for immunizations in dialysis patients based on age and transplant status. Although dialysis patients generally have a reduced immunologic response and develop lower and less sustained antibody titers to immunizations, the CDC recommends vaccinating all dialysis patients. Despite less robust antibody responses, dialysis patients may be protected from infection, and vaccinating dialysis patients may reduce the risk for virus transmission in dialysis units. Altering immunization schedules and vaccine doses may in some cases improve the antibody response in dialysis patients. Dual vaccination (e.g., simultaneous tetanus and hepatitis B) has also been observed to improve antibody responses in dialysis patients. Live vaccines (varicella zoster, intranasal influenza, measles, mumps, rubella, yellow fever, bacillus Calmette-Guérin, and oral *Salmonella typhi*) should not be administered to transplanted and immunosuppressed patients and thus should be given based on clinical circumstances.

Hepatitis B Vaccine

Table 97.1 summarizes the recommendations for vaccination. Because hepatitis B is transmitted via inoculation through exchange of blood products or body fluids and was responsible for infection outbreaks in dialysis units in the 1980s, hepatitis B vaccination is recommended for all dialysis patients, and monitoring for antibody

Table 97.1

Recommended Adult Immunizations for Dialysis Patients

Vaccine	Dosing and Information
Hepatitis B	40 µg of Recombivax HD on three-dose schedule or 40 µg of Engerix-B on four-dose schedule
Hepatitis A	Only if another risk factor is present
Human papillomavirus	Female—3 doses through age 26 years
	Male—3 doses through age 21 years
Influenza	Age ≥19 years; on dose trivalent vaccine yearly
Measles, mumps, rubella	One or two doses if no immunity
Meningococcal	Only if another risk factor is present
Pneumococcal	One or two doses
Tetanus, diphtheria pertussis	One-time dose of Tdap (tetanus, diphtheria, and pertussis); then boost with Td (tetanus and diphtheria) every 10 years
Varicella zoster	Two doses if no evidence of immunity age >60 years; one dose

Based on Centers for Disease Control and Prevention. Recommended Adult Immunization Schedule. http://www.cdc.gov/vaccines/schedules/downloads/adult/mmwr-adult-schedule.pdf.

protection is required. Only 34% to 88% of dialysis patients will develop immunity through vaccination, which is therefore suggested early in chronic kidney disease (CKD) to take advantage of an improved immune response with less severe kidney disease. Vaccine manipulations (increased dose, extra doses, coadministration of immune modulators or other vaccines) may improve the antibody response in dialysis patients. Patients who do not respond to an initial vaccination series should have the series repeated once. Patients who lose antibody titers after an initial response to vaccine should receive a booster dose. The precise timing of monitoring antibody titers is unclear.

Influenza and H1N1 Vaccine

Similar to the case with other vaccines, dialysis patients develop variable responses to influenza; 36% to 90% develop protective antibodies. Response to the H1N1 vaccine is similar with 33% to 64% of dialysis patients developing antibodies. Older studies suggested that hospitalization and secondary pneumonia were more common among dialysis patients with influenza, leading to the recommendation that all dialysis patients receive yearly influenza vaccines. A more recent study suggested only a small benefit of influenza vaccination in dialysis patients but raised the issue of addressing vaccination strategies to maximize dialysis patient vaccine response (e.g., high-dose trivalent vaccine may be preferable in dialysis patients as it is in older adults; see Table 97.1).

Tetanus, Pneumococcal, Human Papillomavirus, and Varicella Zoster Vaccines

There are few studies of antibody response to these vaccines in dialysis patients. Similar to other vaccines, the antibody response tends to be suboptimal and short-lived. The CDC continues to recommend routine vaccination of dialysis patients with these vaccines (see Table 97.1). If the patient was younger than 65 years of age upon initial pneumococcal vaccination, an additional dose should be given 5 years later. A tetanus, diphtheria, acellular pertussis vaccine became available in the United States in 2005 for those 11 to 64 years of age. A single booster vaccine dose is suggested for adults and is given 2 years or less after the initial vaccine in high-risk individuals. There is little information on the safety and efficacy of varicella zoster and human papillomavirus (HPV) vaccines in dialysis patients. The CDC recommends HPV in age-appropriate individuals with end-stage renal disease (ESRD) (see Table 97.1).

Infection Prevention

Probably because of their impaired immune response, including reduced B- and T-cell responses and phagocytosis, dialysis patients have an increased incidence of and are at increased risk of poor outcomes and complications with bacterial infections. Efforts to reduce dialysis access–associated infections may include the local application of antibiotic creams to access exit sites and intranasal application of antistaphylococcal creams in nasal carriers. Antimicrobial prophylaxis should also be considered a preventive strategy.

Diabetic Foot Care

A routine diabetic foot care program, including nursing assessment and patient education, may be associated with improved footwear adequacy and a reduction in neuropathy, ultimately leading to fewer foot ulcers and wounds.

Dental Care

Periodontal disease, premature tooth loss, and xerostomia are more common among dialysis patients and can lead to systemic inflammation and morbidity. Some have implicated periodontal disease as an inflammatory factor contributing to cardiovascular disease in dialysis patients. Gingivitis and periodontitis are manifestations of poor dental health and are more common in dialysis patients. The cause of periodontal disease in dialysis patients is unclear, but impaired humoral responses and possibly bacterial colonization in response to repeated gingival bleeding from heparinization during dialysis have been postulated. Routine dental care (brushing, flossing, use of mouthwashes, and preventive care by dentists and hygienists) is also less common among dialysis patients. In addition, renal osteodystrophy can involve the mandible and maxilla, resulting in tooth mobility, malocclusion, enamel hypoplasia, metastatic soft tissue calcifications, and demineralization. Educating patients about the importance of routine preventive dental care may help to avoid subsequent issues and infections.

Endocarditis Prophylaxis

There are no data on the usefulness of antibiotic prophylaxis to prevent endocarditis in dialysis patients. However, for patients with known valvular abnormalities, prosthetic heart valves, congenital heart abnormalities, a history of endocarditis, or a heart transplant, antibiotic prophylaxis before dental or periodontal procedures is recommended. A single oral dose of amoxicillin (2 g) or clindamycin (600 mg) in those allergic to penicillin 1 hour before the procedure is recommended. Because of the high risk of endocarditis in the setting of a venous catheter, dialysis patients with tunneled catheters should probably be considered for antibiotic prophylaxis despite the lack of such recommendations by the American Heart Association (AHA). The generalized immune-suppressed state of ESRD prompts some to argue for antibiotic prophylaxis for all dialysis patients undergoing invasive procedures and dental treatments. There are reports of peritonitis occurring after colonoscopy with biopsy in peritoneal dialysis (PD) patients. For this reason, many nephrologists suggest antibiotic prophylaxis according to the AHA endocarditis prevention guidelines in PD patients undergoing colonoscopies. All PD patients should undergo such procedures with a dry peritoneum to reduce the risk of bacterial seeding of the peritoneal cavity filled with dextrose-rich dialysate.

Tuberculosis Screening

Tuberculosis (TB) is more common in ESRD patients, ranging from 6 to 25 times higher than in the general population. Dialysis patients also have a higher risk of developing clinical TB after exposure. Thus, it is important to detect latent TB infection and offer treatment. The tuberculin skin test is based on a delayed hypersensitivity response to a purified protein derivative (PPD) of *Mycobacterium tuberculosis* but has limited sensitivity in dialysis patients. T-cell interferon-γ release assays are now available as screening tests for *M. tuberculosis* infection and seem to be more sensitive screening tests for latent TB infection in ESRD patients. Because of the possible spread of TB in a dialysis unit, consideration should be given to screening patients with one of the interferon-γ release assays (QuantiFERON-TB Gold In-Tube or T-SPOT.TB).

Screening

Several screening protocols are recommended in the general population, many of which can be reviewed online at the American Preventive Task Force's website (http://www.uspreventiveservicestaskforce.org). Some of the recommendations for screening for disease in the general population may be applicable to dialysis patients, but many will not be, in large part because dialysis patients have a lower expected survival, making development of the disease for which screening is suggested unlikely. When considering screening in general, therefore, it is important to consider not only the risk of that disease in the population being screened but also the likelihood that the patient to be screened will live long enough to benefit from screening. For populations such as those on dialysis, a poor prognosis will limit the cost-effectiveness of screening. In addition, one must understand the positive and negative predictive value of the tests chosen to use for screening. Some diseases to be considered for screening in dialysis patients include cancer, falls and frailty, abdominal aortic aneurysms (AAAs), alcohol abuse, cognitive impairment, depression, and hearing and vision loss.

Cancer Screening

Table 97.2 shows recommended cost-effective cancer screening in dialysis patients. The suggested screening varies from the American Cancer Society recommendations

Table 97.2

Suggested Cancer Screening in End-Stage Renal Disease Patients: Individualized, Considering Expected Survival, Risk Factors, and Transplant Status

Cancer*	Recommended Screening
Breast	Yearly mammogram beginning age 40 years and on transplant list Clinical breast examination every 3 years age 20–39; yearly for age >40 years
Colorectal	Beginning age 50 years: yearly fecal occult blood test (FOBT) or fecal immunochemical test (FIT) for those on transplant lists and flexible sigmoidoscopy, colonoscopy, double-contrast barium enema, or virtual colonoscopy per transplant evaluation protocols Positive FIT or FOBT result requires additional evaluation
Cervical	Begin screening at age 21 years; 21–65 years, yearly Pap smears* for those on the transplant list Consider HPV† DNA and HPV vaccine in transplant candidates
Prostate	Age 50 years, annual PSA and DRE for men on transplant list Age 45 years if African American or have father or brother with prostate cancer before the age of 65 years
Renal cell	Yearly CT or MRI in patients on dialysis >3 years and on transplant list

*For all of these cancers, consider screening in high-risk patients with long expected survival times.
†CT, Computed tomography; DRE, digital rectal examination; HPV, human papillomavirus; MRI, magnetic resonance imaging.
Data from Holley JL, Screening, diagnosis, and treatment of cancer in long-term dialysis patients. *Clin J Am Soc Nephrol* 2007;2:604-610; Holley JL. General medical care of the dialysis patient: core curriculum 2013. *Am J Kidney Dis* 2013;61:171-183; Choudhury D, Luna-Salazar C. Preventive health care in chronic kidney disease and end-stage renal disease. *Nat Clin Pract Nephrol* 2008;4(4):194-206; Butler AM, Olshan AF, Kshirsagar AV, et al. Cancer incidence among US Medicare ESRD patients receiving hemodialysis 1996-2009. *Am J Kidney Dis* 2015;65(5):763-772; and American Cancer Society. American Cancer Society Guidelines for the Early Detection of Cancer. http://www.cancer.org/healthy/findcancerearly/cancerscreeningguidelines/american-cancer-society-guidelines-for-the-early-detection-of-cancer.

for cancer screening in the general population because the poor overall survival of dialysis patients limits the cost-effectiveness of some cancer screening. Some cancers, notably bladder and ureteral; renal cell (in the setting of acquired cystic disease); HPV-associated cancers such as cervical, uterine, and tongue; and hepatitis-associated liver cancer are more common in dialysis patients with standardized incidence ratios of 1.5 to 24.1 (Table 97.3). Generally, breast, lung, and colon cancer are not more common among dialysis patients. Stool Hemoccult testing results in dialysis patients are more likely to be positive, probably because of multiple reasons for gastrointestinal blood loss in dialysis patients. Thus, colonoscopies may be more common in this population. Hypothetical analyses to screen for cervical, breast, colon, and prostate cancer in dialysis patients have shown less than 5 days of life saved with screening. Dialysis patients who are not transplant candidates and those 50 to 70 years of age and of white ethnicity are least likely to benefit from cancer screening. Cancer screening among dialysis patients should be individualized and based on the patient's expected survival, risk for the cancer to be screened, and kidney transplant status. Most transplant programs incorporate cancer screening into their transplant evaluation process.

Table 97.3

Cancer Incidence in End-Stage Renal Disease: Literature Summary

Cancer	SIR	Risk Factors in ESRD
Renal cell	3.6–24.1	Acquired cystic disease
Bladder and ureter	1.5–16.4	Analgesic abuse, Balkan nephropathy
Bladder and ureter	1.5–16.4	Oral cyclophosphamide
Tongue	1.2–1.9	Human papillomavirus
Cervical and uterine	0.9	Human papillomavirus
	2.7–4.3	
Liver	1.4–4.5	Hepatitis B and C
Thyroid and other endocrine organs	2.2–2.3	
Breast (women)	0.8–1.42	
Lung or bronchus	0.5–1.28	
Colon or rectum	1.0–1.27	
Pancreas	1.08	
Prostate	0.5–1.08	

ESRD, end-stage renal disease. SIR, standardized incidence ratio.
Data from Holley JL. Screening, diagnosis, and treatment of cancer in long-term dialysis patients. *Clin J Am Soc Nephrol* 2007;2:604-610; Holley JL. General medical care of the dialysis patient: core curriculum 2013. *Am J Kidney Dis* 2013;61:171-183; Choudhury D, Luna-Salazar C. Preventive health care in chronic kidney disease and end-stage renal disease. *Nat Clin Pract Nephrol* 2008;4(4):194-206; and Butler AM, Olshan AF, Kshirsagar AV, et al. Cancer incidence among US Medicare ESRD patients receiving hemodialysis 1996-2009. *Am J Kidney Dis* 2015;65(5):763-772.

Falls and Frailty

Falls

Falls occur more commonly among dialysis patients than in the general population, reportedly at a rate of 1.6 falls per dialysis patient-year versus 0.6 to 0.8 falls per patient-year in the geriatric population. Hip fracture is a common result of a fall and is four times more frequent among dialysis patients. Hip fractures are associated with higher mortality; thus, preventing falls in dialysis patients could theoretically reduce mortality and morbidity. Risk factors for falls in dialysis patients include age, comorbid conditions, a history of falls, and mean systolic blood pressure. Dialysis-associated hypotension and fatigue may also contribute to falls, which are among the most common adverse events in hemodialysis (HD) units. Screening for fall propensity by routinely asking dialysis patients about falls (previous fall is a risk factor for future falls); fostering exercise programs to increase muscle strength; and ensuring normal 25 vitamin D levels, which is associated with improved muscle strength, may help to reduce the likelihood of falls. Formal testing for fall risk and investigation of the home for environmental fall risk factors may prove useful in individual cases. The American Preventive Task Force assigns level B evidence (should offer or provide) to screen for fall risk in those older than 65 years in the general population and recommends exercise or physical therapy as well as vitamin D supplementation in an attempt to prevent falls.

Osteoporosis and Bone Mineral Density

The primary risk of falls is hip fracture. The benefits of bone densitometry as screening for osteoporosis in the dialysis population is unclear. Although abnormalities of bone mineral are more common in ESRD patients, the complex nature of the abnormalities makes bone densitometry results difficult to interpret. Moreover, common treatments for osteoporosis, such as bisphosphonates, are not recommended in dialysis patients.

Frailty

In the geriatric population, the frailty phenotype predicts disability, hospitalization, and mortality. Frailty is recognized as a clinically useful marker for complex cumulative stresses on a biologic model that leads to functional decline with attendant morbidity and mortality. Frailty is associated with hospitalization and death in dialysis patients and was seen in 67% of dialysis patients in the Dialysis Morbidity and Mortality Wave 2 Study. Identifying frailty among dialysis patients could potentially lead to interventions designed to forestall functional decline and its consequences.

Abdominal Aortic Aneurysm

Depending on patient age, gender, and tobacco use, the American Preventive Task Force recommends screening for AAA. The best evidence (level B—should offer or provide) for AAA screening is in men 65 to 75 years of age who have ever smoked. Level C evidence (selectively offer screening) is reported in men 65 to 75 years of age who have never smoked. Women who have never smoked should not be screened, and there is insufficient evidence to recommend screening for AAA in women who have smoked. There are no comparable data in dialysis patients. Thus, similar to cancer screening in dialysis patients, it seems prudent to screen only dialysis patients with long expected survival and high risk for AAA.

Alcohol Abuse

There is little information about alcohol abuse in the dialysis population. One study in an urban HD group found 27.6% of patients scored in the alcoholism range on the MAST (Michigan Alcoholism Screening Test) with the estimate in the general population ranging from 5% to 10%. Alcohol dependence at the time of ESRD diagnosis is associated with reduced survival in those undergoing kidney transplantation. Additional study of alcohol abuse in dialysis patients is needed, including validation of commonly used screening tests such as the MAST or CAGE (ever thought about Cutting down, have people Annoyed you by criticizing your drinking, have you ever felt bad or Guilty about drinking, do you ever have an Eye opener?).

Cognitive Impairment

The American Preventive Task Force does not recommend screening for cognitive impairment in the general population because of insufficient evidence of efficacy. Cognitive impairment is three times more common in the dialysis population, affecting 16% to 38% of patients undergoing neuropsychological testing. Between 30% and 55% of ESRD patients 75 years of age and older have cognitive impairment as do 10% to 30% of young or middle-aged ESRD patients. "Mild cognitive impairment" generally describes impairment greater than that seen with normal aging but not meeting the criteria for dementia. Dementia is defined as progressive and chronic cognitive dysfunction with impaired memory and loss of function in at least one other cognitive domain such as reasoning, attention or executive function, orientation, language, or the skills required for planning and sequencing tasks. The decline observed from one's baseline cognitive level must be severe enough to interfere with independence and daily activities of living. Cerebrovascular disease in ESRD likely contributes to the high rate of cognitive decline and dementia. Additional risk factors for dementia include anemia and albuminuria, age, nonwhite race, and female gender. Because of the high incidence of cognitive impairment in dialysis patients, screening may be useful for decision making, identifying potentially treatable causes, and possibly improving outcomes. Most important, recognizing cognitive impairment can serve as an impetus and direction for ACP with dialysis patients and their families.

Many screening tests for dementia exist. The use of such tests will depend on the clinical condition being considered, the time available for testing, and the frequency of anticipated testing. Table 97.4 illustrates some available dementia screening tests and the time required to administer the test. Although the Mini-Mental State Examination (MMSE) is the best known of the screening tests, it does not evaluate executive function, and because deficits in executive function are a feature of vascular dementia, the MMSE is probably not the screening test of choice in dialysis patients in whom vascular dementia may be likely. Most screening tests are sensitive but lack specificity. Uremia, delirium, and depression should be excluded as reversible treatable causes of cognitive impairment before diagnosing dementia.

Depression

Depression occurs in 20% to 30% of dialysis patients, impacting quality of life, adherence with treatments, functional status, and symptoms such as pain. Higher mortality rates and more frequent hospitalizations are seen in depressed dialysis patients. The American Preventive Task Force recommends screening for depression

Table 97.4

Dementia Screening Tests

| Instrument | Administration | |
	Time (min)	Comments
Mini-Mental State Exam	7–10	Norms available; does not test executive function
Montreal Cognitive Assessment	10	Evaluates executive function
Clock Drawing Task	1–3	Evaluates executive function; less cultural bias
Mini-Cog	3–4	Clock drawing + three-word recall
KDQOL Cognitive Subscale	1–2	Self-report, validated in ESRD

ESRD, End-stage renal disease; KDQOL, Kidney Disease Quality of Life.
Reprinted with permission from Holley JL. General care of dialysis patients. *Am J Kidney Dis* 2013;61(1):171-183.

in the general population when staff-assisted depression care supports are in place (grade B evidence).

Vision

Ocular diseases such as cataracts, optic neuropathy, macular degeneration, subconjunctival calcification, and microvascular and diabetic retinopathy occur more commonly in CKD patients. Regular ophthalmologic examination and monitoring may prevent complications such as retinal detachment, hemorrhage, and vision loss. Patients with diabetes should continue to have regular eye examinations and treatment for retinopathy. Heparin anticoagulation during HD is considered safe without an increased risk of retinopathy.

Hearing

Sensorineural hearing loss occurs more commonly in dialysis patients, affecting 46% to 77% of these patients. Factors contributing to hearing loss in dialysis patients include hypertension, diseases such as vasculitis and Alport syndrome, electrolyte disturbances, exposure to radiocontrast and ototoxic medications such as aminoglycosides, and possibly vitamin D and nerve conduction dysfunction. High-frequency hearing loss is most common and is not related to dialysis vintage. Amplification with hearing aids is the primary treatment for hearing loss. Because Medicare does not cover the cost of hearing aids, financial constraints may complicate treatment for some dialysis patients. Vestibular dysfunction has also been seen in dialysis patients, especially in those exposed to high total doses of aminoglycosides.

Health Care Counseling

Exercise, weight loss and dietary counseling, tobacco use and cessation, and sexual dysfunction and contraception are all areas of preventive care addressed primarily by health care counseling. Each of these is relevant to ESRD patients, and many are addressed in other chapters (see Section XVI, Nutritional Management of Dialysis Patients; Section XVI, Rehabilitation and Psychosocial Issues).

Exercise

Regular exercise can potentially improve physical functioning, control of diabetes and blood pressure, and enhance psychosocial well-being and cardiovascular risk reduction, leading to improved overall health-related quality of life. Nephrologists rarely assess dialysis patients' activity levels, and only 13% of dialysis patients report achieving the recommended level of physical activity (moderate intensity 3 days/wk for 30 minutes each session). Lack of time and motivation, fatigue, and dyspnea are common barriers to exercise among dialysis patients. Formal studies of exercise's effects on dialysis patients showed a 12% improvement in physical performance and health-related quality of life, most pronounced in patients with the lowest levels of function at the start of the study. Dialysis unit exercise programs may provide opportunities for regular activity that lead to improved physical performance and functioning, in turn reducing the likelihood of frailty and falls. An enthusiastic and dedicated dialysis facility staff is integral to the success of such programs.

Obesity and Weight Loss

Obesity is an increasing problem in dialysis patients, affecting 30% of the population. Obesity can be a barrier to kidney transplantation, a complication of PD, and a factor associated with improved survival in HD patients. There is limited information about successful weight loss programs in dialysis patients. Bariatric surgery is increasingly considered by morbidly obese patients and has been reported as a successful strategy in dialysis (pretransplant) patients, although the mortality rate was 3.5% higher in dialysis patients compared with non-ESRD patients.

Tobacco Use and Cessation

Although there is no information on smoking cessation among dialysis patients, in the general population, most adult smokers want to stop, and even brief, repetitive cessation counseling from health care providers is effective. Thus, routine inquiry and counseling about tobacco cessation should be incorporated into health care counseling for dialysis patients who smoke. In the general population, 30% of those who stop smoking used medications as a part of their cessation strategy. Dose reduction of bupropion to 150 mg every 3 days versus 150 mg daily in nondialysis patients is recommended based on pharmacokinetic data. Varenicline should be dosed at 0.5 mg/day in dialysis patients.

Contraception and Sexual Dysfunction

Although sexual dysfunction is common in women (30%–80% experience) and men (70% report erectile dysfunction) on dialysis, most patients do not discuss these issues with their nephrologists or other care providers. Because sexual dysfunction can negatively impact patients' quality of life, this area of health care counseling in dialysis patients likely deserves more attention. See Chapter 58, Metabolic Abnormalities: Evaluation of Sexual Dysfunction.

Although ESRD may be considered a relatively effective contraceptive because of reduced fertility in women on dialysis, pregnancy can occur, and thus premenopausal women on dialysis should be counseled about the possibility of pregnancy and effective means of contraception, especially if they have regular menstrual periods. If conception is deemed possible, angiotensin-converting enzyme inhibitors and angiotensin receptor blockers should be discontinued because of the risk of fetal malformations with their use at the time of conception. Available contraceptive methods include intrauterine devices (probably should be avoided in women on PD because of the risk of infection), barrier methods, and hormonal therapies. There is little information about specific contraceptive methods in women with ESRD but the risks and benefits of each in the general population likely also apply to dialysis patients.

Advance Care Planning and Palliative or Supportive Care

Advance Care Planning

Advance care planning is a process of communication among patients, their families, and health care providers addressing goals of care within the context of the patient's values. Development and completion of advance directives (e.g., designation of a health care surrogate or proxy, living wills) may be one outcome of ACP but is not a requisite component of the ACP process. In many states, the Physician Orders for Life-Sustaining Treatment (POLST) form may be applicable and completed as desired by patients and families to ensure a patient's wishes for life-sustaining care are followed. POLST are actual orders signed by a provider (physician or in some cases nurse practitioner or physician's assistant) and generally include sections on resuscitation status; guides for overall aggressiveness of care (maximizing comfort, wishes for selective treatments, complete life-sustaining care) in terms of intubation, vasopressors, antibiotics; and choices for medically administered nutrition such as feeding tubes and intravenous hydration. Designation of a surrogate decision maker and the patient or surrogate's signatures as well as the signing health care provider complete the document. In states accepting POLST forms, they are legally binding orders for care and the degree of that care as directed by the patient and his or her health care proxy.

Advance care planning should be part of the routine and periodic care of each dialysis patient. The process of ACP should begin early in the course of CKD because ACP will be important in dialysis modality or conservative management selection when CKD stage 5 is reached. In addition, ACP will form the basis of the end-of-life care desired by the patient and his or her family and loved one. For patients and families to make informed decisions about their care, including whether or not to begin dialysis, an estimate of prognosis is needed and should be provided by the nephrologist or primary providers discussing treatment, including options for dialysis. Tools exist for predicting survival on dialysis and use comorbidity such as the Charlson Comorbidity Index, patient age, serum albumin level, functional status, and the surprise question ("Would you be surprised if this patient died in the next 6 months?"), yielding sensitivity of around 85%. When asked, most patients desire information on prognosis and require it to make informed decisions about their health care wishes. The Renal Physicians Association Clinical Practice Guideline, Shared Decision-Making in the Appropriate Initiation of and Withdrawal from Dialysis, is a clinically useful guide with toolkits to aid nephrologists in these aspects of care.

Supportive (Palliative) Kidney Care

Although supportive care is not classically defined as preventive care, in many respects, it is since anticipating and treating symptoms, fostering ACP, and planning for end-of-life care are the primary tenets of supportive care and represent opportunities for preventive care. Supportive care is appropriate for anyone with a chronic illness and should begin early in the course of that illness, accompanying curative care (Fig. 97.1). The increasingly elderly CKD population is focusing attention on conservative care without dialysis for some patients, and supportive care is clearly indicated for this group as well as for dialysis patients with their high symptom burden. Time-limited trials of renal replacement therapy are advocated in cases of unclear patient and family wishes and prognosis. End-of-life care is one aspect of supportive care that includes hospice care, which is appropriate for any patient thought to have 6 months or less of remaining life. Hospice has been underused in ESRD patients but is appropriate for any patient withdrawing from dialysis and for those in CKD stage 5 opting out of dialysis. Some are advocating consideration of

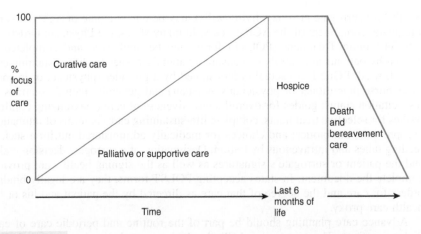

Figure 97.1

Palliative care can be provided simultaneously with curative care. End-of-life and hospice care are components of palliative care with hospice care occurring in the last 6 months of life. Bereavement care for the family and loved ones extends beyond the death of the patient. (Adapted from Lynn J. Living long in fragile death: the new demographics shape end of life care. *Hastings Center Rep* 2005;Spec No:S14-S18.)

"palliative dialysis" for patients unwilling or not ready to stop dialysis. Involvement of palliative care specialists when available is encouraged, particularly by nephrologists and dialysis care providers with little experience in kidney supportive care. The Coalition for Supportive Care of Kidney Patients (www.kidneysupportivecare.org) and the RPA Clinical Practice Guideline, *Shared Decision-Making in the Appropriate Initiation of and Withdrawal from Dialysis,* are invaluable resources for supportive care for CKD and ESRD patients.

Monitoring: Lipids, Glucose, Anemia, and Bone and Mineral Disorders

Monitoring disease states and control of therapeutic interventions is another aspect of preventive care. In the case of ESRD patients, anemia and bone and mineral disorders are monitored routinely in dialysis units (see Chapter 50, Anemia in Patients with End-Stage Kidney; Chapter 51, Iron Use in ESRD Patients). Chapter 64 reviews monitoring needs in patients with diabetes, which includes glucose control and the complications of diabetes such as retinopathy and neuropathy. Chapter 56 discusses monitoring and managing lipid disorders. In addition, dialysis accesses are monitored for function and complications, and these issues are reviewed in the relevant chapters (see Section IX, Complications During Hemodialysis).

CHAPTER 98

Application of Telemedicine to Patients With End-Stage Renal Disease

Spencer Westcott • Mark Kaplan, MD •
Mahesh Krishnan, MD, MPH, MBA, FASN

Telemedicine in End-Stage Renal Disease: Overview of the Opportunity and Issues

By their very nature, nephrologists are very data focused. Dialysis itself is and always will be a very data-intensive procedure, as evidenced by the meticulous detailed flowsheets and laboratory data that are generated on hundreds of thousands of patients a year. Given the hunger for increasingly more data, it should come as no surprise that the use of telemedicine fits naturally into the practice of dialysis. Surveys reveal great interest in telemedicine among nephrologists for patient care, yet few are using this technology today. Elsewhere in health care, virtual medical consultations have more than doubled in the past 5 years to more than 75 million served. This trend is not likely to be going away; the question is: When will dialysis have its moment, and what does it take to implement such a program?

For the sake of clarity, we chose to define the specific term *teledialysis* to differentiate the concept from the use of electronic approaches by nephrologists for virtual consultation outside the dialysis setting. Teledialysis then refers to the ability to remotely monitor patients undergoing dialysis. In addition to the monitoring, teledialysis should also include the use of two-way communication, such as by audio or video. This may be monitoring of patients in free-standing dialysis clinics or at home or even patients receiving renal replacement therapy in the hospital. Principles from this guidance may be further expanded to include patient monitoring in the case of peritoneal dialysis (PD), self-dialysis, and home dialysis.

The general framework required for teledialysis parallels the way intensive care units have been monitored by a centrally located physician for some time through an electronic intensive care unit (eICU) system. This ability to monitor outcomes and communicate on demand has been proven to be effective, has been associated with improved patient outcomes and positive experiences for patients and caregivers in the hospital setting, and informs the use of similar programs in the outpatient setting such as dialysis.

The need is high today and will be greater if not essential in the future. In various parts of the world, a nephrologist is required to be in the facility when treatments are being delivered. This regulatory requirement is historic and may reflect previous issues requiring a physical presence such as the use of acetate-based dialysate, with frequent profound episodes of hypotension. This regulatory requirement does not exist in other regions such as the United States.

Given that the world is increasingly facing a nephrologist supply issue, this regulatory requirement becomes a rate-limiting factor to opening free-standing and rural dialysis units. Coupled with the shortage is an increased demand on nephrologists' time. Teledialysis may provide a necessary mitigation to allow the nephrology community to continue to provide high-quality dialysis care to an ever-growing population.

The Health Care System in the United States Presents Particular Challenges

Given the increased use of telemedicine in the United States, examining the challenges provides a useful framework for anyone considering implementing a teledialysis program.
- Physician reimbursement:
  - **Medicare:** Reimbursement for dialysis rounding is limited to originating sites and must either be outside the metropolitan statistical area or in an area with a health professional shortage. The vast majority of dialysis patients have traditional Medicare; therefore, the Centers for Medicare & Medicaid Services has tremendous influence on the reimbursement for teledialysis.
  - **Medicaid:** Reimbursement for telemedicine varies by state. Trends indicate reimbursement for telemedicine is on the rise.
  - **Private insurance:** There are no consistent standards governing private payers; however, states continue to pass parity laws requiring telemedicine reimbursement by private payers.
- **ESRD Conditions for Coverage (CMCs):** Medicare CFCs certify the facility as qualifying for Medicare payment. At least one in-person rounding visit per month is required of physicians.
- **Health Insurance Portability and Accountability Act (HIPAA):** Take care to ensure HIPAA guidelines are followed at all times, including technology hardware and software selection, as well as in-center patient care.
- **Licensure:** Physicians are required to be licensed in the state where the patient is located, not where the physician is located.
- **Malpractice:** The American Medical Association recommends the following to minimize potential risk associated with telemedicine:
  - Define the minimum requirements to establish the doctor–patient relationship.
  - Determine who owns the huge amounts of data available to both patients and physicians.
  - Require medical liability carriers to write telemedicine and data-related risks in policies.

Similar variants of these issues no doubt occur in every country of the world. A deep understanding of the health care delivery system and regulatory concerns in any country where teledialysis may be implemented is a must.

A Framework for Implementation of a Teledialysis Program

As mentioned earlier, there are two specific aspects of teledialysis. The first is a variant on traditional telemedicine, which in this context is defined by remote rounding and recommendations. Here, the essential capability is for a clinician to remotely interact with the patient and remote caregiver to allow diagnosis and treatment. The second aspect focuses on the ability to achieve a virtual presence by the remote clinician with the same fidelity as if the provider were physically present in the remote site. To achieve this goal, one relies on remote access to an electronic medical record (EMR); telemetrics that provides either real-time streaming or batched submission of data from a dialysis machine or ancillary device such as a blood pressure (BP) cuff or remote stethoscope; and some type of virtual presence, which could be videoconferencing.

We define the framework of teledialysis with the following components. First, there needs to be a remote user (either a clinic in the case of in-center dialysis or the patient's home in the case of monitoring home modality patients) who serves as the originating site for the teledialysis program. Next, a central monitoring facility or physician's office is designated as the receiving site, which is contacted by the originating site to provide care. This is described in Fig. 98.1.

Having defined the framework of the teledialysis system, we move to defining specific use cases or scenarios against which the system needs to function. Each of these use cases defines the specific equipment and personnel needed, as well as to potentially dictate the ratio of remote to receiving sites.

Routine Nonemergent Nephrologist Rounding Use Case

A routine use case involves the remote scheduled rounding by a nephrologist. In this scenario, the nephrologist contacts the dialysis unit at a predetermined frequency, which could be monthly. The remote dialysis unit originates a call to the central monitoring station or physician's office. A wireless two-way mobile video

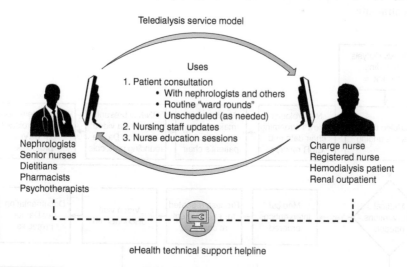

Figure 98.1

Conceptual model of teledialysis. (Modified from http://www.ehealthservices .eu/piloting_services/tele_dialysis.)

connection or robot is used to conduct "rounds" on each patient on dialysis. The remote nephrologist uses a combination of the audio and video feeds, EMR, and remote telemetric feeds from the dialysis device to conduct rounds. Notes and findings are then entered into the EMR. The logical flow for such an interaction is detailed in Fig. 98.2.

The use of remote stethoscopes and other technology that closely mimics in-person visits may be useful for chronic visits.

Emergent Use Case

The first use case can be defined as the emergent consultation request. Specifically, a remote dialysis unit has an acute issue that requires immediate intervention by a trained nephrologist. Such emergent situations require regional definition but could include acute hypotensive events, dialyzer reactions, seizures, and cardiac arrest. Communications in this scenario may be fundamentally by phone, augmented by access to the patient's electronic records. In a more complex system, real-time telemetric data detailing vital signs and run sheet parameters may be used, supplemented by video connections allowing the remote nephrologist to be virtually present in the dialysis unit and gather the needed information for both diagnosis and treatment. Although this may be as simple as an Internet-enabled camera, this communication may be as complex as to involve a remote robot, with the ability to "see" the patient and gather some vital information, through the use of a remote microphone, stethoscope, and so on. A sample flow for such a situation is:

1. The dialysis clinic registered nurse (RN) or internist identifies an emergent patient situation.
2. A call is placed to the central nephrologist in the monitoring station.
3. The central nephrologist reviews streaming data or real-time data at the central site.

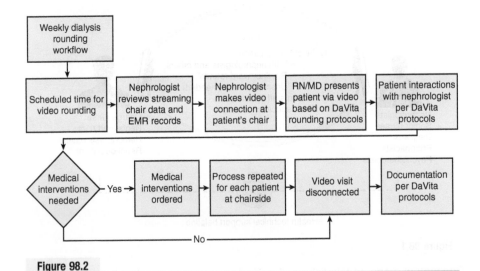

Figure 98.2

Logical diagram of teledialysis. EMR, Electronic medical record.

4. The central nephrologist makes a video connection to the RN or internist at the patient's bedside.
5. The central nephrologist conducts virtual assessment and medical interventions.
6. The central nephrologist documents in the EMR.

Home and Peritoneal Dialysis: Remote Monitoring Use Case

Adaptations of the above use cases can be used for home hemodialysis (HD) and PD. Because these patients have much less frequent direct contact with their caregivers today, there is a significant opportunity for remote monitoring to identify instances when interventions from caregivers may improve the overall health of patients and ultimately prevent hospitalization episodes or other adverse events. The primary application today is remote monitoring of patients' vital signs and overall health, but this population has the potential for video and voice interventions in the future. Baseline remote monitoring metrics include:

- Weight
- BP
- Pulse and heart rhythm
- Symptomatic questions
  Additional measures for future consideration include:
- Temperature
- Glucose levels
- Treatment and machine alarm data
- Video chat or secure message chat

Because home dialysis patients are typically younger than traditional in-center patients, they are more likely to already have smartphones or tablets today. As capabilities are developed to leverage these existing connectivity points, this has the potential to significantly reduce the cost of delivering telemedicine to these patients, which strengthens the business case for broader adoption.

Other Miscellaneous Use Cases

Other use cases for teledialysis include building trust with high-risk patients, follow-up on missed rounding because of schedule or timing conflicts, discussion of and review of medications (including viewing medication and bottles), updated history and physical examinations, and reviewing future appointments. Because of legal and compliance restrictions, video interactions may be limited to credentialed caregivers.

Integrated Kidney Care (Global Capitation) Use Case

The goal of integrated care is to improve the quality of patient care at lower cost. Telemedicine can be a helpful tool in this model to improve the efficiency of care delivery while retaining or improving outcomes through increased and immediate access. In the future, telemedicine may be used to transform the dialysis center into a comprehensive care center or ESRD medical home. Typically, dialysis centers are not credentialed to provide additional services; however, centers in the future may provide patients with multiple rounding consultations while receiving their dialysis treatment. Given the significant comorbidities that exist with dialysis patients and the transportation challenges for many patients, the dialysis center of the future could be a one-stop shop for comprehensive patient care. Telemedicine will likely play an important role in delivery of that care.

Teledialysis Technology Requirements

Technology changes so quickly that best practice recommendations quickly go out of date. That said, constant change and increased investment in telemedicine technology is much more of an opportunity for teledialysis than a concern, including improved bandwidths and connections, new technologies, and increased access to smartphones. There are foundational elements that will likely be a necessary part of teledialysis in the coming years.

Bandwidth, Resolution, and Frame Rate Requirements:

- Minimum: 256 kbps of circuit bandwidth (may lead to poor experience)
- Preferred minimum: 512 kbps; 1 Mbps (HD)
- Preferred: 4 Mbps or higher
- See Table 98.1.

Information Technology Security Requirements

- Comprehensive code review, including end-to-end secure transfer of data
- Encryption of data in transit using Transport Layer Security (TLSv1) or a similar secure protocol when using Transmission Control Protocol/Internet Protocol (TCP/IP). If User Datagram Protocol (UDP) is used, standard encryption such as Datagram Transport Layer Security (DTLS) should be used.
- Encryption of data at rest using Advanced Encryption Standard (AES)-256 encryption or similar encryption algorithm. Second, all backup data will be encrypted using a similar encryption method.
- Use a single port (TPC or UDP) for call signals and media streaming (no dynamic ports)

Table 98.1

Bandwidth/Resolution/Frame Rate Requirements

Bandwidth	Resolution	Frame Rate	Notes
384 Kbps	CIF	30 fps	Not recommended
512 Kbps	4CIF	15 fps+	Recommended min SD
768 Kbps	4CIF	30 fps	
1 Mbps	HD720	15 fps+	Recommended min HD
2 Mbps	HD720	30 fps	
4 Mbps	HD720	60 fps	Preferred
6 Mbps	HD1080	30 fps	

Hardware and Video Requirements

Hardware and Functionality

When researching full digital and camera carts versus tablets, one should consider the benefits and tradeoffs of functionality and cost. For example, tablets cost significantly less, take up less space, and may be easier to manage in more confined treatment areas at many inpatient centers. Different carts and tablets provide varying flexibility for multifunction, including rounding, EMR, telemetric, and video intervention. Rounding "robots" may be useful in hospital settings because of their mobility, but they require significant upfront costs and may be cumbersome to store, maintain, and upgrade.

Video

A video link is preferred and can be integrated or delivered by split monitor. Installation should preferably be one camera per dialysis station with the ability for the nephrologist or data access technician to focus in on a specific station on his or her screen. This may be facilitated by the use of in-ceiling or camera microphones to allow the originating site to communicate with the receiving central monitoring site to facilitate two-way communication. Alternatively, this may be done by phone.

Other

Digital hardware is advancing rapidly, which will give physicians more control rather than fully relying on clinic teammates. As an example, consider the use of digital stethoscopes that connect through the video conferencing software without additional software required.

Dialysis Machine Data

Teledialysis requires a clear understanding of how the needed data elements will flow from remote to originating site. In one approach, data flow as shown in Fig. 98.3.

Dialysis Machine Data

At present, there is an absence of consistency in the data format that can be streamed from various dialysis machines. This results in the need for a custom interface for each type of dialysis machine. This lack of consistency is neither efficient nor effective. Solving this issue as a dialysis community is important for large-scale implementation and adoption of teledialysis.

A global data model is being defined by the dialysis community in conjunction with HL7 to set the minimum data elements for dialysis machine streaming data. Dimensions of this data model include mandatory and optional date fields, unified field names with crosswalk to each machine type, and the frequency of data transmission. Alarm data are an additional real-time parameter that can be monitored remotely. Although reacting to alarms is a local clinic responsibility, it may be beneficial to have the alarms centrally monitored in a remote monitoring application.

Data workflow draft

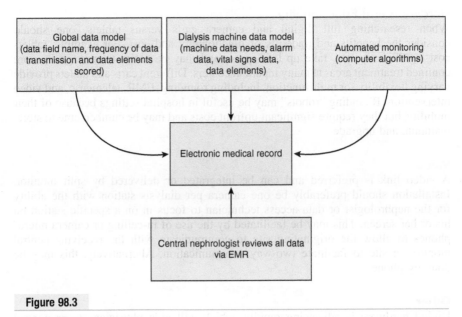

Figure 98.3

Draft of teledialysis workflow. EMR, Electronic medical record.

A sample minimum data set for dialysis data streaming may include the following:
1. Vital signs data
2. Sample data elements include:
   a. Treatment duration
   b. Pretreatment BP sit
   c. Postreatment BP sit
   d. Posttreatment BP Stand
   e. Posttreatment BP Stand
   f. Pulse
   g. Liters processed
   h. Average blood flow rate
   i. Dialysate flow rate
   j. Volume removed
   k. Lowest blood flow rate

Nontechnology Teledialysis Requirements
Policy and Procedures

Given the complexity of the medical and regulatory parameters that govern the use of teledialysis, it is crucial to have a solid set of policies and procedures to ensure success. Essential policies and procedures include a scope of service template, a quality review policy template, a physician credentialing policy template, a chairside physician communication policy template, and a complaint response policy. Given that regulations around scope of practice and telemedicine are country and even state specific, proper attention toward the appropriate regionalization of these policies and procedures is critical.

Documentation is another regulatory aspect that requires formalized evaluation and description. Two common models exist. The first is consultative only; it includes no documentation other than the originating site stating that it contacted the central nephrologist. The second is where the receiving site documents in the local EMR. Although either may be acceptable, the second is preferable to ensure continuity of care in a patient centric informatics environment.

Program Management and Implementation

A proper program management framework is critical to program success. Best practices in program management include (but are not limited to):

1. **Getting buy-in from nurses early in the process.** This can be done by highlighting how teledialysis can improve the efficiency and effectiveness of their work, improve clinical outcomes, or save time. Having participating nurses comfortable with the technology and pilot testing is key to ensuring that nurses are motivated to keep patient adherence high, especially when it comes to patient compliance with remote monitoring data.

2. **Actively involved administrative staff.** This could include dedicated and detailed support to supervise nurses, ensure adherence, and answer challenges nurses face during rollout, which helps increase the viability and sustainability of the program.

3. **Engaged physicians** who are excited about testing new technology for patient care, especially if there are reimbursement hurdles

4. **A dedicated project manager.** This should include one dedicated staff member responsible for data collection and liaising with hospitals to ensure collection of admissions data. The project manager is ideally responsible for collecting and publishing monthly data on specific types of hospitalizations, readmissions, and patient churn.

5. **Technical support.** The project manager may need to be supplemented with a technical representative who makes sure remote monitoring patients are installing and using the devices properly.

6. **Legal and compliance.** To review the regulatory, HIPAA, credentialing, and other factors that create risk with telemedicine.

7. **Measurement of success.** To ensure that any investment in telemedicine is worthwhile, it is important to measure success. Metrics may come from multiple sources such as:
   - Providers (e.g., dialysis center or hospital, physicians)
   - Technology partner
   - Individuals via feedback
   - Potential metrics to track include:
     - Experience of telemedicine visit via survey or interview (patient, physician, facility): Was video important for the intervention?
     - Visit frequency, quality, and length of time
     - Nature of visit (e.g., was a hospitalization or missed treatment avoided?)

Training

As with any new endeavor, staff and physician training is essential to the smooth operation of a telemedicine program. At least one member of the remote dialysis unit should be trained in the facile operation of the equipment. Nurses need to be trained in the types of issues that may or may not be amenable to teledialysis. Nephrologist training includes training on the technology system as well as training on documentation.

Paper and soft copy instructions and reference materials on use cases, metrics tracking, cleaning and maintenance, and support are helpful resources, as well as clear training and reminders on HIPAA protection, logging out of EMR systems on a tablet that is multiuse, and other risks to regulatory and corporate policies and procedures.

Examples of Teledialysis in Use Today

The concept of teledialysis is not theoretical. There are examples of teledialysis being used in dialysis clinics today. For example, the DaVita Colombia dialysis clinics are testing a teledialysis system to allow remote dialysis clinics to be connected and monitored by a centrally located nephrologist. As a result of this innovative new approach, patients can avoid having to travel great distances to receive dialysis. Another example is in Scotland, where a satellite dialysis unit is monitored from a central hospital. (http://news.bbc.co.uk/2/hi/uk_news/scotland/highlands_and_islands/8634562.stm). One of the oldest programs for teledialysis exists in the northern reaches of Finland, where remote rural units are monitored from a central university hospital using video and other communications media.

Conclusions

As the number of dialysis patients increases and the number of nephrologists continues to be rate limiting, teledialysis has the potential to allow nephrologists to continue to care for patients in multiple settings. In implementing a teledialysis program, it is fundamental to have a clear understanding of the local regulations and the technology and nontechnology requirements. The most common use cases for teledialysis can then be mapped against these requirements to ensure that the program is successful. Future efforts to standardize dialysis streaming and other data sets will continue to improve the efficiency and efficacy of teledialysis toward the goal of improving the lives of patients with renal disease.

INDEX

Note: Pages followed by *b, t,* or *f* refer to boxes, tables, or figures, respectively.